EMERGENCY MEDICINE

EMERGENCY MEDICINE

Edited by

HAROLD L. MAY, M.D.

Assistant Clinical Professor of Surgery
Harvard Medical School
Associate in Surgery
Brigham and Women's Hospital
Boston, Massachusetts

A WILEY MEDICAL PUBLICATION
JOHN WILEY & SONS
New York • Chichester • Brisbane • Toronto • Singapore

Production Supervisor: Rosalind Straley
Editorial Supervisor: Megan Thomas
Copyeditor: Harriet Serenkin
Illustrator: Harriet Greenfield
Cover design: Wanda Lubelska

Library of Congress Cataloging in Publication Data:

Main entry under title:

Emergency medicine.

  (A Wiley medical publication)
  Includes index.
  1. Emergency medicine—Addresses, essays,
lectures. I. May, Harold L. II. Series.

RC86.7.E579 1984   616'.025   83-10349
ISBN 0-471-86328-9

Printed in the United States of America

10 9 8 7 6 5 4 3

To Aggie, Jeannette, Alison, and Margie
with deep affection

CONTRIBUTORS

Americo A. Abbruzzese, M.D.
Gastroenterologist
Winthrop Community Hospital
Winthrop, Massachusetts

Frederick W. Ackroyd, M.D.
Associate Professor of Surgery
Harvard Medical School
Associate Visiting Surgeon
Massachusetts General Hospital
Boston, Massachusetts

Paul Allen, M.D.
Assistant Professor of Anesthesia
Harvard Medical School
Associate in Anesthesia
Brigham and Women's Hospital
Boston, Massachusetts

Joseph S. Alpert, M.D.
Professor of Medicine
University of Massachusetts Medical School
Director, Division of Cardiovascular Medicine
University of Massachusetts Medical Center
Worcester, Massachusetts

Kenneth A. Arndt, M.D.
Associate Professor of Dermatology
Harvard Medical School
Dermatologist-in-Chief
Beth Israel Hospital
Boston, Massachusetts

St. George T. Aufranc, M.D.
Attending Surgeon
New England Baptist Hospital
Associate Staff Physician
New England Deaconess Hospital
Boston, Massachusetts

Jonathan Bates, M.D.
Senior Associate in Ambulatory Medicine
Children's Hospital Medical Center
Boston, Massachusetts

Joseph R. Benotti, M.D.
Assistant Professor of Medicine
Assistant Director, Cardiac Catheterization Laboratories
University of Massachusetts Medical Center
Worcester, Massachusetts

Don C. Bienfang, M.D.
Assistant Professor of Ophthalmology
Harvard Medical School
Interim Chief of Neuroophthalmology
The Massachusetts Eye and Ear Infirmary
Boston, Massachusetts

David C. Brooks, M.D.
Chief Resident in Surgery
Brigham and Women's Hospital
Boston, Massachusetts

John F. Burke, M.D.
Helen Andrus Benedict Professor of Surgery
Harvard Medical School
Chief of the Trauma Services
Massachusetts General Hospital
Boston, Massachusetts

Edmund B. Cabot, M.D.
Instructor in Surgery
Harvard Medical School
Associate in Surgery
Director of Surgical Emergency Services
Brigham and Women's Hospital
Boston, Massachusetts

Elliott L. Cohen, M.D.
Chairman, Department of Emergency Medicine
Lahey Clinic Medical Center
Burlington, Massachusetts

John J. Collins, Jr., M.D.
Professor of Surgery
Harvard Medical School
Chief, Division of Thoracic and Cardiac Surgery
Brigham and Women's Hospital
Boston, Massachusetts

Nathan P. Couch, M.D.
Associate Professor of Surgery
Harvard Medical School
Surgeon
Brigham and Women's Hospital
Boston, Massachusetts

Stephen P. Dretler, M.D.
Assistant Professor of Surgery
Harvard Medical School
Assistant Urologist
Massachusetts General Hospital
Boston, Massachusetts

David E. Drum, M.D., Ph.D.
Associate Professor of Radiology (Nuclear Medicine)
Harvard Medical School
Radiologist
Brigham and Women's Hospital
Boston, Massachusetts

Roger H. Emerson, Jr., M.D
Instructor in Orthopedic Surgery
Harvard Medical School
Assistant in Orthopedic Surgery
Massachusetts General Hospital
Chief, Division of Orthopedics
The Cambridge Hospital
Boston, Massachusetts

Paul Feldon, M.D.
Assistant Professor of Orthopedic Surgery
Tufts University School of Medicine
Chief of Hand Surgery
St. Elizabeth's Hospital
Boston, Massachusetts

Edwin G. Fischer, M.D.
Assistant Professor of Surgery
Harvard Medical School

Senior Associate in Surgery (Neurosurgery)
Children's Hospital Medical Center
Brigham and Women's Hospital
Boston, Massachusetts

John H. Fisher, M.D.
Associate Professor of Surgery
Harvard Medical School
Senior Associate in Surgery
Children's Hospital Medical Center
Boston, Massachusetts

Howard S. Frazier, M.D.
Professor of Medicine
Harvard Medical School
Director, Center for the Analysis of Health Practices
Harvard School of Public Health
Physician
Beth Israel Hospital
Boston, Massachusetts

Gerald H. Friedland, M.D.
Associate Professor of Medicine
Albert Einstein College of Medicine
Director, Medical Service I
Montefiore Medical Center
Bronx, New York

Klaus Geiger, M.D.
Professor of Anesthesia
Department of Anesthesiology and Intensive Care Medicine
University of Heidelberg
Head, Respiratory and Intensive Care Unit
Klinikum Mannheim
Mannheim, Federal Republic of Germany

Samuel Z. Goldhaber, M.D.
Instructor in Medicine
Harvard Medical School
Associate in Medicine
Brigham and Women's Hospital
Boston, Massachusetts

Robert M. Goldwyn, M.D.
Clinical Professor of Surgery
Harvard Medical School
Head, Division of Plastic Surgery
Beth Israel Hospital
Senior Surgeon
Brigham and Women's Hospital
Boston, Massachusetts

Irving H. Gomolin, M.D., C.M.
Assistant Professor of Medicine
University of Connecticut School of Medicine
Farmington, Connecticut
Assistant Director of Medical Services
Hebrew Home and Hospital
Hartford, Connecticut

Stephen V. Hall, M.D.
Director, Cardiac Anesthesia
Baystate Medical Center
Springfield, Massachusetts

Joseph M. Healey, Jr., J.D.
Associate Professor of Community Medicine and Health Care
Department of Community Medicine and Health Care
University of Connecticut School of Medicine
Farmington, Connecticut

Gerald B. Healy, M.D.
Associate Professor of Otolaryngology
Harvard Medical School
Associate Professor of Otolaryngology
Boston University School of Medicine
Otolaryngologist-in-Chief
Children's Hospital Medical Center
Boston, Massachusetts

Stephen E. Hedberg, M.D.
Clinical Assistant Professor of Surgery
Harvard Medical School
Associate Visiting Surgeon and
Senior Endoscopist in Gastrointestinal Surgery
Massachusetts General Hospital
Boston, Massachusetts

Norman K. Hollenberg, M.D., Ph.D.
Professor and Director of Physiologic Research
Department of Radiology
Harvard Medical School
Senior Associate in Medicine
Brigham and Women's Hospital
Boston, Massachusetts

Robert W. Hussey, M.D.
Associate Professor of Orthopedic Surgery
Medical College of Virginia
Chief, Spinal Cord Injury Service
Richmond Veterans Administration Medical Center
Richmond, Virginia

Edward E. Jacobs, Jr., M.D.
Clinical Instructor in Otolaryngology
Harvard Medical School
Associate Surgeon in Otolaryngology
Massachusetts Eye and Ear Infirmary
Boston, Massachusetts

Carol B. Jankowski, R.N., M.Ed.
Associate in Radiology (Nuclear Medicine)
Harvard Medical School
Senior Research Associate
Brigham and Women's Hospital
Boston, Massachusetts

Kirtly Parker Jones, M.D.
Instructor in Obstetrics and Gynecology
Harvard Medical School
Assistant in Obstetrics and Gynecology
Brigham and Women's Hospital
Boston, Massachusetts

Leonard B. Kaban, D.M.D., M.D.
Associate Professor of Oral and Maxillofacial Surgery
Harvard School of Dental Medicine
Associate in Surgery
Children's Hospital Medical Center
Associate in Surgery
Brigham and Women's Hospital
Boston, Massachusetts

Gary P. Kearney, M.D.
Clinical Assistant Professor of Surgery
Harvard Medical School
Associate in Surgery
Brigham and Women's Hospital
Boston, Massachusetts

J. Kenneth Koster, Jr., M.D.
Assistant Professor of Surgery
Harvard Medical School
Assistant in Surgery
Brigham and Women's Hospital
Boston, Massachusetts

Dennis M.D. Landis, M.D.
Assistant Professor of Neurology
Harvard Medical School
Assistant Neurologist
Massachusetts General Hospital
Boston, Massachusetts

David C. Lewis, M.D.
Professor of Medicine and Community Health
Donald G. Millar Distinguished Scholar in Alcoholism
Studies
Chairman, Department of Community Health
Director, Center for Alcohol Studies
Brown University
Providence, Rhode Island

Alan Lisbon, M.D.
Instructor in Anesthesia
Harvard Medical School
Associate Director of Respiratory Surgical Intensive Care
Unit
Beth Israel Hospital
Boston, Massachusetts

Frederick H. Lovejoy, Jr., M.D.
Associate Professor of Pediatrics
Harvard Medical School
Associate Physician-in-Chief
Children's Hospital Medical Center
Director, Massachusetts Poison Control System
Boston, Massachusetts

Inder V. Malhotra, M.D.
Assistant Professor of Anesthesia
Harvard Medical School
Co-Director of Clinical Anesthesia
Beth Israel Hospital
Boston, Massachusetts

Harold L. May, M.D.
Assistant Clinical Professor of Surgery
Harvard Medical School
Associate in Surgery
Brigham and Women's Hospital
Boston, Massachusetts

Michael A. McGuigan, M.D., C.M.
Assistant Professor of Pediatrics and Pharmacology
Faculty of Medicine
University of Toronto
Medical Director, Poison Information Centre
The Hospital for Sick Children
Toronto, Ontario, Canada

Kevin M. McIntyre, M.D., J.D.
Assistant Professor of Medicine
Harvard Medical School
Department of Medicine

Peter Bent Brigham Hospital and
Veterans Administration Medical Center
West Roxbury, Massachusetts

John B. Mulliken, M.D.
Associate Professor of Surgery
Division of Plastic and Maxillofacial Surgery
Harvard Medical School
Associate in Surgery
Children's Hospital Medical Center and
Brigham and Women's Hospital
Boston, Massachusetts

Edward A. Nalebuff, M.D.
Clinical Professor of Orthopedic Surgery
Tufts University School of Medicine
Chief of Hand Service
New England Baptist Hospital
Boston, Massachusetts

Russell Nauta, M.D.
Chief Resident in Surgery
Brigham and Women's Hospital
Boston, Massachusetts

Peter T. Nieh, M.D.
Assistant Professor of Surgery
University of Connecticut Health Center
Farmington, Connecticut
Senior Staff Urologist
Veteran's Administration Hospital
Newington, Connecticut

Nicholas O'Connor, M.D.
Instructor in Surgery
Harvard Medical School
Associate Surgeon
Brigham and Women's Hospital and
Children's Hospital Medical Center
Boston, Massachusetts

Roger V. Ohanesian, M.D.
Clinical Instructor of Ophthalmology
University of California at Irvine
Irvine, California
Chief of Ophthalmology
South Coast Medical Center
Attending Physician
San Clemente General Hospital
South Laguna, California

CONTRIBUTORS

Robert T. Osteen, M.D.
Assistant Professor of Surgery
Harvard Medical School
Associate in Surgery
Brigham and Women's Hospital
Boston, Massachusetts

Robert C. Pascucci, M.D.
Instructor in Anesthesia (Pediatric)
Harvard Medical School
Associate Director, Multidisciplinary Intensive Care Unit
Children's Hospital Medical Center
Boston, Massachusetts

Lynn M. Peterson, M.D.
Assistant Professor of Surgery
Harvard Medical School
Surgeon
Brigham and Women's Hospital
Boston, Massachusetts

Reed E. Pyeritz, M.D., Ph.D.
Assistant Professor of Medicine and Pediatrics
The Johns Hopkins University School of Medicine
Physician and Director of Clinical Services in Division of Medical Genetics
The Johns Hopkins Hospital
Baltimore, Maryland

Peter Reich, M.D.
Associate Professor of Psychiatry
Harvard Medical School
Chief of Psychiatry
Brigham and Women's Hospital
Boston, Massachusetts

Donald T. Reilly, M.D., Ph.D.
Clinical Instructor of Orthopedic Surgery
Harvard Medical School
Assistant in Orthopedic Surgery
Brigham and Women's Hospital
Boston, Massachusetts

Malcolm P. Rogers, M.D.
Assistant Professor of Psychiatry
Harvard Medical School
Assistant Director, Psychiatric Service
Brigham and Women's Hospital
Boston, Massachusetts

David S. Rosenthal, M.D.
Associate Professor of Medicine
Harvard Medical School
Clinical Director, Hematology Division
Brigham and Women's Hospital
Boston, Massachusetts

Donald H. Rubin, M.D.
Assistant Professor of Medicine and Microbiology
University of Pennsylvania
Hospital of the University of Pennsylvania
Philadelphia, Pennsylvania

Alfredo A. Sadun, M.D., Ph.D.
Assistant Professor of Ophthalmology
Harvard Medical School
Massachusetts Eye and Ear Infirmary
Boston, Massachusetts

John H. Sanders, M.D.
Assistant Professor of Surgery
Northwestern University Medical School
Associate Attending Surgeon
Northwestern Memorial Hospital
Chicago, Illinois

Anthony P. Scapicchio, M.D.
Clinical Instructor in Surgery
Harvard Medical School
Boston, Massachusetts
Director, Ambulatory Services and Emergency Services
Mount Auburn Hospital
Cambridge, Massachusetts

Albert L. Sheffer, M.D.
Associate Clinical Professor of Medicine
Harvard Medical School
Director, Allergy Clinics
Brigham and Women's Hospital and
Beth Israel Hospital
Allergy Section Chief
New England Deaconess Hospital
Boston, Massachusetts

Gary L. Simpson, M.D., Ph.D., MSc (Oxon)
Assistant Professor of Medicine
Department of Medicine
University of New Mexico School of Medicine
Albuquerque, New Mexico

Harold S. Solomon, M.D.
Assistant Professor of Medicine
Harvard Medical School
Associate Physician
Brigham and Women's Hospital
Boston, Massachusetts

Robert S. Stern, M.D.
Assistant Professor of Dermatology
Harvard Medical School
Associate Dermatologist
Beth Israel Hospital
Boston, Massachusetts

William Strauss, M.D.
Instructor in Medicine
Harvard Medical School
Director of the Heart Station
Veterans Administration Hospital
West Roxbury, Massachusetts

Phillip G. Stubblefield, M.D.
Associate Professor of Obstetrics and Gynecology
Harvard Medical School
Associate Gynecologist
Massachusetts General Hospital
Boston, Massachusetts

Lewis Sudarsky, M.D.
Instructor in Neurology
Harvard Medical School
Staff Neurologist
Veterans Administration Medical Center
West Roxbury, Massachusetts,
Beth Israel Hospital, and
Brigham and Women's Hospital
Boston, Massachusetts

David J. Sugarbaker, M.D.
Resident in General Surgery
Brigham and Women's Hospital
Research Fellow in Gastroenterology

Beth Israel Hospital
Boston, Massachusetts

Joseph Upton, M.D.
Assistant Professor of Surgery
Harvard Medical School
Assistant in Surgery
Children's Hospital Medical Center and
Brigham and Women's Hospital
Boston, Massachusetts

Paul H. Wise, M.D.
Instructor in Pediatrics
Harvard Medical School
Director, Emergency and Primary Care Services
Children's Hospital Medical Center
Boston, Massachusetts

Lee A. Witters, M.D.
Assistant Professor of Medicine
Harvard Medical School
Assistant Physician
Massachusetts General Hospital
Boston, Massachusetts

Marshall A. Wolf, M.D.
Associate Professor of Medicine
Harvard Medical School
Associate Physician-in-Chief
Brigham and Women's Hospital
Boston, Massachusetts

Anthony E. Young, M.A., M.Chir.
Consultant Surgeon
St. Thomas' Hospital
London, England

W. B. Jerry Younger, M.D.
Assistant Professor of Medicine
Harvard Medical School
Associate in Medicine
Massachusetts General Hospital
Boston, Massachusetts

PREFACE

The battlefields of Korea and Vietnam taught us lessons about the delivery of medical care that allowed us to save the lives of many critically injured people in the 1950s and 1960s. Those lessons and other revolutionary insights that were gained at about the same time made it possible for victims of sudden death to be resuscitated by lay persons. These developments have led us to focus our attention during the past two decades on the improvement of emergency medical services. The process of developing an emergency medical service system has begun, emergency medical technicians and paramedical personnel have been trained, and a new specialist—the emergency physician—has emerged.

An unexpected by-product of this movement was the realization that many graduating medical students and practicing physicians were not as well prepared as the emergency medical technicians to provide competent initial care for many common emergencies. Many medical schools have therefore developed courses to ensure that graduating physicians would be competent and confident in dealing with common emergencies. Such a course gave birth to this book. Many of the contributors to *Emergency Medicine* have been participants in the course that has been offered at Harvard Medical School for its fourth-year medical students for the past 9 years. This book has been written not only for medical students, residents, and emergency physicians, but for any physician who is called upon, sometimes unexpectedly, to provide emergency care, especially when confronted with an emergency outside his or her speciality.

There were two questions in our minds during the preparation of the book: (1) What does the physician need to know in order to provide effective initial care for the emergency? (2) What does the physician have to be able to do? To provide answers to these questions, we divided the book into five parts. Part I focuses on the basic principles of life support by discussing the major pathophysiologic mechanisms that cause death or life-threatening emergencies. It presents the major clinical manifestations and discusses in detail the approach to

the management of these problems in the emergency room. Part II discusses trauma by defining the injuring mechanisms and the body's responses to injury and by discussing the evaluation and initial management of the critically injured patient and the management of the specific injuries. Part III discusses acute disorders, arranged by organ system (e.g., acute disorders of the skin, acute genitourinary disorders); by general category (e.g., acute metabolic disorders, poisoning); and by age group (e.g., pediatric emergencies). Part IV discusses the medicolegal implications of emergency medical care.

Part V is a "book within a book." In it are described and illustrated the common medical procedures carried out in the emergency room setting. One of the resources used by a surgeon-in-training to learn how to perform an operation is the illustrated operation atlas. Following the example of a good atlas, the procedure section not only describes how to perform a procedure but also how to avoid some of its common pitfalls.

The discussion of each emergency is presented in the context of emergency room practice, although the emergency may occur and have to be dealt with at another location. It focuses on what the primary physician does in evaluating and providing initial management for the patient rather than on what the consultant may have to do in providing definitive care. There are many emergencies that can be managed definitively by the primary or emergency physician, and the discussion here is aimed at providing the information that will be needed.

We hope that *Emergency Medicine* will be helpful to those who use it. It can serve as a reference during the management of situations that may be acute, but not urgent; however, it can be helpful in urgent or life-threatening situations only if the appropriate sections have been read and understood before the emergency.

No book of this size and scope is ever written and produced without a great expenditure of effort by many people. I am deeply indebted to the contributors who were diligent in writing their chapters, many of whom made a considerable investment of time. Harriet Greenfield faithfully kept completion of the illustrations a high priority in spite of many other demands on her time. Dr. Herbert Abrams, Chief of the Radiology Department of Brigham and Women's Hospital, Boston, and Dr. Donald Trunkey, Chief of the Surgical Service of the San Francisco General Hospital, generously gave permission for the use of their slides. Dr. William Bennett encouraged, advised, and gave constructive criticism during the early phases of this project. Executive Editor Robert Hurley and the staff of John Wiley & Sons have been most supportive and helpful in overseeing the production of this book. Special thanks must go to Rosalind Straley who supervised its production with such dedication, skill, and good humor. Many secretaries have been painstaking in preparing the manuscript, as well as patient and helpful in coordinating the communication that has been necessary and in attending to countless other details. Most important, we thank our families who, through no choice of their own, have shared the sacrifice of time that has been involved in the preparation of this book.

Harold L. May

CONTENTS

PART I
LIFE SUPPORT

PART II
ACUTE INJURIES

PART III
OTHER ACUTE DISORDERS

29. SKIN MANIFESTATIONS OF ACUTE DISORDERS   565

Robert S. Stern and Kenneth A. Arndt

30. ACUTE NEUROLOGIC DISORDERS   583

Dennis M.D. Landis

31. ACUTE NONTRAUMATIC EYE DISORDERS 599
*Alfredo A. Sadun
and Don C. Bienfang*

32. ACUTE NONTRAUMATIC DISORDERS OF THE EAR, FACIAL STRUCTURES, AND UPPER AIRWAY 613
*Edward E. Jacobs, Jr.,
and Leonard B. Kaban*

33. THE ACUTE ABDOMEN 653
Lynn M. Peterson

41. PSYCHIATRIC EMERGENCIES   787
Malcolm P. Rogers and Peter Reich

42. POISONING   805
*Michael A. McGuigan
and Frederick H. Lovejoy, Jr.*

43. DRUG OVERDOSE AND WITHDRAWAL   823
David C. Lewis and Irving H. Gomolin

44. PEDIATRIC EMERGENCIES   845

*Paul H. Wise, Jonathan Bates,
and John H. Fisher*

PART IV
MEDICOLEGAL CONSIDERATIONS

45. MEDICOLEGAL CONSIDERATIONS OF EMERGENCY MEDICAL CARE   883

*Elliott L. Cohen, Joseph M. Healey, Jr., and
Anthony P. Scapicchio*

PART V
EMERGENCY PROCEDURES

RESUSCITATION 897

ASPIRATION AND DRAINAGE TECHNIQUES AND DIAGNOSTIC PROCEDURES 965

SPECIAL PROCEDURE   1025

EMERGENCY MEDICINE

LIFE SUPPORT

PART I

1

CLINICAL DEATH AND RESUSCITATION

Robert C. Pascucci
William Strauss
Gary L. Simpson
Kevin M. McIntyre
Harold L. May

Clinical death, the reversible transition between life and biologic death, is the ultimate emergency. It begins when the last agonal breath has been taken and the heart has stopped beating. The patient looks like a corpse—unresponsive, with dilated pupils, and without breath or heartbeat. If rescuers do not intervene, disintegration within the various organs and tissues makes resuscitation impossible.

The idea that death can be reversed is not new. Since antiquity, people have struggled to find ways to resuscitate those who have died. Until relatively recently, many of the methods that were used were those that had been practiced for over 1,000 years, but within the past 4 decades the pioneering efforts of Claude Beck, V.A. Negovsky, and others have led to an increased understanding of the pathophysiology of cardiac arrest and to the development of clinically effective methods of its management. Direct compression and defibrillation of the heart through the open chest had made resuscitation possible within the hospital under special conditions. But it was not until 1959, when Kouwenhoven, Jude, and Knickerbocker described external chest compression, that resuscitation became feasible for many potential victims of sudden death occurring outside of the hospital.

In 1978 there were 1,928,000 deaths in the United States. Of these, 729,500 (37.8%) were caused by heart disease, 397,000 (20.6%) by cancer, 175,600 (9.1%) by cerebrovascular diseases, and 105,500 (5.5%) by accidents. Many of these deaths were expected and unavoidable; that is, body defenses had deteriorated and were exhausted, either because of advanced age or irreparable pathology. But 650,000 victims die annually of ischemic heart disease in the United States, and about 350,000 of these deaths occur outside of the hospital, usually within 2 hours after onset of symptoms. Most such deaths are caused by ventricular fibrillation. In these patients, clinical death is often the first symptom of the disease.

Recent reports from communities with a highly developed approach to cardiac arrest victims—communities with large numbers of lay persons trained in cardiopulmonary resuscitation (CPR), a rapid emergency medical service response system, and well-trained paramedical personnel—have demonstrated that more than 40% of the patients documented to have ventricular fibrillation outside the hospital can be successfully resuscitated if CPR is provided promptly. Since the community must be thought of as the ultimate coronary care unit, an aggressive, continuing, and broadly supported effort to train a large segment of the population in these techniques is required if the full potential of the life-saving measures is to be realized. It is clear that basic life support (BLS) is a holding action, maintaining the victim for a limited period of time. It must be followed by definitive therapy if the outcome is to be successful. Although initial efforts are focused on establishing adequate ventilation and circulation when these have been lost, the true aim of resuscitation has to be to maintain the viability of the brain.

PATHOPHYSIOLOGIC CONSIDERATIONS

Cells can live and function only as they release energy from the glucose molecule. This process of cellular respiration, which requires oxygen, involves the release of hydrogen from organic compounds and storage of free energy in the high-energy phosphate molecule, adenosine triphosphate (ATP), from which it can be readily released. The by-product of this energy-yielding aerobic process of cellular respiration is carbon dioxide. Whenever the supply of oxygen is deficient, whether caused by decreased perfusion of the cell, as in shock, or by a critical decrease in the oxygen content of the blood for whatever reason, energy transformation becomes seriously impaired. Lactic acid can no longer be dehydrogenated and glucose has to be broken down anaerobically, which provides a poor yield of ATP. During aerobic glycolysis, the production of ATP is 19 times as great as it is under anaerobic conditions.

As the energy available to the cell decreases, its vital functions deteriorate. Sodium leaks into the cell, and the level of potassium in the blood rises progressively because the gradient necessary to retain potassium within the cell and sodium in the extracellular fluid can no longer be maintained. Synthesis of protein and enzymes stops because energy is no longer available, and, finally, the structural elements of the cell break down and the cell is destroyed. As death continues, the resulting metabolic end products accumulate as waste from the dying cells.

Although other organs can get some of their energy from

metabolism of fat and proteins, the brain's energy requirements must be met entirely by glucose. Safar points out that brain oxygen stores are depleted within less than 10 seconds of circulatory arrest (the time that it takes for unconsciousness to develop) and that brain glucose stores will last only about 5 minutes for subsequent anaerobic energy metabolism. Beyond this point, energy production ceases and irreversible cellular changes begin. This has led to the observation that after circulatory arrest of more than 5 minutes (under normal conditions), it is unlikely that complete functional restoration of all neurons can occur unless effective resuscitative measures are employed.

The Terminal Patient

There is wide variation in the sequence of events that accompanies death and in the duration of its stages, depending on the underlying pathology and the physiologic state of the person before the terminal event. Sudden cardiac arrest caused by ventricular fibrillation leads within seconds to clinical death, in which neither pulse nor respiration can be detected in the unresponsive patient. In the patient dying in shock from loss of blood or progressive respiratory insufficiency, however, clinical death is preceded by a preterminal state that may last for many hours. In spite of the differences of mechanisms, there are many similarities and characteristic stages, which have been well described by Negovsky, Safar, and others.

PREAGONAL PERIOD

In victims of sudden cardiac arrest from ventricular fibrillation (e.g., as a result of electrical shock) there is virtually no preagonal period, but in other conditions in which death is not instantaneous, the hemodynamic and respiratory disorders that are predominating influences during the preagonal period lead to hypoxia and tissue acidosis. The energy supply during this time is basically aerobic, but functional impairment of the body organs aggravates the disturbance of circulation as ventilation–perfusion relationships in the lungs deteriorate, the ability of the liver to excrete toxic wastes is disrupted, and the kidneys eventually stop functioning. Hypoxia causes reflex stimulation of life-ensuring systems—chemoreceptors, angioreceptors, the respiratory and vasomotor centers, and the reticular formation of the brain stem—in an effort to compensate for failing functions and to preserve the higher centers in the central nervous system (CNS). The rate and depth of breathing, heart rate, and cardiac output increase, while the arterial blood pressure rises in response to constriction of the peripheral and splanchnic blood vessels. At the same time, the capillary network of the brain dilates in an effort to increase the blood supply to the vital structures of the brain. However, in the dying patient, the activation of the compensatory mechanisms is followed by the equally important inhibition of the brain cortex, which defends the higher structures of the central nervous system from maximum exhaustion. The cortical neurons, the most sensitive of all of the cells of the body to hypoxia, are the first to go out of action. The energy expenditure of the central nervous system is lessened; cortical functions are suspended while energy resources are concentrated on the vital regulation of function of the internal organs. The patient first loses rational mentation and then loses consciousness.

TERMINAL PAUSE

The sudden cessation of respiration after a sudden period of tachypnea—the terminal pause—is a response to an increase in the tone of the vagus nerves as they are stimulated by hypoxia. Oxidative processes are repressed and glycolyitic processes increase. The duration of the terminal pause varies from 5 or 10 seconds to 3 or 4 minutes.

AGONY

Agony, which begins after the terminal pause, is the last chaotic and primitive manifestation of life. The brain has switched completely to anaerobic glycolysis and its highest function has failed, relieving the bulbar centers from the regulatory influence of the cerebral cortex. Thus free, these lower centers organize one last effort in the dying patient's struggle for life. The almost extinct processes of respiration and circulation are temporarily reactivated. Sometimes there is a short-term regaining of consciousness. Decerebrate rigidity and general tonic spasms may be observed. Because of the anaerobic glycolysis that energizes this period, incompletely oxidized metabolic products rapidly accumulate. Respiration is at first weak, then increases considerably, and after reaching a maximum, gradually weakens and ceases. All of the respiratory muscles, including the accessory ones, are involved during inhalation. The cardiac contractions temporarily increase in frequency, and the blood pressure may reach a level of 30–40 mm Hg. If energetic therapy is not immediately started, cardiac activity and respiration cease and clinical death sets it.

CLINICAL DEATH

Clinical death has been defined by Negovsky as "the period of respiratory, circulatory, and brain arrest during which initiation of resuscitation can lead to recovery with prearrest central nervous system (CNS) function." It begins either with the last agonal inhalation or the last cardiac contraction. The patient is without pulse or blood pressure and is completely unresponsive to the most painful stimulus; the pupils are widely dilated. Some reflex reactions to external stimulation are preserved. During intubation, for example, respiration may be restored in response to stimulation of the receptors of the superior laryngeal nerve, the nucleus of which is located in the medulla oblongata near the respiratory center.

The duration of clinical death depends on the length of time the cerebral cortex survives in the absence of circulation and respiration. Under normal temperature conditions this period does not, as a rule, exceed 3–6 minutes. Signs of the alteration of cells begin the moment clinical death sets in and, with time, disorders increase. The character and length of the preceding period of dying have considerable effect on the duration of clinical death. In sudden death from ventricular fibrillation in a previously healthy person, the period of clinical death is usually 4–6 minutes; however, when the pathologic process has been tempestuous, the period of clinical death is shortened even though the preceding events may have progressed rapidly. When the terminal stage has been lengthy, the period of clinical death shortens even more; if the patient spends a long time (several hours) in severe hypotension, resuscitation becomes impossible even a few seconds after the cessation of cardiac activity because of exhaustion of all energy resources and of severe morphologic damage.

For the same reason, age also affects the length of the period of clinical death. Resuscitation is much more likely to be successful after the cardiac arrest of a young, healthy person than after that of an elderly person. Isolated cases have been described in which it has been possible to resuscitate children after 10 or even 12 minutes of clinical death, resulting in complete restoration of vital functions.

Terminal states that develop in cases of hypothermia have specific features. The main property of hypothermia—increase of the resistance of the higher sectors of the brain to hypoxia through slowing of metabolic processes and reduction of the energy demand—creates conditions for prolonged brain survival on energy provided by glycolysis. Hypothermia is successfully used to prolong clinical death and is also a factor favorably affecting restoration of the higher sectors of the brain. Experimental investigations carried out in the laboratory have shown that moderate hypothermia (body temperature 24–26°C, 75.2–78.8°F) during dying enables the period of clinical death to be prolonged up to 1 hour (Negovsky). On a background of deep hypothermia (8–10°C, 46.4–50°F) the duration of clinical death has been prolonged up to 2 hours.

BIOLOGIC DEATH AND BRAIN DEATH

Biologic death, which sets in after clinical death, is an irreversible state of cellular destruction. Tissues of the body vary in their ability to survive anoxic and metabolic results, and hence some organs irretrievably "die" sooner than others. During early biologic death, when irreversible changes have already occurred in the brain cortex and full restoration of the function of the central nervous system is impossible, it is occasionally possible to restore the activity of the heart and of the respiratory and certain subcortical centers. Successful cardiopulmonary resuscitation may thus occur despite less successful brain resuscitation, leading to the survival of a person with significant brain damage or, in the worst cases, to the condition known popularly as *brain death.*

The determination of when biologic death has occurred may frequently fall to the emergency physician and in some circumstances is difficult. Legal criteria for certification of death vary from state to state and nation to nation, and many jurisdictions lack a definition compatible with modern techniques of life support. The President's Commission for the Study of Ethical Problems in Medicine and Biomedical and Behavioral Research, recognizing the need for a uniform statute to provide a clear and socially accepted basis for making determinations of death, in July 1981 proposed this model:

Uniform Determination of Death Act

An individual who has sustained either (1) irreversible cessation of circulatory and respiratory functions, or (2) irreversible cessation of all functions of the entire brain, including the brain stem, is dead. A determination of death must be made in accordance with accepted medical standards.

The fulfillment of the first criterion is generally the easier to determine. If, despite optimal cardiopulmonary resuscitation and support for a reasonable period of time, the patient is unable to develop and sustain spontaneous circulation, the patient is dead. Most determinations of death in the emergency setting will be made on this basis.

Fulfillment of the second criterion is more problematic. Guidelines to assist in the medical determination of cessation of brain function have been published, including those of the Ad Hoc Committee of the Harvard Medical School (1968) (Table 1.1), the United States Collaborative Study of Cerebral Death (1976) (Table 1.2), and the Conference of Royal Colleges and Faculties of the United Kingdom (1976) (Table 1.3). The most recent (1981) statement of currently accepted medical standards has been published as a supplement to the recommendations of the President's Commission. An outline of these

TABLE 1.1 Harvard Criteria for Brain Death

1. *Unreceptive and unresponsive.* "Even the most intensely painful stimuli evoke no vocal or other response. . . ."

2. *No movements or breathing.* "Observation covering a period of at least one hour by physicians is adequate to satisfy the criteria of no spontaneous muscular movements or spontaneous respiration or response to stimuli. . . . The total absence of spontaneous breathing may be established by turning off the respirator for three minutes and observing whether there is any effort on the part of the subject to breathe. . . ." (This requires that carbon dioxide tension be normal and the patient be breathing room air for 10 minutes before the test.)

3. *No reflexes.* "The pupil will be fixed and dilated and will not respond to a direct source of bright light. . . . Ocular movement (to head turning and to irrigation of ears with ice water) and blinking are absent. . . . There is no evidence of postural activity (decerebrate or other). . . . Swallowing, yawning, vocalizing are in abeyance. . . . Corneal and pharyngeal reflexes are absent. . . . As a rule the stretch or tendon reflexes cannot be elicited."

4. *Flat electroencephalogram.* "Of great confirmatory value is the flat or isoelectric electroencephalogram. . . ." (Technical guidelines including 5 μV/mm or higher gains, absence of response to pinch or noise, and 10-minute minimum recording time are added.) "All of the above tests shall be repeated at least 24 hours later with no change." Hypothermia (temperature below 32.2°C, 90°F) and central nervous system depressants such as barbiturates must be excluded. "In situations where . . . electroencephalographic monitoring is not available, the absence of cerebral function has to be determined by purely clinical signs . . . or by the absence of circulation as judged by standstill of blood in the retinal vessels, or by absence of cardiac action. . . ."

SOURCE: A definition of irreversible coma: Report of the Ad Hoc Committee of the Harvard Medical School to examine the definition of brain death. *J Am Med Assoc* 1968; 205:337–340.

guidelines is presented in Table 1.4. All have their limitations, and all should be recognized as guidelines for the exercise of good medical judgment rather than as absolute criteria to be used in a blind "checklist" fashion. The essence of the determination is satisfactory assurance that there is no cerebral or brainstem function remaining, that complicating conditions have been ruled out, and that the patient can no longer survive as an individual, independent being. Satisfactory resolution of these issues frequently requires an extended period of observation, and determination of death on a neurologic basis can rarely be attained in the emergency department setting.

Mechanisms of Rapid Death

There are two broad categories into which cardiac arrest can be divided—*primary cardiac arrest,* in which sudden cessation of cardiac function is the first manifestation of acute decompensation, and *secondary cardiac arrest,* in which factors external to the heart cause cardiac arrest as a complication of some other process.

PRIMARY CARDIAC ARREST

A number of disease states predispose to sudden cardiac dysrhythmias or loss of cardiac function. Poor coronary perfusion accompanied by imbalance of myocardial oxygen supply and demand is the most common cause of such an arrest. This mechanism, unfortunately, is seen in patients who have reasonably healthy hearts. Electrical shock, for example, can cause death from a sudden cardiac dysrhythmia even if the damage it causes to other body systems is minimal. Chronic congestive heart failure from valvular disease, myocarditis, or other disease of heart muscle, and ventricular scarring and fibrosis from previous infarction all can lead to primary cardiac arrest. In

TABLE 1.2 Criteria for Cerebral Death (Brain Death) Proposed by the Collaborative Study of Cerebral Death

Prerequisite
  All appropriate diagnostic and therapeutic procedures have been performed.
Criteria
  Each criterion must be present for 30 minutes at least 6 hours after the onset of coma and apnea.
  1. Coma with cerebral unresponsivity (see Definition 1)
  2. Apnea (see Definition 2)
  3. Dilated pupils
  4. Absent cephalic reflexes (see Definition 3)
  5. Electrocerebral silence (see Definition 4)
Confirmatory test
  Absence of cerebral blood flow
Definitions
  1. *Cerebral unresponsivity.* A state in which the patient does not respond purposively to externally applied stimuli, obeys no commands, and does not phonate spontaneously or in response to a painful stimulus
  2. *Apnea.* The absence of spontaneous respiration, manifested by the need for controlled ventilation (i.e., the patient makes no effort to override the respirator) for at least 15 minutes
  3. *Cephalic reflexes.* Pupillary, corneal, oculoauditory, oculovestibular, oculocephalic, ciliospinal, snout, cough, pharyngeal swallowing
  4. *Electrocerebral silence.* An electroencephalogram with an absence of electrical potentials of cerebral origin over 2 μV from symmetrically placed electrode pairs over 10 cm apart and with interelectrode resistance between 100–10,000 Ω

SOURCE: An appraisal of the criteria of cerebral death: A summary statement: A collaborative study. *J Am Med Assoc* 1976; 237:982–986.

TABLE 1.3 Criteria for the Diagnosis of Brain Death

A. Conditions under which the diagnosis of brain death should be considered.
   1. The patient is deeply comatose.
      a. There should be no suspicion that this state is due to depressant drugs.
      b. Primary hypothermia as a cause of coma should have been excluded.
      c. Metabolic and endocrine disturbances that can be responsible for or can contribute to coma should have been excluded.
   2. The patient is being maintained on a ventilator because spontaneous respiration had previously become inadequate or had ceased altogether. Relaxants . . . and other drugs should have been excluded as a cause of respiratory failure.
   3. There should be no doubt that the patient's condition is due to irremediable structural brain damage. The diagnosis of a disorder that can lead to brain death should have been fully established.
B. Diagnostic tests for confirmation of brain death.
   All brainstem reflexes are absent.
   1. The pupils are fixed in diameter and do not respond to sharp changes in the intensity of incident light.
   2. There is no corneal reflex.
   3. The vestibulo-ocular reflexes are absent.
   4. No motor responses within the cranial nerve distribution can be elicited by adequate stimulation of a somatic area.
   5. There is no gag reflex or reflex response to bronchial stimulation by a suction catheter passed down the trachea.
   6. No respiratory movements occur when the patient is disconnected from the mechanical ventilator for long enough to ensure that the arterial carbon dioxide tension rose above the threshold for stimulation of respiration.
C. Other considerations
   1. *Repetition of testing.* The interval between tests must depend upon the primary pathology and the clinical course of the disease. . . . In some conditions the outcome is not so clearcut, and in these cases it is recommended that the tests should be repeated. The interval between tests depends upon the progress of the patient and might be as long as 24 hours. . . .
   2. *Integrity of spinal reflexes.* It is well established that spinal cord function can persist after insults that irretrievably destroy brainstem functions. . . .
   3. *Confirmatory investigation.* It is now widely accepted that electroencephalography is not necessary for the diagnosis of brain death. . . . Other investigations such as cerebral angiography or cerebral blood-flow measurements are not required for the diagnosis of brain death.
   4. *Body temperature.* . . . It is recommended that it should not be less than 35°C before the diagnostic tests are carried out.
   5. *Specialist opinion and the status of the doctors concerned.* Only when the primary diagnosis is in doubt is it necessary to consult with a neurologist or neurosurgeon. Decision to withdraw artificial support should be made after all the criteria presented above have been fulfilled and can be made by any of the following combination of doctors:
      a. A consultant who is in charge of the case and one other doctor.
      b. In the absence of a consultant, his [or her] deputy, who should have been registered for 5 years or more and who should have had adequate experience in the care of such cases, and one other doctor.

SOURCE: Conference of Royal Colleges and Faculties of the United Kingdom: Diagnosis of brain death. *Lancet* 1976; 2:1069–1070.

TABLE 1.4 Criteria for Determination of Death

An individual presenting the findings in *either* section A (cardiopulmonary) *or* section B (neurologic) is dead. In either section, a diagnosis of death requires that *both* cessation of functions, as set forth in subsection 1, *and* irreversibility, as set forth in subsection 2, be demonstrated.

A. An individual with irreversible cessation of circulatory and respiratory functions is dead.
    1. Cessation is recognized by an appropriate clinical examination.
    2. Irreversibility is recognized by persistent cessation of function during an appropriate period of observation and/or trial of therapy.
B. An individual with irreversible cessation of all functions of the entire brain, including the brain stem, is dead.
    1. Cessation is recognized when evaluation discloses findings of a *and* b:
        a. Cerebral functions are absent.
        b. Brain stem functions are absent.
    2. Irreversibility is recognized when evaluation discloses findings of a *and* b *and* c:
        a. The cause of coma is established and is sufficient to account for the loss of brain functions.
        b. The possibility of recovery of any brain functions is excluded.
        c. The cessation of all brain functions persists for an appropriate period of observation and/or trial of therapy.

SOURCE: Guidelines for the determination of death: Report of the medical consultants on the diagnosis of death to the President's Commission for the Study of Ethical Problems in Medicine and Biomedical and Behavioral Research. *J Am Med Assoc* 1981; 246:2184–2186.

many such cases, the pumping function of the heart is so weakened that resuscitation from arrest is impossible.

Sudden loss of cardiac pumping function occurs in association with several patterns of cardiac electrical activity. Ventricular fibrillation, ventricular standstill or asystole, and electromechanical dissociation are three patterns associated with clinical death.

Ventricular Fibrillation

Ventricular fibrillation causes the majority of sudden deaths in patients with preexisting myocardial ischemia. Electrical activity is random and uncoordinated; there is no sequencing of atrial, nodal, and ventricular depolarization. Although the fibrillating myocardium is quite active and its metabolic demands remain high, there is no effective cardiac output and no coronary perfusion; ischemia intensifies as the condition persists. Although myocardial ischemia and spontaneous ectopy are the most common causative factors, external influ-

ences on the heart, including electrical shock, electrolyte abnormalities, hypothermia, drugs, and excess circulating catecholamines, can precipitate ventricular fibrillation.

Ventricular Asystole

Ventricular asystole, a less commonly seen condition, is a pulseless state with cardiac standstill and an isoelectric electrocardiogram (ECG). Its presence usually indicates a severe condition with widespread myocardial damage, and resuscitation is often difficult or impossible. Asystole may develop as the endpoint of a prolonged period of ventricular fibrillation. Less commonly, it may result from increased parasympathetic tone from extraordinary vagal stimulation, with consequent depression of rhythm and conduction. Predisposing conditions, aside from generalized ischemic disease, include Stokes-Adams syndrome (focal ischemia in the conduction system) and dependence on an electrical pacemaker. Electrocution, massive drug overdose, and electrolyte abnormalities may also result in asystole.

Electromechanical Dissociation

Electromechanical dissociation, in which relatively normal cardiac electrical activity is present but is not accompanied by appropriate mechanical contraction, is unusual as a presenting rhythm but frequently appears during resuscitative efforts. Inadequate perfusion pressure is present and volume and pharmacologic support may be required to restore normal circulation. Cardiomyopathy, severe hypocalcemia, and intravascular volume depletion may lead to electromechanical dissociation. Pericardial tamponade may mimic electromechanical dissociation, but it is easily diagnosed and treated by surgical drainage of pericardial fluid.

SECONDARY CARDIAC ARREST

Although the heart may be quite healthy, failure or dysfunction in another organ system may, after a variable period of time, lead to secondary cardiac arrest. Correction of the primary problem must occur simultaneously with the resuscitation of the heart; the severity of the primary disease and the length of time it has been present will determine the ultimate prognosis of the patient.

Respiratory failure, whatever its cause, may lead to arterial hypoxemia and hypercarbia. Cardiac activity may initially be stimulated by such abnormalities, but if they remain uncorrected, the patient becomes acidotic, the myocardium is unable to sustain tone or contraction, and asystole ensues. Acute hypoxia or anoxia causes a very rapid deterioration to cardiac arrest, usually within 2–3 minutes. If hypoxia is prevented by administration of oxygen but ventilation is interrupted and the victim is allowed to become hypercarbic and acidotic, the process is somewhat prolonged; cardiac arrest will not usually occur until the arterial pH falls below 6.8.

Sudden loss of blood volume, such as in massive traumatic hemorrhage, will result in cardiac arrest. The initial circulatory compensation for such loss is by vasoconstriction and tachycardia; peripheral vascular beds are shut down, and the reduced blood volume is circulated more and more rapidly to the essential organs. Although an adequate perfusion pressure can be maintained by such adjustments for a short period of time, this pressure gradually diminishes as losses continue and intravascular volume is depleted. Cardiac output is no longer able to meet metabolic demands of the vital organs, including the heart itself, and cardiac arrest ensues.

Central nervous system failure may occur acutely from trauma, intracranial hemorrhage, or rapid increases in intracranial pressure. Brainstem output to the heart and respiratory muscles is altered, and their function becomes erratic, depressed, and ultimately terminated.

Metabolic derangements, embolic phenomena, extremes of temperature, toxins, and *acute anaphylactic reactions* all can lead to sudden cessation of cardiorespiratory function. It is the goal of the rescuer to begin resuscitation as early as possible in this period of clinical death in order to avoid the onset of irreversible organic changes and to prevent progression to biologic death.

Resuscitation

There are three goals of resuscitation: (1) basic life support, providing temporary perfusion and oxygenation of vital tissues; (2) restoration of spontaneous cardiac activity and establishment of circulatory self-sufficiency; (3) correction of the underlying disease state, while supporting and protecting all organ systems and assisting them in recovery to as near their prearrest state as possible. Appropriate intervention during clinical death can achieve these goals. Energy production is restored to various tissues, and cells can resume their customary functions. The length of time the patient spends in clinical death, together with the patient's state of health preceding it, will determine the extent of recovery possible.

The initial phase of resuscitation of the patient is restoration of effective pulmonary ventilation and maintenance of such ventilation until the patient is able to do so on his or her own.

Basic life support begins with opening of the airway and provision of expired-air ventilation.

Normally, inhaled air has an oxygen content of 20.94 vol%, and carbon dioxide content of 0.04 vol%; exhaled air contains approximately 15.5 vol% oxygen and 4 vol% carbon dioxide. During resuscitation efforts, hyperventilation by the rescuer can increase the oxygen content of his or her exhaled air; oxygen content may reach 18 vol% with carbon dioxide levels falling concurrently to 2 vol%. This will result in an enriched inspired oxygen concentration (FiO_2) delivery to the patient. Furthermore, air can be exhaled with an approximate force of 70 cm H_2O and with tidal volumes of 1,000–1,250 ml. It has been found that positive pressure artificial ventilation (PPAV), properly applied, without respiratory adjuncts, can produce arterial partial pressures of oxygen (PaO_2) greater than 75 mm Hg (with oxygen saturation of hemoglobin approximately 90%) and $PaCO_2$ of 30–40 mm Hg. A number of animal and clinical studies have proven these pulmonary parameters to be sufficient for sustained ventilatory support and tissue oxygenation.

The use of CPR technique by all strata of medical and lay personnel during the past 2 decades has revolutionized the management and prognosis of CPR. When applied as currently recommended, external cardiac compression (ECC) can produce 20–40% of normal cardiac output (approaching 1–1.5 liters/min), with mean arterial pressures of 30–40 mm Hg. Antegrade blood flow requires a peripheral arterial–venous pressure gradient. As will be discussed, it currently is believed that during ECC this pressure gradient results from differential vascular collapse and reflects the unequal transmission of intrathoracic pressure into the extrathoracic arteries and veins.

When the technique of "cardiac massage" was introduced initially, its effectiveness was thought to rely upon the anatomical arrangement of the structures of the mediastinum. The prevalent notion held that displacement of the sternum posteriorly resulted in compression of the chambers of the heart against the posterior mediastinal compartment and the vertebral column, leading to the generation of forward blood flow.

Evidence accumulated in recent years, however, has shown convincingly that antegrade arterial blood flow can be produced by increases in total intrathoracic pressure, although compression of the heart may contribute in some cases. A number of observations support the phasic increase of intrathoracic pressure as the driving force in CPR. It has been demonstrated, for example, that during CPR the heart cannot function as an unidirectional pump since all cardiac valves are grossly incompetent. Angiographic studies have shown the left ventricle to have a small and relatively fixed volume throughout the external compression cycle. Finally, hemodynamic monitoring during CPR has found essentially equal pressures in the superior vena cava, right atrium, pulmonary artery, left ventricle, and aorta. Therefore it has been postulated that the pressure gradient required for cerebral perfusion during ECC is extrathoracic, that is, formed because of the persistent patency of thick-walled arteries throughout the compression cycle, coupled with the concurrent collapse of jugular veins and the competent closure of intraluminal valves near the termination of the internal jugulars. Thus, the present concept of ECC effectiveness views the heart as a passive conduit for blood with antegrade arterial blood flow produced by generalized elevations in intrathoracic pressure during the compression phase; the importance of an adequate compression time (50–60% of cycle duration) during ECC has been reemphasized.

As successful cardiopulmonary resuscitation continues, the tissues of the body are reperfused and reoxygenated and normal metabolism and function can begin to return. The various tissues resume function at differing rates. Cardiac function is restored rather quickly. Ventricular complexes and then nodal and sinus rhythms appear. As myocardial acidosis is corrected and tone is restored, contractility improves and the heart can once again resume its pumping function. Respiratory function may follow soon afterward, and initial gasping progresses first to a periodic breathing pattern and then to a more normal respiratory cycle. Vasomotor tone and brainstem recovery occur as the respiratory and cardiac rhythms stabilize, and restoration of brainstem reflexes ensues. Cerebral cortical activity recovers more slowly, with an isoelectric electroencephalogram (EEG) giving way to a slow EEG rhythm; a sluggish process of awakening continues, and recovery—not necessarily to baseline function—progresses over days to weeks. Cerebral blood flow is restored, but there is often a spotty pattern of reperfusion and diffuse cerebral edema. Areas of brain with relatively high metabolic demand may, because of regional differences in blood flow, receive inadequate perfusion. This imbalance of demand and flow is referred to as the *no reflow phenomenon* and may be secondary to edema, blood sludging, or vasospasm.

Such areas of hypoperfusion after resuscitation from a hypoxic–ischemic event are seen not only in brain but in other tissues as well, and they may be the basis of the *postresuscitation syndrome*. This syndrome has been shown to include persistent cardiac and respiratory dysfunction (secondary to preexisting disease, edema, and contusion injury from resuscitation), central nervous system abnormalities, and renal and gastrointestinal (GI) dysfunction. Attention to management of each of these areas is begun by the emergency physician and continued by the physician specializing in multidisciplinary critical care.

BASIC LIFE SUPPORT

Basic life support (BLS) techniques are designed to provide sufficient ventilatory and circulatory support to prevent brain damage. The techniques are applied until recovery has occurred or until advanced life support (ALS) procedures can be instituted. The success of resuscitative efforts is related directly to the time required for recognition of cardiopulmonary arrest, the time required to initiate BLS, and the degree to which standards for BLS are followed. Guidelines for life-support techniques originate from the National Conference on Cardiopulmonary Resuscitation and Emergency Cardiac Care.

Recognition of Cardiopulmonary Arrest

Cardiopulmonary arrest is recognized when a person is unresponsive, has ashen gray skin, and lacks adequate respiratory motions. Carotid and femoral pulses are absent; pupils become dilated and after a short time become unresponsive to light. The approximate sequence of sentinel events following abrupt cessation of effective cardiac output includes loss of consciousness (at about 10–15 seconds) and pupillary dilation (at 30–45 seconds), followed by irreversible cerebral cortical damage occurring within 5–10 minutes.

The presence of spontaneous respiration does not exclude the possibility of cardiac arrest. Normal respiratory motion may persist for approximately 1 minute after catastrophic loss of cardiac function. Cardiopulmonary arrest may masquerade as major motor seizures as a result of cerebral hypoxia. Unconscious patients should be assumed to have cardiopulmonary arrest until their vital functions are documented. The time of onset of cardiopulmonary arrest must be noted in order to guide subsequent therapeutic interventions.

The basic Airway, Breathing, Circulation schema constitutes the foundation of CPR. Once the victim's unresponsiveness has been established, a call for help has been made, and the patient has been positioned supine on a firm surface, the sequence of events discussed below is instituted immediately.

Airway Control

The upper airway must be patent for successful pulmonary ventilation. In the unconscious patient, muscular flaccidity allows the mandible and hyoid bone to recede, thus dropping the tongue and epiglottis against the posterior wall of the pharynx. Anatomical hypopharyngeal obstruction results (Fig. 1.1). One of the following maneuvers can be used to relieve this predictable obstruction.

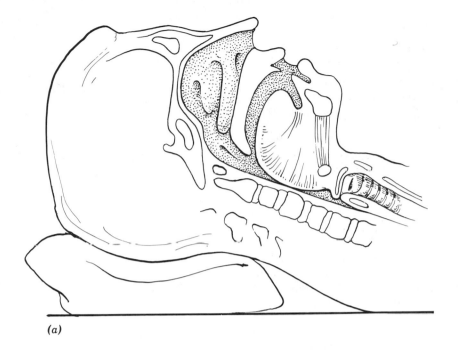

(a)

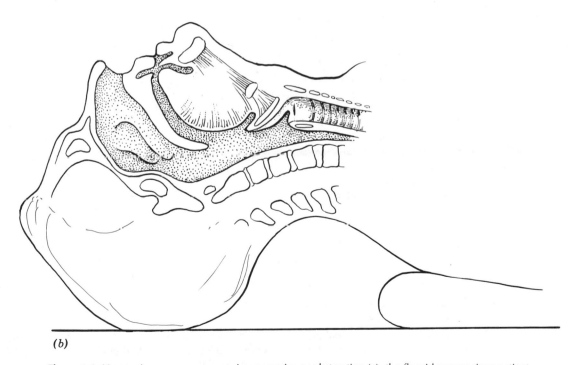

(b)

Figure 1.1 Upper airway management. In upper airway obstruction (a), the flaccid unconscious patient loses muscle tone, thus allowing the mandible, tongue, and associated structures to fall posteriorly, obstructing the airway. (b) Simply tilting the head posteriorly may be sufficient to open the airway.

HEAD-TILT (WITH CHIN-LIFT OR NECK-LIFT) METHOD

The head-tilt procedure is the initial and integral step in opening the upper airway; it should be augmented with either the chin-lift (Fig. 1.2a) or neck-lift (Fig. 1.2b) maneuver. Considerable clinical experience has demonstrated the effectiveness of both adjunctive maneuvers when applied in combination with head-tilt. However, recent studies have suggested that the chin-lift method may be the superior technique, particularly in the resuscitation of an unconscious, apneic patient.

The *head-tilt–chin-lift* method is performed by grasping the anterior portion of the patient's lower jaw with the fingertips of one hand while the other hand is placed on the patient's forehead. The mandible is then displaced forward by lifting the chin as the head is simultaneously tilted backward with the other hand. Care should be taken to avoid compression of the submental soft tissues since this may itself obstruct the airway. The chin should be lifted until the teeth are nearly, but not completely, opposed.

To accomplish the *head-tilt–neck-lift* method, the rescuer positions one hand under the patient's neck and the other hand on the forehead. Gentle forward flexion of the neck with simultaneous backward extension of the head can provide sufficient stretching of the tissues of the anterior neck to restore upper airway patency. The lifting hand should be positioned near the occiput to minimize the risk of hyperextending the cervical spine. Both methods force the mandible forward, thus elevating the tongue and epiglottis away from the posterior pharyngeal wall. In addition, the normal cervical curvature is reestablished and the lumen of the pharynx, which has been narrowed by flexion of the cervical vertebrae, is widened.

The *modified mandible-thrust* method has application in trauma patients in whom the stability of the vertebral column is uncertain. To avoid extension or lateral rotation of the neck, the head is grasped between the palms of both hands and held in a neutral position (Fig. 1.2c). The fingers of both hands are placed behind the angles of the mandibles bilaterally, and the jaw is displaced forward without tilting the head. If the upper airway is not cleared, the head can be extended backward slightly and the maneuver repeated.

CHECK FOR FOREIGN BODIES

Use of any of the methods discussed may be all that is required for successful resuscitation if upper airway obstruction is the sole problem. The rescuer should check for airway patency and presence of spontaneous ventilation by observing chest motion and by listening and feeling for air movement at the mouth and nose. If spontaneous respirations are not detected, a cursory check for foreign bodies in the mouth should be

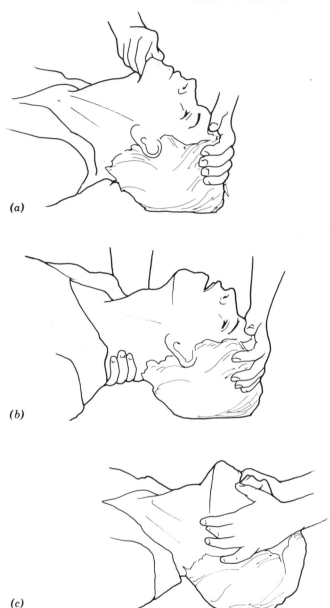

(a)

(b)

(c)

Figure 1.2 Various methods for opening the airway: (a) head-tilt, chin lift; (b) head-tilt, neck lift; (c) mandible or jaw thrust.

made, and artificial pulmonary ventilation should be begun immediately. Careful explorations of the oropharynx for potential foreign body obstruction should not be performed initially unless its presence is known or strongly suspected. One exception to this rule would be the removal of loose dentures.

Breathing

Exhaled air, artificial pulmonary ventilation (by either mouth-to-mouth, mouth-to-nose, or mouth-to-stoma techniques) can provide sufficient ventilatory support for long durations. Although mechanical airways (see advanced life support section) may serve as valuable respiratory adjuncts if readily available, time should not be wasted in locating them.

MOUTH-TO-MOUTH VENTILATION

To perform mouth-to-mouth artificial ventilation, the rescuer maintains the patient's neck extension using one of the techniques described above and occludes the patient's nostrils between the thumb and forefinger of the hand that is positioned on the forehead (Fig. 1.3a). (Use of the mandible-thrust method dictates that the patient's nostrils be sealed with the rescuer's cheek.) The rescuer then opens his or her mouth widely, inhales deeply, forms a seal over the patient's mouth with his or her lips, and forcibly blows into the patient's mouth, while watching for a corresponding rise of the chest wall. The rescuer removes his or her mouth, listens for passive expiration, and notes the gradual fall of the anterior chest wall. If the rescuer is convinced that adequate ventilation can now be achieved, a total of four consecutive full breaths is delivered to ensure full pulmonary inflation and then the rescuer proceeds directly to the third aspect of basic life support—circulation.

MOUTH-TO-NOSE VENTILATION

Mouth-to-nose ventilation may be required in certain instnces such a massive facial trauma or trismus. The rescuer initially performs a head-tilt maneuver by placing one hand on the patient's forehead and extending the chin upward with the heel of the other hand positioned under the jaw. The mouth is occluded with the palm of the hand. The rescuer's mouth is sealed around the patient's nose as ventilation is delivered. The patient's mouth should be allowed to open during the exhalation phase since the soft palate may impede air flow through the nasopharynx.

MOUTH-TO-STOMA VENTILATION

Mouth-to-stoma ventilation is preferable in patients with established tracheostomy stoma and mandatory in patients with a tracheostomy tube in place. No neck distention maneuvers are required. During all phases of the ventilatory cycle, the rescuer seals the patient's nose and mouth with one hand. The need for this maneuver is obviated if the tracheostomy tube is provided with an inflatable cuff. All other aspects of artificial ventilation through tracheostomy stoma are identical with those of the mouth-to-mouth technique.

RECOGNITION AND MANAGEMENT OF FOREIGN BODY AIRWAY OBSTRUCTION IN THE UNCONSCIOUS PATIENT

Assuming the procedures outlined above have been applied properly, marked airway resistance to the initial ventilatory effort or failure of the patient's chest wall to rise should alert the rescuer to the possible presence of a foreign body obstructing the upper airway. Materials such as dentures, tooth fragments, and vomitus, as well as a variety of intrinsic or induced structural abnormalities, may cause airway obstruction. To remove foreign bodies, the rescuer may employ one or a combination of the following manual maneuvers. Each method is described in the context of resuscitating the supine, unconscious patient.

Back Blows

While in a kneeling position beside the patient, the rescuer should roll the patient toward him or herself until the patient's chest is resting against the rescuer's thigh. A rapid series of four sharp blows should be delivered forcefully with the heel of the hand to a point between the scapulae (Fig. 1.4). This maneuver is performed with the assumption that the foreign body may be impacted at the level of the epiglottis. The patient is then returned to the supine position, the foreign body is removed digitally if possible, as described below, the head is repositioned, and artificial ventilation is instituted once again.

Manual Thrusts (Cough-Creating Thrust Maneuver)

The manual thrust maneuver may be applied to the supine patient's upper abdomen or midchest. For the *abdominal approach,* the rescuer kneels either astride or alongside the patient at the approximate level of the pelvis. The heel of one hand is placed against the patient's abdomen at a point midway between the umbilicus and the lower margin of the thoracic cage. The rescuer's other hand is positioned on top of the first (Fig. 1.5). The rescuer's shoulders are aligned directly over his or her hands, and the rescuer delivers four successive thrusts in an inward and upward direction.

For the *chest approach,* the rescuer kneels beside the patient and positions his or her hands in the exact manner as when administering external cardiac compression (i.e., with the heel of one hand resting on the sternum about 4–7 cm above the xiphoid process and the heel of the other hand placed on top of the heel of the first—see section on circulation). The rescuer's shoulders form a vertical plane over his or her hands,

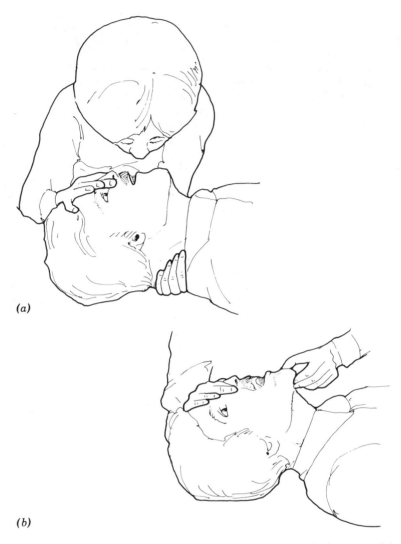

(a)

(b)

Figure 1.3 Mouth-to-mouth ventilation. The rescuer maintains anterior displacement of the jaw by a suitable technique throughout the respiratory cycle.

and the rescuer delivers a series of four successive thrusts directly downward.

The result of properly applied manual thrusts is the generation of substantial intrathoracic and, consequently, intraluminal pressures that frequently can dislodge a foreign body blocking the glottic opening. After completion of the manual thrust maneuver, the foreign body is removed, the head is repositioned, and positive pressure ventilation is reinstituted.

The Finger Sweep

Kneeling beside the supine victim, the rescuer grasps both the victim's tongue and mandible between the thumb and fingers of one hand and lifts upward (the tongue–jaw lift). The index finger of the rescuer's other hand is inserted into the patient's mouth and is directed along the buccal wall to a level deep in the throat at the base of the tongue. Obstructing foreign

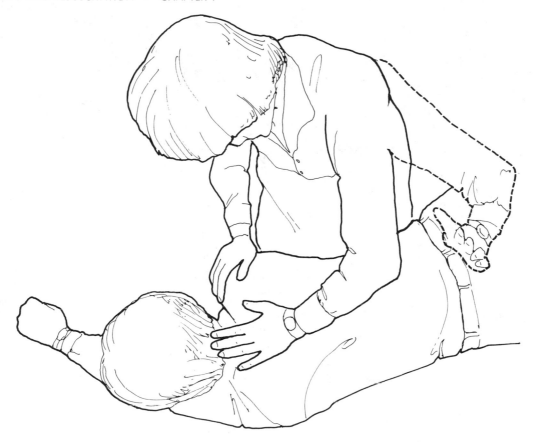

Figure 1.4 Back blows in the unconscious patient. Sharp, firm blows are essential.

bodies may be retrieved by using a hooking motion with the index finger. Once the foreign body has been dislodged and removed, the victim's head should be positioned properly and artificial ventilation should be begun immediately.

OBSTRUCTED AIRWAY IN THE CONSCIOUS PATIENT

Foreign body, upper airway obstruction frequently may result from aspiration of a food bolus while dining—the so-called cafe coronary. The incidence of this type of obstruction is associated with excessive alcohol consumption, loose-fitting dentures, and individuals who speak animatedly or inhale while swallowing. When complete airway obstruction occurs, the victim is unable to speak, cough, or breath. Supraclavicular muscle contractions may be noted before the rapid develop-

ment of pallor, cyanosis, and loss of consciousness. If the victim is conscious and in an upright (sitting or standing) position, both the back blow and manual thrust maneuvers may be applied to relieve such an obstruction.

Back blows should be delivered as described above but with the rescuer positioned beside and slightly behind the victim. In addition, the rescuer should place a supporting hand on the victim's sternum and flex the victim forward (head down if possible) before striking the four rapid blows (Fig. 1.6). The *manual thrust* maneuver may be applied to the upper abdomen (the Heimlich maneuver) or to the midchest when the victim is upright and conscious. To perform either variation, the rescuer positions himself or herself behind the victim and encircles the victim with his or her arms. For the abdominal approach the thumb side of the fist is placed against the victim's epigastrium at a point midway between the umbilicus and the

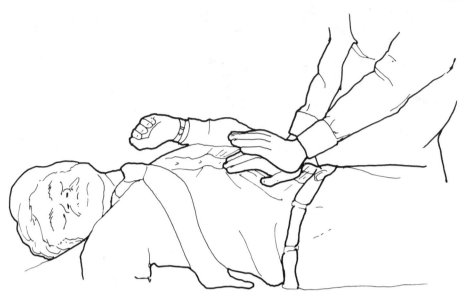

Figure 1.5 Abdominal thrusts. The force of the thrust must be directed inward, upward, and in the midline to ensure effectiveness and minimize risk to abdominal structures.

lower thoracic cage (Fig. 1.7a); for the midchest approach the thumb side is placed against the midpoint and center of the patient's sternum. The fist is grasped securely with the rescuer's other hand (Fig. 1.7b). A series of four quick thrusts is delivered in an upward direction from the upper abdominal position or in an inward or backward direction from the midchest position.

Several points regarding the management of foreign body upper airway obstruction deserve emphasis. There have been no laboratory or clinical studies reported to date that have demonstrated conclusively the superiority of any one maneuver in relieving foreign body airway obstruction. Considerable controversy remains concerning the choice and sequencing of these clearance procedures. Table 1.5 outlines the recommendations of the National Conference on Standards and Guidelines for Cardiopulmonary Resuscitation and Emergency Cardiac Care for the management of foreign body airway obstruction, using the three general maneuvers described above. By necessity, the recommendations are based in large part on retrospective surveys of anecdotal reports of obstruction episodes. Finally, for trained individuals proficient in their execution, several advanced techniques may be used either for removing foreign bodies under direct laryngoscopy (e.g., using conventional instruments such as the Kelly clamp or Magill forceps), or for circumventing the obstruction through cricothyrotomy (e.g., with positive-pressure, transtracheal catheter

ventilation), or rarely through emergent tracheostomy. These techniques are discussed in detail in Chapter 2.

Circulation

Once upper airway patency and the absence of spontaneous respiration have been established, four successive full breaths are delivered. Circulatory status is then ascertained by palpating the carotid or femoral arteries. The carotid artery has the obvious advantage of accessibility and should be the primary site of cardiovascular assessment. It is extremely important to maintain the head-tilt position, with one hand on the victim's forehead, while the other hand gently palpates for the carotid pulse, which should lie just lateral to the thyroid cartilage. Unless the carotid pulse is detected unquestionably, the rescuer should proceed immediately to external cardiac compression.

EXTERNAL CARDIAC COMPRESSION

After the absence of a carotid pulse has been established, the patient should be placed supine on a firm flat surface. If the patient is lying in bed, a backboard or suitable substitute should be placed between the patient and the mattress. The rescuer assumes a position alongside and parallel to the patient's thorax.

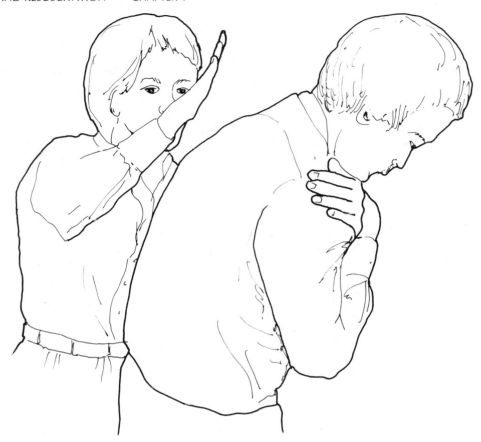

Figure 1.6 Back blows in the conscious patient.

The correct hand position on the sternum may be determined by one of two methods. The rescuer can locate the lower sternal notch with the index finger of the hand nearest the patient's feet and then place the opposite hand on the sternum adjacent to the previously positioned index finger. Alternatively, the rescuer can palpate the xiphosternal angle with the index and middle fingers of one hand and then place the longitudinal axis of the heel of the other hand along the longitudinal axis of the sternum. Regardless of the method, the heel of the hand ultimately should rest approximately 4–7 cm above the xiphoid process. Next, the heel of the palpating hand is placed on top of the heel of the lower hand, and the rescuer positions himself or herself squarely over the vertical axis of the hands (Fig. 1.8a). To prevent needless rib fracture and costochondral separation, at no time should the fingers of either hand subsequently come in contact with the chest wall. A useful safeguard is to interlock the fingers of both hands (Fig. 1.8b). With arms straight and shoulders directly over the vertical axis of the hands, the rescuer exerts downward pressure sufficient to depress the sternum 4–5 cm. The compression stroke should be executed firmly and smoothly, terminated by a sustained pause (constituting at least 50% of the total cycle duration) at the point of maximal sternal depression, and followed by an equally smooth upward motion of the rescuer's torso to the resting position. Recoil of the thoracic cage during the relaxation phase produces a relatively negative increment in intrathoracic pressure, which in turn enhances passive filling of the pulmonary vascular reservoir. During all phases of the compression cycle, the rescuer's hands should never lose contact with the patient's sternum.

Although a variety of compression-to-ventilation rates have been advocated, several studies have confirmed the efficacy

(a)

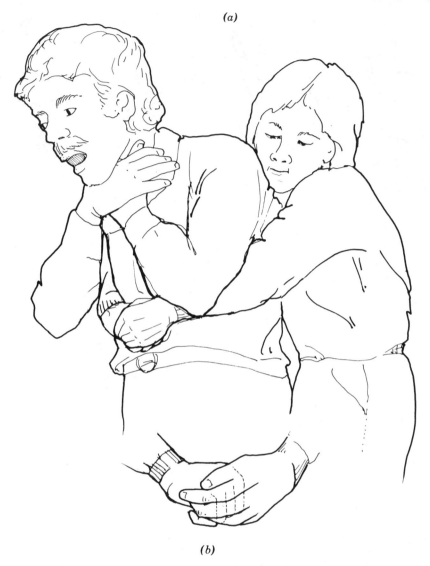

(b)

Figure 1.7 Abdominal thrusts in the conscious patient (the Heimlich maneuver). The rescuer presses his or her fist against the abdomen (a) and grasps the fist securely with the other hand (b) before applying forceful inward and upward thrusts.

of alternating ECC and artificial ventilation at a rate of 15:2 for single-rescuer resuscitations—that is, 15 compressions of the chest (at a rate of 80/min) followed by two rapid lung inflations. When two rescuers, one for ventilation and one for cardiac compression, are engaged in resuscitation, the compression rate should be 60/min, with one ventilation during the upswing of every fifth compression—a ratio of 5:1. It is the obligation of the rescuer providing ventilation to interpose ventilatory efforts without requiring interruption of external cardiac compression by the other rescuer. This coordination is greatly facilitated if the rescuer providing cardiac compression continues a verbal cadence of compressions. Rescuers should be able to exchange functions without interruption of BLS.

TABLE 1.5 Management of Foreign Body Airway Obstruction

Recommended Sequences

1. For the concious choking victim
   a. Identify complete airway obstruction (ask victim if he [or she] is able to speak).
   b. Apply four back blows in rapid succession.
   c. Apply four manual thrusts.
   d. Repeat four back blows and four manual thrusts until they are effective or until the victim becomes unconscious.

2. For the choking victim who becomes unconscious
   The rescuer should call for help, open the airway, and attempt to ventilate. If he [or she] is unsuccessful at ventilation, he [or she] should quickly perform the following:
   a. If a second person is available, he [or she] should activate the EMS system.
   b. Apply four back blows in rapid succession.
   c. Apply four manual thrusts.
   d. Apply the finger sweep. Dentures may need to be removed to improve the finger sweep.
   e. Reposition the head, open the airway, and attempt to ventilate. If the victim cannot be ventilated,
   f. Repeat steps b, c, and d.

3. For the victim who is found unconscious and the cause is unknown
   If the rescuer has found an unconscious victim, he [or she] should establish unresponsiveness, call for help, open the airway, establish breathlessness, and attempt to ventilate. If he [or she] is unable to ventilate, he [or she] should quickly perform the following sequences:
   a. Reposition the head, try again to ventilate. If unsuccessful and a second person is available, he [or she] should activate the EMS system.
   b. Apply four back blows in rapid succession.
   c. Apply four manual thrusts.
   d. Apply the finger sweep. (Rescuer may need to remove dentures to improve finger sweep.)
   e. Reposition the head and attempt to ventilate; if the victim cannot be ventilated,
   f. Repeat the sequence: b, c, and d as described previously.

Recommendations of the 1979 National Conference on Standards and Guidelines for Cardiopulmonary Resuscitation (CPR) and Emergency Cardiac Care (ECC) for the Management of Foreign Body Airway Obstruction. *J Am Med Assoc.* 1981; 244:453–508.

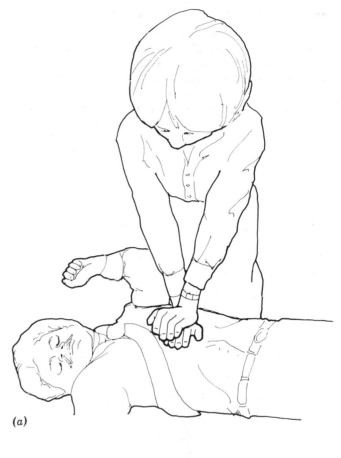

(a)

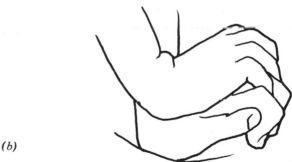

(b)

It is of extreme importance that cardiac compression and ventilation should *never* be interrupted for longer than 5 seconds except under the extreme necessity of executing advanced life support procedures (i.e., endotracheal intubation, intracardiac injection, and subclavian or internal jugular vein catheterization) or because of an absolute need to move the patient. In these limited and restricted circumstances, CPR should not be interrupted for more than 30 seconds.

Figure 1.8 Closed-chest compression. The rescuer works from the patient's side (*a*), keeping arms straight and leaning over the patient to maximize thrust directly downward and to minimize effort required. (*b*) Hands must be located in such a position as to focus the compressive force on the midline of the sternum. Fingers should be kept off the chest, allowing all force to come through the heel of the hand.

Monitoring Effectiveness of Basic Life Support

As mentioned earlier, pupillary response and carotid and femoral pulses may provide some indication of the effectiveness of cardiopulmonary support. However, we must be mindful that a variety of drugs (e.g., atropine or ganglion-blocking agents), as well as intrinsic ocular pathology (e.g., cataracts in elderly patients) may interfere with the pupillary light reflex. In addition, the femoral artery may be more subject to transmitted pressure waves from external cardiac compression, and thus assessment of circulatory adequacy at that site may be deceiving.

Complications of Basic Life Support Procedures

When BLS procedures are properly applied, the inherent risks are clearly acceptable in the context of cardiac arrest. However, awareness of potential complications of CPR may be crucial in the postresuscitation management of the patient.

GASTRIC DISTENTION AND REGURGITATION

Gastric distention is a common complication of CPR, specifically during expired air artificial ventilation. Its occurrence is more likely in the presence of partial or total upper airway obstruction or with the use of high ventilation pressures that exceed esophageal opening pressures. Gastric distention predisposes to regurgitation (with or without pulmonary aspiration) and may limit diaphragmatic excursion sufficiently to compromise pulmonary ventilation. Unless marked distention of the stomach prevents adequate ventilation, it is currently recommended that no attempt should be made to relieve the distention because of the attendant risk of inducing regurgitation and aspiration. If ventilation is compromised, ECC should be interrupted momentarily, the victim rolled onto his or her side, and moderate pressure applied over the epigastrium to expel the entrapped air. If regurgitation occurs at any time during the resuscitation attempt, the victim should be rolled onto his or her side and the regurgitated material allowed to drain from the mouth. Residual vomitus should be wiped from the mouth, the victim repositioned, and BLS reinstituted immediately.

EXTERNAL CARDIAC COMPRESSION

Even when external cardiac compression is properly applied it may result in serious complications. Reported complications include rib and sternal fractures, costochondral separation, pulmonary contusions, lacerations of the esophagus, stomach, inferior vena cava, liver, and spleen, pneumothorax, hemothorax, hemopericardium, flail chest, subcutaneous emphysema, and bone marrow and fat embolization. Although rib fractures occur frequently, particularly in elderly patients, little or no compromise of pulmonary ventilation seems to result unless tension pneumothorax is produced. It is important to note that the vast majority of these complications can be avoided by strict adherence to proper technique.

MANUAL THRUST MANEUVERS

All variations of the manual thrust maneuver have been associated with serious complications. These include rib fractures, hepatic and splenic trauma, gastric rupture, and regurgitation and aspiration. The most frequent causes have been the inappropriate or overzealous use of the thrust maneuver, particularly the abdominal approach.

ADVANCED CARDIAC LIFE SUPPORT

The provision of basic life support—airway maintenance, ventilatory assistance, and external chest compression—is the first step toward facilitating survival for the victim of cardiopulmonary arrest. Progression to advanced life support, using adjunctive equipment, more specialized techniques, and various medications, is the logical next step in continuing resuscitation. Advanced cardiac life support (ACLS) may be applied by trained individuals operating within an emergency medical services system in the community, in transport, and in the hospital setting.

The resuscitation of a victim of cardiac arrest or other catastrophic cardiovascular event is a continuum progressing from the initial life-sustaining techniques of BLS, to the more definitive therapies and stabilization represented by ALS, and finally to the postresuscitative measures that attempt to treat the underlying pathophysiologic disturbances and prevent recurrence of the arrest. The central focus of the following sections will be on those medications or techniques used primarily in the initial resuscitative efforts. The demarcation from therapies more commonly used in the critical care unit setting, however, is at times indistinct. Some brief discussion of the latter type of support will be included, but the major emphasis will be on the initial resuscitative measures most commonly used in the emergency room or by paramedics at the scene of a cardiac arrest.

The discussion of ACLS is presented in detail in the ACLS text published by the American Heart Association.

Airway and Ventilatory Support

OXYGENATION

An essential aspect of resuscitation is the attainment of optimal ventilation and oxygenation. Supplemental oxygen should be used as soon as it can be made available. Although ventilation with the rescuer's exhaled breath may provide an alveolar partial pressure of oxygen (P_{AO_2}) of 80 mm Hg, there will nevertheless be arterial hypoxemia because of diminished cardiac output, intrapulmonary shunting, and ventilation–perfusion (V–Q) mismatch (see Chapter 2). With supplemental oxygen, this hypoxemia can usually be corrected. The administered concentration of oxygen will begin at 100%; after patient stabilization, lower concentrations will be used, guided by measurement of the arterial partial pressure of oxygen (P_{AO_2}).

AIRWAY ADJUNCTS

Frequently, despite appropriate airway positioning with techniques such as the chin lift or jaw thrust, there is still soft tissue obstruction to airflow. This can usually be relieved by an oropharyngeal or nasopharyngeal airway (Procedures 2 and 3). Proper placement of these devices is crucial to their successful use, however. The oral airway must be of the proper size and must be positioned such that the patient's tongue is completely encircled by the concavity of the airway; if it is not, gagging and worsened airway obstruction may ensue. Oral airways are not well tolerated by awake or semiconscious patients, and in these people a nasopharyngeal airway is a better choice. Nasopharyngeal airways are not commonly used in children because their adenoid beds, through which the nasal airway must pass, are frequently large, vascular, and likely to hemorrhage if damaged.

Masks

A well-fitting, properly applied mask is a great help to the rescuer, although some training and experience is required in its use. The mask and its appropriate connections can be used to supply higher concentrations of oxygen. If ventilatory assistance is required, the mask may be used for mouth-to-mask ventilation, or it may be attached to a resuscitation bag for more sophisticated support (Procedure 1). Desirable features in mask design include the following:

1. *The use of transparent material,* allowing the rescuer to assess lip color and to see vomitus or other foreign material in the patient's airway.

2. *The ability to conform to the patient's face* and to provide a tight seal, often accomplished with an air-cushion rim around the mask's perimeter.

3. *A standard 15-mm/22-mm connector* to allow the use of additional airway equipment.

4. *A comfortable fit* for the rescuer's hand.

5. *Availability in the appropriate size and shape* for the patient. Most adults can be assisted adequately with a standard medium-sized (No. 4) oval-shaped mask. Specific considerations for children will be addressed later.

6. *An oxygen insufflation inlet,* which is necessary if oxygen supplementation during mouth-to-mask ventilation is required.

Ventilating Circuits

If the patient's spontaneous ventilation is inadequate, assistance may be provided using a manual ventilating circuit, commonly referred to as a "bag." These devices allow the experienced rescuer to ventilate the patient's lungs with considerably greater ease and control than provided by the exhaled-air technique used in BLS. A good deal of practice is required for their proper use, however. In the hands of an inexperienced individual, successful alveolar ventilation is unlikely, and complications are not infrequent.

There are two broad categories into which these manual resuscitators may be grouped—self-refilling and non-self-refilling units. The self-refilling units, also referred to as *bag–valve–mask* devices or *Ambu bags,* have the great advantage of operating independently of a fresh gas source. They are usually compact and highly portable and can be used at an accident site and in transport without the need for an attendant oxygen source.

The following design features are common to many of the self-refilling units (Fig. 1.9):

1. *A fresh-gas inlet,* through which fresh gas enters the reservoir bag during the refilling phase. Entry through this inlet is frequently controlled by a flap valve, allowing gas flow into, but not out of, the reservoir bag. It is through this valve that room air and supplemental oxygen, if provided, are entrained.

2. *A nipple for oxygen connection,* located close to the inlet valve.

3. *A reservoir bag,* usually of rubber or silicone rubber construction. The bag may be opaque or transparent and should be easy to clean and sterilize without damage to its material. Adult and pediatric sizes are commonly available.

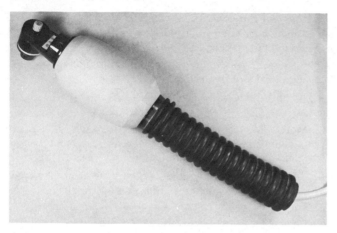

Figure 1.9 The manual resuscitator (self-refilling bag) has a reservoir tail for oxygen accumulation attached. One-way valves direct the flow of gas to the patient and prevent rebreathing of exhaled gases.

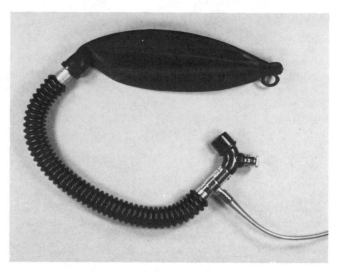

Figure 1.10 The Mapleson system (non-self-refilling bag). Finer control of FiO_2, inflating, and end expiratory pressures is possible. Adequate fresh-gas flow is essential to ensure carbon dioxide removal.

4. *A nonrebreathing valve* to direct flow to the patient during inspiration and to the atmosphere during exhalation. Construction of this valve should be simple, reliable, and rugged. Since the patient may vomit during resuscitation, we should be able to disassemble, clean, and accurately reassemble the valve quickly and easily without dealing with many small parts or confusing connections. The valve casing should be transparent to allow visual inspection of its function.

   A pop-off feature is often provided to avoid inadvertent high airway pressures; there should be provision made for manual overriding of the pop-off if higher pressures are required.

5. *A reservoir tail,* an additional length of large-bore flexible tubing that can be attached to the reservoir bag at the fresh-gas inlet. This attachment allows oxygen from the supply tubing to accumulate within it during the inspiratory and pause phases of the ventilatory cycle thus providing a volume of gas with a high oxygen content to the reservoir bag when next it refills. Without such an attachment, the self-refilling system can deliver 40–50% oxygen at best; with it, the delivered oxygen concentration can approach 100%.

Although the self-refilling units have the advantage of independence from an oxygen source, they lack flexibility for the experienced operator in that they give little sense of the patient's thoracic compliance and, with the exception of the most recent models, do not allow application of positive end expiratory pressure (PEEP). Accordingly, rescuers more adept

in the use of respiratory equipment frequently prefer a non-self-refilling circuit. Variously described as the *Magill circuit,* the *Mapleson circuit,* the *anesthesia bag,* or *black bag,* these nonself-refilling systems are all modifications of a T-piece system first described in 1937 by Philip Ayre (Fig. 1.10).

The following are essential features of the T-piece circuit:

1. *A fresh gas inlet,* which is attached by tubing to the fresh gas source, usually 100% oxygen in the resuscitation situation, with flow rate adjusted as detailed below.
2. *A patient connection* with standard 15-mm/22-mm sizing.
3. *Reservoir tubing,* which is usually corrugated rubber tubing of approximately 1.5 in. diameter. This serves as a conduit for the patient's exhaled breath to the reservoir bag.
4. *A reservoir bag,* which is commonly a soft, collapsable rubber product; a variety of sizes is available.
5. *An exhalation valve,* which may be as simple as an open-tailed reservoir bag with a clip to control gas exhaust or may be a more complex valve located elsewhere in the circuit.

The use of the T-piece circuit allows more precise control of FiO_2. An airway pressure manometer is easily inserted into the circuit, and with pressure monitoring and some experience, a wide variety of ventilatory patterns, inflating and end-expiratory pressures, and airway control is feasible. Proper adjustment of the fresh-gas flow rate to ensure adequate removal of carbon dioxide from the circuit is essential. A flow rate of two to three times the exhaled minute volume is typical; in adult patients, this may require flow rates of 10–20 liters/min.

Esophageal Obturator Airway

The recently developed esophageal obturator airway is widely used in the prehospital phase of emergency care. It is designed to be inserted blindly through the patients mouth into the esophagus and to allow ventilation of the lungs without distension of the stomach or regurgitation of gastric contents (Procedure 5). Once the device has been positioned, the balloon on the distal end is inflated, occluding the esophagus. Ventilation is then begun, and gas flows from the mask and upper tube, through the pharynx, and into the trachea. A newer modification, the esophageal gastric tube airway, allows decompression of the stomach during resuscitation. Should a patient arrive in the emergency room with one of these in place, it is best to leave the esophageal portion in until endotracheal intubation can be accomplished.

Endotracheal Intubation

In most instances of cardiorespiratory arrest, there is no primary abnormality of the upper airway, and ventilation can be accomplished with simple airway restoration and bag and mask techniques. Endotracheal intubation (Procedure 4), although eventually performed, should not be the first priority in initial resuscitation; ventilation and oxygenation come first. Attempts at endotracheal tube placement by those who are inexperienced in so doing are usually unsuccessful and may compromise the ongoing resuscitation attempts. The procedure should be reserved for those well practiced in its completion, and even then it should not be attempted until all necessary equipment (proper sized endotracheal tube, laryngoscope and blade, suction and suction catheters, etc.) and assistance are available.

Once satisfactory placement of an endotracheal tube is accomplished, good airway control is almost assured and the risks of gastric distension and regurgitation are diminished. Better regulation of FiO_2, airway pressures, and ventilatory pattern is offered, and prolonged support of the patient into the postresuscitative period is facilitated. Since the most common complication of endotracheal intubation is a malfunctioning or blocked endotracheal tube, constant surveillance of ventilation and tube function is essential.

Transtracheal Airway

Rarely, an airway cannot be established by the methods described. In such cases, an emergency cricothyrotomy and catheter insertion or tracheostomy (if skilled personnel are present) may be required. These procedures are detailed later in the text (Procedures 7, 9, 10). The tracheostomy will function in the same manner as an endotracheal tube, allowing adequate lumen size for suctioning and conventional ventilation. The cricothyroid puncture, with insertion of a 14- or 16-gauge catheter (the over-the-needle type is preferable), is an emergency technique that may be life saving. In general, oxygenation is usually easily accomplished through such a catheter, but carbon dioxide removal is more difficult. Intermittent insufflation of 100% oxygen from a high-pressure source (15–20 psi), with care being taken to stop insufflation just when the chest starts to rise, is the recommended technique. Normally, exhalation of the gas so insufflated occurs passively through the larynx and upper airway; if exit of gas seems impeded, a second catheter of similar size may be inserted into the cricothyroid membrane to allow for gas escape.

Support of Circulation

Chest compressions during ACLS are performed in the same manner as in BLS. It is important that the rescuer coordinating the resuscitation ensure that compressions are not unduly interrupted while adjunctive procedures are performed.

ELECTROCARDIOGRAPHIC MONITORING

Electrocardiographic (ECG) monitoring is essential during resuscitation, both as a diagnostic tool and as a guide to the most effective therapy. It should be initiated as soon as possible during a resuscitative sequence, though precedence must always be given to good BLS as initial management.

The ECG monitoring is available in several forms. Many defibrillators currently marketed have built-in ECG monitoring circuitry and "quick-look" paddles. Such units sense the patient's ECG pattern from the defibrillator paddles upon their application and display it on a screen for immediate review; appropriate therapy can then be administered. The quick-look system has its greatest usefulness in the setting of ventricular fibrillation (VF); the rhythm can be diagnosed and without delay an appropriate shock applied and its effect assessed. For continuous monitoring, however, the quick-look system is not appropriate and a standard ECG machine or monitoring unit with display screen must be employed.

The most ominous ECG tracing to be seen initially is that of complete cardiac standstill. As resuscitation progresses and spontaneous cardiac activity returns, ventricular fibrillation may be displayed; with successful defibrillation, a regular sinus rhythm appears. The presence of a stable sinus rhythm, however, does not imply that adequate cardiac output is present since mechanical contraction may be poor and the heart may be unable to develop a pressure, a condition known as *electromechanical dissociation*. Futher discussion of the diagnosis and management of these specific patterns of cardiac arrest, along with representative ECGs, is included in the clinical settings section of this chapter.

DEFIBRILLATION

In the usual unmonitored situation, BLS should be instituted while a defibrillator is brought to the scene. Because of the overwhelming incidence of ventricular tachycardia or fibrillation as the cause of arrest, in the early 1970s "blind" defibrillation was recommended as soon as a defibrillator was available. However, as noted, current defibrillators with quick-look paddles enable visualization of the rhythm disturbance upon arrival of the defibrillator. As soon as ventricular fibrillation is documented, defibrillation as described below should be performed.

Precordial Thump

In the clinical situation in which the patient's cardiac rhythm is observed to degenerate to ventricular fibrillation, for example, in the emergency room while a patient with suspected myocardial infarction is being evaluated, a precordial thump should be employed. A sharp blow using the fleshy outside of a closed fist is delivered to the sternum from a height of 8–12 in. If this successfully results in sinus rhythm, a bolus of lidocaine should be given. However, if VF persists, proceed to BLS and to defibrillation as soon as the defibrillator is available.

Electrical Defibrillation

Electrical defibrillation involves passing an electrical current through a fibrillating heart, depolarizing the disorganized contracting myofibrils at once, and allowing for uniform repolarization and subsequent organized cardiac electromechanical activity. Although a more complete discussion of defibrillation, including the factors influencing success, is presented in the procedure section (Procedure 15), the following provides a summary of the technique.

While awaiting arrival of a defibrillator, effective BLS must, of course, be maintained. Upon arrival of the monitor–defibrillator, turn the power on, apply appropriate conductive material to paddles, and apply these to the chest to determine the patient's rhythm. If VF is present, turn on defibrillator power (separate control) and ensure that the defibrillator is not in synchronous mode. Select the energy level (200–300 J), charge the capacitor, and place the paddles on the chest in appropriate locations. *Check to ensure* that no personnel are in contact with the patient and apply firm pressure to paddles while depressing the discharge button or buttons. If no muscle twitch has occurred, recheck the equipment—especially the "synch" switch used for elective synchronous cardioversions.

After the shock has been given, reapply the paddles and observe the rhythm. If VF persists, immediately repeat defibrillation at the same energy level. If still unsuccessful, resume CPR, place an intravenous line, administer epinephrine and sodium bicarbonate (see below), and reshock the patient with 360 J delivered.

VENOUS ACCESS

The establishment of a reliable intravenous route of suitable caliber is an essential part of ACLS. The choice of site is determined by the experience of the rescuer and the anatomy of the patient. Peripheral veins may be used because of convenience, particularly during the arrest situation when access to the neck and chest is restricted by BLS rescue procedures. Cannulation of such veins may be difficult, however, if vasoconstriction or venous collapse is present. Central venous cannulation, although somewhat more difficult technically, offers more secure access and is preferable for drug administration because of proximity to the heart. Sites frequently chosen are the internal jugular, the subclavian, and the femoral veins (Procedure 11). Venous cannulation should not be allowed to interfere with ongoing resuscitative efforts. Certain drugs can be administered by alternative routes if intravenous lines cannot be established quickly. The intratracheal, sublingual, and intracardiac routes are detailed later in this text. Table 1.6 summarizes the use of resuscitation drugs.

CORRECTION OF ACIDOSIS

Acidosis is often present in victims of cardiorespiratory arrest, particularly if the arrest condition has persisted for more than a few minutes. When acidosis is present, there are two components contributing to the acid load. *Respiratory acidosis* results from failure of carbon dioxide elimination; carbon dioxide production continues, but the gas cannot be removed because of pulmonary and cardiac failure, and the $Paco_2$ rises. *Metabolic acidosis* develops concomitantly with tissue hypoperfusion and conversion to anaerobic forms of metabolism. Acidosis must be corrected and pH restored to near normal during the course of ACLS.

Adequate Ventilation

By ensuring adequate alveolar ventilation, carbon dioxide removal can be accomplished and a major component of depressed pH managed. Residual metabolic acidosis can be offset by administration of sodium bicarbonate ($NaHCO_3$), although several cautions must be observed in its administration (see below). If alveolar ventilation is not adequate, the carbon dioxide released from the drug will not be excreted, and correction of the acidosis will not be attained.

Sodium Bicarbonate

Current recommendations for administration of sodium bicarbonate are outlined below. The actual amount of bicarbonate required in each case is inversely related to the effectiveness and speed of initiating resuscitation. Arterial blood gases should be obtained as soon as possible, and dosages subsequent to the first are given based on a calculation of the patient's base deficit (milliequivalents per liter of base deficient from plasma) (see Chapter 11).

ADMINISTRATION. In earlier resuscitative training, excessive emphasis was probably placed on the use of $NaHCO_3$ to correct acidosis. More recently, the realization has come that not only does use of bicarbonate extract a cost (sodium load, potential metabolic alkalosis), but that a large portion of metabolic acidosis can be corrected by restoration of adequate alveolar ventilation. If the period of cardiac arrest was brief, it is likely that $NaHCO_3$ is not required. The $NaHCO_3$ is supplied as prefilled 50-ml syringes containing either 50 mEq (8.4% solution) or 44.6 mEq (7.5% solution). The initial dose for both adult and pediatric patients should be approximately 1 mEq/kg. This is given intravenously slowly and, for infants, should be diluted with equal volumes of 5% dextrose in water. As noted, further administration should be guided by blood gas determinations of pH and P_{CO_2}. A convenient formula is $NaHCO_3$ (mEq) = $0.3 \times$ wt(kg) $\times$ base deficit (mEq/liter). If such laboratory determinants are unavailable, then one half the initial dose every 10–15 minutes is appropriate.

PRECAUTIONS. The sodium and osmolar load are high, and excessive administration of the drug may result in hypernatremia, hyperosmolarity, and metabolic alkalosis. The intravenous line must be cleared before and after administration since admixture with epinephrine will inactivate the catecholamine whereas mixture with calcium preparations results in precipitation of calcium salts.

VOLUME REPLACEMENT

Initial intravenous fluids are usually simple crystalloids such as 5% dextrose in water. Such solutions are inappropriate, however, for rapid expansion of circulatory blood volume, for which isotonic crystalloids (Ringer's lactate, 0.9% saline), colloids, or blood are used. Assessment must be made quickly of adequacy of circulating blood volume, and appropriate measures must be taken to restore losses or remove excesses. Collapsed jugular and peripheral veins, dryness of mucous membranes, absence of normal secretions (tears, saliva), and peripheral vasoconstriction, when combined with an appropriate clinical history, suggest dehydration and volume deficit.

Initial support of deficient intravascular volume is possible by simple elevation of the patient's legs, which encourages venous return to the central circulation. In profound hypovolemia with subsequent cardiac arrest (e.g., massive hemorrhage secondary to trauma), the application of medical antishock garments (MAST suits, Procedure 7) may dramatically improve the patient's condition and allow additional time for fluid administration. If their use has been beneficial, their subsequent deflation and removal must be cautiously achieved but not until appropriate volume support has been begun.

A continuing controversy exists as to the proper place of colloids versus isotonic crystalloids in restoration of intravascular volume. Proponents of crystalloid solutions point out their ready availability, low cost, ease of administration, and freedom from risks of hepatitis and allergic or anaphylactic reactions. Proponents of colloid regimens point out their ability to better sustain intravascular volume and oncotic pressure, and some recent studies document shorter resuscitation times and better survival with colloid usage. Further investigation will be needed to clarify the specific advantages of each component in fluid resuscitation. The specific modalities of volume therapy, including the advantages and disadvantages of various fluids and specialized indications for the same, will be covered in greater detail in the sections on shock and critical injuries.

Volume challenges should be given as needed until cardiac function and blood pressure are restored or until there is evidence of volume overload. A useful approach is to begin volume administration with Ringer's lactate or normal saline. If the quantity of fluid required is in excess of 20–30% of the patient's estimated blood volume (i.e., in excess of 1–2 liters for adults, or 20–30 ml/kg for children), colloid—usually as 5% albumin—is added. Specific blood components are administered as needed to correct deficits in hemoglobin, coagulation factors, and

TABLE 1.6 Resuscitation Drugs

Drug	Initial Dose[a]	Repeat Dosage	How Supplied	Comments
NaHCO₃ (Sodium bicarbonate)	50–100 mEq bolus (1–2 mEq/kg), IV, IC	25–50 mEq (0.5–1 mEq/kg) every 10 min or 0.3 × wt (kg) × base deficit (mEq/liter)	44.5 mEq in 50 ml (7.5%) 50 mEq in 50 ml (8.4%) 50-ml ampules	Indications: Metabolic acidosis. Cautions: Avoid excessive administration; dilute 1:1 with D₅W for infants.
Epinephrine	0.5–1-mg bolus (10 µg/kg) IV, IT, IC	Same, every 5 min as necessary. Infusion: 0.025–0.1 µg/kg/min (may go up to 0.5 µg/kg/min in pediatric patients)	1 mg in 1 ml (1:1,000) ampul 1 mg in 10 ml (1:10,000) (100 µg/ml) Infusion: 1 mg in 500 ml D₅W (2 µg/ml)	Indications: Asystole, to stimulate cardiac activity; fine ventricular fibrillation, to coarsen before electroshock; to increase vascular tone and perfusion pressure. Cautions: Avoid in recurrent ventricular fibrillation occurring after successful defibrillation
Norepinephrine (Levophed)	32–48 µg/min or 0.05–0.5 µg/kg/min, IV; titrate to desired blood pressure response	—	4 mg in 4 ml Dilute before using: e.g., 8 mg in 500 ml D₅W (16 µg/ml)	Indications: Hypotension, especially if peripheral resistance is low; cardiogenic shock. Cautions: Exogenous or endogenous catecholamines may produce artifactually low cuff blood pressure; extravasation may yield tissue necrosis
Isoproterenol (Isuprel)	2–20 µg/min or 0.05–0.5 µg/kg/min, IV; titrate to desired heart rate response (rarely used as bolus)	—	1 mg in 5 ml Dilute before using: e.g., 1 mg in 500 ml D₅W (2 µg/ml)	Indications: Bradycardia. Cautions: Vasodilator; may lower blood pressure; may precipitate tachyarrhythmias; increases myocardial oxygen requirement
Dopamine	2–20 µg/kg/min, IV; variable depending on desired effect	—	200 mg in 5 ml Dilute before using: e.g., 200 mg in 500 ml D₅W (400 µg/ml)	Indications: Low-output state; impaired renal perfusion. Cautions: Tachydysrhythmias, excessive vasoconstriction, hypersensitive response in patients on monoamine oxidase (MAO) inhibitors or with pheochromocytoma
Dobutamine	2.5–10 µg/kg/min, IV	—	250 mg in 20 ml Dilute before using: e.g., 250 mg in 500 ml D₅W (0.5 mg/ml)	Indications: Short-term therapy for refractory heart failure. Cautions: Tachycardia and dysrhythmias
Atropine	0.5 mg (0.02 mg/kg), IV, IT	Same; repeat every 3–5 min to maximum of 2 mg (0.08 mg/kg)	0.4 mg in 1 ml 1 mg in 1 ml 1 mg in 10 ml	Indications: Bradycardia with hypotension; bradycardia with ventricular ectopy; severe bradycardia (<50 beats/min). Cautions: Tachycardia not well tolerated in coronary disease

Drug	Dose	Repeat	Concentration	Indications / Cautions
CaCl₂ (Calcium Chloride)	250–500 mg (10–20 mg/kg), IV	Same; repeat every 5–10 min as necessary	1 g in 10 ml (10%) (100 mg CaCl₂ per ml)	*Indications:* Hypotension; electromechanical dissociation; hyperkalemia *Cautions:* May aggravate digoxin toxicity; extravasation may yield tissue necrosis; rapid administration may produce bradycardia; may precipitate coronary vasospasm in susceptible patients
Calcium gluconate	1–1.5 g (30–60 mg/kg), IV	Same; repeat every 5–10 min as necessary	1 g in 10 ml (10%) (100 mg/ml)	*Indications:* Same as CaCl₂ *Cautions:* Slightly less sclerotic; requires hepatic metabolism to release calcium ion
Lidocaine	50–75 mg (1 mg/kg), IV, IT	Same, every 15–20 min as necessary or Infusion: 1–4 mg/min (15–50 µg/kg/min)	50 mg in 5 ml (1%) 100 mg in 5 ml (2%) 100 mg in 10 ml (1%) 1 g in 25 ml (4%) 2 g in 50 ml (4%) 1 g in 5 ml (20%) Use solutions without epinephrine	*Indications:* Ventricular tachycardia or ectopy *Cautions:* Metabolism slowed in congestive failure; avoid in high degrees of AV block; rapid administration may cause seizures
Bretylium	For VF: 5 mg/kg, IV bolus followed by countershock For VT: 5–10 mg/kg IV over 10–20 min; IM	10 mg/kg, repeated up to maximum of 30 mg/kg Same dosage every 6–8 hr or infusion of 2 mg/min	500 mg in 10 ml	*Indications:* Ventricular tachycardia of fibrillation, especially if refractory to other antiarrhythmics *Cautions:* For VF: Must be followed by DC countershock; orthostatic hypotension, especially if less than 5 mg/kg dosage is given; nausea, vomiting in the awake patient if given too fast; avoid in patients with aortic or pulmonic stenosis
Procainamide (Pronestyl)	100 mg (1.5 mg/kg) bolus over 1 min or 20 mg/min or 17 mg/kg over 1 hr	Same bolus every 5 min until adverse effects or suppression of ventricular ectopic arrhythmia, or 1 g total 2.8 mg/kg/hr maintenance (1.4 mg/kg/hr in renal failure)	1,000 mg in 10 ml 1,000 mg in 2 ml	*Indications:* Suppression of PVC, VT, or VF refractory to therapy with lidocaine *Cautions:* Monitor for ↓BP or QRS widening after each dose; avoid in patients with digitalis intoxication with disturbances of AV conduction
Dextrose	0.5–1.0 g/kg, IV	Same, as necessary	50% (25 g in 50 ml) and 25% (250 mg/ml) solution	*Indications:* Hypoglycemia (documented or suspected) *Cautions:* Hypertonic solution—administer slowly
Naloxone (Narcan)	0.4 mg (10 µg/kg), IV	Same, repeat three times	0.4 mg in 1 ml 0.02 mg in 1 ml	*Indications:* Suspected narcotic overdose

aRoutes: IV, intravenous; IT, intratracheal; IC, intracardiac. These routes are given in order of preference. The IT drugs should be diluted to 10 ml with sterile water. Avoid IC route if possible.

platelets in aliqots of 10–20 ml/kg. When direct measurements of central venous or pulmonary capillary wedge pressure are available, further volume infusion is guided by these data and the clinical course; the goal is to achieve optimal cardiac output and perfusion pressure without excess intravascular fluid.

CARDIOTONIC DRUGS AND VASOPRESSORS

The majority of the cardiotonic and vasopressor agents clinically used exert their actions by directly or indirectly affecting adrenergic sympathetic activity. The effects of these sympathomimetic agents can be grouped into several broad classes—peripheral excitation of certain smooth muscles and peripheral inhibition of other types of smooth muscles, cardiac stimulatory activity, metabolic effects, and CNS stimulation. As initially described by Ahlquist, the body's organ systems appear to respond to these agents as if there were two different types of tissue receptors—alpha and beta. The response of vascular smooth muscle to alpha-receptor stimulation is contraction, whereas the response to beta-receptor stimulation is relaxation. This pattern, however, is not applicable in other sites in which the beta response is stimulatory (e.g., heart) or in which both alpha and beta are stimulatory (e.g., intestinal smooth muscle). In addition, end organs, such as the smooth muscle of skeletal muscle blood vessels, may exhibit both alpha and beta responses: low concentrations of epinephrine activate beta receptors with resultant vasodilation, whereas higher concentrations result in alpha response and vasoconstriction. We should remember that most sympathomimetic agents affect both alpha and beta receptors, but that the range of alpha to beta effects varies considerably from almost pure beta (e.g., isoproterenol) to pure alpha (e.g., methoxamine or phenylephrine).

More recently it was discovered that it is possible to differentiate two distinct patterns for different organs in their response to beta stimulants. Certain agents more selectively affect the heart and small intestine and are called beta$_1$, whereas the other agents exert their response primarily on bronchial and vascular smooth muscle and are called beta$_2$. This beta selectivity is generally dose dependent and is not consistent at higher dose ranges. One final point must be kept in mind concerning the pressor activity of these agents: Pressor responses are the result of multiple complex and diverse direct and indirect interactions that make the elucidation of the actions of an agent at times difficult. Table 1.7 lists the major cardiovascular actions of the sympathomimetic agents commonly used during resuscitations.

Epinephrine

Epinephrine has become a mainstay of cardiac resuscitation and is often the prime factor in a successful outcome. The drug is a sympathomimetic amine with alpha and beta effects, both of which contribute to restoration of spontaneous cardiac activity.

INDICATIONS. The beta$_1$ effects of epinephrine on the heart are those of increased rate and contractility. In the arrest situation, such beta$_1$ stimulation can be employed in several ways. Epinephrine can restore spontaneous contractility to a flaccid heart, converting a flat-line ECG to a fibrillatory pattern or to a coordinated rhythm. It can increase the vigor and intensity of ventricular fibrillation (conversion of fine to coarse ventricular fibrillation) making it more amenable to termination by electrical shock; this may, however, worsen the imbalance between myocardial oxygen supply and demand.

One of the goals of cardiac resuscitation is restoration of myocardial perfusion. Since coronary perfusion is dependent on diastolic and mean arterial pressures (MAP) rather than on systolic pressure, an agent is needed to raise perfusion pressure during the relaxation phase of chest compression. Epinephrine, through its alpha-vasoconstrictive effects, promotes an increase in peripheral vascular resistance, thus providing the needed rise in mean arterial pressure and restoring coronary perfusion. The importance of this alpha-adrenergic stimulation for successful resuscitation has been pointed out in several studies, whereas administration of a pure beta agonist has been shown to be ineffective.

ADMINISTRATION. Although epinephrine is customarily given intravenously, alternative routes of administration have been shown to be effective. If an intravenous line cannot promptly be established, a standard dose of epinephrine, preferably diluted in 5–10 ml of sterile water, can be instilled into the endotracheal tube and distributed across the tracheobronchial tree by ventilation. Rapid onset and sustained duration of effect may be attained using this technique. Atropine and lidocaine have also been administered successfully by the endotracheal route; calcium and bicarbonate, however, should not be so given. The intracardiac route of injection is prone to complications such as laceration of a coronary artery, accidental injection into the myocardial wall, and pneumothorax; it should be regarded as a technique of last resort.

Epinephrine is most frequently administered as a bolus medication, although it is occasionally given as a continuous infusion for ongoing support. Epinephrine is available as 1-ml ampuls containing 1 mg/ml (1/1,000) or as prefilled syringes diluted to 1 mg/10 ml (1/10,000). The most common method of administration during resuscitation is by intravenous bolus using a dose of 0.5–1.0 mg (5–10 ml of the 1/10,000 solution) for adults or 0.01 mg/kg (1 ml/10 kg of the 1/10,000 solution)

TABLE 1.7 Drugs Useful in Resuscitation

Desired Effect	Drug	Effectiveness	Mechanism of Action[a]	Other Effects/Cautions
Increase in heart rate	Atropine	↑ ↑ ↑	Parasympathetic blockade	Administer full dose; lower doses may cause cardiac slowing
	Isoproterenol	↑ ↑ ↑	Beta₁ stimulation of heart	Increased myocardial oxygen consumption. Peripheral vasodilatation, ↓ diastolic pressure (Beta₂ effect); may compromise coronary perfusion
Increase in myocardial contractility	Epinephrine	↑ ↑ ↑	Beta₁ stimulation	Effect varies with dose; larger doses allow alpha effect (vasoconstriction) to predominate
	Isoproterenol	↑ ↑ ↑	Beta₁ stimulation	Same as above
	Dopamine	↑ ↑	Beta₁ stimulation; release of endogenous norepinephrine	Low dose: renal–splanchnic dilation; middose: beta₁ action added; high dose: alpha effects predominate
	Dobutamine	↑ ↑	Beta₁ stimulation	Predominantly a beta₁ drug
	Calcium	↑ ↑ ↑	Direct cellular action	Vasoconstriction; rapid administration may produce bradycardia
	Norepinephrine	↑ ↑	Beta₁ stimulation	Much more prominent alpha effect at relatively low doses
Vasoconstriction; increased mean BP	Epinephrine	↑ ↑ ↑	Alpha stimulation	Predominant effect at higher doses
	Norepinephrine	↑ ↑ ↑	Alpha stimulation	More prominent alpha effect than epinephrine
	Dopamine	↑ ↑	Alpha stimulation	Higher doses only
	Phenylephrine	↑ ↑ ↑	Alpha stimulation	No direct cardiac effect; may cause reflex slowing of heart
	Ephedrine	↑ ↑	Indirect (through release of norepinephrine) and direct alpha stimulation	Similar to epinephrine
	Calcium	↑ ↑ ↑	Direct cellular action	As above
Vasodilation	Isoproterenol	↑ ↑ ↑	Beta₂ stimulation	Has prominent beta₁ effects as well
	Dopamine	↑ ↑	Some beta₂ effect; renal–splanchnic vasodilation	Depends on dose used
	Nitroprusside	↑ ↑ ↑ ↑	Direct relaxation of both arteriolar and venous smooth muscle	Rapid onset/offset; tachyphylaxis may occur; prolonged use may lead to accumulation of thiocyanate and cyanide (CN⁻).
	Nitroglycerin	↑ ↑ ↑	Direct relaxation of vascular smooth muscle, predominantly venous and pulmonary arterial	Rapid onset/offset

[a]Alpha stimulation results in vasoconstriction through increased vascular muscle tone. Beta₁ stimulation results in an increase in cardiac rate and contractility (positive chronotropy and inotropy). Beta₂ stimulation results in bronchodilation and vasodilation through relaxation of smooth muscle. Blockade of these receptors (alpha, beta₁, beta₂) can be selectively accomplished by other drugs and will result in effects opposite to those seen with receptor stimulation.

for pediatric patients. Preferably, this should be given into a central line and may be repeated every 5 minutes. The medication may also be given by continuous infusion in a dose of 0.025–0.1 µg/kg/min (4 mg/500 ml D$_5$W = 8 µg/ml).

PRECAUTIONS. Admixture with bicarbonate solutions may inactivate the epinephrine. Extravasation may lead to tissue necrosis.

Norepinephrine

Norepinephrine is a potent peripheral vasoconstrictor (alpha-receptor stimulating) agent that generally causes an elevation of blood pressure. It is also a powerful inotropic (beta-receptor stimulating) agent. Its major impact in humans is usually upon the blood vessels, although in patients in cardiogenic shock (in which vasoconstriction may already be extreme), an important mechanism by which hypotension is corrected may be through an increase in cardiac performance. The initial response of the coronary circulation to norepinephrine may be vasoconstriction, but this response is transient and coronary vasodilation usually occurs, probably as a result of increased myocardial metabolic activity. Thus coronary artery blood flow may be increased both by dilation of the coronary arterial bed and by an increase in perfusion pressure.

Norepinephrine influences heart function both directly and indirectly. Cardiac output may increase or decrease, depending upon the level of systemic arterial blood pressure, the functional state of the left ventricle, and reflex responses such as carotid baroreceptor-mediated cardiac slowing. Cardiac output often increases when optimal blood pressure is restored, very likely as the result of improved coronary perfusion. Norepinephrine produces a slightly more rapid blood pressure response than other catecholamines. It has the disadvantage of causing renal and mesenteric vasoconstriction, whereas dopamine, at low infusion rates, characteristically causes vasodilation in these areas.

INDICATIONS. Hemodynamically significant hypotension or cardiogenic shock are the principal indications for norepinephrine. In the resuscitative situation, the drug can be useful when profound hypotension remains despite restoration of adequate cardiac rhythm. Although other sympathomimetics such as epinephrine or dopamine are often used for similar situations, norepinephrine can be particularly effective when total peripheral resistance is low. Such an inappropriate decline in systemic arterial resistance may be seen in the course of acute myocardial infarction and patients will usually respond promptly to α-adrenergic receptor agonists.

ADMINISTRATION. Norepinephrine is administered by intravenous infusion only, titrated to the desired blood pressure. It is available as 4-ml ampuls containing 4-mg norepinephrine base, and 1 or 2 ampuls should be diluted in 500-ml D$_5$W or 5% dextrose in normal saline (not plain normal saline). Two ampuls (8 mg) in 500 ml yields a concentration of 16 µg/ml; the use of this concentration in the postarrest patient is advised. The solution should be administered through a catheter well advanced into a vein (see Precautions). A microdrop administration set, in which 60 drops equals one milliliter, may be used. After observing the response to an initial dose of 2–3 ml/min (0.05–0.5 µg/kg/min), adjust the rate of flow to establish and maintain a low–normal blood pressure (usually above 90 mm Hg systolic) or, in previously hypertensive patients, a slightly higher than normal pressure. After the patient has been transferred out of the emergency room to the critical care unit, the drug may be continued for hours to days, but should gradually be tapered; blood pressure should be closely monitored. Abrupt cessation of therapy may result in acute severe hypotension.

PRECAUTIONS. Because standard blood pressure measurements are often inaccurate in patients with severe vasoconstriction, intraarterial pressure monitoring may be necessary for accurate determination of arterial pressure. Norepinephrine is contraindicated in patients with hypotension due to hypovolemia except as an emergency measure to maintain coronary and cerebral perfusion until proper replacement therapy is available. When hypovolemia is present, extreme degrees of vasoconstriction may occur and result in a critical decrease in organ blood flow even when a "normal" blood pressure is recognizable clinically. When continuous hemodynamic monitoring is not being used, blood pressure should be monitored every 2 minutes until the desired level is achieved then every 5 minutes as long as the agent is in use in order to avoid overcorrection of the blood pressure.

Myocardial oxygen requirements may be significantly increased as contractility and left ventricular wall tension are increased. This condition may be particularly deleterious in patients with myocardial ischemia or infarction. Constant monitoring should be carried out to detect cardiac rhythm disturbances. Heart rate and cardiac output may decrease, especially if the blood pressure is raised to unnecessarily high levels. Ischemic necrosis and sloughing of superficial tissues may result if extravasation of norepinephrine is allowed to occur at the site of injection. Phentolamine, 5–10 mg in 10–15 ml of saline solution, should be infiltrated as soon as possible into the area of extravasation to prevent necrosis and sloughing. Some investigators routinely add phentolamine to the norepinephrine infusion as a prophylactic.

Isoproterenol

Isoproterenol is a synthetic catecholamine with nearly pure beta activity. As such, it exerts potent cardiac stimulation by means of positive inotropic and chronotropic effects. The administration of isoproterenol results in a marked augmentation of cardiac output. Other actions are dilation of skeletal muscle, renal and mesenteric arterial beds, and bronchodilation. The vasodilation—chiefly of the skeletal muscle vessels—results in a drop in systemic vascular resistance. Although systolic blood pressure is usually maintained secondary to augmentation of cardiac output, mean and diastolic pressure, and therefore coronary perfusion pressure, usually decrease. This latter effect can be critical in patients after infarction or with ongoing ischemia. Since isoproterenol infusion results in increase in heart rate and contractility—two primary determinants of myocardial oxygen consumption—isoproterenol has the potential to decrease supply (perfusion pressure) while increasing demand (oxygen consumption) to the ischemic myocardium. This combination may be deleterious, especially in the situation of cardiac arrest.

INDICATIONS. Currently, the primary indication for using iso-proterenol is for the treatment of atropine-refractory, hemo-dynamically significant bradydysrhythmias, such as high-degree heart block, profound sinus or functional bradycardia. Its use should generally be that of a holding action until a temporary pacemaker can be inserted.

ADMINISTRATION. A solution of isoproterenol (Isuprel) should be prepared by diluting 1 mg with either 250 ml D$_5$W (4 μg/ml) or 500 ml (2 μg/ml). This should be infused slowly and cautiously at an infusion rate, usually 2–20 μg/min (0.05–0.5 μg/kg/min), sufficient to achieve the desired heart rate. Generally, 60–70 beats/min is satisfactory, although occasionally a more rapid rate may be desirable.

PRECAUTIONS. Because of its potent positive inotropic and chronotropic properties, isoproterenol has the potential to provoke serious ventricular dysrhythmias, including ventricular

fibrillation, as well as to increase markedly myocardial oxygen consumption. It therefore must be used with extreme caution in patients who have had a recent myocardial infarction. It is generally contraindicated if tachyarrhythmias are already present, especially if such dysrhythmias are secondary to digitalis toxicity. If significant hypotension occurs, we can combine with or switch to infusions of dopamine or epinephrine.

Dopamine

Dopamine hydrochloride has both alpha- and beta-receptor stimulating actions, as well as dopamine-receptor stimulating actions. It differs from epinephrine, norepinephrine, and isoproterenol in that it specifically dilates renal and mesenteric blood vessels in doses that may not produce an increase in heart rate or blood pressure (1 to 2 μg/kg/min). This effect is not blocked by β-adrenergic blocking drugs. Its actions differ with the dosage given, and individual responses may differ at the same dosage level. At doses from 2–10 μg/kg/min, dopamine generally has a beta-receptor stimulating action on the heart with resultant increase in cardiac output. At doses greater than 10 μg/kg/min, dopamine has an alpha-receptor stimulating action that results in peripheral vasoconstriction and may begin to cause renal arterial constriction. At doses above 20 μg/kg/min, the alpha-receptor stimulating action may reverse the dilation of renal and mesenteric vessels and result in a decline in renal and mesenteric blood flow. Differences in response of renal and mesenteric vascular beds, as well as dose-related differences in responses, have been attributed to dopamine-specific receptors. These receptors have been labeled *dopaminergic*.

INDICATIONS. The primary indications for dopamine are cardiogenic shock and hemodynamically significant hypotension. Such a situation would exist after an effective cardiac rhythm has been established. Hemodynamically significant hypotension may be defined as a systolic arterial pressure of less than 90 mm Hg with accompanying poor tissue perfusion.

ADMINISTRATION. Dopamine is supplied as 5-ml ampuls containing 40 mg/ml of dopamine. This 200-mg ampul must be diluted in 250 or 500 ml D$_5$W or D$_5$NS (800 μg/ml or 400 μg/ml). A premixed solution has recently been made available. Avoid alkaline intravenous solutions (NaHCO$_3$) that will deactivate the drug. The dose is variable, dependent on the desired action. For hypotensive therapy, the usual initial infusion rate is 2–5 μg/kg/min, which is increased until satisfactory responses of blood pressure and urine output are obtained.

Although most patients will respond to infusion rates well below 20 μg/kg/min, the lowest infusion rate that results in satisfactory perfusion should be the goal of therapy. An occasional patient will have a beneficial response to rates as high as 50 μg/kg/min. To optimize the hemodynamic response, it may be necessary to monitor left ventricular filling pressure, cardiac output, and total peripheral resistance.

PRECAUTIONS. Tachydysrhythmias may result from dopamine therapy and require reduction in dosage or discontinuation of the drug. An undesirable degree of vasoconstriction may result from high doses. On the other hand, blood pressure may be decreased because of the renal vasodilating effect of small doses of dopamine. The desired hemodynamic–heart rate effect may be obtained by combining dopamine therapy with isoproterenol, epinephrine, or norepinephrine. Hemodynamic monitoring may substantially improve our ability to optimize therapy. Ectopic heart beats, nausea, and vomiting are among the more frequent adverse effects of dopamine. Angina pectoris has been reported. Dopamine may produce cutaneous tissue necrosis and sloughing similar to that produced by norepinephrine. Extravasation of the agent must be avoided or, if it occurs, treated promptly as described above for norepinephrine.

Monamine oxidase inhibitors such as isocarboxazid (Marplan), pargyline hydrochloride (Eutonyl), tranylcypromine sulfate (Parnate), and phenelzine sulfate (Nardil) potentiate the effects of dopamine. Therefore, people who have been receiving these agents should be given no more than one-tenth of the usual dopamine dosage. Because dopamine may result in serious acute hypertension in patients with pheochromocytoma, it is contraindicated in this setting. The drug should not be discontinued abruptly but should be tapered gradually.

Dobutamine

Dobutamine is intended for short-term intravenous use in the treatment of patients with refractory heart failure. It is a direct β-adrenergic receptor stimulating agent and increases myocardial contractility. It differs from norepinephrine in that it produces little systemic arterial constriction at usual dose level. It differs from isoproterenol in that tachycardia is not as problematic. Renal and mesenteric blood flow usually will increase as cardiac output increases.

Dobutamine may be used with nitroprusside with further enhancement of cardiac output. The use of nitroprusside results in a decrease in peripheral arterial resistance and the use of dobutamine may maintain coronary perfusion. Such combined usage of these drugs would usually be reserved for postresuscitation stabilization.

INDICATIONS. Dobutamine may be useful in patients with refractory congestive heart failure, particularly when it is a result of temporary depression of ventricular function and myocardial contractility. Dopamine, however, continues to be the agent of choice for some clinicians, in part because of its effect on renal circulation and in part because of greater experience with the agent.

ADMINISTRATION. A low-dose level of 0.5 μg/kg/min of dobutamine may be effective. The usual dosage range is 2.5–10.0 μg/kg/min. Dobutamine is supplied as a vial containing 250 mg of the drug, which is dissolved into 10 ml of sterile water and is further diluted with 250- or 500-ml D_5W (1 mg/ml or 0.5 mg/ml).

PRECAUTIONS. Dobutamine may cause tachycardia and dysrhythmias, especially at dosage levels in excess of 20 μg/kg/min. Evidence of the effect of dobutamine on myocardial infarction size remains conflicting, and caution in its use in this setting is advisable.

ANTIARRHYTHMIA AGENTS

Antiarrhythmic agents obviously play an integral role in many resuscitation situations. Lidocaine remains the mainstay for maintainance of a stable rhythm after electrical defibrillation. A new agent, bretylium, offers similar use, as well as enhances the success rate for electrical defibrillation. Procainamide is commonly used in the critical care unit for postarrest stabilization; a brief discussion of its properties is warranted because of its occasional use in the emergency room.

Lidocaine

Ventricular ectopy is not an unusual finding during a resuscitative sequence. Specific treatment of premature or ectopic ventricular beats in an otherwise stable patient is given only for unusually frequent beats or for those occurring in a particularly worrisome pattern. An unstable patient with myocardial ischemia, however, is much more prone to progress from simple ventricular premature beats to ventricular tachycardia or fibrillation, and in these patients treatment with an antiarrythmic agent should be given promptly.

INDICATIONS.   Lidocaine has been shown to be an effective agent in suppressing undesirable automaticity. Its onset of action is rapid. Its duration of action is brief but may be prolonged by use of a continuous infusion of drug. Rapid suppression of ventricular ectopic beats may be obtained. The drug is also indicated in ventricular tachycardia and ventricular fibrillation that has recurred after a successful defibrillation or that has been refractory to defibrillation. Correction of the underlying cause of the arrhythmia (hypoxemia, hypercarbia, myocardial ischemia, electrolyte imbalance, etc.) must be accomplished as well for successful stabilization of the cardiac rhythm.

ADMINISTRATION.   A solution of lidocaine, typically 20 mg/ml (2%), should be prepared for intravenous infusion. Prefilled syringes are widely available for bolus injections. The customary treatment is to begin with a bolus dose of approximately 1 mg/kg and then to immediately initiate a continuous infusion of the drug at 2–4 mg/min (15–50 μg/kg/min). If there is no preexisting coronary disease and if the underlying cause of the dysrhythmia is corrected, the infusion may be tapered rapidly or, perhaps, may not be required.

PRECAUTIONS.   Dosage should be reduced in low cardiac output states and in hepatic failure because of decreased drug metabolism and possible excessive accumulation. Toxic manifestations are usually seen first in the central nervous system (slurring of speech, tinnitus, sleepiness, feeling of impending doom) and can progress to frank seizures; these may be controlled with a short-acting barbiturate (e.g., thiopental) or diazepam, as dictated by the clinical situation. Lidocaine in large doses can diminish myocardial contractility.

Bretylium

Bretylium tosylate was initially introduced and evaluated as an antihypertensive agent. The unacceptable incidence of orthostatic hypotension associated with oral administration precluded its use for this condition; however, it soon became apparent that it possesses unique pharmacologic and electrophysiologic properties as an antiarrhythmic agent.

Pharmacologically, it is an adrenergic blocking agent, preventing norepinephine release from peripheral adrenergic nerve terminals. When the drug is first administered an initial release of norepinephrine is seen; it subsequently prevents further norepinephrine release and prevents the uptake of circulating norepinephrine into these same nerve terminals thereby potentiating the actions of circulating catecholamines.

Experimental work, including models of induced myocardial infarction, as well as electrically induced ventricular fibrillation, has documented the efficacy of bretylium for defibrillation. Investigations have demonstrated that bretylium markedly changed the ventricular fibrillation threshold (VFT) and prevented electrically induced VF (Bacaner). Further interesting observations provided by these and similar studies were that bretylium was able to induce spontaneous reversion to sinus rhythm of the electrically induced VF and that the improvement in VF threshold was more pronounced than with quinidine, procainamide, lidocaine, or propranolol. Additionally, these experimental studies as well as clinical trials have noted that bretylium appears more effective alone than when other antiarrhythmics are already present in the serum. The exact mechanism of antiarrhythmic efficacy is poorly understood. In infarcted canine hearts, bretylium has appeared able to reduce the disparity in action potential duration and refractory period between normal and ischemic tissue. This disparity is felt to be a probable source for reentrant ventricular arrhythmias in the myocardial infarction period.

Clinical studies have demonstrated results similar to those found in the laboratory: Bretylium has been demonstrated to be effective in suppressing ventricular ectopic activity, especially ventricular tachycardia and ventricular fibrillation, in a variety of conditions including acute myocardial infarction, chronic ischemic disease, hypertensive disease, and valvular heart disease. It has proven to be effective as an adjunct to electrical defibrillation in cases resistant to defibrillation alone. There has been some suggestion, as yet poorly documented, that bretylium is superior to lidocaine in this regard. It has been reported that a group of patients who had high-grade ventricular ectopic activity refractory to at least one other antiarrhythmic agent were successfully treated with bretylium (Amsterdam et al). In another study in which a large group of patients was treated with the agent, it was demonstrated that only two factors influenced a successful outcome: administration soon after onset of the dysrhythmia and the withholding of other antiarrhythmic agents during its use. This latter finding, borne out by other clinical as well as experimental studies, seems to be related to the antagonistic hemodynamic and electrophysiologic activities of other antiarrhythmic agents. It should be noted, however, that many cardiologists have successfully used the drug following the use of other agents. A fascinating observation by a group of Italian cardiologists was their ability to defibrillate five out of seven patients by means of external cardiac massage and bretylium alone. This successful chemical defibrillation has been uniquely possible only with bretylium.

The above noted success in treating high-grade ventricular

arrhythmias with bretylium has suggested its potential use as a prophylactic agent in the face of an acute myocardial infarction. Although it is unquestionably effective, the reported incidence of up to 30% of orthostatic hypotension associated with bretylium, albeit mild, has tempered the ready acceptance for this indication.

The initial response to parenteral administration is an increase in cardiac output and mean systemic pressure and fall in left ventricular filling pressure. This short-lived (10–20 minutes) enhancement of left ventricular performance is the result of norepinephrine release from nerve endings and is followed by a delayed hypotensive effect secondary to peripheral adrenergic blockage. Up to 88% of patients may develop hypotension; and, although this is the most common side effect, it is generally mild and does not require discontinuation of the drug. It is most marked when the patient is volume depleted, when other antecedent cardiac depressant antiarrhythmics have been used or when doses less than 5 mg/kg have been used. Underdosing results in unabated peripheral dilatation without the balancing augmentation of cardiac output.

INDICATIONS.   The prime indications for the use of bretylium are therapy for ventricular tachycardia (VT) and fibrillation, especially if they are refractory to other antiarrhythmic agents and/or electrical countershocks. It also may provide suppressive therapy for recurrent VT or VF and may possibly serve as a prophylactic antiarrhythmic in situations of acute myocardial infarctions.

Well-conducted clinical comparisons of bretylium against other agents are not available. Indeed such controlled studies are extremely difficult if not impossible to conduct. However, in the laboratory setting with electrically induced VF it clearly is superior to the other drugs and appears unique in its ability to chemically defibrillate directly. Bretylium should no longer be considered a drug of last resort but rather one of first or second choice, perhaps selected soon after other agents have failed and preferably used by itself.

ADMINISTRATION.   Bretylium is available as a 500-mg ampul (10 ml). The dosage for ventricular fibrillation is 5 mg/kg undiluted, given rapidly intravenously and followed by countershock. If this is unsuccessful, 10 mg/kg is given, repeated if necessary every 15 minutes up to a maximum total initial dose of 30 mg/kg. Each dosage must be followed by direct current (DC) countershock. For refractory or recurrent ventricular tachycardia, 500 mg should be diluted to 50 ml with saline and given 5–10 mg/kg over 10–20 minutes. This may be repeated every 6–8 hours or alternatively given as a drip of 2 mg/min. Bretylium may be given intramuscularly.

PRECAUTIONS.   Orthostatic hypotension is the most common adverse reaction and may be treated by putting the patient in Trendelenburg's position or administering fluids. Very rarely, pressors, at lower than normal dosages, are required. Nausea and vomiting may occur in the awake patient if the infusion rate is too fast. Potentially, bretylium may exacerbate ventricular tachydysrhythmias caused by digitalis toxicity because of its known catecholamine releasing activity. However, this effect should be transient, and bretylium seems to be a reasonable choice for intractable VT or VF. A relative contraindication is administration to patients who cannot compensate for peripheral vasodilation by an increase in stroke volume, for example, severe aortic or pulmonic stenosis or pulmonary hypertension.

Procainamide

Although chronic administration of procainamide is somewhat hampered by the short duration of action of the oral preparation, this agent is an effective therapy for ventricular as well as some supraventricular arrhythmias. In the critical care setting, it is most useful for treatment of ventricular ectopic activity not fully suppressed by lidocaine.

Procainamide's direct electrophysiologic activities on the heart are very similar to those of quinidine. The adrenergic effects (e.g., vagolytic), however, are somewhat weaker than those of quinidine. Both agents are effective for rhythm disturbances arising on the basis of either an ectopic focus or secondary to a reentry mechanism.

INDICATIONS.   Indications for use of procainamide are suppression of premature ventricular contractions, ventricular tachycardia, or fibrillation that is refractory to therapy with lidocaine.

ADMINISTRATION.   Procainamide is a very versatile agent that can be given intravenously by bolus injection or slow infusion, intramuscularly, or orally. Although the intravenous route is preferred in the critical care setting, the drug is well absorbed, albeit more slowly, intramuscularly. Several dosage schedules have been proposed. Commonly, 100-mg boluses (1.5 mg/kg) injected over 1 minute are repeated every 5 minutes until either arrhythmia suppression occurs, adverse effects appear (see below), or a total loading dose of approximately 1 g (15 mg/kg) is achieved. A second method is to infuse 20 mg/min (0.3 mg/

kg/min) up to the same total loading dose as above followed by a constant infusion of 1–4 mg/min (15–50 µg/kg/min). Finally, some authorities have suggested a loading dose of 17 mg/kg over 1 hour followed by a maintenance infusion of 2.8/ mg/kg/hr (1.4 mg/kg/hr in patients with impaired renal function).

PRECAUTIONS. Blood pressure (BP) and ECG should be monitored after each loading bolus for hypotension or prolongation of PR, QRS, or QT intervals. Although the hypotension usually responds to slowing the infusion rate, prolongation of the QRS complex by more than 50% of its initial width signifies a toxic blood level and may herald atrioventricular conduction disturbances including high-degree heart block and asystole. This is especially true in patients with digitalis intoxication. Administration of procainamide should be avoided for the treatment of ventricular arrhythmias associated with marked disturbances of atrioventricular conduction.

OTHER AGENTS

Atropine

INDICATIONS. Resuscitation of the patient may result in restoration of regular sinus rhythm but a slow heart rate. This sinus bradycardia in itself is not bothersome. Frequently, however, there is accompanying hypotension or ventricular ectopy; if these are severe or if the bradycardia itself is extreme, treatment with atropine sulfate is indicated to increase the heart rate by vagal blockade.

ADMINISTRATION. Atropine is usually given intravenously, although the intratracheal and sublingual routes are alternatives. Sublingual injection of atropine has been used by many with good effect. The tongue is well vascularized, and its venous return to the heart is direct and rapid. Intramuscular administration, although normally effective, cannot be used in the resuscitative situation because of peripheral vasoconstriction and unpredictable uptake from the muscle depot. Caution must be taken to avoid administration of too small a dose since low doses of atropine may cause further slowing of the heart rate. This effect is thought to result from central vagal stimulation and perhaps from an additional direct action on the heart. The standard adult dosage is 0.5 mg, repeated every 3–5 minutes until the desired effect is obtained, to a maximum dose of 2

mg. The pediatric dose is 0.02 mg/kg. Available concentrations vary; the most frequent concentrations are 0.4 or 1 mg/ml.

PRECAUTIONS. Tachycardia is not well tolerated in patients with severe coronary disease.

Calcium

The contractile state of myocardial tissue is in part controlled by alterations in the intracellular concentration of the calcium ion. The myocardium seems especially dependent on external calcium as a source of intracellular calcium; therefore, transmembrane calcium flux serves as an important regulatory function. Administration of calcium produces an increase in myocardial contractility and perhaps in ventricular automaticity as well.

INDICATIONS. The usefulness of calcium is most evident in the presence of electromechanical dissociation, in which cardiac electrical activity is reasonably normal but mechanical cardiac output is lacking. Assuming adequate intravascular volume has been restored, a dramatic increase in cardiac output and blood pressure is often seen after administration of calcium. Successful use of the drug for restoration of an electrical rhythm in ventricular standstill has been less well proven, although this use is still recommended by many. If citrated blood products are rapidly administered during the course of a resuscitative event, the plasma ionized calcium level may fall precipitously secondary to chelation of circulating calcium ions by the citrate. This may lead to a transient but severe hypotensive state that is easily reversed by calcium administration.

The use of calcium in advanced life support is not without controversy. Dangerously high levels of serum calcium have been demonstrated after administration of acceptable doses of calcium chloride. It must be used with caution in the digitalized patient because of the synergism between the two agents. This is especially true when there is ventricular tachycardia secondary to digitalis toxicity.

ADMINISTRATION. Calcium is commonly supplied as one of three different salts: calcium chloride ($CaCl_2$), calcium gluceptate, and calcium gluconate. This last preparation is less frequently available because of its instability. The chloride salt provides the most direct source of calcium ion and produces the most rapid effect; the gluceptate and gluconate salts require hepatic degradation to release free calcium ions. During resuscitation, when immediate effect is essential, calcium chloride is the best choice. It is highly irritating to tissue and veins, however, and must be injected into a relatively large vein and precautions must be taken to avoid extravasation. If only small peripheral veins are available, calcium gluceptate or calcium gluconate should be used. The amount of elemental calcium per molecule varies from salt to salt: 27 mg Ca^{2+} per 100 mg salt for calcium chloride, 18 mg Ca^{2+} per 100 mg salt for calcium gluceptate, and 9 mg Ca^{2+} per 100 mg salt for calcium gluconate. Suggested dosages (in milligrams of the complete salt) are as follows: Calcium chloride can be administered in 250–500 mg/dose for adults, repeated every 5–10 minutes as needed; 10–20 mg/kg/dose for children. Calcium chloride is available as a 10% solution (100 mg/ml). Calcium gluconate can be administered in 1–1.5 g/dose (adult) and 30–60 mg/kg dose (pediatric), repeated every 5–10 minutes as needed. This is also supplied as a 10% solution (100 mg/ml).

PRECAUTIONS.   Both preparations should be given slowly intravenously, ensuring that any previously administered bicarbonate has cleared the line. Overly rapid administration may result in bradycardia in the situation of a beating heart. Calcium chloride is sclerotic if extravasated. Calcium salts must be used with caution in the digitalized patient.

Nitroprusside

Although vasodilators are primarily used in the intensive care unit setting, they have been found to be occasionally useful in the emergency room for postarrest stabilization. In the clinical setting of severe acute or chronic ventricular dysfunction that may exist after myocardial infarction or cardiac arrest, vasodilator therapy has been shown to be of potential benefit. Sodium nitroprusside, a rapidly acting agent, produces both arterial and venous dilatation. It represents the primary parenteral vasodilator for therapy for acute left ventricular dysfunction because of its ease of administration and balanced effects on both preload and outflow resistance (commonly, albeit incorrectly, referred to as afterload).

Arterial dilatation results in a reduction in outflow impedance of the left ventricle. Such drugs are able to reduce the resistance to left ventricular ejection, thereby increasing forward cardiac output and improving tissue perfusion. Venodilatation results in reduction in left ventricular filling pressure with two beneficial effects: The decrease in left ventricular end diastolic volume and, therefore, end diastolic pressure reduces myocardial oxygen consumption, while the reduction in the mean ventricular filling pressure decreases the hydrostatic pressure in the pulmonary capillaries, thus decreasing transudation of fluid and reducing pulmonary congestion.

The effects of nitroprusside on hemodynamics and ventricular performance are dependent on the underlying status of myocardial function. Nitroprusside dilates both the venous (capacitance) system and arterial (resistance) vessels. It has been emphasized that normal individuals or patients with well-preserved left ventricular function are quite sensitive to changes in preload and are relatively insensitive to changes in outflow impedance. Administration of nitroprusside to these patients would result in venous pooling with little balancing augmentation of stroke volume by reduction in afterload. The result would be a fall in cardiac output and reflex tachycardia secondary to barocenter stimulation. As discussed in Chapter 3, patients with depressed left ventricular function are little affected by changes in filling pressures (i.e., flat portion of Starling's curve), but they are extremely sensitive to changes in outflow resistance. Patients with reduced cardiac output, such as after myocardial infarction, have elevated systemic vascular resistance. Reduction in this outflow resistance will be accompanied by a rise in stroke volume and little or no change in blood pressure. Since mean systemic pressure is little changed, there is little stimulus to the barocenters to produce reflex tachycardia. Additionally, it has been shown that the reflex response of patients with heart disease is blunted. Nitroprusside should be administered with caution, starting at a low dose. Generally, reflex tachycardia in response to nitroprusside infusion represents excessive reduction in blood pressure or inadequate left ventricular filling pressure.

INDICATIONS.   Most patients surviving resuscitation are in an extremely tenuous state, often secondary to depressed left ventricular function. The potential benefits of vasodilator therapy are increased cardiac output and reduction in left ventricular end diastolic pressure (LVEDP) secondary to improved emptying and venous pooling. The reduction in pulmonary congestion and myocardial oxygen consumption that result from a lower LVEDP can be critical in patients with ischemic heart disease postarrest. A reduction in mortality from 85 to 40% in patients with cardiogenic shock who received vasodilator therapy has been reported.

The potential uses of vasodilator therapy during or immediately following resuscitation include any situation in which cardiac output is significantly reduced. This is especially true in cases in which valvular regurgiation (e.g., aortic or mitral regurgitation) or left-to-right shunting (e.g., postinfarct ventricular septal defect) exists. Less commonly, a marked pressure load may be imposed upon a relatively normal ventricle, as in hypertensive crisis. In such a situation nitroprusside has become the treatment of choice.

ADMINISTRATION. Nitroprusside has quite rapid onset of action, and changes in administration rate are apparent within minutes. The infusion rates, initially recommended for starting therapy, of 50 μg/min (0.5 μg/kg/min) are reasonable for hypertensive crisis but may be excessive for patients with left ventricular failure. In patients in the latter situation, the infusion should begin at 10 μg/min, with 5–10 μg/min increments every 5 minutes. Most patients with severely impaired pump performance will respond to 50–100 μg/min total dose, although an occasional patient requires a significantly higher dosage. Patients with hypertensive crisis can require 400–1,000 μg/min or more. The pediatric dosage is 0.5–8.0 μg/kg/min, with an average dosage of 3 μg/kg/min. Nitroprusside is available as 50-mg dihydrate vials; the drug should be dissolved in 5 ml D_5W and mixed with 250–1,000 ml D_5W. Although it appears that the reconstituted solution can be used for longer than the recommended period of 4 hours, the mixture should be prepared at the time of use and not stored.

PRECAUTIONS. Hypotension is the most frequently encountered side effect of nitroprusside and is generally secondary to excessive dosage. Retching, vomiting, apprehension, and muscular twitching have been reported, usually after overly rapid infusion, and respond to slowing the infusion rate. Worsening of ventilation–perfusion mismatch has been noted in patients treated with nitroprusside.

Nitroprusside is converted to thiocyanate by a hepatic enzyme, and thiocyanate is cleared by the kidneys. Signs and symptoms of nitroprusside toxicity generally represent thiocyanate toxicity and include nausea, tinnitus, blurred vision, and delirium. Although a blood level determination for thiocyanate is available, this is generally not necessary unless high dosages are used for a prolonged period, especially in patients with renal dysfunction.

Dextrose

INDICATIONS. Hypoglycemia may accompany cardiorespiratory collapse, particularly in young infants and elderly patients, and will delay successful resuscitation if not corrected. A simple chemical strip test can quickly provide a crude but clinically useful estimate of blood glucose level on just a few drops of blood, and appropriate therapy may then be given.

ADMINISTRATION. Dextrose is supplied as 50% dextrose in water ($D_{50}W$) (500 mg/ml), which is usually diluted to 25% dextrose in water ($D_{25}W$) for administration intravenously as a slow bolus. The usual dose is 0.5–1 g/kg.

Naloxone

INDICATIONS. Persistently constricted pupils during effective CPR, together with a clinical history suggestive of narcotic overdose, will prompt the administration of naloxone (Narcan). Naloxone, which is an essentially pure narcotic antagonist, will produce rapid dramatic improvement if opioid overdose is present; in the absence of narcotics it will cause no detrimental change in the patient's condition.

ADMINISTRATION. The adult dose is 0.4 mg and the pediatric dose is 0.01 mg/kg. This may be repeated at 2–3 minute intervals; if no response occurs after three doses, narcotic depression is not likely to be present. Naloxone is supplied in ampuls of 0.4 mg/ml and 0.02 mg/ml (Narcan Neonatal).

PRECAUTIONS. If effective, the dose may need to be repeated every 45–60 minutes until the original narcotic drug has been eliminated, as the duration of action of naloxone is relatively short.

OTHER PROCEDURES

Emergency Pacemaker Implantation

Although the actual technique for insertion of a temporary pacemaker is discussed in detail in the procedure section (Procedure 16), a brief description of the life-threatening situations requiring such a technique is appropriate here. The primary indication for an emergency pacemaker is profound bradyarrhythmia with resultant cardiac output inadequate to support tissue perfusion. Such bradycardic states may arise from conduction system disease and complete heart block, from excessive parasympathetic tone, or as a slow junctional or idioventricular escape mechanism following electrical defibrillation.

Pacemaker implantation is frequently used as a last resort during asystole. Since this condition usually results from profound myocardial damage or severe underlying metabolic derangement, the low incidence of success is not unexpected. Similarly, an attempt at emergency pacemaker insertion is often made in the presence of electromechanical dissociation. However, since this condition represents the inability of the heart to generate an organized and effective contraction despite an adequate intrinsic electrical mechanism, the addition of an artificial electrical stimulus provides little benefit.

One to two milligrams of atropine given intravenously is mandatory in each of the above situations before introduction of the pacemaker. This quick and relatively safe drug trial may accelerate even the most profound bradyarrhythmia and provide adequate cardiac output. Frequently, if the results with atropine have been unsuccessful an infusion of isoproterenol is useful while the more definitive pacemaker is being readied and inserted.

For any of the above situations, the actual techniques are the same: either transvenous insertion of an endocardial lead or transthoracic insertion of a pacing stylet. The former can be carried out by using balloon-tipped floatation catheters or semi-floating hockey stick-shaped catheters, either of which can be introduced blindly with electrocardiographic confirmation of location. Alternatively, a standard bipolar pacing catheter can be passed blindly from the femoral vein, although fluoroscopic guidance is usually preferable. Transthoracic pacing involves introducing a pacing stylet through an intracardiac needle. Although this technique is the easiest to ensure ventricular capture during cardiac arrest, the clinical situations during which it is usually used have resulted in a dismal record of success.

Internal Cardiac Compression

Anatomical or mechanical restrictions inherent to the underlying disease state of the patient may render external cardiac compression impossible or ineffective. Marked chest deformities, such as severe pectus excavatum or carinatum, chest wall instability, and pericardial tamponade, are examples of clinical situations in which emergency thoracotomy and internal cardiac compression (ICC) may be required. It should be emphasized that conventional external CPR must be applied initially; only if this is ineffective should internal compression be considered. Use of this procedure requires a knowledge of indications, experience with the mechanics of emergency thoracotomy, as well as the actual technique of ICC, and readily available thoracic surgical backup.

Monitoring During Advanced Cardiac Life Support

ELECTROCARDIOGRAPHIC MONITORING

As already discussed, ECG monitoring is essential during resuscitation, both as a diagnostic tool and as a guide to the most effective therapy. It should be initiated as soon as possible during a resuscitative sequence. Initially, the "quick look" paddles should be used, if available, but the standard ECG machine or monitoring unit with a display screen should be attached as soon as possible during the resuscitation.

BLOOD PRESSURE

Blood pressure must be monitored as soon as ECG rhythm and pulse have been restored. Palpation of the pulse in one of the major arteries is a reasonable guide to adequacy of chest compression. The presence of a "good pulse," however, is mainly a reflection of systolic pressure and does not indicate adequacy of mean arterial pressure or blood flow. Indirect measurement of blood pressure, such as by cuff and manometer, or direct measurement, using an intraarterial catheter, will serve as a guide to further therapy (Procedure 14). Cohn and others have emphasized that in the vasoconstricted patient, secondary to either endogenous or exogenous catecholamines, determinations that rely on the Korotkoff sounds (cuff or Doppler) may be artifactually significantly lower than true intraarterial pressure. Although introduction of an intraarterial line can be quite useful once the patient is stabilized and transferred to an intensive care unit, in the emergency room, attainment by palpation of an adequate large vessel pulse such as the carotid or femoral artery is a reasonable goal.

AUSCULTATION

The stethoscope is one of the simplest and yet most versatile monitoring tools available. Adequacy of ventilation is easily and continuously monitored by chest auscultation, allowing early diagnosis of complications of resuscitation such as pneumothorax or malposition of the endotracheal tube.

TEMPERATURE MEASUREMENT

Temperature measurement is appropriate in all resuscitative attempts but is particularly so in pediatric and geriatric patients and in those who have been exposed to temperature extremes. Moderate-to-severe hypothermia can delay the patient's return to spontaneous cardiac rhythm and must be corrected before resuscitative efforts can truly be called unsuccessful.

LABORATORY INVESTIGATIONS

Laboratory investigations will guide ongoing therapy. The most useful initial measurements include arterial pH and blood gases (Procedure 13), the hematocrit, serum glucose, sodium, potassium, and calcium (total calcium or, if available, ionized calcium). If abnormalities are noted, they may be treated, and the success of such treatment may be monitored by repeated measurements. Blood gas analyses, in particular, should be repeated every 5–10 minutes until they have stabilized.

DOCUMENTATION

Timely charting, whereby all measured vital signs, interventions performed, and laboratory data are recorded, will be helpful to those personnel assuming care of the patient after resuscitation.

Sequencing Events in Cardiopulmonary Resuscitation

The sequence in which the various therapeutic modalities described above will be applied varies from patient to patient. Clearly, good basic support of oxygenation, ventilation, and circulation is essential as a first step. Next is ECG diagnosis of heart rhythm, followed by specific therapy guided by ECG diagnosis and response. Ventricular asystole signifies a severe metabolic deficit or myocardial insult. In such circumstances, the usual sequence is to attempt to restore some spontaneous cardiac activity using epinephrine, calcium, bicarbonate (to correct acidosis), and perhaps atropine; these drugs are frequently given in "rounds" while CPR continues. If recovery of fibrillatory activity is accomplished, defibrillation may then be performed to achieve a sinus rhythm. Once stable sinus rhythm is attained, attention is given to suppressing further dysrhythmias, to optimizing blood pressure, cardiac output, and rate, and to minimizing the workload on the heart. Correction of underlying disorders (hypovolemia, hypothermia, hypoglycemia, sepsis, electrolyte disturbances, etc.) must be attempted simultaneously. Once stabilized, the patient may be transported to an intensive care setting for follow-up care.

Termination of Cardiopulmonary Resuscitation

The decision to terminate unsuccessful resuscitative efforts is always a difficult one, particularly if the patient is a child or young adult. Inability to restore adequate cardiovascular performance after sufficient time and effort is the most certain basis for this decision. Criteria for brain death can rarely be attained in the emergency room resuscitation, but absence of reactive pupils, lack of spontaneous activity and response to deep pain, and absent brainstem reflexes are ominous prognostic signs.

During resuscitative efforts, the patient's family must be regarded as high priority. Physicians and nurses, despite hectic circumstances and time constraints, must spend some moments with the family, offering whatever support is possible and ensuring that they understand as fully as possible what has happened to their loved one. Issues of guilt will arise and appropriate reassurance must be given. Although the patient's family must be consulted and feelings and concerns regarding prolongation of efforts considered, under no circumstances should the family feel that they have made the decision to terminate support. Referrals to appropriate social service agencies and arrangements for follow-up care for the family can be made as needed; the patient's primary physician must be contacted since his or her assistance will be invaluable.

IMMEDIATE POSTRESUSCITATION SUPPORT

The smooth transition from successful resuscitation to ongoing critical care is the joint province of the emergency service, the transport team, and the ultimate primary caretakers. Care must be taken to ensure continued patient monitoring and continuity of therapy during this transition to prevent or immediately rectify further decompensation.

Evaluation and Stabilization

Once resuscitation has been completed, efforts must be directed toward evaluation and stabilization of the patient. A careful history and physical examination must be performed, emphasizing the establishment of the precipitating cause of the cardiac arrest and the identification of concurrent illnesses or injuries. Special attention must also be paid to completion of a neurologic examination, defining current level of function and identifying neurologic deficits for comparison with prearrest status.

Diagnostic studies required for ongoing management should be completed; for example, a chest film (for tube and line placement as well as disease), full ECG, blood and other samples for a complete blood count (CBC), urinalysis, electrolytes, and cardiac enzymes. If blood transfusion or surgery is anticipated, samples for cross match should be dispatched to the blood bank.

Stabilization will include correction of metabolic deficits and initiation of necessary medications (antibiotics, diuretics, etc.). Respiratory support will include optimizing ventilatory support with appropriate adjustments of FiO_2, positive end expiratory pressure, and mechanical assistance. Oxygen supplementation should be provided to all patients, even if they seem quite stable and are without respiratory compromise, to maximize myocardial oxygenation. Cardiovascular support should include continued monitoring and pharmacologic suppression of arrythmias. Vasoactive and sympathomimetic drugs should be used to provide adequate cardiac output with minimal cardiac work.

The emergency room physician must decide which facilities are available to provide ongoing care. Transportation to the continuing care facility should occur only after reasonable stability has been achieved and all people involved are prepared.

Transport

Transportation of the patient is best accomplished with a physician and nurse in attendance at all times. If necessary travel is only within the hospital, the emergency room or intensive care staff, perhaps aided by the anesthesiologist, should be able to provide this service. If interhospital movement is necessary, a transport team may be provided by the referral center (especially in pediatric facilities); if not, the responsibility for the patient's safe transport rests with the referring physician.

The physician must be certain that adequate equipment is provided for the movement of the patient. A continuous ECG monitor, stethoscope, and blood pressure cuff are basic necessities; more sophisticated monitoring may also be required. Appropriate airway support equipment, including laryngoscope with blade, spare endotracheal tube, mask, ventilating circuit, and adequate oxygen supply should be available. A full E-cylinder of oxygen (Fig. 1.11) (approximately 2,200 psi) contains 660 liters of oxygen; at a typical flow rate of 10 liters/min, 66 minutes of oxygen are available. Resuscitation drugs and a defibrillator, if necessary, should be at hand. In a busy hospital, security personnel are often helpful in clearing corridors, holding emergency elevators, and the like.

Intensive Care

Continued observation of the postarrest patient should be in a critical care setting in which appropriate nursing and physician personnel and necessary monitoring and therapeutic equipment are available. Ongoing care is frequently organized in a problem-oriented manner since multisystem disease is commonly found either as cause for or as a result of the cardiopulmonary arrest.

CARDIORESPIRATORY SYSTEM

Appropriate ventilatory support is provided, guided by physical examination, chest films, and arterial blood gases; the presence of pulmonary edema is noted and treated. Cardiotonic or vasoactive drug therapy, diuresis, or fluid loading may be required; such decisions may be guided by more invasive monitoring of central venous pressure, pulmonary artery and capillary pressure, and determinations of cardiac output.

RENAL–METABOLIC SYSTEMS

Urinary output may be monitored by use of an indwelling catheter; the etiology of a reduced urine output must be investigated to assess whether prerenal factors or true renal dysfunction are responsible. Overall balance of intake and output, including daily weights, will be helpful in fluid management. Abnormalities in electrolytes, serum proteins, and enzymes should be noted and treated.

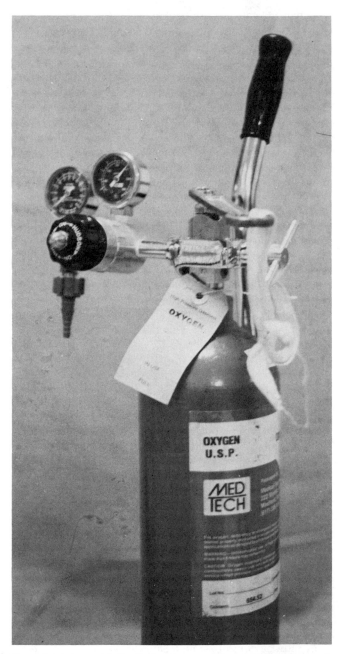

Figure 1.11 A portable E-cylinder of oxygen. Note that the tank wrench, essential for access to the tank contents, is tied to the regulator apparatus to preclude loss.

HEMATOLOGIC–GASTROINTESTINAL SYSTEMS

Stress ulceration and gastrointestinal bleeding should be anticipated and prophylactic therapy given; hepatic dysfunction and intestinal ileus are not uncommon after an anoxic–ischemic event. Blood should be examined to ensure adequacy of circulating red blood cells, white blood cells, and platelets. Assessment of the coagulation system by measuring prothrombin time (PT), partial thromboplastin time (PTT), and perhaps bleeding time is essential; abnormalities are frequently found, particularly after massive transfusion, and correction may be required. Infectious diseases should be sought out and appropriately treated.

CENTRAL NERVOUS SYSTEM

Unfortunately, many patients have successful restoration of cardiorespiratory function but are left with severe central nervous system sequellae. Because of this, efforts are being made to improve the brain-oriented care given to critically ill patients. In emergency medical care, the concept of cardiopulmonary–cerebral resuscitation (CCPR) is being developed to emphasize the need for protection of the brain during and after severe cardiopulmonary decompensation.

The primary injury to the brain—a hypoxic–ischemic event—has already occurred by the time we are called upon to care for the victim. Our goal in brain-oriented resuscitation is to avoid further injury to the brain, to provide optimal conditions for its healing, and, if possible, to ameliorate the damage done. One of the results of brain injury is brain swelling. Significant brain swelling within the closed intracranial vault will lead to excessive pressure on and further damage to brain tissue. Our therapies are directed toward minimizing brain edema, as well as minimizing the volume of the other contents of the intracranial vault.

Continuing critical care for patients at risk for cerebral edema includes *dehydration,* using osmolar or other agents, to maintain a serum osmolarity in the 300–310-mosm range; *hyperventilation,* with PaCO$_2$ controlled in the 25–30 mm Hg range to decrease cerebral blood flow; *steroids,* possibly, to minimize edema; *positioning,* with the head midline and at a 30 degree upward tilt; *seizure control,* usually with diphenylhydantoin, to minimize increases in cerebral metabolic rate; *muscle paralysis* as needed to avoid coughing and bucking and to ease ventilation; and *temperature control* to avoid fever. *Intracranial pressure* is monitored directly with an appropriate device. If initial measures are insufficient to control intracranial pressure, *barbiturates* in moderately high doses may be added; active *hypothermia* may also be used to minimize cerebral metabolism and blood flow.

Clearly, this multiplicity of therapeutic maneuvers, not all of which have been proven to be of value, is beyond the scope of initial emergency care. None is indicated until good cardiorespiratory function is assured. The awareness of possible therapies, however, will allow initiation of some of these maneuvers in the emergency room, as well as their continuation in the intensive care unit. Careful attention to positioning, ensurement of good oxygenation and modest hyperventilation, administration of steroids and osmotic agents, and fluid restriction, if appropriate, can all be begun as soon as the patient has stabilized. Investigation of the early use of barbiturates— a therapy not without risk of cardiovascular depression—is currently underway in a number of centers.

Successful resuscitation of a patient, followed by his or her ultimate return to family, friends, and a productive life, is one of the most rewarding experiences we may have. The extension of life support into the community, which can be accomplished by thorough training of nurses, paramedics, police and fire personnel, and the general public, is essential for such resuscitation to be effective. Early administration of basic life support to patients, followed by their entry into an efficient emergency medical service (EMS) system and subsequent receipt of advanced cardiac life support, can only be accomplished by community involvement, education, and support. It has been estimated that full implementation of potential lifesaving mechanisms in the community may save 100,000–200,000 lives each year in the United States; this will come only when each person living within a community has learned his or her own role in providing critically needed life support.

RESUSCITATION OF THE INFANT AND CHILD

Cardiopulmonary arrest is a rare occurrence in children. The heart of a young, healthy child without coronary disease or ischemia is able to withstand a great deal more insult than that of the adult. Respiratory disease, however, is both more common and more severe in the pediatric patient and frequently leads to critical airway compromise. The child's airway passages are small in diameter and easily obstructed by foreign bodies, secretions, and edema. The progression from such compromise to respiratory failure, hypoxemia, acidosis, and subsequent cardiac arrest can occur with frightening speed. Rapid attention to and alleviation of airway disease in children, then, is crucial to successful resuscitation; once the airway is restored and gas exchange normalized, cardiac stabilization is usually accomplished with ease.

The clinical history is of great importance in sorting out the etiology of a pediatric arrest; an accurate and complete review of the antecedent events will often suggest a specific diagnosis not apparent from the examination alone. The following are several circumstances to be suspected:

1. *Foreign bodies.* Toys, peanuts, balloons, and plastic covers may all cause suffocation.
2. *Infection of the airway.* As in croup and epiglottitis (see Chapter 43).
3. *Accidents and trauma.* Including multiple trauma, near drowning, and poisonings.
4. *Sudden infant death syndrome (SIDS).* Typically occurs in a child 3–4 months old, although there is risk during the child's entire first year.

If a specific problem is suspected, direct attention to it during CPR will often speed the success of the resuscitation.

As an arbitrary convention, the resuscitation literature has defined anyone younger than 1 year old as an infant, anyone 1–8 years old as a child, and anyone over 8 years old as an adult. Although adult techniques of resuscitation may indeed be applied to a typical 9 year old, medication dosages should continue to be based on a per kilogram basis until true adult size and weight are achieved.

Basic Life Support

Assessment of a patient's responsiveness is accomplished easily—vigorous stimulation (shake and shout) should produce awakening and a cry. If not, further therapy is needed and help should be summoned.

POSITIONING

The circumstances in which a child is found will often suggest whether trauma has occurred; if so, caution must be taken in positioning the child in order to avoid further damage, particularly if spinal injury is suspected. If the child is face down, he or she must be rolled over as a unit, carefully avoiding twisting of the spinal column.

AIRWAY

Correction of airway obstruction may be the only therapy required for some children. The diagnosis of obstruction is easily made if the child is still conscious and struggling: Great efforts at chest wall movement will be accompanied by retractions (suprasternal and intercostal), nasal flaring, and agitation, yet little or no air movement will be felt or heard at the mouth or nose. Stridor may or may not be present, depending on the degree of obstruction and vigor of respiratory efforts.

Relief of soft tissue airway obstruction can be accomplished by the same techniques as used in adults; the head-tilt, neck-lift or the head-tilt, chin-lift technique (Fig. 1.12) is recom-

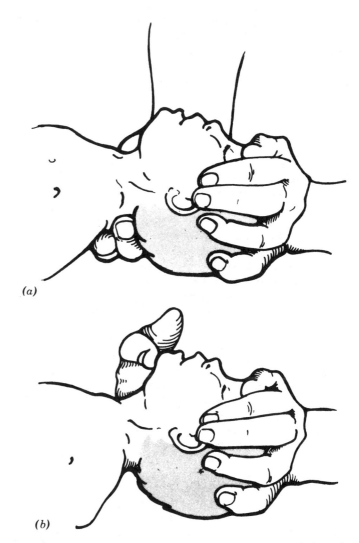

(a)

(b)

Figure 1.12 Airway control in the infant and child. (a) Head-tilt, neck-lift and (b) head-tilt, chin-lift methods are shown. Care must be taken to avoid extreme hyperextension and to avoid undue pressure on the trachea. (Used with permission from Standards and guidelines for cardiopulmonary resuscitation (CPR) and emergency cardiac care (ECC). *JAMA* 244:473, 1980.)

mended. In our experience, a straight anterior thrust of the jaw by forceful dislocation of the mandible at the angles of the jaw seems to work best (Fig. 1.13). The head should be slightly elevated (a folded towel under the occiput works nicely) and gently extended; extreme hyperextension, because of the child's collapsable trachea, will worsen, rather than improve, the situation.

Foreign material (toys, food, loose teeth) should be removed from the oropharynx under direct vision. If airway obstruction is felt to be secondary to an aspirated foreign body, the obstruction may be partial or complete. *Complete* airway obstruction owing to a foreign body may be relieved with back blows or chest thrusts. The infant should be placed face down on the rescuer's forearm, head lower than trunk, to allow gravity to assist in expulsion of the object (Fig. 1.14); the forearm may be rested on the rescuer's thigh for greater support. For the infant, four back blows are delivered in rapid succession between the infant's shoulder blades; the infant is then turned as a unit, face up, and four chest thrusts are delivered in a manner similar to that detailed later for external cardiac compression. If the object is dislodged into the upper airway, it can be carefully removed. The patency of the airway is again tested; if obstruction persists, these procedures are repeated. The technique for the child is similar; if the victim is too large to be comfortably held on the rescuer's forearm, the child may be draped across the thighs with the head lower than the trunk. The abdominal thrust is not recommended for infants and children because of the ease with which liver or spleen damage can occur.

If the foreign body is causing *partial* airway obstruction but the child is moving some gas with his or her own efforts, it is best *not* to attempt dislodgement of the foreign body (it may then totally occlude the airway) but rather to arrange for more sophisticated management such as bronchoscopy. Oxygen should be administered as soon as it is available since despite severe airway obstruction, hypoxemia can often be averted by inhalation of supplemental oxygen, even before the obstruction is fully relieved.

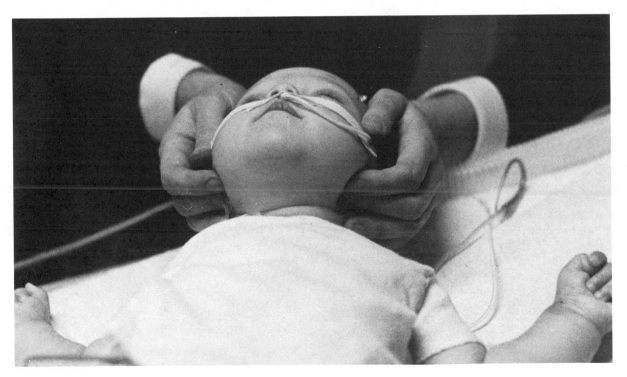

Figure 1.13 Straight anterior thrust of the jaw by forceful dislocation lifts the mandible and associated tissues away from the trachea, thus opening the airway. The rescuer should be able to feel a "click" as the jaw moves forward.

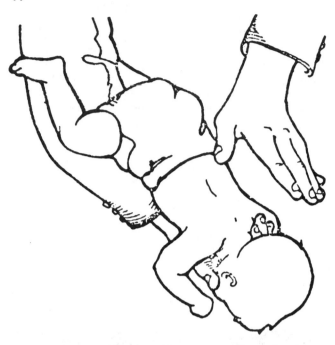

Figure 1.14 Back blows in the infant. The lowered head allows gravity to assist in expulsion of foreign material. (Used with permission from Standards and guidelines for cardiopulmonary resuscitation (CPR) and emergency cardiac care (ECC). *JAMA* 244:475, 1980.)

BREATHING

Successful relief of airway obstruction will be signified by the return of airflow through the nose and mouth of the victim who is still attempting to breathe. Should simple relief of airway obstruction not be adequate to restore gas exchange, rescue breathing must begin. The general technique used is that used in adult cardiopulmonary resuscitation. An airtight seal must be obtained using the rescuer's mouth; frequently the child's nose and mouth will be covered. Four "staircase" breaths are administered to reexpand the lungs and ensure airway adequacy. Breaths should be gentle; there should be adequate force and volume to see the chest rise. Excessive pressure and volume will cause gastric distension, thereby hindering lung expansion and making regurgitation more likely. If adequate chest expansion is not obtained, airway obstruction persists and the rescuer must repeat the procedures of opening the airway and attempting to ventilate once again. If the rescuer is still unable to ventilate the child, a foreign body must be suspected and attempts must be made to dislodge it as previously described.

Once chest expansion is attained, the pulse is checked (see below); if adequate circulation is present, the rescue breathing alone should be continued. The younger infant requires a faster ventilatory rate than the older child; typical rates are 30–40 breaths per minute for the newborn and infant, 20–30 breaths per minute for the young child, and 12–20 breaths per minute for the older child.

CIRCULATION

If the child's pulse is not palpable, circulatory support must be provided. As the child's carotid artery is difficult to palpate and the precordial impulse is not always reliable, the best arteries to examine are the brachial and the femoral arteries.

External chest compression is applied in a fashion analogous to that in adult cardiopulmonary resuscitation. As the heart may be higher in the chest in infancy, the proper area of compression in infants is the midsternum or slightly below; in older children, the site is further down toward the lower half of the sternum. The rescuer is positioned by the victim's side. Sternal compression may be provided by a few fingers, one hand, or two hands as required (Fig. 1.15a). Proper depth of compression varies from 0.5–1 in. in the infant to 1–1.5 in. in the older child; a pulse should be palpable if compression is adequate. The child must be placed on a firm surface for the technique to be successful. If two rescuers are available, a comfortable and effective technique for the newborn and small infant is for the rescuer who is performing chest compressions to surround the victim's chest with his or her hands, compressing the sternum with the thumbs while supporting the child's vertebral column from behind with the fingers (Fig. 1.15b).

The rate of compression will vary from approximately 120 compressions per minute in the newborn and small infant to 80 in the older child. The recommended ratio of compressions to ventilations is 5:1, even if one-person cardiopulmonary resuscitation is required. Should a second rescuer be available, compressions should be counted out loud by the rescuer performing them, and ventilations should be interspersed without interrupting the cadence.

Advanced Life Support for Children

AIRWAY AND VENTILATORY SUPPORT

The general technique of airway management in children is similar to that in adult cardiopulmonary resuscitation. *Hypoxemia* develops more rapidly in children when ventilation is interrupted because of their smaller functional residual capacity and hence decreased oxygen reserves; the provision of

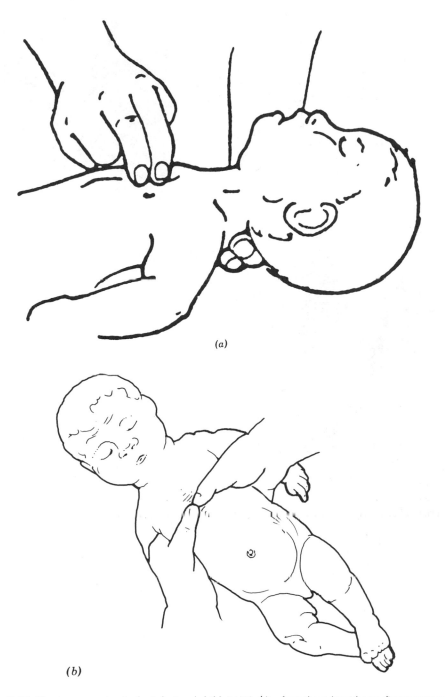

(a)

(b)

Figure 1.15 Chest compression in the infant and child. (a) Working from the side with two-finger compression. (Used with permission from Standards and guidelines for cardiopulmonary resuscitation (CPR) and emergency cardiac care (ECC). *JAMA* 244:473, 1980.) (b) An alternative position for chest compression when two rescuers are available; particularly useful in the hospital setting.

supplemental oxygen is crucial. *Airway adjuncts* and *masks* are used in a manner analagous to that in adult resuscitation. In children, oral airways are preferable to nasopharyngeal airways. The child's adenoid bed is highly vascular, and the risk of epistaxis and adenoid bleeding with a nasopharyngeal airway is great. The child's face is of such a contour that triangularly shaped masks, such as the Trimar or Rendell-Baker-Soucek (Fig. 1.16), are often more appropriate than the ovoid adult mask. In addition to providing a better fit, such masks have significantly less dead space, thus allowing a greater portion of each breath to participate in alveolar gas exchange.

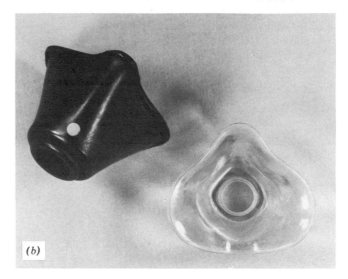

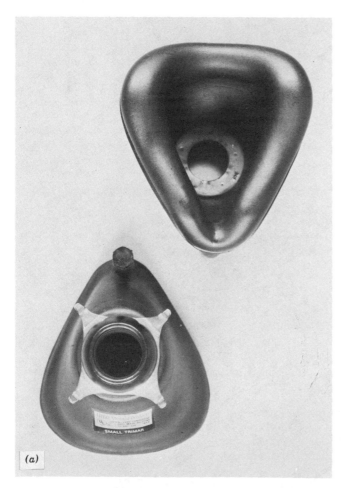

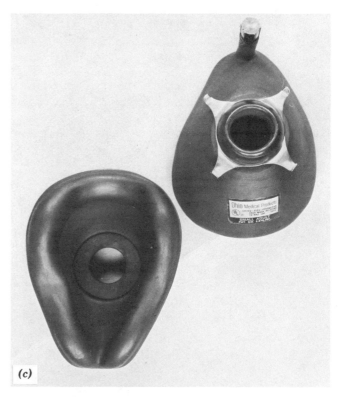

Figure 1.16 The (a) Trimar and (b) Rendell-Baker-Soucek masks are somewhat triangular and will fit a child's face well. The conventional mask (c) has a more oval shape. Final choice is made by the rescuer based on ability to obtain a good fit and personal comfort.

VENTILATING CIRCUITS

Ventilating circuits of both the self-refilling and nonself-refilling types are available with reservoir bags ranging in size from 500 ml to several liters. The choice of reservoir size will depend on the size of the patient and the rescuer's hand; smaller bags tend to give better control of ventilation and a better "feel" for the patient's compliance. Particular attention must be paid to the size of each breath and the pressure required to achieve good ventilation. Adequate chest expansion and air entry should be documented by auscultation of the chest; appropriate ventilation will achieve lung aeration without causing gastric distension. The lowest effective inflating pressures should be used. An *airway pressure manometer* may be inserted in the circuits to allow measurement of these pressures; most children can be effectively ventilated with peak pressures of 18–25 cm H_2O.

LARYNX

The larynx of the infant and child is positioned at a slightly higher level than that of the adult, corresponding to vertebral levels C-3–C-4 rather than C-5–C-6. The epiglottis is shorter and more U shaped as well, particularly in the neonate. Because of these characteristics, laryngeal exposure and endotracheal intubation are more easily accomplished using a straight laryngoscope blade (e.g., Miller) rather than a curved one. The straight blade is allowed to lift the epiglottis directly, allowing visualization of the vocal cords and insertion of an appropriately sized endotracheal tube (Procedure 4).

The narrowest point of the adult upper airway is the glottis; the narrowest point in a child (up to approximately 10 years of age) is the subglottic region. Thus a cuff is not required on the endotracheal tube in the infant to 10-year-old age bracket. Trauma to the subglottic region by an endotracheal tube that fits too snugly must be avoided since severe long-term consequences may result. The correctly sized tube is one that achieves a good seal but still allows a slight leakage of gas around it. Typical inside diameters (ID) of tubes are as follows: premature infant: 2.5 mm; term newborn: 3 mm; 6 month old: 3.5 mm; 1 year old: 4 mm; 18 months–2 years old: 4.5 mm (Table 1.8). A good rule of thumb for children 2 years or older is that the proper size may be found by adding 16 to the patient's age (in years) and then dividing that sum by 4. A more rapid but rough estimate of proper tube size is to choose one the same size as the child's little finger. Should the initially chosen tube be too large or too small, a tube either 0.5 mm smaller or larger will usually fit properly. Once intubation has been accomplished, careful positioning and secure taping are essential to ensure good ventilation of both lungs; the ideal

TABLE 1.8 Pediatric Resuscitation Endotracheal Tube Sizes

Age	Tube Size[a]	Laryngoscope Blade
Premature newborn	2.5 mm ID	Miller 0
Term newborn	3.0 mm ID	Miller 0 or 1
6 months	3.5 mm ID	Miller 1
1 year	4.0 mm ID	Miller 1, Wis-Hipple 1.5
18 months	4.5 mm ID	Miller 1, Wis-Hipple 1.5
2 years and above	$\dfrac{16 + \text{age (years)}}{4}$	Miller 1 or 2 Wis-Hipple 1.5 Macintosh 2 or 3

[a]Uncuffed tube < 10 years old or < 6 mm ID; cuffed tube > 10 years old or > 6 mm ID

positioning places the tip of the endotracheal tube 1.5–2 cm above the carina. If the tube is poorly placed, a shift in position of only 1 cm will frequently cause the tip of the tube either to pass the carina and lodge in a mainstream bronchus or to migrate proximally and leave the trachea.

VENOUS ACCESS

Obtaining and securing an intravenous line is often difficult in a small child. The techniques and landmarks for venous cannulation are identical in children and adults. The internal and external jugular veins and the femoral vein can usually be cannulated percutaneously, even in small infants; the subclavian vein, popular in adults, is somewhat more difficult to enter in children. To avoid interruption of cardiopulmonary resuscitation, sites remote from the neck and chest may be preferable. The brachiocephalic vein in either arm is often useable. The saphenous vein may be cannulated percutaneously or by surgical cutdown (Procedure 11) as it courses along the medial aspect of the ankle; the usual point of entry into the vein is 1 cm above and 1 cm anterior to the medial malleolus of the tibia. Access to the central circulation and the use of a larger-bore catheter may be obtained by entering the femoral vein, located just medial to the femoral artery; careful attention to asepsis, particularly in this area, is required in order to minimize complications.

The size of the catheter chosen will depend on vessel size and on resuscitation requirements. Most infants will have veins of sufficient diameter to allow at least a 22-gauge catheter to be used; the older infant and child will allow those of 20-, 18-, or 16-gauge catheters to be used without difficulty. In general, a catheter unit will be more secure than a butterfly-type device, although the latter is acceptable for initial therapy and stabilization. Delay in accomplishing access should be minimized; the rescuer should not hesitate to perform or request surgical cutdown if percutaneous attempts fail. If venous access is unavoidably delayed, epinephrine, lidocaine, or atropine are effective by the intratracheal route, as previously described for adult resuscitation.

A standard maintenance intravenous fluid for the pediatric patient should usually include some dextrose and salt, given at an hourly rate of 4 ml/kg for the first 10 kg of body weight, an additional 2 ml/kg for the next 10 kg, and 1 ml/kg more for each kilogram over 20. Maintenance sodium (Na^+) is usually 2–3 mEq/kg/day; maintenance potassium (K^+) is 1–2 mEq/kg/day. An example of such calculations is given below:

ity to vasoconstrict. A child can be drastically hypovolemic and still have a relatively normal blood pressure; when the volume loss finally exceeds the ability to compensate, however, the subsequent loss of blood pressure is catastrophic, and loss of cardiac output with subsequent cardiac arrest occurs within minutes.

It is inappropriate, then, to be reassured that a child is doing well and is not hypovolemic simply because the blood pressure is adequate. Volume replacement must be begun early, guided by clinical history, physical examination, degree of tachycardia, and response to volume challenge. Restoration of spontaneous circulation to the victim of cardiac arrest cannot occur until hypovolemia is corrected.

Patient's weight	36 kg	
Fluid administration	First 10 kg at 4 ml/kg/hr	= 40 ml/hr
	Second 10 kg at 2 ml/kg/hr	= 20 ml/hr
	Next 16 kg at 1 ml/kg/hr	= 16 ml/hr
	Proper rate	= 76 ml/hr or 1,824 ml/day
Electrolyte composition	Na^+ (2–3 mEq/kg/day)	= 72–108 mEq/day
	K^+ (1–2 mEq/kg/day)	= 36–72 mEq/day

The proper solution for this child is one that will give approximately 75–100 mEq of sodium in approximately 1,800 ml of fluid per day. Commonly available solutions include 5% dextrose in quarter-normal (0.225% NaCl, 38.5 mEq Na^+ per liter) or half-normal (0.45% NaCl, 77 mEq Na^+ per liter) saline. Potassium may be added as needed after assessment of renal function and measurement of serum electrolytes; it frequently is omitted during emergency resuscitation. For the child in our example, D_5 0.225% NaCl at 75 ml/hr, with 20 mEq potassium chloride added per liter, would be the usual choice. This maintenance solution and rate assumes normal hydration and renal function. Such a solution is *not* appropriate for rapid infusion as a correction for hypovolemia. Specific volume replacement should be given with a more isotonic solution (normal saline or Ringer's lactate) or colloid, as discussed below.

PHARMACOLOGIC AND CIRCULATORY SUPPORT

The child subjected to ongoing loss of circulatory blood volume, as in hemorrhagic shock, responds somewhat differently than the adult under similar circumstances. As losses continue, the adult will become tachycardic and gradually lose blood pressure over some time; the lowering of blood pressure can be used as an indicator of the need for volume replacement. The child will also become tachycardic; blood pressure, however, is much better preserved than in the adult, owing to the child's highly responsive sympathetic nervous system and abil-

Volume replacement in the child is usually given in aliquots of 10–20 ml/kg, using isotonic crystalloid or a colloid solution. Typically, we begin with a crystalloid such as Ringer's lactate; once replacement has exceeded 20–30 ml/kg, colloids are usually used. Five percent albumin or a similar purified plasma protein fraction may be used; if a coagulopathy must be corrected, fresh-frozen plasma or platelets may be administered. The "normal" hematocrit in newborns is in the range of 45–50% and by 3 months of age it may have dropped to 30%. As red blood cell production resumes it will rise to approximately 35% by 1 year of age and remain there until puberty, when it rises again to typical adult levels. If the patient's measured hematocrit is significantly low, red blood cells may be given, usually as packed red blood cells, as a portion of the volume replacement.

"Doses" of colloids and red blood cells, as with other volume-replacement solutions, are in boluses of 10 ml/kg; repeat infusions are given as needed, guided by clinical response and laboratory measurements. Careful attention must be given, especially in the small child, to ensure that excess volume administration is avoided; a useful technique is to administer all volume challenges with a syringe rather than by gravity drip.

DRUG THERAPY

Drug therapy in pediatric cardiopulmonary resuscitation is not greatly different than that in adult resuscitation. Typical dosages are given in the previous section on advanced cardiac

TABLE 1.9 Pediatric Emergency Drugs: Typical Dilutions for Infusion Pump Use

Standard Drips	Strength	Starting Dose
Dopamine	30 mg in 100 ml D_5W	Body weight in kg in ml/hr (5 μg/kg/min)
Epinephrine	1 mg in 100 ml D_5W	Body weight in kg in ml/hr (0.17 μg/kg/min)
Isoproterenol	1 mg in 100 ml D_5W	Body weight in kg in ml/hr (0.17 μg/kg/min)
Lidocaine	120 mg in 100 ml D_5W	Body weight in kg in ml/hr (20 μg/kg/min)
Norepinephrine	1 mg in 100 ml D_5W	Body weight in kg in ml/hr (0.17 μg/kg/min)

life support and the starting doses are given in Table 1.9. An estimation of body weight is usually adequate for purposes of initial resuscitation; general weight guidelines are offered in Table 1.10.

Particular attention should be paid to restoring normal body *temperature;* the cold infant will remain acidotic and poorly perfused. *Hypoglycemia* is common, with similar manifestations, and must be corrected. *Hypocalcemia* is frequently found in the neonate. Patients who have received large volumes of blood products over a short period of time will often exhibit transient severe hypocalcemia, caused by the chelation of circulating calcium ions by the citrate contained in the blood bank anticoagulant. A dramatic response to calcium administration is seen in this circumstance. If *drug ingestion* is suspected, naloxone should be given; if an organophosphate

TABLE 1.10 Pediatric Resuscitation: Average Weights for Age

Age	Weight (kg)	Weight (lb)
Term newborn	3–4	6–9
6 months	7–8	15–18
1 year	9–11	20–24
18 months	10–12	22–26
2 years	11–14	24–30
3 years	15	33
5 years	20	44
8 years	25	55
10 years	30	66
15 years	50	110

ingestion is likely, large doses of atropine (0.02 mg/kg, repeated several times) are appropriate.

Sodium bicarbonate, if needed, should be diluted 1:1 with D_5W or sterile water and administered slowly to a neonate or young infant. Rapid administration of concentrated bicarbonate solution causes dramatic osmolar and pH shifts and may be associated with intracranial hemorrhage in such young patients.

MONITORING

General monitoring planning and techniques are similar to those used in adult resuscitation. Auscultation to determine blood pressure is frequently difficult in children. The systolic blood pressure can be approximated by palpation of the pulse distal to the occluding cuff. A more accurate technique is the use of a Doppler flow probe to indicate return of arterial flow; simple, inexpensive devices are available for this purpose and are no more difficult to use than a stethoscope. Use of the proper-sized cuff is essential; a cuff size of approximately two-thirds the length of the child's upper arm is appropriate.

Temperature measurement is by rectal thermometer. If mild to moderate hypothermia is present, warming of the room, blankets, radiant heating, and warming of intravenous fluids may help in its correction; more severe hypothermia requires core rewarming, as discussed later in this chapter.

Laboratory measurements are as in adult resuscitation, and special attention should be paid to serum glucose and calcium levels. Arterial blood samples for gas analysis and pH determination are equally important and should be repeated every 5–10 minutes throughout the resuscitation; persistent metabolic acidosis usually suggests hypoperfusion and will often respond to volume infusion. Urine output is carefully followed by insertion of an indwelling urinary catheter; if a conventional Foley catheter of small enough size is unavailable, an infant feeding tube makes a good substitute.

CONTINUING THERAPY

Once stabilization of the child has been attained, arrangements should be made for his or her transfer to an intensive care unit guided by a pediatrician or, if possible, to a pediatric medical center. Many tertiary-level pediatric hospitals are able to provide a transport service; an experienced pediatric nurse and physician are sent by ambulance or, if necessary, by air to the community hospital and accompany the child on the trip to the pediatric center, providing ongoing care en route. Experience has shown that such provision of intensive care in transport has resulted in a better long-range outcome for the children involved.

Immediate postresuscitation support, as in adults, should concentrate on maximizing cardiorespiratory performance, correcting underlying disease states, and preventing further damage to organ systems. Dopamine seems to have gained greatest popularity for its support of renal blood flow and modest inotropy and vasotonic effect. If more vigorous support is required to maintain adequate systemic blood pressure, epinephrine may be used; these children usually have a poor prognosis. Isoproterenol is useful for its bronchodilation and positive chronotropy. Cardiac output is relatively more dependent on heart rate in the child, and coronary disease is usually absent; deliberate attempts to attain a tachycardia are useful in supporting cardiac output and do not usually carry the same risk of myocardial oxygen supply–demand imbalance as is present in the adult.

As discussed earlier, primary cardiac arrest or dysrhythmia is not common in the child. An underlying disease process, frequently of the respiratory system, is usually present. Attention to its accurate diagnosis and swift correction are essential in the postresuscitative period to avoid recurrence of cardiopulmonary collapse. Proper application of measures such as continuous positive airway pressure and mechanical ventilation should be begun during acute resuscitation and continued in later support.

Organ system support and prevention of further damage are begun as early as possible. Renal failure can often be averted or ameliorated by judicious volume administration and the use of dopamine and, if necessary, diuretics. Prevention of cerebral swelling and intracranial hypertension, as previously outlined, may avert secondary central nervous system damage and allow a good outcome.

The decision to terminate unsuccessful resuscitative efforts is particularly difficult in the child, from both medical and emotional viewpoints. Cardiovascular unresponsiveness despite prolonged efforts is the most certain basis for this decision, and—particularly in a child—implies massive prior cardiovascular insult. Assessment of cerebral damage and function is based on the same principles as in adults. Clearcut absence of cerebral circulation for prolonged periods of time at normal temperature and a physical examination demonstrating deep unconsciousness, lack of spontaneous respirations, lack of all brainstem reflexes, and fixed and dilated pupils for more than 30 minutes despite adequate cardiovascular and respiratory support are ominous signs and will support a decision to cease resuscitation. Unfortunately, even such conditions are not foolproof indicators of cerebral death. If there is any doubt, it is best to complete cardiorespiratory resuscitation and, if stability is attained, to assess neurologic function more carefully over the succeeding 24 hours with repeated examinations and indicated laboratory testing to support an appropriate decision.

Whether or not the resuscitation is successful, support of the family must be provided throughout the resuscitation period and into the subsequent hours, days, and months. Parents will often feel great guilt over the illness or loss of their child. "If only we had brought him to the doctor sooner, he would have been all right" is a universal thought and fear of every parent whose child is seriously ill. The family unit and its individual members must be sustained throughout the patient's illness; if this is not accomplished, resuscitation of the pediatric patient has been, in a real way, incomplete.

CLINICAL SETTINGS

Ventricular Fibrillation

Multiple studies have documented that in the majority of cases of sudden death, the initial rhythm disturbance discovered is ventricular fibrillation. One representative sample shows that from a total of 426 out-of-hospital arrests, 72% of patients were in ventricular fibrillation and the remainder were evenly divided amongst asystole, idioventricular rhythm, and other bradycardic states (Liberthson et al). Although there has been recent suggestion that the bradycardic–asystolic events are more likely to occur when evidence of acute ischemia or infarction is lacking, it appears certain that from 65 to 95% of cases of sudden death occur secondary to ventricular fibrillation.

Elucidation of the factors predisposing to sudden death has been somewhat difficult. Although there is no question that more than 90% of cases have severe obstructive coronary artery disease noted by catheterization or autopsy, it is less clear as to the role of acute myocardial infarction. It has recently been reported that 44% of infants had suffered an acute infarction as diagnosed by new Q-wave development on the ECG coupled with serum enzymatic determinations; 34% were felt to have had an ischemic event on the basis of enzymatic abnormalities coupled with abnormalities of the ST-T wave segments; and 22% were felt to have had a primary arrhythmic event. These percentages are remarkably similar to those in the sample mentioned above, in which results relied on ECG changes exclusively. In another study it was similarly noted that in only approximately one-third of the cases could a certain diagnosis of infarction be made (Cobb et al). A disturbing feature of this report was the fact that the patients who had suffered a definite transmural infarct had an improved long-term prognosis compared to those who had not. The difficulty in confirming an acute infarction obviously results from the trauma of resuscitation and defibrillation and the lack of pathologic markers for infarction less than 6–12 hours old.

The risk factors predisposing to sudden death are the same as those for coronary artery disease in general, for example, cigarette smoking, hypertension, and hypercholesterolemia. Although 33 to 66% of sudden death victims have had a known history of antecedent cardiovascular disease, only 25% had prodromal symptoms lasting more than 30 minutes. Another 25% had symptoms lasting only minutes, and fully 50% of the cases collapsed without any prodromal symptom at all. It has been noted that despite the high incidence of prior cardiac disease in this study population, sudden cardiac death was the initial manifestation of disease in 33% of the cases.

Although coronary artery disease is the major disease state predisposing to sudden death, other conditions can occur, for example, mitral valve prolapse, myocarditis, and cardiomyopathies, especially idiopathic hypertrophic subaortic stenosis (IHSS).

DIAGNOSIS

The diagnosis of ventricular fibrillation depends on the ECG demonstration of a chaotic ventricular rhythm lacking any evidence of organized depolarization (Fig. 1.17). Depending on the amplitude of these waveforms, the terms *coarse VF,* generally signifying more recent onset, and *fine VF* have been used. The latter may frequently require drug therapy before defibrillation is successful.

MANAGEMENT

As discussed in the section on defibrillation, electrical countershock is the definitive therapy for ventricular fibrillation and should be carried out as soon as a defibrillator is available. Although cases of successful pharmacologic defibrillation by means of bretylium have been reported, countershock remains the mainstay of therapy. When electrical defibrillation has been unsuccessful, drug therapy may be helpful. Epinephrine may be useful especially to "coarsen" fine VF. Other potentially useful drugs are sodium bicarbonate, if clinically indicated, and antiarrhythmics such as lidocaine, bretylium, or procainamide. After each pharmacologic intervention, repeat countershock is performed and CPR is continued.

PROGNOSIS

Those patients who survive out-of-hospital cardiac arrest remain at continued high risk. Both the Seattle heart watch and the Detroit experience indicate 1- and 2-year mortalities of approximately 16% and 33%, respectively. It has been documented that the majority of the subsequent mortality was due to recurrent ventricular fibrillation. Although attempts at reducing the high risk to survivors of out-of-hospital ventricular fibrillation by medications and/or coronary revascularization surgery have been carried out, the results thus far have been inconclusive. Despite an occasional optimistic report, most of the series has been hampered by either study design or the small number of patients treated. Currently, attempts are being made to further stratify this group into high- and lower-risk subpopulations by measurement of left ventricular function and possibly by electrophysiologic testing. It is hoped that such investigations will improve the long-term prognosis of these patients.

Asystole and Severe Bradyarrhythmias

Asystole, the total absence of electromechanical cardiac activity, and several profound bradyarrhythmias (Fig. 1.18), for example, slow junctional rhythm, idioventricular or agonal rhythm, and third-degree heart block with inadequate ventricular escape rate, may be lumped together in discussing their impact on sudden death. Although the ventricular tachyarrhythmias are unquestionably the most common initial rhythm disturbance, the incidence of bradycardic–asystolic arrest is not insignificant, representing approximately 30% of present-

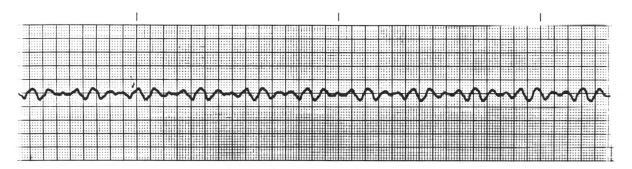

Figure 1.17 Ventricular fibrillation.

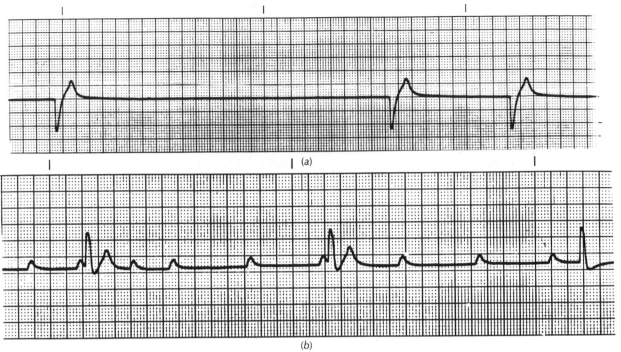

Figure 1.18 Bradyarrythmias. (a) Slow, idioventricular rhythm; usually associated with no effective cardiac output and carries a poor prognosis. (b) Complete heart block with slow ventricular escape rate.

ing rhythm disturbances in several large series. The impact of such statistics is accentuated by the dismal results in achieving successful resuscitation.

It has long been felt that asystole usually represents the end point of a long-standing derangement. Although profound metabolic abnormality, especially hypoxemia, can undoubtedly predispose to these rhythm disturbances, long-standing severe coronary artery disease still remains the most usual common denominator. In the examination of survivors of sudden death, it was noted that the patients felt to have had a primary arrhythmic event, that is, without evidence of either acute myocardial ischemia or infarction, were older and had three times the incidence of history of prior myocardial infarction. The incidence of complete heart block or asystole in that subgroup was 35% in contrast to 4–5% for those patients with evidence of acute ischemia or infarction. Another study reported on a small group of patients who expired by sudden death while wearing ambulatory monitoring equipment (Clark et al). Instead of the expected high-grade ventricular tachyarrhythmias, these patients were found to have gradually developed brady-

cardia without known prodrome, culminating in asystole or agonal rhythm. All eight patients had severe coronary artery disease, and the implication was made that profound bradycardic–asystolic rhythms may represent severe diffuse myocardial ischemia.

Another predisposing factor for this form of cardiac arrest may be excessive vagal tone. Asystole secondary to generalized parasympathetic discharge is not an uncommon occurrence with induction of anesthesia or during surgical procedures. Similar situations may occur with stimulation of various organs such as bladder, anus, esophagus, or carotid sheath.

DIAGNOSIS

Ventricular asystole is documented by total absence of ventricular electrical activity. A variant of this is profoundly slow idioventricular rhythm with an occasional ventricular escape beat seen (Fig. 1.18). Third-degree heart block without functioning ventricular escape pacemaker activity will be seen as just a series of P waves.

MANAGEMENT

Since it is well documented that high levels of vagal tone may result in cessation of both ventricular and supraventricular pacemaker activity, it is advisable to administer 1–2 mg of atropine intravenously soon after initiating resuscitation of the patient documented to have asystole, heart block, or slow idioventricular rhythm. Epinephrine is a crucial drug for the resuscitation of patients with asystole or profound slow ventricular escape rhythms; sodium bicarbonate and calcium chloride may also be required. Rarely has countershock or ventricular pacing been successful, and these should probably be used only as a final effort. The treatment of heart block relies on increasing the heart rate to a suitable level by means of atropine, followed, if necessary, by isoproterenol and temporary pacemaker insertion.

PROGNOSIS

Despite equal response from the emergency medical system, the initial resuscitative success and subsequent clinical course of patients suffering from bradycardic–asystolic arrest is drastically worse than that experienced by patients with ventricular tachycardia or fibrillation. In a group of 352 patients who suffered out-of-hospital arrests, 31% were found to be in bradycardic–asystolic arrest: 9 of these 108 patients were initially resuscitated and admitted to the hospital alive. None survived to be discharged (Myerberg).

Electromechanical Dissociation

Electromechanical dissociation (EMD) represents organized electrical activity as documented by the ECG (Fig. 1.19), coupled with the absence of pulse or other evidence of effective myocardial contraction. Certain catastrophic events, such as massive pulmonary embolism, can produce this condition; however, it more commonly represents profound myocardial ischemia or rupture of the myocardial free wall postinfarction. Since Ca^{2+} transport is an essential aspect of electromechanical coupling, administration of Ca^{2+} may be helpful. However, the prognosis is often grave and resuscitation unsuccessful.

It is imperative to realize that severe cardiac tamponade may exactly mimic the findings of electromechanical dissociation. The potentially life-saving technique of diagnostic and therapeutic emergency pericardiocentesis can only be successful if the index of suspicion for this condition is high.

Electrical Shock

Victims of electrical current accidents and those struck by lightning account for 1,000–1,500 deaths annually in the United States. Although utility linemen and construction workers constitute a major proportion of the total number of electrocution fatalities, approximately one-third of such fatalaties result from occurrences in the home or in mundane work settings. Victims of electrical current accidents frequently suffer severe thermal injuries, and, in addition, may sustain traumatic injuries from resulting falls. Alternating current can produce tetanic muscular contractions preventing the victim from releasing contact with the current. Since this is a generalized effect, tetany of thoracic respiratory musculature may lead to anoxic arrest. Furthermore, a massive convulsive phenomenon may occur, resulting in prolonged respiratory paralysis even after current contact has been terminated. Victims of low-voltage exposure frequently develop ventricular fibrillation. Victims of massive current exposure or persons struck by lightning commonly suffer asystolic arrest.

Clearly, the immediate intervention must be the removal of the victim from contact with the current source *without* touching the victim directly. Because of the diversity of potential injuries that may be associated with electrical shock, initial assessment must include the aspects of thermal and traumatic injury evaluation detailed in subsequent chapters. However, the primary consideration remains the emergent detection and prompt management of cardiopulmonary insufficiency or failure. When indicated, BLS resuscitation, as previously described, should be implemented immediately. Expeditious transport of the patient to an appropriate burn or trauma facility is imperative.

A variety of factors, including the pathway of current through the body, grounding, and the amplitude and duration of contact to the current source, influence the extent and severity—and consequently the prognosis—of primary electrical injury.

Trauma

A major concern in trauma patients should be avoidance of further injury. Cervical spine instability should be suspected, particularly if there is evidence of cranial or facial injury. If BLS resuscitation is necessary in these circumstances, the modified mandible-thrust method should be used to establish upper airway patency. Care also should be taken to maintain head–neck–chest alignment during CPR. Rapid transport of victims to emergency medical facilities is of paramount importance.

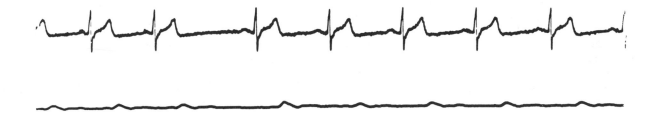

Figure 1.19 Electromechanical dissociation. The presence of electrical activity, even if reasonably normal in appearance, does not necessarily imply adequate mechanical performance. Despite electrical complexes, the arterial pressure wave (lower trace) reveals no effective perfusion.

Drowning and Near Drowning

It has been estimated that there are approximately 7,000 drowning fatalities and 50,000 near-drowning victims annually in the United States; roughly one-third of the fatalities are children. A variety of circumstances may surround the submersion. Submersion may occur in fresh or salt water and during warm or cold weather. Younger children may drown when left unattended in the bathtub or wading pool; they may wander away from parents who are engaged in other activities and may later be found submerged in an unprotected pond or pool. Older children and adults are more commonly drowned by an accident occurring while they are swimming or engaged in other water sports.

Initial resuscitation at the scene of the accident is crucial; it is imperative that the victim be reached in the water quickly and that artificial ventilation be begun immediately, even before the victim can be removed from the water. In cases of suspected neck injury, the victim's neck must be maintained in a neutral position during all motion; the head, neck, and torso must be aligned and moved as a unit; airway patency must be obtained by jaw thrust or chin lift without head tilt. Once the patient can be placed on a firm surface, full BLS is begun and continued during transport to the emergency room; the rapidity and efficacy of BLS are key factors in the patient's ultimate prognosis.

ASSESSMENT

An accurate history must be sought in the initial management of the near-drowning victim. Although firm prognostic significance cannot easily be attached to each individual criteria, some estimate of the patient's prognosis may be possible if all factors are known. Specific information to be ascertained includes the following:

1. *Circumstances causing submersion.* Was there trauma or drug ingestion involved? Was the patient able to swim? Did anyone see the actual submersion event?
2. *Length of submersion.* This should be estimated as closely as possible.
3. *Temperature of the water.* Cold water, with resultant hypothermia, will have a protective effect and will affect prognosis.
4. *Need for resuscitation at the site.*
5. *Provision of effective CPR.* How quickly was it begun? Was good BLS continued, if needed, until the patient's arrival at the emergency facility?
6. *Duration of resuscitation required* to achieve spontaneous heart rate and respirations.
7. The *need for resuscitation on arrival* at the emergency room. In general, patients still requiring CPR on arrival at the hospital have a poorer prognosis than those who do not.

The near-drowning patient is best viewed as one who has suffered a particular form of hypoxic–ischemic injury in which there is multisystem involvement. During resuscitation, steps must be taken to address each of these systems individually and to initiate appropriate forms of therapy. Since cerebral damage can frequently result from prolonged submersion, assessment of the patient's neurologic function should be performed as early as possible to serve as a baseline for future reference. Those patients who arrive in the emergency room awake or with minimally blunted consciousness, even if having required initial resuscitation, will generally do well without intensive neurologic care; those who arrive in a coma will require special cerebral resuscitative measures.

A rapid assessment of neurologic function should include several observations. Evaluation of brainstem reflexes (pupillary size and reaction, oculocephalic response, presence of cough and/or gag), and investigation for lateralizing signs, which might suggest trauma and intracranial bleeding, are essential. The comatose patient may be assessed for eye-opening, verbal, and motor responses, as scored against the Glasgow Coma Scale (Table 1.11); patients with lower scores require more intensive intervention for cerebral protection.

The patient's temperature must be measured with a thermometer capable of low readings. If severe hypothermia is present, special techniques for rewarming, discussed later in this chapter, may be required.

MANAGEMENT

Cardiovascular System

Advanced cardiac life support will proceed as usual. Volume status should be assessed and adequate intravascular volume ensured without overhydration. Dysrhythmias may be prominent if hypothermia is present; most patients with dysrhythmias will respond to warming and conventional measures. Restoration of adequate mean arterial pressure to ensure cerebral perfusion is crucial. Anoxic–ischemic injury to the heart is not uncommon, and pressor support is often required.

Respiratory System

Aspiration of water and foreign material may have occurred, although the presence of large amounts of water in the lungs is unusual. Fresh water—a hypotonic fluid—is rapidly absorbed into the circulation, whereas salt water—a hypertonic solution—tends to bring fluid from the circulation into the lungs.

TABLE 1.11 Glasgow Coma Scale[a]

Eyes	Open	Spontaneously	4
		To verbal command	3
		To pain	2
	No response		1
Best motor response	To verbal command	Obeys	6
	To painful stimulus	Localizes pain	5
		Flexion—withdrawal	4
		Flexion—abnormal (decorticate rigidity)	3
		Extension (decerebrate rigidity)	2
		No response	1
Best verbal response		Oriented and converses	5
		Disoriented and converses	4
		Inappropriate words	3
		Incomprehensible sounds	2
		No response	1
Total			3–15

[a]The Glasgow Coma Scale, based upon eye-opening, verbal, and motor responses, is a practical means of monitoring changes in level of consciousness. If response on the scale is given a number, the responsiveness of the patient can be expressed by summation of the figures. *Lowest score is 3; highest is 15.*

Surfactant washout is thought to be more severe with fresh water than with salt water. Both forms of aspiration will predispose to atelectasis, alveolar collapse, and potential pneumonitis, and initial management should include ventilation with an adequate FiO$_2$, using PEEP of 4–6 cm H$_2$O to prevent alveolar collapse. Consideration should be given to antibiotic coverage if aspiration is documented, particularly if contaminated water was involved.

Gastrointestinal and Renal Systems

The gastrointestinal tract, the liver, and the kidneys may have suffered anoxic–ischemic damage. Mucosal sloughing and stress ulceration are not uncommon; a nasogastric tube should be passed and antacids administered. Monitoring of urine output through an indwelling catheter is appropriate as acute tubular necrosis is not uncommon. Electrolyte abnormalities may be present and require correction, although electrolyte changes secondary to aspiration require inhalation of a large volume of water and are actually quite rare.

Hematologic System

Hemolysis may be present after massive fresh water aspiration but there is seldom need for treatment of this in the emergency setting. If a coagulopathy is present, appropriate diagnostic studies should be requested and treatment given as needed.

Central Nervous System

Brain-oriented resuscitation is carried out in the fashion previously outlined. Initial cardiopulmonary stability must be obtained to ensure restoration of oxygenation and perfusion to the brain; more sophisticated measures of cerebral protection are not indicated until these are ensured. An attempt should be made to use the minimal amount of fluids required to resuscitate the patient since dehydration will be part of later management. Mannitol, an osmotic diuretic, may be administered in a dose of 0.5–1 g/kg in order to speed excretion of excess free water. Modest hyperventilation, with PaCO$_2$ in the 30–34 torr range, can be maintained throughout resuscitation and transport to an intensive care facility. Steroids, such as dexamethasone in doses of 1 mg/kg, are used by some to reduce cerebral edema. With such initial management, brain preservation is maximized and secondary damage from intracranial hypertension is made less likely.

PROGNOSIS

Cessation of unsuccessful resuscitation efforts is a difficult decision. Presence of relatively good prognostic signs (hypothermia, early provision of CPR, young age) favor more prolonged attempts. Rewarming of the profoundly hypothermic patient must be accomplished before resuscitation can truly be termed unsuccessful. Although overall mortality and morbidity figures remain poor for those near-drowning patients arriving in coma, more investigation into provision of good cardiopulmonary–cerebral resuscitation may improve our results with this unfortunate group of patients.

Hypothermia

Victims of cardiopulmonary arrest may also be victims of hypothermia, and it is not infrequent that severe lowering of body temperature has been the precipitating event for the cardiovascular collapse.

A complete discussion of the physiology of hypothermia and the considerations related to restoration of normothermia is beyond the scope of this chapter. There are excellent reviews of the subject available; see the selected references at the end of this chapter.

Accidental hypothermia ensues when a person loses heat to the environment in excess of his or her ability to produce it. It may be seen to result from cold water immersion, from prolonged exposure to the elements, or—particularly in the elderly and infirm—from living in homes that are underheated because of rising fuel costs. In general, a rectal temperature of less than 35°C (95°F) is indicative of "clinical hypothermia"; a temperature of less than 33°C (91.4°F) is "severe hypothermia." Hypothermia may further be subdivided by duration of cold exposure into acute (6 hours or less), subacute (6–24 hours), and chronic (greater than 24 hours) hypothermia. For our current purpose, we will consider resuscitation from acute, severe hypothermia of victims with no medical predisposition for its development.

The effects of severe hypothermia on various organ systems follow some general patterns. As body temperature drops, the *basic metabolic rate* (BMR) progressively increases to produce more heat; *shivering*, a key mechanism for heat production, is maximal at 35°C (95°F) but gradually decreases as the patient cools and the ability to sustain heat production is lost. Most shivering ceases at 31–32°C (87.8–89.6°F), and muscular rigidity and loss of voluntary motion set in below 30°C (86°F). Normal *consciousness and mentation* are present to 34°C

(93.2°F), although fatigue will begin to set in somewhat before then. Between 32 and 34°C (89.6–93.2°F) consciousness begins to cloud, and by 26–27°C (78.8–80.6°F) patients are unconscious, pupils are unreactive and deep tendon reflexes are absent; the EEG becomes isoelectric at 17°C (62.6°F). *Respiratory efforts,* initially stimulated, begin to slow as body temperature drops, and usually cease between 28 and 30°C (82.4–86°F); bronchorrhea and pulmonary edema may develop. *Extracellular fluid* begins to accumulate, and a cold-induced diuresis occurs as the temperature drops; the severely hypothermic patient is often *intravascularly volume depleted* despite the presence of tissue edema. Most significant from the viewpoint of ACLS are the effects of cold on the *cardiovascular* system. Although heart rate is initially increased with the increased metabolic rate, as cooling progresses from 34°C through the 28–30°C range (93.2° through 82.4–86°F), progressive bradycardia ensues. There is a great risk of *ventricular fibrillation* in the 28–32°C (82.4–89.6°F) range, particularly if the heart is irritated in any way; lower temperatures give rise to spontaneous ventricular fibrillation and, ultimately, asystole. There is a characteristic ECG finding in hypothermic patients who maintain a spontaneous rhythm—a "J" or "Osborn" wave, a rounded positive deflection occurring immediately after the QRS complex, sometimes mistaken for a T wave (Fig. 1.20).

ASSESSMENT

Patients with severe hypothermia may well appear irreversibly dead—they are often cold and stiff and have no palpable pulse, audible heart sounds, or discernable respiratory efforts. Their pupils may be fixed and dilated, and they may be in a deep coma. Electrocardiographic activity may be bizarre, and asystole or ventricular fibrillation are not uncommonly found. Many instances of successful resuscitation of such patients have been recorded in the literature, however. The maxim, "Do not assume the patient is dead until he or she is warm and dead," has become a commonly quoted rule of thumb in dealing with victims of severe hypothermia.

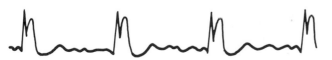

Figure 1.20 The "J" or "Osborn" wave seen in patients with hypothermia.

MANAGEMENT

As initial resuscitation of the victim begins, the emergency room physician must quickly establish the diagnosis and possible etiology of the hypothermia. A brief review of the history, especially regarding duration of exposure, mechanism of injury, and resuscitation efforts before the patient arrived in the emergency room, may be helpful in judging the patient's prognosis and response. The diagnosis is established by measurement of the rectal temperature; since this may be well below the usual range, a special low-reading thermometer should be available. Continuous monitoring of temperature throughout the resuscitation period will then be required. The ECG, once obtained, will likely demonstrate either bradycardia with an unusual pattern or ventricular fibrillation or asystole.

If an organized rhythm is present, the physician must assess whether sufficient spontaneous cardiac output is present; if not, continued circulatory support must be given, volume status optimized, and rewarming begun. The risk of precipitation of sudden ventricular fibrillation is great, especially as therapy continues and the patient is warmed through the 28–32°C (82.4–89.6°F) range of maximum ventricular irritability. Careful handling of the patient is essential; sudden changes in body position or jarring the patient or bed may induce fibrillation. If attempts at placement of a central line (CVP) are made, great care must be taken not to enter the heart; catheter stimulation, again, may provoke ventricular fibrillation.

If ventricular fibrillation or asystole is present, vigorous rewarming must be begun at once. The hypothermic heart is unresponsive to countershock and is poorly responsive to conventional drug therapy. Such efforts are not indicated until the patient can be rewarmed.

A variety of techniques for rewarming have been described, and debate continues over advantages and disadvantages of each. The methods may be divided into *active* (provision of heat) and *passive* (prevention of losses); active methods may further be divided into *surface,* or *external,* rewarming and *core,* or *internal,* rewarming. Although gentle, passive rewarming techniques are probably appropriate for patients with milder or more chronic hypothermia, these techniques will have little use for patients with severe hypothermia and cardiopulmonary arrest. Our discussion, then, will deal only with active provision of heat.

Surface rewarming has been accomplished by immersion in hot water, heated thermal blankets, plumbed garments, and simple heating pads or hot water bottles. There is some risk to the technique. Warming of the extremities will produce peripheral vasodilation; this will cause increased return of cold blood from the periphery to the heart, resulting in a further drop in core temperature—a phenomenon known as *afterdrop*. In addition, the rapid vasodilation of peripheral vessels in the presence of reduced intravascular volume may lower perfusion pressure. These difficulties can be overcome by application of heat directly to the thorax and abdomen alone, allowing the extremities to remain cold until core temperature has begun to rise.

More invasive methods of core rewarming have been successfully used. Intragastric and intracolonic provision of heat, either by fluid-filled balloon catheters with closed-loop circulation of a warm fluid or by warm enemas and gastric lavage, are useful for core rewarming. *Inhalation therapy*, with provision of maximal warming (to 43–44°C, approximately 110°F) and humidity of inspired gas, will both prevent respiratory heat loss and provide heat gain. *Diathermy* offers the ability to heat tissues below the subcutaneous fat layer; the risk of burns and the need for personnel experienced in its application are limiting factors.

Peritoneal lavage with warm solutions is effective in core rewarming and requires a minimum of equipment usually available at community hospitals; the risk is somewhat greater than that of other techniques but, in experienced hands, is still low. *Extracorporeal blood rewarming* is the most efficient and direct technique for restoration of heat to the core; it can be accomplished in most cases using a simple femoral vein–femoral artery circuit and a standard cardiopulmonary bypass unit. It is the therapy of choice in centers equipped for and experienced in its use.

In summary, the following techniques for accomplishing rapid rewarming have been described; each should be considered and used if thought reasonable:

1. *Warming room* and providing reasonable humidity
2. *Warming intravenous fluids*
3. *Surface warming of trunk only* with radiant heat or heating blanket (set to as high a temperature as possible without burning the patient (40–43°C, 104–110°F)
4. *Heated humidification* of inspired gases (to 43–44°C, approximately 108–110°F; this is considerably higher than usual settings and must be closely monitored)
5. *Gastric and colonic warming,* either by lavage or by fluid-filled balloon catheters
6. *Diathermy,* if equipment and skilled personnel are available
7. *Peritoneal lavage*
8. *Extracorporeal warming* with appropriate circuits and heat exchangers

Often the restoration of heat to the body core will result in spontaneous reversion to a sinus rhythm as the heart rewarms; if not, conventional drug and countershock therapy may be used. Acid–base balance may require particular attention; acidosis is likely to be present and some bicarbonate may be required but caution is needed to avoid overmedication. Fluid shifts will make volume management more difficult, and measurement of central venous pressure will likely be necessary.

PROGNOSIS

Successful resuscitation, because of the protective effects of hypothermia on the brain and other tissues, is frequently followed by complete recovery. Efforts should thus be continued until the patient is warmed or capabilities for warming and resuscitation are exhausted without success. The resuscitation of the hypothermia victim is often a great strain on the resources and personnel of the entire hospital; the reward is often the return of the victim to a useful and productive life.

SUGGESTED READINGS

Ahlquist RP: A study of adrenotropic receptors. *Am J Physiol* 1948; 153:586.

American Heart Association: Standards and guidelines for cardiopulmonary resuscitation (CPR) and emergency cardiac care (ECC). *J Am Med Assoc* 1980; 244:453.

Amsterdam EA, Mansour EJ, Hughes LL, et al: Present status of glucagon and bretylium tosylate, in Russek HI, Zohman B (eds): *Changing Concepts in Cardiovascular Disease.* Baltimore, The Williams & Wilkins Co, 1972, Chap 20, pp 215–235.

Antman EM, Stone PH, Muller JE, et al: Calcium channel blocking agents in the treatment of cardiovascular disorders. Part I: Basic and clinical electrophysiologic effects. *Ann Intern Med* 1980; 93:875–885.

Antonaccio MJ (ed): *Cardiovascular Pharmoacology.* New York, Raven Press, 1977.

Bacaner MD: Bretylium tosylate for suppression of induced ventricular fibrillation after experimental myocardial infarction. *Nature* 1968; 220:494.

Bacaner MD, Schrienemachers D: Bretylium tosylate for the suppression of ventricular fibrillation after experimental myocardial infarction. *Nature* 1968; 220:494.

Bangs CC, Hamlet MP, Mills WJ: Help for the victim of hypothermia. *Patient Care,* December 15, 1977, 46–68.

Bishop RL, Weisfeldt ML: Sodium bicarbonate administration during cardiac arrest. *J Am Med Assoc* 1976; 235:506–509.

Black PM: Brain death. *N Engl J Med* 1978; 299:338–344, 393–401.

Black PM: Guidelines for the diagnosis of brain death, in Ropper AK, Kennedy SK, Zervas NT (ed): *Neurological–Neurosurgical Intensive Care*. Baltimore, University Park Press, 1983.

Braunwald E: Control of myocardial oxygen consumption. Physiologic and clinical considerations. *Am J Cardiol* 1971; 27:416–432.

Brown DC, Lewis AJ, Criley JM: Asystole and its treatment: The possible role of the parasympathetic nervous system in cardiac arrest. *JACEP* 1979; 8:448–452.

Campbell NPS, Webb SW, Adgey AAJ, et al: Transthoracic ventricular defibrillation in adults. *Br Med J* 1977; 2:1379.

Carden E, Friedman D: Further studies of manually operated self-inflating resuscitation bags. *Anesth Analg* 1977; 56:202–206.

Cascho JA, Crampton RS, Cherwek ML, et al: Determinants of ventricular defibrillation in adults. *Circulation* 1979; 60:231–240.

Chatterjee K, Mandel WJ, Vyden JK, et al: Cardiovascular effects of bretylium tosylate in acute myocardial infarction. *J Am Med Assoc* 1973; 223:757.

Chatterjee K, Parmley WW: Role of vasodilator therapy in heart failure. *Prog Cardiovasc Dis* 1977; 19:301.

Cobb LA, Baum RS, Alvarez H, Schatter WA: Resuscitation from out of hospital ventricular fibrillation: 4 year follow up. *Circulation* 1975; 52, Suppl III, 223.

Cobb, LA, Werner JA, Trobaugh GB: Sudden cardiac death: A decade's experience with out of hospital resuscitation. *Mod Concepts Cardiovasc Dis* 1980; 49:31.

Cohn JN, Franciosa JA: Vasodilator therapy of cardiac failure. *New Engl J Med* 1977; 297:27–31, 254–58.

Collinsworth KA, Kalman SM, Harrison DC: The clinical pharmacology of lidocaine as an anti-arrhythmic drug. *Circulation* 1979; 50:1217–1230.

Cranefield PF: Ventricular fibrillation. *N Engl J Med* 1973; 289:732–736.

DelGuercio LRM, Feins NE, Cohn JD, et al: Comparison of blood flow during external and internal cardiac massage in man. *Circulation* 1965; 31 (suppl 1):171–180.

Dorsch JA, Dorsch SE: *Understanding Anesthesia Equipment*. Baltimore, The Williams and Wilkins Co, 1975.

Ellrodt G, Chew CY, Singh BN: Therapeutic implications of slow-channel blockade in cardiocirculatory disorders. *Circulation* 1980; 62:669–679.

Ewy GA: Cardiac arrest and resuscitation: Defibrillators and defibrillation. *Curr Probl Cardiol* 1978; 2:1–71.

Fillmore SJ, Shapiro M, Killip T: Serial blood gas studies during cardiopulmonary resuscitation. *Ann Intern Med* 1970; 72:465–469.

Forrester JS, Diamond G, Chatterjee K, et al: Medical therapy of acute myocardial infarction by application of hemodynamic subsets (first of two parts). *N Engl J Med* 1976; 295:1356–1362.

Forrester JS, Diamond G, Chatterjee K, et al: Medical therapy of acute myocardial infarction by application of hemodynamic subsets. *N Engl J Med* 1976; 295:1356–1362, 1404–1413.

Gettes LS: Electrophysiology of cardiac arrhythmias, in Eliot RS, Wolf GL, Forker AD (eds): *Cardiac Emergencies*. Mt Kisco, NY, Futura Publishing Co Inc, 1977.

Gilman AG, Goodman LS, Gilman A, et al (eds): Cardiovascular Drugs, in *The Pharmacological Basis of Therapeutics*, ed 6. New York, Macmillan Inc, 1980.

Goldberg LI: Dopamine—clinical uses of an endogenous catecholamine. *N Engl J Med* 1974; 291:707–710.

Goldstein S, Landis JR, Leighton R, et al: Characteristics of the resuscitated out of hospital cardiac arrest victim with coronary heart disease. *Circulation* 1981; 64:977.

Greenblatt DJ, Bolognini V, Koch-Weser J, et al: Pharmacokinetic approach to the clinical use of lidocaine intravenously. *J Am Med Assoc* 1976; 236:273–277.

Gregory GA: Resuscitation of the newborn. *Anesthesiology* 1975; 43:225.

Guidelines for the Determination of Death: *J Am Med Assoc* 1981; 246:2184–2186.

Harnett RM, Sias FR, Pruitt JR: *Resuscitation from Hypothermia: A Literature Review*. US Department of Transportation, United States Coast Guard, report No. CG-D-26-79 1979. National Technical Information Service, Springfield, VA 22151.

Harrison DC: Practical guidelines for the use of lidocaine. *J Am Med Assoc* 1975; 233:1202–1204.

Haugen RK: The cafe coronary: Sudden deaths in restaurants. *J Am Med Assoc* 1963; 186:142–143.

Heimlich HJ: A life-saving maneuver to prevent food-choking. *J Am Med Assoc* 1975; 234:398–401.

Jacobs HB: Emergency percutaneous transtracheal catheter and ventilator. *J Trauma* 1972; 12:50–55.

Jude JR, Kouwenhoven WB, Knickerbocker GG: Cardiac arrest. Report of application of external cardiac massage on 118 patients. *J Am Med Assoc* 1961; 178:1063–1070.

Kerber RE, Sarnat W: Factors influencing the success of ventricular defibrillation in man. *Circulation* 1979; 60:226–230.

Kitchen MG III, Kastor JA: Pacing in acute myocardial infarction indications, methods, hazards and results, in Brest AN, Wiener L, Chung EK, et al (eds): *Innovations in the Diagnosis and Management of Acute Myocardial Infarction. Cardiovascular Clinics Series*. Philadelphia, FA Davis Co, 1975, Vol 7, No 1.

Koch-Weser J: Drug therapy: Bretylium. *N Engl J Med* 1979; 300:473–477.

Kouwenhoven WB, Jude JR, Knickerbocker GG: Closed-chest cardiac massage. *J Am Med Assoc* 1960; 173:1064–1067.

Kuller LH: Sudden death—definition and epidemiologic considerations. *Prog Cardiovasc Dis* 1980; 23:1–12.

Landsam AA, McAuliff JP, et al: Differentiation of receptor systems activated by sympathomimetic amines. *Nature* 1967; 214:597.

Liberthson RR, Nagel EL, Hirschman JC, Nussenfeld SR: Primary ventricular defibrillation: Prognosis and follow up. *New Engl J Med* 1974; 291:317.

Livesay JJ, Follette DM, Fey KH, et al: Optimizing myocardial supply/demand balance with a-adrenergic drugs during cardiopulmonary resuscitation. *J Thorac Cardiovasc Surg* 1978; 76:244–251.

Lown B, Crampton RS, DeSilva RA, et al: The energy for ventricular defibrillation—too little or too much? *N Engl J Med* 1978; 298:1252–1253.

Lown B, Neuman J, Amarasingham R, et al: Comparison of alternating current with direct current electroshock across the closed chest. *Am J Cardiol* 1962; 10:223–233.

Luce JM, Cary JM, Ross BK, et al: New developments in cardiopulmonary resuscitation. *J Am Med Assoc* 1980; 244:1366.

McIntyre KM: Cardiopulmonary resuscitation (CPR) and the ultimate coronary care unit, editorial. *J Am Med Assoc* 1980; 244:510–511.

McIntyre KM, Lewis JA (eds): *Textbook of Advanced Cardiac Life Support*. Dallas American Heart Association, 1981.

Mason DT, Vera Z, Miller RR, et al: Treatment of tachyarrhythmias, in Mason DT (ed): *Cardiac Emergencies*. Baltimore, The Williams & Wilkins Co, 1978.

Mattar JA, Weil MH, Shubin H, et al: Cardiac arrest in the critically ill: II. Hyperosmolal states following cardiac arrest. *Am J Med* 1974; 56:162–168.

Myerburg RJ, Conde CA, Sung RJ, et al: Clinical electrophysiologic and hemodynamic profile of patients resuscitated from prehospital cardiac arrest. *Am J Med* 1980; 68:568.

Nagel EL, Hirschman JC, Nussenfeld SR, et al: Telemetry—medical command in coronary and other mobile emergency care systems. *J Am Med Assoc* 1970; 214:332–338.

Negovsky VA: *Current Problems of Reanimatology*. Moscow, Mir Publishers, 1975.

Orlowski JP: Cardiopulmonary resuscitation in children. *Pediatr Clin North Am* 1980; 27:495.

Palmer RF, Lasseter KC: Drug Therapy: Sodium Nitroprusside. *New Engl J Med* 1975; 292:294.

President's Commission for the Study of Ethical Problems in Medicine and Biomedical and Behavioral Research: *Defining death; medical, legal, and ethical issues in the determination of death*. Washington, DC, Government Printing Office, 1981.

Redding JS: The choking controversy: Critique of evidence of the Heimlich maneuver. *Crit Care Med* 1979; 7:475–479.

Redding JS (ed): Second Wolf Creek Conference on CPR. *Crit Care Med* 1981; 9:5.

Reuler JB: Hypothermia: Pathophysiology, clinical settings and management. *Ann Intern Med* 1978; 89:519.

Roberts JR, Greenberg MI, Baskin SI: Endotracheal epinephrine in cardiorespiratory collapse. *JACEP* 1979; 8:515–519.

Roberts JR, Greenberg MI, Knaub MA, et al: Blood levels following intravenous and endotracheal epinephrine administration. *JACEP* 1979; 8:53–56.

Safar P, *Cardiopulmonary Cerebral Resuscitation*. Philadelphia, WB Saunders Co, 1981.

Safar P: Cardiopulmonary-cerebral resuscitation, in Shoemaker WC, Thompson WL (ed): *Critical Care: State of the Art*. Fullerton, CA, The Society of Critical Care Medicine, 1981, vol II.

Safar P: *Respiratory Therapy*. Philadelphia, FA Davis Co, 1965, chaps 3 and 4.

Safar P, Benson DM, Berkebill PE, et al: Teaching and organizing cardiopulmonary resuscitation, in Safar P (ed): *Public Health Aspects of Critical Care Medicine and Anesthesiology*. Philadelphia, FA Davis Co, 1974, pp 162–191.

Safar P, Bleyaert A, Nemoto EM, et al: Resuscitation after global brain ischemia–anoxia. *Crit Care Med* 1978; 6:215–227.

Safar P, Elam J (eds): *Advances in Cardiopulmonary Resuscitation*. New York, Springer-Verlag New York Inc, 1977.

Schofferman J, Oill P, Lewis AJ: The esophageal obturator airway: A clinical evaluation. *Chest* 1976; 69:67–71.

Sellick BA: Cricoid pressure to control regurgitation of stomach contents during induction of anesthesia. *Lancet* 1961; 2:404–406.

Singh BN, Collett JT, Chew CY: New perspectives in the pharmacologic therapy of cardiac arrhythmias. *Prog Cardiovasc Dis* 1980; 22:243–301.

Singh BN, Ellrodt G, Peter CT: Verapamil: A review of its pharmacological properties and therapeutic use. *Drugs* 1978; 15:169–197.

Sodium bicarbonate in cardiac arrest, editorial. *Lancet* 1976; 1:946–947.

Steen PA, Tinker JH, Pluth JR, et al: Efficacy of dopamine, dobutamine, and epinephrine during emergence from cardiopulmonary bypass in man. *Circulation* 1978; 57:378–384.

Sung RJ, Elser B, McAllister RG Jr: Intravenous verapamil for termination of re-entrant supraventricular tachycardias. *Ann Intern Med* 1980; 93:682–689.

Tacker WA Jr, Ewy GA: Emergency defibrillation dose: Recommendations and rationale. *Circulation* 1979; 60:223–225.

Taylor G, Tucker WM, Greene HL, et al: Importance of prolonged compression during cardiopulmonary resuscitation in man. *N Engl J Med* 1977; 296:1515–1517.

Todres DI, Rodgers MC: Methods of external cardiac massage in the newborn infant. *J Pediatr* 1975; 86:781.

Tuttle RR, Mills J: Dobutamine: Development of a new catecholamine to selectively increase cardiac contractility. *Circ Res* 1975; 36:185.

White RD, Gilles BP, Polk BV: Oxygen delivery by hand-operated emergency ventilation devices. *JACEP* 1973; 2:105–108.

Winkle RA, Glantz SA, Harrison DC: Pharmacologic therapy of ventricular arrhythmias. *Am J Cardiol* 1975; 36:629–650.

Wyman MG, Lalka D, Hammersmith L, et al: Multiple bolus technique for lidocaine administration during the first hours of an acute myocardial infarction. *Am J Cardiol* 1978; 41:313–317.

Yakaitis RW, Otto CW, Blitt CD: Relative importance of alpha- and beta-adrenergic receptors during resuscitation. *Crit Care Med* 1979; 7:293–296.

Yakaitis RW, Redding JS: Precordial thumping during cardiac resuscitation. *Crit Care Med* 1973; 1:22–26.

2

RESPIRATORY DISTRESS

Alan Lisbon
Klaus Geiger
Stephen V. Hall
Inder V. Malhotra

Patients seen in the emergency room who are complaining of difficulty in breathing require rapid attention and continuous observation by medical personnel. This applies even to those patients who do not appear to be acutely distressed, since unrecognized early respiratory insufficiency can progress to frank respiratory failure and death within minutes. Successful management of acute respiratory insufficiency requires early recognition, quick assessment, and rapid administration of oxygen and appropriate ventilatory care. Therapy consists first of support, then of correction of the physiologic derangement. Once the life-threatening emergency is controlled, a more thorough diagnostic assessment may begin in preparation for transfer of the patient to a critical care area of the hospital.

Since the care of patients with respiratory insufficiency requires an understanding of the anatomy of the airways and lungs and of the pathophysiology of respiratory failure, this chapter will begin with a brief review of these two subjects. Some symbols and their approximate normal values that are useful when dealing with patients with respiratory distress are listed in Table 2.1.

ANATOMIC AND PATHOPHYSIOLOGIC CONSIDERATIONS

The airway extends from the mouth and nostrils to the terminal bronchioles and serves to conduct gases for exchange in the alveoli (Fig. 2.1). The airway may be divided at the vocal cords into a supraglottic portion, consisting of the mouth, nostrils, and pharynx, and a subglottic portion, consisting of the trachea and its subsequent branches. The trachea begins at the vocal cords and extends for 10–11 cm, dividing into the right and left mainstem bronchi opposite T-5 posteriorly and the Louis' angle anteriorly. In children, the trachea bifurcates opposite the third costal cartilage. The narrowest part of the upper airway is at the vocal cords in the adult and at the cricoid cartilage in the child. These two areas are common spots at which foreign bodies become caught and cause obstruction. The right bronchus is 2.5 cm long and is shorter but greater in diameter and more in line with the trachea than is the left bronchus. Foreign bodies or too enthusiastically placed endotracheal tubes are therefore more likely to be lodged in the right mainstem bronchus.

Distal to the mainstem bronchi, the airways continue to branch and serve as conductive airways until the terminal bronchioles. In the respiratory bronchioles, alveolar ducts, sacs, and alveoli, gas exchange takes place. The ducts are surrounded by smooth muscle fibers as far as the respiratory bronchioles. Throughout the lung are elastic fibers that provide support and cause passive collapse of the lung during exhalation.

The common causes of respiratory distress are listed in Table 2.2. Most acute and chronic lung diseases are produced by the following pathophysiologic mechanisms:

1. Abnormal control of respiration
2. Abnormal relation of ventilation to perfusion
   a. Increased dead space to tidal volume
   b. Increased right-to-left shunt
3. Changes in lung mechanics
   a. Decreased compliance
   b. Increased airway resistance
4. Changes in chest wall mechanics or mechanics of breathing

Ventilation

Minute ventilation is that volume of gas that enters the respiratory tree in one minute. Normal ventilation is controlled by the medullary respiratory center in the floor of the fourth ventricle and by the peripheral chemoreceptors near the carotid arteries. A decrease in pH or increase in carbon dioxide of the blood or cerebrospinal fluid (CSF) perfusing the medullary respiratory center will cause an increase in ventilation, as will a reduction in a partial oxygen pressure (PO_2) in the blood supplied to the carotid chemoreceptors.

During quiet inspiration, the diaphragm, innervated by cervical roots 3, 4, and 5, descends, thus creating a negative pressure gradient between the mouth and alveoli and causing gas to be drawn into the lungs. The amount of gas drawn into the respiratory tree in one breath is the *tidal volume* (V_T). Expiration is passive and occurs because of elastic recoil in the lung. Ventilation may be augmented both in inspiration and expiration by the use of the intercostal muscles, abdominal musculature, and accessory muscles of respiration in the neck.

TABLE 2.1 Some Symbols and Formulas Used in Respiratory Therapy

Symbol or Abbreviation	Variable	Approximate Normal Values (70 kg Resting Adult)
FiO_2	Fraction of inspired oxygen (60% = 0.6)	0.21 (air), 1 (100% O_2)
PAO_2	Alveolar oxygen tension	100 mm Hg (FiO_2 0.21, P_B 760 mm Hg)
$PACO_2$	Alveolar carbon dioxide tension	40 mm Hg
PaO_2	Arterial oxygen tension	75–100 mm Hg (FiO_2 0.21) 500–600 mm Hg (FiO_2 1.0)
$PaCO_2$	Arterial carbon dioxide tension	40 mm Hg
$P\bar{v}O_2$	Mixed venous oxygen tension	40 mm Hg
$P\bar{v}CO_2$	Mixed venous carbon dioxide tension	42–45 mm Hg
A-aDO_2	Alveolar–arterial oxygen difference	10–15 mm Hg
A-a$DO_2{}^1$	Alveolar–arterial oxygen difference (at FiO_2 1)	50–75 mm Hg
Q	Cardiac output	5 liters/min
P_B	Barometric pressure	760 mm Hg at sea level
V_T	Tidal volume	500 ml (7 ml/kg)
V_D	Dead space ventilation	2 ml/kg
V_D/V_T	Dead space to tidal volume ratio	0.3

Disorders of the central nervous (CNS) and neuromuscular systems, such as sedative drug overdose, head trauma, cervical spine injury, or ascending polyneuritis, act to decrease ventilation but do not directly affect the lungs. These diseases disrupt ventilatory control, not end organ function (Table 2.3).

The portion of gas that enters the alveoli is termed *alveolar ventilation,* and it is this gas that takes part in exchange. Gas that is excluded from exchange is *dead space ventilation* (V_D), usually expressed as a fraction of the tidal volume (V_D/V_T). Alveolar ventilation and the partial pressure of carbon dioxide in arterial blood ($PaCO_2$) are inversely related. The adequacy of alveolar ventilation is measured clinically by the $PaCO_2$.

Ventilation is not uniform throughout the lung. There are regional differences in ventilation even in the normal lung; the dependent portions of the lung receive more ventilation per unit volume than do those that are nondependent.

DEAD SPACE

The airway-conducting system, which ends with the respiratory bronchioles, composes the anatomical dead space. The average value for anatomical dead space (in milliliters) approximately equals the body weight (in pounds). In the healthy adult man, the dead space volume is about 150 ml; in healthy young women it may be as low as 100 ml; in healthy older men it may be as high as 200 ml. In addition to anatomical dead space, the physiologic dead space includes alveoli devoid of blood flow (alveolar dead space) (Fig. 2.2). In a healthy man at rest, the physiologic dead space equals the anatomical dead space and is approximately 30% of tidal volume (normal range V_D/V_T ratio 0.2–0.3). Elevation of V_D/V_T implies increased wasted ventilation and an increased energy expenditure in breathing.

The physiologic dead space may be approximated by the following equation:

$$V_D/V_T = (PaCO_2 - PECO_2)/PaCO_2,$$

where $PaCO_2$ is the partial pressure of CO_2 in arterial blood and $PECO_2$ is the partial pressure of mixed expired CO_2. With ventilation in excess of perfusion, the physiologic dead space will be increased. This may occur in the normal lung in the upright position as a result of the effect of gravity on the distribution of pulmonary blood flow. Increased dead space occurs in pathologic conditions such as the following:

1. Fall in cardiac output (hemorrhage, hypotension)

2. Occlusion of the pulmonary arteries (pulmonary embolus, decreased capillary blood flow secondary to high mean airway pressure)

3. Advanced obstructive pulmonary emphysema

WORK OF VENTILATION

The work expended in effective ventilation depends on the compliance of the lungs and chest wall and the airway resistance.

Compliance

Compliance describes the elastic attributes of the chest wall (muscles, tendons, connective tissue) and the lungs (elastic fibers, surfactant). Lung compliance is the change in lung volume per change in airway pressure. The effective compliance is defined as tidal volume (V_T) divided by peak airway pressure in a ventilated patient. The normal value for an adult when supine is 50 ml/cm H_2O. Disease states with decreased compliance are commonly called *restrictive ventilatory diseases*. Low compliance implies an increased work of breathing. Patients with low compliance commonly breathe shallowly and rapidly.

Compliance is decreased in conditions associated with the following:

1. Decreased elastic recoil of the lung (atelectasis, pneumonia, pulmonary congestion with and without edema, pulmonary fibrosis, and increased alveolar surface tension)
2. Decreased elastic recoil of chest wall (kyphoscoliosis, obesity, abdominal distension)
3. Intrathoracic space-occupying process (pleural effusion, pneumothorax)

Airway Resistance

Airway resistance is proportional to the pressure drop between the alveoli and the mouth divided by the flow rate. Airway resistance is increased in any condition that causes obstruction; thus, disease states with decreased flow rates, for example, tracheal stenosis, epiglottitis, and bronchial asthma, are commonly called *obstructive ventilatory diseases*. Patients with these diseases commonly breathe slowly and deeply.

An increase in airway resistance results in an increase in work of breathing to maintain effective alveolar ventilation. Increase in expiratory resistance requires forced expiration to overcome the resistance to airflow. Increase in expiratory resistance may increase intrathoracic pressure, which in turn may decrease venous return and cardiac output.

Perfusion

Almost complete equilibrium is achieved between the perfusing blood and the alveolar gas under ordinary circumstances.

Abbnormalities in pulmonary perfusion, such as those occuring in pulmonary embolism or fat embolism, can contribute substantially to derangements in respiratory function. The pulmonary vascular system is normally a low-pressure system (pulmonary artery pressure, PAP = 25/8 mm Hg; mean pulmonary artery pressure, $\overline{PAP}$ = 8 mm Hg), and pulmonary vascular resistance is one-fifth that of systemic resistance. The pulmonary vascular resistance is affected by intraalveolar pressure, lung volumes, and cardiac output. Decreased pulmonary arterial pH as well as decreased alveolar oxygen tension (PAO_2) and arterial hypoxemia lead to vasoconstriction. With localized areas of decreased PAO_2 there are localized areas of va-

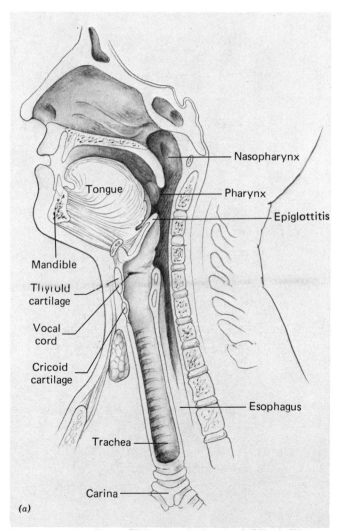

Figure 2.1 (a) Upper and (b) lower airways.

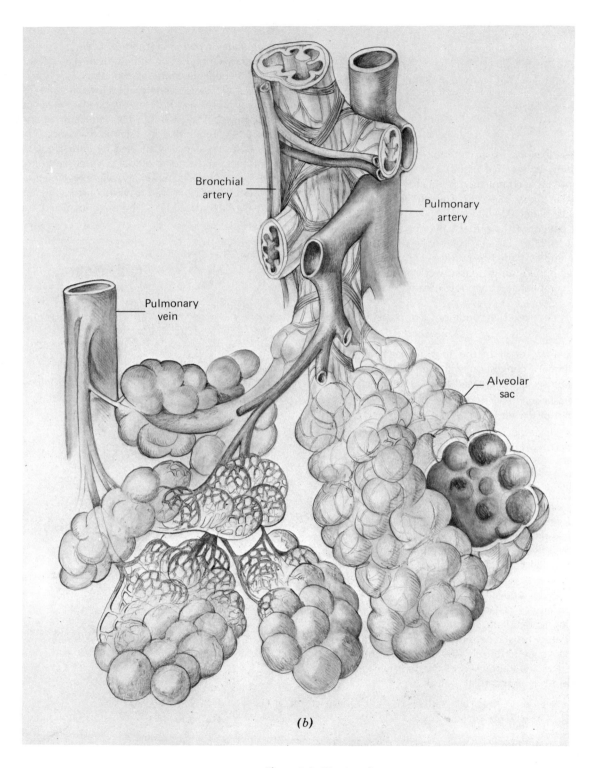

Figure 2.1 *(Continued)*

TABLE 2.2 Common Causes of Respiratory Failure in the Emergency Room

Abnormal Control of Respiration
  Depressed respiratory drive in obtunded patient
    Intracranial injury
    Increased intracranial pressure
    Drug poisoning
  Neuromuscular disorders
    Cervical trauma
    Myasthenia gravis
    Polyneuritis
    Poliomyelitis
Changes in Lung Mechanics and/or Mechanics of Breathing
  Increased airway resistance
    Partial or total obstruction of upper airway
      Tongue
      Foreign material
      Epiglottitis
      Laryngeotracheobronchitis
      Angioneurotic edema
      Laryngeal trauma
      Laryngeal malignancy
      Laryngeal nerve palsy
      Tracheal stenosis
    Lower airway obstruction
      Asthma
      Infectious tracheobronchitis
      Aspiration tracheobronchitis
      Chronic obstructive pulmonary disease
  Decreased compliance
    Alveolar collapse and interstitial edema
    Pulmonary edema with acute left ventricular failure
    Pulmonary edema with increased capillary permeability
    ARDS (trauma, shock, drowning, massive pneumonia, aspiration, sepsis)
    Impaired chest wall mechanics
      Pneumothorax
      Flail chest
      Pleural effusion
Abnormal Relation of Ventilation to Perfusion
  Pulmonary edema with acute left ventricular-failure
  Pulmonary edema with altered capillary permeability (trauma, shock, DIC, aspiration, sepsis)
  Pneumonia
  Pulmonary embolus
    Fat embolus
  Atelectasis
  Pulmonary hemorrhage

soconstriction so that compensation is attempted by matching perfusion to ventilation.

SHUNT

Shunt, like dead space, consists of an anatomical and a physiologic portion and is that part of the output of the right ventricle that does not participate in gas exchange. The anatomical shunt is the 3–5% of the cardiac output in healthy people that bypasses ventilated alveoli through the Thebesian venous system of the left ventricle, through bronchial vein–pulmonary vein anastomoses, and through direct channels between the pulmonary arteries and veins. The anatomical shunt increases in disease states associated with hypertrophy of bronchial vessels, such as chronic bronchitis, bronchiectasis, and cystic fibrosis, or the perfusion of nonventilated areas that may occur in a pulmonary arteriovenous fistula.

In a physiologic right-to-left shunt, a sizable fraction of pulmonary venous blood comes from lung areas in which pulmonary ventilation is greatly decreased relative to perfusion (Fig. 2.2). This blood shows a deficit in O_2 content. Venous admixture reduces arterial P_{O_2} by adding venous blood with low P_{O_2} (40 mm Hg) to arterialized blood leaving the pulmonary capillary bed with P_{O_2} of 100 mm Hg. The Pa_{CO_2} is not significantly altered by venous admixture because the difference between the P_{CO_2} of mixed venous blood (Pv_{CO_2} 46 mm Hg) and pulmonary capillary blood, which is in equilibrium with alveolar CO_2 tension (PA_{CO_2} 40 mm Hg) is small and any increase of Pa_{CO_2} will immediately stimulate the respiratory center. This increases the minute ventilation and returns the Pa_{CO_2} to normal. The physiologic shunt increases with all lung and airway diseases associated with low ventilation–perfusion ratios. These diseases include pneumonia, atelectasis, pulmonary edema, and pulmonary hemorrhage.

The perfusion of the lung (Q) is not uniform; perfusion is greater at dependent portions of the lung. If ventilation (V) is compared to perfusion (V/Q), we see that even in the normal lung, ventilation is in excess of perfusion at the apex of the upright lung, and perfusion is in excess of ventilation at the base of the lung.

Many lung diseases cause V/Q mismatch with poor transfer of oxygen and carbon dioxide between the alveolar space and pulmonary venous blood. Areas with high V/Q have ventilation in excess of perfusion (increased dead space). Those with low V/Q have perfusion in excess of ventilation (increased shunt). The amount of V/Q abnormality can be estimated from calculating the physiologic dead space and the alveolar–arterial oxygen gradient (A-aD_{O_2}), which is described below.

Arterial Blood Gases

Arterial blood gases are of paramount importance in the management of patients with respiratory distress. Respiratory failure is defined as hypoxia with or without hypercapnia. The diagnosis can be made only by the measurement of the Pa_{O_2} and the Pa_{CO_2} in the laboratory. The normal arterial blood gases are shown in Table 2.4.

TABLE 2.3 Mechanisms of Respiratory Failure

Location of Pathology	Example	Pathophysiology	PaO_2	ABG $PacO_2$	pH
CNS	Epidural hematoma Drug overdose	Abnormal control Possible abnormal V/Q	−	↑	↓
Cervical cord	Cervical spine fracture	Abnormal control	−	↑	↓
Peripheral nerve	Guillain-Barré	Abnormal control	−	↑	↓
Neuromuscular junction	Myasthenia	Abnormal control	−	↑	↓
Chest wall	Flail chest	Change in Chest wall mechanics and mechanics of breathing	− ↓	− ↑	− ↓
Pleural cavity	Pneumothorax	Change in Chest wall mechanics and mechanics of breathing	↓	− ↑	− ↓
Upper airway	Foreign body infection	Abnormal V/Q	↓	↑	↓
Lower airway	Asthma, COPD	Abnormal V/Q lung mechanics	↓	↓ − ↑	↑ − ↓
Lung	Pulmonary edema	Abnormal V/Q Change in lung mechanics	↓	− ↑	− ↓
Pulmonary vasculature	Pulmonary embolism	Abnormal V/Q	↓	↓	↑

ARTERIAL OXYGEN TENSION

The relationship between the arterial oxygen tension (PaO_2) in the blood and the oxygen tension simultaneously present in alveolar gas (A-aDO_2), and the inspired oxygen fraction (FiO_2), provides information about the mechanism that underlies the disturbance in gas exchange. Normal values for PaO_2 vary considerably with age and are influenced by altitude and ambient oxygen concentration at which the measurement is performed. In healthy people who are measured at sea level, PaO_2 should be 95 mm Hg or higher. The regression of PaO_2 with age is as follows:

- Sitting: $PaO_2 = 104 − 0.27 \times$ age (years) mm Hg

- Supine: $PaO_2 = 103 − 0.42 \times$ age (years) mm Hg

Values of PaO_2 below normal represent hypoxemia. The PaO_2 may be decreased by ventilation perfusion mismatch, increased right-to-left shunting, alveolar hypoventilation without supplementary oxygen, diffusion impairment, and increased O_2 consumption. Increased O_2 consumption relative to O_2 transport is a less frequent cause of hypoxemia and occurs only in the presence of abnormally increased right-to-left shunting (Table 2.5).

Oxygen Transport

Oxygen is carried in the blood primarily in combination with hemoglobin (Hb) with each fully saturated gram of hemoglobin carrying 1.34 ml of oxygen. Only a small amount of oxygen, 0.03 ml/100 ml blood/mm Hg, is carried in solution. The oxyhemoglobin saturation curve, which shows the relationship between the hemoglobin saturation and PaO_2, may be shifted by various factors such as pH, temperature, anemia, or concentration of 2,3-diphosphoglycerate (2,3-DPG) (Fig. 2.3). We strive to stay on the knee of the oxyhemoglobin saturation curve so that small changes in PaO_2 do not cause sharp swings in hemoglobin saturation. A PaO_2 of at least 60–65 mm Hg is usually sufficient for this.

The amount of oxygen delivered to the tissues depends on the concentration of hemoglobin, its saturation, and the cardiac output. Blood flow to vital organs may be increased to compensate for hypoxemia.

ARTERIAL CARBON DIOXIDE TENSION

Carbon dioxide exists in the blood in the following three forms:

1. As bicarbonate
2. In combination with the NH_2 group of hemoglobin as carbamino compounds

Normal

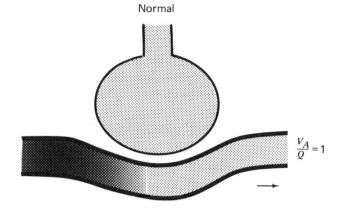

$$\frac{V_A}{Q} = 1$$

Deadspace

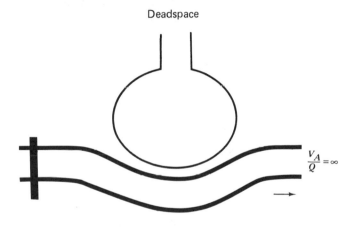

$$\frac{V_A}{Q} = \infty$$

Shunt

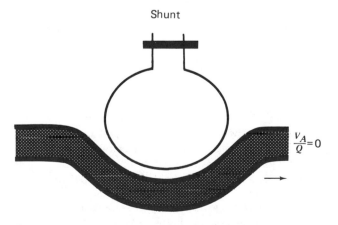

$$\frac{V_A}{Q} = 0$$

Figure 2.2 Ventilation perfusion relationships.

TABLE 2.4 Normal Blood Gases

Age	P_{O_2}	P_{CO_2}	pH
< 50	> 90		
< 60	> 80		
< 70	> 70	38–42	7.38–7.42
< 80	> 60		
< 90	> 50		

3. Dissolved in solution in which it is 20 times more soluble than oxygen

The normal arterial CO_2 tension ranges between 38 and 42 mm Hg. Alterations in Pa_{CO_2} reflect changes in alveolar ventilation or changes in the rate of CO_2 production. In respiratory failure, the adequacy of alveolar ventilation is expressed by the Pa_{CO_2}, not by any other value.

When CO_2 production is constant, hyperventilation associated with anxiety, pain, or hypoxia leads to hypocapnia (decreased Pa_{CO_2}) and respiratory alkalosis. Clinically, this may be seen in patients with mild pulmonary insufficiency, pulmonary embolism, and sepsis. By contrast, hypoventilation caused by decreased respiratory rate and tidal volume associated with central nervous system depression or increased pulmonary physiologic dead space associated with acute lung disorders results in hypercapnia (increased Pa_{CO_2}) and respiratory acidosis (Table 2.6). Increased CO_2 production caused by fever or increased circulating catecholamines during respiratory distress can lead to a rise in Pa_{CO_2} unless minute alveolar ventilation concurrently increases.

ARTERIAL pH

In the blood, carbon dioxide combines with water to form carbonic acid. This is a weak acid that dissociates to yield

TABLE 2.5 Causes of Hypoxemia

Decreased alveolar P_{O_2}
  Deficiency of ambient Fi_{O_2}
  Hypoventilation
  Venous admixture
Increased shunt
Decreased mixed venous oxygen content
  Increased metabolic rate
  Low cardiac output
  Anemia
  Abnormal hemoglobin
Diffusion impairment

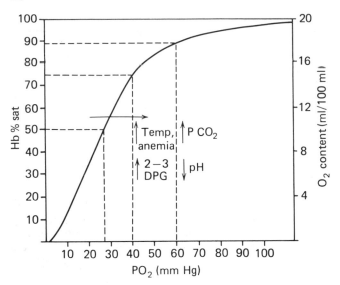

Figure 2.3 The oxyhemoglobin dissociation curve. The curve may be sifted to the right by fever, increasing PCO_2, decreasing pH, anemia, and 2, 3-DPG.

hydrogen ions according to the following modified Henderson–Hasselbalch equation:

$$pH = pK' + \log \frac{([HCO_3])}{k \cdot PaCO_2}$$

where pK' is the dissociation constant, [HCO_3] is the bicarbonate concentration, and k is a constant. The normal arterial

TABLE 2.6 Causes of Hypoventilation

Depression of respiratory centers
 Drug poisonings
 CNS trauma
 Elevated PCO_2
Interruption of ventilatory motor nerves or neuromuscular junction
 Muscle relaxants
 Myasthenia gravis
 Ascending polyneuritis
 Anterior horn disease
Disease of respiratory muscles
Abnormal thorax mechanics
 Kyphoscoliosis
 Arthritis
 Emphysema
Abnormal lung mechanics
 Pleural effusion
 Pneumothorax
 Fibrosis
 Pneumonia
 Obstruction of respiratory tract

pH is 7.38–7.44. Deviations of arterial pH outside the normal range are referred to as acidemia (decreased pH) or alkalemia (increased pH). Alterations in arterial pH can be caused by changes in the plasma concentration of $PaCO_2$, metabolic acids, or carbonic acid. Severe acidemia (pH < 7.20) depresses myocardial contractility, causes CNS depression, predisposes the myocardium to arrythmias, impairs circulatory barostasis, and promotes hyperkalemia.

In patients with respiratory acidemia, the $PaCO_2$ increases acutely and the arterial pH falls. If there is an acute fall in $PaCO_2$, the pH will rise, yielding a respiratory alkalemia. Patients with respiratory insufficiency may have changes in plasma concentrations of metabolic acids in addition to changes in $PaCO_2$. When metabolic and respiratory changes in the acid–base balance occur simultaneously, it is helpful to refer to a nomogram, such as that of Siggaard-Andersen, to determine how much each component contributes to the overall acid–base derangement (see Fig. 11.1). An estimate can be made by knowing that each acute 10 mm Hg increase in $PaCO_2$ above 40 mm Hg will decrease the pH by 0.07. Similarly, a 10 mm Hg decrease in $PaCO_2$ below 40 mm Hg will increase the pH by 0.10. When the pH is appropriately adjusted for a $PaCO_2$ of 40 mm Hg, the pH will reflect only the metabolic components of the acid–base imbalance.

INITIAL EVALUATION AND EMERGENCY ROOM MANAGEMENT

Evaluation of the Patient

The evaluation of the patient with respiratory distress must proceed rapidly and concurrently with therapy. The emergency room physician must not hesitate to call colleagues in anesthesia, surgery, or medicine to assist early on with patient care.

When the patient is seen initially, it is useful to obtain a brief history. It is important to know if the condition is acute or chronic. Is there a past history of respiratory problems? Has trauma occurred? What was the nature of events that preceded the acute episode? What medications or drugs does the patient use? Does the patient have any allergies? In life-threatening circumstances, however, the urgency of the situation may make it impossible or unwise to take time to obtain any history until the necessary resuscitation has been accomplished.

Recognition of early respiratory insufficiency can be difficult. All patients with respiratory complaints who appear restless or slightly tachypneic need close scrutiny. Although agitation and tachypnea may be due to anxiety in some patients, the so-called hyperventilation syndrome they present with is frequently an early sign of respiratory insufficiency. Restlessness may be a sign of hypoxemia, even in the absence of cyanosis. Acute hypercapnia may be manifest as apprehension or confusion, and may be followed by coma. Tachypnea is a common sign of impending or established respiratory failure in patients with acute pneumonias (viral, bacteria, or chemical) or acute exacerbations of chronic obstructive lung disease, pulmonary edema, pulmonary embolism, or asthma. Serial measurements of respiratory rate, pulse rate, and blood pressure are important in the early detection of respiratory insufficiency in this group of patients. Progressive tachypnea, tachycardia, and hypertension or sudden hypotension and bradycardia are signs of worsening respiratory failure.

Severe respiratory insufficiency is usually readily recognized. Patients are markedly tachypneic, agitated, and gasping for air. Noisy labored breathing, using the muscles of the neck and abdomen to assist inspiration and expiration, is a sign of upper or lower airway obstruction. Flaring of the nasal alae and sternal and intercostal retractions may also occur. Cyanosis should be assumed to represent inadequate pulmonary blood gas exchange until proven otherwise by arterial blood gas measurements. Severe respiratory insufficiency can be associated initially with hypertension and tachycardia or with hypotension and bradycardia. Hypotension and bradycardia are ominous signs usually seen in the most severely hypoxemic and acidemic patients.

Respiratory insufficiency in the comatose patient can be easily overlooked. Marked hypoventilation and apnea are readily recognized in patients with severe CNS depression, but clinical recognition of moderate hypoventilation can be very difficult in these patients. Significant partial airway obstruction causing serious hypoxemia, hypercapnia, and acidemia can exist in patients who superficially appear to have adequate ventilation. In patients with acute intracranial pathology and elevated intracranial pressure, hypoxemia and hypercapnia will cause cerebral vasodilation that can lead to further increased intracranial pressure, uncal herniation, and death. *The reliance on clinical signs for the detection of respiratory insufficiency in the obtunded patient is hazardous. The importance of the early placement of an endotracheal tube and measurement of arterial blood gases cannot be overemphasized.*

Initial Management—General Measures

OXYGEN ADMINISTRATION

Once respiratory insufficiency is suspected or recognized in a patient, certain therapeutic measures must be undertaken immediately; more accurate assessment can be completed under less urgent conditions. The early administration of supplemental oxygen is essential. Carbon dioxide retention and acidemia are much better tolerated in the absence of hypoxia, and correction of hypoxemia may make a very agitated patient quite manageable. The primary goal of oxygen therapy is to raise oxygen tension in arterial blood to levels that existed in the patient before the acute episode or at least to above 60 mm Hg.

Patients who are in respiratory distress but are breathing spontaneously should be given oxygen by face mask. If respiratory control is normal, the patient with a ventilation–perfusion imbalance (e.g., pneumonia, moderate asthma, or pulmonary embolism) can usually be satisfactorily oxygenated by face mask or nasal cannulas. If the ventilation–perfusion imbalance is associated with a significant degree of right-to-left shunt, however (e.g., adult respiratory distress syndrome or pulmonary edema), adequate oxygenation cannot usually be achieved by simple increase of the FiO_2. Although there may be an initial response to high concentrations of oxygen, it is likely that additional therapeutic modalities will be required.

Special care is required in providing O_2 when respiratory insufficiency is caused by acute ventilatory failure superimposed on chronic failure, such as in chronic obstructive lung disease. In patients with chronic elevation of $PaCO_2$, the respiratory control mechanism is dependent primarily on a hypoxic drive; administering O_2 in uncontrolled amounts may lead to rapid worsening of alveolar hypoventilation, rise in $PaCO_2$, fall in pH, and death. In these patients, O_2 administration is begun at 24% with frequent monitoring of arterial blood gases.

Oxygen must always be administered at the lowest possible dose—that which provides maximum benefit with minimal risk. Exposure to more than 50% oxygen for longer periods than 24 hours poses a significant risk of oxygen toxicity with the development of interstitial and alveolar edema, impairment of the phagocytic function of macrophages, and finally fibrosis. In the presence of airway obstruction (e.g., secondary to a mucous plug or airway closure), the inhalation of 100% oxygen, even for short periods of time, can cause absorption atelectasis. In this situation the oxygen flows rapidly from the alveolus to the capillary because of the large diffusion gradient between the alveolus and capillary. After the oxygen has left the alveolus only the partial pressure as a result of carbon dioxide and water vapor remain. (The nitrogen has been replaced by oxygen.) The remaining pressure may be insufficient to maintain the alveolus in an open state. This collapse of the alveoli may occur even when the FiO_2 is considerably less than 1, but it takes a longer time because the nitrogen remains in the alveolus longer, functioning as a splint to keep the alveolus open. The use of positive end expiratory pressure (PEEP) may eliminate the need to deliver such high concentrations of oxygen. Drying out of secretions is common if the inspired oxygen is not adequately humidified, and for this reason attention must always be given to the humidification of oxygen.

Methods of Administration

Nasal cannulas (prongs) are probably the most common and least expensive method of oxygen administration (Fig. 2.4). They have the further advantage of being well tolerated and allow the patient to be active without interruption of oxygen administration. The disadvantages are that the cannulas are relatively easily dislodged and that oxygen flow rates in excess of 6 liters/min delivered by cannulas tend to dry the nasal mucosa. For this reason, flow rates less than 6 liters/min are normally used (Table 2.7). An effective FiO_2 as high as 0.40 has been reported with the use of this appliance. As with the simple oxygen mask, FiO_2 depends upon the proportion of the patient's ventilation-to-oxygen flow rate. Each liter flow of oxygen provides an additional inspired oxygen concentration of approximately 4%. It should be noted that gastric rupture has been associated with nasal prongs used concurrently with nasogastric tubes.

The standard *plastic face mask* is normally fitted loosely to the face; this allows room air to be drawn in with each inhalation, and exhaled gas to be vented through holes in the body of the mask. Since oxygen flow to the mask is needed to "wash" carbon dioxide from the mask, the minimal flow rates used with plastic masks are between 6 and 10 liters/min, with a resulting FiO_2 of 0.35–0.65. The oxygen concentration delivered is inversely proportional to the patient's own ventilation, that is, the larger the patient's tidal volume or the higher the inspiratory flow rate, the more room air is drawn in and mixed with oxygen. In general, the plastic face masks are light and comfortable for the patient.

The *Venturi mask* (Venti mask) is specifically designed to deliver a relatively low but precise FiO_2. Short of intubation, it is probably the best available device for providing a controlled oxygen concentration. It uses the Bernoulli principle of entrainment of ambient air around an oxygen jet, delivering a fixed oxygen concentration for inspiration. The commonly available masks provide FiO_2 values of 0.24, 0.28, 0.35, and 0.40. A prime indication for the use of this type of mask is in the treatment of patients with chronic obstructive pulmonary disease. These masks fit loosely and the Venturi produces a relatively high total gas flow to the mask, serving to flush the dead space of the mask and thereby preventing rebreathing. Patients must be cautioned not to block the air inlet ports. The recommended oxygen flow rates to the mask are listed in Table 2.7.

The *face hood* is less efficient for administration of high oxygen concentration than is the Venturi mask, but it is useful when high humidity in the form of mist is required. The gas flow must be equal to or greater than the patient's minute volume; otherwise room air is drawn into the hood, diluting the final concentration of humidity and oxygen. Whenever a high concentration of humidity and oxygen is needed, the heated aerosol generator is indicated, whether attached to the face hood or another type of face mask.

The *partial rebreathing mask,* which combines the simple mask with the reservoir bag, can be used for administration of relatively high oxygen concentrations (0.45–0.70). The mask is designed in such a way that the first part of the expired tidal volume, primarily dead space air that is high in oxygen concentration, together with its water vapor, enters the reservoir bag during expiration. There it mixes with the oxygen that constantly flows into the neck of the mask and is directed into the reservoir during expiration. The mixture from the reservoir bag is rebreathed with the next inhalation. The oxygen flow rate to the mask is adjusted so that the reservoir never completely collapses during expiration. The mixture from the reservoir bag is rebreathed with the next inhalation. Adequate oxygen flow (9–10 liters/min) must be used to prevent carbon dioxide accumulation. With such a flow rate and a well-fitted mask, the resulting FiO_2 will be in the range of 0.40–0.65.

The *nonrebreathing mask* is similar to the partial rebreathing mask except for the fact that it is provided with a one-way valve between the reservoir and the mask. The valve is arranged in such a way that no part of the patient's exhaled volume can enter the reservoir bag. During exhalation the oxygen flow fills the reservoir bag; on inspiration the patient receives oxygen from the source gas, as well as from the reservoir bag, making it possible for the inspired oxygen concentration to approach 90%, provided the mask fits well about the face.

The devices described above can only be used if the patient is breathing spontaneously. If the patient is not breathing or if severe hypoventilation is present, mouth-to-mouth ventilation or an *air mask bag unit* (Ambu bag or hand resuscitator) (discussed in Chapter 1) may be used while preparations for insertion of an endotracheal tube are being made. If care is taken to keep the patient's neck extended and the mask tightly applied to the patient's face (Procedure 1) (Fig. 2.4), effective ventilation can be provided by this device. As soon as possible, this type of unit should be attached to an oxygen source in order that oxygen-enriched air may be provided to the patient. When assisting a patient's ventilation, we must remember that some assemblies such as the commonly used Ambu bag do not deliver supplemental oxygen unless the bag is manually

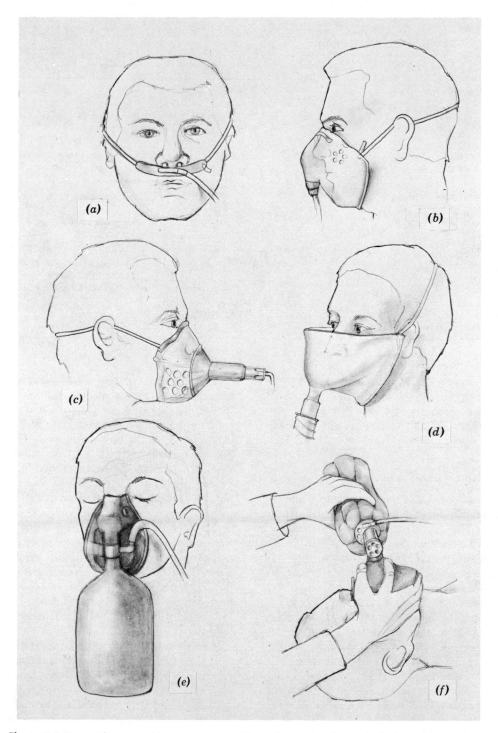

Figure 2.4 Types of oxygen therapy apparatus: (a) nasal cannula; (b) standard plastic face mask; (c) Venturi mask; (d) face hood; (e) rebreathing mask; (f) bag and mask combination.

TABLE 2.7 Forms of Oxygen Therapy

Type of Equipment	Flow (liters/min)	O_2 Concentration (%)	Characteristics
Nasal cannula (prongs)	1–6	24–44	Confortable; easily dislodged; low humidity
Mask without reservoir	6–10	40–60	Light, easy to use; minimal discomfort
Venturi mask			Accurate delivery; can be humidified; sometimes uncomfortable
24 or 28%	4	24 or 28	
35 or 40%	8	35 or 40	
Mask with partial rebreathing reservoir	9–10	45–70	
Mask with nonrebreathing reservoir	9–10	Up to 90	Adequate humidity possible; expensive
Face hood	6–12	30–55	Well tolerated; good humidity
Canopy tent		Variable up to 50	Good humidity; patient inaccessible; more appropriate for children
T-tube adaptor for use with endotracheal or tracheostomy tubes		Can vary to achieve any concentration	

emptied during each breath. If a patient is allowed to breathe without assisted ventilation with this type of unit, the patient will inspire room air through the expiratory port of the one-way valve rather than the oxygen-enriched gas within the self-inflating bag.

ESTABLISHING A SATISFACTORY AIRWAY

Patients with respiratory distress require immediate examination of their upper airway. If partial upper airway obstruction is suspected and breathing is spontaneous, supplemental oxygen is administered before the airway is examined. In the supine obtunded patient, the falling back of the tongue is a frequent cause of airway obstruction (Fig. 2.1). If there are no signs or suspicions of high cervical dislocations or fracture, the patient's head is extended and the jaw pulled or pushed forward by pressure behind the angles of mandible, as described in Chapter 1, to provide as clear an airway as possible. If cervical trauma is suspected, the patient's head is not extended but is held in a neutral position while the jaw is pulled forward. The head and neck should be immobilized in a four-post collar until further work up rules out cervical pathology. If the patient is unconscious, an oropharyngeal airway should be inserted in order to maintain an open air passage between the tongue and posterior pharynx. Attempts to insert this airway in the alert patient may cause gagging and vomiting.

After a few breaths of oxygen have been given to the patient, the oropharynx can be quickly examined and cleared of all foreign material. The patient's face is turned to the side and the jaws firmly opened with steady pressure. If the jaws are tightly clenched, the physician's index finger can be inserted between the teeth and the buccal mucosa into the space behind the patient's last molar teeth and then be used as a wedge to pry the jaws open. Liquid material can be removed by suctioning; remaining solid material is carefully removed manually. Oropharyngeal suctioning should not last more than 15 or 20 seconds at one time since it can seriously aggravate hypoxemia and acidemia. Gentle, precise movements are essential during laryngoscopy or suctioning of the oropharynx. Careless, forceful probing often causes struggling, gagging, and retching and can result in serious oropharyngeal trauma, vomiting, and aspiration of gastric contents. This is especially true in hypoxic patients since they have depressed laryngeal reflexes.

The removal of foreign material (food, blood, dentures, etc.) from the upper airway can be life saving if performed quickly. However, if a cursory laryngoscopy reveals no obvious cause of obstruction, persistent laryngoscopy is unwise since it is unlikely to reveal a remediable cause of obstruction to the untrained eye. If epiglottitis (see below) is suspected as the cause for upper airway obstruction, the examiner must limit intraoral manipulation for fear of converting a partial obstruction into a total one unless the examiner is prepared to insert an endotracheal tube or perform cricothyrotomy immediately.

If the patient still has respiratory distress after the oropharynx has been quickly cleared of secretions, and it sounds as if there may still be foreign material in the tracheobronchial tree (whether it be tenacious mucus, purulent material, aspirated gastric juice, blood, or other material), and the patient is unable to cough effectively, nasotracheal suctioning should be quickly performed under sterile conditions (Procedure 6). The suction should not be applied for longer than 5 or 10 seconds at one time, in order to avoid depletion of the oxygen supply. Nasopharyngeal suctioning should not be one of the initial procedures if the patient has pulmonary edema.

Endotracheal Intubation

Apneic or grossly hypoventilating obtunded patients require immediate controlled ventilation after the upper airway has been cleared of all foreign bodies. If the airway remains inadequate after proper positioning of the head and mandible and insertion of the oropharyngeal airway, ventilation is controlled with a self-inflating bag–mask unit until arrangements can be made for endotracheal intubation (Procedure 4). The unit should be connected to an oxygen source when possible. Tracheal intubation with a cuffed tube facilitates ventilation and protects the airway from gross aspiration of gastric contents. Gastric distention is also avoided. If prolonged intubation will be necessary, a large, low-pressure, high-compliance cuff should be used in order to minimize the risk of tracheal pressure necrosis from the pressure of the balloon.

In most patients, oral intubation can be accomplished with direct visualization of the glottis. Suction apparatus must always be available. Although intubation usually occurs under urgent conditions, the placement of the tracheal tube must be done with precision. Furious thrusts with a tracheal tube can cause serious laryngeal trauma and can frequently lead to endobronchial or esophageal intubations. If difficulty is encountered during intubation, it is generally wise to reinstitute controlled ventilation by face mask until help arrives. A misplaced tracheal tube is far more hazardous than a partially obstructed airway. Once the tracheal tube has been secured in place, excessive hyperventilation of the patient should be avoided, especially in a patient with a $Paco_2$ greater than 60 mm Hg before intubation. A sudden reduction in $Paco_2$ can precipitate hypotension, cardiac arrhythmias, and seizures.

The general indications for endotracheal intubation are as follows:

1. Airway maintenance
2. Prevention of aspiration
3. Pulmonary toilet
4. Institution of controlled ventilation
5. Provision of Fio_2 > 60% or PEEP therapy

Cricothyrotomy

In situations in which there is apparent upper airway obstruction and if none of the above procedures performed during the first 60 seconds is successful in relieving the obstruction, cricothyrotomy should be performed (Procedure 9). This procedure requires only seconds to perform and is far simpler and less risky than the standard tracheotomy. If a satisfactory airway is obtained during the initial resuscitation by means of orotracheal tube, nasotracheal tube, or cricothyrotomy, then tracheotomy can be performed later if necessary, without hurry in the operating room.

If the patient's larynx has been traumatized directly, cricothyrotomy should not be performed. In these patients, intubations need not be difficult and should be attempted first. If placement of an endotracheal tube is not possible, several large-bore needles are inserted through the cricothyroid membrane and oxygen is given by insufflation (Procedure 7). This procedure may sustain a patient's life until a tracheotomy can be performed. Should the above measures fail or if large-bore needles are not available, an emergency tracheotomy should be performed (Procedure 10). The physician who has never performed this is cautioned not to attempt to do so in emergency situations unless simpler procedures are ineffective and a trained surgeon is not available.

INTRAVENOUS ACCESS

A plastic intravenous cannula is inserted into all patients with respiratory distress to allow administration of drugs and fluids. At the time of insertion, a blood sample is sent to the laboratory for complete blood count (CBC), electrolytes, blood urea nitrogen (BUN), and glucose. If the patient is suspected of drug overdose, a blood sample is sent for toxicologic analysis. In patients with trauma or surgical disease, a blood sample is sent to the blood bank so that it may be typed and cross matched.

MONITORING AND MEASUREMENTS

Arterial Blood Gases

While oxygen is being administered and the airway is being established, a member of the emergency room team should obtain a sample of arterial blood for analysis (Procedure 13).

During the course of emergency room management of patients with acute respiratory insufficiency, serial blood gas measurements are obtained every 15–30 minutes to monitor changes in respiratory function. In patients who are likely to require prolonged intensive care, the percutaneous insertion of a radial artery cannula will facilitate serial arterial blood gas measurements and will allow continuous monitoring of the arterial pressure. The adequacy of the ulnar circulation should be ascertained before placement of the cannula by performance of an Allen test (Procedure 14).

Vital Signs

All patients with acute respiratory insufficiency require frequent or continuous monitoring of blood pressure, pulse, and respiratory rate. A flowchart should be used to follow the various parameters. The patient's cardiac rhythm should be monitored continuously by use of an electronic monitor. A standard 12-lead electrocardiogram (ECG) is taken for most patients as a baseline and also to assist in detecting those cases in which the underlying cause for respiratory insufficiency is cardiac.

Central Venous Pressure or Pulmonary Capillary Wedge Pressure

Not infrequently, respiratory insufficiency is caused by derangement of cardiovascular function. In addition, measures that are used to combat respiratory failure sometimes have an adverse effect on the cardiovascular system. In these situations, central venous pressure (CVP) or pulmonary capillary wedge pressure (PCWP) must be monitored. The central venous line can be placed when the patient is in the emergency room (Procedure 12). The CVP is helpful in assessing a patient's volume status and provides a convenient route for the administration of cardiotonic drugs. It cannot be used safely, however, if there is left ventricular failure or intrinsic pulmonary disease, nor is the CVP an accurate monitor when PEEP is being used. In these situations a Swan-Ganz catheter should be inserted in order to monitor the PCWP. This catheter should be inserted when the patient is in the intensive care unit or operating room.

Vital Capacity

In patients in whom impending respiratory insufficiency is suspected, the measurement of vital capacity is helpful. The vital capacity is defined as the maximum expired volume after a maximal inspiration. It is best measured with the patient sitting upright. The measurement is simple, and all that is needed is a spirometer, a one-way valve, and a snug face mask or mouthpiece. The normal vital capacity in young, healthy men is approximately 70 ml/kg, but most patients can tolerate a vital capacity as low as 20 ml/kg without any appreciable respiratory difficulty. Patients with a vital capacity less than 10 ml/kg will eventually become exhausted when breathing spontaneously and will require mechanical ventilatory support. Serial vital capacity measurements are essential in managing patients with ascending polyneuritis or myasthenia gravis.

Alveolar–Arterial Oxygen Difference

Determination of the alveolar–arterial oxygen difference (A-aDo$_2$) is an important diagnostic procedure in the early detection of imminent respiratory insufficiency since this value changes before the patient has lost the ability to maintain adequate oxygenation. The A-aDo$_2$ can be measured at any inspired O_2 concentration, but it correlates best with changes in intrapulmonary shunting when measured after a patient has inspired 100% O_2 for 15–20 minutes. The A-aDo$_2$ obtained on 100% O_2 (A-aDo$_2{}^1$) is calculated by the following equation:

$$A\text{-aDo}_2{}^1 = P_B - P_{H_2O} - Paco_2 - Pao_2$$

where P_B is barometric pressure and P_{H_2O} is tension of water vapor in the lung (47 mm Hg at 37°C). The normal A-aDo$_2{}^1$ is 50–75 mm Hg. A rough approximation of the percentage of shunt can be made by dividing the A-aDo$_2{}^1$ by 20.

In the absence of CO_2 retention and acidemia, most patients breathing spontaneously with an A-aDo$_2{}^1$ of less than 350 mm Hg can be managed by administering high concentrations of oxygen by face mask. An A-aDo$_2{}^1$ above 350 mm Hg is generally an indication for intubation and mechanical ventilation.

Foley Catheter

Most patients who are in severe respiratory distress or who require endotracheal intubation will also require an in-dwelling bladder catheter. This prevents urinary retention and allows close monitoring of urinary output and volume status.

INITIAL DIAGNOSTIC STUDIES

Chest Radiograph

As soon as the necessary life support systems have been started a chest film should be taken, not only as an aid for diagnosis and management, but also to confirm the position of any tubes that may have been placed. This should be a portable film. The endotracheal tube tip should be at least 2 cm above the carina.

Gram Smear and Cultures

Whenever pulmonary or systemic infection is suspected, sputum cultures and blood cultures for aerobic and anaerobic organisms should be obtained. A Gram stain of the sputum should always be performed (see Chapter 28).

AIRWAY CARE

In the patient with respiratory insufficiency, the airway must be kept as patent and as free of secretions as possible so that gas exchange may be maintained at a maximum level. Chest physiotherapy is useful in clearing secretions and preventing airway closure and atelectasis.

Humidification

Water is a major therapeutic agent in the treatment of patients with bronchopulmonary disease. Secretions from bronchopulmonary infection and irritation may cover the mucosal surfaces of the respiratory tract with a dry coat that further compromises the airway. The water aerosol, which "rains out" in the airways, dilutes tenacious secretions, moistens dry crusts, and irritates the tracheal bronchial lining, thus stimulating coughing and expectoration of the diluted secretions. When a thickened secretion is the main problem, the primary need is for some form of humidification. Dry oxygen has an intensely drying effect on the mucosa of the respiratory tract. Oxygen should be given in humidified form when possible.

Mechanical Ventilation

Mechanical ventilation is mandatory for patients who are unable to maintain adequate oxygenation in spite of the use of the modalities of therapy previously described. It must be stressed that mechanical ventilation is generally a supportive tool. The respiratory muscles of patients who are laboring to get air in and out of their lungs require as much as 40% of the total oxygen used, contrasted with the 1–3% of oxygen used by patients during normal respiratory activity. Assisted or controlled ventilation provides these struggling patients with more available oxygen and, at the same time, significantly reduces their work of breathing while other measures are applied to reverse the underlying pathophysiologic processes, if such a reversal is possible.

Table 2.8 lists some of the clinical indications for initiation of mechanical ventilation. Sometimes the indications are clear-cut and the decision is obvious when the patient is first seen. More often, however, the decision is made by following the

TABLE 2.8 Physiologic and Biochemical Criteria for Institution of Controlled Ventilation

PaO_2 less than 70 mm Hg while breathing more than 60% oxygen
$A\text{-}aDO_2$ greater than 350 mm Hg while breathing 100% oxygen
$PaCO_2$ increasing above 60 mm Hg
pHa decreasing below 7.25 mm Hg
Vital capacity less than 10 ml/kg
V_D/V_T greater than 0.6 (performed in ICU)

response of arterial blood gases, repeated frequently (every 15 or 20 minutes) after oxygen therapy has been begun in the emergency room. The physician should be guided by the clinical situation rather than by a number. As previously noted, some patients with incipient respiratory failure initially hyperventilate in an effort to compensate for the derangements. This leads to an initial reduction in $PaCO_2$. The sudden rise of $PaCO_2$ above 40 mm Hg in these patients often signals the overwhelming of the compensatory mechanisms. Death may occur rapidly if mechanical ventilation is not begun quickly. On the other hand, a $PaCO_2$ of 60 mm Hg or above in a patient with chronic obstructive pulmonary disease (COPD) is an indication for mechanical ventilation only if there is evidence that the $PaCO_2$ is rising rapidly because of a superimposed acute problem that is producing acute respiratory acidosis. In the patient with COPD, a PaO_2 of 50–60 mm Hg is usually adequate.

Once a patient with COPD is intubated and placed on mechanical ventilation, it may be difficult to wean him or her from ventilatory support at a later time. Before the patient is placed in this situation, the appropriateness as well as the indications for mechanical ventilation must be discussed with the patient, the family, and the physician (see below).

TRANSPORT OF PATIENTS WITH RESPIRATORY INSUFFICIENCY TO THE INTENSIVE CARE UNIT

After the life-threatening emergencies have been dealt with and the patient's condition has been stabilized, transfer of the patient from the emergency room to the intensive care unit (ICU) can be considered. Safe transfer for these patients requires careful coordination between emergency room and intensive care unit personnel. Before transfer, the intensive care unit must have prepared a bed and equipment space and obtained the necessary monitoring and ventilatory equipment. During transfer, the patient should be accompanied by a physician, nurse, and respiratory therapist. The safety of the transfer depends upon continuation of all monitoring and therapeutic measures that were instituted in the emergency room. Ventilation can be continued manually with Ambu bag and oxygen supplied from a small portable tank. Continuous ECG and arterial monitoring need not be interrupted since many portable battery powered multichannel monitors are available. A battery powered direct current (DC) defibrillator and resuscitation kit with all drugs and equipment necessary for treatment of cardiopulmonary arrest must accompany the transport of critically ill patients with respiratory failure. A summary of the management of respiratory distress is given in Table 2.9.

UPPER AIRWAY OBSTRUCTION

The causes of acute upper airway obstruction are shown in Figure 2.5. Upper airway obstruction is life threatening and patients require immediate therapy. Its onset may either be insidious or acute. Acute respiratory insufficiency caused by upper airway obstruction may occur in all age groups. It is most commonly seen, however, in infants and young children.

TABLE 2.9 Essentials of Emergency Room Management of Respiratory Insufficiency

1. Early recognition of signs
    a. Dyspnea
    b. Tachypnea
    c. Labored respirations
    d. Stridor
    e. Wheezing
    f. Rales
    g. Cyanosis
    h. Obtundation
    i. Apnea
2. Quick assessment of primary cause
    a. Cardiopulmonary arrest
    b. Upper airway obstruction
    c. Lower airway obstruction
    d. Pulmonary edema
    e. Inadequate central respiratory drive
    f. Impaired chest wall mechanics
3. Early therapeutic intervention
    a. Clearing of upper airway
    b. Supplemental inspired oxygen
    c. Intubation and controlled ventilation
    d. Insertion of chest tube for tension pneumothorax
4. Early measurements of cardiopulmonary function
    a. Systemic blood pressure and heart rate
    b. Arterial blood gases
    c. Hemoglobin, BUN, serum glucose, and electrolytes, type and cross match
    d. Chest film
    e. 12-lead ECG
    f. Central venous or pulmonary arterial pressure catheter

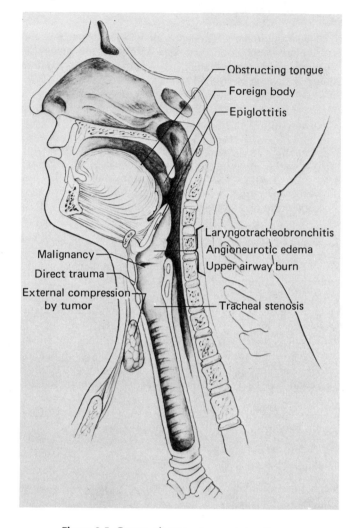

Figure 2.5 Causes of upper airway obstruction.

The increased susceptibility of children can be explained to a large extent by the smaller diameter of the airway. A 1-mm reduction in a 5-mm airway causes an increase in resistance to airflow 100 times greater than a 1-mm reduction in a 12-mm airway.

The patient with upper airway obstruction may present with shortness of breath, hoarseness, and progressive stridor. The cause is usually evident from a brief history. Gurgling sounds may be heard in the upper airway. The patient may have difficulty in clearing secretions. Partial obstruction may progress to total obstruction with remarkable rapidity. Complete airway obstruction demands immediate intervention with laryngoscopy, endotracheal intubation, or cricothyrotomy and resuscitation, if necessary. If the situation is not life threatening, the following, more leisurely course, can be followed: provide humidified oxygen; obtain a brief history; examine the patient's head, neck, oropharynx, and lungs; determine the arterial blood gases; and insert an intravenous cannula. Consultations with an anesthesiologist and otolaryngologist may be helpful. Indirect and direct laryngoscopy need not be performed immediately unless the presence of a foreign body or cervical trauma is suspected or insertion of an endotracheal tube is intended. Lateral neck films (with a physician and facilities for intubation available) may be helpful.

Foreign Bodies in the Upper Airway

The occlusion of the airway by a foreign body occurs commonly and is the sixth leading cause of accidental death in the United States. Obstruction of the airway may occur while the patient is eating at a restaurant, giving name to the so-called cafe coronary. There is a strong association of this entity with the ingestion of alcohol and the wearing of dentures. Choking may also be caused by a swallowing dysfunction secondary to esophageal motility disorders or pseudobulbar disease.

Whereas food is a common foreign body in an adult, a child may obstruct the airway with any object that he or she places into the mouth. Children commonly choke on a foreign object while simultaneously eating and running.

Airway obstruction caused by a foreign body may be partial or complete. If partial, the patient will cough and show inspiratory stridor. Patients with partial airway obstruction who are coughing and able to speak should not be interfered with since they will be able to clear their airways more effectively than by externally applied maneuvers.

Patients with complete obstruction are *unable to speak or breathe*. They may place their hands at their necks to show they are choking, and then become pale and rapidly progress to unconsciousness with cyanosis. The victim of choking may not be noticed until he or she has progressed to unconsciousness and is found lying on the ground. The care of patients with foreign body obstruction in the upper airway is discussed in Chapters 1 and 44.

Patients with complete airway obstruction who are brought to the emergency room are usually in extremis and have probably suffered hypoxic brain injury if obstruction has been longer than 4–6 minutes. The obstruction should be immediately removed under direct laryngoscopy using Magill forceps. Full cardiopulmonary resuscitation will probably be necessary.

In caring for patients who claim to have aspirated or swallowed a foreign body but do not appear to be in respiratory distress, lateral neck films may be helpful in locating the site of enlodgement. A thin, flat coin may rest in the sagittal plane if it is caught between the vocal cords or in the larynx, or it may be in the coronal plane if it is in the esophagus. Bronchoscopy may be necessary to remove foreign bodies located below the cords; this is best performed in the operating room.

Once the foreign body has been removed, follow-up care consists of a chest film to rule out aspiration or the existence of another foreign body. The film may not show the object but may show hyperinflation distal to the obstruction. If the object removed was sharp, laryngoscopy is in order to look at the patient's vocal cords and upper airway. The patient should be watched for fever, soreness, and dysphagia as signs of perforation or ulceration. Patients with repeated patterns of choking and aspiration of foreign bodies deserve workup for tracheoesophageal fistula, Zenker's diverticulum, esophageal webs, neurologic disorders, or abnormalities of esophageal motility.

Infectious Causes of Upper Airway Obstruction

EPIGLOTTITIS

Epiglottitis and croup are infectious causes of life-threatening upper airway obstruction. Epiglottitis is caused by bacteria, typically *Haemophilus influenzae* or β-hemolytic streptococci. It occurs most frequently in children over 2 years, but it may also occur in infants and adults.

Diagnosis

The course is fulminant and is characterized by upper respiratory tract infection occurring for fewer than 24 hours and a temperature greater than 39°C (102°F). Patients present with dysphagia and drooling and are in respiratory distress. The patient prefers to sit leaning forward. Coughing is frequently absent, and stridor is less prominent than with croup. There is leukocytosis with a left shift.

If the diagnosis is in doubt, the patient may be accompanied to the x-ray department by an anesthetist for lateral soft tissue neck films before the direct examination. Films should not be obtained if they will delay definitive treatment.

Therapy

The diagnosis of epiglottitis is confirmed by direct examination, but this should not be performed in the emergency room since it may lead to further swelling and complete obstruction. Examination should be performed in the operating room with an experienced laryngoscopist present. Laryngoscopy will show a cherry-red epiglottis with surrounding edema. Conservative therapy dictates endotracheal intubation at this time, using an endotracheal tube 1 mm smaller than usual, since patients with epiglottitis are notorious for the development of sudden complete airway obstruction. The endotracheal tube is removed when there is a significant air leak around the tube. This usually occurs within 2–3 days. In children, dexamethasone, 0.5 mg/kg, should be given before extubation; the initial antibiotic of choice is ampicillin 100 mg/kg. Management of patients with this condition is discussed in Chapter 44.

Epiglottitis occurs in adults but is usually not as fulminant as in children. It can be severe when associated with *H. influenzae.* Diagnosis is suggested by sore throat, respiratory distress, muffled voice, and cervical adenopathy. The patient's temperature will be about 38.5°C (101°F) and white blood cell count will be about 15,000–20,000. The adult disease is more slowly moving than it is in children; a sore throat develops approximately 2 days before respiratory distress. Therapy is humidified oxygen, broad-spectrum antibiotics, and airway management when indicated.

CROUP

As indicated in Chapter 44, croup differs from epiglottitis in that it is a viral illness caused by parainfluenza, influenza, or Respiratory syncytial (RSV) viruses. The child who presents with croup is usually under 3 years old and has had an upper respiratory tract infection for more than 24 hours. The patient presents with rhinorrhea and low-grade fever and progresses to having a high-pitched barking cough with inspiratory stridor. The patient shows retractions, nasal flaring, tachypnea, and dyspnea. White blood cell count is usually normal and there is some lymphocytic predominance.

Humidified oxygen in a croup tent remains the mainstay of croup therapy since hypoxemia is found in a majority of patients with croup. Racemic epinephrine, 1 part in 7 through a micronebulizer, and dexamethasone (Decadron), 0.5 mg/kg intravenously, may be added. Endotracheal intubation can usually be averted by these measures.

LUDWIG'S ANGINA

Ludwig's angina (Fig. 32.9e) is a rare and virulent infection that consists of inflammation of the soft tissues of the sublingual space. There may be extension to the submaxillary or soft tissues of the neck. It may begin as trauma to the interior of the mouth, as oral infection, or as tonsillitis. Frequently, streptococci or gas-producing bacteria are the causative organisms. The disease is most frequently seen in children and young adults. The airway is compromised by displacement of the tongue superiorly and posteriorly. There is boardlike swelling in the submaxillary and submental areas and induration of the

floor of the mouth. There may be trismus secondary to spasm of the internal pterygoid muscles. Temperature and white blood cell count are both elevated. Therapy consists of semielective tracheostomy, appropriate antibiotics, and warm packs applied to the infected area. Should an abscess form, incision and drainage are indicated after the airway is secured.

Respiratory Injury after Burns

Respiratory compromise after burns may be either of the upper or lower airways and may be due to thermal or inhalation injury. Thermal injury is most common after steam burns and causes respiratory embarrassment secondary to edema of the upper airway, including epiglottis, vocal cords, and upper trachea. The upper airway rapidly cools the air and thus protects the lung parenchyma. Inhalation injury is caused by smoke and other noxious products of incomplete combustion. These substances produce mucosal damage and sloughing, paralysis of cilia, bronchospasm, loss of surfactant, atelectasis, and edema.

DIAGNOSIS

Initially, the burn patient with a respiratory component presents with hoarseness, wheezing, and production of carbonaceous sputum. Ninety-five percent of these patients will have burns on their faces with injection of the mouth and pharynx. Many will have been burned while they were in a closed space. Chest examination may show rales or bronchial breath sounds. Some patients show no signs of pulmonary compromise at admission but develop signs of respiratory distress 24–72 hours later. This latter group of patients will have previously been admitted to the hospital for therapy for their burns. Their management is discussed in Chapter 25.

The frequent monitoring of blood gases is mandatory since burn patients are hypoxemic. Available oxygen is decreased and extraction and consumption are increased. Early on, the cardiac output is decreased. These patients may be further compromised by high levels of carboxyhemoglobin. The chest films may reveal little or may show diffuse or patchy infiltrates. The xenon 133 lung scan may shown early inhalation injury before physical or radiologic signs are manifest.

THERAPY

Patients with mild upper airway obstruction should be treated with dexamethasone, 10 mg intravenously. More severe obstruction dictates endotracheal intubation; if it is performed early it may prevent the need for emergency cricothyrotomy or tracheostomy. The protection of the airway becomes increasingly more difficult as the patient's face and pharynx become more swollen. An endotracheal tube should be placed early, when it may be done easily, to prevent the performance of a tracheostomy when such placement becomes impossible. Tracheostomy introduces a serious additional source of sepsis. Arterial blood gases dictate the need for mechanical ventilation or PEEP. Patients with carbon monoxide intoxication are treated with controlled ventilation and 100% oxygen. The transfusion of packed red blood cells improves oxygen-carrying capacity and content. Oxygen should be humidified for the burn patient, and chest physiotherapy should be ordered.

Tracheal Stenosis and Tracheal Tumors

Respiratory distress secondary to narrowing of the tracheal lumen may have iatrogenic causes, such as previous tracheostomy or endotracheal intubation, or there may be encroachment of the laryngeal or tracheal lumen because of narrowing by tumor or extrinsic tracheal compression. Stenosis after tracheostomy usually occurs at the level of the tracheostomy from cicatricial healing of the stoma. Tracheomalacia may be found at the level of the cuff.

DIAGNOSIS

Patients with tracheal stenosis and tracheal tumors present with shortness of breath, wheezing, and stridor. They have difficulty in clearing secretions, which leads to obstruction. Hemoptysis is seen in patients with tracheal tumors, but it is a late sign. Diagnosis is aided by lateral soft tissue neck films and bronchoscopy. A chest film should be obtained to rule out other causes of tracheal obstruction or pneumonitis. Fluoroscopy is useful in revealing tracheomalacia.

THERAPY

Therapy consists of administration of humidified oxygen. Dexamethasone, 8–10 mg intravenously, may reduce swelling. Arterial blood gases are a necessity. Patients will first show tachypnea and hyperpnea, but they may tire because of consequent retention of carbon dioxide. Should an elevation of $Paco_2$ become apparent, the patient will require endotracheal intubation. An assortment of pediatric and standard endotracheal tubes should be made available as soon as the diagnosis is suspected. It is hoped that patients can be stabilized before bronchoscopy and surgery so that tracheal reconstruction may be done only as an elective or semielective procedure.

Laryngeal Trauma

Damage to the larynx may occur from direct trauma to the neck or, functionally, from damage to the laryngeal nerves.

Laryngeal trauma commonly occurs in association with automobile accidents when the victim is thrown forward and hits the neck on the steering wheel or dashboard. The patient may present with dysphagia, cough, hemoptysis, or neck pain. Physical examination may reveal a deformity of the neck contour, laryngeal tenderness, or bony crepitus. Should laryngeal damage be suspected, indirect and/or direct laryngoscopy is indicated. If there are signs of increasing dyspnea, gentle endotracheal intubation or tracheostomy must be performed (as discussed in Chapter 19).

The indirect causes of laryngeal dysfunction are varied and include damage to the laryngeal nerves by trauma, injury during surgery, malignant neoplasms, central nervous system dysfunction, and infection. The innervation of the larynx is from the vagus through the superior and recurrent laryngeal nerves. Transection of both the superior and recurrent laryngeal nerves will place the vocal cord in the cadaveric position midway between adduction and abduction. Complete section of the recurrent laryngeal nerve blocks both the abductors and the adductors, and the tensing action of the cricothyroid then causes the cords to adduct. Incomplete recurrent laryngeal nerve palsy causes paralysis of abduction before adduction so that the cord is brought to midline. If the partial recurrent nerve paralysis is bilateral, the cords meet at midline and airway obstruction occurs. Immediate treatment consists of endotracheal intubation, with succinylcholine 1.5 mg/kg if necessary, or cricothyroidotomy.

Angioneurotic Edema and Hypersensitivity Reactions

Edema of the upper airway may be caused by hereditary, allergic, or nonallergic factors. The allergic angioneurotic edemas and hypersensitivity reactions are discussed in Chapter 7. Hereditary angioneurotic edema is caused by the absence of C1 esterase inhibitor.

DIAGNOSIS

Patients with hereditary angioneurotic edema present with edema of the extremities, face, and airway and with recurrent abdominal pain. There may be submucosal edema of the upper respiratory tract. The precipitating event may be trauma, extremes of temperature, or emotional stress. Indirect laryngoscopy should be performed to evaluate the patient's airway.

THERAPY

Therapy for acute exacerbations is difficult, and although epinephrine (0.3–0.5 ml 1:1,000 subcutaneously) or hydrocortisone (1–5 mg/kg) should be tried, there may be little response to these agents. Compromise of the airway usually develops over several hours, and there is a change in voice or dysphagia. This is an indication for endotracheal intubation by an expert laryngoscopist since further trauma to the airway and larynx may rapidly lead to complete obstruction. Intubation can usually be performed on a nonemergency basis.

ACUTE LOWER AIRWAY OBSTRUCTION

Acute increases in lower airway resistance, which occur in patients with acute asthmatic crises or in patients with acute tracheobronchitis and chronic obstructive pulmonary disease (COPD) can lead to serious and life-threatening emergencies.

Asthma

Asthma is characterized by intermittent episodes of dyspnea and tachypnea while the patient is at rest with wheezes, rales, and rhonchi. The episodes vary in severity, ranging from mild dyspnea to a gasping, wheezing, hypoxemic struggle. What begins as a mild episode can rapidly progress to a severe attack, including hypoxemia, progressive hypercapnia, and metabolic and respiratory acidemia. Every patient admitted to the emergency room with an acute attack of asthma must receive critical attention and aggressive therapy. Status asthmaticus is a severe attack of asthma that does not respond to repeated dosages of epinephrine or theophylline.

Asthma attacks are usually triggered by exposure to airborne allergens or by tracheobronchial infection, but they may be precipitated by overuse of aerosols, termination of steroid therapy, or emotional stress. The pathology consists of narrowing and plugging of small bronchi and bronchioles caused by increased bronchoconstrictor tone, mucosal hypertrophy, and abundant viscous mucus. The involvement of the small bronchi and bronchioles is nonuniform. Hypoventilation of normally perfused alveoli distal to obstructed airways results in increased intrapulmonary shunting and decreased PaO_2. Mild hypoxemia appears during moderate degrees of airway obstruction and worsens as the obstruction becomes increasingly severe. Although the physiologic dead space of the lung increases during an acute asthma attack, carbon dioxide retention does not appear except during prolonged severe airway obstruction. Asthmatic patients with moderate airway obstruction are usually hypocapnic as the result of hyperventilation stimulated by hypoxemia and anxiety. Carbon dioxide retention develops as fatigue sets in and is an urgent indication for intervention with intubation and mechanical ventilation.

DIAGNOSIS

The diagnosis of acute asthma is usually easily established by symptoms and physical findings alone. A brief history is important to establish what medications, if any, the patient has already administered to him or herself. Questioning the patient may also uncover a history of heart disease, raising the possibility that the patient may have "cardiac" asthma as a manifestation of acute left ventricular failure. The emergency room physician must rule out pulmonary embolus, a foreign body, or pneumothorax as a cause of wheezing.

Most patients will have a PaO_2 less than 70 mm Hg and a $PaCO_2$ less than 40 mm Hg during an asthmatic attack. A $PaCO_2$ greater than 50 mm Hg in an asthmatic patient, especially associated with a pH less than 7.3, usually indicates that the patient is tiring, is critically ill, and should be hospitalized in an intensive care unit. Serum electrolytes should be measured since asthma can sometimes be associated with hyponatremia secondary to inappropriate antidiuretic hormone secretion. In addition, patients who are receiving cortisone may have reduced serum potassium. Serum theophylline levels should be measured in any patient who has been receiving any form of this medication.

If sputum is being produced, it should be examined by Gram stain since infection is one of the common precipitating factors of asthma. As soon as possible after the initial therapy has been started, a chest film should be taken to identify any associated pathology.

During a moderate asthmatic attack, the forced expiratory volume during the first second of exhalation (FEV_1) is reduced to 1,000–1,200 ml (in contrast to the normal FEV_1 of 3,000–4,000 ml) because of increased airway resistance. The FEV_1 will be less than 1,000 ml in patients experiencing severe asthma attacks and may be less than 500 ml in patients with status asthmaticus.

THERAPY

The emergency treatment of asthma requires the correction of hypoxemia, reduction of bronchoconstrictor tone, correction of metabolic acidemia, hydration, and mobilization of airway secretions. While arrangements are being made to alleviate bronchospasm, it is essential to give the patient high concentrations of humidified oxygen. Ideally, the gas should be saturated with water vapor using a heated humidifier. For asthmatic patients, nebulizers should only be used with great caution when airway secretions cannot be thinned by humidifier therapy alone since the droplets of water generated by a nebulizer may irritate distal airways and aggravate bronchospasm.

Hydration

An intravenous cannula should be inserted when the blood specimen is obtained for electrolyte determination. Patients with asthma rapidly become dehydrated from respiratory water loss and from the exhaustion and breathlessness that makes it difficult for them to take fluids orally during an attack. Their sputum becomes thick and tenacious. Five percent dextrose in water (D_5W) may be given until serum electrolyte values are known. In the emergency room, 100–200 ml of fluid can be given every hour. In the average adult patient who requires hospitalization for asthma, the fluid intake should be continued at 3,000–3,500 ml/day to ensure adequate loosening of secretions. If the patient is only moderately distressed, the fluids may be given orally. Care must be exercised, however, because the theophyllines often lead to gastric irritation and vomiting.

Drug Therapy

Reduction in bronchoconstrictor tone is accomplished with β-adrenergic stimulants and theophyllines. Electrocardiographic monitoring should be established before bronchodilator therapy is begun since both the β-adrenergic stimulants and the theophyllines can cause serious cardiac arrhythmias. The medication record must be constantly reviewed during the management of patients with a severe asthma attack.

Epinephrine, the most commonly used adrenergic stimulant, is usually given subcutaneously in a dose of 0.3–0.5 ml of 1:1,000 dilution. Severely acidotic patients may fail to show improvement after receiving epinephrine, but correction of the pH to greater than 7.2 with intravenous bicarbonate will usually restore its effectiveness.

Terbutaline, a newer drug with greater specificity for bronchial muscle beta receptors, can be given in dosages of 0.25–0.5 mg subcutaneously every 4 hours. Because of its specificity for bronchial muscle, its incidence of causing cardiac arrythmias is less than that of epinephrine or isoproterenol. An additional advantage is that terbutaline is longer acting than epinephrine.

For patients with severe asthma *aminophylline* is the most immediately effective drug for the rapid relief of bronchoconstriction. It is given in a slow intravenous infusion of 4–7 mg/kg over a 15–30-minute period. Subsequently, infusions of 1 mg/kg/hr will suffice for most patients. The serum level of theophylline should be monitored to ensure therapeutic levels (10–20 μg/ml) and to avoid toxicity. Many physicians find it useful to mix 500 mg aminophylline in 500 ml D_5W and give both the loading dose and maintenance dosages from this mixture. This treatment will also begin rehydration of the patient.

Inhalation Therapy

In patients suffering from an acute asthmatic attack, intermittent positive pressure breathing (IPPB) is often useful as a vehicle for the delivery of aerosolized medications. In adults, 0.5 ml 1:200 isoproterenol in 5 ml normal saline or 0.5 ml 1:200 isoetharine in 5 ml normal saline may be given over a 15-minute period. Because of its powerful $β_2$-adrenergic stimulating effect (smooth muscle relaxation) isoproterenol is a potent bronchodilator. However, its $beta_1$ receptor (cardiac stimulation) action combined with its vasodilation effect sometimes results in such an increase in cardiac output and pulmonary perfusion that the ventilation–perfusion ratio is reduced (pulmonary perfusion is increased more than the bronchodilatation that improves ventilation). As a result, the hypoxemia may paradoxically worsen. Furthermore, the risk of cardiac arrhythmias is increased by $beta_1$ stimulation in the presence of hypoxia. In spite of these potential risks, extensive clinical experience with isoproterenol has proved that it can still be used effectively as an aerosol bronchodilator with a wide range of safety. Correction of hypoxemia with oxygen and continuous ECG monitoring should minimize the possibility of induction of cardiac arrhythmias by isoproterenol.

Isoetharine has gained wide acceptance as a bronchodilator. Through its $beta_2$ specificity it relaxes bronchial smooth muscles but has a much less stimulating action on the heart than does isoproterenol. Isoetharine combined with the topical vasoconstrictor effect of phenylephrine (Bronkosol) produces relaxation of bronchospasm and, at the same time, shrinkage of swollen mucous membranes. Phenylephrine may cause excessive tachycardia or other cardiac arrhythmias, and if it is given to patients with hypertension, cardiac disease, acute coronary occlusion, or hyperthyroidism, it must be given with great caution.

In the subacute or chronic situation, isoproterenol, isoetharine, or racemic epinephrine can be given by hand-bulb nebulizers, inert cartridges, or IPPB. The technique for use of the hand-bulb or cartridge nebulizers is as follows: After maximal expiration, aerosol is inhaled slowly to full inspiration, and the breath is held for several seconds. The cycle is repeated after a pause of 1 minute for a total of 2–4 inhalations. For the hand-bulb nebulizer, 2.25% racemic epinephrine of 1:200 isoproterenol should be used; for the powered nebulizers or IPPB, 0.5–1 ml 1:200 isoproterenol or 2.25% racemic epinephrine is diluted with 2–4 ml saline or water, which is enough for 10–15 minutes of treatment. The aerosolization of β-adrenergic agents may also be useful in the therapy for severe asthma in patients who have been intubated.

Sodium Bicarbonate

Patients with very severe asthmatic crises will frequently develop lactic acidosis as the result of hypoxemia and the intense struggle to breathe. The severity of the lactic acidosis is often compounded by a concurrent respiratory acidosis. Correction of the metabolic component with sodium bicarbonate will improve myocardial and central nervous system function and improve pulmonary circulation and will augment the beneficial effects of endogenous and exogenous catecholamines during the crisis. It must be given with care, and the patient's response must be carefully monitored in order to avoid the precipitation of metabolic alkalosis.

Chest Physiotherapy

In some asthmatic patients, part of their airway obstruction is caused by tenacious secretions in the respiratory tract. For these patients, physical methods of sputum removal should be used as an adjuvant to the bronchodilators. Vigorous percussion and postural drainage is not usually tolerated during the acute attack, but the use of pillows to elevate the patient's hips, if well tolerated, can be helpful in mobilizing secretions.

Corticosteroids

Patients who do not respond to the therapy discussed above within 4–8 hours or who have been on maintenance steroid therapy should be given large doses of steroids early, although the clinical effect of this form of therapy is delayed 12–24 hours. Steroids are also indicated in patients with profound eosinophilia, poor cardiac status that may limit other modalities of treatment, or a rapid downhill course. The asthmatic patient may need a plasma 17-hydroxycorticosteriod concentration in excess of 100 μg/100 ml. This may be obtained by intravenous hydrocortisone succinate, 4 mg/kg every 3–4 hours. The asthmatic patient who is dependent on steroids may need even larger dosages to achieve this blood level as a result of a markedly elevated metabolic clearance rate of cortisol.

Hospital Admission

Asthmatic patients should be admitted to the hospital if their asthma attack fails to break within 8 hours, FEV_1 is less than 1 liter, there is carbon dioxide retention, they exhibit an inability to retain fluids or medications, or this is their first time on steroid therapy.

Intubation and Mechanical Ventilation

A few patients who progress to status asthmaticus fail to respond to the aforementioned treatments and require intubation and controlled ventilation while they are in the intensive care unit. Intubation should be performed by experienced personnel. Undue laryngeal and tracheal stimulation will aggravate an already dangerous bronchospasm. Mechanical ventilation is accomplished with a volume-controlled ventilator since airway pressures of 50 cm H_2O or higher are often required. Pressure-limited ventilators will be inadequate and should not be used for these patients. Since patients should be paralyzed with pancuronium bromide, 0.05–0.1 mg/kg, this support should be given when the patient is in an intensive care unit. After institution of controlled ventilation, 1–2 mg doses of diazepam or morphine sulfate may be given for sedation. Sedatives should never be administered to a patient experiencing a severe asthma attack before intubation and mechanical ventilation.

Acute Respiratory Insufficiency in Patients with Chronic Obstructive Pulmonary Disease

Bronchitis or emphysema alone may be the cause of chronic obstructive pulmonary disease (COPD); however the two usually coexist. Emphysema is associated with destruction of respiratory bronchioles and alveoli. This damage can cause obstruction of distal airways, obliteration of small pulmonary vessels, and increased physiologic dead space. Chronic bronchitis is characterized by mucous gland hypertrophy and increased mucus secretion in the bronchi and bronchioles. The excessive mucus production and impaired clearing (diminished cough and ciliary activity) result in obstruction of both large and small airways. Infection of the bronchi and bronchioles is frequently, but not always, present. Increased intrapulmonary shunting occurs in patients with severe COPD as a result of patchy hypoventilation of well-perfused regions of the lung, most commonly at the lung bases. Increased work of breathing is mainly as a result of increased airway resistance.

Chronic hypoxemia and hypercapnia cause pulmonary arterial constriction and hypertrophy, which, superimposed on the obliteration of small pulmonary vessels, leads to failure of the right side of the heart (cor pulmonale). Progressive hypoventilation causes increasing hypoxemia and carbon dioxide retention, which progresses to somnolence and coma. These patients may present with papilledema as a sign of increased intracranial pressure because of increased $Paco_2$. Cardiac arrhythmias and gastrointestinal bleeding are additional complications associated with carbon dioxide retention.

Respiratory failure in patients with chronic obstructive pulmonary disease is usually precipitated by some identifiable cause. Although infection is by far the most common underlying factor, cardiac decompensation, trauma, oversedation, surgery, or pulmonary embolism may be responsible. Treatment must involve the correction of these conditions.

INITIAL DIAGNOSIS

A careful evaluation is mandatory when a patient with suspected chronic obstructive pulmonary disease comes to the emergency room in respiratory distress. The patient must be examined carefully to determine whether or not there is evidence of congestive heart failure or pulmonary infection. An arterial blood sample should be drawn immediately while the patient is breathing room air and is in a sitting position. Serum electrolytes are drawn concurrently to help distinguish between acute and chronic carbon dioxide retention. Patients with chronic carbon dioxide retention will have a hypochloremic hypokalemic alkalosis and high serum bicarbonate concentrations. Normal serum chloride and bicarbonate concentrations suggest that the patient with acutely decompensated chronic lung disease was previously normocapnic. An ECG should be taken to document the presence or absence of cor pulmonale and cardiac arrhythmias. A chest film is usually necessary since the auscultatory findings in this group of patients are not usually diagnostic.

THERAPY

Oxygen Therapy

It is essential that patients with acutely decompensated chronic obstructive pulmonary disease not be overtreated with O_2 since excessive inspired concentration may depress respiratory drive and cause CO_2 retention sometimes to the point of CO_2 narcosis. After the initial arterial sample is drawn, 24% O_2 is administered by Venturi mask. A PaO_2 of 50–60 mm Hg is adequate since small increases in a PaO_2 below 60 mm Hg will produce large changes in arterial O_2 content. The Venturi mask may be changed to deliver 28% or 35% O_2 if necessary. Arterial blood gases must be repeated to monitor the response to supplemental O_2.

Mobilization of Secretions

Aggressive therapy to improve oxygenation and ventilation without resorting to intubation and controlled ventilation is vitally important in the patients with COPD and requires an almost continuous nursing effort. Chest physiotherapy and water aerosol therapy are instituted in the emergency room, in addition to frequent encouragement from the nurses to cough and raise sputum.

Bronchodilators

Beta adrenergic stimulators can be given subcutaneously or by aerosol in patients with bronchospasm. Although isoproterenol is effective, its use is being superseded by terbutaline and metaproterenol, which have more specific bronchodilator action and less cardiac stimulation. Terbutaline may be given 2.5–5 mg orally four times a day or 0.25–0.5 mg subcutaneously. Isoproterenol or isoetharine may be used as aerosols, or aminophylline may be given intravenously as described for asthma treatment. This group of patients is more sensitive than patients with asthma to the side effects of bronchodilators. Atrial and ventricular arrhythmias are not uncommon after administration of these drugs. Corticosteroids are not used routinely, but they may be given intravenously in patients with acute exacerbation of bronchitis associated with wheezing.

Digitalis and Diuretic

The patient should be digitalized if there is evidence of biventricular insufficiency. Patients with cor pulmonale and right ventricular failure usually do not respond to digitalization but may respond to diuretic therapy and treatment of the lung disease. Adequate serum potassium must be assured before digitalization.

Treatment of Potassium Depletion and Hypochloremia

As discussed in Chapter 11, potassium chloride is given as needed to correct the hypochloremia and potassium depletion of chronic respiratory acidosis. This is of even greater importance in patients who have been on chronic diuretic therapy since most diuretics induce metabolic alkalosis, thereby decreasing the sensitivity of the respiratory center and increasing carbon dioxide retention.

Antibiotic Therapy

Respiratory infection is a frequent precipitating factor of acute respiratory insufficiency in these patients; the most frequent organisms are *Streptococcus pneumoniae, H. influenzae,* and viral agents. If there are signs of infection—fever, increased cough, increased amounts or thickening of sputum—antibiotic therapy should be initiated after a Gram stain of the sputum has been obtained and cultures have been taken. Ampicillin, tetracycline, or erythromycin, 1–2 g/day, can be given for 7–10 days.

Intubation and Controlled Ventilation

Aggressive therapy to improve oxygenation and ventilation without resorting to intubation and controlled ventilation in an intensive care unit is vitally important in these patients. Intubation and controlled ventilation are instituted only if serial arterial blood gas measurements and vital signs indicate imminent cardiopulmonary collapse. A controlled volume ventilator is used since high inspiratory pressures are often required and sudden changes in total pulmonary compliance may occur. Although arterial hypoxemia is corrected immediately, hypercapnia should be corrected slowly over a period of hours. Rapid reduction of the $PaCO_2$ can lead to seizures, hypotension, and serious cardiac arrhythmias. The eventual goal is usually not a $PaCO_2$ of 40 mm Hg, but rather a higher $PaCO_2$ estimated to be near the patient's usual value.

Hypotension is a common complication of mechanical ventilation in patients with COPD. Hypovolemia as the result of poor fluid intake and fever is usually obscured by the neurosympathetic and adrenergic response to hypercapnia and stress. Institution of controlled ventilation relieves the stress and reduces the $PaCO_2$, resulting in reduced neurosympathetic tone, and unmasking hypovolemia. Furthermore, mechanical ventilation impedes venous return by increasing mean intrathoracic pressure, especially in severely emphysematous patients. Intravascular volume replacement should be instituted with careful monitoring of the central venous or pulmonary artery and pulmonary capillary wedge pressures.

PROGNOSIS

The decision to intervene with intubation and controlled ventilation sometimes imposes an unpleasant dilemma for the emergency room physician. Institution of controlled ventilation in patients with terminal COPD may create a ventilator-dependent person whose existence until death is completely tied to physicians, nurses, machines, and tubing. It is impossible to predict with complete accuracy which patients will benefit and which patients will suffer from intervention with mechanical ventilation. The presence of an acute reversible contributing cause of acute respiratory failure in patients with a history of moderate daily physical activity usually suggests a good prognosis.

PULMONARY EDEMA

Pulmonary edema is the abnormal accumulation of fluid in the extravascular spaces of the lung. This space consists of the interstitial tissue space and the alveolar gas space. Pulmonary edema can be caused by increased capillary hydrostatic pressure, increased capillary endothelial permeability, and alterations in the balance of osmotic and oncotic forces. In normal lungs, salt and water pass freely across the pulmonary capillary endothelium into the interstitium and then back again in response to hydrostatic and osmotic forces. At the arterial end of the capillary, the sum of capillary hydrostatic pressure and

pulmonary interstitial osmotic pressure is greater than the capillary osmotic pressure. The net flux of salt and water is out of the capillary into the pulmonary interstitium. As the blood passes toward the venous end of the capillary, the capillary hydrostatic pressure and interstitial osmotic pressure decrease whereas the capillary osmotic pressure increases. At the venous end of the capillary, the net flux of fluid is back into the vessel. Protein, including albumin and some globulins, cross the endothelial barrier and eventually appear in the pulmonary lymph. The total protein concentration in normal pulmonary lymph is between 50 and 80% of the plasma–protein concentration.

A net outflow of fluid and protein from the capillary to the interstitial space exists which has been estimated to be approximately 20 ml/hr in healthy people. The rich lymphatic drainage of the lung easily accommodates this small net outflow. Pulmonary lymphatic drainage can increase up to 10 times in response to increased interstitial fluid accumulation.

Alteration in the delicate balance of osmotic and hydrostatic forces and membrane permeability can result in massive transudation of fluid and protein out of the capillaries and into the pulmonary interstitium. Eventually, fluid and protein will cross the alveolar walls into the alveoli as the lymphatic drainage is overwhelmed. The accumulation of fluid in the pulmonary extravascular spaces leads to a decrease in pulmonary compliance, narrowing of small peripheral airways, and alveolar flooding and collapse.

Vital capacity and the resting end expiratory lung volume or functional residual capacity (FRC) are reduced as small airway closure and alveolar collapse occur. The dependent portions of the lung where blood flow is greatest are the first to be affected. Arterial hypoxemia develops as blood continues to perfuse nonventilated alveoli. Whereas perfusion persists in nonventilated segments of lung, ventilation is shifted to relatively less-well-perfused segments, causing an increase in physiologic dead space. Respiratory rate and minute ventilation must increase to compensate for this. The combination of stiffer lungs and increased demand for minute ventilation results in markedly increased work of breathing in patients with pulmonary edema.

Hypoxemia is an early finding in patients with pulmonary edema. Hypoventilation and carbon dioxide retention usually do not occur until exhaustion has set in during the preterminal phase of pulmonary edema.

Cardiac Pulmonary Edema

The most common cause of increased intracapillary hydrostatic pressure is left ventricular failure. When there is an increase in capillary hydrostatic pressure there is a proportional increase in fluid transudation. Lymphatic drainage increases. In previously normal lungs, no significant accumulation of extravascular fluid occurs until the left atrial pressure exceeds 25–30 cm H_2O. When an abrupt increase in intracapillary pressure occurs and is large enough to exceed circulatory compensatory mechanisms, pulmonary edema develops. Common causes of acute left ventricular failure include acute myocardial injury, arrythmias, valvular disease, anemia, excessive administration of blood and fluid while resuscitating patients in shock, and the intravascular absorption of massive amounts of water during fresh water drowning.

DIAGNOSIS

Diagnosis of cardiac pulmonary edema is usually established on the basis of historical information and the physical findings of cyanosis, tachypnea, and moist pulmonary rales. Occasionally, pink froth may be apparent in the patient's mouth and nostrils. A grossly elevated A-aDO_2[1] is present.

Chest Film

Although the treatment of acute pulmonary edema should begin when the diagnosis is suspected, a chest film should be obtained as soon as possible. The radiographic changes of pulmonary edema occur in a standard sequence. The first change is redistribution of intrapulmonary blood flow to the upper lobes of the lung. With increasing venous pressure, there is decreased flow to the lower lobes caused by increasing interstitial edema. Apparent blood flow to the upper zones of the lung increases.

The changes that occur with interstitial pulmonary edema have been summarized as follows (Fig. 2.6):

1. *Perivascular cuffing.* The well-defined pulmonary arteries lose their definition and become blurred.
2. *Perihilar hazing.* With increasing interstitial edema, the hilar borders become ill defined.
3. *Septal lines.* Edema collects in the lymphatics, which are normally not visible. They appear as sharp, linear densities that extend from the pleural surface toward the center of the chest.
4. *Subpleural fluid.* Fluid may accumulate in the subpleural space.
5. *Alveolar pulmonary edema.* As the volume and pressure of interstitial fluid become greater than the ability of the pulmonary lymphatics to cope with it, fluid moves into the alveolus. The density of this fluid appears the same as that

of pneumonia, but it is highly gravity dependent. It will vary as the patient's position varies.

THERAPY

The therapy for acute pulmonary edema is aimed at increasing oxygenation and ventilation, decreasing left ventricular filling, and improving left ventricular function.

If significant hypotension is not present, the patient should be placed in an upright sitting position. This position increases vital capacity and decreases venous return to the heart. Oxygen is given by mask or nasal cannulae, and arterial blood gases are obtained. Positive pressure ventilation may be applied with bag and mask to decrease venous return and decrease intrapulmonary shunt. If there is no improvement after appropriate drug therapy and assisted positive pressure ventilation, intubation with controlled ventilation is indicated.

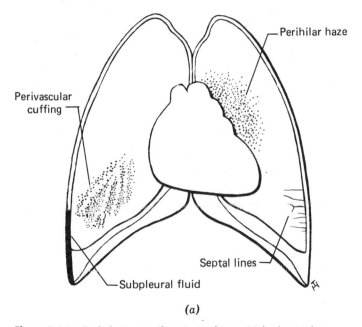

(a)

Figure 2.6 (a) Radiologic manifestations of interstitial edema. (b) Interstitial edema; the pulmonary vessels are blurred and the hilum of the lung has lost its sharp border. (c) Septal lines in chronic failure of the left side of the heart, which extend from pleural surface to center of thorax. (d) Segmental alveolar edema. (e) Alveolar pulmonary edema. The edema fluid is collected centrally in the alveoli around the hilum. Note the clarity of the periphery of the lungs. (Used with permission form Dr. Herbert Abrams, Chief of Radiology, Brigham and Women's Hospital, Boston, MA)

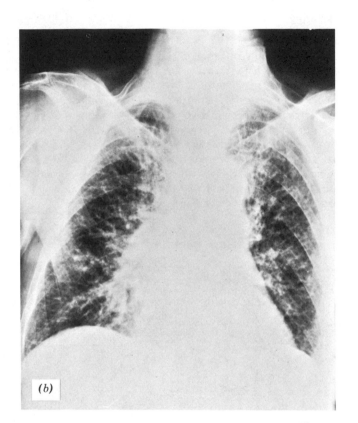

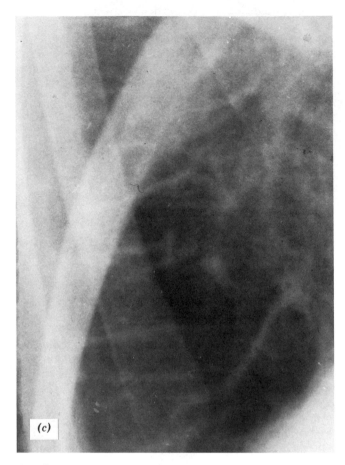

Figure 2.6 (*Continued*)

Intravenous Access

An intravenous solution of D_5W to keep the vein open is begun in order that intravenous medications may be administered easily.

Morphine

In the absence of obvious contraindications (e.g., severe COPD or hypotension), 0.1–0.3 mg/kg of morphine sulfate is administered intravenously in 2–3 mg boluses in order to help allay anxiety and to produce venodilatation with resulting decreased venous return to the heart. The cardiac output is maintained, and in some patients it may actually increase. If the peripheral vasodilatory effect of morphine causes hypotension in some patients, this is quickly remedied by lowering the patient from the sitting position and by elevating the patient's legs. Morphine is a potent respiratory depressant, and ventilation must be closely monitored.

Diuretic Therapy

In most patients, intravenously administered furosemide, 20–40 mg bolus, produces a brisk diuresis within 20–30 minutes. It can cause immediate prediuretic hemodynamic improvement by increasing systemic venous capacitance. If diuresis fails to occur with the first dosage of furosemide, the patient should receive second or third dosages of the drug, doubling the dosage each time it fails to produce the desired diuresis. Diuretic therapy must be used judiciously because profound diuresis occasionally leads to severe reduction in intravascular

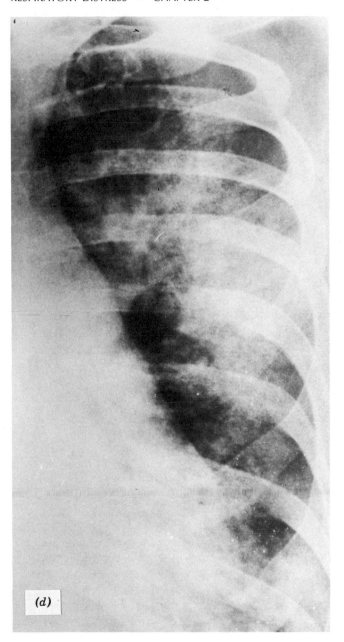

(d)

Figure 2.6 (*Continued*)

volume, producing a reduction in cardiac output and systemic hypotension. An in-dwelling urethral catheter should be inserted.

Vasodilators and Phlebotomy

The reduction of venous return can be accomplished by vasodilators, such as nitroglycerin (NTG), and may strikingly increase cardiac output in those people who do not respond sufficiently to furosemide. Nitroglycerin, by increasing venous capacitance, acts as a pharmacologic phlebotomy. The use of the agent intravenously demands intraarterial and pulmonary arterial monitoring. A drip is made of 25–50 mg NTG mixed in 250 ml D_5W. The dose given is indicated by reduction in pulmonary capillary wedge pressure and increase in cardiac output. An α-adrenergic agent such as phenylephrine (Neo-Synephrine) may be needed to support systemic blood pressure. It is obvious that these measures are only necessary in patients with severe congestive heart failure. Less ill patients, however, may benefit from the application of topical nitrates, such as nitropaste or sublingual NTG, as adjunctive therapy.

Phlebotomy will also reduce venous return but has fallen out of favor as pharmacologic methods have become available to unload the heart. The removal of blood is best done with the use of sterile donor collection bags so that erythrocytes removed by venesection can be packed and subsequently returned to the patient.

Aminophylline

Aminophylline is sometimes useful in treating patients with heart failure. It works directly on the bronchial smooth muscle to reverse the bronchospasm induced by hypoxia and thereby improves the ventilation–perfusion ratio. Since aminophylline is a potent renal vasodilator, it acts as a mild diuretic by increasing the glomerular filtration rate. In addition, it may augment left ventricular function. Its major disadvantage is that it may cause cardiac arrhythmias if given too rapidly intravenously. For this reason, it is recommended that 4–6 mg/kg be diluted in 50–100 ml 5% D_5W and infused over 15–30 minutes, followed by a constant infusion of up to 1 mg/kg/hr.

The patient who fails to respond to the above measures will require further therapy in an intensive care unit including intubation, mechanical ventilation, and PEEP therapy.

Pulmonary Edema Caused by Changes in Capillary Permeability and Osmotic Pressure— Adult Respiratory Distress Syndrome

Many patients with acute respiratory insufficiency present with edematous lungs in the absence of acute left ventricular failure. Although the causes are varied, the pathophysiology is similar

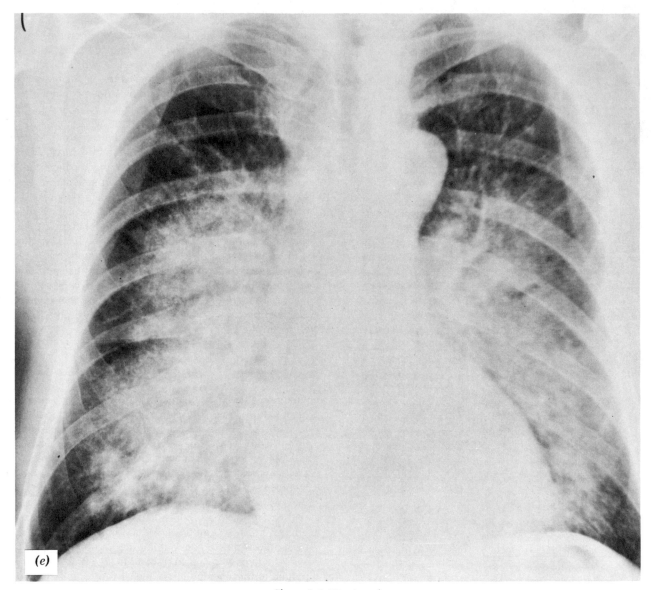

(e)

Figure 2.6 *(Continued)*

and involves increased pulmonary capillary permeability with changes in the balance of osmotic forces, causing a net flux of water into the pulmonary interstitium. Hyaline membranes may be found. The causes include traumatic shock, septic shock, viral pneumonitis, bacterial pneumonitis, salt and fresh water aspiration, gastric acid aspiration, smoke and toxic fume inhalation, oxygen toxicity, fat embolism, disseminated intravascular coagulation, massive transfusion, and pulmonary contusion. All patients with major trauma should be closely observed for development of this type of pulmonary lesion— adult respiratory distress syndrome (ARDS)—during the first few days of their hospitalization. Typically, there are 12–24 hours of latency between the initial physiologic insult and the appearance of symptoms and radiologic changes of respiratory insufficiency. Awareness of this delay in onset is crucial when evaluating victims of smoke and toxic fume inhalation and of near drowning. In general, near-drowning victims should be admitted to the hospital for observation. If victims of smoke or toxic fume inhalation are completely asymptomatic after 12 hours of observation, they are advised of the possibility of delayed onset of symptoms and are discharged to be observed by friends or family over the ensuing 24 hours. Smoke or fume inhalation victims with persistent cough or tachypnea should be admitted to the hospital for further observation.

DIAGNOSIS

The onset of ARDS is manifest by progressive tachypnea, dyspnea, hypoxemia, decreased compliance, and increasing pulmonary infiltrates on chest films. This insidious onset contrasts with the rather sudden appearance of symptoms and radiographic changes in patients with pulmonary edema secondary to acute left ventricular failure. Occasionally, left ventricular failure may occur in patients with respiratory insufficiency caused by massive pulmonary capillary leakage because of the associated cardiovascular compromise secondary to coronary heart disease or trauma to the chest and heart. In this situation, the diagnosis of left ventricular failure requires measurement of the left side of the heart filling pressures. If the necessary monitoring facilities exist in the emergency room, a triple lumen Swan-Ganz catheter is inserted to measure the pulmonary capillary wedge pressure (PCWP). Usually these facilities are not available and the assessment of PCWP is deferred until the patient is transferred to the intensive care unit or operating room.

THERAPY

The general therapy for patients with ARDS consists of maintaining adequate oxygenation, ventilation, cardiac output, and renal function. The institution of mechanical ventilation is frequently associated with hypotension in patients with acute respiratory insufficiency and pulmonary capillary leakage. Fluid losses as a result of trauma, fever, inanition, and massive transudation of protein-rich fluid out of the intravascular space into the lung result in hypovolemia and oliguria. Replacement of losses with blood, colloid, and crystalloid solutions is required. A central venous pressure catheter (or pulmonary artery catheter) is placed, and its intrathoracic position demonstrated by chest roentgenogram before replacement of fluid deficits is undertaken. Once mechanical ventilation has been instituted, the patient is best managed in an intensive care unit.

An in-dwelling bladder catheter is inserted to allow hourly monitoring of urine output. If patients with oliguria do not respond to the increased intravascular volume while the CVP rises above 10 cm H_2O or the PCWP rises above 15 mm Hg in patients with previously normal myocardial function, diuretics are indicated. Before administering a diuretic, a sample of urine, if available, should be sent for analysis of sodium and potassium concentrations and osmolality. This information will be obscured by drug-induced alterations in renal tubular function in oliguric patients who are given diuretics, especially when furosemide or ethacrynic acid are used. The lack of a response to diuretics strongly suggests that acute renal failure exists.

In the absence of a pulmonary artery catheter or measurements of cardiac output, the use of inotropic agents should be reserved for those patients with severe hypotension, elevated central venous pressures, and oliguria. A continuous infusion of dopamine, 2–10 μg/kg/min, isoproterenol, 0.5–4 μg/min, or epinephrine, 0.5–4 μg/min as indicated, may be used to resuscitate these patients. The ECG must be scrupulously observed for arrhythmias and signs of myocardial ischemia.

Overhydration must be avoided because of the abnormal tendency of these patients to sequester fluid in their lungs. If a diuretic is administered, its hemodynamic effects must be carefully monitored. Serum electrolytes, BUN, and osmolality must be followed closely. Osmolality can be maintained in the range of 300–310 if BUN and blood sugar are normal. If serum potassium is low, it may be replaced by the use of small volumes of concentrated potassium chloride administered very slowly into the central circulation. In the absence of abnormal fluid losses, fluid should be restricted to 20–25 ml/kg/day. The contribution of nebulizers to water balance must be taken into account, recognizing the fact that patients on ventilators do not have insensible water loss from the lungs. It has been shown that in a patient in whom an arterial line, Swan-Ganz catheter, and peripheral intravenous line are in place, it is almost impossible to keep fluids below 750 ml/day even if no fluids are ordered. Extreme care is therefore necessary.

A nasogastric tube is placed because of the tendency of patients on mechanical ventilators to develop adynamic ileus. Because of the high incidence of stress ulceration and erosive gastritis, antacids should be ordered.

Steroids have been advocated for the treatment of patients with ARDS but their ultimate usefulness has yet to be demonstrated. It is thought that sodium methylprednisolone administered intravenously, 30 mg/kg every 6 hours for 48 hours, may protect the lung membranes from chemical effects of white blood cell aggregates and fatty acids.

ASPIRATION

Aspiration of gastric content occurs quite commonly in patients with decreased consciousness, whether it is secondary to drug overdose, caused by depressed laryngeal function, or caused by neurologic compromise. The extent of damage depends on the pH of the aspirated fluid. Maximum damage occurs at a pH of 1.5. Above pH 2.5, the effects of the aspirate are similar to those of distilled water. The pH of a normal fasting stomach is 1.3–2.

In patients with aspiration, hypoxemia occurs acutely because of reflex airway closure and, subsequently, because of decreased surfactant activity and interstitial and alveolar edema. There may be obstruction because of large food particles distributed throughout the airways. Acid aspiration causes a chemical burn with loss of alveolar capillary integrity with exudation of fluid and protein into the alveoli. There is decreased compliance with increased wet-to-dry lung weights. There are changes in the pulmonary vasculature with increased pulmonary artery pressure and elevated pulmonary artery resistance. Cardiac output falls. The portions of the lung affected by these changes are those most dependent at the time of aspiration.

Therapy

Prevention is the most important measure in the care of patients who are at risk for aspiration. A patient with depressed consciousness should be nursed on his side. It is helpful when positioning these patients to bring the lower part of the shoulder back and the upper part of the leg forward. Anyone who vomits should be turned to the side, placed in Trendelenburg position, and have the oropharynx suctioned. Sellick's maneuver (pressure applied to the cricoid cartilage) can prevent aspiration as a result of regurgitation and should be performed on all patients in danger of imminent cardiac arrest or at risk of aspiration before intubation. Intubation is necessary to prevent further aspiration and to allow correction of hypoxemia and provision of mechanical ventilation. Oxygen and mechanical ventilation are provided according to arterial blood gases and the usual criteria for instituting mechanical ventilation; PEEP is added as necessary. Endotracheal suctioning stimulates coughing, removes aspirated material, and allows a check on the pH of the aspirate. Bronchoscopy is useful for removing large particles. Chest physiotherapy will help to raise debris and secretions.

Much of the treatment of pulmonary aspiration is controversial. There is little place for bronchial lavage. Steroids are advocated by some, but studies showing efficacy are not well controlled. The rationale for the use of steroids is their ability to decrease inflammation, stabilize lysosomal membranes, and prevent leukocyte aggregation. Prophylactic antibiotics are probably of little benefit and may lead to superinfection. The complications of aspiration—pneumonia, empyema, and lung abscess—are not necessarily prevented by prophylactic antibiotics, and it is recommended that they be withheld pending the results of sputum Gram stains, cultures, and x-ray films. The time interval between aspiration and development of clinical signs is quite variable (minutes to hours), and patients demand close observation in an intensive care environment.

NEAR DROWNING

When water enters the larynx, it triggers intense laryngospasm in an attempt to prevent pulmonary aspiration. Drowning without aspiration accounts for 10–20% of drowning deaths. If the person is rescued quickly and laryngospasm is controlled, drowning will be prevented and recovery will be complete and rapid. If, however, the victim remains in the water, he or she may swallow large amounts of fluids. This causes vomiting and gasping with aspiration of water into the lungs. The victim may also aspirate water directly without swallowing or vomiting.

There are several differences between drowning in sea water and drowning in fresh water. Sea water is hypertonic (Na, 509 mEq/liter; K, 11.3 mEq/liter; C1, 56 mEq/liter) and draws more fluid into the lungs than does fresh water. Fresh water is hypotonic and is absorbed into the circulation with resulting increase in intravascular volume. Sodium, chloride, and calcium content increase after immersion in sea water and decrease after immersion in fresh water. Potassium increases in both, by absorption in sea water and by hemolysis in fresh water. The change in electrolytes, however, is not usually the cause of death.

Therapy

In near-drowning victims at the beach, the first priority should be given to ventilation. Laryngospasm will usually break from hypoxia, but if it is severe cricothyrotomy may be necessary. Intubation is preferred if facilities are available. Oxygen should be administered. As discussed in Chapter 1, cardiopulmonary resuscitation (CPR) should be instituted for those victims without a heart beat and continued even if things look hopeless, at least until the patient has arrived in the emergency room.

This holds particularly for children who are victims of near drowning in cold water.

Even if the patient is alert and breathing on arrival in the emergency room, he or she should be admitted since it may take up to 48 hours for the signs and symptoms of pulmonary edema or aspiration to emerge clinically. Victims of more severe near drowning should be treated as if they were patients after cardiac arrest with respiratory failure. A nasogastric tube should be passed and stomach contents aspirated. Chest films, ECG, arterial blood gases, complete blood cell count (CBC), prothrombin time (PT), partial thromboplastin time (PTT), platelet count, and electrolytes should be obtained.

Victims of severe near drowning in fresh water will require mechanical ventilation for 48–72 hours since surfactant is destroyed and it will take this long for it to reconstitute. Diuretics, such as furosemide, will decrease blood volume. Victims of salt water near drowning may have massive pulmonary edema in the presence of hypovolemia and normal cardiac function.

Severe near drowning is a multisystem catastrophe. There is a severe metabolic acidemia. Cerebral edema and disseminated intravascular coagulation (DIC) must be suspected and treated if diagnosed. Decadron, 10 mg intravenously to start and 4 mg intravenously every 6 hours, and lasix may be useful in combatting cerebral edema. Hemolysis may cause severe hemoglobinemia with acute renal failure.

PULMONARY VASCULAR OBSTRUCTION

Pulmonary Embolism

It is estimated that pulmonary embolism (PE) causes approximately 200,000 deaths per year in the United States, making it the third most frequent cause of death in this country. Approximately one-third of all clinically significant cases occurs in patients with cardiac disease and about one-third occurs in patients in the immediate postoperative period. Other predisposing conditions include peripheral venous disease, hip fractures in elderly patients, malignancy, systemic infection, pregnancy, and oral contraceptive use. Approximately 90% of pulmonary emboli originate in the veins of the lower extremity; other sites are pelvic veins, upper extremity veins, and the right side of the heart.

DIAGNOSIS

The clinical course of PE depends on the size of embolus, the number of episodes, the previous state of pulmonary circulation, and the previous condition of the lungs and heart. The characteristic picture of acute pulmonary embolism is a result of a combination of a fall in cardiac output and hypoxemia due to ventilation of unperfused lung (increased V/Q). Compliance may fall as a result of release of vasoactive substances and terminal airway closure. Pulmonary artery pressures are elevated, and pulmonary vascular resistance is increased, particularly after recurrent microembolization.

Dyspnea and sudden chest pain are common presenting symptoms. The pain is usually sharp and pleuritic in nature, but the discomfort sometimes closely mimics that of myocardial infarction. Rather frequently the patient is apprehensive and has a vaguely defined sense of impending doom. Hemoptysis is present in only about one-third of patients. Similarly, the physical signs are usually not specific. Tachypnea is found in most patients. A pleural rub may be present. Tachycardia is common, and there may be accentuation of the pulmonic component of the second heart sound. There can be evidence of failure of the right side of the heart with massive embolism;

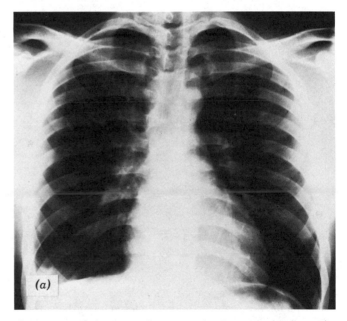

(a)

Figure 2.7 Radiologic manifestations of pulmonary embolism. The patient is a 17-year-old male with recurrent episodes of hemoptysis and chest pain on his right side. (a) Chest film shows a peripheral infiltrate in the right costophrenic angle and a freely layering right pleural effusion. (b) The V/Q scan shows a large segmental defect at the left base with ventilation and a defect at the right base. (c) The pulmonary and angiogram shows multiple filling defects in the lower lobe branches.

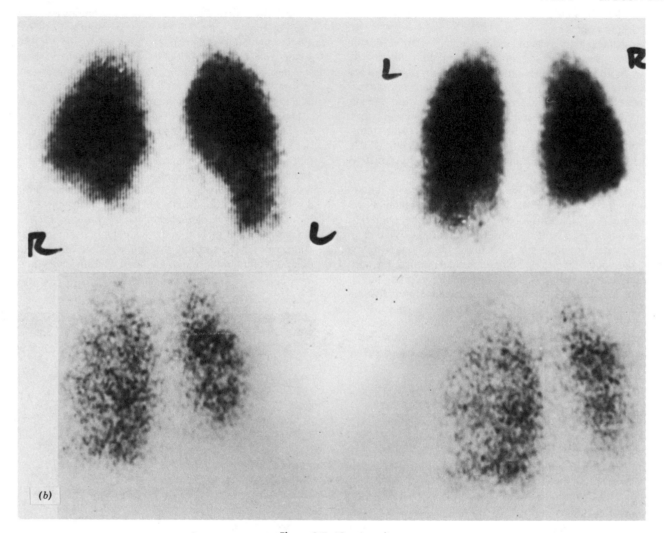

Figure 2.7 *(Continued)*

there may be hypotension or shock. Although most pulmonary emboli originate in leg veins, clinical evidence of phlebitis may be found in only one-third or fewer of such patients. Homan's sign, traditionally associated with lower leg thrombophlebitis, is seldom helpful in making the diagnosis. A more helpful clinical sign is the unequal dorsiflexion of the ankle or the complaint of pain in the calf when the patient is asked to dorsiflex the ankles. Measurement of the calves and thighs may show asymmetry. Impedance plethysmography, while noninvasive, correlates well with venography.

The most helpful laboratory test in the preliminary diagnosis of PE is the measurement of blood gases. In most patients with significant pulmonary emboli, the Pa_{O_2} on room air is below 80 mm Hg and Pa_{CO_2} is often normal or low because of hyperventilation—the usual response to pulmonary embolism.

The ECG is not a reliable diagnostic aid, but it may show sinus tachycardia and ST segment and T-wave changes. Those patients with massive emboli may demonstrate tall P waves in the inferior leads, a rightward or leftward shift in the QRS axis, and T-wave inversions in the right precordial leads indicative of right ventricular strain. Right bundle branch block and ventricular arrythmias may develop.

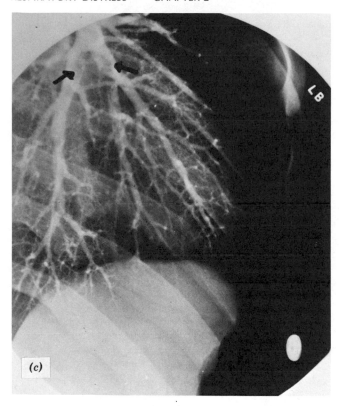

Figure 2.7 *(Continued)*

The chest film is normal in at least one-half the patients with pulmonary embolism, and only in about one-fourth does it show the classic peripheral wedge-shaped consolidation said to be characteristic of pulmonary infarction. A primary role of the chest film therefore, becomes that of excluding other intrathoracic pathology that so often presents with a clinical picture similar to that of pulmonary emboli (e.g., congestive heart failure, pneumothorax, or pneumonia). Since infiltrates that do occur secondary to pulmonary embolism usually are delayed in appearance for at least 12 hours, a near-normal chest film is a frequent finding in a patient with acute pulmonary embolism (Fig. 2.7).

If pulmonary embolism is suspected on clinical grounds, the next diagnostic step should be to obtain a pulmonary V/Q scan. In patients presenting with symptoms that are consistent with the diagnosis of pulmonary embolism but that provide negative findings on a chest roentgenogram, a V/Q scan may show areas of ventilation with perfusion mismatch. A normal V/Q scan usually excludes a pulmonary embolus. False positives, that is, areas of V/Q mismatch, may be seen in patients with chronic lung disease. Pulmonary angiography, combined with catheterization of the right side of the heart to provide hemodynamic data, remains the most specific and accurate procedure for the diagnosis of pulmonary embolus. Pulmonary angiography should be performed in patients who have a strong clinical story and positive V/Q scan, have previous history of pulmonary parenchymal disease, and are at high risk for anticoagulation.

THERAPY

Once the diagnosis of PE is established, anticoagulation with heparin (150 U/kg intravenous loading dose followed by approximately 20 U/kg/hr by continuous infusion or 75–125 U/kg intravenously every 4 hours) should be started to maintain the PTT 2–2.5 times greater than control. Although heparin in adequate dosages may prevent thrombus formation or propagation, it cannot prevent fragmentation or detachment of a nonadherent thrombus. Adjuvant measures in the treatment of pulmonary embolism include bed rest, treating hypoxemia if necessary with humidified oxygen, warm soaks and elevation for thrombophlebitis, and symptomatic relief of pain. In patients with recurrent episodes of pulmonary emboli despite adequate anticoagulation when pulmonary blood flow is obstructed by 50% or more or when heparin therapy is contraindicated (active bleeding, recent stroke, or coagulopathy), interruption of the inferior vena cava should be performed either by placement of an umbrella filter or by surgical clipping.

In patients with significant hypoxemia, mechanical ventilation should be instituted. Hemodynamic monitoring and support of the circulation as well as pulmonary vasodilators are necessary to prevent right heart insufficiency deteriorating into right heart and subsequent left heart failure. In rare instances of patients with massive pulmonary embolism who do not respond to intensive medical therapy, pulmonary embolectomy on cardiopulmonary bypass should be considered. Diagnosis and management of pulmonary embolism is discussed in more detail in Chapters 3 and 4.

SUGGESTED READINGS

Bates DV, Macklem PT, Christie RV: *Respiratory Function in Disease.* Philadelphia, WB Saunders Co, 1971.

Bendixen H, Egbert L, Hedley-Whyte J, Laver MB, Pontoppidan H: *Respiratory Care.* St. Louis, The CV Mosby Co, 1965.

Burton GG, Gee GN, Hodgkin JE: *Respiratory Care: A Guide to Clinical Practice.* Philadelphia, Lippincott, 1977.

Dalen JE, Alpert JS: Natural history of pulmonary embolism. *Prog Cardiovasc Dis* 1975; 17:259–270.

Diener CF, Burrows B: Further observation on the course and prognosis of chronic obstructive lung disease. *Am Rev Respir Dis* 1975; 11:719.

Hedley-Whyte J, Burgess GE III, Feeley TW, Miller MG: *Applied Physiology of Respiratory Care.* Boston, Little Brown & Co, 1976.

Lockhart CH, Battaglia JD: Croup and epiglottitis. *Pediatr Ann* 1977; 6:262.

Macklem PT: Tests of Lung Mechanics. *NEJM* 1975; 293:339.

McPherson SP: *Respiratory Therapy Equipment.* St. Louis, Mosby, 1977.

Modell JH, Graves SA, Ketover A: Clinical course of 91 consecutive near-drowning victims. *Chest* 1976; 70:231–238.

Nunn JF: *Applied Respiratory Physiology.* London, Butterworths, 1977.

Pruitt BA Jr, Erickson DP, Morris A: Progressive pulmonary insufficiency and other pulmonary complications of thermal injury. *J Trauma* 1975; 15:369.

Rinaldo JE, Rogers RM: Adult Respiratory-Distress Syndrome. *NEJM* 1982; 306:900.

Sasahara AA, Sharma GVRK, Parisi AF: New development in the detection and prevention of venous thromboembolism. *Am J Cardiol* 1979; 43:1214.

Shapiro BA, Harrison RA, Trout CA: *Clinical Application of Respiratory Care.* Chicago, Yearbook, 1979.

Shapiro BA, Harrison RA, Walton JR: *Clinical Application of Blood Gases.* Chicago, Yearbook, 1977.

Staub NC: Pulmonary edema. Physiologic approaches to management.*Chest* 1978; 74(5):559.

Van Arsdel PP, Paul GH: Drug therapy in the management of asthma. *Ann Intern Med* 1977; 87:68–74.

Wynne JW, Modell JH: Respiratory aspiration of stomach contents. *Ann Intern Med* 1977; 87:466–474.

3
SHOCK

Joseph R. Benotti
John J. Collins, Jr.

Shock, the common pathway by which a variety of insults may cause death unless prompt and well-conceived intervention is undertaken, is a state of reduced tissue perfusion that results in cellular hypoxia and widespread organ failure. Effective management requires an understanding of the basic physiologic disturbances associated with shock and demands rapid correction of these derangements in the critically ill patient. An orderly approach to diagnosis and therapy is essential.

PATHOPHYSIOLOGY OF SHOCK

Tissue hypoperfusion causes disruption of structure and function of the cell because its energy needs are not met. As described in Chapter 1, cellular processes requiring energy are normally sustained by production of adenosine triphosphate (ATP). This high-energy compound is produced by mitochondrial oxidative phosphorylation, a process that requires continuous oxygen delivery by the blood stream. When blood flow and oxygen delivery are critically reduced, cellular function must rely on the inadequate amount of ATP produced by anaerobic metabolism of glucose to pyruvic acid. To maintain this anaerobic pathway with its limited production of ATP, pyruvate must be further reduced to lactic acid. Insufficiency of energy supply leads to cellular injury and necrosis that, in turn, causes potassium and phosphate leakage, activation and release of intracellular proteolytic enzymes, and further damage. The end result is widespread organ failure and metabolic acidosis.

Cardiac Output

In all types of shock, except some instances of septic shock, the cardiac output is reduced. Understanding the aberrations that reduce cardiac output is essential to efficient management of shock states.

The cardiac output is determined by the heart rate and stroke volume. Both ventricles invariably have the same rate of contraction, but the determinants of stroke volume must be considered independently for the right and left ventricles. Furthermore the structural characteristics of the right and left ventricles are quite different, and therapy for inadequate function of one or the other may not be the same. In general, stroke volume of each ventricle is determined by filling pressure (preload), contractility, and outflow resistance (afterload).

PRELOAD

Preload, the filling pressure, is the atrial pressure that provides the driving force for ventricular filling in diastole. It is dependent on total blood volume, venous tone, and the competence of the heart—specifically the right or the left ventricle—as a pump. Since preload is increased by such maneuvers as blood transfusion or by increasing venous tone, the ventricular volume at the end of diastole is greater and the cardiac output is increased (Fig. 3.1, curve A). An abrupt decline in preload, resulting from sudden loss of blood volume or a lessening of venous tone, results in a decline in cardiac output.

CONTRACTILITY

Contractility refers to the vigor with which the ventricles contract to generate pressure and eject blood into the aorta or pulmonary artery. The most common cause for depression of contractility is myocardial infarction. In patients with uncomplicated myocardial infarction (Fig. 3.1, curve B), in spite of a reduction in myocardial contractility, the cardiac output can be maintained at a satisfactory level by a compensatory increase in preload. In patients with congestive failure (curve C), the myocardial contractility is so reduced that cardiac output can be satisfactorily maintained only if left ventricular filling pressure is considerably elevated beyond normal range. At this level pulmonary congestion and, not infrequently, pulmonary edema occur. If more than 40% of the ventricular muscle fibers are damaged or destroyed by myocardial infarction, although the ventricle may be operating at the apex of its function curve (point D) with marked elevation of the left ventricular filling pressure, an adequate cardiac output cannot be delivered. Cardiogenic shock is the result. Some pathologic conditions causing depressed contractility are irreversible in the acute stage. In others, the use of inotropic agents such as digoxin and dopamine is therapeutically useful because contractility may be increased, for example, by moving from curve C to curve B.

AFTERLOAD

Afterload is the impedance against which the ventricle must eject blood into the great vessels. As afterload increases, the

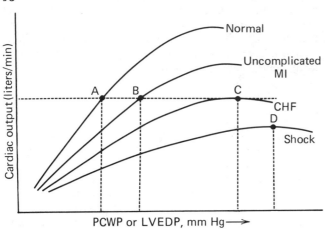

Figure 3.1 Schematized ventricular function curves in normal patients, patients with acute uncomplicated myocardial infarction, patients with acute myocardial infarction with congestive heart failure, and patients with acute myocardial infarction complicated by cardiogenic shock. With progressively more cumulative ventricular injury, the heart requires a greater left ventricular end diastolic pressure (LVEDP) or pulmonary capillary wedge pressure (PCWP) to maintain cardiac output at or above a critical level. This is represented by the line connecting points A, B, and C. The cost of maintaining this cardiac output is a progressive elevation in PCWP, a diminution in pulmonary compliance, an increase in the work of breathing, arterial hypoxemia, and dyspnea. In patients with cardiogenic shock, the ventricle operates at the apex of its depressed function curve (point D). Nonetheless only an inadequate cardiac output can be maintained despite severe pulmonary congestion; tissue hypoperfusion, renal failure, and shock ensue. (Used with permission from Mason DT, et al., in Eliot R: *The Acute Cardiac Emergency*, Futura Publishing Company, 1972, p. 137.)

resistance to ventricular emptying rises. Unless preload or contractility increases, the cardiac output declines. For example, systemic hypertension is most often accompanied by an increase in total peripheral resistance that could reduce cardiac output. This is likely if left ventricular performance is not supported by an increase in preload or in the force of cardiac contraction. Aortic stenosis increases the impedance to ventricular ejection because of a narrowed aortic valve orifice and requires more vigorous ventricular contraction to sustain the cardiac output. In a similar fashion, pulmonary embolism raises the impedance to the ejection of blood by the right ventricle, and increases in right ventricular contractility and filling pressure are required to maintain the cardiac output.

The rate and rhythm of contraction of the heart may impair output when they are outside of rather wide limits. Impairment of contractility or compliance may cause significant narrowing of the range of rate and rhythm in which the cardiac output remains adequate. The normal heart will tolerate rates from 35–180 beats/min in a variety of rhythms, but hearts with valve or muscle abnormalities may require more physiological rates and synchronous atrial and ventricular contraction.

Compensatory Mechanism

Compensation for a tendency toward reduced cardiac output is rapid in onset and involves several physiologic responses.

NEUROHUMORAL

Inadequate cardiac output is detected as a decline in pulse pressure by the baroreceptors of the carotid and aortic sinuses. In turn, they stimulate the vasomotor center of the medulla, resulting in increased sympathetic discharge to the heart and peripheral vasculature. More intense baroreceptor activation elicits epinephrine release from the adrenal medulla and more intense sympathetic activation. Sympathetic stimulation of the heart, mediated by beta$_1$ receptor activation by norepinephrine, results in an increase in heart rate and myocardial contractility. Stimulation of peripheral blood vessels by activation of the alpha receptors in vascular smooth muscle results in vasoconstriction that, at the arteriolar level, increases total peripheral resistance to preserve central blood pressure and maintain sufficient coronary and cerebral perfusion pressure to deliver flow to these vital organs. Vasoconstriction at the venular level reduces the reservoir capacity of the venous circulation, thus increasing venous return and cardiac filling. As a result, cardiac output rises.

RENAL

Declining perfusion to the kidneys activates the renin–angiotensin–aldosterone mechanism. Angiotensin II, a mediator of this sequence, is a potent vasoconstrictor and enhances renal retention of salt and water as does aldosterone, which is released from the adrenal cortex. In addition, activation of this mechanism enhances renal potassium excretion. The net effect is renal conservation of sodium and water to restore blood volume, venous return, and cardiac output. Assuming normal renal and adrenal function and no diuretic use, the urine produced is low in sodium (less than 10 mEq/liter) and high in potassium under these circumstances.

Volume depletion activates the release of antidiuretic hormone (ADH) from the posterior pituitary gland. ADH increases the permeability of the distal renal tubule to water, thereby enhancing renal water reabsorption and urine concentration. The net effect is preservation of total body water and excretion of maximally concentrated urine (at least 600 mosm/liter).

METABOLIC

Intense sympathetic stimulation activates glycogenolysis and elevates blood sugar. Lipolysis in adipose tissue is stimulated so that free fatty acids are liberated into the blood stream. Cortisol released from the adrenal cortex augments these responses, potentiates the responsiveness of the kidney to various salt- and water-retaining hormones, and augments the cardiovascular response to sympathetic stimulation.

Classification of Shock

An orderly approach is facilitated by classification of shock according to the initiating cause of reduced peripheral perfusion. Many attempts have been made to classify the shock syndrome. A simple and useful scheme includes the following:

- Hypovolemic shock
    Absolute hypovolemia
    Relative hypovolemia
- Cardiogenic shock
- Obstructive shock

All hypoperfusion syndromes fit reasonably well into one of these categories, thereby establishing guidelines for rational theraputic interventions.

HYPOVOLEMIC SHOCK

Absolute Hypovolemia

Hypovolemia may be due to an absolute deficiency in the total circulating blood volume. Hypovolemic shock results in inadequate cardiac output and shock because of deficient cardiac filling or preload.

Volume depletion can result from a variety of causes. The *loss of whole blood* because of acute hemorrhage in excess of 1 liter in the average-sized adult can result in tissue hypoperfusion and shock. *Plasma loss* associated with thermal wounds is the immediate cause of shock in patients with major burns. Similar losses within the gut and peritoneum are responsible for shock as a presenting manifestation or complication of pancreatitis, bowel obstruction, or intraabdominal catastro-

phes such as bowel infarcts resulting in peritonitis. *Extracellular fluid loss* in the form of crystalloid as a result of protracted vomiting, diarrhea, gastrointestinal fistulous output, or excessive renal salt loss because of salt-losing nephropathy or overzealous diuretic therapy can result in volume deficiency to the point of frank shock. *Pure water deficits* as a result of insensible losses from respiration or sweating can precipitate hypovolemia and hypernatremia in the obtunded febrile patient. A similar syndrome can result in shock and hypernatremia in patients with diabetes insipidus who, through obtundation, are deprived of their thirst mechanism.

Relative Hypovolemia

Neurogenic shock is due to a failure in preload because of increased vascular capacitance resulting from sudden cessation of venous tone. Although the blood volume is usually normal, the patient in neurogenic shock is in relative hypovolemia because the circulating blood volume is insufficient to fill the exanded capacity of the vasodilated circulatory system. The decline in arteriolar tone due to sympathetic interruption prevents the increase in peripheral resistance that normally accompanies a reduction in preload and cardiac output. The net result is a decline in cardiac output and peripheral resistance, producing significant hypotension.

SEPTIC SHOCK

Septic shock, via a complex and incompletely understood mechanism, adversely affects preload, contractility, and vascular resistance to cause cardiovascular collapse. Patients with severe hypovolemia and cardiac problems usually have reduced cardiac output and are vasoconstricted, but many patients with septic shock have a normal or increased output.

CARDIOGENIC SHOCK

Cardiogenic shock results from an inadequate cardiac output despite the presence of a sufficient total blood volume. This syndrome can be due to a number of derangements affecting heart rate or rhythm, myocardial contractility, mechanical obstruction in the valves or great vessels, or restriction of ventricular filling. In practice, cardiogenic shock is usually the result of left ventricular failure. Of course, since the heart represents two pumps in series, failure of either the right or left pumping chamber can result in inadequate circulation throughout the entire system. The most common causes of cardiac deterioration are coronary disease and valvular disease; these entities affect left ventricular pumping capability far more often than that of the right ventricle.

Myocardial infarction depresses overall ventricular contractility. If the cumulative damage is in excess of 40% of the ventricular muscle mass, the heart is unable to sustain sufficient cardiac output to support life.

The normal heart tolerates extreme tachycardia (200 beats/min) or bradycardia (35 beats/min) very well for long periods of time with little or no alteration in cardiac output. In a setting of cardiac disease, however, rapid tachyarrhythmias compromise diastolic filling and critically reduce the cardiac output. Bradyarrhythmias can have similar consequences.

OBSTRUCTIVE SHOCK

Congestive heart failure due to chronic elevation of afterload (hypertension, aortic stenosis, or other chronic outflow obstruction) is common, but acute circulatory shock as a result of increased afterload from such causes is uncommon. When present, it is usually rapidly fatal. Massive pulmonary embolism is not often classified as a cause of cardiogenic shock since the heart may be completely normal. However, as a result of the acute increase in afterload of the right ventricle and the acute decrease in preload of the left ventricle, acute massive pulmonary embolism causes shock due to the sudden reduction in cardiac output. Though the pump and blood vessels may be physically intact and intrinsically normal, states in which the circulatory system are encumbered by external forces preventing proper cardiac function may be termed *obstructive shock*. Such shock may be observed, for example, in the occurence of pulmonary embolism, pericardial tamponade, or dissecting aneurysm with arterial luminal obstruction.

ASSESSMENT AND MANAGEMENT OF THE PATIENT IN SHOCK

Rapid Evaluation

A rapid assessment of circulatory adequacy by observation and palpation is often possible within a few moments of encountering a patient in the emergency room. If a patient is alert with good skin color and warm hands and feet and has a slow regular pulse, it is unlikely that circulatory inadequacy exists. On the other hand, if the patient shows impairment of consciousness, cold extremities, a weak, thready pulse, and a pallor of the mucus membranes, it seems very probable that circulatory inadequacy exists. This initial impression is sufficient evidence to begin those interventions designed for the early management of circulatory insufficiency or circulatory shock.

During the performance of those measures designed to combat circulatory inadequacy, it may become evident that certain peripheral organ systems are not functioning properly as a result of a lack of blood supply. The early signs of organ system failure are manifested by dysfunction of the central nervous system, cardiovascular system, or renal system. Central nervous system manifestations of inadequate circulation—confusion, agitation, or coma—may occur as manifestations of inadequate cerebral oxygenation. The cardiovascular signs of inadequate circulation and of the compensatory sympathetic stimulation include arterial hypotension, narrowed pulse pressure, tachycardia, a rapid, thready pulse, and diminished heart sounds. In addition, there are pallor, sweating, and acrocyanosis, the peripheral cyanosis reflecting the increased extraction of oxygen by the tissues because of the sluggishness of the circulation. The most common manifestation of inadequate perfusion of the kidneys is oliguria or anuria, which may occur very early in the course of circulatory shock, even before the blood pressure declines. Restoration of renal blood flow is rapidly accompanied by improvement of urinary output. Therefore, the urine output is useful in assessing the adequacy of circulatory support with administration of volume expanding solutions and/or vasopressor drugs.

Initial Management

Once shock has been diagnosed, it is necessary to intervene promptly in order that the patient not progress to an irreversible state of shock and in order that permanent damage not result to vital organs. Immediately after making the diagnosis, certain measures may be taken as an initial therapeutic effort.

CONTROL OF VENTILATION AND OXYGENATION

Since the fundamental derangement in shock is inadequate oxygen delivery to peripheral organs, maximizing the oxygen content of blood delivered to these organs is of paramount importance. Because of blood loss and/or cutaneous vasoconstriction, the patient may be pale but not cyanotic despite a significant degree of arterial undersaturation. Therefore, all patients presenting in shock require supplemental oxygen via nasal cannula or face mask. If there is a problem with the airway or with the mechanics of ventilation, further measures (described in Chapter 2) must be immediately undertaken.

INTRAVENOUS ACCESS

Depending on the severity of shock and its cause, two or three large intravenous catheters (at least 18 gauge but preferably 15 gauge) should be inserted (Procedure 11). The most important criteria for adequate intravenous access in shock is that it should be rapidly available, of large size, and accurately placed so that extravasation is not a problem. One of the catheters should be advanced into the superior vena cava to be used for constant monitoring of central venous pressure (CVP) (Procedure 12).

At the time of catheter insertion blood should be drawn for typing and cross matching, complete blood count, and electrolytes. Any additional tests that are indicated, for example, glucose, creatinine, or amylase, should be ordered at the same time.

CORRECTING THE INITIATING CAUSES OF SHOCK

If the cause of shock is not corrected rapidly, other treatment may be of no avail. Sometimes the cause is immediately apparent and correctable. If there is obvious hemorrhage that can be stopped by pressure or by some other immediately available method, the blood loss should be stopped. If internal bleeding is so massive that replacement of blood and fluid will not be able to keep up with the loss, an operation should be performed as quickly as possible even though the patient is in shock. If blood loss can be replaced more rapidly than it is lost, the patient should be brought into the best possible condition before an operation is performed.

POSITIONING

If there is evidence of hypovolemia or neurogenic shock, the legs can be elevated to about 30 degrees with the torso horizontal. This will help to drain the large capacitance veins of the lower extremity that contain as much as 30% of the blood volume. In patients with dyspnea and evidence of cardiogenic shock, on the other hand, the legs should be kept flat and the head should be elevated 30 degrees to minimize pulmonary vascular congestion.

FLUID RESUSCITATION

Appropriate fluid therapy is vital in all forms of shock. In shock states characterized by volume depletion, it is definitive therapy. In all forms of shock, however, it is an important supportive aspect of overall therapy.

Blood

When shock results from blood loss, blood replacement to restore the existing deficit, as well as specific measures to stop the bleeding, constitute definitive therapy. Although whole blood is specific therapy for acute hemorrhage, its use carries some disadvantages. Specifically, it takes at least 30–45 minutes to obtain appropriately typed and cross-matched blood, and there is a definite risk of transmitting infectious disease (viral hepatitis and malaria) with transfused blood. The risk of transmitting hepatitis is lessened by using packed red cells and concomitant colloid or crystalloid administration in place of whole blood.

Banked blood slowly loses its oxygen-carrying capacity; red cells lose potassium to the medium, and the pH of the medium declines. Platelets and most clotting factors lose their activity in banked blood. The preservative chelates calcium. Because of these changes in banked blood, the following precautions must be observed when massive transfusion (in excess of 5–6 units) is required: (1) Regular measurement of the serum potassium and pH are mandatory. This is necessary to prevent hyperkalemic acidosis, which is a major risk in the shocked patient who may at the same time be developing renal failure; (2) an ampule of calcium gluconate or lactate should be administered with every 6–8 units of banked blood to prevent hypocalcemia; (3) the administration of 1–2 units of fresh frozen plasma for each 6–8 units of banked blood transfused is necessary to prevent dilutional coagulopathy.

In circumstances of life-threatening exsanguination, it is reasonable to administer unmatched O-negative blood in an attempt to restore circulatory function. However, in almost all circumstances, the patient can be sustained with infusions of synthetic plasma expanders and/or dextran while sufficient time is taken to procure typed and cross-matched blood since the transfusion with group O unmatched blood carries a definite risk. The risk of transfusion can be lessened by the use of type specific uncross-matched blood in such emergencies. With only a 5-minute delay, most blood banks should be able to deliver unmatched whole blood of the same ABO and Rh group as the recipient.

Colloids

Colloids are solutions containing substances of high molecular weight that cannot readily diffuse through normal capillary membranes. Substances most commonly used in shocked patients include plasma, albumin, synthetic plasma expanders, and dextran.

Plasma was originally obtained from a number of donors and was provided in the form of pooled plasma. Because of the high risk of transmitting serum hepatitis with this preparation, its use has largely been abandoned.

Synthetic plasma expanders are commercial intravenous solutions of macromolecules in a physiologic electrolyte solution. These are readily available, and there is no risk of transmitting hepatitis or other blood-borne infections.

Dextran is available as clinical dextran or low molecular weight dextran. Both of these compounds are effective plasma expanders; they also decrease blood viscosity and may improve microcirculatory flow. These compounds may interfere with platelet function, alter coagulation mechanisms, or interfere with cross-match reactions. Hence, blood must be drawn for typing and cross-matching before the administration of dextran. It is ill-advised to administer dextran before any contemplated surgery because of the risk of bleeding. The administration of dextran will result in a high urine specific gravity. Therefore, the high urine specific gravity will not reflect the status of volume depletion. Finally, no more than 1 liter of dextran should be given per 24 hours.

Crystalloids

Crystalloid solutions (saline, lactated Ringer's) are primary modes of initial therapy in all forms of hypovolemic shock if blood or colloid solutions are not instantaneously available. Although their distribution is not restricted to the intravascular compartment, a sufficient quantity of the solution remains within the vascular space to partially restore peripheral perfusion. These solutions are clearly indicated as definitive therapy when hypovolemia results in the loss of protein-free fluid. Examples of such losses include protracted vomiting and inappropriate renal salt and water loss.

Regarding the use of crystalloid solution, it should be remembered that diffusion of noncolloid salt solutions out of the intravascular compartment is relatively rapid so that a volume of up to four times the amount of intravascular volume loss must be infused as crystalloid solution to restore circulatory blood volume. Furthermore, there are theoretical advantages to buffered salt solution such as lactated Ringer's, and concern about accumulation of lactate has not proved to be clinically important. Finally, it should be remembered that there is no place for the use of salt-free crystalloid solutions (dextrose and water) in primary resuscitation.

Although crystalloids can expand the intravascular volume temporarily, they dilute the remaining red cells and protein, thus reducing the oxygen-carrying capacity, buffering ability, and colloid oncotic pressure of the blood. In disease states in which the capillaries may have a greatly increased permeability, these solutions may leave the intravascular spaces so rapidly that little or no transient volume expansion is provided. Furthermore, excessive administration of such fluids can cause additional edema in the lungs and interfere with movement of oxygen and nutrients to cells, thus increasing the likelihood of later respiratory failure.

DRUG THERAPY

When the cause of shock is clearcut and is rapidly corrected, most patients respond quickly to fluid resuscitation. However, in patients with cardiogenic, bacteremic, and neurogenic shock, definitive therapy often requires the use of vasoactive drugs. Furthermore, in any patient with shock in whom there is evidence of continuing hypotension and central nervous system and/or myocardial hypoperfusion despite the initiation of apparently appropriate fluid therapy, drugs to enhance cardiovascular function are indicated. These agents are catecholamine derivatives that act on either alpha or beta receptors. Alpha receptors, contained in vascular smooth muscle and activated by norepinephrine, mediate arteriolar vasoconstriction as well as increases in venous tone. The stimulation of alpha receptors results in an elevation in total peripheral resistance and an increase in venous return to the heart. Beta receptors, stimulated by norepinephrine released from cardiac sympathetic nerves, mediate increases in heart rate and myocardial contractility. These are specified as $beta_1$ receptors. As pointed out in Chapters 1 and 2, other beta receptors, categorized as $beta_2$ receptors, mediate smooth muscle dilatation whether in the peripheral vasculature or in the smooth muscle lining the bronchioles. Stimulation of $beta_1$ receptors results in a rise in heart rate, an increase in myocardial contractility, and an overall increase in cardiac function. Most vasoactive compounds act through stimulation of these adrenergic receptors.

Sympathetic stimulation, which is not only important as a compensation for shock of any etiology but also as the mechanism by which most vasoactive drugs act, depends upon the maintenance of pH in a rather narrow physiologic range. The hallmarks of shock are tissue ischemia and metabolic acidosis. As the pH declines, the capacity of the heart and peripheral vasculature to respond to adrenergic stimulation declines. To maximize sympathetic compensation and preserve cardiovascular function, the metabolic acidosis often must be corrected with specific alkali therapy in the form of intravenous sodium bicarbonate.

Norepinephrine

Norepinephrine (Levophed) acts on alpha receptors in the arteriolar and venular smooth muscle to increase total peripheral resistance and venous tone. It acts on cardiac beta receptors (beta$_1$ receptors) to increase the heart rate and improve myocardial contractility. The result is enhanced venous return, increased cardiac output, and increased total peripheral resistance. The net effect is a more optimal perfusion pressure for maintenance of blood flow to the heart and brain. This comes about at the expense of cutaneous, skeletal muscle, and renal, and splanchnic perfusion. It must be borne in mind that though norepinephrine will optimize the delivery of blood to the heart and brain, it will not improve and, indeed, will aggravate the existing tissue ischemia in other organs. For this reason norepinephrine must be used in conjunction with the replacement of existing fluid loss, and ongoing losses must be checked.

Patients with hypotension and shock who are not responding to vigorous fluid replacement should be treated with norepinephrine in the emergency room. For this purpose, 4 ml of norepinephrine is added to 1,000 ml 5% dextrose or 5% dextrose and saline solution and administered through a well-secured intravenous plastic cannula, preferably in a large vein, in order to avoid the risk of extravasation and tissue necrosis. Two to three milliliters are administered rapidly, and the flow rate is adjusted to establish and maintain a low normal blood pressure (80–100 mm Hg systolic).

Extravasation of norepinephrine solution into the subcutaneous tissue is treated by infiltration of 5–10 ml phentolamine (an α-adrenergic blocking drug) as soon as possible around the site of extravasation.

Isoproterenol

Isoproterenol increases cardiac rate and myocardial contractility through beta$_1$ receptor stimulation. It also affects skeletal muscle vasodilation through beta$_2$ receptor activation. The net effect is tachycardia, elevation in cardiac output, and a tendency toward arrhythmia. The blood pressure may not rise because of the combination of increased cardiac output as well as a decline in total peripheral resistance. Isoproterenol's major use is to speed up the heart rate in circumstances of shock associated with bradycardia. It is also effective in the management of septic shock. Because isoproterenol increases myocardial oxygen consumption, it may provoke malignant arrhythmias and does not predictably increase perfusion pressure. Its use is contraindicated in cardiogenic shock resulting from myocardial infarction, except when required to temporarily increase heart rate.

One milligram isoproterenol (5 ml) is diluted in 500 ml 5% dextrose (1:500,000 fluid concentration) and infused at a rate of 0.25–2.5 mg/min titrated to maintain heart rate at 70–110 beats/min and blood pressure at a low normal range (80–100 mm Hg systolic). For the treatment of septic shock, shock secondary to bradycardia and/or heart block, or shock due to pulmonary embolism, treatment with isoproterenol should be instituted in the emergency room or as soon as the diagnosis is made.

Metaraminol

Metaraminol (Aramane) is a potent vasopressor and functions to deplete norepinephrine by displacement. Its actions are almost identical to those of norepinephrine except that it does not appear to reduce renal blood flow as much as norepinephrine.

The treatment of hypotension and shock with metaraminol can be instituted in the emergency room while defects in the circulating blood volume are being corrected. Ten milliliters metaraminol is added to 500 ml sodium chloride or 5% dextrose solution at the rate of infusion titrated to restore the arterial blood pressure to a low-normal range.

Methoxamine

Methoxamine (Vasoxyl) is, for all practical purposes, a pure α-adrenergic receptor stimulating agent. It is a potent vasopressor with little, if any, direct effect on the heart. It is most useful in elevating peripheral resistance and venous tone when hypotension and organ hypoperfusion are associated with inadequate sympathetic tone and a "relative" increase in the capacitance of the vascular tree. This agent is useful in "spinal" shock associated with spinal cord trauma or spinal anesthesia. It also may be useful in elevating the total peripheral resistance and aortic perfusion pressure in other circumstances where hypotension seems to be associated with an inadequate degree of vasoconstriction and a well maintained cardiac output.

Methoxamine is available in a solution (20 mg/ml) for intramuscular or intravenous administration. The usual intravenous dose for hypotensive emergencies is 3–5 mg (0.15–0.25 ml) injected slowly. To maintain a more prolonged effect, the intravenous dose may be supplemental by 10–20 mg (0.5–1.0 ml) methoxamine intramuscularly (IM).

Sodium Bicarbonate

With prolonged shock, metabolic acidosis becomes severe and the pH declines below 7.2. This causes depression of cardiac contractility and decreases responsiveness of the vascular smooth muscles to catecholamine. The result is a decline in blood pressure as cardiac output and total peripheral resistance decline. Definitive therapy for this acidosis requires restoration of tissue perfusion so that the liver can metabolize lactic acid to sodium bicarbonate and the base deficit can be corrected. However, if the pH declines below 7.2, it is appropriate to administer sodium bicarbonate to correct the acidosis consequent to organ hypoperfusion. It is reasonable to give 2 ampules (44 mEq/ampule) of sodium bicarbonate and then immediately repeat the arterial blood gas and pH determinations.

The results should be available within several minutes, and, if the pH is still below 7.2, an additional 2 ampules of sodium bicarbonate should be administered intravenously. It is important that the arterial pH be checked after each administration of sodium bicarbonate so that too rapid a correction of the acidosis does not occur. This could result in a delayed but profound alkalosis, especially when the excessive body stores of lactic acid are metabolized to sodium bicarbonate after successful resuscitation of the shock state. At this point the pH may abruptly rise above 7.5 with significant physiologic consequences. Alkalosis results in cerebral vasoconstriction and also compromises the ability of the red cells to give up oxygen to the tissues. The net result is diminished tissue oxygenation. These complications can result in central nervous system symptoms as severe as those accompanying the initial shock and acidosis.

The replacement dose of sodium bicarbonate for the treatment of the metabolic lactic acidosis of shock can be calculated according to the following guidelines: Dose (in milliequivalents) = estimated lean total body weight in kilograms $\times$ 0.6 liter H_2O/kg lean body weight $\times$ (25-measured serum bicarbonate concentration) mEq/liter $\times$ 0.5. The physiologic basis of this formula is that total body water is 60% of lean body mass and the bicarbonate distribution spare is 50% of the total body water. After having calculated the total bicarbonate replacement dose, we give only 50% of this dose and then recheck the arterial pH before further bicarbonate administration. This avoids overcorrection of the base defect with resultant alkalosis since it allows for the generation of bicarbonate ion from lactate ion as the acidosis is reversed by other therapy directed at improving the tissue function.

Monitoring

The patient with shock invariably demonstrates rapid changes in all major physiologic and biochemical parameters. Furthermore, more subtle changes may reflect the first manifestation of clinical improvement or deterioration; these changes are complex and intimately related. To recognize such changes, a flow sheet is required. On this sheet all parameters are simultaneously recorded and correlated so that subtle changes can be detected at the earliest possible moment. Specific parameters that must be followed continuously or at periodic intervals of several minutes to a few hours include the following: blood pressure, pulse, central venous pressure, urine output, and pulmonary status.

BLOOD PRESSURE

Since therapy of shock is essentially the reversal of organ underperfusion and perfusion is a function of blood pressure, continuous measurement of the blood pressure assumes paramount importance. Resuscitation from hypovolemia is reflected by a rise in the cuff mean and pulse pressure as the stroke output of the heart increases in response to fluid administration. In the presence of sustained hypotension (systolic cuff pressure below 100 mm Hg), peripheral cuff blood pressures may underestimate central aortic pressure. This is due to the profound compensatory sympathetic vasoconstriction accompanying sustained hypotension. In fact, it is dangerous to assume that the blood pressure that is unobtainable by cuff technique is, in fact, low. Although the so-called unobtainable blood pressure or pulse is usually associated with severe hypotension, 5–10% of the patients with such a finding actually have a normal or high blood pressure. For this reason, accurate measurement of the arterial pressure in profoundly vasoconstricted patients requires cannulation of a radial or brachial artery with a large bore (16-gauge) cannula of sufficient length to be positioned in the axillary artery. Since peripheral arterial pulses may be difficult to palpate in this group of patients, percutaneous insertion of a radial catheter may be difficult. A cutdown is usually required (Procedure 14). Alternatively, the femoral artery can be cannulated percutaneously with a similar sized cannula. The femoral approach is particularly advantageous. In the absence of preexisting peripheral vascular disease, this is a rapid, safe, clean approach that does not require cutdown and direct vascular exposure. In the patient with relatively normal arteries it does not jeopardize the distal extremity and does not put the patient at risk from central nervous system events caused by a catheter malposition proximal to the takeoff of the blood vessels to the head or inadvertent air or clot embolization. However, the femoral approach to continuous monitoring of blood pressure should not be used in infants or small children.

Intraarterial pressure recording is usually not required in the emergency room and is most appropriately performed by experienced personnel in the critical care unit.

PULSE

In the treatment of shock, it must be remembered that the primary concern is the blood flow throughout the body, especially to the brain and heart. Unfortunately, a poor correlation often exists between blood flow and blood pressure, especially when vasopressor drugs are used to raise the pressure. For this reason, at the same time that the blood pressure is being closely monitored, the urine output and other clinical indications of blood flow—the warmth and color of the skin and the quality of the pulse—must be carefully and frequently observed. The rhythm is continually monitored by the *electrocardiogram* (ECG) and displayed on an oscilloscope. The rhythm is also intermittently, but frequently, monitored by direct palpation. Successful resuscitation results in an increase in the pulse amplitude and a decline in the pulse rate. As cardiac stroke volume is restored, the pulse volume rises; as reflex sympathetic compensation abates, the pulse rate declines. Continuous ECG monitoring allows the instantaneous detection, diagnosis, and treatment of various arrhythmias (described in Chapter 5).

CENTRAL VENOUS PRESSURE

Pivotal to the correct diagnosis and management of the patient in shock is rapid and accurate measurement of the central venous pressure (CVP). It is most appropriate to obtain this information as soon as possible, preferably by cannulation of the central venous system in the emergency room. This can be accomplished via percutaneous cannulation or cutdown of the brachial vein or via percutaneous cannulation of the femoral, subclavian, or external jugular vein by an experienced physician.

Central venous pressure is a function of the blood volume and blood flow in the central veins, the sympathetic tone to the capacitance vessels (the venules), the competence of the right ventricle as a pump, and the intrathoracic pressure. It normally ranges between 3 and 8 cm of saline. In hypovolemic shock the central venous pressure is always below 5 cm and often approaches 0 cm. It may also be low or low normal in patients with cardiogenic shock with acute left ventricular failure. Here the right ventricle is able to pump blood into the pulmonary circuit, but the left ventricle is unable to pump blood from the pulmonary to the systemic circuit without an excessive filling pressure to stretch the left ventricle and elevate its preload.

In the presence of low central venous pressure, fluid administration that produces a rise in CVP to normal levels can be taken as an indicator of the restoration of blood volume.

Should the central venous pressure be normal upon initial determination in the presence of what appears to be hypovolemic shock, a diagnostic and therapeutic trial of rapid fluid administration is undertaken. From 200 to 500 ml of crystalloid are rapidly administered (over 5–10 minutes) in 50-ml boluses. In response to this infusion, the central venous pressure will either rise abruptly to abnormal levels (greater than 12 cm of saline) or remain in the low-normal range. An abrupt rise in the central venous pressure in the presence of signs of improving organ perfusion suggests that the volume resuscitation is nearly adequate and that the rate of fluid administration should be slowed to prevent volume overload and the development of pulmonary congestion.

Should the central venous pressure abruptly rise in response to a volume push in the face of persisting organ hypoperfusion or hypotension, we must suspect the following conditions:

1. The unmasking of left ventricular dysfunction that may have antedated or, in fact, have given rise to the initial hypotensive episode. Often patients will develop shortness of breath, an increase in the respiratory rate, and basilar rales. Fluid administration must be terminated and further therapy governed by the pulmonary capillary wedge pressure measured by Swan-Ganz catheterization of the pulmonary artery in the intensive care unit.

2. The presence of acute pulmonary embolism as a cause of shock (usually the central venous pressure will be elevated upon presentation).

3. The presence of pericardial tamponade, the classical manifestation of which (elevated jugular venous pressure) is obscured by concomitant volume depletion. We may anticipate this situation in patients who present with open thoracic or upper abdominal trauma. These patients may have hemopericardium and tamponade concomitant with hypovolemia to the point of exsanguination.

Should the central venous pressure remain constant or rise only slightly (less than 5 cm H_2O) while the blood pressure and/or signs of peripheral organ perfusion improve, we may conclude that hypovolemia was, indeed, the precipitating event; fluid replacement should continue at a rapid rate until all signs of organ underperfusion abate and the central venous pressure stabilizes in the normal range.

If the central venous pressure remains low and evidence of peripheral hypotension persists after rapid volume administration, we should suspect that losses are profound with much more fluid required for resuscitation or that the losses (e.g., occult gastrointestinal, intrathoracic, or retroperitoneal bleeding) are ongoing.

There are four errors that are commonly made in the use of the CVP for monitoring of shock:

1. Failure to check the position of the catheter by x-ray film before making treatment decisions based on the results of CVP measurements.
2. The attempt to assess the adequacy of circulating volume on the basis of one measurement alone. It is much more important to consider the first measurement as a baseline to which subsequent values can be compared as the response to therapy is continuously followed.
3. Reliance on the CVP to detect fluid overloading when crystalloid solutions are administered. Gross overloading with salt solution may occur with a normal CVP.
4. The attempt to assess left ventricular function by means of the CVP. The left ventricular filling pressure can be rising in spite of a normal central venous pressure. The CVP cannot be used as a substitute for measurement of the pulmonary capillary wedge pressure, which is the true index of the filling pressure of the left ventricle.

PULMONARY CAPILLARY WEDGE PRESSURE

In the presence of left ventricular failure the CVP is an inaccurate guide for therapy. For this reason, patients in cardiogenic shock should be transferred to the intensive care unit as soon as possible in order that their pulmonary capillary wedge pressure (PCWP) can be monitored. The PCWP accurately reflects the left ventricular filling pressure except in the presence of mitral stenosis. Although this procedure can be performed without flouroscopic guidance, it is advantageous to place the catheter under direct visualization using a portable flouroscopy unit. This ensures proper placement and insures accuracy in the PCWP measurement. In addition, it lessens the likelihood of kinking of the tube or of having redundant catheter loops in the right ventricle that may cause arrhythmias.

URINE OUTPUT

Decreased renal perfusion and reduction in the glomerular filtration rate are hallmarks of almost all forms of shock. The two exceptions are shock associated with diabetic ketoacidosis and hyperosmolar nonketotic coma where glycosuria may obligate fluid for the renal tubules despite a reduction in the glomerular filtration rate. Fluid resuscitation, through increasing the cardiac output, increasing mean arterial pressure, and decreasing renal vasoconstriction, elevates the glomerular filtration and the urine production rates. In order to assess this parameter, a Foley catheter should be aseptically introduced into the bladder to follow the hourly urine output. The initial sterile urine specimen obtained should be sent for urinalysis, culture, sodium concentration, and urine osmolarity, as well as specific gravity. Hypovolemic shock should be associated with low urine sodium (less than 10–12 mEq/liter) and high urine osmolarity (greater than 400 mosm/kg) as long as there is no glycosuria or renal tubular dysfunction as a result of intrinsic renal disease, previous diuretic therapy, deficiency of the antidiuretic hormone, or adrenal cortical insufficiency.

As long as the central venous pressure is low and urine flow is less than 20 ml/hr, vigorous fluid administration is appropriate. An increase in the hourly urine flow and the urine sodium concentration and a decline in the urine osmolarity signify that therapy is proceeding to a successful conclusion.

PULMONARY STATUS

Frequent monitoring of the respiratory rate, chest examination, and the blood gases is essential in the management of the patient in shock. With rapid fluid administration, especially in elderly patients with preexisting cardiac disease, the left ventricular diastolic and pulmonary capillary pressures may rise rapidly leading to pulmonary congestion and edema. A rise in the respiratory rate, the development of basilar rales, and blood gases showing hypoxemia, hypocarbia, and respiratory alkalosis suggest the development of congestive heart failure. Treatment with supplemental oxygen, diuretics, digoxin, and vasodilators is instituted according to the principles outlined in Chapter 6.

The patient in shock is always at risk for the development of pulmonary failure. This complication may be due to the aspiration of gastric contents before and during the initial resuscitation, generalized sepsis, pulmonary contusion sustained as a result of chest trauma, fat embolism, or the cumulative effects of circulatory insufficiency on the alveolar–capillary unit (adult respiratory distress syndrome).

Such complications develop after successful initial resuscitation and stabilization usually after 72 hours of hospitalization. Persistent fever, a rising respiratory rate, dyspnea, progressive arterial hypercarbia and hypoxemia despite administration of supplemental oxygen, and the appearance of diffuse, bilateral alveolar infiltrates on the chest roentgenogram heralds the development of adult respiratory distress syndrome. Treatment includes intubation and ventilatory support usually with positive and expiratory pressure, diagnosis, and specific antimicrobial therapy for any concurrent pulmonary infection. General supportive measures are indicated as outlined in Chapter 2.

CLINICAL SETTINGS

Absolute Hypovolemia

HYPOVOLEMIC SHOCK

The patient presenting with hypovolemic shock requires accurate, complete, and swift evaluation to maximize the chance for successful therapeutic outcome. The overall presentation is predicted upon the precipitating insult; the nature, duration, and severity of the volume depletion; and the presence or absence of underlying disease. Obviously, pertinent history, physical examination, and preliminary therapy are simultaneously undertaken.

Diagnosis

The patients appear pale with cool and clammy extremities and may, in fact, display acrocyanosis because of slowed circulation and the more complete extraction of oxygen from hemoglobin. They are anxious, sometimes agitated, confused, or frankly obtunded depending upon the duration and severity of central nervous system hypoperfusion. Blood pressure is reduced, or at least the pulse pressure is narrowed, and there is tachycardia resulting from the sympathetic discharge. The patient who is not frankly hypotensive in the supine position can be stressed to demonstrate an orthostatic decline in blood pressure. If the patient sits up briefly, the blood pressure often declines by at least 10–20 mm Hg and the pulse rises by 10–15 beats/min. Such a posturally induced rise in pulse and decline in blood pressure indicate extravascular volume depletion in excess of 500 ml. The narrowed pulse pressure and tachycardia are manifest as a rapid, thready pulse. In fact, because of profound vasoconstriction and reduced cardiac stroke output, the patient's pulse may not be palpable at the radial, brachial, or dorsalis pedia arteries. Usually, however, the pulse will be weak but palpable in the carotid, femoral, or brachial arteries. Reduced stroke output of the heart results in a softening of the heart sounds; indeed, they may really be inaudible over the precordium. Because of the low central venous pressure resulting from volume depletion, the jugular veins are collapsed.

Diagnosis of hypovolemic shock is obvious when the patient presents in such a state of cardiovascular collapse. Further acquisition of data is directed at elucidating the precipitating event. Obvious external or gastrointestinal bleeding suggests hemorrhagic shock, whereas a history of anticoagulant use may suggest spontaneous retroperitoneal hemorrhage. A history of trauma may suggest hemothorax or hemoperitoneum (see Chapter 12). Patients in shock who also have fever, abdominal pain, abdominal tenderness, and decreased or absent bowel sounds present the picture of hypovolemic shock secondary to peritonitis. Such could result from pancreatitis, volvulus, strangulated hernia, empyema of the gallbladder, perforated duodenal ulcer, bowel infarction, or a variety of other catastrophes resulting in peritonitis with secondary sepsis and extensive third space fluid loss (see Chapter 33).

When the cause of the volume depletion is less obvious, the history assumes greater importance. Previous vomiting or diarrhea suggests volume depletion resulting from excessive gastrointestinal fluid losses, such as can result from gastroenteritis. Frank shock from such losses is more common in children since the extracellular fluid volume is more susceptible to such losses (see Chapter 43). A history of polyuria may suggest salt-losing nephritis, diabetes insipidus, or diabetes mellitus with ketoacidosis. Finally, excessive diuretic therapy can eventuate in volume depletion to the point of shock.

Therapy

The principles involved in the therapy for hypovolemic shock have previously been discussed. It must be emphasized that it is urgent to establish sufficient intravenous access to accomplish rapid fluid resuscitation and correction of acute losses. Furthermore, with hemorrhagic shock not only must existing losses be corrected with whole blood or packed cells and colloid or crystalloid infusion, but also vigorous attempts must be made to stop ongoing losses. It must be emphasized that in injuries to the chest, abdomen, or extremities vascular access must be established in an area where there is no question about the integrity of the proximal venous anatomy (see Chapter 12). For example, in circumstances of open chest injury, the vascular access should be established in the lower extremities; and, conversely, in circumstances of abdominal injury, the vascular access should be established in the upper extremities. In all cases of hypovolemic shock where blood loss has resulted from open trauma, closed trauma, or intestinal hemorrhage, early surgical consultation should be sought so that definitive therapy can be undertaken as soon as indicated.

In circumstances of shock resulting from intraabdominal catastrophe with resulting peritonitis, several measures must be undertaken simultaneously. In addition to the establishment of reliable vascular access and the rapid infusion of an adequate volume of colloid or crystalloid solution, nasogastric intubation should be established, a central venous pressure line should be positioned within the right atrium or the great veins of the chest, broad spectrum antibiotics as outlined in the section on septic shock should be administered, and early surgical consultation should be obtained.

Shock resulting from vomiting, diarrhea, or excessive renal

losses of fluid and electrolytes requires the infusion of isotonic saline or lactated Ringer's solution until the central venous pressure has normalized, the pulse is slower, and the blood pressure has been stabilized. After the extracellular volume defect is corrected by appropriate fluid administration, the normally perfused kidney will be able to correct the more subtle osmotic and electrolyte derangements and therapy need not be directed at a precise correction of osmotic and electrolyte derangements.

Relative Hypovolemia

BACTEREMIC SHOCK

Bacteremic, or septic, shock is a syndrome of inadequate tissue perfusion due to adverse cardiocirculatory effects of bacterial infection. This condition results from gram-negative sepsis in about two-thirds of patients and from gram-positive sepsis in the remainder. In approximately one-fourth of all patients with a gram-negative bacteremia, the complete syndrome of septic shock may develop. The epidemiology of this syndrome is significant. It occurs most often in men over age 40. In those under 40, women with obstetric or gynecologic problems predominate. Most patients have at least one of the following medical conditions: cirrhosis, leukemia, alcoholism, diabetes mellitus, metastatic carcinoma, lymphoma, burns, urinary or biliary tract infections, prior surgery, or manipulation of the genitourinary or gastrointestinal tracts. If such conditions are associated with antimetabolite therapy, corticosteroid therapy, or irradiation, the potential for septic shock is enhanced. Some common gram-positive organisms usually implicated include staphylococci, pneumococci, and clostridia. The pathophysiology of this syndrome is multifactorial, but for gram-negative organisms it is closely related to the release of endotoxin, a polysaccharide, into the circulation. The initial response to bacteremia is usually a diminution in the peripheral vascular resistance and an increase in the cardiac output. Nonetheless, the increment in cardiac output is insufficient to compensate for the fall in vascular resistance. The net result is hypotension and a pooling of blood into the body's microvascular beds, ineffective cardiac output, and tissue anoxia.

Diagnosis

It is not difficult to recognize the fully developed bacteremic shock syndrome. Nonetheless, early or atypical manifestations of bacteremic shock may cause considerable confusion. This diagnosis must be entertained in any elderly patient demonstrating unexplained mental changes, hyperventilation, high fever, hypothermia, clinical evidence of hypoglycemia, or unexplained hypotension. In the early stages of this syndrome, in conjunction with the drop in peripheral vascular resistance and rise in cardiac output, the patient may demonstrate "warm shock," which includes the presence of a full pulse pressure, warm dry skin, mild hypotension, and little or no change in urinary output. Blood gases at this time usually demonstrate an elevation in the pH and hypocarbia. In time, untreated and, unfortunately, many treated patients progress to the syndrome of "cold shock." At this juncture, hypotension is more profound and the patient is usually clammy, cold, pale, and peripherally cyanotic. The pulse is weak and thready, and the urine output is markedly decreased. As a manifestation of the tissue hypoperfusion, metabolic acidosis supervenes with the reduction in the arterial pH due to a reduction in bicarbonate stores. Central venous pressure is usually low. There is usually an elevation of the white count with a shift to the left. The platelet count may be normal or decreased with evidence of disseminated intravascular coagulation and, as a manifestation of hemoconcentration, the hemoglobin and hematocrit may be initially elevated. Blood cultures, though not invariably, are usually positive.

The differential diagnosis includes stroke, aortic dissection, hemorrhage, myocardial infarction or pulmonary embolism, and in some circumstances, pericardial effusion with tamponade.

Management

All patients suspected of having septic shock should have a central venous pressure line positioned and urinary output monitored. Blood should be drawn for culture, electrolyte, blood urea nitrogen (BUN), and creatinine determinations. Hypotension should be treated initially with colloid fluid replacement therapy; if manifestations of peripheral hypoperfusion do not correct, isoproterenol or dopamine therapy should be instituted in order to restore cardiac output and peripheral perfusion. Cultures of blood, urine, any fluid collections in the various serous body cavities, or wound exudates should be rapidly obtained, and institution of intravenous broad-spectrum antibiotic therapy should not be delayed. Such therapy would include a broad-spectrum drug that is effective against a variety of gram-negative organisms such as gentamycin in a dose of 1.7 mg/kg with the frequency of subsequent doses determined by the creatinine clearance. In addition, a bacteriocidal antibiotic that is effective against most gram-positive organisms, including penicillin-resistant staphylococci, such as nafcillin 6–12 gm/day in divided doses, depending upon the underlying renal function, should be administered. Supplemental oxygen or mechanically assisted ventilation should be provided based upon the patient's clinical state and the results of arterial blood gas determinations. The presence of purulent material in serous body cavities or an abscess requires emergency drainage by operative exploration or percutaneous catheter placement to hasten resolution of septic shock.

NEUROGENIC SHOCK

The maintenance of venous return, cardiac output, and arterial pressure depends upon modulation of venous tone, cardiac performance, and peripheral arteriolar resistance by the sympathetic nervous system. Sympathetic discharge is constantly maintained to preserve the tautness of the vascular system and enable it to maintain venous pressure and venous return despite fluctuations in the total blood volume.

Abrupt cessation of sympathetic outflow, as occurs in injuries to the cervical or upper thoracic spinal cord, can result in hypotension and, in the extreme circumstance, evidence of organ hypoperfusion. With the interception of venous tone, the volume of the capacitance circuit increases, venous pressure declines, and cardiac output fails. Because of a failure of sympathetic arteriolar tone, total peripheral resistance declines. Because mean arterial pressure is equal to the product of cardiac output and total peripheral resistance it, too, must decline.

Diagnosis

Patients with spinal shock often have a history of trauma; they are often hypotensive, but because total peripheral resistance is also reduced, they demonstrate warm, well-perfused extremities. Sweating should not be present below the injured spinal cord segment. The presence of cool, cyanotic extremities indicates that cardiac output is profoundly depressed and vigorous fluid administration should be instituted promptly. Urine output may be inappropriately high because of failure of compensatory renal vasoconstriction.

Management

Treatment includes the following: (1) excluding the presence of internal bleeding into the chest, mediastinum, retroperitoneum, pelvis, or abdomen; (2) vigorous fluid resuscitation with saline at 200–400 ml/hr to restore blood pressure; (3) vasopressor therapy with methoxamine or metaraminol to increase venous and arteriolar tone via α-adrenergic mediated vasoconstriction and restore blood pressure.

A word of caution is in order: The patient presenting with head trauma and who develops shock may have occult spinal cord injury and/or occult bleeding. Furthermore, if there is a history of concomitant head trauma or concussion along with the spinal cord injury and significant internal bleeding is not present, α-adrenergic vasopressors rather than fluids are more appropriate to restore blood pressure in order to retard the development of intracranial edema.

CARDIOGENIC SHOCK

Cardiogenic shock, most commonly seen in the setting of acute myocardial infarction, is defined by the following criteria: (1) widespread evidence of peripheral ischemia; (2) oliguria—urine output less than 20 ml/hr; (3) reduced cardiac output (cardiac index less than 2.5 liters/min/m²); (4) inadequate left atrial filling pressures as defined by a PCWP of at least 15–16 mm Hg; (5) and evidence of acute myocardial infarction by ECG.

Diagnosis

The patient is often a middle-aged or elderly man with a history of chest pain, weakness, or shortness of breath. He may or may not have a known history of cardiac disease or hypertension. Initial examination is directed at detecting organ hypoperfusion as defined above, looking for evidence of cardiac dysfunction—that is, a third heart sound, a summation gallop, or heart murmurs suggestive of mitral regurgitation or ventricular septal defect—and looking for evidence of pulmonary congestion and edema. The ECG is crucial in that it displays evidence of acute transmural or subendocardial myocardial infarction in the vast majority of patients. The diagnostic features of cardiogenic shock are discussed in Chapter 4.

Management

Therapy is directed at stabilizing the patient. After a widebore intravenous catheter is inserted and an ECG has been obtained, the patient is placed on a continuous ECG monitor. He is given low flow oxygen via a face mask or nasal cannula. Blood gases are obtained 10–15 minutes after starting supplemental oxygen therapy in order to document the adequacy of arterial oxygenation, to make sure that the patient is not retaining carbon dioxide (as many patients with heart attacks are heavy smokers and have a history of chronic obstructive pulmonary disease) and to detect the presence of a metabolic (lactic) acidosis resulting from tissue ischemia and anaerobic glycolysis. Furthermore, slight hypoxia with a respiratory alkalosis may suggest the presence of incipient pulmonary congestion long before rales or frank signs of pulmonary edema are manifest. The management of cardiogenic shock is discussed in Chapter 4.

Should frank hypotension (blood pressure less than 100 systolic) persist after a fluid challenge by rapid infusion of 100–200 ml of normal saline, the patient is started on dopamine to maintain cardiac output sufficient to perfuse the coronary arteries and central nervous system. The initial dose of dopamine is 2 mg in 500 ml D$_5$W run at 4–8 μg/kg/min. Should the blood pressure not be restored to a level of 100 mmHg systolic after a few minutes of infusion at this rate, the dose is increased. Should the patient remain hypotensive despite a dopamine infusion rate of 15–20 μg/kg/min, the patient is started on norepinephrine to elevate the systolic blood pressure above 90 mm Hg. Persistent hypotension and pressor requirements despite administration of 200–300 ml of saline or in the presence of frank pulmonary congestion require catheterization of the pulmonary artery. Specifically, right heart catheterization with a Swan-Ganz balloon-tipped, thermodilution catheter in the coronary care unit is mandatory in order to rule out structural complications of myocardial infarction, measure cardiac output and PCWP and to decide on a further course of therapy. These hemodynamic parameters are absolutely essential to rule out a component of relative volume depletion that could have resulted from vomiting, nitrate or morphine administration, previous diuretic therapy, or inadequate fluid intake associated with acute infarction. Furthermore, these hemodynamic measurements, as well as continuous online intraarterial recording of the blood pressure, are mandatory to monitor the patient's response to inotropic drug administration.

The placement of Swan-Ganz catheters and arterial monitoring lines should be done under aseptic conditions after the patient has arrived in the coronary care unit.

See also Chapters 4 and 5 for a more complete discussion of the treatment of cardiogenic shock.

Obstructive Shock

Inadequate cardiac output and tissue hypoperfusion result from conditions in which the heart cannot adequately empty in systole (pulmonary embolism) or fill in diastole (pericardial tamponade)

PULMONARY EMBOLISM

Patients with a debilitating illness such as cancer or cardiovascular disease, patients who have been on bed rest for any reason, or patients who have sustained trauma to the lower extremities can develop deep venous thrombosis. Should a clot break loose from within the leg veins, it is carried to the right side of the heart and impacts in the pulmonary artery tree. If

this embolus obstructs more than 40–50% of the pulmonary arterial cross-sectional area, acute pulmonary hypertension, right ventricular failure, and shock can ensue. With the acute reduction in pulmonary arterial cross-sectional area, pulmonary vascular resistance abruptly rises. The resulting abrupt increase in impedance to right ventricular emptying precipitates a decline in cardiac output since the right ventricle cannot empty against this sudden load. As cardiac output declines, the right ventricle dilates and fails and the mean right atrial pressure rises.

Diagnosis

As described in Chapter 2, the patient presents with a history of dyspnea, pleuritic chest pain, cough, or hemoptysis. He may or may not display evidence of venous thrombosis of the lower extremity. On examination there is evidence of widespread organ hypoperfusion and tachypnea. The patient is hypotensive, tachycardiac, and diaphoretic. The neck veins are distended since the central venous pressure is elevated because of acute right ventricular failure. This is in sharp contrast with a patient with hypovolemic shock who has a low central venous pressure and collapsed neck veins. It is also in contradistinction to the patient in cardiogenic shock who may have low-normal or distended neck veins. Because of pulmonary hypertension, the pulmonic component of the second heart sound is intensified, the second heart sound may be widely split, or there may be a right parasternal lift and a pulmonary ejection murmur. Other diagnostic features are discussed in Chapter 2.

Management

The treatment of pulmonary embolism is divided into three areas: (1) measures to improve ventilatory function and gas exchange; (2) measures to prevent subsequent, life-threatening embolism; (3) measures to relieve the obstruction to right ventricular outflow and improve right ventricular function in order to reverse shock.

Embolic obstruction of the pulmonary arteries of any clinical significance is invariably accompanied by ventilation perfusion mismatch and an increase of the ventilatory dead space to total volume ratio. The patient complains of dyspnea and there is invariably some degree of hypoxia and respiratory alkalosis. In more severe cases, cyanosis is evident. The administration of supplemental oxygen to increase the percentage of oxygen in the inspired air will alleviate or correct severe hypoxemia in almost all cases. If ventilation is compromised and carbon dioxide retention develops, intubation and mechanical respiratory assistance are required to correct hypercarbia and respiratory acidosis (described in Chapter 2).

When pulmonary embolism is first clinically suspected, before the performance of confirmatory diagnostic procedures, the patient must be protected from the development of a subsequent and likely fatal pulmonary embolism. Accordingly, the patient should receive 4,000–8,000 units of heparin immediately by intravenous bolus. This is followed by the administration of heparin intravenously by continuous infusion to maintain the activated partial thromboplastin time at two and one-half to three times control value. This is usually accomplished by a dose of heparin in the range of 1,000–2,000 units/hr. This therapy prevents the formation and propagation of large occlusive thrombi in the deep veins of the legs and thighs thereby reducing the likelihood of a subsequent embolic event. Should the patient subsequently develop a documented pulmonary embolism despite the administration of anticoagulant therapy in a dose that appropriately prolongs the partial thromboplastin time, definitive prophylactic therapy is indicated to protect the patient from a subsequent embolic event. This therapy involves measures designed to mechanically obstruct the migration of thrombi from the large veins of the thigh and pelvis and through the inferior vena cava. This is accomplished by placing a clip around the inferior vena cava just below the level of the renal veins through a retroperitoneal surgical approach. This procedure requires the administration of general anesthesia and is relatively contraindicated in high-risk patients. In such patients definitive prophylactic therapy can be accomplished by the positioning of an umbrella filter under fluoroscopic guidance in the vena cava just below the level of the renal veins. This procedure can be performed under local anesthesia through an internal jugular or femoral venous cutdown.

If the patient has evidence of tissue and organ hypoperfusion as a result of pulmonary embolism, measures to improve right ventricular function and acutely relieve the obstruction to right ventricular outflow must be undertaken in order to reverse the shock state. Intravenous streptokinase promotes more rapid lysis of pulmonary emboli by the fibrinolytic system and hastens hemodynamic improvement. Isoproterenol can improve the function of the acutely pressure-overloaded right ventricle and enable it to maintain a satisfactory cardiac output despite the resistance to emptying offered by the emboli in the pulmonary artery. It is administered in a dose sufficient to maintain the systolic blood pressure above 85–90 mm Hg, to restore urine output, and to alleviate other evidence of organ hypoperfusion. Should isoproterenol fail to correct the shock state rapidly, the patient can be sedated with morphine so that external cardiac massage can be administered without undue discomfort. This improves the function of the failing right ven-

tricle and, at the same time, may break up large emboli lodged in the main or first-order pulmonary arteries, thereby rapidly relieving the obstruction to right ventricular outflow and restoring peripheral perfusion. At the same time, preparations should be underway to perform pulmonary embolectomy, usually under cardiopulmonary bypass, to relieve the obstruction to right ventricular outflow and restore the cardiac output to normal.

AIR EMBOLISM

Air or gas embolism to the right ventricular cavity or pulmonary artery can also present as cardiovascular collapse. It should be suspected when a predisposed patient suddenly develops systemic hypotension, tachycardia, or tachypnea. A peculiar to-and-fro murmur over the pericardium may suggest this diagnosis. Conditions predisposing to lethal air or gas embolism of the right side of the heart include transfusions in bottles pressurized with air, vaginal gas insufflation, insertion of central catheters by the subclavian or internal jugular approach, and craniotomy in the sitting position. In this latter circumstance, negative intrathoracic and venous pressure may draw air into open veins.

A fatal air or gas embolism on the right side of the heart results from obstruction of flow in the right atrium and pulmonary outflow tract. Conditions that determine the severity of shock and the likelihood of developing cardiac arrest are the volume and solubility of the gas, the underlying cardiovascular status of the patient, and the position of the patient. In man, probably over 300 ml of gas must rapidly enter the venous system in order to precipitate cardiovascular collapse.

Treatment

The treatment of a gas embolism on the right side of the heart involves the following: (1) administration of 100% oxygen by intermittent positive pressure ventilation; (2) positioning the patient head down and left side down in order to facilitate the exit of foam into the right heart from the pulmonary outflow tract; (3) use of isoproterenol, as previously outlined, and (4) if cardiac arrest supervenes, opening the chest to perform open-chest cardiac resuscitation including needle aspiration of air from the right ventricle.

PERICARDIAL TAMPONADE

As the pericardium distends with fluid, intrapericardial pressure rises and tends to throttle the ventricle in diastole so that it can no longer be filled by the blood returning to the central circuit at a normal central venous pressure. Consequently, the venous return is impaired, pulse rises, venous tone rises, and the central venous pressure rises. If further fluid accumulates in the pericardial space, further cardiac filling is retarded despite the compensatory rise in central venous pressure to maintain the pressure gradient for ventricular filling in diastole. At this point the cardiac output abruptly declines, and the patient develops circulatory collapse.

Diagnosis

The patient with pericardial tamponade appears acutely distressed and is diaphoretic, tachycardic, and frankly hypotensive. He may be cyanotic. However, the hallmark of tamponade is profound distention of the neck veins resulting from the inordinate elevation of the intrapericardial pressure.

Treatment

Rapid intravenous access is established, and colloid or whole blood is administered to maximize the central venous pressure and preserve the gradient for ventricular filling in diastole. At the same time provision is made to perform therapeutic pericardiocentesis to remove the fluid that has collected in the pericardium and to reduce pericardial pressure. In this way venous return can be restored and cardiac output can be maintained. In the presence of tamponade in the setting of closed or open thoracic trauma, immediate provision for thoracotomy and pericardiotomy should be made since the cause of the pericardial tamponade may indeed be atrial or ventricular laceration or a tear in one of the great vessels requiring immediate surgical attention.

SUGGESTED READINGS

Ahlquist RP: A study of adrenotropic receptors. *Am J Physiol* 1948; 153:586.

Ahlquist RP: Agents which block adrenergic β-receptors. *Ann Rev Pharmac* 1968; 8:259–272.

Braunwald E (ed): Beta-Adrenergic Blockade: A New Era in Cardiovascular Medicine: Proceedings of an International Symposium, New York, NY. *Excerpta Medica: International Congress Series No. 446.* Symposium held October 3–4, 1977. Princeton, NJ, *Excerpta Medica,* 1978.

Braunwald E, Frahm CJ: Studies on Starling's law of the heart. *Circulation* 1961; 24:633.

Burton AC: *Physiology and Biophysics of the Circulation.* Chicago; Year Book Medical Publishers Inc, 1965.

Cardiovascular drugs, in Gilman AG, Goodman LS, Gilman A, et al (eds): *The Pharmacological Basis of Therapeutics,* ed 6. New York, Macmillan Inc, 1980, pp 761–833.

Cohn JN, Luria MH: Studies in clinical shock and hypotension: The value of bedside hemodynamic observations. *J Am Med Assoc* 1964; 190:891–896.

Crowell JW, Guyton AC: Cardiac deterioration in shock: II. The irreversible stage. *Int Anesthesiol Clin* 1964; 2:171.

Gorlin R, Sonnenblick E: Regulation of performance of the heart. *Am J Cardiol* 1968; 22:16.

Guyton AC: Regulation of cardiac output. *Anesthesiology* 1968; 29:314.

Haller JA Jr, Ward MJ, Cahill JL: Metabolic alterations in shock: The effect of controlled reduction of blood flow on oxidative metabolism and catecholamine response. *J Trauma* 1967; 7:727.

Hurst JW, Logue RB, Schlant RC, et al (eds): *The Heart, Arteries, and Veins.* New York, McGraw-Hill Book Co, 1978, pp 1942–1987.

Levine HJ (ed): *Clinical Cardiovascular Physiology.* New York, Grune & Stratton Inc, 1976.

Linman JW: Physiologic and pathophysiologic effects of anemia. *N Engl J Med* 1968; 279:812.

MacLean LD: Shock and metabolism. *Surg Gynecol Obstet* 1968; 127:299.

Mikulic E, Cohn JN, Franciosa JA: Comparative hemodynamic effects of inotropic and vasodilator drugs in severe heart failure. *Circulation* 1977; 56:528–533.

Moore FD, Lyons JH, Pierce EC, Morgan AP Jr, Drinker PA, MacArthur JD, Dammin GJ (eds): *Post-Traumatic Pulmonary Insufficiency.* Philadelphia, WB Saunders Co, 1969.

Shires GT: Shock and metabolism. *Surg Gynecol Obstet* 1967; 124:284.

Simeone FA: Hemorrhagic shock: Metabolic effects. *Science* 1963; 141:536.

Skillman JJ, Lauler DP, Hickler RB: Hemorrhage in normal man. Effect on renin, cortisol, aldosterone, and urine composition. *Ann Surg* 1967; 166:865.

Thal AP, Brown EB Jr., Hermneck AS, Bell HH: *Shock, a Physiologic Basis for Treatment.* Chicago, Year Book Medical Publishers Inc, 1971.

Thal AP, Wilson RF, Kalfuss L, Andre J: The Role of Metabolic and Humoral Factors in Irreversible Shock, in Mills LC, Moyer JH (eds): *Shock and Hypotension.* New York, Grune & Stratton Inc, 1965.

Weiner L: Rational therapeutic approach to cardiogenic shock, in Melmon KL (ed): *Cardiovascular Drug Therapy.* Cardiovascular Clinic Series, No 2, Philadelphia, FA Davis Co, 1974, vol 6.

Weiner N: Norepinephrine, epinephrine and the sympathomimetic amines, pp 138–175; Drugs that inhibit adrenergic nerves and block adrenergic receptors, pp 176–210, in Gilman AG, Goodman LS, Gilman A et al (eds): *Goodman and Gilman's The Pharmacological Basis of Therapeutics* ed 6. New York, Macmillan Inc, 1980.

Wiggers CJ: *Physiology of Shock.* Cambridge, Harvard University Press, 1950.

4

CHEST PAIN

Samuel Z. Goldhaber
Marshall A. Wolf

Myocardial infarction, pulmonary embolus, and aortic dissection account for approximately 33% of all deaths among adults in the United States and for more than 90% of all sudden deaths. Thus the patient with chest pain presents a special challenge to the emergency room physician: to distinguish those patients with one of these treatable life-threatening emergencies from the many patients with a sometimes equally painful but clinically less significant cause of chest discomfort. In particular, the physician must decide whether the patient has myocardial ischemia or infarction since this carries a significant risk of preventable sudden death.

Approximately 600,000 people in the United States die from *myocardial infarction* and ischemia annually. More than 50% of these deaths are the result of a fatal arrhythmia, usually ventricular fibrillation. These arrhythmic deaths, which are most frequent during the initial phase of the ischemic event, can be prevented. The 30–50% reduction in the hospital mortality of myocardial infarction achieved by coronary care units is a result of the almost complete elimination of primary arrhythmic fatalities. Experience of coronary care units has clearly demonstrated that treatment of ventricular fibrillation is not nearly as successful as its prevention by the initiation of antiarrhythmic therapy before the onset of sustained, hemodynamically compromising arrhythmias. The physician in the emergency room situation dealing with patients with chest pain must promptly identify those patients with myocardial infarction and initiate prophylactic antiarrhythmic therapy.

Pulmonary embolus and *aortic dissection* are the other two most common chest emergencies where prompt recognition is essential to improved survival. Neither of these entities is nearly as common as myocardial infarction; pulmonary embolus probably causes or contributes to no more than 50,000 deaths annually in the United States, and thoracic aortic dissection probably causes no more than a few thousand deaths annually. Diagnosis may be extremely difficult in patients with pulmonary embolus since neither the signs nor the symptoms of this problem are specific; a high index of suspicion and a willingness to pursue the diagnosis actively are essential. Aortic dissection is frequently confused with myocardial infarction and often remains undiagnosed until autopsy. A persistently normal electrocardiogram (ECG) or a new murmur of aortic insufficiency in a patient with severe, prolonged chest pain should suggest the possibility of dissection.

The other causes of pain in the chest are either far less threatening or far less common than are myocardial infarction, pulmonary embolus, and aortic dissection. Chest wall pain syndrome, among the most common reasons for patients to seek emergency care, can usually be identified with a careful history and physical examination. Pericarditis, which occasionally is confused with acute myocardial infarction, often can be distinguished on the basis of the effect of varying position on the pain and the characteristic ECG changes. Esophageal discomfort may be very difficult to distinguish from ischemic pain; a history of dysphagia, heartburn, or discomfort occurring during swallowing or during or after meals is often the only diagnostic clue that permits its distinction from ischemic pain.

EVALUATION OF THE PATIENT

The patient presenting with chest pain must be seen promptly. A brief history and physical examination should suffice to identify most of the patients with a significant likelihood of myocardial infarction. A secure intravenous access should be established. The patient's cardiac rhythm should be monitored and stabilized. Prophylactic antiarrhythmic therapy should be given if the patient is very early in the course of infarction or if immediate transfer to a coronary care unit is not possible.

History

The characteristics of the chest discomfort often suffice to permit an initial triage decision (Table 4.1). Thus, the middle-aged man with several hours of substernal squeezing discomfort radiating to the chin and inner aspect of the left arm almost invariably merits admission to the coronary care unit, whereas the patient with needlelike recurrent pain in the area of the cardiac apex almost never does.

The pain of coronary ischemia is usually described as pressing, aching, constricting, or heavy. In some patients it may be experienced as a sense of fullness under the sternum, occasionally with accompanying nausea. Only rarely is it burning and almost never is it knifelike or stabbing. It is often described as frightening.

The pain of coronary ischemia is usually experienced as a diffuse discomfort in the center of the chest. Chest wall pain is usually more sharply localized, frequently to the costochondral junction. Pain sharply localized to the area of the

TABLE 4.1 Differential Diagnosis of Chest Discomfort

Cardiovascular
  Angina
  Myocardial infarction
  Pericarditis
  Dissecting aortic aneurysm
  Pulmonary embolism
Pulmonary
  Pleurisy of unknown etiology
  Pneumonia
  Pneumothorax
  Mediastinal emphysema
Gastrointestinal
  Reflux esophagitis
  Esophageal spasm
  Esophageal rupture
  Peptic ulcer
  Gallbladder disease
  Pancreatitis
Neuromusculoskeletal
  Chest wall pain and tenderness
  Tietze's syndrome
  Herpes zoster

cardiac apex is unusual in ischemic disease and is more consistent with hyperventilation, chest wall pain, or anxiety. Radiation of pain to the inner aspects of the arms and the jaw is common with ischemic pain, and radiation to the back is rather uncommon. Intraabdominal processes infrequently cause pain that radiates to the arms. Aortic dissection frequently is accompanied by pain in the back and occasionally by pain in the flanks.

The effect of various maneuvers, positions, and interventions on the severity of the discomfort may be useful in differential diagnosis. Chest wall pain can often be reproduced by directly compressing the painful area or by stretching or compressing the costochondral junction. Pains that increase with respirations are much more likely to be due to irritation of the pleural surfaces or to inflammation of the chest wall than to coronary ischemia. An exception to this rule is a patient presenting with postmyocardial infarction pericarditis after a painless infarction. Discomfort that is worse when the patient is supine or lying on the left side and that is relieved when the patient sits up and leans forward is suggestive of pericardial inflammation. Patients with ischemic pain are often much more comfortable sitting than lying down, in contrast to patients with functional chest discomfort, who often are more comfortable lying down.

Significant relief from antacids may point toward esophageal irritation or peptic disease. An increase in the pain with swallowing suggests esophageal spasm, pericardial inflammation, or mediastinitis.

Prompt relief with nitroglycerine is consistent with either coronary ischemia or esophageal pain. For diagnostic purposes, it is important to establish that such relief occurred within a minute or two of taking the nitroglycerine; relief occurring less rapidly is not suggestive of coronary ischemia.

If the pain is recurrent, the circumstances under which the discomfort appeared may be useful in differential diagnosis. Discomfort that appears on exposure to cold is suggestive of coronary artery disease. Similarly, discomfort that appears during exertion, especially if this involves walking uphill or prolonged exertion with the arms, is suggestive of coronary disease. Discomfort appearing after large meals may be due to either coronary disease or gastrointestinal problems. Angina is more likely to occur early in the day or in the initial aspects of an activity, for example, the patient who requires a nitroglycerine as he approaches the first tee and then plays 18 holes without further difficulty. Mild exertion in unfamiliar surroundings is more likely to cause angina than more vigorous exertion under circumstances in which the patient feels comfortable, familiar, and unstressed.

It must be emphasized that the initial triage decision often depends on a skillful history. In many patients with significant cardiovascular problems, the physical examination and screening laboratory tests will be normal. It is entirely appropriate to initiate therapy on the basis of a "good" history alone.

Physical Examination

Certain aspects of the physical examination are useful in the initial triage of the patient with chest pain. Blood pressure should be determined in both arms, and the presence or absence of both carotid pulses should be noted since these signs may provide the only clue to a proximal aortic dissection. The respiratory rate should be carefully measured since tachypnea in the presence of a clear chest is often the only clue to an underlying pulmonary embolus. The temperature may prove useful since myocardial infarction is rarely accompanied by a temperature greater than 38.5°C (102°F), whereas pneumonia may produce considerably higher temperatures. Chest palpation may elicit subcutaneous emphysema or point tenderness. The former may be the only clue to mediastinal emphysema; the latter, if it reproduces the patient's symptoms exactly, may obviate the need for an extensive diagnostic workup. The presence of bibasilar rales in the absence of cardiomegaly is suggestive of myocardial infarction. A friction rub may help localize the discomfort to the pleura or pericardium. Retrosternal dullness is often an early sign of pericardial effusion. Careful palpation of the heart in forced expiration may demonstrate a faint anterior heave; the development of this finding in a patient with chest pain is virtually diagnostic of myocardial infarction. The absence of a fourth heart sound would make the diagnosis of myocardial infarction somewhat suspect. A new murmur of aortic insufficiency may be the first clue to aortic dissection. A to-and-fro friction rub argues for pericardial rather than acute ischemic disease, although occasionally patients with transmural infarcts involving the epicardium may have a rub within the first few days of their infarct. Abdominal tenderness, guarding, rebound, and the absence of bowel sounds would all be unusual in the patient with an intrathoracic process. Absent femoral pulses may be the only clue to an aortic dissection. Calf or thigh tenderness or inequality in the size of the lower extremities would increase the likelihood of pulmonary embolic disease.

Laboratory Evaluation

Although electrocardiogram and serum enzymes are often abnormal by the time the patient with a myocardial infarction presents in the emergency room, both are normal sufficiently often that the patient with a suggestive history should not be detained in an unmonitored facility while awaiting these results. The diagnosis of pulmonary embolus can be excluded by a normal lung scan; false positive scans are common enough that pulmonary angiography is often necessary to establish this diagnosis. Although widening of the aortic shadow on a lateral or anteroposterior (AP) chest film is often seen in the patient with a thoracic aortic dissection, a normal chest film does not rule out a dissection; aortic angiography is mandatory to establish the diagnosis and to determine the extent of the dissection.

CLINICAL SETTINGS

Coronary Heart Disease

Coronary heart disease is the result of an imbalance between the need of the myocardium for oxygen and the ability of the coronary blood vessels to satisfy this need. During the past 5 years, it has become apparent that many patients with angina have components of both obstructive coronary disease and coronary spasm. Both mechanisms can contribute to decreased myocardial blood flow, resulting in an imbalance in myocardial oxygen demand and supply. If such an imbalance occurs transiently at a time of unusual exertion or stress, the patient may experience discomfort termed *angina pectoris*. Myocardial

infarction is the result of a more prolonged imbalance accompanied by tissue necrosis.

DIAGNOSIS

History

The pain of coronary ischemia is usually localized to the center of the chest. It may radiate to the neck or the inner aspects of one or both arms, more often the left. It rarely radiates to the back and is rarely localized to the inframammary as opposed to the substernal or subxiphoid regions. The quality of the discomfort is usually pressing or constricting. Often it is likened to the tightness of a clenched fist, the so-called Levine sign. It occasionally is described as a sense of indigestion or an expanding feeling under the breast bone. It may be difficult to describe; the patient who complains of a discomfort in the center of the chest unlike anything he or she has experienced before and that is difficult to classify is a strong suspect for coronary disease. The discomfort is infrequently described as burning; it is almost never knifelike, stabbing, or changed by swallowing or respiration. The patient is often more comfortable sitting or standing than lying supine; the patient with functional chest pain often prefers to lie down and rest. If the patient has been having recurrent episodes of this discomfort, it often has a pattern, being precipitated by cold weather, exertion, especially following large meals, walking up hills, or emotional stress. Certain features of the history suggest a component of coronary spasm, such as nonexertional angina, especially angina that occurs like clockwork in the middle of the night to awaken the patient from sleep. Patients whose angina is precipitated by cold exposure or who have associated conditions involving spasm of blood vessels, such as migraine headaches or Raynaud's phenomenon, are likely to have an element of coronary spasm contributing to the angina. If a patient's angina worsens with beta blockade, the possibility of coronary spasm should be considered. Angina pectoris usually lasts not less than 1 or 2 minutes nor more than 20 or 30 minutes. The discomfort of myocardial infarction may be as brief as that of angina pectoris, but it is frequently more prolonged and more severe, requiring opiates rather than nitroglycerine for relief.

Physical Examination

The physical examination is often completely normal (except for an S_4 gallop) in the patient with angina or with an uncomplicated acute myocardial infarction. A dyskinetic ventricular heave, best appreciated in forced expiration, can be found in about 30% of patients sometime during the first few days after their infarction. The development of a new loud systolic murmur suggests either acute disruption of the mitral valve apparatus or ventricular septal rupture. The presence of a pleural or pericardial rub, different blood pressures in the two arms, or a new murmur of aortic regurgitation would suggest that the chest pain may not be a result of myocardial infarction. An elevated jugular venous pulse in the presence of clear lung fields raises the possibility of right ventricular infarction, especially in patients with inferior or posterior infarction. When these findings are associated with hypotension, differentiation of right ventricular infarction from cardiac tamponade, pericardial constriction, and pulmonary embolus is imperative.

Electrocardiogram

The patient with angina pectoris often has accompanying ST-T abnormalities on the electrocardiogram. These may take the form of ST depression or T-wave inversion. The patient with angina caused by coronary spasm may have ST elevation with reciprocal ST depression that is indistinguishable from an acute transmural infarction. However, an empiric trial of sublingual nitroglycerine or bucchal nifedipine may rapidly reverse the coronary spasm, resulting in an ECG that reverts dramatically, within minutes, from acute transmural ischemia to normal. The patient with myocardial infarction may have no ECG abnor-

malities whatsoever but more commonly has characteristic findings. Fairly early in the course of a myocardial infarction the T waves may become tall and peaked resembling those seen in hyperkalemia (Fig. 4.1). These hyperacute T waves are usually a very transient phenomenon, rarely lasting more than a few hours, and are probably seen only several times a year in a busy emergency room. More commonly, patients present with one of three ECG patterns: subendocardial ischemia (Fig. 4.2), intramural infarction (Fig. 4.3), or transmural infarction (Fig. 4.4a). In subendocardial infarction, which is usually seen in older patients with rather large hemodynamically compromising infarcts, there are widespread ST depressions. In an intramural infarct, there are localized T-wave inversions without QRS abnormalities. In transmural infarction, we see the evolution of classic ST elevation (Fig. 4.5a), T-wave inversion, and Q-wave development (Fig. 4.5b). The differentiation between acute transmural infarction and acute pericarditis (Fig. 4.5) by ECG may be difficult.

Laboratory Evaluation

When myocardial tissue is damaged or destroyed there are accompanying characteristic abnormalities in several serum enzymes (Fig. 4.6). Serial determinations of these various enzymes have proved extremely useful in the diagnosis of acute

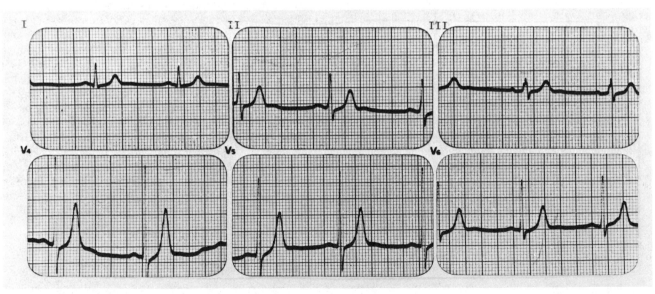

Figure 4.1 Leads I, II, III, V₄, V₅, V₆ are shown. Tall, peaked, symmetrical (hyperacute) T waves, best seen in leads V₄ and V₅, can occasionally be the earliest sign of myocardial infarction.

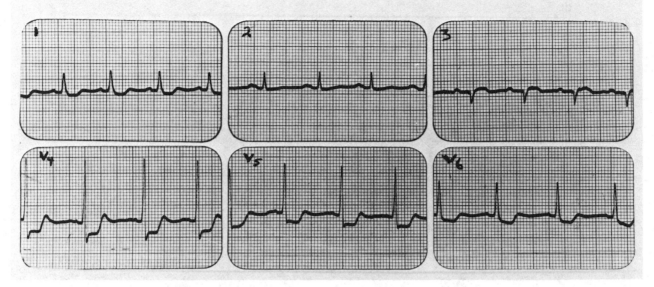

Figure 4.2 Leads I, II, III, V₄, V₅, V₆ are shown. There is subendocardial ischemia, with 1 mm ST-segment depression in lead I and 2-4. mm ST-segment depression in leads V₄–V₆. The persistence of these ST-segment depressions would differentiate infarction from angina.

myocardial infarction in the hospital setting. It must be emphasized, however, that as many as 25% of the patients who develop changes of an acute myocardial infarction in a coronary care unit (CCU) have normal serum enzymes at the time they are seen in the emergency room and that the decision to admit a patient to the coronary care unit should not usually be delayed until the enzyme determinations are completed. Other diagnostic tests for myocardial infarction that depend on the variable uptake of radioactive substances by normal and ischemic or infarcted myocardium, such as the thallium and technetium pyrophosphate scans, respectively, are of little use in the emergency evaluation of a patient's chest pain.

INITIAL THERAPY

Myocardial Infarction

The patient with a "good history" for prolonged coronary pain whose physical examination is not suggestive of aortic dissection or pulmonary embolus should be prepared for transfer to the CCU at this point. Further delays in the emergency room area while ECGs and chest films are being obtained are unnecessary and often inappropriate. Although most of the patients with myocardial ischemia or infarction will have char-

acteristic changes in their ECG at this time, 15–25% do not. Similarly, although the chest film may show a wedge-shaped infiltrate consistent with pulmonary infarction or widening of the aortic root suggestive of aortic dissection, the yield of these abnormalities does not justify delaying admission of the coronary suspect to a CCU.

Before leaving the emergency room, certain measures are appropriate (Table 4.2). The patient is likely to be quite frightened; some gentle reassurance may considerably reduce anxiety. Oxygen should be administered; some patients find a nasal cannula much less confining and stressful than a face mask. A secure intravenous route should be established. The cardiac rhythm should be monitored. Pain should be relieved; in the absence of known hypersensitivity, morphine is the agent of choice for this purpose. 2 to 3 mg intravenously may suffice; two or three such doses may be required. By using small increments, it is possible to reduce the likelihood of severe hypotension, vagotonia, or respiratory depression. The hypotension seen with morphine is a result of venous pooling and usually responds to elevating the feet; vagotonia may require atropine 0.3–1 mg. Naloxone (Narcan), a narcotic antagonist, will rapidly reverse respiratory depression from morphine or meperidine. One ampule (0.4 mg) can be given as an intravenous bolus. If significant improvement is not obtained within

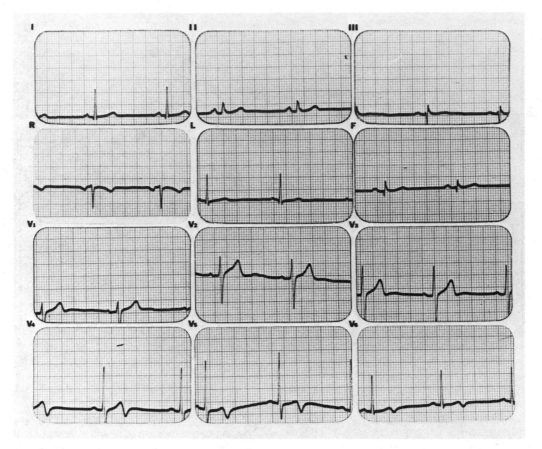

Figure 4.3 12-lead electrocardiogram demonstrates biphasic T waves in V_4–V_6 in a patient who has sustained an intramural infarction. There are no pathological Q waves and no loss of R waves. Therefore, no electrocardiographic evidence exists for transmural infarction.

several minutes, an additional ampule can be given. Failure to obtain significant improvement after 2–3 doses suggests that respiratory depression cannot be accurately attributed to excessive narcotic administration. Nitrous oxide administered as a 35–60% mixture with oxygen is an alternative analgesic available in some institutions.

Prophylactic antiarrhythmic therapy is appropriate before transfer to the CCU unless the patient is bradycardic. Lidocaine is the agent of choice (Table 4.3). Lidocaine 1–1.5 mg/kg administered intravenously as a bolus will provide therapeutic blood levels that can, in most instances, be maintained with a 2 mg/min infusion. In the patient who is having ventricular arrhythmias, these should be suppressed before transfer to the CCU. If an initial bolus of lidocaine does not suppress the arrhythmia, two to three additional boluses of a 0.5 mg/kg may be administered at 1–2 minute intervals. At any given dose of lidocaine, serum levels will tend to be higher than usual in patients with heart failure, liver disease, or coadministration of propranolol. If the ventricular arrhythmia still persists, intravenous procainamide is probably the agent of second choice. From 50–100 mg should be given intravenously every 3–5 minutes to a maximum of 1 g while monitoring the patient's blood pressure and the width of the QRS complex. Should both of these drugs fail to suppress the arrhythmia, the patient should be transferred to the CCU in which alternative antiarrhythmic drugs, such as bretylium, and/or overdrive suppression with a temporary transvenous right ventricular pacemaker can be used.

The patient with sinus bradycardia who is hypotensive or having ventricular irritability should have his or her heart rate increased. Intravenous atropine, 0.3–0.4 mg, usually suffices. A second dose may be given 4–5 minutes later if the first dose does not increase the heart rate appropriately. Patients with first- and second-degree atrioventricular (AV) block may also respond to atropine. Patients with complete heart block infrequently respond to atropine, and a transvenous pacemaker is usually required. While preparations for a transvenous pacemaker are being made, an isoproterenol infusion should be started and titrated to maintain an acceptable ventricular rate.

Patients with atrial fibrillation may be treated medically if the rhythm is well tolerated. Patients with atrial fibrillation with a rapid ventricular rate and those with atrial flutter, especially if they are experiencing continuing pain and/or hypotension, almost always require emergency control of the ventricular rate. If the patient does not have heart failure or heart block, intravenous verapamil can be used emergently to slow the rate of atrial fibrillation and atrial flutter. In approximately 30% of cases, verapamil will convert atrial flutter to sinus rhythm. Unfortunately, in the setting of acute myocardial infarction, many patients have contraindications to verapamil. Such patients often require emergency cardioversion. Five-milligram increments of intravenous diazepam (Valium) may be given at 2–3-minute intervals until the patient is drowsy. Alternatively, an ultrashort-acting barbiturate may be used. Atrial flutter usu-

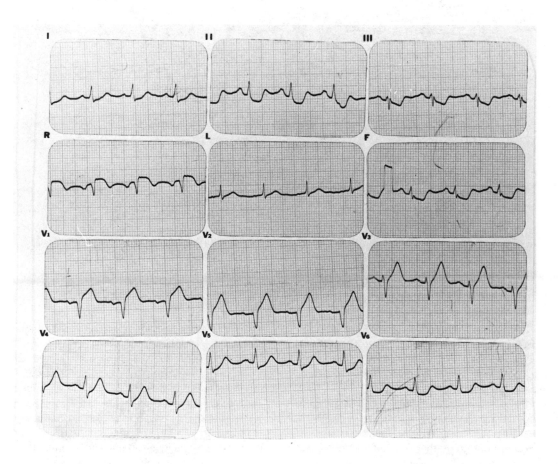

Figure 4.4a 12-lead electrocardiogram from a 67 year old woman demonstrates acute transmural anteroseptal infarction with ST-segment elevation in V_1, V_2. There is reciprocal ST-segment depression inferiorly (II, III, AVF) and laterally (V_6). (Tracing kindly supplied by Dr. L. Frederick Kaplan, Leonard Morse Hospital, Natick, MA).

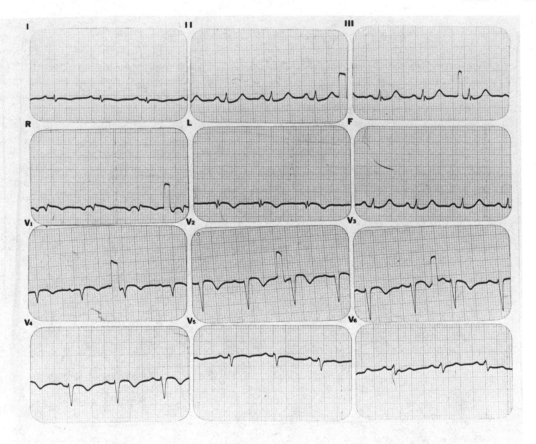

Figure 4.4b 12-lead electrocardiogram demonstrates evolution of transmural infarction in the same patient as in Figure 4.4a. This tracing was taken 2 days later. Note development of Q waves and the new loss of R waves in V_1, V_2. T-wave inversion has developed in leads V_1–V_4. The reciprocal ST-segment depression inferolaterally has resolved.

ally reverts with less than 25 Watt seconds (WS). Atrial fibrillation frequently requires 100–200 WS for reversion. A digitalis drug and procainamide or quinidine should be administered to prevent recurrences of the arrhythmias. The treatment of these arrhythmias is discussed in Chapter 5.

Some patients who present with hypotension respond to volume or to pressors (see Chapter 3). In particular, treatment of right ventricular infarction may require volume expansion. Those patients who respond to neither of these measures usually have had extensive myocardial damage and have an extremely grave prognosis. The patient who is hypotensive should be placed in a supine position with feet slightly elevated. A dopamine or norepinephrine (Levophed) drip may be started

while the patient is being transported to the intensive care unit (ICU). For norepinephrine, one or two 4-mg ampules are diluted in 1 liter of D_5W and infused at a rate sufficient to raise the systolic blood pressure to 90–100 mm Hg. If the patient fails to respond to 40–50 μg/min, further increases in the dosage usually are not successful. Occasionally such patients do respond to other vasopressors, such as metaraminol (Aramine) or epinephrine, or to inotropic stimulants, such as dobutamine. In hypotensive patients, arterial and Swan-Ganz catheters should be inserted. Those patients with low wedge pressures should be given a saline infusion to see if this will restore their blood pressure to normal limits and permit tapering of the pressors. Right ventricular infarction should be considered in patients

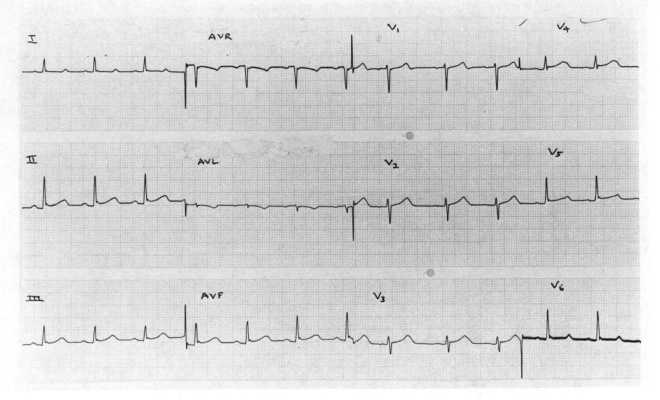

Figure 4.5a 12-lead electrocardiogram demonstrates acute pericarditis in a 57 year old man after aortic valve replacement. There is ST-segment elevation in leads I, II, III, AVF, V_2–V_6 with reciprocal ST-segment depression in endocardial lead aVr. Leads II, III, AVF have PR segments that suggest slight (0.5 mm) downward sloping depression.

with hypotension, neck vein distension, clear lung fields, and low pulmonary capillary wedge pressure. Proper therapy includes fluid administration.

Some patients who fail to respond to pressors and volume can be saved by intraaortic balloon pumps and/or emergency surgery. Intravenous or intracoronary thrombolytic therapy remain investigational procedures. Future therapy may be focused on limitation of infarct size with agents such as beta blockers and nitrates, followed by myocardial reperfusion with thrombolytic agents.

Angina

Patients with a new onset of angina or with a new unstable pattern of angina may be hospitalized for further evaluation and therapy. Myocardial infarction should be excluded if the diagnosis is uncertain. In anginal patients, ideal care can often be given in a monitored "step down" or intermediate care unit. Therapy can be instituted with beta blockade, nitrates, or calcium channel blocking agents. The number of medications and the dosages need to be titrated to the patient's response to therapy. Hospitalization provides an opportune time for patient and family education, psychological support and counseling, and institution of diet and exercise plans. Almost all patients with angina will undergo at least limited exercise testing after they have been stabilized. Patients with refractory angina or those with markedly positive exercise tests will usually have cardiac catheterization recommended to assess hemodynamics and define coronary anatomy. In patients with unstable angina refractory to medical treatment, the insertion of an intraaortic

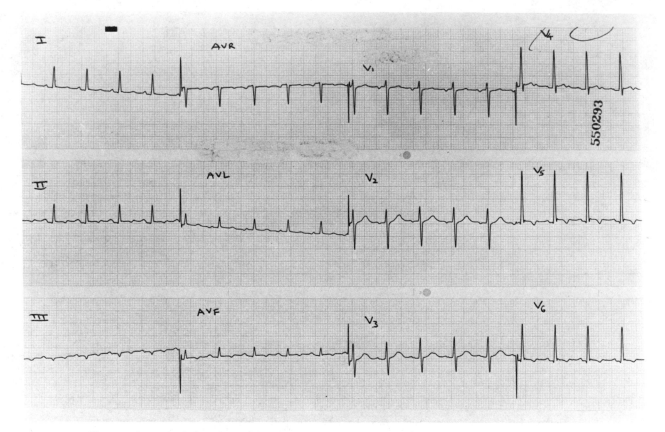

Figure 4.5b 12-lead electrocardiogram demonstrates evolution of acute pericarditis in same patient as in Figure 4.5a, four days later. The inferolateral (II, III, AVF, V₄–V₆) T waves have inverted and the ST segments have returned toward normal.

balloon pump often relieves symptoms and permits a safer, more easily tolerated cardiac catheterization.

The three major classes of drugs used to treat angina are nitrates, beta blockers, and calcium channel blocking agents. At this time, the preferred agent with which to initiate antianginal therapy has not been clearly established. Whereas patients with refractory angina are generally given all three classes of agents if clinically tolerated, patients with more moderate angina are often given only one or two of the three classes of agents.

The *nitrates* are potent vasodilators that exert their strongest effect on the venous system (capacitance vessels) and a lesser effect on the arterial circulation (resistance vessels). The nitrates dilate the large epicardial coronary arteries, even if these vessels are atherosclerotic. Nitrates relieve angina largely by decreasing cardiac work through peripheral venodilatation.

Venodilatation leads to reduced venous return to the heart; there is a subsequent decrease in left ventricular end systolic and end diastolic volumes. In addition, right atrial, pulmonary artery, left atrial, and left ventricular pressures decline after nitrate administration, causing an improvement in the oxygen supply–demand ratio in the heart. Nitrates are also associated with a reflex tendency toward sinus tachycardia.

Nitrates can be administered sublingually, orally, topically, or intravenously. Oral administration is probably the most convenient. Common side effects include headaches and postural

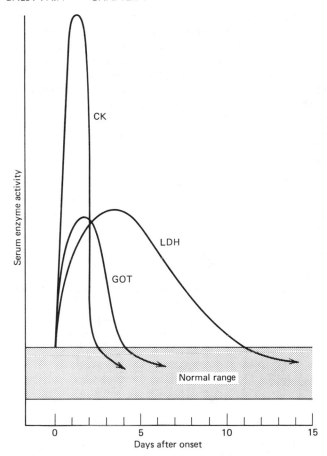

Figure 4.6 Time course of release of cardiac enzymes during acute myocardial infarction. Creatine phosphokinase (CK) is released first, followed by glutamic-oxaloacetic transaminase (GOT) and lactic dehydrogenase (LDH).

dizziness related to orthostatic hypotension. The dose of nitrates is usually limited by hypotension or headache. Sublingual nitroglycerin can be administered in doses of 0.3–0.6 mg. Sublingual nitroglycerin has a duration of action of 30 minutes and is most useful in treatment of anginal episodes rather than for chronic prevention of anginal attacks. Isosorbide dinitrate is a longer-acting agent with a duration of action of approximately 2 hours after sublingual administration and 4–6 hours after oral administration. Isosorbide dinitrate is given in widely varying doses of 5–80 mg, depending on the patient's response and tolerance. Topical nitroglycerin preparations include an

TABLE 4.2 Initial Management of Patients with Acute Myocardial Infarction

1. Reassurance
2. Cardiac monitor
3. Secure intravenous line
4. Oxygen, usually by nasal cannula.
5. Pain control, usually with intravenous morphine.
6. Antiarrhythmic prophylaxis or treatment with lidocaine as drug of choice (see Table 4.3 for dosage regimens).
7. Frequent clinical assessment of hemodynamic status.
8. Treat patients with fluid overload with intravenous furosemide.
9. Treat patients with hypotension with fluids, if appropriate (e.g., right ventricular infarction) or pressors (but avoid isoproterenol). Treat patients with marked hypertension with nitroprusside. Do not let blood pressure deviate more than 30 mm Hg from baseline.
10. Maintain sinus rhythm and treat patients with aggressively marked bradycardia, rapid atrial fibrillation, or rapid atrial flutter (see text).
11. Transfer expeditiously from emergency room to coronary care unit.

ointment (given in dosages of 1–3 in. every 4–6 hours) or the more recently introduced nitroglycerin discs. Intravenous nitroglycerin may be particularly useful for patients with refractory chest pain because of unstable angina (or myocardial infarction). A nitroglycerin infusion is initiated at a low dosage

TABLE 4.3 Lidocaine Dosage Regimens

Loading dose	1–2 mg/kg by slow intravenous infusion (up to 50 mg/min) *or* 100 mg given over 2 min at 10-min intervals *or* 50 mg over 1 min, given 4 times, 5 min apart *or* 20 mg/min infused for 10 min
Maintenance dose	2–4 mg/min for 24 hr
To raise concentration acutely	Give a 50-mg bolus over 1 min and simultaneously increase infusion rate to no more than 4 mg/min. Reduce dosage and consider ordering serum levels in patients who have lidocaine infusions > 24 hr and/or heart failure, liver disease, or coadministration of propranolol.

(e.g., 25 μg/min) and increasing concentrations are then given, with titration to the patient's response. Optimal monitoring of this treatment necessitates an arterial line; a Swan-Ganz line in this setting often adds additional valuable information.

Beta blockers decrease myocardial oxygen consumption at rest and reduce the amount of oxygen required for a given state of exercise. Myocardial contractility, blood pressure, and heart rate decrease with beta blocker therapy. Currently, six beta blockers have been released by the Food and Drug Administration (FDA). Two of the six (propranolol and nadolol) have been approved specifically for the treatment of angina (Table 4.4). All six beta blockers share a common set of contraindications: asthma, heart block, and uncompensated congestive heart failure. Beta blockers are usually given until symptomatic relief is obtained or side effects, most commonly bradycardia or congestive heart failure, appear. It should be noted that after

TABLE 4.4 Orally Administered Antianginal Agents

Drug	Peak Blood Concentration After Administration	Primary Route for Metabolism	Plasma Half-Life	Usual Dose	Primary Side Effects	Miscellaneous Comments
Beta blocking agents						
Propranolol*	1–1.5 hr	Hepatic	4 hr	10 mg qid–80 mg qid (may also be given bid)	Myocardial depression; bronchospasm, fatigue, depression	
Metoprolol	1–2 hr	Hepatic	5–7 hr	50 mg bid–200 mg bid	Myocardial depression; fatigue, depression	Cardioselective in dosages up to 100 mg/day; approved only to treat hypertension
Nadolol*	3–4 hr	Renal	14–24 hr	40–320 mg once daily	Myocardial depression; bronchospasm, fatigue, depression	Does not cross the blood–brain barrier; therefore CNS side effects may be less frequent
Atenolol	2–4 hr	Renal	6–9 hr	50–200 mg once daily	Myocardial depression; bronchospasm in higher doses, fatigue, depression	Cardioselective; approved only to treat hypertension; does not cross the blood–brain barrier; therefore, CNS side effects may be less frequent
Timolol	1–2 hr	Hepatic	3–4 hr	10 mg bid–30 mg bid	Myocardial depression; bronchospasm, fatigue, depression	Approved for reduction of cardiovascular mortality and reinfarction in survivors of acute myocardial infarction; approved for treatment of hypertension
Pindolol	1–2 hr	Hepatic	3–4 hr	5 mg tid–30 mg bid	Myocardial depression; bronchospasm	Has intrinsic sympathomimetic activity
Calcium channel blocking agents						
Nifedipine	1–2 hr	Renal	4–5 hr	10 mg tid–20 mg qid	Headache, dizziness, nausea, hypotension, peripheral edema	Minimal effects on AV and SA node
Verapamil	1–2 hr	Renal with substantial first-pass metabolism in the liver	3–7 hr	80 mg tid–120 mg qid	Nausea, constipation; cardiac depressant effects are more likely in patients taking concomitant beta blocker therapy	Depression of AV and SA node; negative inotrope
Diltiazem	0.5–1 hr	Hepatic	3–4 hr	30 mg qid–60 mg qid	Less AV block and less negative inotropy than verapamil; less hypotension than nifedipine	Low incidence of side effects

*Propranolol and nadolol are the only two beta blocking agents approved by the Food and Drug Administration for treatment of angina.

abrupt cessation of therapy, propranolol has been associated with an exacerbation of unstable angina and acute myocardial infarction.

The nitrates and beta blockers complement each other. Nitrates tend to reduce left ventricular volume, which tends to be increased with beta blockade. On the other hand, the bradycardic effect of beta blockers compensates for reflex tachycardia often induced by nitrates.

The *calcium channel blocking agents* nifedipine, verapamil, and diltiazem have been approved by the FDA for the treatment of angina. These agents inhibit slow calcium channel activity in vascular smooth muscle and myocardium. They cause both coronary artery and peripheral arterial dilatation. Verapamil, in contrast to nifedipine, can cause depression of atrioventricular conduction and sinoatrial node chronicity, in addition to a negative inotropic effect (Table 4.4). Diltiazem has a lower incidence of side effects than either nifedipine or verapamil.

PROGNOSIS

Myocardial Infarction

An important study from Stanford examined the question of whether patients in whom myocardial infarction is excluded have a better prognosis after hospitalization than those surviving infarction. Somewhat surprisingly, the rate of myocardial infarction was almost identical in both groups at 6 months and again at 28 months of follow-up. Cardiomegaly, congestive heart failure, and angina in patients after discharge from the hospital tended to increase the risk of morbidity and mortality in both groups.

Of the patients admitted to the hospital with myocardial infarction, approximately 33% will go on to develop life-threatening complications. These are evenly divided between arrhythmias and severe congestive heart failure and shock. The experience of many CCUs has demonstrated that almost all of the patients with potentially life-threatening arrhythmias can be saved through the aggressive use of antiarrhythmic drugs. These fatal arrhythmias are most likely to occur in the earliest stages of acute myocardial infarction. In the future, severe congestive heart failure and shock may be prevented by measures designed to limit infarct size. Thus, prompt arrival in the emergency room and prompt recognition of the patient with myocardial infarction are the keys to reducing mortality from myocardial infarction. In patients who have had a myocardial infarction, three large well-conducted randomized trials have shown that survival is more than 25% improved and the risk of recurrent infarction is reduced in patients given long-term prophylactic timolol, metoprolol, or propranolol instead of placebo after postmyocardial infarction stabilization.

Careful studies have clearly demonstrated that the long-term prognosis of subendocardial infarction is comparable to that of transmural infarction. In these studies, the distinction between subendocardial and nontransmural infarction (Figs. 4.2 and 4.3) was not made. Although not yet studied, it may be that the prognosis of nontransmural infarction (as defined in this chapter) is significantly better than the prognosis of either subendocardial or transmural infarction. It seems that subendocardial infarction is an unstable event associated with a great risk of later infarction and high late mortality rate. This suggests that an aggressive management approach is warranted in patients with subendocardial infarction.

Angina

The prognosis for patients with angina depends in large part on the severity of the clinical syndrome, which usually reflects the extent of coronary disease. In low-risk patients who show good exercise performance, have minimal or no symptoms, and have a normal or only mildly positive exercise test, mortality from coronary disease may be as low as 2% annually. In high-risk patients, who have symptoms causing limitation in physical activity, poor exercise performance, and markedly positive exercise tests, the risk of death may be as high as 25% annually. Coronary artery bypass grafting has been shown to prolong life in patients with obstructive left main coronary artery disease or its anatomical equivalent. In a randomized multicenter European study, survival was improved in patients with three vessel disease who underwent bypass surgery.

The role of emergency bypass surgery in patients with unstable angina has been studied extensively by a multicentered National Cooperative Study Group. There was no advantage to performing immediate emergency bypass surgery in patients with unstable angina (patients with left main coronary artery disease were excluded from this study). Initial medical stabilization was found to benefit patients with one, two, and three vessel disease and the subgroups with ST segment elevation during pain or with left anterior descending coronary artery disease. Initial medical stabilization was followed by elective surgery in patients who failed to respond satisfactorily to medical therapy. It has also been shown that intraaortic balloon counterpulsation reduces morbidity and mortality in patients with unstable angina who do not respond adequately to medical therapy.

Pulmonary Embolus

Pain, especially pleuritic pain, is a common presenting manifestation of pulmonary embolic disease even though many patients with pulmonary embolus experience dyspnea in the absence of pain. In patients with underlying coronary disease, the discomfort may occasionally mimic that of myocardial infarction. Much more commonly, however, the discomfort is pleuritic, and in the emergency room setting it presents the dilemma of distinguishing pleuritic discomfort accompanying pulmonary infarction from pleuritic pain accompanying a variety of other causes of pleural irritation.

The patient with pulmonary embolus frequently has a clear predisposing factor, such as recent surgery, pregnancy, thrombophlebitis, severe congestive heart failure, or birth control pills. In addition to pain, the episode is almost always accompanied by tachypnea, and a patient with marked tachypnea with a clear chest on examination is highly suspect for emboli. A friction rub is heard in 20–30% of patients with pulmonary infarction, and hemoptysis is almost as common. It should be pointed out that the diagnosis of pulmonary embolus has a tendency to be overlooked in older patients or in patients with concomitant pneumonia.

DIAGNOSIS

The diagnosis of pulmonary embolus is usually suspected on the basis of the patient's history and the clinical setting. Except in the presence of massive embolus with acute strain on the right side of the heart, physical examination is of limited help in confirming the diagnosis. Most patients with significant emboli have a respiratory rate of greater than 20/min. A pleural rub is heard in about 20% of patients.

The patient who does not have dyspnea, tachypnea, or signs of thrombophlebitis is unlikely to have pulmonary embolus. Sinus tachycardia is the most common ECG finding; less than 20% of patients develop a rightward shift of the QRS axis and T-wave inversions in the right precordial leads indicative of right ventricular strain. The chest film is normal in many patients with pulmonary infarction and only in about 25% of patients does it show the classic peripheral wedge-shaped consolidation characteristic of pulmonary infarction. Arterial blood gases have also been used for screening, and a combination of reduced P_{O_2} and reduced P_{CO_2} have been seen in many patients with pulmonary embolic disease. However, studies of relatively healthy populations have shown that it is possible to maintain normal arterial oxygenation despite embolization. Radioisotopic lung scans are the definitive screening procedure. False negatives are rare when multiple views are obtained, and the false-positive rate can be considerably reduced if simultaneous ventilation studies are performed. The definitive diagnostic procedure remains the pulmonary angiogram, and it becomes especially important in patients with pneu-

monia or congestive heart failure who have indeterminate lung scans.

THERAPY

The patient who is suspected of having a pulmonary embolus should have a lung scan performed. Should this procedure be delayed, the patient should usually be heparinized while waiting for diagnostic studies. From 5,000–10,000 units should be given as an intravenous injection followed by an intravenous infusion of approximately 1,000 units per hour, the infusion rate being adjusted to produce a partial thromboplastin time (PTT) of $2–2\frac{1}{2}$ times normal. If a patient with pulmonary embolus cannot be safely anticoagulated, interruption of the inferior vena cava with a filter or clip will be necessary. Diagnosis and management of pulmonary embolus are discussed in Chapters 2 and 3.

Aortic Dissection

DIAGNOSIS

The pain of aortic dissection is often extremely severe, unrelenting, and poorly responsive to analgesics. It is often described as "ripping" or "tearing" but may lack these distinguishing characteristics and be difficult to differentiate from the pain of myocardial infarction. It often begins more suddenly than the pain of myocardial infarction, which is usually gradual in onset. It is more likely to go to the back than is the pain of myocardial infarction, and occasionally, as the dissection extends, it may move from the chest to the upper part of the back to the lower part of the back to the flank. Dissection is usually seen in the setting of hypertension or Marfan's syndrome.

The physical examination may be helpful in suggesting the diagnosis of aortic dissection. The loss of a carotid pulse, the appearance of a murmur of aortic insufficiency, the development of a rapidly increasing pericardial effusion, and the presence of a marked difference in the blood pressure in the two upper extremities or in the upper extremities and the lower extremities are all suggestive of aortic dissection. Often the patient is pale and diaphoretic and is obviously in considerable distress; the appearance suggests shock while the blood pressure remains high. Unless the dissection involves one of the coronary arteries, the ECG usually does not change. Chest film may show widening of the aortic shadow, but this is not an invariable finding and cannot be used to rule out a dissection. Angiography is the diagnostic procedure of choice both for establishing the diagnosis of aortic dissection and for defining its extent.

INITIAL THERAPY

Although many thoracic aortic dissections may eventually require surgical intervention, the initial treatment for all patients is medical. The blood pressure should be promptly lowered. Beta blocking agents, which diminish the rate of blood pressure rise, are also indicated since they decrease the extent of further dissection.

The patient with a thoracic aortic aneurysm, especially one involving the proximal aorta, requires prompt angiography and surgery. While awaiting surgery, the patient's blood pressure should be lowered. A trimethaphan (Arfonad) or nitroprusside drip combined with small doses of intravenous propranolol (Inderal) is effective in lowering the blood pressure, as well as the rate of rise of blood pressure (dp/dt), thus decreasing the shear on the aorta in an effort to prevent further extension of the dissection. A 500-mg ampule of trimethaphan diluted to 500 ml in D_5W administered with a constant infusion pump at the rate of 1–4 ml/min usually provides adequate blood pressure lowering. The blood pressure must be carefully monitored during the infusion. Propranolol is given in 0.5–1 mg increments every few minutes to a maximum of 5–6 mg unless bronchoconstriction, severe bradycardia, or congestive heart failure develops.

Chest Wall Pain

DIAGNOSIS

Pains arising from the chest wall, which the patient often fears are a symptom of heart disease, can often be diagnosed on the basis of the history and physical examination. Most of these pains are a result of costochondritis, a bruised or fractured rib, a pulled muscle, or a pinched nerve. They are usually experienced as a discrete pain rather than a diffuse compression or squeezing discomfort. Frequently they are knife-like or pinching. The duration is either extremely brief, lasting a few seconds, or of much greater duration than that due to coronary heart disease, lasting several hours to days. The pain is sometimes precipitated by movements involving the chest or upper extremity and may be confused with one of the pleuritic syndromes.

Physical examination can usually confirm the diagnosis. The patient is asked to localize the discomfort with one finger. Pressure by the examiner on this site usually precipitates the patient's symptoms. Sometimes it is necessary to have the patient move his or her upper extremity and/or trunk against resistance in order to reproduce the symptoms.

Treatment consists of reassurance alone, or in those cases with persistent discomfort, local heat, rest, and analgesics.

Pericarditis

DIAGNOSIS

The pain of pericarditis arises from inflammation of the adjacent parietal pleura and is increased by positions or activities that increase the friction between the pleural surfaces. It may be aggravated by lying on one side or the other, by swallowing, by coughing, or by taking deep breaths. Rarely, it occurs synchronously with each heart beat. It may be relieved when the patient sits up and leans forward. The pain is usually greatest in the anterior chest and sometimes in the substernal area, mimicking the pain of myocardial ischemia, but more often, it is greatest in the precordial area. Occasionally when the diaphragmatic pleura is involved, it may be localized at the tips of the shoulders and the neck. The discomfort may either be a dull persistent aching or may have a sharper, more pleuritic quality.

Physical examination may reveal retrosternal dullness on percussion as a manifestation of accompanying effusion and, more characteristically, a to-and-fro friction rub. The rub may be extremely transient and often is incomplete; that is, rather than having the classic three components, only one or two of the components may be heard. Patients with acute and/or large effusions may have signs of tamponade, including jugular venous distention and a pulsus paradoxus in excess of 10 mm Hg.

Chest film may be normal; if there is an accompanying effusion, it may show apparent enlargement of the heart. The ECG is extremely useful in suggesting and confirming the diagnosis (Fig. 4.5). The characteristic changes are elevation of the ST segments in both the precordial and standard limb leads with reciprocal ST depressions in the endocardial leads (aV$_r$ and sometimes III or V$_1$ or both). Depression of the PR segment reflecting inflammation of the atrial myocardium is also seen in acute pericarditis. As the condition progresses, the T waves, which initially are peaked and upright, invert. Finally the ST segment returns to normal, but it does not become depressed. The ECG changes are distinguished from those of ischemic heart disease by the absence of ST-T depression. They are sometimes confused with the pattern of early repolarization, a normal ECG variant. Early repolarization can be distinguished on the basis of stability of its pattern through serial ECGs, through the more localized ST elevations, and by the absence of abnormalities of atrial repolarization. A few patients may demonstrate electrical alternans; this is most common in patients with malignant effusion and tamponade. Echocardiography may confirm the presence of an effusion as well as quantitate its amount. The diagnosis and treatment of pericarditis are discussed in Chapters 3 and 20.

Other Conditions Associated with Chest Pain

SPONTANEOUS PNEUMOTHORAX

The pain of pneumothorax may be minimal or may be extremely severe. It is usually sudden in onset and is often knifelike and accompanied by shortness of breath and a feeling of considerable apprehension. The discomfort is usually localized to one or the other sides of the chest rather than being in the midline as is myocardial disease, and it may be accompanied by either considerable dyspnea or a marked diminution in exercise tolerance. Breath sounds may be reduced over the involved hemithorax, but this finding may be absent in partial pneumothorax. Spontaneous pneumothorax is discussed in Chapter 20.

PLEURISY

Inflammation of the parietal pleura produces discomfort that is aggravated by respiration or coughing. It is usually knifelike and rather superficial, as opposed to the dull deep pain of myocardial ischemia. In those patients in whom history and/or chest film fail to demonstrate an inflammatory cause for the discomfort, pulmonary embolus must be strongly considered. Lung scan is indicated if the patient is postoperative or postpartum, is taking birth control pills, or has thrombophlebitis.

MEDIASTINAL EMPHYSEMA

Air under increased pressure in the mediastinal space can provide severe discomfort. This usually results from rupture of a pulmonary alveolus with dissection of the air into the mediastinum or from a perforation of the esophagus or trachea. A characteristic crunching occurs with each heart beat, and the chest film shows air shadows in the mediastinum and often in the soft tissues of the neck.

ESOPHAGEAL PAIN

Esophageal pain is usually the result of the reflux of gastric contents into the esophagus with secondary spasm of the musculature of the lower esophagus. Frequently it is experienced as a burning sensation; it may also produce squeezing or gripping discomfort similar to that felt with myocardial ischemia. The association of the discomfort with ingestion of alcoholic beverages, spicy foods, chocolate, and coffee or tea and with relief after taking antacids may be helpful in identifying the discomfort as originating in the esophagus. A history of dysphagia is also useful in identifying the patient with esophageal pain. Nitroglycerine may relieve the secondary spasm, and this may be a source of confusion with anginal discomfort.

Rupture of the lower end of the esophagus either as the result of severe esophagitis or neoplasm can produce severe discomfort that is usually aggravated by swallowing. A chest film may demonstrate free air in the mediastium. It may be precipitated by a vomiting or coughing spell, especially in elderly men. Prompt surgical treatment is essential.

INTRAABDOMINAL DISEASE

Pancreatitis, duodenal ulcer, and gallbladder disease may all cause lower substernal discomfort. Abdominal tenderness or guarding, elevated serum amylase, elevated amylase clearance, and calcification in the pancreatic bed are all useful in identifying the patient with pancreatitis. A history of discomfort that is relieved with food or antacids, hematemesis, epigastric or right upper quadrant tenderness or guarding, guaiac positive stools, or free air under the diaphragm all are useful in distinguishing peptic disease from myocardial ischemia. Referral of pain to the back, especially to the right subscapular region, discomfort over the right upper quadrant, and acholic stools are useful in identifying the patient with a biliary origin of discomfort (see Chapter 33).

SELECTED REFERENCES

Bell WR, Simon TL, DeMets DL: The clinical features of submassive and massive pulmonary emboli. *Am J Med* 1977; 62:355–360.

Beta-Blocker Heart Attack Study Group: The beta-blocker heart attack trial. *J Am Med Assoc* 1981; 246:2073–2074.

Beta-Block Heart Attack Trial Research Group: A randomized trial of propranolol in patients with acute myocardial infarction. I. Mortality results. *J Am Med Assoc* 1982; 247:1707–1714.

Braunwald E: Mechanism of action of calcium channel blocking agents. *N Engl J Med* 1982; 307:1618–1627.

Cannom DS, Levy W, Cohen LS: The short- and long-term prognosis of patients with transmural and nontransmural myocardial infarction. *Am J Med* 1976; 61:452–458.

Davidson DM, DeBusk RF: Prognostic value of a single exercise test 3 weeks after uncomplicated myocardial infarction. *Circulation* 1980; 61:236–242.

Epstein SE, Kent KM, Goldstein RE, Borer JS, Rosing DR: Strategy for evaluation and surgical treatment of the asymptomatic or mildly symptomatic patient with coronary artery disease. *Am J Cardiol* 1979; 43:1015–1025.

European Coronary Surgery Study Group: Coronary artery bypass surgery in stable angina pectoris: Survival at two years. *Lancet* 1979; 1:889–892.

Fabricius-Bjerre N, Munkvad M, Knudsen JB: Subendocardial and transmural myocardial infarction: A five year survival study. *Am J Med* 1979; 66:986–990.

Fortuin NJ, Weiss JL: Exercise stress testing. *Circulation* 1977; 56:699.

Goldhaber SZ, Hennekens CH, Evans D, Newton E, Godleski JJ: Factors influencing the correct antemorten diagnosis of major pulmonary embolism. *Am J Med* 1982; 73:822–826.

Harper RW, Kennedy G, DeSanctis RW, Hutter AM Jr: The incidence and pattern of angina prior to acute myocardial infarction: A study of 577 cases. *Am Heart J* 1979; 97:178–183.

Harrison DC: Should lidocaine be administered routinely to all patients after acute myocardial infarction? *Circulation* 1978; 58:581.

Hillis LD, Braunwald E: Coronary artery spasm. *N Engl J Med* 1978; 299:695–702.

Hillis LD, Braunwald E: Myocardial ischemia (3 parts). *N Engl J Med* 1977; 296:971,1034,1093.

Hjalmarson A, Herlitz J, Malek I, Ryden L, Vedin A, Waldenstrom A, Wedel H, Elmfeldt D, Holmberg S, Nyberg G, Swedberg K, Waagstein F, Waldenstrom J, Wilhelmsen L, Wilhelmsson C: Effect on mortality of metoprolol in acute myocardial infarction. A double-blind randomized trial. *Lancet* 1981; 2:823–827.

Hutter AM, DeSanctis RW, Flynn T, Yeatman LA: Nontransmural myocardial infarction: A comparison of hospital and late clinical course of patients with that of matched patients with transmural anterior and transmural inferior myocardial infarction. *Am J Cardiol* 1981; 48:595–602.

Kent KM, Rosing DR, Ewels CJ, Lipson L, Bonow R, Epstein SE: Prognosis of asymptomatic or mildly symptomatic patients with coronary artery disease. *Am J Cardiol* 1982; 49:1823–1831.

Langou RA, Geha AS, Hammond GL, Cohen LS: Surgical approach for patients with unstable angina pectoris: Role of the response to initial medical therapy and intraaortic balloon pumping in perioperative complications after aortocoronary bypass grafting. *Am J Cardiol* 1978, 42:629–610.

Leinbach RC: Right ventricular infarction. *J Cardiovasc Med* 1980; 5:499–504.

Levy W, Cannom DS, Cohen LS: The nontransmural myocardial infarction in perspective. *Cardiovasc Rev Rep* 1981; 2:1285–1294.

Lie KI, Wellens HJ, vanCapelle FJ, et al: Lidocaine in the prevention of primary ventricular fibrillation: A double-blind randomized study of 212 consecutive patients. *N Engl J Med* 1974, 291:1324.

Lorell BH, Leinbach RC, Pohost GM, et al: Right ventricular infarction. Clinical diagnosis and differentiation from cardiac tamponade and pericardial constriction. *Am J Cardiol* 1979; 43:465.

Mahony C, Hindman MC, Aronin N, Wagner GS: Prognostic differences in subgroups of patients with electrocardiographic evidence of subendocardial or transmural myocardial infarction. The favorable outlook for patients with an initially normal QRS complex. *Am J Med* 1980; 69:183–186.

Norwegian Multicenter Study Group: Timolol-induced reduction in mortality and reinfarction in patients surviving acute myocardial infarction. *N Engl J Med* 1981, 304:801–807.

Ochs HR, Carstens G, Greenblatt DJ: Reduction in lidocaine clearance during continuous infusion and by administration of propranolol. *N Engl J Med* 1980; 303:373.

Oliva PB: Pathophysiology of acute myocardial infarction, 1981. *Ann Intern Med* 1981; 94:236–250.

Ratliff NB, Hackel DB: Combined right and left ventricular infarction: pathogenesis and clinicopathologic correlations. *Am J Cardiol* 1980; 45:217–221.

Rude RE, Muller JE, Braunwald E: Efforts to limit the size of myocardial infarcts. *Ann Intern Med* 1981; 95:736–761.

Schroeder JS, Lamb IH, Hu M: Do patients in whom myocardial infarction has been ruled out have a better prognosis after hospitalization than those surviving infarction? *N Engl J Med* 1980; 303:1–5.

Slater EE, DeSanctis RW: The clinical recognition of dissecting aortic aneurysm. *Am J Med* 1976; 60:625–633.

Takaro T, Hultgren HN, Lipton MJ, Detre KM, and participants in the study group: The VA cooperative randomized study of surgery for coronary arterial occlusive disease. II. Subgroup with significant left main lesions. *Circulation* 1976; 54:III-107–III-117.

Unstable angina pectoris: National cooperative study group to compare medical and surgical therapy. II. In-hospital experience and initial follow-up results in patients with one, two and three vessel disease. *Am J Cardiol* 1978; 42:839–848.

Unstable angina pectoris: National cooperative study group to compare medical and surgical therapy. IV. Results in patients with left anterior descending coronary artery disease. *Am J Cardiol* 1981; 48:517–524.

Unstable angina pectoris study group: National cooperative study group to compare medical and surgical therapy. III. Results in patients with S-T segment elevation during pain. *Am J Cardiol* 1980; 45:819–824.

Weintraub RM, Aroesty JM, Levine FH, Markis JE, LaRaia PJ, Cohen SI, Kurland GF: Medically refractory unstable angina pectoris. I. Long-term follow-up of patients undergoing intraaortic balloon counterpulsation and operation. *Am J Cardiol* 1979; 43:877–882.

5
ARRHYTHMIAS

Marshall A. Wolf
Samuel Z. Goldhaber

The patient with a rapid or slow heart rate presents a unique diagnostic and therapeutic challenge to the emergency room physician who must identify the nature of the arrhythmia, determine whether it is primary or the result of other illness, estimate the hemodynamic consequences of the arrhythmia, and develop an effective treatment plan. Fortunately, most patients tolerate tachycardia and bradycardia sufficiently well to permit an ordered approach to these tasks. Those patients with a hemodynamically compromising arrhythmia and some patients with underlying heart disease require more immediate therapy. This is especially important if the patient has an acute myocardial infarction or critical valvular heart disease.

Patients with rate and rhythm disorders present in a variety of ways to the emergency room. Many come in because they are bothered by palpitations. Others, especially those with underlying heart disease, are not able to compensate for the increased cardiac oxygen consumption or the decreased cardiac output associated with the arrhythmia and may present with chest pain, hypotension, syncope, or congestive heart failure. A minority have their arrhythmia noted incidentally while they are being seen in the emergency room for unassociated illnesses.

EVALUATION OF THE PATIENT

History

The medical history may elucidate both the nature and cause of a patient's arrhythmia (Table 5.1). A history of previous episodes of arrhythmia and the patient's response to therapy can be extremely helpful. A detailed medication history should be obtained, and special attention should be paid to digitalis drugs, antiarrhythmic medications, diuretics, and psychotropic and antihypertensive medications. A history of rheumatic heart disease or other valvular heart disease may markedly influence the type and timing of treatment. A history suggesting recent myocardial infarction should accelerate the pace of both evaluation and treatment. Symptoms suggesting cardiac decompensation would also mandate prompt therapy. Symptoms of thyroid dysfunction, pulmonary embolic disease, gallbladder disease, and pneumonia should also be sought.

Physical Examination

The physical examination is probably more important in terms of evaluating the response of the patient to the arrhythmia and possible etiologies of the arrhythmia than for the differential diagnosis of the type of arrhythmia. Some aspects of the physical examination are crucial in the emergency setting (Table 5.2); these include determination of the blood pressure, respiratory rate, venous pressure, temperature, thyroid examination, evaluation of the lungs, especially for signs of chronic obstructive pulmonary disease, pneumonia, and congestive heart failure, and edema. In patients with sinus tachycardia, a stool for occult blood is mandatory. The examination of the heart itself is often difficult in patients with tachycardia since the rapid heart rate precludes careful analysis of the heart sounds and murmurs; therefore patients who are initially seen during a tachycardia should have a repeat cardiac examination after the heart rate has been controlled. Occasionally, we may detect flutter waves or signs of atrioventricular (AV) dissociation, such as cannon A waves or the cascade of varying heart sounds that is sometimes seen with ventricular tachycardia. It should be emphasized that these may be difficult observations to make and, especially with critically ill patients, are rarely worth a prolonged investment of time.

Laboratory Evaluation

The extent of appropriate laboratory investigation is in large part a function of the nature of the arrhythmia. Thus, patients with atrial fibrillation should have thyroid function tests, whereas those with paroxysmal atrial tachycardia (PAT) with block should have digoxin and digitoxin levels and serum electrolytes performed. Diuretic therapy predisposes to hypokalemia that is arrhythmogenic. Both hypomagnesia and hypercalcemia increase the tendency to digitalis toxicity. Anemia and acid–base disorders frequently precipitate arrhythmias. Additional laboratory tests are discussed in the sections on the individual arrhythmias.

Electrocardiogram

An electrocardiogram (ECG) should be obtained as soon as rapid heart action is noted since tachycardia may often be paroxysmal, cease abruptly, and remain undocumented if the ECG is deferred until the history and physical examination are completed. This initial ECG, in addition to the standard 12-lead tracing, should include a rhythm strip from a lead in which

TABLE 5.1 Common Precipitants of Arrhythmias

Heart Disease
  Ischemic
  Valvular
  Cardiomyopathy
  Congenital
  Degenerative (fibrocalcific)
Pulmonary Disease
  Pneumonia
  Thromboembolism
  Chronic obstructive pulmonary disease
Medications
  Digitalis
  Antiarrhythmics
  Diuretics
  Psychotropics—tricyclics, phenothiazines, lithium
  Antihypertensives
  Alcohol
  Caffeine
  Thyroid hormone
  Clofibrate
Miscellaneous
  Stress
  Thyroid disease
  Gallbladder disease
  Electrolyte disorders
  Acid–base disorders
  Anemia
  Exercise

atrial activity can be appreciated (usually lead II or V_1). If none of the standard leads clearly shows atrial activity, recordings from additional leads should be obtained (Table 5.3). Often chest leads, with the chest electrode positioned high along either the right or left sternal border, may show atrial activity when none is apparent in the standard leads.

TABLE 5.2 Pertinent Physical Examination in Patients with Arrhythmia

Vital signs—blood pressure, pulse, respiratory rate, temperature
Jugular venous pressure and pulse contour—check for cannon and flutter waves
Thyroid examination
Cardiopulmonary examination
Stool for occult blood in patients with sinus tachycardia
Carotid sinus massage (unless contraindicated)

TABLE 5.3 Electrocardiographic Leads to Detect Atrial Activity[a]

Lewis lead	Right arm electrode at RUSB in second ICS
	Left arm electrode at RLSB in fourth ICS
	Record on lead I
Golub lead	Right arm electrode at RUSB in second ICS
	Left arm electrode at LLSB in fourth ICS
	Record on lead I
Esophageal lead	This lead is swallowed and positioned at the level of the left atrium
Right atrial lead	Insert transvenously

[a]RUSB, right upper sternal border; RLSB, right lower sternal border; LLSB, left lower sternal border; ICS, intercostal space.

The initial ECG should include the response to carotid sinus massage (CSM) or some other vagotonic maneuver. Although CSM is often invaluable in the diagnosis and treatment of tachyarrhythmias, it is not without hazard. It should only be performed by a physician experienced in the procedure and is relatively contraindicated in a patient with carotid artery bruits or a history of cerebral vascular insufficiency or stroke. It is important that the ECG be monitored continually during the CSM, which may produce transient AV dissociation or interruptions of the arrhythmia that are crucial to diagnosis. The physician performing CSM should continuously observe the patient's rate response. Duration of massage should never exceed 3 seconds and should be terminated immediately when slowing is perceived. It is preferable to perform CSM several times for brief periods while attempting to determine the patient's sensitivity to the manuever rather than for a prolonged period that may induce cerebrovascular ischemia. Rarely, prolonged asystole results from the procedure; asking the patient to cough usually results in an immediate resumption of heart action.

In addition to obtaining an ECG promptly, it is often useful to obtain previous ECGs on the patient because evidence of previous myocardial infarction or accelerated AV conduction may be of crucial importance in understanding the present episode of arrhythmia. The presence of bundle branch block in the earlier tracing may be useful in distinguishing between a ventricular tachycardia and a supraventricular tachycardia. Finally, the presence of new ST-T abnormalities consistent with ischemia may be critical in terms of the etiology of the present episode and in the choice of therapy.

ELECTROCARDIOGRAM ANALYSIS

Although a detailed discussion of ECG analysis is beyond the scope of this book, certain principles that should be kept in mind are mentioned. It is important to analyze ECGs in a thorough systematic manner; this approach avoids overlooking any potentially useful information. The usual procedure begins with assessment of rate. At standard speed (25 mm/sec) on standard paper, the rate between two QRS complexes can be estimated by noting the number of large (5 mm) boxes between the QRS complexes. The rate is 300, 150, 100, 75, 60, 50 beats/min for 1, 2, 3, 4, 5, 6 large (5 mm) boxes, respectively. Alternatively, the number of small boxes (1 mm) between QRS complexes can be divided into the constant 1,500 to determine the rate. Rhythm is usually determined next; normal sinus rhythm is defined as QRS complexes following P waves, between 60–100 beats/min. In analyzing ECGs for rhythm it is important to find the P waves (if present), which are usually seen best in leads II, III, AVF, and V_1. Sinus arrhythmia, a slightly irregular sinus rhythm, is very common and often occurs with phasic variations in the respiratory cycle. The QRS axis is normally 0–100 degrees in adults under 40 years of age and varies from -30 to 90 degrees in elderly patients. The PR, QRS, and QT intervals are assessed next. The normal PR interval is 0.12–0.20 seconds. The normal QRS interval is 0.06–0.10 seconds. The normal QT interval varies with heart rate. For a heart rate of 70, the range is 0.33–0.40 seconds. Between heart rates of 45–110, the upper and lower limits of the QT interval increase by 0.02 seconds for every 10 beats/min of decrease in heart rate below 70 beats/min and, conversely, decrease by 0.02 seconds for every 10 beats/min of increase in heart rate above 70 beats/minute. This rule of thumb for "corrected" QT intervals is only valid between heart rates of 45–110 beats/min. The morphology of P wave, QRS complex, and T wave are then examined carefully, followed by a search for U waves, delta waves, bundle branch block, and intraventricular conduction defects.

The following are key observations in arrhythmia diagnosis:

1. Is the ventricular rhythm regular or irregular (RR interval)?
2. Is the atrial rhythm regular or irregular (PP interval)?
3. What is the atrial rate?
4. How are the atrial and ventricular complexes related?
   a. Coupled or independent?
   b. Which is the pacemaker?
5. What is the response to carotid sinus massage or other vagal maneuvers?

In approaching the ECG from a patient with a tachyarrhythmia, it is almost always possible, on the basis of a few simple observations, to determine the nature of the arrhythmia. The rate of atrial and ventricular activity should be carefully measured. The regularity of the atrial and ventricular activity should be established; often recordings taken at the onset or termination of an arrhythmia may be crucial in determining whether the atria are driving the ventricles or vice versa. The result of CSM should be critically examined since this may produce alterations in atrioventricular (AV) or ventriculoatrial (VA) conduction that permit distinction between supraventricular and ventricular tachycardia. If CSM fails to slow the heart rate, pharmacologic slowing of the rate can usually be achieved with edrophonium, propranolol, or verapamil. The use of these medications is discussed in detail in the section on paroxysmal supraventricular tachycardia. Using the observations discussed here, it is usually possible to classify the arrhythmia quickly.

IRREGULAR VENTRICULAR RESPONSE

If the ventricular response is irregular (Fig. 5.1a), we are usually dealing with atrial fibrillation (AF), multifocal atrial tachycardia (MAT), sinus rhythm with multiple atrial or ventricular premature beats (APB; VPB), a supraventricular tachycardia (SVT) with varying AV block, or an unusual form of ventricular tachycardia, torsade de pointes. In atrial fibrillation and MAT, the atrial activity is quite chaotic; in supraventricular tachycardia with frequent premature beats or variable AV conduction, the underlying atrial mechansim is usually quite regular. The distinction between atrial fibrillation and MAT is often made on the basis of atrial rate (much slower in MAT), as well as on the difference in the nature of the atrial mechanism. Most ventricular tachycardias, which are sometimes slightly less regular than the supraventricular tachycardias, are nonetheless predominantly regular, especially with rapid rates, and should not cause confusion with atrial fibrillation or MAT. Torsade de pointes, an unusual form of ventricular tachycardia usually seen in patients with underlying QT prolongation, is irregular but usually easily identified on the basis of its characteristic morphology. Torsade de pointes should not be confused with ventricular fibrillation, which is discussed in Chapter 1.

REGULAR VENTRICULAR MECHANISM

If the ventricular mechanism is regular and the QRS is narrow (less than 0.11 seconds), the response to carotid sinus pressure frequently provides the critical information for differential diagnosis (Fig. 5.1b). If AV block results from this maneuver and the atrial mechanism continues with unchanged rate, we are either dealing with atrial flutter or PAT with block. The distinction between these two is usually made on the basis of heart rate since the atrial mechanism in PAT with block rarely exceeds 220 beats/min and the flutter rate in a patient who has not been treated with quinidine or procainamide rarely is

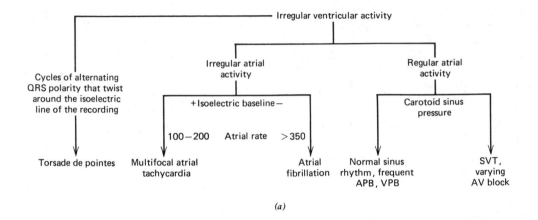

Irregular ventricular activity

Cycles of alternating QRS polarity that twist around the isoelectric line of the recording

Irregular atrial activity

+ Isoelectric baseline −

100 − 200   Atrial rate   > 350

Regular atrial activity

Carotoid sinus pressure

Torsade de pointes

Multifocal atrial tachycardia

Atrial fibrillation

Normal sinus rhythm, frequent APB, VPB

SVT, varying AV block

(a)

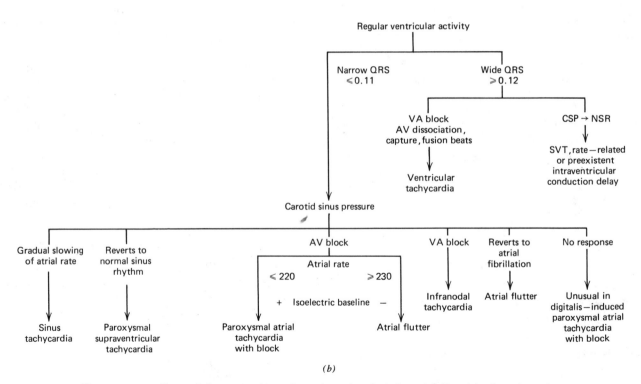

Regular ventricular activity

Narrow QRS ≤ 0.11

Wide QRS ≥ 0.12

VA block AV dissociation, capture, fusion beats

CSP → NSR

Ventricular tachycardia

SVT, rate—related or preexistent intraventricular conduction delay

Carotid sinus pressure

Gradual slowing of atrial rate

Reverts to normal sinus rhythm

AV block

Atrial rate

≤ 220   ≥ 230

+   Isoelectric baseline   −

VA block

Reverts to atrial fibrillation

No response

Sinus tachycardia

Paroxysmal supraventricular tachycardia

Paroxysmal atrial tachycardia with block

Atrial flutter

Infranodal tachycardia

Atrial flutter

Unusual in digitalis—induced paroxysmal atrial tachycardia with block

(b)

Figure 5.1 (a) Differential diagnosis of irregular tachycardia. (b) Differential diagnosis of regular tachycardia. csp, carotid sinus pressure; NSR, normal sinus rhythm.

slower than 230 beats/min. If carotid sinus pressure terminates the arrhythmia, it is almost always paroxysmal supraventricular tachycardia (PSVT) (synonymous with PAT), although a few cases of ventricular tachycardia responding in a similar fashion have been described. If the atrial rate gradually slows in response to carotid sinus pressure and then gradually reaccelerates, the underlying mechanism is almost certainly sinus tachycardia. If a regular atrial mechanism converts to atrial fibrillation, it is likely that the original mechanism was atrial flutter. If no change in the atrial or ventricular rate is observed with carotid sinus pressure, it is unlikely that the underlying mechanism is digitalis-induced PAT with block. This lack of response may be seen with all the other regular tachycardias.

REGULAR VENTRICULAR RESPONSE WITH WIDE QRS

If the ventricular mechanism is regular and the QRS is wide (greater than 0.11 seconds), the arrhythmia is either ventricular tachycardia or a supraventricular tachycardia with either preexistent intraventricular conduction delay or rate-related intraventricular conduction delay (Table 5.4). The presence of capture or fusion beats or the demonstration of AV dissociation is diagnostic of ventricular tachycardia. A QRS width greater than 0.14 seconds, left axis deviation of the QRS axis, and a QRS configuration in V_1 other than rsR' all suggest ventricular origin of the arrhythmia. If carotid sinus massage terminates the arrhythmia, it is much more likely to be supraventricular in origin. Occasionally, carotid stimulation evokes VA block, which is diagnostic of ventricular tachycardia.

BRADYARRHYTHMIAS

The bradyarrhythmias present much less of a diagnostic challenge than do the tachyarrhythmias. However, they still require the same type of systematic approach. We must examine the rate and regularity of the atrial and ventricular activity and then determine their relationship, if any.

In patients with sinus bradycardia, the atrial rate is slow (less than 60) and regular; each P wave is followed by a QRS complex. If patients are asleep or well conditioned, their heart rates may normally be as slow as 40 beats/min. Therefore, as mentioned previously, arrhythmias must be evaluated in clinical context. If the primary pacemaker site is lower than the sinus node but is still within the left atrium, the P waves may become inverted in leads II, III, and AVF and an *ectopic atrial rhythm* will be apparent instead of a normal sinus rhythm. In patients with *sinus node dysfunction,* which may be due to sinus arrest or sinus exit block, a pause devoid of P waves occurs that may either be a multiple of the basic cycle length or may have a more complicated pattern similar to a Wenckebach period at the AV node. Blocked atrial premature beats that are not apparent in the monitoring lead may simulate sinus arrest or sinoatrial exit block.

The *sick sinus syndrome* represents a group of conditions that display sinus node dysfunction. These include sinus arrest, sinoatrial exit block, failure to restore sinus rhythm promptly after cardioversion of atrial flutter, marked sinus bradycardia, chronic atrial fibrillation with a slow ventricular response that is not drug induced, sinus bradycardia with recurrent paroxysmal atrial fibrillation, and the bradycardia–tachycardia syn-

TABLE 5.4 Ventricular Tachycardia versus Aberrant Conduction

Variable	Ventricular Tachycardia	Aberrant Conduction
Rate (beats/min)	100–250	130–210
QRS width (in the absence of drugs)	Often > 0.14 sec (70%)	Often < 0.14 sec
Left axis deviation	Yes	No
rSR' or rsR' in V_1	No	Yes
Monophasic or biphasic QRS in V_1	Yes	No
Rsr' in V_1	Yes	No
R:S < 1 in V_6	Yes	No
AV dissociation	Yes	No
Concordant precordial QRS pattern	Yes	No
Capture or fusion beats	Yes	Infrequent
Termination by CSM	Rare	Yes
Ventricular–atrial block	Occasional	No

drome. The sick sinus syndrome is discussed in detail in Chapter 9.

Patients with first-degree AV block (PR interval greater than 0.20 seconds) have a regular atrial and ventricular rhythm with a prolonged PR interval (Fig. 5.2). In second-degree AV block, the atrial rhythm is regular and there are occasional absent ventricular responses. In the patient with third-degree, or complete heart block, the atrial and ventricular responses are usually regular but dissociated. Complete heart block is characterized by an atrial rate faster than the ventricular rate. Atrioventricular dissociation is characterized by a ventricular rate faster than the atrial rate. Isorhythmic dissociation is characterized by similar atrial and ventricular rates, despite dissociation of atrial and ventricular beating.

Other Diagnostic Techniques

In the emergency setting, more invasive diagnostic techniques for patients presenting with arrhythmias are rarely justified or necessary. Occasionally, passage of an intraatrial lead permits appreciation of atrial activity that may not be apparent on a surface ECG. On rare occasions, cardioversion may be required for both diagnostic and therapeutic purposes, but this should be used cautiously if there is any possibility that the arrhythmia may be a manifestation of digitalis intoxication since cardioversion may exacerbate digitalis intoxication.

INITIAL MANAGEMENT—GENERAL MEASURES

Most patients with tachyarrhythmias tolerate their rhythm disturbance well unless they have significant underlying heart disease. In patients who are well compensated it is appropriate to take adequate time to reassure the patients, to take a careful history, to perform a physical examination, and to perform diagnostic maneuvers sufficient to elucidate the mechanism of the arrhythmia before attempting therapy. In those patients who

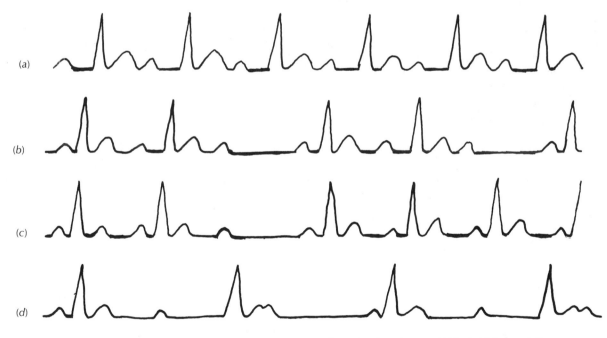

Figure 5.2 Atrioventricular block. The PR interval is prolonged in first-degree AV block (a) but each P wave is followed by QRS complex. In second-degree AV block, occasional P waves are blocked at the AV node and no QRS complex follows. In Wenckebach AV block (b) there is a gradual lengthening of the P–R interval in the beats preceding the dropped beat; in Mobitz-type II block (c), the PR interval is constant, and occasional beats are completely blocked. In complete heart block (d) there is no relationship between the atrial and ventricular activity, and the atrial rate is faster than the ventricular rate.

are seen in the midst of an acute myocardial infarction or with arrhythmia-induced acute cardiac decompensation, it may be necessary to treat the arrhythmia more promptly. If the arrhythmia is a response to rather than the cause of congestive heart failure, successful treatment may require correction of the underlying congestive heart failure (CHF) directly, and therapeutic maneuvers aimed at the rhythm disturbance alone may be unsuccessful. If the arrhythmia is paroxysmal rather than sustained, antiarrhythmia medication or carotid sinus massage is preferable to cardioversion. Many of the arrhythmias will respond to several different therapeutic approaches; in selecting among them, the physician's familiarity with the agent, as well as its safety and convenience, is an important criterion. The ECG monitoring should be continuous during the course of emergency treatment, and frequent observations, including rhythm strips, should be recorded. Careful attention must be paid to changes in heart rate during treatment since small increments in heart rate may be crucial in identifying those patients who are digitalis intoxicated and those who have other problems for which the treatment selected is inappropriate.

TACHYARRHYTHMIAS

Intravenous antiarrhythmic drugs are frequently prescribed for treatment of patients with tachyarrhythmias (Table 5.5). Dosage decisions in the emergency room must often be based on clinical signs of toxicity or efficacy without the benefit of confirmatory laboratory blood tests. However, even when antiarrhythmic blood levels are readily available (Table 5.6), much caution must be exercised in their interpretation. Generally, the mean and two standard deviations of clinically effective therapeutic blood levels for a large number of patients are calculated to establish the therapeutic range. However, any individual patient may have effective or toxic blood levels that are above or below the established therapeutic range. Despite a nominally subtherapeutic or toxic blood level of antiarrhythmic drug, no firm conclusions should be drawn unless the laboratory values are correlated with what is occurring clinically. These same principles are equally important in the interpretation of blood levels of digitalis glycosides. In less urgent situations, oral rather than intravenous antiarrhythmic agents may be used to control tachyarrhythmias (Table 5.7).

Cardioversion is often the treatment of choice for patients with poorly tolerated rhythm disturbances. Since this modality does not prevent recurrences of arrhythmias, antiarrhythmic drugs should be given to stabilize the patient after reversion. Diazepam (Valium) given in 2.5–5-mg intravenous increments until the patient is drowsy, often provides amnesia for the procedure. Atrial flutter and ventricular tachycardia often re-

vert with low energies (1–10 WS); atrial fibrillation often requires 50–150 WS for reversion. In the patient with ventricular tachycardia and a sinusoidal pattern that makes distinction of the QRS and T waves uncertain, we can either use low energies in the defibrillation modes or high energy (150 WS) cardioversion. Cardioversion enhances digitalis effect; if there is uncertainty as to whether or not the patient is digitalis intoxicated, a 1–2 WS discharge can be used. If this elicits ventricular irritability or other signs of digitalis intoxication, the procedure can be postponed; if emergency reversion is indicated, lidocaine can be used to suppress the ventricular irritability. Indicators for cardioversion are discussed in the sections on the specific arrhythmias.

Pacemaker therapy can be lifesaving, and this technique should be available to physicians dealing with patients with arrhythmia. In addition to its original use for patients with heart block, it has proven useful in dealing with patients with supraventricular tachycardias and bradycardias (tachycardia–bradycardia syndrome), and some patients with ventricular irritability and an associated bradycardia. Some patients with supraventricular tachycardia can be reverted with rapid pacing.

Elective temporary pacemaker placement is usually done through a subclavian vein under fluoroscopic or electrocardiographic guidance. This approach is quite safe in experienced hands but can have considerable morbidity if improperly performed; medical management with atropine and/or isoproterenol may be preferable to pacemaker implantation by inexperienced personnel.

Atrial Fibrillation

Atrial fibrillation is an exceedingly common arrhythmia, both in patients with and without underlying heart disease. It is common in patients with left atrial enlargement, especially mitral valve disease, and can be seen as a result of congestive heart failure of any etiology. It may occur after pneumonectomy and during the course of pneumonia, pneumothorax, atelectasis, or pulmonary embolism. It is a classic complication of thyrotoxicosis, and every patient with this arrhythmia should have his or her thyroid function assessed. Occasionally, it seems to occur as a response to stress or drinking alcoholic beverages.

DIAGNOSIS

The atrial rate in atrial fibrillation usually exceeds 350 beats/min and is grossly irregular. Atrial activity is continuous (Fig. 5.3). The constant atrial activity (versus the isoelectric baseline seen in patients with multifocal atrial tachycardia) can often

TABLE 5.5 Tachyarrhythmias

Rhythm	Rate (beat/min)	ECG Signs	Etiology	Response to CSM	Drug	Comments
Atrial fibrillation	300–600 (atrial); ventricular rate slower	Constant irregular atrial activity; often best seen in lead V_1; ventricular response is usually irregular	Thyrotoxicosis, stress, left atrial enlargement, mitral valve disease, lung disease, alcohol	AV block increased and ventricular response decreased	Digitalis for rate control except in patients with an accessory pathway; propranolol or verapamil for rate control; quinidine, procainamide, cardioversion	A regularized ventricular response or group beating suggests AV block or digitalis toxicity; a ventricular response > 200 suggests an accessory pathway
Multifocal atrial tachycardia	100–150	Discrete P waves of at least three distinct morphologies; irregular variations in P–P intervals, isoelectric baseline	Pulmonary disease; electrolyte or acid–base disorders	May transiently decrease rate of atrial activity	Maintenance digitalis or digitalis for CHF; quinidine	These patients are at risk for digitalis toxicity; treat underlying medical condition
Torsade de pointes	160–280, but usually 200–240	Cycles of QRS complexes that twist around isoelectric line of recording	QT prolongation; hypokalemia; liquid protein diets	No effect	Isoproterenol; ventricular or atrial overdrive pacing; bretylium	Quinidine, disopyramide, procainamide are contraindicated; must differentiate from ventricular fibrillation
Sinus tachycardia	100–200	A P wave precedes each QRS complex at a regular PR interval	Physical exertion, fever, thyrotoxicosis, anemia, AV fistula, CHF, elevated levels of circulating catecholamines	Gradual slowing	Beta blockade (usually inadvisable); treat underlying condition	Search for underlying etiology
PSVT (AV nodal reentry)	140–200, but usually, 150–180	Atrial and ventricular depolarizations usually occur simultaneously; therefore P waves are usually buried within QRS complexes and are not apparent	Fig. 5.6 and 5.7. Usually initiated by atrial premature beat (APB), alcohol, stress, caffeine	Either no effect or abrupt conversion to sinus rhythm	Vagal maneuvers; intravenous verapamil, propranolol, digitalis, edrophonium	Often occurs in young healthy people without organic heart disease; AV block excludes this diagnosis

	Rate	ECG features	Associated conditions	Effect of carotid sinus pressure	Treatment	Comments
PSVT (accessory pathway)	150–240, often over 200	Usually a narrow QRS complex is closely followed by an inverted P wave	Fig. 5.8. Usually the AV-node serves as slow antegrade pathway and AV bypass tract as retrograde fast pathway	Either no effect, slight slowing or abrupt conversion to sinus rhythm	Intravenous propranolol, procainamide, verapamil, lidocaine	If CSP → AV block, this diagnosis is excluded
Atrial flutter	230–400, usually 250–330	Sawtooth F–P baseline; usually 2:1 AV response	Organic heart disease or lung disease	AV block increased and decreased ventricular rate, atrial rate unchanged (usually); atrial fibrillation (occasionally)	Intravenous verapamil converts 30% to sinus rhythm; digitalis for rate control; quinidine; cardioversion; rapid atrial pacing	Rate control is more difficult than in patients with atrial fibrillation
PAT with block* (digitalis induced)	90–220 (average rate 180)*	Isoelectric T–P baseline with upright and diminutive P waves in limb leads	Digitalis; an automatic atrial tachycardia with features of PAT and atrial flutter; provoked by hypokalemia	AV block increased but atrial rate unchanged	Withhold digitalis and give potassium if potassium level is low	Begins and terminates with gradual change in rate and abrupt change in P wave
PAT with block (not induced by digitalis)	140–250	Isoelectric T–P baseline with upright and diminutive P waves in limb leads	Organic heart disease; corpulmonale	AV block increased but atrial rate unchanged; occasionally no response	Administer digitalis; treat underlying condition	Begins and terminates with gradual change in rate and abrupt change in P wave
Ventricular tachycardia	100–250, often 130–170	See Table 5.4	Acute MI; cardiomyopathy; primary VT, without organic heart disease	No effect	Lidocaine; procainamide; bretylium; cardioversion	Usually requires aggressive workup and therapy; may degenerate to ventricular fibrillation

*This arrhythmia usually has a slower rate and is approximately three times more common than PAT with block that is not induced by digitalis.

TABLE 5.6 Antiarrhythmic Drugs Approved for Intravenous Use

Dosage Information	Lidocaine	Procainamide	Bretylium	Phenytoin	Verapamil
Therapeutic range (µg/ml)	2–6	4–10	0.5–1.5	10–18	?
Usual loading dose[a]	1–2 mg/kg over several minutes	Up to 1,000 mg at up to 50 mg/min	5 mg/kg initially, up to 30 mg/kg over 45–90 min	Up to 1,000 mg at up to 50 mg/min	2.5 mg increments over 2 min; dose limited by hypotension usually after 15–20 mg
Usual maintenance therapy[a]	2–4 mg/min	1.5–6 g/day	5–10 mg/kg, up to 30 mg/kg/day	200–400 mg/day	Oral dosage of 240–480 mg/day
Dosage interval	Continuous infusion	3–4 hr	6–8 hr, up to 30 mg/kg/day	12–24 hr	Intravenous dose is repeated only to maintain control of ventricular rate
Side effects	CNS	Hypotension with loading dose, GI, lupuslike syndrome (chronic)	Hypotension, enhances digitalis toxicity	CNS, asystole	AV block, CHF, neurologic, GI, hypotension
Reasons to decrease dosage	Prolonged infusion, CHF, liver disease	Renal disease	Renal disease	Liver disease	Liver disease

[a]These values represent first approximations only; adjustments will often be required based on close monitoring of clinical status.

best be appreciated in an anterior chest lead, especially V_1. Occasionally, after a patient has been in atrial fibrillation for a prolonged period of time, the voltage of the atrial activity decreases, and it may be difficult to appreciate atrial activity without an esophageal or intraatrial lead. The patient with atrial fibrillation usually has both irregular atrial activity and irregular ventricular response.

Although accessory pathways will be discussed in detail in the section below on paroxysmal supraventricular tachycardia, it is worth noting the importance of identifying the rare patient with atrial fibrillation and accelerated ventricular conduction antegrade through an accessory pathway (e.g., Wolff-Parkinson-White syndrome). Such patients usually have a very rapid (200–300 beats/min) irregular ventricular heart rate with a wide QRS complex. The gross irregularity rhythm should distinguish atrial fibrillation through an accessory pathway from rapid ventricular tachycardia. If the diagnosis is suspected, digitalis should be withheld because it may accelerate antegrade conduction through an accessory pathway. The consequences of such an increase in ventricular rate are often serious and sometimes life threatening.

A final diagnosis worth considering is digitalis toxicity in the presence of atrial fibrillation. Increased AV block in combination with increased automaticity is a hallmark of digitalis toxicity. A regularized ventricular response, group beating,

accelerated junctional rhythm, and increased ventricular ectopy can all suggest digitalis toxicity in the presence of atrial fibrillation.

TREATMENT

The treatment of atrial fibrillation may be directed at terminating the arrhythmia and/or increasing the AV block so that the ventricular response is slower. In patients who do not require immediate restoration of sinus rhythm, initial therapy is usually directed at decreasing the ventricular response, either with a digitalis preparation, propranolol (0.5–1 mg intravenously in increments to a maximum of 3–5 mg), or verapamil (5–15 mg intravenously over 5–20 minutes). Increments of digoxin or ouabain are given at 1–2-hour intervals until appropriate rate reduction is obtained. Digitalis slows AV conduction and decreases the ventricular response. The earliest manifestation of digitalis intoxication may be acceleration of the ventricular rate. If the patient's rate is increasing rather than decreasing with increments of digitalis, a presumptive diagnosis of digitalis toxicity can be made, especially if there is an associated increase in ventricular ectopic activity. As mentioned above, acceleration of the ventricular rate with digitalis drugs is also seen in patients with Wolff-Parkinson-White syndrome and atrial fibrillation.

TABLE 5.7 Frequently Used Oral Antiarrhythmic Agents

Dosage Information	Quinidine	Procainamide	Disopyramide	Propranolol	Verapamil
Therapeutic plasma concentration range (µg/ml)	2–6	4–10	2–5	0.02–1	
Loading dose (mg)[a]	600–1,000	500–1,000	200–400	Given intravenously in 0.5–1 mg increments to avoid first-pass hepatic extraction; maximum of 0.1 mg/kg	Given intravenously in 2.5 mg-increments q 2 min; dose limited by hypotension
Usual maintenance dosage (mg/day)[a]	1,200–2,000	1,500–6,000	400–800	Usually 40–160 but up to 1,000	240–480
Usual dosage interval (hr)	6	3–4	6	6	6–8
Time of peak concentration after oral dose (hr)	1–1.5 for sulfate; 3–4 for gluconate	45–90 min for standard capsule; up to 4 hr for sustained release capsule	1–2	1–1.5	1–2
ECG changes	↑ QRS, ↑ QT	↑ QRS, ↑ QT	Slight ↑ QT	↑ PR; ↓ ventricular response in AF	—
Common side effects	GI	GI, lupuslike syndrome	Anticholinergic, CHF	Neurologic, CHF, may exacerbate bradyarrhythmias in sick sinus syndrome	Neurologic, GI, AV block, CHF
When to reduce dosage and consider measuring blood levels in patients	Liver disease, CHF, age > 60 yr	Renal disease	Renal disease	Liver disease	Liver disease

[a]These values represent first approximations only; determinations of proper dosage require close and frequent observations of the patient, using ambulatory monitoring techniques as needed.

In the emergency setting, termination of atrial fibrillation would usually be done with cardioversion in patients in the midst of an acute myocardial infarction who have continuing pain or hypotension or in patients with fulminant pulmonary edema as a result of arrhythmia. It must be emphasized that cardioversion must be supplemented with other antiarrhythmic modalities or atrial fibrillation may recur. In most instances, procainamide or quinidine would be given before cardioversion in order to prevent recurrences of this rhythm. Cardioversion energies in excess of 50 WS are usually required for successful reversion of atrial fibrillation. Often, in a patient whose digitalis status is unknown, a 1- or 2-WS test dose may be used initially since if this produces ventricular irritability or an acceleration in the ventricular rate, we would be cautious about proceeding with cardioversion.

The patient with atrial fibrillation and accelerated conduction through an accessory pathway (e.g., Wolff-Parkinson-White syndrome) may respond to intravenous lidocaine (1–2 mg/kg). Otherwise cardioversion is usually needed because the rapid ventricular response (200–300/min) often causes hemodynamic compromise.

Patients who have been fibrillating for more than 24–48 hours may embolize after reverting to sinus rhythm. Therefore, those patients with long-standing atrial fibrillation should be anticoagulated for at least 2 weeks before elective reversion. Contraindications to cardioversion are (1) elderly patients with a slow ventricular response (as a manifestation of the sick sinus syndrome), (2) patients unable to tolerate chronic antiarrhythmic medications, and (3) patients with an enlarged left atrium who repeatedly revert to atrial fibrillation despite multiple cardioversions and trials of antiarrhythmic medication.

During the past 10 years, several studies have established

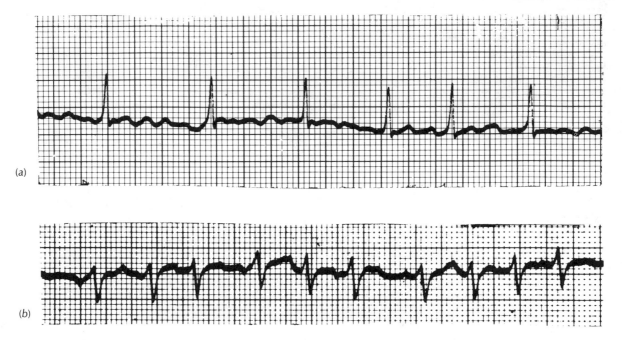

Figure 5.3 In atrial fibrillation (*a*) the atrial activity is continuous and chaotic; in multifocal atrial tachycardia (*b*) the baseline is isoelectric and there are discrete P waves and varying P morphologies and PR intervals.

that chronic atrial fibrillation increases morbidity and mortality. These studies have provided further rationale for aggressive conversion of new onset atrial fibrillation to sinus rhythm and long-term anticoagulation for chronic atrial fibrillation. An autopsy study of patients with atrial fibrillation showed that symptomatic emboli, with pathologic or surgical confirmation, occurred in 41% of patients with mitral valve disease, 35% of patients with ischemic heart disease, and 21% of patients with an otherwise normal heart. In contrast, systemic embolism was found in only 7% of a control group of autopsy patients with ischemic heart disease but without atrial fibrillation. In the Framingham study, the development of chronic atrial fibrillation was associated with a doubling of overall mortality and of mortality from cardiovascular disease.

Multifocal Atrial Tachycardia

Multifocal atrial tachycardia is characterized by a heart rate greater than 100 beats/min and at least three atrial pacemakers with varying PP intervals and varying PR intervals (Fig. 5.3). It is often seen in the setting of severe respiratory failure and is most often confused with atrial fibrillation. The presence of an isoelectric baseline and distinct atrial pacemakers as op-

posed to continuous atrial activity is crucial in distinguishing between these two arrhythmias.

Multifocal atrial tachycardia, like sinus tachycardia, should suggest treatment of the underlying disorder rather than treatment directed at the rhythm disturbance. Digitalis rarely causes this arrhythmia nor is the arrhythmia often responsive to this medication. Occasionally quinidine may prove useful in controlling some of the atrial irritability, but this is rarely indicated.

Torsade de Pointes

Torsade de pointes, an unusual but often serious arrhythmia, is seen in patients with prolongation of ventricular repolarization, manifested in the ECG as QT prolongation. Torsade de pointes occurs occasionally in patients with idiopathic QT prolongation; it is more frequently the result of medications that prolong ventricular repolarization such as quinidine, procainamide, disopyramide, tricyclic antidepressants, and the phenothiazine antipsychotic drugs. Other factors predisposing to torsade de pointes include hypokalemia, hypomagnesemia, subarachnoid hemorrhage, and liquid protein diets.

It is important to differentiate torsade de pointes from ventricular fibrillation, with which it can be confused. Torsade de

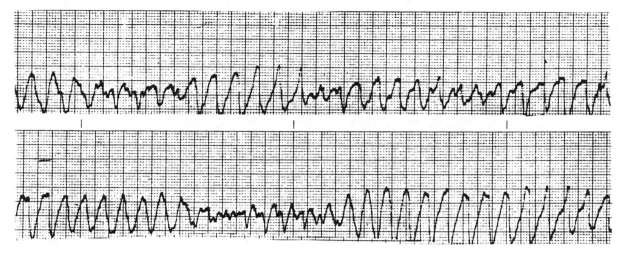

Figure 5.4 Torsade de pointes. The ventricular complexes are wide and vary in a rhythmic undulating pattern.

pointes (Fig. 5.4) is often paroxysmal and is characterized by a rapid and irregular ventricular rate. Cycles of alternating polarity twist around the isoelectric baseline of the recording. The QRS duration is prolonged, and on longer rhythm strips there is a characteristic variation of the QRS voltage in a sinusoidal pattern.

Measures that decrease the QT interval can be successful in managing this arrhythmia. These include correcting any electrolyte abnormalities (such as hypokalemia), isoproterenol infusion, and rapid ventricular "overdrive" pacing. Bretylium appears to be a promising agent. However, drugs such as quinidine and procainamide, that increase the QT interval, are contraindicated. Increasing awareness of torsade de pointes makes documentation of the QT interval imperative before and during antiarrhythmic therapy with quinidine, procainamide, and disopyramide.

Sinus Tachycardia

Sinus tachycardia is rarely a primary problem. It is seen as a normal response to exercise or other physiologic stresses. In patients, it is usually a response to some underlying illness such as hypovolemia, fever, thyrotoxicosis, anemia, electrolyte abnormalities, congestive heart failure, and hypoxia and usually responds best to treatment of the underlying disorder. Treatment that attempts to slow the rate directly with the use of digitalis, propranolol, or other cardioactive drugs may prove hazardous. The diagnosis often can be established if multiple

rhythm strips can be obtained over time since, in contrast to other supraventricular tachycardias, the sinus rate varies in this rhythm. Carotid sinus pressure may produce a gradual slowing and reacceleration, a response that is not seen in the other regular supraventricular tachycardias. Rate measurements are occasionally helpful since it is unusual for sinus tachycardia to exceed 200 beats/min in adults.

Paroxysmal Supraventricular Tachycardia

The paroxysmal supraventricular tachycardias (PSVT) (paroxysmal atrial tachycardia and paroxysmal junctional tachycardia) are rhythms that frequently occur in the absence of underlying heart disease. Their onset is sudden, and most patients experience an uncomfortable thumping in the chest and a feeling of anxiety. Some patients will also experience polyuria during these episodes. Although an occasional patient may be able to identify a specific precipitant for these arrhythmias, such as alcohol, caffeine, or stress, more often paroxysmal SVT occurs in an unpredictable fashion. These arrhythmias are frequent in patients with accelerated AV conduction, either of the Lown Ganong Levine type with a short PR interval and no delta wave or of the Wolff-Parkinson-White type with both a short PR interval and a delta wave. In the latter group, the rate of the atrial tachycardia may exceed 200 beats/min, which is a rate not seen often in adults with PSVT (Fig. 5.5).

Paroxysmal supraventricular tachycardia is usually caused by AV nodal reentry in which a wave of current is continuously

CSP

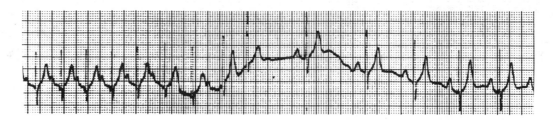

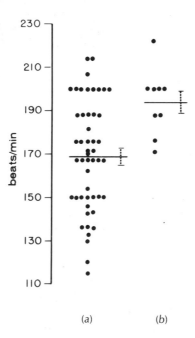

(a)   (b)

Figure 5.5 Paroxysmal supraventricular tachycardia. The tracing demonstrates a regular rhythm with narrow QRS complexes at a rate of 150 beats/min. Carotid sinus pressure (CSP) produces reversion to normal sinus rhythm. The heart rate in AV nodal—heart reentry (a)—is considerably slower than the rate observed in reentry through an accessory pathway—(b) (After Wu et al: *Cardiol,* 41;1045–105, 1978.)

propagated within a closed circuit. For reentry to occur, there must be dissociation of impulses into two pathways, a slow pathway and a fast pathway (Fig. 5.6). An impulse is blocked in the fast pathway and is conducted antegrade down the slow pathway. Meanwhile, excitability recovers in the fast pathway and the impulse can return retrograde through the fast pathway to its point of origin. Continued propagation of the impulse in such a circuit results in a sustained reentrant tachycardia through the AV node (Fig. 5.7).

The possibility of an accessory pathway as part of the PSVT mechanism should be considered, particularly in patients with tachycardias faster than 200 beats/min. In most patients with accessory pathways, which are muscular bridges connecting the atrium and the ventricle, the AV node serves as the slow antegrade pathway and the AV bypass tract serves as the retrograde fast pathway (Fig. 5.8). The AV bypass tracts that conduct impulses only in the retrograde direction are not associated with any ECG manifestations of ventricular preexci-

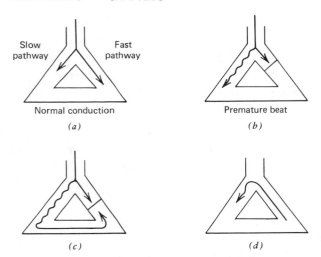

Figure 5.6 Requirements for reentry. (a) Two pathways with differing refractory and conduction patterns linked by a common distal pathway. A normally conducted impulse enters both pathways and is conducted more rapidly down the fast pathway. (b) Disparity in the refractory periods of these pathways allows a premature beat to block in the fast pathway and conduct down the slow pathway. (c) Sufficiently slow conduction within the slow pathway allows the fast pathway to regain excitability. (d) Conduction of the impulse up the fast pathway. Continued propagation of the impulse in the circuit results in a sustained reentrant arrhythmia. (Adapted from Morady F, Scheinman, MM: Paroxysmal supraventricular tachycardia. I. Diagnosis. *Mod Concepts Cardiovasc Dis* 1982; 51:107.)

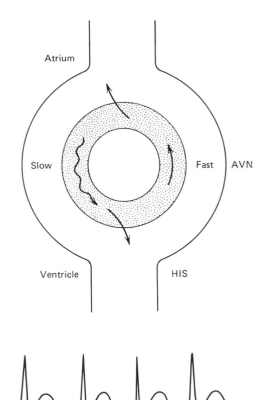

Figure 5.7 Mechanisms of AV nodal reentry tachycardia. Atrioventricular nodal reentrant tachycardia. The reentry circuit is confined to the atrioventricular node (AVN): The slow pathway serves as the antegrade limb of the circuit, and the fast pathway serves as the retrograde limb. Since the ventricles are depolarized through the His-Purkinje axis, the QRS complex (ECG) is narrow unless there is abnormal intraventricular conduction. Atrial and ventricular depolarization usually occur simultaneously, thus the P waves are buried within the QRS complex and are not apparent. (Adapted from Morady F, Scheinman MM: Paroxysmal supraventricular tachycardia. I. Diagnosis. *Mod Concepts Cardiovasc Dis* 1982; 51:108.)

tation (such as the Wolff-Parkinson-White syndrome) and are therefore referred to as *concealed*. Narrow QRS complexes suggest that for the reentry circuit, the AV nodal pathway is antegrade and the accessory pathway is retrograde. Wide QRS complexes, which are less common, suggest that the accessory pathway is antegrade and the AV nodal pathway is retrograde, especially if narrow QRS complexes have been documented on previous tracings of the patient during normal sinus rhythm.

DIAGNOSIS

The diagnosis of PSVT is usually established on the basis of rate and regularity and the response to carotid sinus pressure (Table 5.5). With the exceptions mentioned above, the rate of PSVT in adults is usually in the 140–200 beats/min range. The rhythm tends to be extremely regular, both from lead to lead and from hour to hour. Carotid sinus pressure or other vagal maneuvers frequently terminate PSVT. Such a response is usually considered diagnostic of PSVT, although a few cases of

ventricular arrhythmias terminating with carotid sinus massage have been reported. Atrioventricular block is almost never seen as a response to carotid sinus massage or other vagal maneuvers in patients with PSVT, and its presence would make PAT with block or atrial flutter more likely.

TREATMENT

Treatment of PSVT is usually directed toward changing intraatrial or AV conduction and thus interrupting the reentry path-

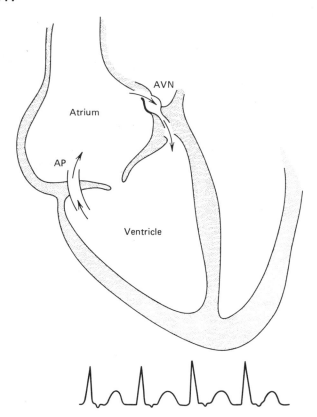

Figure 5.8 Mechanism of reciprocating tachycardia through an AV bypass tract Reciprocating tachycardia involving an AV accessory pathway (AP). The reentry circuit consists of (AVN), atrium, AP, and ventricle. Antegrade conduction through the AVN results in a normal pattern of ventricular depolarization: Rapid retrograde conduction through the AP results in an atrial depolarization that occurs just after ventricular depolarization. The ECG thus shows a narrow QRS complex followed closely by a P wave. (Adapted from Morady F, Scheinman MM: Paroxysmal supraventricular tachycardia. I. Diagnosis. *Mod Concepts Cardiovasc Dis* 1982; 51:109.)

pressure, which may cause retinal detachment, should no longer be employed.

When simple vagal stimulation alone is unsuccessful in terminating PSVT, other measures that sensitize to vagal stimulation or alter AV conduction are used. In otherwise healthy people without organic heart disease, intravenous verapamil is quickly becoming the drug of choice in the emergency room treatment of PSVT. Verapamil, 5–10 mg intravenously over 5–10 minutes, will revert most of these arrhythmias. This agent should be used cautiously in patients with preexistent AV conduction problems, heart failure, or possible digitalis intoxication. Hypotension associated with verapamil therapy is common but transient. Edrophonium hydrochloride (Tensilon) in a dose of 5–10 mg intravenously will often terminate PSVT and carotid sinus massage is often successful after the patient has received edrophonium. Edrophonium can enhance digitalis toxicity and should be used with caution if this is a serious possibility. It also causes a parasympathetic response, including nausea, abdominal cramps, and increased salivation. Vasopressors may terminate PSVT, especially in the patient with mild hypotension. In the elderly, vasopressors may cause chest pain or tachycardia and should be used with careful monitoring of both heart rate and blood pressure. Vasopressors should be given as a diluted intravenous infusion rather than as a bolus and should be stopped when the blood pressure reaches 140/90. Rapid digitalization is also a very effective means of dealing with these arrhythmias. Digoxin 0.50–0.75 mg or ouabain 0.2–0.4 mg given intravenously over 10 minutes often suffices to revert the arrhythmia spontaneously. These drugs also markedly sensitize the patient to carotid sinus pressure and other vagal manuevers. Propranolol given intravenously in 0.5–1 mg increments to a maximum of 3–5 mg is also effective. Cardioversion rarely needs to be used for patients with PSVT unless the patient is hemodynamically compromised or acutely ischemic.

In patients with PSVT, an accessory pathway, and normal QRS complexes (Fig. 5.6), propranolol is the drug of choice because it depresses antegrade AV nodal conduction (Table 5.8). The effect of verapamil on such patients is variable because verapamil's effect on the accessory pathway is variable. To prevent PSVT in these patients, propranolol, 30–120 mg/day, is quite useful.

In patients with PSVT, an accessory pathway, and wide QRS complexes, digitalis should usually be avoided because it shortens the effective refractory period of the accessory pathway (Table 5.8) and may cause the tachycardia to become even faster. In such patients, lidocaine is the drug of choice. Procainamide or quinidine are also effective.

In patients with PSVT and an accessory pathway that is re-

way necessary to maintain the arrhythmia. A variety of modalities are available for this purpose. Vagal stimulation, either with carotid sinus massage or Valsalva maneuver, is frequently effective in reverting these arrhythmias. Often, if initially unsuccessful, vagal maneuvers will be successful after the patient has been digitalized or treated with a vasopressor or parasympathomimetic agent. It should be emphasized that if carotid sinus pressure is applied and is unsuccessful, another modality should be used rather than repeating this maneuver. Eyeball sistant to medications, or especially if the patients have atrial fibrillation or atrial flutter with anomalous conduction, cardioversion should be used. For the very rare cardioversion-resistant tachyarrhythmia associated with accessory pathway, overdrive pacing may be necessary.

Atrial Flutter

Atrial flutter is an easy rhythm to diagnose and a rather difficult one to manage. It appears most often in the setting of organic heart disease or pulmonary disease. Pulmonary embolus also may predispose to this arrhythmia.

DIAGNOSIS

The diagnosis of atrial flutter is established by demonstrating atrial activity at a rate between 230 and 350 beats/min usually with a constant saw tooth pattern as opposed to discrete P waves; atrial activity is often best appreciated in leads II, III, and aV_F (Figure 5.9). Carotid sinus pressure with production of AV block may be necessary to demonstrate the flutter waves since many patients present with 2:1 block and alternative flutter waves are obscured by the QRS complex. If CSM does not reveal the flutter waves by inducing AV block, verapamil, propranolol, or edrophonium can be used diagnostically to increase AV block and expose the flutter waves. Atrial flutter is most often confused with paroxysmal atrial tachycardia with block, which has an isoelectric baseline and diminutive, upright P waves in II, III, and aV_F. Moreover, the atrial rate in PAT with block rarely exceeds 220 beats/min whereas untreated flutter rarely occurs at rates below 230 beats/min. Quinidine and propranolol slow the flutter mechanism and flutter rates below 200 beats/min can occasionally be seen in patients taking these drugs.

TABLE 5.8 **Effects of Antiarrhythmic Drugs on the Effective Refractory Periods of the Normal Atrioventricular and Accessory Pathways**

Drugs	Effective Refractory Period	
	AV Node	Accessory Pathway
Verapamil	Lengthened	Variable
Propranolol	Lengthened	No change
Digitalis	Lengthened	Shortened
Lidocaine	No change	Lengthened
Quinidine	Shortened	Lengthened
Procainamide	No change	Lengthened

TREATMENT

Atrial flutter is often a difficult rhythm to manage with medications and may require cardioversion or rapid atrial pacing for restoration of sinus rhythm. It should be remembered, however, that termination of atrial flutter does not prevent recurrences of atrial flutter. In the treatment of atrial flutter, a digitalis drug is usually used to increase AV block. Digitalization speeds the flutter rate and often converts the rhythm to atrial fibrillation, which is much more easily managed. Propranolol or verapamil may be used to increase AV block. Verapamil converts atrial flutter to sinus rhythm in approximately 30% of cases. Quinidine or procainamide will convert some patients (approximately 25%) to sinus rhythm and is useful in preventing recurrences after cardioversion.

Paroxysmal Atrial Tachycardia with Block

Paroxysmal atrial tachycardia (PAT) with block is a confusing arrhythmia. It is often not paroxysmal, resembles flutter more than PAT, often occurs in the absence of block, and may accelerate and decelerate gradually. Much of this confusion can be eliminated if it is remembered that the arrhythmia is really an ectopic, automatic supraventricular tachycardia (as opposed to a reentry SVT) that blocks. It occurs both as a manifestation of digitalis intoxication and, ironically, as a manifestation of underlying heart disease that responds best to digitalis. PAT with block because of digitalis intoxication is from two to three times as common as PAT occurring in the absence of this medication, and the appearance of this arrhythmia is very strong presumptive evidence of digitalis intoxication. Those patients with digitalis-induced PAT with block are often ill with gastrointestinal (GI), visual, and psychotropic side effects of the medication and, in addition, frequently have ventricular premature beats (VPBs) and other signs of digitalis intoxication.

DIAGNOSIS

In the species of PAT with block not caused by digitalis, the heart rate is usually similar to that observed in patients with paroxysmal atrial tachycardia (140–250 beats/min). The arrhythmia induced by digitalis usually appears at a rate of 140 beats/min or below; it rarely exceeds 220 beats/min. Although carotid sinus pressure usually increases AV block, the atrial rate remains unchanged (Fig. 5.10). CSM often demonstrates the underlying atrial mechanism and serves to differentiate PAT with block from all other arrhythmias except atrial flutter, which is usually faster than PAT with block and which has an undulating baseline. Digitalis-induced PAT with block is more

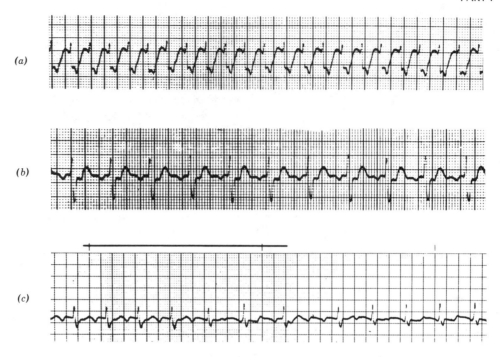

(a)

(b)

(c)

Figure 5.9 Atrial flutter. (*a*) One-to-one, conduction is observed with a ventricular rate of 200 beats/min; the patient was taking quinidine, which caused the atypically slow flutter rate. (*b*) A few minutes later the ventricular rate slowed as the patient went into 2:1 AV block. When carotid sinus pressure was applied (*c*), it was possible to identify the underlying flutter activity.

responsive to CSM than is PAT with block due to other causes such as underlying heart disease. In fact, inability to increase the AV block with CSM makes the diagnosis of digitalis-induced PAT with block unlikely.

TREATMENT

The patient with PAT with block must be hospitalized, and all digitalis preparations must be stopped. Potassium deficits should be corrected promptly with small increments of intravenous potassium chloride. Lidocaine may be useful in suppressing associated ventricular premature contractions and ventricular tachycardia. Cardioversion is extremely hazardous in these patients since it may produce ventricular tachycardia and ventricular fibrillation if the patient is digitalis toxic.

The diagnosis of PAT with block unrelated to digitalis should be made with great caution since the treatment of this arrhythmia (digitalis and/or cardioversion) may prove lethal in the patient with the arrhythmia induced by digitalis. Quinidine may be effective in treating patients with PAT with block that is *not* induced by digitalis.

Ventricular Tachycardia

Ventricular tachycardia (VT), defined as three or more consecutive beats of ventricular origin at a rate greater than 100 beats/min, may occur both as a manifestation of underlying heart disease and in the absence of demonstrable heart disease.

Ventricular tachycardia, especially at rapid rates, can degenerate to ventricular fibrillation (VF). After myocardial infarction, VT is associated with heart failure and ventricular aneurysm. Ventricular tachycardia can be precipitated by electrolyte imbalance, acid–base disorders, alcohol, and medications, especially (and ironically) by antiarrthymic medications.

The mechanism of VT is usually a result of a reentry circuit that is initiated by a ventricular premature beat. Occasionally, VT is initiated from a parasystolic focus that discharges autonomously and that is "protected" from the rest of the ventricle.

Diagnosis of ventricular tachycardia (Fig. 5.11) is often far more difficult than treatment since only a minority of patients have demonstrable AV dissociation or fusion beats (Table 5.4). A regular tachycardia with a rate of 100–250 beats/min and a widened QRS complex is consistent with VT or with SVT with

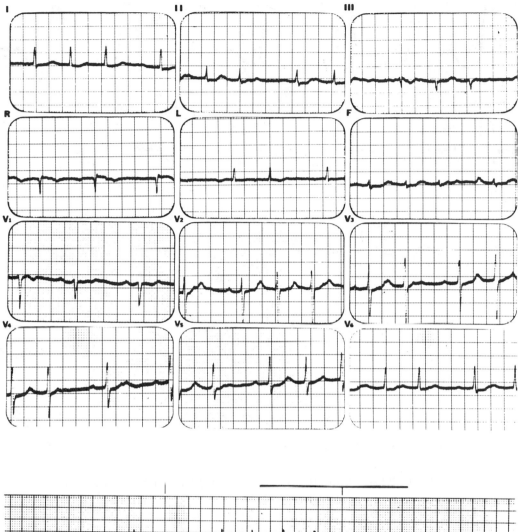

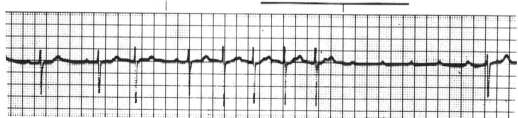

Figure 5.10 Paroxysmal atrial tachycardia with block. The patient had been given digoxin for paroxysmal atrial fibrillation. At first glance the irregular ventricular rhythm may suggest atrial fibrillation, but the underlying regular atrial activity is apparent in the right precordial leads. Carotid sinus pressure (below) clearly demonstrates the underlying regular atrial activity.

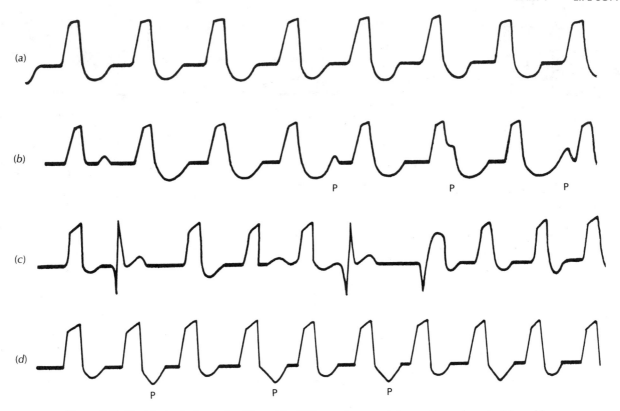

Figure 5.11 Ventricular tachycardia. The wide QRS complexes and the rapid regular rate (a) could represent either VT or a SVT with a preexisting intraventricular conduction delay or rate-related intraventricular conduction delay. The presence of AV dissociation (b), fusion or capture beats (c), or 2:1 VA block (d), permits assignment of the pacemaker to the ventricle.

rate-related intraventricular conduction delay or with preexistent bundle branch block (Table 5.4). Carotid sinus massage may be useful in distinguishing between these two. If it terminates the arrhythmia, it is very likely that the arrhythmia was a SVT. If it fails to terminate the arrhythmia, it may produce increased AV or VA block, both of which can be useful in differential diagnosis. His bundle electrocardiography is often diagnostic but is rarely an emergency procedure. (Torsade de pointes was discussed previously.)

A variant of ventricular tachycardia is *accelerated idioventricular rhythm* (AIVR) in which an ectopic focus fires the ventricles at 60–100 beats/min. AIVR occurs during myocardial infarction, especially during a bradycardic inferior myocardial infarction, and during myocarditis or digitalis toxicity. AIVR is usually benign but may accelerate to ventricular tachycardia.

TREATMENT

Ventricular tachycardia frequently requires prompt treatment since it may be accompanied by hemodynamic compromise and because it may degenerate to ventricular fibrillation. Lidocaine is often effective and a dose of 75–100 mg should be given immediately, followed by additional increments of 25–50 mg to a maximum of 2 mg/kg (Table 5.9). If lidocaine is successful in reverting the arrhythmia, an intravenous drip of 2–4 mg/min should be started to prevent recurrences. Should lidocaine prove unsuccessful in terminating the arrhythmia, another antiarrhythmic measure should be used rather than hoping that an intravenous drip of lidocaine will subsequently prove successful. Intravenous procainamide is the pharmacologic agent of choice for patients who are unresponsive to

TABLE 5.9 Lidocaine Dosage Regimens

Loading dose	1–2 mg/kg by slow intravenous infusion (up to 50 mg/min) *or* 100 mg given 2 times at 10-min intervals *or* 50 mg over 1 min, given 4 times, 5 min apart *or* 20 mg/min infused over 10 min
Maintenance dosage	2–4 mg/min for 24 hr
To raise concentration acutely	50-mg bolus over 1 min and simultaneously increase rate to no more than 4 mg/min

Reduce dosage and consider ordering serum levels in patients who have heart failure, liver disease, or coadministration of propranolol.

lidocaine. It is usually employed by giving 50 mg/min intravenously up to a maximum dose of 1 g with careful monitoring of blood pressure and QRS width. For patients who stabilize or revert on this regimen, a maintenance intravenous infusion of 2–4 mg/min is then used to prevent recurrences. Patients with hemodynamic compromise who are unresponsive to lidocaine and procainamide may be given bretylium, 5 mg/kg intravenously as a bolus. The initial 5 mg/kg dose can be repeated every 5–15 minutes, with dosages as high as 30 mg/ kg over 45–90 minutes. The dose of bretylium is frequently limited by hypotension. Bretylium may also exacerbate digitalis intoxication, which is a contraindication to using bretylium.

Patients with VT are usually very responsive to cardioversion and often require less than 25 WS. It must be emphasized that reversion to sinus rhythm will not prevent recurrences of the arrhythmia and that antiarrhythmic drugs should be given for this reason.

Accelerated idioventricular rhythm may be difficult to suppress but often does not warrant treatment. For patients with myocardial infarction and AIVR, lidocaine or atropine are the most likely agents to be effective.

Rarely, VT will be refractory to medical therapy. In such instances, overdrive pacing or ventricular aneurysectomy may be warranted.

BRADYARRHYTHMIAS

Sinus Bradycardia

A sinus rhythm with a rate of 50 beats/min or below may be a normal finding and is often seen in the well-conditioned athlete. It can also be a sign of sinus node dysfunction or hypothyroidism. Vagally mediated sinus bradycardia may be seen in patients with severe pain, nausea, increased intracranial pressure, and carotid sinus sensitivity. Several medications predispose to sinus bradycardia: beta blockers, parasympathomimetic medications, and antihypertensive medications such as methyldopa (Aldomet) and reserpine.

Treatment depends on whether sinus bradycardia causes symptoms. In those patients who tolerate the arrhythmia poorly and manifest decreased blood pressure, confusion, or increased ventricular irritability, restoration of normal heart rate may be indicated. Intravenous atropine is usually the agent of first choice; 0.2–0.3 mg of atropine intravenously may be sufficient and is less likely to cause complications than the 0.5–1 mg dose usually recommended. Additional 0.2-mg boluses may be given every few minutes to a maximum of 1 mg. If atropine is unsuccessful in increasing the heart rate, isoproterenol can be tried; 1–2 μg of isoproterenol per minute is given by an intravenous infusion with careful monitoring of the heart rate, rhythm, and blood pressure. An occasional patient with an acute myocardial infarction, ventricular irritability, and sinus bradycardia may require a transvenous pacemaker.

Sinus Node Dysfunction

Dysfunction of the sinus node, a common problem in older patients, is often a manifestation of underlying heart disease or a complication of therapy with digitalis or lithium. Sinus node dysfunction presents either as sinus exit block or as sinus arrest (Fig. 5.12). Both sinoatrial block and sinus arrest may be asymptomatic. If they are complicated by syncope, congestive heart failure, or increased ventricular irritability, treatment may be indicated. Atropine and isoproterenol are often less successful in patients with these disorders than in those with sinus bradycardia, and transvenous pacemakers are more often required.

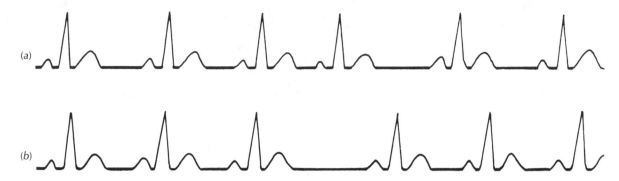

Figure 5.12 Sinus node dysfunction. (a) The gradually decreasing P–P interval preceding a pause is typical of sinus exit block. In sinus arrest (b), the P–P interval tends to be more regular with the exception of the pauses as a result of the occasional failure of atrial capture.

Frequently, especially in elderly patients, sinus node dysfunction or sinoatrial dysfunction is associated with paroxysmal tachyarrhythmias (bradycardia–tachycardia syndrome). This syndrome often necessitates both pacemaker therapy for the bradycardia and antiarrhythmic medication to suppress the tachycardia.

Patients with chronic sinoatrial dysfunction are at relatively high risk from systemic embolism. The risk of embolization remains even after pacemaker implantation. Thus patients with sinus node dysfunction, like those with chronic atrial fibrillation, require chronic anticoagulation.

Atrioventricular Block

The patient with first degree AV block, defined as PR interval prolongation greater than 0.20 seconds in which every P wave is followed by a QRS complex, may have no underlying heart disease but more frequently is taking digitalis or has some fibrosis or ischemia in the region of the AV node. Such patients are predisposed to more advanced degrees of heart block but require no treatment until such advanced degrees of heart block occur.

If some of the P waves are not conducted to the ventricles, the patient has second-degree AV block. This may occur with and without PR interval prolongation and in various ratios between the P waves and QRS complexes. Clinically, it is most useful to subdivide this group into those with Mobitz type I (Wenckebach) second-degree AV block, whose PR interval prolongation gradually increases until a QRS is dropped, and those with Mobitz type II second-degree AV block, who suddenly have a blocked QRS without antecedent increased PR interval (Fig. 5.2). Mobitz type I second-degree AV block is usually a manifestation of AV node dysfunction, although occasionally it is observed in patients with disease in the Purkinje system. It is a common complication of myocardial infarction, especially inferior myocardial infarction, and is also seen in patients with digitalis intoxication. If it progresses to complete heart block, it tends to do so gradually rather than suddenly, and the junctional pacemaker that subsumes the pacing function during complete heart block usually has a heart rate greater than 40 beats/min and is sufficient to avoid severe hypotension or congestive failure. However, Mobitz type II second-degree AV block is more ominous, and the location of the compromised conduction is usually below the AV node. Mobitz type II second-degree AV block can rapidly degenerate to complete heart block with a ventricular response inadequate (< 40 beats/min) to maintain perfusion to vital organs.

The patient with third-degree, or complete heart block (Fig. 5.2), has a regular ventricular rhythm with no relationship between the P waves and the QRS complex. The width of the QRS complex and the heart rate are useful in estimating the location of the ventricular pacemaker since in patients with a junctional pacemaker, the rate is often in the 40–60 beats/min range and the QRS complex is narrow, whereas in the patient with a ventricular pacemaker distal to the AV node, the heart rate is likely to be less than 40 beats/min and the QRS complex wider than 0.11 seconds.

TREATMENT

Atropine in doses similar to those used for sinus bradycardia may improve the AV conduction, especially in Mobitz type I second-degree AV block. Patients who have Mobitz type II second-degree AV block and complete heart block with a slow ventricular escape rhythm may not respond well to atropine or isoproterenol. Patients with complete heart block with a ventricular escape rhythm almost always require transvenous pacing in order to maintain an adequate cardiac output. Patients with an acute myocardial infarction and Mobitz type II AV block should have a prophylactic temporary transvenous pacemaker immediately inserted. Those who progress to complete heart block during their infarction require permanent pacemakers to prevent the likelihood of subsequent sudden death.

Patients with no significant underlying heart disease and junctional escape rhythm often tolerate complete heart block well and no therapy is required. Patients with both junctional escape rhythm and underlying heart disease may not tolerate the loss of atrial preload or the reduced rate and may develop syncope, congestive heart failure, or ventricular irritability. Although these patients occasionally respond to atropine or isoproterenol in the emergency situation, pacemaker therapy is the treatment of choice.

The prognosis for patients with AV block depends on the heart disease associated with the conduction disturbance. The patient with transient AV block because of myocarditis will have an excellent prognosis if recovery from myocarditis is complete. However, the patient with complete heart block because of massive anterior myocardial infarction has a poor long-term prognosis even with pacemaker therapy. Unfortunately, patients with extensive myocardial damage from infarction or cardiomyopathy are vulnerable to further muscle damage and to ventricular fibrillation despite a normally functioning permanent pacemaker.

SELECTED READINGS

Antman EM: *Supraventricular Arrhythmias.* Upper Montclair, NJ: Health Scan Inc, 1981.

Chung EK: Wolff-Parkinson-White syndrome: Current views. *Am J Med* 1977; 62:252–266.

Cohn PF, Wynne J, eds: *Diagnostic Methods in Clinical Cardiology.* Boston, Little Brown and Co, 1982.

DeSanctis RW: Disturbances of cardiac rhythm and conduction, in Rubenstein E, Federman DD (eds): *Scientific American Medicine,* New York, NY, 1982.

DeSilva RA, Graboys TB, Podrid PJ, Lown B: Cardioversion and defibrillation. *Am Heart J* 1980; 100:881–895.

Fairfax AJ, Lambert CD, Leatham A: Systemic embolism in chronic sinoatrial disorder. *N Engl J Med* 1976; 295:190–192.

Giardina E-GV, Fenster PE, Bigger JT Jr, Mayersohn M, Perrier D, Marcus FI: Efficacy, plasma concentrations and adverse effects of a new sustained release procainamide preparation. *Am J Cardiol* 1980; 46:855–862.

Heissenbuttel RH, Bigger JT Jr: Bretylium tosylate: A newly available antiarrhythmic drug for ventricular arrhythmias. *Ann Intern Med* 1979; 91:229–238.

Hinton RC, Kistler JP, Fallon JT, Friedlich AL, Fisher CM: Influence of etiology of atrial fibrillation on incidence of systemic embolism. *Am J Cardiol* 1977; 40:509–513.

Horan MJ, Kennedy HL: Characteristics and prognosis of apparently healthy patients with frequent and complex ventricular ectopy: Evidence for a relatively benign and new syndrome with occult myocardial and/or coronary disease. *Am Heart J* 1981; 102:809–810.

Horowitz LN, Josephson MF, Spielman SR, Greenspan AM, Harken AH: New approaches to diagnosing and treating ventricular tachycardia. *J Cardiovasc Med* 1980; 5:715–728.

Josephson ME: Paroxysmal supraventricular tachycardia: An electrophysiologic approach. *Am J Cardiol* 1978; 41:1123–1126.

Josephson ME, Kastor JA: Supraventricular tachycardia: Mechanisms and management. *Ann Intern Med* 1977; 87:346–358.

Josephson ME, Seides SF: *Clinical Cardiac Electrophysiology: Techniques and Interpretations.* Philadelphia, Lea & Febiger, 1979.

Kannel WB, Abbott RD, Savage DD, McNamara PM: Epidemiologic features of chronic atrial fibrillation: The Framingham study. *N Engl J Med* 1982; 306:1018–1022.

Kastor J: Temporary pacing for patients with postinfarction atrioventricular block. *J Cardiovasc Med* 1982; 7:381–391.

Koch-Weser J: Bretylium. *N Engl J Med* 1979; 300:473–477.

Koch-Weser J: Disopyramide. *N Engl J Med* 1979; 300:957–962.

Koch-Weser J, Klein SW: Procainamide dosage schedules, plasma concentrations, and clinical effects. *J Am Med Assoc* 1971; 215:1454–1460.

Lie KI, Wellens HJ, van Capelle FJ, Durrer D: Lidocaine in the prevention of primary ventricular fibrillation: A double-blind, randomized study of 212 consecutive patients. *N Engl J Med* 1974; 291:1324–1326.

Lown B: Sudden cardiac death—1978. *Circulation* 1979; 60:1593–1599.

Lown B, Graboys TB: Management of patients with malignant ventricular arrhythmias. *Am J Cardiol* 1977; 39:910–918.

Lown B, Levine SA: The carotid sinus: Clinical value of its stimulation. *Circulation* 1961; 23:766–789.

Lown B, Wolf M: Approaches to sudden death from coronary heart disease. *Circulation* 1971; 44:130–142.

Lown B, Wyatt NF, Levine HD: Paroxysmal atrial tachycardia with block. *Circulation* 1960; 21:129–143.

McAnulty JH, Rahimtoola SH, Murphy E, DeMots H, Ritzmann L, Kanarek PE, Kauffman S: Natural history of "high-risk" bundle-branch block. Final report of a prospective study. *N Engl J Med* 1982; 307:137–143.

McGoon MD, Vliestra RE, Holmes DR Jr, Osborn JE: The clinical use of verapamil. *Mayo Clin Proc* 1982; 57:495–510.

Margolis B, DeSilva RA, Lown B: Episodic drug treatment in the management of paroxysmal arrhythmias. *Am J Cardiol* 1980; 45:621–626.

Mauritson DR, Winniford MD, Walker WS, Rude RE, Cary JR, Hillis LD: Oral verapamil for paroxysmal supraventricular tachycardia: A long-term, double-blind randomized trial. *Ann Intern Med* 1982; 96:409–412.

Morady F, Scheinman MM: Paroxysmal supraventricular tachycardia. Part I. Diagnosis. *Mod Concepts Cardiovasc Dis* 1982; 51:107–112.

Morady F, Scheinman MM, Desai J: Disopyramide. *Ann Intern Med* 1982; 96:337–343.

Moss AJ, Davis RJ: Brady-tachy syndrome. *Prog Cardiovasc Dis* 1974; 16:429–452.

Moss AJ, Davis HT, DeCamilla J, Bayer LW: Ventricular ectopic beats and their relation to sudden and nonsudden cardiac death after myocardial infarction. *Circulation* 1979; 60:998–1003.

Rabkin SW, Mathewson FAL, Tate RB: Relationship of ventricular ectopy in men without apparent heart disease to occurrence of ischemic heart disease and sudden death. *Am Heart J* 1981; 101:135–142.

Rosen KM, Barwolf C, Ehsani A, Rahimtoola SH: Effects of lidocaine and propranolol on the normal and anomalous pathways in patients with preexcitation. *Am J Cardiol* 1972; 30:801–809.

Scheinmann MM, Strauss HC, Evans GT, Ryan C, Massie B, Wallace A: Adverse effects of sympatholytic agents in patients with hypertension and sinus node dysfunction. *Am J Med* 1978; 64:1013–1020.

Shine KI, Kastor JA, Yurchak PM: Multifocal atrial tachycardia: Clinical and electrocardiographic features in 32 patients. *N Engl J Med* 1968; 279:344.

Smith WM, Gallagher JJ: Les torsades de pointes: An unusual ventricular arrhythmia. *Ann Intern Med* 1980; 93:578–584.

Waxman HL, Myerburg RJ, Appel R, Sung RJ: Verapamil for control of ventricular rate in paroxysmal supraventricular tachycardia and atrial fibrillation or flutter: a double-blind randomized crossover study. *Ann Intern Med* 1981; 94:1–6.

Wellens HJJ, Bär FWHM, Lie KI: The value of the electrocardiogram in the differential diagnosis of a tachycardia with a widened QRS complex. *Am J Med* 1978; 64:27–33.

Wellens HJJ, Durrer D: Wolff-Parkinson-White syndrome and atrial fibrillation: Relation between refractory period of accessory pathway and ventricular rate during atrial fibrillation. *Am J Cardiol* 1974; 34:777–782.

6

CARDIAC DECOMPENSATION

Joseph S. Alpert

Heart failure in patients seen in emergency rooms is most frequently due to coronary artery disease, but hypertensive heart disease, valvular heart disease, and various forms of myocardial disease (especially alcoholic cardiomyopathy) also are common etiologies. Only rarely does heart failure result from congenital heart disease.

Many factors, which are listed in Table 6.1, can precipitate left ventricular failure. Some patients "slide" into heart failure because of a dietary salt indiscretion. A more specific cause is usually responsible for the decompensation, however. Pulmonary embolism or pneumonia are common causes, but myocardial infarction and severe myocardial ischemia are the most frequent causes.

The major complaints of a patient who presents in an emergency room with heart failure may be symptoms of cardiac decompensation itself or they may be symptoms of another illness that has caused heart failure. The left ventricle, the right ventricle, or both may fail. Failure may be chronic, or acute, or both. It may be mild or severe, and a change (a worsening or an improvement) in the decompensation may occur in minutes, hours, or days.

While general and specific measures are being instituted to reverse the pathophysiologic sequence of left or right ventricular failure, the physician must address a critical question: Why did the patient develop heart failure when he or she did?

Physicians must be able to differentiate the syndromes of left and right ventricular failure by evaluating subjective and objective data to narrow the range of possible diagnoses. Only after physicians have ascertained which side of the heart has failed and determined the etiology of the dysfunction can they prescribe the appropriate therapy.

INITIAL ASSESSMENT

History and Physical Examination

EVIDENCE OF LEFT VENTRICULAR FAILURE

Pulmonary congestion secondary to an increase in the diastolic pressure in the left atrium and left ventricle produces the symptoms of left ventricular failure. Dyspnea on exertion, the earliest symptom, is usually followed by orthopnea and paroxysmal nocturnal dyspnea. The pathophysiologic mechanisms of orthopnea and paroxysmal nocturnal dyspnea are similar: When a patient moves from an erect to a supine position, blood that has been sequestered in the large venous reservoir in the legs returns to the central circulation and the pulmonary vessels; pulmonary vascular pressure increases, fluid accumulates in the interstitial spaces, breathing becomes difficult, and the oxygen level in the blood decreases.

Extremely severe pulmonary congestion results in pulmonary edema, which is discussed in Chapter 2. Symptoms of pulmonary edema include severe dyspnea at rest and a cough productive of frothy sputum. Arterial hypoxemia, the result of ventilation–perfusion mismatches in a congested lung, further depresses left ventricular function, and hypoxemia combined with decreased cardiac output causes extreme fatigue in a patient whose left ventricle has failed.

Rales, indicating accumulation of fluid in the pulmonary interstitium, can be heard at the base of both lungs soon after the left ventricle begins to fail. As the decompensation worsens and pulmonary edema (interstitial and intraalveolar) becomes more severe, rales are apparent over an increasing area of the lung fields; the lungs' ability to supply the body with oxygen decreases, hypoxia increases, and tachypnea results. Hypoxia may progress to such a degree, in fact, that the patient may appear to be cyanotic. Tachycardia is usually present, and left ventricular third heart sounds are common. A few patients, most of whom have a history of bronchial asthma, develop significant wheezing.

Dyspnea, on exertion or at rest, and orthopnea with arterial hypoxemia also frequently accompany chronic obstructive pulmonary disease (COPD). Therefore, the first question that must be answered by the physician evaluating a dyspneic patient is whether the dyspnea is secondary to cardiac or to pulmonary dysfunction. A checklist such as the one in Table 6.2 is often useful in helping a physician distinguish one etiology from the other, but at times the differentiation cannot be made until the patient is admitted to the intensive care unit and his or her pulmonary capillary wedge pressure (PCWP) is measured with a Swan-Ganz (flow-directed balloon) catheter.

EVIDENCE OF RIGHT VENTRICULAR FAILURE

The symptoms and signs of right ventricular failure and conditions that mimic it (constrictive or effusive pericarditis, for example) are manifestations of the resulting systemic venous congestion. Peripheral edema and fatigue (the latter secondary to inadequate cardiac output) are usually the earliest symptoms. Once venous congestion stretches the hepatic capsule, pain is felt in the right upper quadrant. Anorexia, nausea, and

153

TABLE 6.1 Precipitants of Left Ventricular Failure

Factors that impair the heart's ability to perform
    Arrhythmias (atrial fibrillation, heart block)
    Discontinuation of diuretics, digitalis
    Myocardial depression (ischemia, infarction, alcohol, thiamine
    deficiency, bacterial sepsis, drugs)
Factors that increase the load on the heart
    Dietary salt indiscretion
    Infection
    Fever
    Increased physical exertion
    Surgery
    Anemia
    Thyrotoxicosis

malabsorption, secondary to splanchnic venous congestion, eventually develop.

When the right ventricle fails, the patient's neck veins are usually elevated, the liver is frequently enlarged and tender, hepatojugular reflux may be noted, and peripheral edema is often apparent. Ascites occurs only rarely, most commonly in patients with chronic right ventricular failure. Not all signs, however, are present in all patients.

RADIOGRAPHIC SIGNS OF LEFT AND RIGHT VENTRICULAR FAILURE

The earliest roentgenographic sign of left ventricular failure is a "redistribution" of pulmonary venous flow; that is, more blood than normal flows through the vessels in the upper lobes of the lung and less flows through vessels in the lower lobes. As pulmonary venous pressure rises, pulmonary congestion worsens and the chest film reveals Kerley B lines and fluid in the major and minor fissures of the right lung, which are signs of fluid accumulation in the pulmonary interstices (described in Chapter 2). The marginal contours of the pulmonary vessels, normally sharply defined, gradually fade and a perihilar haze develops. Fluffy alveolar infiltrates and pleural effusion appear eventually, and the classic "butterfly" contour associated with pulmonary edema is seen on chest films. Radiographic evidence of heart failure usually does not appear until 12 hours after the left ventricle begins to fail; signs of pulmonary congestion rarely disappear until approximately 1–2 days after the condition is resolved, even though hemodynamic evidence of

TABLE 6.2 Differentiation of Pulmonary and Cardiac Dyspnea

	Pulmonary	Cardiac
History	Industrial exposure; extensive tobacco use; recurrent respiratory infections; previous abnormal pulmonary function tests; daily cough-producing sputum, perhaps purulent	Previous angina, myocardial infarction, or rheumatic fever; previous evidence of abnormal cardiac function such as an abnormal ECG, presence of a murmur, or cardiomegaly seen on film
Physical examination	Increased respiratory rate; increased thoracic AP diameter; clubbing; localized rales; rhonchi; evidence of consolidation	Increased respiratory rate; S_3 and S_4 gallops; diffuse or symmetrical rales; murmur
ECG	Low voltage; poor R-wave progression; RVH	Old or recent MI; LVH except in mitral stenosis where RVH may be present
Chest film	Increased pulmonary volume with large AP diameter and flattened diaphragms; localized consolidation; small heart; normal pulmonary vasculature	Normal pulmonary volume and diaphragm; cardiomegaly; pulmonary vascular redistribution; Kerley-B lines; interstitial or alveolar edema
Pulmonary capillary wedge pressure	Normal (< 12 mm Hg)	Elevated (usually > 20 mm Hg)
Pulmonary function tests	Markedly abnormal (restrictive or obstructive pattern)	Normal or mild abnormalities

resolution is observed earlier. The physician must keep these radiologic "phase lags" in mind when planning therapeutic strategy for a patient with left ventricular failure.

The evidence of right ventricular failure on chest films may be subtle. In fact, nothing abnormal may be evident except a distended azygous vein; the right ventricle is not always enlarged. Abdominal films, however, may reveal an enlarged liver, and the spleen is sometimes larger than normal as well. Ascites may be observed in patients with severe right ventricular failure.

DIAGNOSTIC PROCEDURES FOR LEFT AND RIGHT VENTRICULAR FAILURE

One of the most reliable ways to confirm a diagnosis of left ventricular failure is to determine the patient's *pulmonary venous pressure,* which reflects the filling pressure of the left ventricle. This is most easily done indirectly by measuring the PCWP, which correlates with pulmonary venous pressure in most patients, with a Swan-Ganz catheter. A value greater than 12–15 mm Hg implies that the patient's left ventricle has failed. Insertion of a Swan-Ganz catheter is usually not performed in the emergency room since this can be a time-consuming procedure requiring careful monitoring and even fluoroscopy in selected cases. Insertion of these catheters is usually carried out once the patient has arrived in the intensive care unit.

Central venous pressure (CVP), an accurate reflection of right atrial or right ventricular filling pressure, should be measured in patients with suspected right ventricular failure (Procedure 6). A value greater than 8 mm Hg confirms the diagnosis of right ventricular failure. However, CVP may be normal even when the PCWP is markedly elevated; CVP thus provides no information about left ventricular function.

MANAGEMENT

General Considerations

Management of the patient with cardiac decompensation depends on the severity of the patient's heart failure. Patients with pulmonary edema and heart failure complicating acute myocardial infarction should be rapidly hospitalized in an intensive care unit with minimal emergency room therapy. Patients with mild to moderate degrees of left or right ventricular failure can be given initial therapy in the emergency room and then discharged home with outpatient follow-up (see pages 158–159). In general, patients presenting to the emergency room with heart failure should be placed in a sitting or reclining position,

given supplemental inspiratory oxygen, and connected to an electrocardiographic monitor. An intravenous line should be inserted and kept open with a very slow infusion of 5% dextrose in water. History is elicited, a physical examination is performed, and pertinent laboratory information (for example, chest roentgenogram) is collected. A therapeutic plan is then formulated, and the initial steps of this plan are carried out. At this point, the patient is either admitted or sent home with detailed (frequently written) instructions.

Specific Medications

DIGITALIS

Increasing cardiac output is a major goal of therapy. Digitalis glycosides, the mainstay of treatment of left ventricular failure, affect the heart muscle directly and increase the force and velocity of contraction of both normal and failing hearts; cardiac output increases modestly in patients with heart failure.

TABLE 6.3 Extracardiac Manifestations of Digitalis Preparations

Gastrointestinal
  Anorexia
  Nausea
  Vomiting
  Diarrhea
  Abdominal discomfort
Central nervous system
  Headache
  Drowsiness
  Malaise
  Nightmares
  Disorientation
  Delirium
  Blurred vision
  Altered color vision
  White halos around dark objects
  Diplopia
  Scotomas
  Optic neuritis
Hematologic
  Thrombocytopenia
  Eosinophilia
Skin
  Rashes
  Gynecomastia

Digitalis preparations are particularly valuable for managing left ventricular failure secondary to coronary artery disease, hypertension, valvular heart disease, or any form of cardiomyopathy (except idiopathic hypertrophic subaortic stenosis for which digitalis is contraindicated). Digitalis glycosides are also useful for treating right ventricular failure if it is due to left ventricular failure. Acute or chronic cor pulmonale, pericardial constriction, and tamponade, on the other hand, do not generally respond to digitalis therapy.

Because digitalis preparations have a low therapeutic:toxic dose ratio, toxicity is common. Symptoms are not limited to the heart; in fact, they affect many other parts of the body as well (see Table 6.3). Cardiac toxicity may manifest itself through any type of atrial or ventricular arrhythmia or through a conduction defect (see Chapter 5).

A control electrocardiogram (ECG) should be obtained before digitalis is administered, for the drug causes an ST-T pattern (scooped depression) that may mimic that seen with ischemic heart disease (Fig. 6.1). The physician must ascertain whether the patient is already being treated with digitalis because a loading dose administered to a patient receiving maintenance digitalis therapy can result in toxicity; if doubt exists, a blood sample should be analyzed for serum digoxin or digitoxin levels before digitalis therapy is initiated. In addition, it is essential to determine the patient's renal and hepatic status and the level of serum electrolytes before administering a digitalis glycoside.

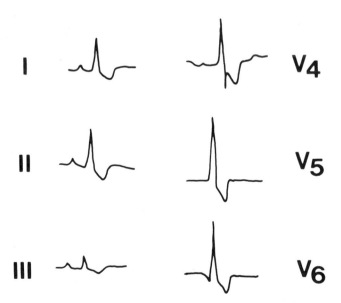

Figure 6.1 Electrocardiographic evidence of digitalis effect.

Digitalizing and maintenance doses of the two most common forms of digitalis are listed in Table 6.4. Because digoxin is excreted in the urine, a patient with renal insufficiency should receive a smaller maintenance dose than the one indicated in the table. Digitoxin, on the other hand, is cleared in the liver; patients with liver disease should receive smaller maintenance doses of this drug. Digoxin is generally the preferred drug; it is more rapidly excreted so dosage can be adjusted more easily. The rate and route of administration for digitalizing a patient depends on the severity of the left ventricular failure. If failure is moderate, a maintenance dose without a loading dose is usually sufficient. The intravenous route is preferable if the patient is unable to eat or is too sick to swallow pills, or if severe right ventricular failure has resulted in abnormal gastrointestinal function.

The physician should carefully explain the dangers and symptoms of digitalis toxicity to patients before they leave the hospital or emergency room. Written instructions are often the best assurance that patients will understand the treatment regimen. Because digitalis intoxication is especially likely if hypokalemia develops, potassium supplements or potassium-sparing drugs should be a part of the therapy if diuretics are also prescribed.

DIURETICS

Salt and water retention is common to all patients with left and right ventricular failure. Therefore, reestablishment of a normal internal milieu by promoting the loss of excess salt and water is another major goal of therapy. Many diuretics are available, all of which should ordinarily be administered orally rather than intravenously because the slower loss of sodium with oral therapy permits a normal hemodynamic status to be attained gradually. Rapid intravenous diuresis, which is rarely necessary, is not desirable since severe hypovolemia or even hypotension may result. Unless a cardiovascular emergency such as pulmonary edema presents (Chapter 2), intravenous diuretic administration should be avoided.

In addition to a decrease in intravascular volume, diuretic therapy frequently produces electrolyte imbalances, some of which can be life threatening. All patients with normal or near-normal renal function should receive potassium chloride or potassium-sparing diuretics (spironolactone, triamterene) in combination with the saluretic diuretics. Frequent measurements of serum potassium level are helpful when diuretic therapy is initiated. If hypokalemia, which often causes muscle weakness, cramping, and abdominal distention, occurs, digitalis intoxication is a risk. Chronic diuretic therapy can also

TABLE 6.4 Most Commonly Used Cardiac Glycosides

| Preparation | Loading Dose | | Usual Daily Maintenance Dose (Oral) | IV Action | | | Principal Excretory Route |
	Oral	IV		Onset	Maximum Effect	Half-life	
Digoxin	1.25–1.50 mg	0.75–1.0 mg	0.25–0.50 mg	15–30 min	1.5–5 hr	36 hr	Kidney
Digitoxin	0.7–1.2 mg	1.0 mg	0.1 mg	25–120 min	4–12 hr	4–6 day	Liver

result in sodium depletion. If this occurs, serum levels of sodium and chloride are low, and symptoms such as muscle weakness and cramping, somnolence, and disorientation develop.

The characteristics of the most commonly used diuretics are summarized in Table 6.5. A thiazide diuretic such as hydrochlorothiazide (Esidrix, 50 mg) or a small dose of furosemide (Lasix, 20–40 mg) is frequently prescribed initially as therapy for outpatients with moderate left or right ventricular failure. Usually diuretic therapy is initiated after admission to the hospital or at outpatient follow-up if signs and symptoms of cardiac decompensation persist after digitalis has been administered, activity has been minimized, and salt intake has been restricted. However, heart failure is frequently so severe that the physicians know when they first see the patient that both digitalis and diuretic therapy will be required. Both therapies can be initiated simultaneously, but the serum potassium level must be monitored closely. Some patients with severe cardiac decompensation require large doses of furosemide or ethacrynic acid each morning. Such patients invariably require hospitalization.

Powerful diuretics must be used cautiously, otherwise they may cause serious complications. Acute sodium depletion associated with the use of loop diuretics (furosemide, ethacrynic acid) occurs most frequently when heart failure is modest or of recent onset. Levels of serum electrolytes are initially normal, but the brisk, induced diuresis results in a decrease in intravascular volume and thus an increase in hematocrit and in blood urea nitrogen (BUN) level. These changes produce symptoms such as weakness, dizziness, and postural hypotension. Therapy consists of either decreasing the dose of diuretic or stopping it completely while increasing fluid and salt intake slightly.

All potent diuretics except the mercurials increase the amount

TABLE 6.5 Most Commonly Used Diuretics for Left or Right Ventricular Failure

Preparation	Mechanism	Usual Dosage	Onset of Action	Duration of Action
Hydrochlorothiazide (Esidrix)	Inhibits sodium reabsorption in the distal tubules	50 mg 1–2 times a day	2 hr	12 hr or longer
Furosemide (Lasix)	Inhibits sodium reabsorption in the loop of Henle	20–120 mg 1 time a day	Oral: 1 hr IV: 5 min	Oral: 6 hr IV: 2 hr
Ethacrynic acid (Edecrin)	Inhibits sodium reabsorption in the loop of Henle	50–100 mg 1 time a day	Oral: 30 min IV: 15 min	Oral: 6–8 hr IV: 3 hr
Spironolactone (Aldactone)	Competitively inhibits renal tubular effects of aldosterone	25 mg 4 times a day	Gradually over 1–2 days	2–3 days after therapy ceases
Triamterene (Dyrenium)	Inhibits sodium reabsorption associated with potassium secretion	100 mg 1–3 times a day	2 hr	12–16 hr

of potassium excreted in the urine. Secondary hyperaldoster-onism, a manifestation of heart failure, further augments the excretion of potassium. The resulting hypokalemia, which predisposes the patient to atrial and ventricular arrhythmias even if digitalis is not being administered, is one of the most common precipitating causes of cardiac arrhythmias associated with diuretic therapy.

Diuretic-induced hypokalemia is frequently associated with hypochloremic alkalosis. Because the appearance of the triad of hypokalemia, hypochloremia, and alkalosis is so common, patients for whom potent diuretics are prescribed should also receive potassium chloride (approximately 40 mEq orally a day) as preventive therapy. If hypokalemia develops, a higher dose of potassium is necessary to correct the electrolyte disorder. Potassium-sparing diuretics (spironolactone, triamterene) and potassium supplements should never be prescribed simultaneously, however, because life-threatening hyperkalemia can result.

Diuretics have some other common complications. When large doses of furosemide and ethacrynic acid are given, they may cause transitory hearing loss. When a thiazide or a potent loop diuretic (furosemide and ethacrynic acid) is given, the serum uric acid level may rise. The thiazides and, occasionally, furosemide can also produce hyperglycemia.

Transfer from the Emergency Room to the Hospital

Patients with pulmonary edema (Chapter 2) or severe heart failure require hospitalization. If no evidence of arrhythmia is present, if the patient is stable, and if the patient is not to be monitored in the hospital, no special precautions are necessary during transfer. If all three conditions are not met, the following precautions must be taken:

1. A physician and a nurse should accompany the patient.
2. The patient should be connected to a portable monitor and an ECG pattern should be clearly visible on the screen.
3. An intravenous catheter should be securely inserted and the fluid (5% dextrose in water) should be dripping slowly.
4. A portable battery-operated defibrillator, a syringe containing 100 mg of lidocaine, and a syringe containing 1 mg of atropine should accompany the patient.
5. Oxygen from a portable tank should be administered nasally to the patient during transfer.
6. Transfer should be as rapid as possible.

SUBSEQUENT THERAPY IN THE HOSPITAL OR AS AN OUTPATIENT

Activity

Bed rest alone markedly improves cardiac decompensation; in fact, bed rest initiates diuresis in many patients. Because deep venous thrombosis is a risk if a patient is in a recumbent position continuously, a bed-to-chair regimen is usually advisable. The patient should be allowed to sit in a comfortable chair for at least 60 minutes two times per day. In addition, it is frequently beneficial to encourage them to flex the soles of their feet against a foot board that has been placed at the end of the bed. Such exercise seems to increase the flow of blood in the deep veins of the legs and thereby helps to prevent the development of venous thrombosis.

Diet

Patients with heart failure have a decreased cardiac output in response to various bodily demands. Even the increased splanchnic blood flow after eating can strain the heart. Therefore, just as bed rest decreases muscular work and thus demands on the heart, light diet prevents excessive increases in splanchnic blood flow. Diets of more than 1,500 calories a day should rarely be prescribed.

Restricting salt is less important now than it was before the powerful loop diuretics became available. Nevertheless, the patient's salt intake at home should be estimated and matched in the hospital diet so that an appropriate diuretic dosage can be determined before discharge. Patients who have experienced severe heart failure can usually be placed initially on a diet containing 2 g sodium a day; the amount of sodium patients are allowed to ingest can be gradually increased until they can tolerate a diet to which no salt is added (4–5 g sodium). Diuretic dosage must, of course, be adjusted appropriately.

Temperature Regulation

Hot, humid weather can significantly increase the demand placed on the heart by increasing the flow of blood to the skin and sweat glands. In order to minimize this demand, patients should be cared for in air-conditioned or fan-ventilated areas. Activity during the hot periods of the day and in areas of the home where excessive heat is likely to accumulate should be avoided.

Monitoring Therapy

Patients with cardiac decompensation require careful monitoring during treatment to ensure that therapy is, in fact, effective. Weight, intake, output, and/or vital capacity should be recorded daily and can be expected to change appropriately during the course of therapy. Urinary output should exceed fluid intake, weight should decline, and vital capacity (in left ventricular failure patients) should increase. If minimal changes in these parameters occur, however, therapy has not been successful, and treatment modalities should be reexamined and more aggressive ones begun.

Outpatient Management

Patients with less severe left or right ventricular failure may be treated as outpatients. The following list summarizes the proper management regimen:

1. A baseline chest film, ECG, complete blood count (CBC), measurements of BUN and electrolytes, and an accurate determination of the patient's weight should be obtained.
2. Gradual digitalization should be initiated. (A daily dose of 0.25 mg of digoxin orally digitalizes a patient in approximately 1 week.)
3. Oral diuretic therapy may also be started. A single daily dose of a thiazide diuretic is adequate for patients with mild decompensation. Furosemide (20–40 mg orally per day) or ethacrynic acid (50 mg orally per day) should only be used to treat severe heart failure. A single intravenous dose of furosemide (40 mg) or ethacrynic acid (50 mg) may be administered in the emergency room to a patient with recurrent heart failure despite oral diuretic therapy, but the daily diuretic dose should also be increased.
4. Oral potassium chloride therapy (40 mEq/day in patients with normal renal function) should be initiated.
5. Patients should be instructed to return to or call the emergency room if they worsen or fail to feel significantly better within 24–48 hours. They should return in 3–4 days for a reexamination; the chest should be x-rayed, serum potassium levels measured, and the patient weighed.
6. It is frequently helpful to have patients record their weight each day at home until their first return visit. If their weight does not decrease by at least 1 kg (about 2 lb), therapy has probably not been successful.
7. A few patients with refractory left ventricular failure respond to vasodilator therapy because it reduces ventricular afterload. The initial dosage should be 10 mg of isosorbide dinitrate orally every 6 hours, which may be increased gradually to 40 mg every 6 hours if the drug is well tolerated. An alternative vasodilator is nitroglycerin ointment; 1.5 cm should be applied every 4 hours to a 20- to 25-cm^2 area and covered with plastic wrap; if the treatment is tolerated, the dosage may be gradually increased to 5 cm every 4 hours. Hydralazine (50 mg two to four times a day) has also been shown to be effective in some patients with refractory left ventricular failure.
8. Valve replacement should be considered for patients with valvular heart disease who develop left or right ventricular failure.

CLINICAL SETTINGS

Coronary Artery Disease

The symptoms of left ventricular failure secondary to coronary artery disease, the most common etiology of cardiac decompensation, may develop and worsen gradually or they may present acutely. Myocardial infarction or left ventricular ischemia triggers heart failure in many patients who usually give histories of recent or past infarction or angina pectoris. Patients who have had an infarction in the past may "slide" into heart failure because of dietary salt indiscretion.

A fourth heart sound is usually prominent, and a third heart sound may be detected as well. The ECG can confirm a suspected diagnosis of acute myocardial infarction or ischemia and can also reveal evidence of previous infarction. The diagnosis of coronary artery disease is discussed in Chapter 4. Chest films may demonstrate either a normal sized heart or an enlargement of the left ventricle. Specific therapy for coronary artery disease is discussed in Chapters 3 and 4.

Mitral Valve Disease

MITRAL STENOSIS

A history of acute rheumatic fever in childhood and a gradual increase in the severity of symptoms resembling those seen in patients with left ventricular failure, which develop over many years, suggests that mitral stenosis is the cause of heart failure. The precordial impulse may not be present, but if it is detected, it appears in only a small area. A right ventricular lift is often detected along the left side of the sternum, and a rumbling murmur is heard at the apex during diastole. The chest film usually demonstrates left atrial and frequently right ventricular enlargement; however, the left ventricle is usually normal in size. Redistribution of blood flow of the pulmonary vessels (or signs of even more severe pulmonary congestion) are also often evident. The ECG may be normal, or it may reflect right ventricular hypertrophy (RVH). Abnormal mitral valve motion produces a characteristic pattern on echocardiography: The diastolic opening slope (E to F slope) of the anterior leaflet is reduced, and anterior movement of the posterior mitral leaflet appears.

MITRAL REGURGITATION

Mitral regurgitation is accompanied by a prominent left ventricular precordial impulse and a loud holosystolic murmur, which tends to be loudest at the apex and radiates to the axilla. A prominent click heard in the first half of systole and close to or fused with the first heart sound when the patient stands is a common sign of prolapse of the mitral valve. Ruptured chordae, which cause acute mitral regurgitation, may produce a murmur similar to the ejection murmur heard with aortic stenosis. If regurgitation is severe, a loud third heart sound is usually present. The chest film demonstrates enlargement of the left atrium and the left ventricle, as well as signs of pulmonary congestion. Left ventricular hypertrophy (LVH) is usually detected on the ECG. Standard therapy for left ventricular failure (as outlined earlier) is initiated. The patient should be considered for mitral valve surgery.

Aortic Valve Disease

Two forms of aortic valve impairment may cause the left ventricle to fail.

A patient with *aortic stenosis* frequently has had an asymptomatic murmur for many years, but the clinical condition deteriorates quickly if syncope, angina, or left ventricular failure develop. Left ventricular failure due to aortic stenosis is accompanied by a thrusting left ventricular precordial impulse, a loud systolic ejection murmur at the base that radiates to the neck, and small carotid pulsations with delayed upstroke. The left ventricle is somewhat enlarged in the chest film, and the ECG demonstrates LVH, often with associated ST-T changes.

Aortic insufficiency, on the other hand, produces a carotid pulsation that seems to bound and collapse and a left ventricular precordial impulse that is quite vigorous. A high-pitched murmur heard in the first half of diastole is most prominent along the left side of the sternum when the patient is seated and exhales deeply. The left ventricle is quite enlarged on the chest film, and the ECG indicates that the left ventricle has hypertrophied. Standard therapy for left ventricular failure (as outlined earlier) is initiated. The patient should be considered for aortic valve surgery.

Primary Myocardial Disease

Symptoms of left ventricular failure usually develop gradually but relentlessly in patients with cardiomyopathy. A left ventricular precordial impulse is often detected over a wide area, prominent third and fourth heart sounds are frequently heard, and an inconsequential murmur resulting from mitral regurgitation (secondary to dilatation or abnormal functioning of the mitral valve apparatus) is common. The chest film indicates that the left ventricle is larger than normal and that the lungs are congested. The ECG may demonstrate LVH, nonspecific ST-T changes, or patterns similar to those of a myocardial infarction (for example, poor R-wave progression). An echocardiogram is frequently useful because it can document whether the left ventricle is significantly dilated and whether the contractility of the left ventricle is diffusely depressed. Therapy for left ventricular failure (as outlined earlier) is employed.

Pulmonary Embolism

A seemingly unexplainable worsening of existing left or right ventricular failure may be caused by pulmonary embolism that is not severe. Massive pulmonary embolism, however, invariably results in cardiovascular collapse, producing many of the same signs as right ventricular failure: elevated neck veins, a right ventricular lift alongside the sternum, and a third heart sound (S_3) that becomes more prominent on inspiration (right ventricular S_3). Arterial hypotension or frank shock is usually present as well.

Although the signs of pulmonary embolism mimic those of right ventricular failure, therapy is not the same for both conditions. Therefore, if there is any reason to suspect pulmonary embolism, a lung scan and a pulmonary angiogram should be used to confirm the diagnosis. Therapy for pulmonary embolism is outlined in Chapters 2 and 3.

Chronic Obstructive Pulmonary Disease

Acute right ventricular failure in patients with COPD is usually precipitated by a respiratory infection. Cyanosis of the lips, skin, and nail beds suggests that marked arterial hypoxemia is present, and breathing is frequently quite rapid. Findings on chest films vary from patient to patient and depend on the extent of pulmonary parenchymal damage and on the type and location of the acute infectious process. Thus, evidence of effusion or consolidation may be found, localized rales may be heard, and bronchospasm causing wheezing may be observed. Although only nonspecific changes on the ECG are common, the chest film reveals the stigmata of COPD (hyperinflation, flattened diaphragm, and sometimes obvious bullae) and superimposed pneumonitic infiltrates. Measurements of arterial blood gases often indicate that P_{O_2} is low, P_{CO_2} is elevated, and pH is low. Therapy for COPD is outlined in Chapter 2.

Conditions that Mimic Right Ventricular Failure

Pericardial constriction and *effusion with tamponade* produce findings similar to those observed in patients with right ventricular failure (jugular venous distention, hepatomegaly, peripheral edema). However, no right ventricular impulse alongside the sternum can be detected and no third heart sound can be heard. Indeed, the first and second heart sounds are barely audible, and it may be impossible to discern the point of maximal impulse. Sinus tachycardia, a narrow pulse pressure, and extremely distended neck veins are frequently present.

A pulsus paradoxus in excess of 10 mm Hg accompanies all but a few cases of pericardial effusion and cardiac tamponade (see Chapter 19), but it is rare with constrictive pericarditis. Patients with tamponade demonstrate cardiomegaly on chest films; patients with pericardial constriction, on the other hand, have normal-sized hearts. Echocardiography is a very sensitive test for determining the presence of fluid in the pericardial space. Therapy for cardiac tamponade is outlined in Chapter 19.

SUGGESTED READINGS

Alpert JS, Rippe JM: *Manual of Cardiovascular Diagnosis and Therapy.* Boston, Little Brown & Co, 1980.

Braunwald E: Clinical manifestations of heart failure, in Braunwald E (ed): *Heart Disease.* Philadelphia, WB Saunders Co, 1980, chap 15.

Braunwald E: Pathophysiology of heart failure, in Braunwald E (ed): *Heart Disease.* Philadelphia, WB Saunders Co, 1980, chap 13.

Braunwald E: Heart failure, in Isselbacher KJ, Adams RD, Braunwald E, Petersdorf RG, Wilson JD (eds): *Harrison's Principles of Internal Medicine.* New York, McGraw-Hill Book Co, 1980, chap 236.

Smith TW, Braunwald E: The management of heart failure, in Braunwald E (ed): *Heart Disease.* Philadelphia, WB Saunders Co, 1980, chap 16.

7

ANAPHYLAXIS

Albert L. Sheffer

Often explosive in onset, *anaphylaxis* is the most emergent allergic catastrophe. Symptoms may vary from mild pruritus to irreversible hypotension and/or fatal pulmonary insufficiency due to laryngeal edema. Resulting from the antigen-induced release of biologically active materials from mast cells or basophils, such reactions may be consequent to sensitization with specific IgE. However, direct mast cell degranulation or alterations in arachidonate or complement pathways may lead to similar clinical manifestations.

Reliable data pertinent to the incidence of anaphylaxis to specific antigens in appropriate populations is not available. A constitutional factor that appears to predispose a person to anaphylaxis is atopy. Five of 15 patients dying of anaphylaxis due to penicillin were asthmatic. Similarly, Levine's studies revealed that the likelihood of involving a skin-sensitizing antibody (IgE) of the type associated with systemic anaphylaxis was three to four times greater in atopic recipients.

The anatomic findings associated with fatal systemic anaphylaxis fall into three patterns. These include acute pulmonary hyperinflation due to airway obstruction and/or laryngeal edema, urticaria, and/or vascular collapse. The successful therapy for the acute anaphylactic reaction is contingent upon the early recognition of symptoms resulting from the aforementioned with prompt institution of therapy.

Thus, an anaphylactic reaction should be considered when an accurate history reveals the abrupt onset of appropriate signs and symptoms in a person administered the requisite antigen. Idiosyncratic or toxic reactions are the only alternative diagnosis when the criteria for an immunologic response can be met. These include a recognized antigen that, upon repeated administration, induces increasingly severe reactions with shortening of the latent period—the time between the administration of the antigen and the onset of symptoms. The triad of pruritic urticaria, throat tightness, as well as respiratory insufficiency and/or syncope with vascular collapse occurring abruptly after drug administration is diagnostic of anaphylaxis.

The pathogenesis of such reactions usually is consequent to IgE-dependent anaphylaxis. These may occur in nonatopic as well as in allergic individuals with personal or family histories of asthma, rhinitis, or eczema. Foods, such as shellfish, nuts, and chocolate; drugs and therapeutic agents, such as penicillin and immunotherapeutic extracts; and Hymenoptera venom from bee, wasp, yellow jacket, hornet, and fire ant, or even specific antigens are recognized precipitants of such life-threatening reactions via IgE mechanisms.

However, anaphylaxis may also result from the administration or formation of immune complexes. In an uncommon complication due to administration of blood, serum, or immunoglobulins, such reactions may result from the transfusion of IgE of donor origin directed against an antigen to which the recipient is exposed at the time of the transfusion. The transfusion of a soluble antigen into a host sensitized to this antigen similarly can precipitate IgE adverse reactions. More commonly, such transfusion reactions are consequent to immune complex formation with the activation of complement leading to vascular and smooth muscle alterations but involving generation of anaphylatoxin with mast cell mediator release. Patients deficient in IgA may possess IgG antibodies to IgA, particularly recipients of multiple transfusions. These antibodies form complexes with IgA and activate complement. IgA comprises 0.5–4% of IgG preparations. Such anti-IgA responses may also occur in people receiving immunoglobulin replacement therapy. Aggregates of immunoglobulin may occur in such preparations and fix complement.

Aspirin and other nonsteroidal antiinflammatory agents, as well as tartrazine, a coloring agent, FD&C yellow dye No. 5, cause anaphylactic responses in approximately 1% of the population. Asthmatics manifest bronchospasm whereas normal people or patients with rhinitis usually manifest urticaria and/or angioedema as the adverse reaction. Nearly 20% of the patients intolerant of nonsteroidal antiinflammatory agents will react to azo dyes such as tartrazine and to benzoate preservatives. Aspirin-intolerant patients should be advised to avoid the drug since documentation can only be confirmed by challenge. Of interest is the apparent tolerance of such aspirin-intolerant people to related compounds such as sodium salicylate or choline salicylate. Skin testing and other in vivo techniques have not demonstrated correlation with clinical disease. Presumably such nonsteroidal antiinflammatory agents inhibit cyclooxygenase, an enzyme participating in the generation of prostaglandin from arachidonic acid. Prostaglandin by-products induce bronchoconstriction and other manifestations consequent to the generation of prostaglandin metabolites, that is leukotrienes. Also implicated in such reactions have been other mediators such as histamine and complement-generated factors.

Anaphylactic-type reactions occur consequent to the administration of various therapeutic and diagnostic agents causing degranulation of the mast cells. Antibody to radiocontrast media has not been demonstrable, and, as a consequence, skin testing is not predictive of such adverse responses. Opiates, curare, and d-tubocurarine, as well as highly charged antibiotics such as polymyxin B, are also histamine-releasing agents from mast cells and basophils. Alterations in complement concentrations have been demonstrated in unconfirmed reports after administration of radiocontrast media, but the pathobiologic mechanism by which this anaphylactic phenomena occurs is not clarified.

Those antigens capable of inducing anaphylaxis in humans include proteins, polysaccharides, and haptenes (Table 7.1). Anaphylactic symptoms may occur after ingestion of food, after administration of therapeutic or diagnostic agents, upon contact of skin or mucous membranes with aerosols or solutions of antigenic substances, after irrigation with antigen of various body orifices or injection of antigen through or into the skin, and on rare occasion during exercise (Table 7.1).

DIAGNOSIS

Anaphylaxis is a clinically defined, life-threatening entity that is often explosive in onset. Symptoms may vary from mild pruritis to irreversible shock and/or fatal pulmonary insufficiency. Usually preceded by a sensation of generalized warmth and pruritus, the acute anaphylactic syndrome may be manifested as one of three clinical patterns. Urticaria and angioedema may occur as distinct entities or in association with one of the other clinical manifestations, that is, respiratory distress and/or profound hypotension. Respiratory distress occurs as a result of upper airway obstruction due to laryngeal edema or severe bronchospasm. The former may be experienced as hoarseness, stridor, dysphagia, or a lump or tightness in the throat. Bronchospasm is usually associated with an audible expiratory wheeze, tightness in the chest, or even absent breath sounds if air flow is significantly reduced. Either of these two

TABLE 7.1 Systemic Anaphylaxis in Humans

Class	Example
I. IgE Mediated	
A. Protein	
1. Antiserum	Tetanus and diptheria antitoxins
2. Hormones–Enzymes	Insulin; ACTH; relaxin; chymotrypsin; trypsin; penicillinase
3. Venom (Hymenoptera)	
4. Allergen extract (pollen, food)	Ragweed; Bermuda grass; buckwheat; egg white; cotton seed
5. Glue	
6. Hemoglobin (guinea pig)	
B. Polysaccharides	
1. Acacia	
2. Dextran	
3. Iron-dextran	
C. Haptenes	
1. Antibiotics	Penicillin; tetracycline; demethylchlortetracycline; chlortetracycline; nitrofurantoin; streptomycin
2. Vitamins	Thiamine; folic acid
D. Exercise-induced reaction	
II. Complement mediated (transfusion reaction with IgA deficiency)	
III. Arachidonate mediated (aspirin)	
IV. Direct mast cell releasing agents (RCM)	
V. Idiopathic	

clinical patterns may proceed rapidly to fatal respiratory failure. Similarly, the third syndrome results from severe hypotension, presenting a sudden loss of consciousness or lightheadedness with fatalities resulting from persistent vascular collapse. Any of these three syndromes—cutaneous, respiratory, or vascular—may be associated with nausea, vomiting, gastrointestinal colic, and/or bloody diarrhea.

TREATMENT

Systemic Reaction Management

Mild wheezing, pruritus, and transient urticaria can usually be managed as described for the *local reaction*. However, the explosive nature of the anaphylactic reaction requires close attention to the maintenance of oxygenation or normotension.

SPECIFIC THERAPY: IMPAIRED ABSORPTION OF ANTIGEN

1. Epinephrine hydrochloride (Adrenalin) 1:1,000, 0.3 ml (300 μg) injected into the injection site.
2. Tourniquet applied proximal to the injection site.
3. In the event of a hymenoptera sting, flick, do not squeeze, the stinger (bee) from the site.

ENHANCED OXYGENATION

1. Epinephrine hydrochloride 1:1,000, 0.5 ml (500 μg) subcutaneously, administered into a nonoccluded extremity.
2. Oxygen by controlled flow.
3. Intermittent positive pressure breathing (IPPB) with isoproterenol 1:200 (Isuprel), 0.5 ml, and saline, 1.5 ml.
4. Aminophylline, 500 mg diluted into 250 ml 5% dextrose and water, administered intravenously over 1 hour.
5. Endotracheal intubation with assisted respiration if effective oxygenation cannot be established in 1–3 minutes in obstruction caused by bronchospasm or upper respiratory obstruction (laryngeal edema).

HYPOTENSION

1. Hydrocortisone sodium succinate, 100 mg administered as an intravenous push and 100 mg added to an intravenous infusion of 250 ml of 5% dextrose in saline. Higher doses may be required.

2. Levarterenol bitartrate (Levophed)—add 4 ml of 0.2% solution to 1,000 ml of 5% dextrose solution. Each milliliter of the dilution contains 4 μg of base administered intravenously in a plastic catheter; adjust the rate to 2 ml/min to maintain a low-normal blood pressure.
3. Dopamine hydrochloride.

Late Reactions (15–60 minutes)

The longer the period (latent) between administration of antigen and onset of symptoms, the less severe are the sequelae. Often these reactions may occur after the patient has left the physician's office. Such patients should be encouraged to return for specific therapy, including epinephrine hydrochloride, 1:1,000, 0.2–0.5 ml injected subcutaneously. However, administration of diphenhydramine (Benadryl), 50 mg orally, and anhydrous theophylline, and/or ephedrine, or similar-acting drugs (i.e., beta agonist) may be all that is warranted.

Aqueous epinephrine hydrochloride is the most valuable drug in the treatment of anaphylaxis. It is seldom necessary to administer it intravenously. Patients prone to such a phenomenon should be advised to carry the medication with them at all times for treating even the slightest reaction.*

Prophylaxis: Normal Recipients

The successful management of anaphylaxis requires anticipation of an adverse reaction whenever a therapeutic program is instituted. Minimization of an anaphylactic reaction can often be accomplished by considering the sensitivity of the recipient and the dose and rate of absorption, as well as the antigenicity of the drug. All patients must be questioned regarding previous drug reactions with specific reference to the drug or test dose to be administered.

A negative history is never a guarantee of a nonreactivity to any former pharmacologic agent. The most insignificant prior reaction must be given careful consideration before that drug or any chemically related medicament is administered. Any history of an adverse drug reaction requires substitution with a chemically unrelated compound for the allergen. Corroboration of a significant drug reaction history by direct skin testing may produce fatal reaction. It is seldom feasible to predict drug hypersensitivity by serologic or skin testing. For this reason, such procedures should be discouraged as routine techniques.

---

*Epi-Pen Center Laboratories, Port Washington, NY or ANA-Kit, Hollister-Stier, Spokane, WA.

Recipients of heterologous serum should always be tested before treatment. Before routine administration of horse serum (recipients without a history of hypersensitivity to the substance), intracutaneous testing with 0.20 ml of a 1:10 dilution of the serum should be negative. If there is a history of previous reaction to horse serum, the intracutaneous test should be preceded by a scratch test of serum diluted 1:1,000 and then a scratch test of undiluted serum before the intradermal testing using the 1:10 dilution. If the history of skin reaction is indicative of reactivity, human tetanus immune globulin should be used to confer passive immunization.

Intravenously infused dye should be administered cautiously. Skin test reactions with radiopaque iodinated contrast agents have correlated poorly with clinical experience. The reactions that do occur may not be immunologically determined or may be cytotoxic reactions. However, routine intravenous administration of a test dose is mandatory in all instances to prevent untoward reactions. Prophylactic administration of prednisone 50 mg every 6 hours for three doses, ending 1 hour before RCM study, and diphenhydramine 50 mg intramusculary, 1 hour before direct mast cell releasing agent (RCM) study has been helpful in preventing adverse reactions to RCM.

People susceptible to anaphylaxis but not capable of being immunologically protected should be identified.* Stinging insect first aid treatment kits containing essential ingredients requisite for anaphylactic first aid should be prescribed to affected people, as well as to those with food and idiopathic anaphylaxis.

Stinging Insect (Hymenoptera) Anaphylaxis

Significant systemic anaphylaxis occasioned by stinging insects of the order Hymenoptera (bees, wasps, hornets, yellow jackets, and fire ants) requires prophylactic injection therapy. It is possible to immunize people who would otherwise be susceptible to fatal systemic anaphylaxis from insect stings by frequent prolonged injections with gradual increments of stinging insect venom extracts. The use of venom sac contents has been of protective value. Protection from fatal anaphylactic reactions is thought to be afforded from the production of blocking (IgG) antibodies and/or reduction in venom-specific IgE, the release of chemical mediators at a concentration too low to cause systemic manifestations and therefore inducing mediator depletion so significant that no systemic reaction occurs when rechallenge occurs, the induction via T lymphocytes

*Medic Alert Foundation, Turlock, CA 95380.

(suppressor), or other mechanisms that may contribute to this induction of tolerance.

"Desensitization" has been used also to effect a tolerant state to a drug required by a sensitized recipient. If such an agent is to be used in spite of a history of anaphylaxis, a positive skin test, or both the risk of fatal anaphylaxis must outweigh treating the patient without the appropriate material. The initiation of such therapy is best accomplished in an area of a hospital equipped to treat anaphylaxis and the attendant manifestations of hypotension and respiratory obstruction. An intravenous infusion must first be established to facilitate the administration of drugs in case of vascular collapse. Equipment and personnel talented in administration of endotracheal intubation and assisted respiration must be available. Scratch and intradermal tests are performed on the flexor surface of the forearm at the least concentration eliciting a slight, less than 5 mm, or no local reaction. In the event of an excessive local reaction or associated systemic manifestations, a tourniquet can be applied proximal to the reaction site and epinephrine injected locally into the site and into the other extremity to prevent systemic manifestations. The material should be gradually increased in concentration by scratch testing. At each top concentration the material should be injected, using one dilution less intracutaneously, repeating the same dosage if no significant reaction occurs subcutaneously, and finally injected intramuscularly in increasing doses so that the initial dose of any route does not exceed the final dose for the previous route. Thirty minutes should be allowed between injections to permit maximum absorption of antigen without accumulation. The aim of such a procedure is to produce a desensitized state similar to that seen in patients experiencing severe anaphylactic reactions. This "desensitized state" is not permanent and must be maintained by the continued multiple-dose antigen administration. When interrupted the patient is presumably sensitive and may experience a severe anaphylactic reaction if rechallenged with the antigen. Fatal anaphylactic reactions have ensued after institution as well as in the midst of apparently successful desensitization programs. This is not a recommended procedure and as mentioned above is considered only when the patient's status dictates the use of a drug to which he or she has been allergic.

ATOPIC RECIPIENTS

Inquiry as to a personal or family occurrence of atopy (hay fever, asthma, or eczema) is imperative. People so afflicted are thought to experience serious drug reactions more frequently than usual. Horse serum or egg vaccine products, penicillin, Hymenoptera stings, and aspirin are less well tolerated by the atopic patient. Treatment and testing of the allergic patient is a common cause of anaphylaxis and is more readily managed if administered in the upper arm. Patients receiving allergy extract injection therapy should be observed for a period of not less than 15 minutes following administration of therapy for evidence of local systemic manifestations. A local reaction greater than 2 cm requires that the patient be detained with appropriate treatment and observation until improvement is evident. Any systemic manifestation should be treated as outlined subsequently.

PRIOR REACTORS

For those people who have experienced well-documented or even suspected mild reaction, substitution therapy is imperative. This includes the use of propoxyphene hydrochloride or acetaminophen for acetylsalicylic acid, lidocaine (Xylocaine) for procaine, and human tetanus immune globulin instead of the heterologous antiserum, the use of which may produce a fatal reaction. Those patients with well-defined reactions to specific medications require no further corroboration. Appropriate facilities for treating an anaphylactic reaction must be readily accessible when skin testing is performed. These include parenterally administerable drugs, epinephrine hydrochloride, aminophylline, diphenhydramine, levarterenol, hydrocortisone sodium succinate, and isotonic saline solution, as well as facilities for endotracheal intubation or tracheostomy. The presence of intravenous infusion established in the vein of the nontested extremity is required. This intravenous infusion is maintained until the appropriate drug has been administered without reactivity for 30 minutes. Initially low-antigen concentration scratch tests are applied with intradermal testing of the highest nonreactive scratch test solution. Negative skin tests cannot be relied upon with security.

The reaction of the penicillin metabolites is a complex phenomenon, now well correlated with various clinical states and metabolic products. The acute anaphylactic symptoms result more often from a minor metabolic product of the parent compounds. The major metabolite is associated with the accelerated anaphylactic symptoms or late reaction. Aged benzyl penicillin skin tests are of predictive value to establish a reactivity to the acute explosive reaction, whereas penicilloyl poly-L-lysine antigen is of predictive value in assessing the accelerated reactions.

Local Reaction Management

The well-defined local reaction occurring at the site of parenterally administered drugs requires specific therapy for preventing discomfort and systemic manifestations. Local reactivity is invariably indicative of subsequent systemic sensitization. Therefore, therapy with the specific or crossreacting drugs should be avoided.

Specific therapy includes the following:

1. Apply a tourniquet proximal to the site of the reaction if an extremity is involved, with relaxation of the occlusion 1 minute every 3 minutes.
2. Epinephrine hydrochloride 1:1,000, 0.2 ml administered subcutaneously into the reaction site.
3. Epinephrine hydrochloride 1:1,000, 0.3 ml administered subcutaneously into the nonoccluded extremity.
4. Diphenhydramine hydrochloride, 50 mg by mouth or intramuscularly depending upon the severity of the local reaction.
5. Theophylline, ephedrine, or beta-2-agonist tablet.
6. Observe the patient until the reaction begins to subside (usually 30–60 minutes).

PROGNOSIS

The prognosis is contingent upon the route of administration, sensitivity of the recipient, duration of the latent period of antigen administration and onset of symptoms, early recognition of adverse reaction, and accessibility of medical management. Patients have succumbed in spite of optimal therapy availability, possibly a result of delay in institution of full therapeutic maneuvers. Once recovery has occurred, prognosis is contingent upon the patient's ability to avoid further administration of the responsible antigen.

SUGGESTED READINGS

Austen KF, Sheffer AL: Vascular responses, the anaphylactic syndrome, in Fitzpatrick TB, Arndt KA, Clark WH, Eisen AZ, VanScott EJ, Vaughn JH (eds): *Dermatology in Internal Medicine.* New York, McGraw-Hill Book Co, 1971, pp 1244–1261.

Hunt KS, Valentine MD, Sobotka AK, Benton AW, Anodio, FJ, Lichtenstein LM: A control trial of immunotherapy in insect hypersensitivity. *N Engl J Med* 1978; 299:157–161.

James LP Jr, Austen KF: Fatal systemic anaphylaxis in man. *N Engl J Med* 1964; 270:597.

Levine BB: Immunologic mechanisms of penicillin allergy. *N Engl J Med* 1966; 275:1115.

Orange RP, Donsky GJ: Anaphylaxis, in Middleton E Jr, Reed CE, Ellis EF (eds): *Allergy Principles and Practice.* Saint Louis, CV Mosby Co, 1978, vol 2, pp 563–573.

Sheffer AL, Austen KF: Exercise induced anaphylaxis. *J Allergy Clin Immunol* 1980; 66:106–111.

Sheffer AL, Wasserman SI: Anaphylaxis in rheumatology and immunology, in Cohen AS (ed): *Science and Practice of Clinical Medicine.* New York, Grune & Stratton Inc, 1978, vol 4, pp 468–470.

Stechschulte DJ, Austen KF. Anaphylaxis, in Zweifach BW, Grant L, McCloskey, RT (eds): *The Inflammatory Process,* ed 2. New York, Academic Press Inc, 1974, vol 3, pp 237–276.

8
HYPERTENSION

Harold S. Solomon
Norman K. Hollenberg

Hypertension, which ranges from a slight to an extreme elevation of blood pressure, is so common that an estimated 30% of visits to practitioners of adult medicine are for its treatment. Hypertensive emergencies, however, are rare; they occur in fewer than 1% of patients with high blood pressure. Although all hypertensive conditions require or benefit from treatment, two groups—*emergent* and *urgent*—must be distinguished because they are more effectively and more safely treated by different methods.

Truly emergent episodes of high blood pressure must be treated within minutes to prevent severe hemorrhagic or neurologic complications. Failure to act can result in rapid clinical deterioration and even death. Less immediately life threatening, but still serious, are urgent conditions for which treatment may be delayed without undue risk for a few hours or days. The distinction between these two classes of hypertension is important because rapidly acting antihypertensive drugs incur risk that must be weighed against potential benefit to the patient. In general, an emergent condition improves dramatically as the patient's blood pressure is reduced. An urgent condition, on the other hand, requires prompt attention, but its course is less threatening and somewhat less affected by a rapid lowering of blood pressure with parenteral medications. Tables 8.1 and 8.2 list emergent and urgent manifestations of hypertension.

The absolute level of blood pressure is only one indication of a hypertensive emergency and must always be interpreted in conjunction with other physical signs of accelerated disease and with the relevant history. Evidence of encephalopathy, a history of high blood pressure, signs and symptoms of cardiovascular complications, eclampsia, or the simultaneous ingestion of tyramine and monoamine oxidase (MAO) inhibitors coupled with an extreme elevation of blood pressure signal the need for immediate treatment.

Urgent conditions include those arising as hypertension progresses and damages small arteries and arterioles. Hemorrhages and infarctions in the eyes, kidneys, heart, or nervous system necessitate lowering the patient's blood pressure. Hospitalization with bed rest, observation, and oral rather than parenteral therapy are usually indicated. Postoperative patients who develop severe hypertension with bleeding, and new patients, even if asymptomatic, whose diastolic blood pressure is above 130 mm Hg are also in need of urgent but not instant treatment.

INITIAL ASSESSMENT

Time is of the essence in hypertensive emergencies. Hence, eliciting a complete medical history should be waived in favor of obtaining a brief relevant history, including information about the current illness, medications the patient is taking, and prior adverse drug reactions. The goal is to identify the secondary cause of the hypertension. Except in rare cases, the patient's blood pressure should be lowered rapidly, but therapy depends to a large extent on the underlying condition. Table 8.3 outlines a suggested course of action.

An intravenous catheter should be inserted and an electrocardiogram (ECG) should be obtained while the history is being taken and the patient is being examined. Blood should be drawn immediately for laboratory studies—a complete blood count (CBC) and measurement of blood urea nitrogen (BUN) and serum creatinine, electrolytes, and glucose. A urine specimen should also be sent to the laboratory for analysis and culture. Therapy should not, however, be deferred until the results of any of these tests are known. Likewise, a posteroanterior x-ray film of the chest should be made but not at the expense of delaying therapy.

The patient's mental status and evidence of any neurologic changes are of paramount importance. Unfortunately, distinguishing immediately among hemorrhagic stroke, occlusive stroke, transient cerebral ischemia, eclampsia, and hypertensive encephalopathy is not always possible; yet therapy depends to some extent on the differential diagnosis. Lowering blood pressure too rapidly, for example, may exacerbate the symptoms of an occlusive stroke or a transient ischemic attack. A cardiovascular catastrophe is always a possible cause of severe hypertension if the patient complains of chest or back pain. Myocardial infarction or ischemia and dissecting aneurysm are the most important diagnoses to consider in the short term. Dissecting aneurysms, which are discussed in Chapter 4, are exceedingly variable in their manner of presentation.

Therapy must often be determined from data gathered rapidly, and sometimes incompletely, at the bedside. Though incomplete, such information is sufficient to guide the initial therapy for most patients, and a more extensive evaluation can usually be safely postponed until a patient's condition has been stabilized. Unless a cause of the hypertensive emergency (for example, eclampsia or ingestion of both tyramine and MAO inhibitors) is uncovered, however, a thorough evaluation of

TABLE 8.1 Hypertensive Emergencies

Malignant hypertension with or without encephalopathy
Acute complications of accelerated hypertension
    Pulmonary edema
    Cerebrovascular accident with hemorrhage or infarction
    Aortic dissection
Hypertension with special causes
    Eclampsia
    Tyramine toxicity
    Pheochromocytoma

TABLE 8.2 Urgent Conditions Associated with Hypertension

Evidence of hemorrhage and exudates in eyegrounds
Myocardial infarction or severe angina
Occlusive stroke or transient ischemic attack
Renal failure or significant renal impairment
Burns, acute glomerulonephritis, or preeclampsia
Postoperative bleeding
New cardiovascular or neurologic symptoms in a previously
hypertensive patient
Newly developed hypertension (diastolic blood pressure greater than
130 mm Hg)

TABLE 8.3 Sequence of Clinical Events in Hypertensive Emergencies

Brief history emphasizing cardiovascular and neurologic systems
and prior medications
Physical examination
Access to circulation
Electrocardiogram (ECG)
Determination of baseline CBC, BUN, creatinine, electrolytes,
glucose levels; urinalysis and urine culture
Parenteral therapy instituted with appropriate agent based on initial
clinical evaluation
Chest film (posteroanterior, not portable anteroposterior)
Admission to intensive or coronary care unit
Reassessment and modification of therapy based on initial
laboratory studies and clinical response; longer-acting agents or oral
therapy begun
Further diagnostic evaluation considered

the patient is mandatory so that the secondary cause of hypertension can be ascertained.

TREATMENT

General Considerations

Parenteral therapy should begin as soon as the physician has enough data to select an antihypertensive agent. The choice of medication depends on several factors, including the clinical setting in which the hypertension presents, the persistence and hemodynamic effects of the drugs available, and the availability of reliable monitoring and an experienced nursing staff. In general, a patient for whom the diagnosis cannot be established at bedside is more safely treated with a drug whose effects dissipate rapidly. If the agent worsens the patient's condition, the therapeutic strategy can then be rapidly altered. Agents such as reserpine and methyldopa, which may alter the level of consciousness, should be avoided. Patients hospitalized in facilities where they cannot be monitored minute by minute should be treated with agents such as diazoxide, intravenous methyldopa, intramuscular reserpine, or hydralazine, whose effects are more prolonged and do not require the constant attention that the more rapidly acting agents (nitroprusside, trimethaphan) do. Although parenteral therapy is mandatory for initial treatment of hypertensive emergencies, oral agents should be substituted as soon as possible.

Parenteral antihypertensives, listed in Table 8.4, are basically of two types: vasodilators and agents that act by interrupting the sympathetic nervous system at some level. All of them reduce either cardiac output or peripheral vascular resistance; some decrease both. These distinctions, which are discussed later in this chapter, are important. The dilators reduce peripheral resistance by dilating peripheral arterioles; they increase heart rate as well. Because nitroprusside acts both as a vasodilator and as a venodilator, it also reduces venous return; cardiac output therefore usually decreases. Diazoxide and hydralazine, which do not reduce venous return, cause increases in cardiac output. Of the agents acting on the sympathetic nervous system, trimethaphan, reserpine, and methyldopa decrease both peripheral resistance and cardiac output; phentolamine reduces peripheral resistance, and propranolol reduces cardiac output.

The most rapidly acting agents with broad application are nitroprusside, trimethaphan, and diazoxide. Hydralazine's onset of action is intermediate; reserpine and methyldopa are somewhat slower. Phentolamine, propranolol, and perhaps the

TABLE 8.4 Hemodynamic Effects of Parenteral Antihypertensives

Agent[a]	Mechanism of Action	Cardiac Output	Peripheral Resistance	Venous Return
Vasodilators				
Nitroprusside (Nipride)	Dilation of arteriolar (resistance) and venous (capacitance) beds	Decreased or unchanged	Decreased	Decreased
Diazoxide (Hyperstat)	Dilation of arteriolar bed only	Increased	Decreased	Increased
Hydralazine (Apresoline)	Dilation of arteriolar bed only	Increased	Decreased	Increased
Agents acting on sympathetic nervous system				
Trimethaphan (Arfonad)	Autonomic ganglionic blockage and direct arteriolar dilatation	Decreased	Decreased	Decreased
Reserpine	Central and peripheral catecholamine depletion	Decreased or unchanged	Decreased	Decreased
Methyldopa (Aldomet)	? Central depression ? False transmission Direct vasodilation	Decreased or unchanged	Decreased	Decreased
Phentolamine (Regitine)	Comparative α-adrenergic inhibition Direct vasodilation	Increased	Decreased	Increased
Propranolol (Inderal)	Comparative β-adrenergic inhibition	Decreased	Increased	Decreased

[a]The drugs of each type are listed in order of decreasing rapidity of action.

new angiotensin antagonists have specific effects that limit their usefulness. Table 8.5 summarizes the route of administration, the usual adult dosage, and the approximate onset and duration of action of the parenteral medications.

Specific Medications

VASODILATORS

Sodium Nitroprusside

Sodium nitroprusside (Nipride), known as a parenteral antihypertensive agent since 1929, has gained widespread use since it became commercially available. Because it is consistently effective and because it combines several useful actions, the drug's popularity is warranted. Nitroprusside is particularly efficacious for treating hypertension complicated by

left ventricular failure. By increasing venous capacitance, it permits blood to pool in the extremities; as a result, vascular resistance, cardiac output, and, therefore, blood pressure decrease. Nitroprusside is also effective for treating hypertensive encephalopathy or stroke because it does not affect the sensorium. It has an immediate onset of action and its effect dissipates very rapidly when the infusion is discontinued. As advantageous as these characteristics are, they are also responsible for the drug's major drawback—the necessity for constant supervision.

Prolonged administration of nitroprusside may result in thiocyanate toxicity, which is manifested by mental confusion and psychosis. In one study, however, continuous use for a mean period of 6 days produced no marked toxic reactions. Nevertheless, if nitroprusside is administered for longer than 72 hours, the patient's serum thiocyanate level should be mea-

TABLE 8.5 Parenteral Antihypertensives

Agent	Route	Dose	Onset	Duration
Vasodilators				
Nitroprusside	IV continuously	20–400 µg/min	<1 min	minutes
Diazoxide	IV rapidly	75–300 mg (–5 mg/Kg)	1–3 min	4–18 hr
Hydralazine	IV or IM	5–20 mg	15 min	2–6 hr
Agents acting on sympathetic nervous system				
Trimethaphan	IV continuously	1–15 mg/min	<1 min	minutes
Reserpine	IM	0.5–5 mg	2–3 hr	4–8 hr
Methyldopa	IV	250–1,000 mg	1–3 hr	4–8 hr
Phentolamine	IV	5–15 mg	<1 min	¼–2 hr
Propranolol	IV slowly	1–5 mg	<1 min	1–2 hr

sured every other day and the dosage reduced if the level exceeds 12 ml/dl. Other side effects—nausea, vomiting, apprehension, sweating, and muscle twitching—may occur acutely but can usually be reversed quite readily by reducing the infusion rate.

Nitroprusside is available in vials containing 50 mg of powder. Sterile 5% dextrose in water (3 ml) should be instilled into the vial, then diluted in 500 ml of 5% dextrose in water to prepare a solution of 100 mg/ml. The usual adult dose averages 2 ml/min (200 µg/min). The dosage should be adjusted as necessary to achieve the desired reduction of blood pressure. Both the bottle containing the solution and the intravenous tubing should be wrapped in aluminum foil to prevent light from altering the nitroprusside; once prepared, the solution, to which no other drugs should be added, should not be kept or used for longer than 4 hours.

Diazoxide

Diazoxide (Hyperstat), a thiazide derivative that lowers blood pressure very rapidly, is effective for 4–12 hours. It acts directly by dilating resistance vessels, but because it does not affect capacitance vessels, its primary action does not interfere with reflex cardiac stimulation. Cardiac output and heart rate, therefore, increase as blood pressure decreases. And because blood pressure is lowered, cardiac work and myocardial oxygen consumption decrease, despite increased cardiac output.

Relatively safe and effective, diazoxide is the drug of choice for treating most uncomplicated malignant hypertension, and it is also widely used to treat eclampsia. (However, it may produce fetal hyperglycemia.) The reflex increase in cardiac output, an effect of both diazoxide and hydralazine, contraindicates administering these drugs to patients with dissecting thoracic aneurysms; altered shear forces at the site of dissection can cause the aneurysm to extend even though blood pressure has been lowered.

Diazoxide is available in ampules containing 300 mg in a 20-ml solution. The selected dose, usually 20 ml (300 mg), should be injected as rapidly as possible into a peripheral vein through a large-bore needle or catheter. The peak antihypertensive effect should occur within 30 seconds, but if a 5-ml (75-mg) dose produces no effect in 1 or 2 minutes, another 20 ml (300 mg) should be given immediately. The dose can be repeated as often as necessary, usually 3–10 hours later.

Hydralazine

Hydralazine (Apresoline) has hemodynamic effects much like diazoxide's; it dilates peripheral arterioles and increases cardiac output and heart rate. It can, however, precipitate or exacerbate angina pectoris in patients who present with coronary insufficiency unless it is administered with a drug (propranolol, reserpine, methyldopa) that interrupts the reflex cardiac stimulation.

Hydralazine has recently become popular for treating chronic congestive heart failure (CHF) because it reduces peripheral resistance, which is elevated in CHF, and thus allows cardiac output to increase. When administered to hypertensive patients, hydralazine has an effect that is immediate, peaks in 30–60 minutes, and persists for several hours. However, its long-term benefits and complications in treating CHF have yet to be evaluated fully.

Headache and tachycardia are common adverse reactions; coronary insufficiency is less frequent. Hydralazine, for the same reason as diazoxide, should not be given to a patient with a dissecting aneurysm.

Hydralazine is supplied in ampules of 20 mg in a 1-ml solution. An initial dose of 5 mg, given intramuscularly or intravenously, can be followed with additional doses of 5–20 mg as needed at 1–4-hour intervals.

SYMPATHETIC BLOCKERS

Trimethaphan

A ganglionic blocker, Trimethaphan (Arfonad) interrupts both sympathetic and parasympathetic functioning and also has a direct vasodilator action that is unrelated to ganglionic blockade. The drug, which dilates both capacitance and resistance vessels, reduces cardiac output. Like nitroprusside, it acts rapidly, its effects dissipate within a minute, and its administration requires constant supervision. Because it dilates capacitance vessels, trimethaphan has an orthostatic effect; elevating the head of a patient's bed therefore enhances the agent's antihypertensive effect. If trimethaphan is chosen as the initial therapeutic agent, longer-acting drugs should also be given as part of the early treatment regimen because tachyphylaxis to trimethaphan occurs after it has been used for 24 hours.

Because trimethaphan reduces cardiac output and consequently shear forces in the aorta, it is an agent of choice for the initial treatment of hypertension associated with dissecting aneurysms of the thoracic aorta. It is also useful for treating most other forms of hypertensive emergency; however, this drug may cause ileus, urinary retention, and blurred vision because of its parasympatholytic effect.

Trimethaphan is marketed in vials containing 500 mg in a 10-ml solution. One ampule added to 500 ml of 5% dextrose in water yields a concentration of 1 mg/ml. An intravenous infusion of 3–4 mg/min (50–60 drops/min) should be adjusted to achieve the desired blood pressure response.

Reserpine

Reserpine (Serpasil) depletes catecholamines in the central nervous system and in peripheral areas. Its effect begins 1–3 hours after administration, and hypotension occasionally complicates its use. Because the usual large parenteral doses commonly cause somnolence, reserpine should not be used to treat patients presenting with neurologic symptoms. Since diazoxide, nitroprusside, and methyldopa have become available, reserpine is used much less frequently than it was in the past.

Reserpine is supplied in ampules containing 5 mg in a 2-ml ampule. A test dose of 0.5 mg (0.2 ml) intramuscularly should be given intially and followed ½ hour later with 5 mg (2 ml) intramuscularly if the test dose is effective and tolerated. If the 5-mg dose produces no response within a few hours, larger doses will not be particularly effective; the drug should therefore be discontinued.

Methyldopa

Methyldopa (Aldomet) has proved to have an antihypertensive effect that is still poorly understood. The formation peripherally of α-methylnorepinephrine from α-methyldopa led to the belief that the effect was due to the formation of a "false neurochemical transmitter." But methyldopa also has a prominent central effect, and it remains unclear whether the drug's antihypertensive property results from central inhibition of sympathetic activity, from action as a peripheral false transmitter, or even from direct vasodilation. Changes in blood pressure vary greatly from patient to patient; some patients respond dramatically within 2 hours, whereas others do not respond at all. Methyldopa is now often chosen as an agent with moderate rate of onset and duration of action.

Methyldopa is particularly appropriate for patients with renal insufficiency. Its primary metabolic product, α-methylnorepinephrine, which normally would be cleared by the kidney, is itself an effective antihypertensive. The drug thus works well if renal clearance is diminished and seemingly has little adverse effect on renal functioning.

Methyldopa does cause somnolence but not nearly to the degree that an equivalent dose of reserpine does. Nevertheless, methyldopa is relatively undesirable for treating patients with neurologic symptoms.

Methyldopa comes in 5-ml vials containing 250 mg. The dose should be added to 100 ml of 5% of dextrose in water and administered in an intravenous drip over a 30-minute period. The usual dose for adults is 250 mg, but up to 3 g may be administered at one time if necessary to reduce blood pressure to the desired level. If there is no effect on blood pressure 2 hours after an initial 250-mg dose, 500–750 mg should be given. The maintenance dose can be repeated every 6 hours.

Phentolamine

Phentolamine (Regitine), a competitive antagonist of norepinephrine, has very limited usefulness; in fact, it is effective only if a patient has pheochromocytoma or hypertension induced by the simultaneous ingestion of tyramine and MAO inhibitors. Some physicians have recommended that a 5-mg test dose of phentolamine be given before any other antihypertensive therapy is instituted, and if the patient's diastolic pressure falls more than 25 mm Hg, the presumptive diagnosis of pheochromocytoma is made. Phentolamine should be given in the operating room if pheochromocytoma is unexpectedly found during surgery and is associated with acute severe hypertension.

Phentolamine is supplied in vials containing 5 mg of powder, and each is accompanied with an ampule of 1 ml of sterile water. The 5 mg of the drug should be diluted in the 1 ml of sterile water to prepare a 5 mg/ml solution, which should be administered intravenously as a bolus. A dose of 5 mg usually effectively reduces blood pressure in 5–10 minutes, but up to 15 mg (3 ml) may be given. The dose may be repeated as often as necessary.

Propranolol

Propranolol (Inderal) is a competitive, β-adrenergic inhibitor that has little antihypertensive effect when given intravenously. Although intravenous propranolol decreases cardiac output, the effect is offset by a reflex increase in peripheral vascular resistance, which is mediated by α-adrenergic responses. Consequently, arterial pressure decreases only slightly.

Propranolol is effective, however, for patients with dissecting thoracic aneurysm, which requires that myocardial contractility be decreased. The drug also partially interrupts the reflex tachycardia produced by diazoxide, hydralazine, and nitroprusside. A patient with pheochromocytoma who is given an alpha blocker (phentolamine, dibenzyline) may also require propranolol to block the β-adrenergic effects of the catecholamine excess, especially if an arrhythmia occurs. Unless such a patient is first given adequate doses of alpha blockers, propranolol, because of its beta blockade, causes a dramatic increase in alpha activity and an increase in blood pressure.

Propranolol is supplied in 1-ml ampules containing 1 mg. The usual dose is 1 mg administered at a rate of 1 mg every 1–5 minutes by slow intravenous infusion. Careful monitoring of heart rate and blood pressure is mandatory. The dosage interval is determined by the heart rate response and can be as often as every 5 minutes. The total dosage should not exceed 0.1 mg/kg in a 4-hour period.

DIURETICS

Much has been written about the benefits of intravenously administering potent diuretics, such as furosemide or ethacrynic acid, to patients being treated with diazoxide. But all antihypertensive drugs, not just diazoxide, may cause sodium retention as a consequence of blood pressure reduction, a fact that the physician must keep in mind during any hypertensive emergency. Intravenous diuretics need not, however, be given the instant that the administration of antihypertensive drugs is begun; the physician can await the BUN and creatinine determination and the results of the urinalysis to select a diuretic and dosage.

Management of Excessive Hypotensive Effect

Occasionally a patient reacts to antihypertensive therapy with too great a reduction in blood pressure. If rapidly acting agents (trimethaphan, nitroprusside) have been used, the hypotension does not require any therapy other than discontinuing the antihypertensive agent. But because the effects of longer-acting drugs cannot be stopped quickly, plasma expanders may be necessary; indeed, they may be lifesaving.

The most common reason for hypotension is a slight, preexisting volume deficit that becomes apparent when an agent that inhibits the sympathetic activity is administered. If hypotension persists once adequate volume has been restored, pressors may be required. Norepinephrine (Levophed) rather than sympathomimetics (ephedrine, mephentermine, amphetamine derivatives) should then be used because the sympathomimetics may be ineffective if a patient has been treated with catecholamine-depleting agents (reserpine, guanethidine).

CLINICAL SETTINGS

Probably the most important factor for the physician to consider when deciding which drug to use is the clinical setting in which the hypertensive emergency presents. Table 8.6 summarizes the relative usefulness of drugs for various conditions. Although guidelines can be given, no hard and fast rules can be made; each patient must be evaluated and treated individually.

Malignant Hypertension

DIAGNOSIS AND PROGNOSIS

The most common hypertensive emergency is the syndrome of malignant hypertension. Blood pressure is dramatically elevated; evidence of papilledema, hemorrhages, and exudates appear in the patient's retinas; and spastic arteriolar changes can be observed. The condition may present alone or it may coexist with other clinical problems. An increasing number of patients with mild or moderate hypertension are being adequately treated, and consequently the de novo appearance of

TABLE 8.6 Selection of Parenteral Antihypertensive Agents

Agent	Setting							
	Acute Pulmonary Edema	Encephalopathy	Dissecting Aneurysm; Other Chest Pain	CVA Thrombosis and Hemorrhage	Malignant Hypertension Including Renal Causes	Pheochromocytoma	MAO Inhibitors and Tryamine	Toxemia or Eclampsia
Vasodilators								
Nitroprusside	1	2	3	1	2	2	2	?
Diazoxide	2	1	X	2	1	2	2	1
Hydralazine	3	3	X	2	3	3	3	2
Agents acting on sympathetic nervous system								
Trimethaphan	2	2	1	1	1	2	2	X
Reserpine	3	X	2	3	3	3	3	X
Methyldopa	3	X	2	3	3	3	3	3
Phentolamine	0	0	0	0	0	1	1	0
Propranolol	0	0	2	0	0	2	2	0

X, usually contraindicated; 0, not useful; 1, usual first choice in acute setting; 2, frequently useful in acute setting; 3, occasionally useful in acute setting, frequently useful for long-term therapy; ?, unknown usefulness.

malignant hypertension as an outgrowth of progressive, untreated essential hypertension seems to be decreasing. Today malignant hypertension occurs more often as a complication of another disease, such as renal failure or renal artery stenosis. The appearance of malignant hypertension in patients over the age of 60 years who have never been known to be hypertensive before is almost invariably a result of atherosclerotic renal artery disease in either or both renal arteries.

Antihypertensive drugs have greatly improved the survival rate of patients with malignant hypertension. Most studies conducted before the agents were available reported a 95% 1-year mortality rate if the condition were untreated. Vigorous therapy can now achieve a 50% 5-year survival rate. Cautious optimism is nevertheless the wisest attitude for a physician to adopt when discussing prognosis with a patient and family.

THERAPY

If a patient with malignant hypertension presents with failing vision, left ventricular failure, or headache or any other neurologic symptom, parenteral treatment is mandatory. Although bed rest and oral therapy are at times permissible for patients who do not demonstrate these symptoms, treatment usually begins with parenteral agents. Diazoxide is usually the agent of choice, but trimethaphan, nitroprusside, intramuscular reserpine, or intravenous methyldopa may be used; the selection of the drug ultimately depends on the desired rate of blood pressure reduction.

Because malignant hypertension is so often a complication of progressive renal disease, the patient's renal functioning must also be considered before a therapeutic decision is made. Severe renal insufficiency may require early dialysis to relieve fluid overload or the signs and symptoms of uremia. Many patients with mild or moderate renal insufficiency, on the other hand, experience a temporary worsening of renal function after blood pressure is reduced, but the condition usually improves. Acute renal failure, frequently with oliguria, may accompany malignant hypertension. Occasionally a patient with refractory malignant hypertension appears to be near death even though all the usual therapeutic measures have been employed. Bilateral nephrectomy and hemodialysis may be considered, but these procedures are extreme and the risks must be carefully weighed when deciding whether a bilateral nephrectomy should be performed because recovery of renal function may occur as long as 6 months after dialysis is initiated. Minoxidil, a drug that often has intolerable long-term side effects, has been effective for treating patients with severe hypertension and end-stage renal disease when other therapies have been ineffective.

A few patients require surprisingly small doses of antihypertensive medications after the initial malignant phase is treated, but careful out-patient follow-up is obviously mandatory. Because malignant hypertension can complicate every known form of high blood pressure, a complete diagnostic evaluation should be performed as soon as feasible.

Acute Pulmonary Edema

DIAGNOSIS

Hypertensive patients who develop acute pulmonary edema often improve greatly if arterial blood pressure and thus the afterload on the heart are reduced. Decreasing systemic vascular resistance, which is elevated in all but a few patients with hypertension and CHF, results in an increase in cardiac output and a decrease in cardiac work. The two agents of choice in this setting are nitroprusside and trimethaphan. They decrease peripheral vascular resistance and affect the capacitance vessels in such a way that venous return decreases. The myocardium consequently works against less resistance, and the reduction of venous return reverses the pulmonary edema.

The cause of acute pulmonary edema in the presence of hypertension is extremely important, for if the patient has suffered an acute myocardial infarction or has a history of coronary artery disease, special caution is required when dilators are used to reduce blood pressure. Although nitroprusside has been reported to be beneficial in treating acute myocardial infarction and cardiogenic shock, too rapid or too great a reduction of pressure with vasodilators may reduce coronary artery perfusion and increase myocardial ischemia.

THERAPY

Opiates, intravenous diuretics, oxygen, and rotating tourniquets are all effective for treating congestive heart failure while blood pressure is being reduced with dilators. Digitalis should be administered to any patient for whom it has not been previously prescribed, but its effect may be minimal if blood pressure is extremely high.

Some physicians would include diazoxide as an agent of choice for treating hypertension associated with pulmonary edema. However, because coronary insufficiency may underlie the condition and because the unpredictable lowering of pressure with diazoxide may result in adverse consequence, we elect to use nitroprusside first and trimethaphan only if nitroprusside is ineffective.

Hypertensive Encephalopathy

Hypertensive encephalopathy, the most serious complication of accelerated hypertension, mandates the immediate lowering of blood pressure. Although blood pressure is virtually always greater than 250/130 mm Hg, papilledema is not always present. On the other hand, some physicians have reported that hypertensive encephalopathy may develop at even lower blood pressure levels in patients with acute glomerulonephritis or eclampsia.

DIAGNOSIS

Acute, though generally reversible, neurologic signs and symptoms may result from severe hypertension. Headache, photophobia, somnolence, vomiting, visual impairment, and other transient focal neurologic disturbances (e.g., seizures) are among the manifestations of this type of encephalopathy. Because visual disturbances are the most frequent presenting symptom, it is not surprising that an ophthalmologist or an optometrist is often the first to make the diagnosis.

Hypertensive encephalopathy must be differentiated from other syndromes of hypertension and neurologic dysfunction, including cerebral hemorrhage, occlusive stroke, rapidly growing brain tumors, pseudotumor cerebri, cerebral torulosis, and acute lead encephalopathy. Improvement of neurologic abnormalities when a patient's blood pressure is lowered is the hallmark of hypertensive encephalopathy. Spinal fluid proteins are elevated, and the spinal fluid is often mildly xanthochromic; superficial hemorrhages, multiple small thrombi, edema, and necrotizing arteritis in the brain are seen during autopsy of a patient who has died from this condition.

THERAPY

Diazoxide is the drug of first choice if the diagnosis of hypertensive encephalopathy is certain. If another neurologic diagnosis (such as stroke) that could be worsened by lowering the patient's blood pressure is a possibility, one of the more rapidly dissipating agents, nitroprusside or trimethaphan, should be used. These two drugs are preferable if the diagnosis has not been established beyond doubt because their effects are short-lived and thus can be controlled by discontinuing or reducing the dosage if the patient's neurologic status deteriorates as blood pressure decreases. The effects of diazoxide, on the other hand, persist for 4–12 hours and cannot be easily counteracted. Neither reserpine, which induces obtundation and may lower the patient's seizure threshold, nor methyldopa,

which causes drowsiness and thus may obscure neurologic findings, should be given.

While efforts are made to lower blood pressure, precautions should be taken to prevent seizures and to control them and protect the patient if they do occur. Patients at risk for seizures should be restrained in the lateral recumbent, not the supine, position; side rails of the bed should be padded, suction should be available, and intravenous diazepam (Valium) should be at the bedside.

Cerebral Vascular Accident

The differential diagnosis to be considered is the same as that for hypertensive encephalopathy. If hemorrhage is suspected, a neurologist should be consulted and surgery considered. If cerebral thrombosis is likely, blood pressure should cautiously be reduced to the lowest level possible without precipitating or aggravating neurologic symptoms. The agent of choice in this setting is trimethaphan or nitroprusside, again because the effect of each dissipates rapidly.

Dissecting Aortic Aneurysm

DIAGNOSIS

Any patient who presents with acute chest pain, back pain, or midline abdominal pain and with hypertension may be suffering a dissection of thoracic aorta; care must therefore be taken to establish or exclude the diagnosis (see Chapter 4). Dissection should be considered if chest pain is atypical for coronary pain, is absolutely midline, radiates to the back or abdomen, or is described as "tearing" or "burning." The ECG of a patient with chest pain and dissection may demonstrate left ventricular hypertrophy (LVH) without myocardial infarction or ischemia. A posterior anterior film of the chest usually reveals a widened mediastinum. Neurologic symptoms suggesting an occluded carotid or vertebral artery, especially if evidence of vascular obstruction elsewhere is also found, are another indication of dissection. In addition, if a murmur or aortic insufficiency is heard or if clinical signs of pericardial tamponade present, dissection is highly likely.

THERAPY

Today, antihypertensive drugs are generally the preferred mode of therapy for dissection during its acute phase because medical management results in a better survival rate than does surgical intervention. The goal of therapy is to lower both blood pressure and the rate at which the left ventricle generates pressure in order to lessen the shear forces at the site of dissection and prevent it from extending. Trimethaphan is the parenteral drug of choice; intramuscular reserpine, intravenous methyldopa, oral propranolol, or guanethidine may be given at the same time; and diuretics should be administered simultaneously. Because the renal arteries may be included in the area of dissection, urinary output must be carefully monitored. Only after the patient's condition has been stabilized and blood pressure lowered should angiography and surgery be considered.

Severe Preeclampsis or Eclampsia

DIAGNOSIS

The presence of hypertension, seizures, and proteinuria in the third trimester of pregnancy consititues a severe form of hypertension, eclampsia. It is important to remember that this syndrome can occur with blood pressure elevation that would be modest in a nonpregnant patient, from 150/100 upwards. Ultimately, interrupting the pregnancy reverses the syndrome. Secondary forms of hypertension such as pheochromocytoma, or renal artery stenosis, should be considered.

THERAPY

Reducing blood pressure and interrupting the pregnancy are mandatory for a pregnant patient with severe hypertension and seizures (eclampsia). Although magnesium sulfate, administered intramuscularly, has been popular with obstetricians for many years, diazoxide has been used with increasing frequency as its effectiveness has become apparent. Diazoxide can cause hyperglycemia in the fetus, but this condition does not seem to pose clinical problems. Trimethaphan should not be used because ganglionic blockade results in fetal ileus and stops labor; reserpine should also be avoided because it increases the likelihood of seizures.

Pheochromocytoma

DIAGNOSIS

Patients with pheochromocytoma, a rare cause of hypertensive crisis, may present with characteristic episodic symptoms referable to the sympathetic nervous system (sweating, syncope, headaches, palpitation) or they may present with relatively sustained or episodic hypertension. Any patient with severe hypertension may therefore have a pheochromocytoma, but the diagnosis is more likely if the patient has a history of hyperparathyroidism, medullary carcinoma of the thyroid, or pheochromocytoma. Evidence of neurofibromatosis or the other phakomatoses also suggests that the hypertension is due to pheochromocytoma.

THERAPY

In the past the administration of 5 mg of phentolamine intravenously before any other drug was given was recommended as a diagnostic test. Pheochromocytoma could be confirmed if the patient's systolic blood pressure fell more than 35 mm Hg or diastolic more than 25 mm Hg. (Such changes suggest a catecholamine excess.) This procedure was necessary because the antihypertensive agents made it impossible to determine levels of catecholamine metabolites in the urine accurately and thus made pheochromocytoma difficult to diagnose if treatment had already been initiated. However, more recently developed laboratory methods allow catecholamines, metanephrines, and vanillylmandelic acid (VMA) to be measured after most drugs have been administered, and the precaution is no longer essential.

A patient with a pheochromocytoma responds to antihypertensive drugs as other hypertensive patients do, and nitroprusside, trimethaphan, or diazoxide can confer benefits. These agents may produce tachycardia and signs of a β-adrenergic excess, conditions that necessitate the addition of propranolol to the therapeutic regimen. Propranolol, however, is contraindicated as a first agent because it can exacerbate α-adrenergic reflex effects (hypertension) in a patient with pheochromocytoma and actually cause an increase in pressure.

Tyramine Ingestion by Patients on Monoamine Oxidase Inhibitors

Hypertensive crises may occur in patients who are taking MAO inhibitors, such as pargyline (Eutonyl), tranylcypromine (Parnate), isocarboxazid (Marplan), and phenelzine (Nardil), though use of these drugs is becoming increasingly rare. A dramatic outpouring of catecholamines is triggered by the ingestion of sympathomimetic agents such as ephidrine, amphetamines, tyramine, phenylephrine, and foods and beverages containing tyramine (e.g., Chianti wine, certain beers, unpasteurized cheeses, pickled herring). The treatment of hypertension in this setting is the same as for pheochromocytoma.

SUGGESTED READINGS

Dissecting Aortic Aneurysm

DeBakey ME, Henly WS, Cooley DA, et al: Surgical management of dissecting aneurysms of the aorta. *J Thorac Cardiovasc Surg* 1965; 49:130.

Hirst AEN, Johns VJ Jr, Kime SW Jr: Dissecting aneurysm of the aorta: A review of 505 cases. *Medicine* 1958; 37:217

Wheat MW, Palmer RF, Bartley TD, Seelman RC: Treatment of dissecting aneurysms of the aorta without surgery. *J Thorac Cardiovasc Surg* 1965; 50:364.

Malignant Hypertension

Kincaid-Smith P, McMichael J, Murphy EA: The clinical course and pathology of hypertension with papilledema (malignant hypertension). *Q J Med* 1958; 27:117.

Sokolow M, Perloff D: Five-year survival of consecutive patients with malignant hypertension treated with antihypertensive agents. *Am J Cardiol* 1960; 9:858.

Wagener HP, Keith NM: Cases of marked hypertension, adequate renal function and neuroretinitis. *Arch Intern Med* 1924; 34:374.

Hypertensive Encephalopathy

Finnerty FA Jr: Hypertensive encephalopathy. *Am J Med* 1972; 52: 672.

Severe Hypertension with Renal Insufficiency

Lazarus JM, Hampers CL, Bennett AH, et al: Urgent bilateral nephrectomy for severe hypertension. *Ann Intern Med* 1972; 76:713.

Mroczek WJ: Malignant hypertension: Kidneys too good to be extirpated. *Ann Intern Med* 1974; 80:754.

Wilson C, Byron FB: Renal changes in malignant hypertension: Experimental evidence *Lancet* 1939; 1:136.

Wood JW, Blythe WB, et al: Management of malignant hypertension complicated by renal insufficiency. *N Engl J Med* 1967; 277:57. Followup study. *N Engl J Med* 1974; 291:10.

Treatment of Hypertensive Emergencies

AMA Committee on Hypertension: The treatment of malignant hypertension and hypertensive emergencies. *J Am Med Assoc* 1974; 228:1673.

Bhatia SK, Frolich ED: Hemodynamic comparison of agents useful in hypertensive emergencies. *Am Heart J* 1973; 85:367.

Koch-Weser J: Hypertensive emergencies. *N Engl J Med* 1974; 290:211.

Pheochromocytoma

Crago RM, Eckholdt JW, Wiswell JG: Pheochromocytoma: Treatment with alpha and beta adrenergic blocking drugs. *J Am Med Assoc* 1967; 202:870.

Ross EJ, Prichard BNC, Kaufman L, et al: Preoperative and operative management of patients with pheochromocytoma. *Br Med J* 1967; 1:191.

9
SYNCOPE

Samuel Z. Goldhaber
Joseph R. Benotti

Syncope, a common chief complaint in emergency medicine, can be defined as a temporary loss of consciousness. Often, the terms *fainting spell* or *blackout spell* are used. In an emergency ward setting, the patient has usually regained consciousness by the time the physician is making an initial assessment of the problem. Assessment is complicated by the range of diagnoses and prognoses that are possible—from completely innocuous to life threatening (Table 9.1).

PATHOPHYSIOLOGY

Central nervous system tissue essentially has no capacity to store or generate glucose or high-energy phosphate compounds under anaerobic conditions. Consequently, the brain must receive adequate amounts of oxygen and glucose at a constant rate via the cerebral arterial system to provide the energy required for neuronal function. Cerebral blood flow averages 50 ml/100 g of brain tissue per minute under normal conditions. When cerebral blood flow falls below a critical threshold value of 30 ml/100 g of brain tissue per minute, syncope occurs within seconds. Irreversible brain damage can occur in less than 5 minutes unless a critical threshold of cerebral perfusion is maintained. Since cerebral perfusion is related directly to the blood pressure, any cardiovascular condition responsible for episodic hypotension can result in syncope, especially if the reflex increase in systemic vascular resistance is inadequate.

There is little α-adrenergic innervation of the cerebral arterioles. Consequently, under circumstances characterized by intense generalized (shock) or regional (exercise) vasoconstriction, arterial pressure and perfusion to the central nervous system are preserved at the expense of blood flow to the kidneys, skin, nonexercising skeletal muscle, and splanchnic bed. The cerebral arterial circuit is capable of autoregulating perfusion such that, in the absence of cerebrovascular disease, perfusion is maintained relatively constant over a wide range of arterial pressure. However, atherosclerosis in the carotid and/or vertebrobasilar systems increases the resistance to flow and impairs the capacity of these vessels to vasodilate and maintain flow as perfusion pressure drops. Consequently, elderly patients with cerebral atherosclerosis may be more likely to faint as a result of any cardiovascular insult.

IMPAIRED CARDIAC FILLING

Orthostatic Hypotension

When a person stands, there is pooling of blood in the venous capacitance vessels of the lower extremities. This is partially prevented by tissue pressure, the pumping action of skeletal muscles, and the inhibition of retrograde venous flow by venous valves. The net effect, however, is diminished venous return resulting in diminished stroke volume, decreased cardiac output, and a fall in systolic blood pressure. The drop in arterial pressure stimulates the baroreceptors in the aorta and carotid sinus. The carotid sinus, a fusiform structure located at the bifurcation of the common carotid artery, may be palpated 2–3 cm below the angle of the jaw posterior to the anterior belly of the sternocleidomastoid muscle. Afferent impulses from the carotid sinus are transmitted to vasomotor (pressor) sympathetic and cardioinhibitory (depressor) parasympathetic centers in the medulla via the glossopharyngeal nerve. Decreased pressure on the carotid sinus, as occurs with orthostatic hypotension, causes decreased parasympathetic outflow and increased sympathetic outflow. The efferent impulses mediated through sympathetic pathways cause peripheral vasoconstriction, an increase in heart rate, and a rise in catecholamine and renin levels. As a result of these mechanisms, there is, under normal circumstances, increased venous return to the heart, augmented ventricular stroke volume (due to increased venous return and increased inotropic effect), increased cardiac output, and a rise in systolic blood pressure. When this orthostatic blood pressure regulating mechanism fails, syncope occurs, characterized by a drop in systolic pressure, an initial rise in diastolic pressure, tachycardia, and then a drop in diastolic pressure. In this form of syncope, there is an initial lack of venous return, diminished cardiac output, and a decrease in cerebral perfusion. Tachycardia, pallor, and sweating are due to sympathetic stimulation. The common causes of orthostatic hypotension are listed in Table 9.2.

Hypotension of Pregnancy

Pregnant women often have marked fluctuations in cardiac output that may depend on body position. When women in their third trimester are supine they may experience a decrease

181

TABLE 9.1 Causes of Syncope

I. Impaired cardiac filling
  A. Orthostatic hypotension
  B. Cardiac tamponade
  C. Drug effect (e.g., nitrates)
II. Impaired cardiac ejection
  A. Impaired cardiac contractility
    1. Myocardial infarction
    2. Cardiomyopathy
    3. Drug toxicity (e.g., diuretic-induced hypotension)
  B. Dysrhythmias
    1. Tachydysrhythmias
      a. Atrial
        i. Fibrillation
        ii. Flutter
        iii. Paroxysmal atrial tachycardia
        iv. Wolff-Parkinson-White Syndrome
        v. Sick sinus syndrome (as part of the bradycardia–tachycardia syndrome)
        vi. Hyperkalemia
      b. Ventricular
        i. Tachycardia
        ii. Fibrillation
        iii. Syndromes associated with delayed repolarization (prolonged QT interval)
        iv. Artificial pacemaker failure
        v. Drugs causing ventricular dysrhythmias
          a. Toxicity from antidysrhythmic medication
          b. Digitalis toxicity
          c. Phenothiazines
          d. Tricyclic antidepressants
    2. Bradydysrhythmias
      a. Complete heart block
      b. Artificial pacemaker failure
      c. Sick sinus syndrome
      d. Hypersensitive carotid sinus syndrome
      e. Sinus bradycardia with myocardial ischemia
      f. Drug toxicity (e.g., sinus bradycardia induced by sympatholytic agents such as aldomet or by lithium toxicity)
  C. Valve and vessel obstruction
    1. Atrial outflow obstruction
      a. Right and left atrial myxomas
      b. Tricuspid and mitral stenosis (usually rheumatic)
      c. Obstruction of valvular prosthesis

    2. Ventricular outflow obstruction
      a. Left ventricle
        i. Supravalvular stenosis
        ii. Valvular stenosis
        iii. Subvalvular stenosis
      b. Right ventricle
        i. Pulmonic stenosis
        ii. Tetralogy of Fallot
    3. Pulmonary vascular obstruction
      a. Pulmonary embolism
      b. Pulmonary hypertension (primary and secondary)
      c. Eisenmenger's complex
      d. Positive end expiratory pressure
III. Interference with cerebral blood flow or metabolism
  A. Extracranial large artery obstruction
    1. Carotid and vertebral artery stenosis
      a. Stroke
      b. Transient ischemic attack
    2. Pulseless disease
    3. Subclavian steal syndrome
  B. Hyperventilation syndrome
  C. Hypoglycemia
  D. Acceleration
  E. Drug toxicity
    1. Insulin
    2. Barbiturates
    3. Alcohol
  F. Diffuse spasm of cerebral arterioles (e.g., hypertensive encephalopathy)
IV. Combinations—Miscellaneous
  A. Common faint
  B. Swallowing syncope
  C. Micturition syncope
  D. Defecation syncope
  E. Weight lifter's syncope
  F. Glossopharyngeal nerve syncope
  G. Cough syncope

Adapted from Dunn MI, Carley JE: Syncope, in Eliot RS, Wolf GL, Forker AD (eds): *Cardiac Emergencies,* Mount Kisko, NY, Futura Publishing Co Inc, 1977, pp 96–97. Used with permission.

TABLE 9.2 Causes of Orthostatic Hypotension

I. Volume depletion
   A. Blood loss
   B. Massive diuresis
   C. Postgastrectomy dumping syndrome
II. Venous obstruction or pooling
   A. Pregnancy
   B. Prolonged standing
   C. Prolonged bed rest
   D. Postexercise vasodilatation
   E. Spinal anesthesia
   F. Drug induced
      1. Antihypertensive drugs
      2. Diuretics
      3. Nitrates
      4. Phenothiazines
      5. L-dopa
III. Neurologic disease
   A. Diabetic neuropathy
   B. Alcoholic neuropathy
   C. Pernicious anemia
   D. Tabes dorsalis
   E. Amyloid disease
   F. Pyridoxine deficiency
   G. Multiple sclerosis
   H. Guillain-Barré syndrome
   I. Syringomyelia
   J. Postsympathectomy syndrome
   K. Porphyria
   L. Drug induced (e.g., vincristine)
IV. Endocrine disease
   A. Hyperaldosteronism
   B. Addison's disease
   C. Pheochromocytoma
   D. Simmonds' disease
V. Idiopathic (e.g., Shy-Drager syndrome) (see Table 9.3)

Adapted from Dunn MI, Carley JE: Syncope, in Eliot RS, Wolf GL, Forker AD (eds): *Cardiac Emergencies.* Mount Kisko, NY, Futura Publishing Co Inc, 1977, p 99. Used with permission.

in cardiac output and stroke volume due to uterine obstruction of inferior vena cava blood flow. These findings can be reversed by the lateral decubitus position.

Postexercise Syncope

Postexercise syncope primarily occurs in teenagers who have engaged in vigorous, strenuous activity in a warm environ-

ment. With exercise, there is a marked increase in cardiac output, and maximum vasodilatation occurs. When the exercise is terminated, the cardiac output decreases rapidly, but the vasodilatation persists, resulting in both an expanded vascular bed and decreased cardiac output, which causes hypotension and syncope.

Idiopathic Orthostatic Hypotension

Chronic idiopathic orthostatic hypotension is also known as *primary autonomic insufficiency* and *primary orthostatic hypotension* (Table 9.3). It is a primary degenerative disorder that impairs the autonomic nervous system and can either be preganglionic or postganglionic in origin. The *Shy-Drager syndrome* (chronic preganglionic autonomic insufficiency) involves degeneration of the afferent limb of the reflex arc despite normal resting levels of norepinephrine. Chronic postganglionic autonomic insufficiency is associated with degeneration of the sympathetic ganglia and abnormally low resting levels of norepinephrine. In both syndromes, the response to upright posture is abnormal, with inadequate peripheral vasoconstriction, inadequate acceleration of heart rate, and little if any rise in norepinephrine levels. During the Valsalva maneuver, there is a greater than normal decline in arterial pressure and a reduced or absent overshoot following Valsalva release.

TABLE 9.3 Signs and Symptoms of Idiopathic Orthostatic Hypotension

1. Orthostatic hypotension
2. Anhidrosis
3. Impotence
4. Reversed diurnal urinary output
5. Heat intolerance
6. Diarrhea
7. Loss of temperature regulation
8. Tremor
9. Loss of muscle tone
10. Drowsiness
11. Square wave response of blood pressure to Valsalva maneuver
12. Absence of blood pressure rise with supine exercise
13. Increased urinary output and renal blood flow in supine position

Adapted from Dunn MI, Carley JE: Syncope, in Eliot RS, Wolf GL, Forker AD (eds): *Cardiac Emergencies,* Mount Kisko, NY, Futura Publishing Co Inc, 1977, p 100. Used with permission.

Cardiac Tamponade

With the rapid accumulation of a small amount of pericardial fluid or the gradual accumulation of a large amount of fluid, cardiac tamponade and syncope may occur. The high intrapericardial pressure impairs venous return by compressing the heart, causing marked reduction in stroke volume, cardiac output, and cerebral perfusion. Venous and right atrial pressure rise (often to 20 mm Hg or more), systolic arterial pressure falls, pulse pressure narrows, and pulsus paradoxus occurs (with peak arterial systolic pressure decreasing 15–20 mm Hg during inspiration). With extreme tamponade, pulsus alternans may be found.

IMPAIRED CARDIAC EJECTION

Impaired Ventricular Contractility

Impaired ventricular contractility can cause a decrease in stroke volume, cardiac output (the product of stroke volume and heart rate), cerebral perfusion, and ultimately syncope. The most obvious example is massive myocardial infarction, which is discussed in detail in Chapter 4. Severe cardiomyopathy and drug toxicity (such as large doses of beta blockers in the setting of heart failure) should also be considered.

Dysrhythmias

Of the dysrhythmias that cause syncope, ventricular tachycardia and ventricular fibrillation are most ominous (Chapters 1 and 5). These ventricular dysrhythmias, alone or in combination with an acute chest pain syndrome, may herald acute myocardial infarction that presents with syncope (Chapter 4).

STOKES-ADAMS DISEASE

Stokes-Adams disease is a broad term that refers to cardiac syncope from transient cerebral ischemia due to a sudden deleterious change in heart rate, heart rhythm, or atrioventricular conduction. When the eponym *Stokes-Adams* is used, it usually refers to transient complete heart block with ventricular asystole during syncopal attacks. However, the term actually encompasses supraventricular and ventricular dysrhythmias with and without atrioventricular block. The atrioventricular block most likely to lead to such attacks is Mobitz Type II second-degree atrioventricular block and/or third-degree (complete) atrioventricular block. The most common cause of atrioventricular block in elderly patients is idiopathic sclerosis producing damage of the cardiac conduction system (Lenegre's

disease) or fibrocalcific degeneration of the myocardium and the conduction system (Lev's disease). At times, electrolyte disorders or the toxic effects of drugs superimposed upon relatively mild degenerative cardiac conduction system disease will precipitate Stokes-Adams attacks. A more complete list of causes of heart block is provided in Table 9.4.

SICK SINUS SYNDROME

Sick sinus syndrome refers broadly to a subset of the Stokes-Adams syndrome. However, in common usage the sick sinus

---

TABLE 9.4 Causes of Complete Heart Block

I.   Structural lesions of the heart
   A. Congenital complete heart block
   B. Infectious disease
      1. Acute rheumatic fever
      2. Diptheria
      3. Syphilis
      4. Mumps
      5. Toxoplasmosis
   C. Connective tissue disease
      1. Systemic lupus erythematosus
      2. Dermatomyositis
      3. Rheumatoid arthritis
      4. Ankylosing spondylitis
      5. Marfan's syndrome
   D. Valvular heart disease
      1. Valve calcification (e.g., aortic stenosis)
      2. Endocarditis involving the conduction system
   E. Degenerative disease
      1. Fibrocalcific degeneration of the myocardium and conduction system (Lev's disease)
      2. Idiopathic sclerosis of the conduction system (Lenegre's disease)
      3. Myotonia dystrophy
      4. Friedrich's ataxia
      5. Progressive muscular dystrophy
   F. Ischemia
      1. Coronary artery disease with or without infarction
      2. Coronary spasm
   G. Neoplastic disease
      1. Lymphoma
      2. Rhabdomyosarcoma
      3. Lymphangioendothelioma
      4. Metastatic tumors
      5. Mesothelioma

(continued)

TABLE 9.4 (Continued)

H. Metabolic disease
 1. Hemachromatosis
 2. Gout
 3. Myxedema
 4. Hyperthyroidism
I. Trauma
 1. Surgical heart block
 2. Nonpenetrating chest injury
J. Diseases of unknown etiology
 1. Reiter's syndrome
 2. Sarcoidosis
 3. Amyloidosis
 4. Paget's disease
II. Electrolyte disorders
 A Hyperkalemia
 B. Acidosis
III. Toxic effects of drugs
 A. Digitalis glycosides
 B. Antidysrhythmic agents
 1. Quinidine
 2. Procainamide
 3. Lidocaine
 4. Diphenylhydrantoin
 5. Beta blockers
 6. Verapamil
 C. Tricyclic antidepressants

Adapted from Pomerantz B, O'Rourke RA: The Stokes-Adams syndrome. *Am J Med* 1969; 46:941–960. Used with permission.

syndrome encompasses a large but specific group of cardiac dysrhythmias (Table 9.5). The sick sinus syndrome is characterized by recurrent supraventricular tachydysrhythmias in patients with underlying sinus bradycardia and/or bradydysrhythmias. Automaticity of lower pacemakers is often depressed in the sick sinus syndrome, and conduction disturbances are common in the atria, AV node, bundle branches, and ventricles. The *bradycardia–tachycardia syndrome* is a subset of the sick sinus syndrome. Syncope occurs in the sick sinus syndrome because of decreased heart rate (from bradydysrhythmias) and/or decreased stroke volume (tachydysrhythmias).

Delayed Repolarization Syndromes

In 1957, Jervell and Lange-Nielsen reported on four congenitally deaf siblings with QT prolongation, fainting attacks, and three sudden deaths at ages 4, 5, and 9 years old. Subsequent

TABLE 9.5 Sick Sinus Syndrome

I. Bradydysrhythmias
 A. Sinus bradycardia with or without atrial premature depolarizations
 B. Sinoatrial block
 C. Sinus arrest and atrial standstill⁻
 D. Temporary asystole following tachycardia or following electrical cardioversion of atrial tachydysrhythmia
 E. Atrial fibrillation with a slow ventricular response that is not drug induced
II. Tachydysrhythmias
 A. Atrial fibrillation
 B. Atrial flutter
 C. Supraventricular tachycardia
III. Bradycardia–tachycardia syndrome

studies indicate that this syndrome has autosomal recessive inheritance. Several years later, two additional families were described with similar cardiac findings, normal hearing, and the genetics of autosomal dominance with varying expression. Much more common are the secondary causes of delayed repolarization, which are outlined in Table 9.6.

TABLE 9.6 Etiology of Delayed Repolarization Syndromes

A. Primary (idiopathic) prolonged QT syndrome
 1. Jervell and Lange-Nielsen type—autosomal recessive inheritance with congenital neural deafness
 2. Romano-Ward type—autosomal dominance with normal hearing
 3. Sporadic type—noninherited disorder with normal hearing
B. Secondary types of QT interval syndromes
 1. Drug-induced causes—antidysrhythmic agents, phenothiazines, tricyclic antidepressants, lithium, and prenylamine
 2. Metabolic abnormalities—electrolyte imbalance, chronic alcoholism, hepatic dysfunction, and liquid protein diet
 3. Central nervous system lesions—cerebral vascular thrombosis, intracerebral hematoma, subarachnoid hemorrhage, head trauma, and cerebral tumors
 4. Autonomic system dysfunction—radical neck surgery, carotid endarterectomy, and vagotomy
 5. Coronary heart disease—acute myocardial or subendocardial infarction
 6. Mitral valve prolapse
 7. Miscellaneous—congenital heart block, pheochromocytoma, and cardiac ganglionitis

From Moss AJ, Schwartz PJ: Delay repolarization (QT or QTU prolongation) and malignant ventricular arrhythmias. *Modern Concepts Cardiovasc Dis* 1982; 51:85–90. Reprinted with permission of the American Heart Association.

Hypersensitive Carotid Sinus Syndrome

There are two major forms of carotid sinus hypersensitivity. The more common *vagal (cardioinhibitory)* form is manifested by sinus bradycardia, sinus arrest, atrioventricular block, or occasionally asystole. The less common *vasodepressor type* of carotid sinus hypersensitivity is manifested by hypotension without significant bradycardia or atrioventricular block. The vagus nerve probably mediates both types of hypersensitive carotid sinus syndrome; therefore, the distinction between the two forms of this disorder may be somewhat artificial. Some patients exhibit both vagal and vasodepressor types of syndromes.

VALVE AND VESSEL OBSTRUCTION

Atrioventricular Valve Obstruction

Mitral or tricuspid obstruction may result from rheumatic stenosis of the valve or from thrombus formation on a prosthetic valve. Myxoma of the atrium can produce syncope by obstructing the flow of blood from atrium to ventricle.

Ventricular Obstruction

AORTIC STENOSIS

Left ventricular outflow obstruction is associated with syncope that can occur at rest or, more often, with exertion. In severe valvular aortic stenosis, the afterload is markedly increased, and therefore the ability of myocardial fibers to shorten is decreased. Obstruction to cardiac output develops and increases gradually, as does compensatory left ventricular hypertrophy. In the majority of patients with aortic stenosis, the cardiac output at rest remains normal. However, during exertion, the cardiac output often fails to rise normally. Postexertional syncope suggests that decreased venous return and failure to fill a very stiff left ventricle are important causes of syncope in this disorder.

HYPERTROPHIC OBSTRUCTIVE CARDIOMYOPATHY

Hypertrophic obstructive cardiomyopathy is commonly referred to as *idiopathic hypertrophic subaortic stenosis* (IHSS). The left ventricle is hypertrophied, and the cavity is small. In contrast to obstruction produced by a fixed orifice (as in patients with valvular aortic stenosis) in which there is impedance to left ventricular ejection throughout systole, hypertrophic obstructive cardiomyopathy is characterized by dynamic obstruction that usually appears well after ejection has begun. Hypertrophied, bizarrely shaped, and abnormally arranged myocardial cells are often present in the septum but are rare or absent in the left ventricular free wall. Disproportionate (asymmetric) septal hypertrophy is present in most patients with this syndrome. There is a pressure gradient within the body of the left ventricle, which is separated from a subaortic chamber by the thickened septum and the anterior leaflet of the mitral valve that abuts the septum. The pressure gradient may be quite labile. When ventricular volume is reduced by decreased preload, decreased afterload, or increased myocardial contractility, the anterior mitral valve leaflet apposes the septum, and dynamic obstruction is produced. With IHSS, syncope frequently can occur in patients without a pressure gradient between the body of the left ventricle and the subaortic chamber. This suggests that, as with aortic stenosis, failure to fill a very stiff left ventricle may be a crucial factor in causing syncope.

Pulmonary Vascular Obstruction

Syncope may be a presenting symptom of pulmonary embolism. This disorder, if severe, will precipitate acute right ventricular failure (with an increase in right ventricular end-diastolic pressure and right atrial mean pressure) and a decreased stroke volume, which in turn causes decreased cardiac output. In these patients, there is almost always more than 50% obstruction of the pulmonary arterial circulation and acute cor pulmonale. The right atrial mean pressure correlates well with the severity of pulmonary vascular obstruction.

Other causes of pulmonary vascular obstruction include right-to-left shunting in the Eisenmenger's syndrome and chronic pulmonary hypertension (either primary or secondary). In mechanically ventilated patients, postive end-expiratory pressure can also cause syncope by decreasing pulmonary blood flow and cardiac output.

INTERFERENCE WITH CEREBRAL BLOOD FLOW

On a pathophysiologic basis, syncope has a less rapid onset than epilepsy. With epilepsy, there is a sudden spread of an electric discharge. With syncope, the failure of the cerebral circulation is more gradual.

Extracranial Large Vessel Disease

Severe atherosclerosis of the aortic arch and its main branches may predispose patients to syncope. Neurologic symptoms frequently accompany carotid artery stenosis and pulseless disease. Fainting may result from exercise of an upper extremity when there is marked proximal obstruction of the ipsilateral subclavian artery. This occurs because of retrograde flow down the vertebral artery into the subclavian artery distal to the obstruction (subclavian steal syndrome), which compromises the cerebral circulation.

Hyperventilation Syndrome

The overbreathing is usually the result of an underlying anxiety but may be due to central stimulation from drugs. The hyperventilation results in hypocapnia and alkalosis, which in turn leads to cerebral arterial vasoconstriction and diminished flow. The reflex increase in cerebral vascular resistance can decrease cerebral blood flow as much as 40% within 2 minutes. This decrease in cerebral blood flow approaches but usually does not attain the threshold required for a syncopal episode. With diminished cerebral perfusion there is a progressive decrease in oxygen delivery to the brain as evidenced by diffuse slowing of brain wave activity on the electroencephalogram.

Acceleration

Acceleration may produce syncope in airplane pilots by causing venous pooling, and thus a marked fall in cardiac output.

COMBINED MECHANISMS

The *common faint,* also referred to as *vasovagal syncope, vasodepressor syncope,* or *vasomotor syncope,* occurs because of inappropriate neurogenic reflexes that temporarily reduce cerebral perfusion. With the common faint, vagal activity increases, blood flow in the muscles increases acutely (because of peripheral vasodilatation), and arterial pressure drops suddenly.

As blood pools in the extremities, cerebral blood flow decreases. The final common pathway is a decrease in blood flow to the brain below a critical level required to maintain consciousness. Hyperventilation usually accompanies vasodepressor syncope. This leads to a decrease in arterial P_{CO_2} that in turn causes increased cerebral vasoconstriction, thereby further impairing cerebral perfusion.

During cardiac catheterization, decreases in pulmonary vascular resistance, systemic vascular resistance, heart rate, and cardiac index were noted in all patients with vasovagal syncope. Despite decreased mean arterial pressure, the heart fails to compensate by increasing cardiac output. The autonomic nervous system's inappropriately increased parasympathetic activity has been referred to as *acute circulatory disorganization.*

The psychological factors associated with the common faint suggest that the threat or occurrence of actual or symbolic physical injury may cause the pooling of blood in peripheral muscles as part of a defensive "fight or flight" reaction. Normally, when muscle contraction does not promptly ensue, this neurogenic vasodilatation is promptly counteracted. However, in the common faint, circulatory preparation for flight persists inappropriately. A conflict may develop between the flight or fight reaction, which mobilizes for massive motor activity, by increasing sympathetic activity and increasing blood flow to peripheral muscles, to deal with threat or danger, and the "conservation or withdrawal reaction," which serves to conserve energy and reduce engagement with a threatening, unsupportive environment by enhanced vagal activity. The latter reaction may be a holdover from lower organisms, which by sham death, hibernation, and blending with the background make themselves less conspicuous to predators. Normally, one type of autonomic reaction (fight or flight versus conservation or withdrawal) should inhibit the other. It has been postulated that in patients with the common faint, there is uncertainty as to which autonomic reaction is more useful. As psychic conflict and uncertainty peak, both sets of responses may become activated simultaneously and produce inappropriately decreased cardiac output in combination with decreased systemic vascular resistance. The result is usually a benign faint, but the same set of circumstances may lead to dysrhythmia and sudden death.

Several other combined mechanisms that cause syncope have been described and should be kept in mind by the emergency ward physician. A detailed discussion of these forms of syncope is beyond the scope of this chapter, but they include swallow (deglutition) syncope, micturition syncope, defecation syncope, weight lifter's syncope, glossopharyngeal nerve syncope, and cough syncope.

INITIAL EVALUATION AND MANAGEMENT OF THE PATIENT WITH SYNCOPE

Occasionally, the physician will witness an acute syncopal episode. In such cases, the physician should immediately determine whether pulse or respiration are impaired. Usually, there will be no cessation of respiration. In the few seconds necessary to assess adequately the carotid or femoral pulse, the syncopal episode will often begin to resolve spontaneously and the strength of the pulse will improve. Under most circumstances, pallor resolves, breathing becomes quicker and deeper, the eyelids flutter, and the patient's awareness of physical weakness and perception of the surrounding environment return simultaneously.

The initial management of syncope (Fig. 9.1) usually consists of checking vital signs and maintaining the patient in the legs-up–head-down position. On rare occasions, cardiopulmonary resuscitation may be required. More often, however, pulse and respiration are restored spontaneously. If appropriate, blood is drawn for serum glucose and hematocrit; intravenous access may be warranted to administer fluids and medication. If syn-

cope could be due to hypoglycemia, narcotics, or tricyclic antidepressants, then 50–100 ml of a 50% dextrose in water solution can be administered intravenously, followed by 1 ampule each of naloxone or physostigmine, respectively. If there is evidence of cyanosis or lung disease, room air arterial blood gases are obtained and supplemental oxygen is administered. The cautions that should be observed in administering oxygen to patients with chronic lung disease are discussed in Chapter 2. Elevation of the legs may be useful to maximize cerebral blood flow. To avoid a recurrence of syncope, overcrowding by well-meaning personnel or by curiosity seekers should be discouraged, tight clothing should be loosened, and the patient should be cautioned against assuming the upright position too quickly.

In most instances, however, the patient will present with a history of syncope that has resolved before arrival in the emergency ward. The busy emergency ward physician should resist the temptation to gloss over the history quickly in order to proceed with physical examination and laboratory evaluation, which are both more easily obtained. Investigating eyewitness accounts from friends, relatives, or bystanders in addition to ambulance paramedics is worth the extra effort. The history may provide important information that helps to separate the transient benign faint from seizures or from impending sudden death. The history may also be useful in defining various types of cardiac syncope. For example, whereas cardiac dysrhythmias often occur at rest, obstruction to cardiac output is more likely to occur with exertion. The ten questions in Table 9.7 may be useful in initial assessment.

During the physical examination of the syncopal patient, careful attention should be given to signs of trauma. The pulse and blood pressure are obtained with the patient in the supine, sitting (legs dangling), and standing (if possible) positions in order to detect postural hypotension. If examination of the radial and apical pulse and review of the electrocardiogram (ECG) demonstrate dysrhythmias, the patient is monitored and admitted for observation. A careful but abbreviated cardiopulmonary examination is performed to look for signs suggestive of cardiac tamponade, valvular heart disease (especially aortic stenosis), hypertrophic obstructive cardiomyopathy, pulmonary hypertension, or pulmonary embolism. After taking vital signs and assessing mental and emotional status, a careful and thorough neurologic and cardiac examination should be completed. Focal neurologic deficits should be sought out. If transient, the possibility of a postictal Todd's paralysis should be considered, as well as a transient ischemic attack. Attention should be given to neck, head, and peripheral arterial pulses to assess their strengths and the presence of bruits. If appropriate, the physical examination can then proceed with several

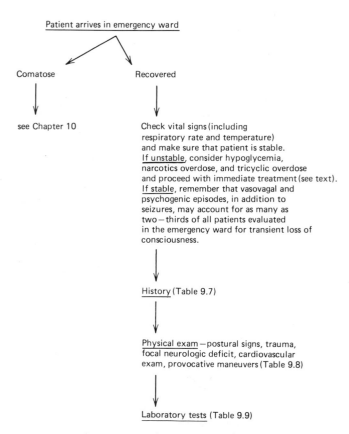

Figure 9.1 Initial management of syncope.

TABLE 9.7 Questions to Ask in the Evaluation of Syncope

1. Was the onset of syncope *sudden* (as in many forms of obstruction to cardiac output) or *relatively gradual* (as in the common faint or orthostatic hypotension)? Was there any warning at all of the impending spell (e.g., aura in epilepsy versus prodrome of giddiness in syncope)?

2. What was the patient doing at the time of the syncopal episode?

3. What was the *duration* of the syncopal episode?

4. What was the patient's *position* at the onset of the syncopal episode (e.g., moving from supine to standing position and then experiencing orthostatic hypotension)? The simple faint usually occurs when the patient is standing, in contrast to seizures, which can occur in any position, including sleep.

5. What *associated symptoms* (e.g., palpitations) occurred before, during, and subsequent to the episode? (e.g., nausea, pain, and fright suggest the common faint, whereas palpitations, both before and after the syncopal episode, may suggest a dysrhythmia.)

6. Was *trauma* associated with the syncopal event, either causing the syncope (cerebrovascular) or as a result of the syncope (e.g., sudden fall to the ground after cardiac syncope)?

7. What *drugs or medications* was the patient taking?

8. Does the patient have a *history of syncope* or is this the first episode?

9. What is the patient's *past medical history*?

10. What was the *emotional context* in which the patient had syncope (i.e., does it suggest the common faint or hyperventilation)?

provocative maneuvers that may provide further clarification (Table 9.8).

In patients who present to the emergency ward with syncope, the laboratory evaluation can range from a spun fingerstick hematocrit and 12-lead ECG (both ideally accomplished within

TABLE 9.8 Provocative Maneuvers for the Assessment of Syncope

Observation of whether a rapid change from supine to standing position reproduces the patient's symptoms

Assessment of heart rate and blood pressure response to carotid sinus pressure (in a patient without symptoms or signs suggestive of carotid atherosclerosis)

Hyperventilation (to reproduce symptoms of syncope or light-headedness and thus to help detect the hyperventilation syndrome)

Arm exercise and elevation (to detect a possible subclavian steal syndrome)

Valsalva maneuver (to elicit signs of obstructive hypertrophic cardiomyopathy)

5 minutes at minimal expense) to a sophisticated technologically oriented investigation that requires subspecialty consultation and hospitalization and costs many thousands of dollars. The simple evaluation may be appropriate in a young patient who presents with a history typical of the common faint (see discussion below). The more extensive evaluation may be appropriate for a patient with an unreliable history whose etiology for syncope remains uncertain (Table 9.9).

In a recent study from the Brigham and Women's Hospital, 198 patients were identified who presented with transient loss of consciousness. Vasovagal or psychogenic etiologies accounted for 40% of the patients, and seizures accounted for 29% of the patients. Even with long-term follow-up, however, the cause of loss of consciousness remained uncertain in 13% of the patients. It is encouraging that history and physical examinations were sufficient for a diagnosis in 85% of the patients in whom a diagnosis could be established.

TABLE 9.9 Laboratory Tests for the Assessment of Syncope

Tests that can usually be completed within 1 hour
  Complete blood count
  Blood for typing and cross matching
  Electrolytes and glucose
  Renal and liver chemistries
  Cardiac enzymes
  A 12-lead ECG (with careful analysis for possible myocardial infarction, bundle branch block, atrioventricular block, sick sinus syndrome, and prolonged QT interval)
  Continuous electrocardiographic monitoring
  Chest roentgenogram
  Arterial blood gases
Tests that usually require several hours or subspecialty consultation
  Echocardiogram (to exclude hemodynamically significant aortic stenosis, mitral stenosis, hypertrophic cardiomyopathy, pericardial effusion, impaired myocardial contractility, atrial myxoma, prosthetic valvular dysfunction)
  Lung scan (to exclude pulmonary embolism)
  Computerized tomography of the head (to exclude certain cerebrovascular etiologies of syncope such as hemorrhagic stroke)
  Carotid Doppler and ophthalmodynanometry (to help evaluate possible obstructive atherosclerotic carotid disease)
  Toxicology studies of blood, urine, and/or stomach contents
  Drug levels of known chronic medications (such as digoxin, quinidine, procainamide, theophylline)
Tests that usually require several days to schedule
  Exercise treadmill test (for evaluation of dysrhythmia)
  Holter monitoring
  Electroencephalography

CLINICAL SETTINGS

The Common Faint

The common faint is the most usual cause of syncope. Such a faint is likely to occur during a painful, frightening, and emotion-laden experience. Situations in which a person is expected to demonstrate courage despite potentially painful or frightening experiences are especially likely to lead to fainting. In the medical context, such faints are associated with procedures ranging from simple venipuncture to cardiac catheterization. Dental procedures, which can involve more fear than actual pain, can also precipitate the common faint. Stressful emotional situations such as hearing unpleasant news about a close relative, arguments with a co-worker or spouse, or school examinations are typical settings for the common faint. It is often found that the patient who faints has discontinued regular eating and sleeping patterns for days to weeks before the faint. The patient is frequently fatigued, overworked, and emotionally distraught. For these reasons, it is important for emergency ward personnel to keep psychological factors in mind when obtaining a history of a syncopal episode.

DIAGNOSIS

The common faint is best diagnosed by carefully reviewing or observing premonitory symptoms and signs. Epigastric discomfort, nausea, blurred vision, and a vague feeling of unawareness are frequent symptoms. Pallor, yawning, sighing, hyperventilation, diaphoresis, impaired hearing, and mydriasis are frequent signs.

MANAGEMENT AND PROGNOSIS

An actual faint can often be aborted if a patient who is in an upright position will sit down or lie down promptly when the prodrome begins. The common faint is usually self-limited and benign. Appropriate management is usually conservative. The patient is placed in a recumbent position with legs elevated. Inhalation of spirits of ammonia and stimulation of the face with cold water are usually not warranted. If the syncopal episode persists, treatment may occasionally be necessary with atropine and drugs that quickly increase systemic vascular resistance such as aramine or norepinephrine. In most instances, however, reassurance and maintenance of a calm demeanor are sufficient to manage the common faint. The prognosis in patients who experience the common faint is usually excellent. Efforts toward management of underlying psychological turmoil are often worthwhile.

Orthostatic Hypotension

Orthostatic hypotension is a common cause of syncope. In younger patients, the clinical setting is usually relative volume depletion from activities such as jogging or sunbathing or from acute illnesses causing vomiting and diarrhea. In older patients, the clinical setting can be profound dehydration (e.g., sepsis) or is often medication related (e.g., common antihypertensive medications such as alphamethyldopa or hydralazine). Bleeding, whether occult or obvious, can also cause orthostatic hypotension.

DIAGNOSIS

The diagnosis of orthostatic hypotension can usually be made by taking a careful history. Confirmation of the diagnosis can be made by taking "orthostatic blood pressure and pulse" while reproducing the patient's symptoms. A patient with orthostatic hypotension will usually have a 10-mm Hg *decrease* in systolic blood pressure and 10-beat/min *increase* in heart rate when moved from the supine to standing position. In such patients, blood loss must be excluded as the cause of syncope. Virtually every patient with orthostatic hypotension should have a rectal examination to help exclude gastrointestinal bleeding.

MANAGEMENT AND PROGNOSIS

The management of orthostatic hypotension will include volume repletion, orally or intravenously (if appropriate), in addition to a search for possible precipitants such as medications. The prognosis depends on the etiology but in most cases is good.

Carotid Sinus Hypersensitivity

Carotid sinus hypersensitivity tends to occur in the elderly and is more frequent in men than in women. Common predisposing factors include arteriosclerosis, hypertension, and diabetes mellitus. Rarely, local scars, lymph nodes, and tumors involving the carotid body predispose to a hypersensitive carotid sinus. Turning the head or wearing a tight collar can precipitate hypotension, bradycardia, dizziness, and syncope.

DIAGNOSIS

The clinical context is the best clue to carotid sinus hypersensitivity. A classic example is syncope in a driver who approaches a busy intersection and looks carefully to the far right and far left. Carotid sinus massage can be done under ECG monitoring in an attempt to reproduce symptoms. During carotid sinus massage, a pause greater than 3 seconds or a decline in diastolic blood pressure of at least 50 mm Hg may indicate a hypersensitive carotid. However, this test must be used with caution for two reasons: First, it may, on rare occasions, precipitate either hemiparesis or death due to sinus arrest without any ventricular escape. Second, although it is a sensitive test, it is not very specific. This provocative maneuver should probably not be used on patients with a carotid bruit, suspected digitalis toxicity, or severe heart disease of any cause. Both carotids should be palpable. The patient should be supine. The carotid sinus massage should be gentle and should not exceed 5 seconds. If the test is positive, it should be repeated after an atropine infusion and with blood pressure monitoring. If the test is negative, it should be repeated with blood pressure measurement.

MANAGEMENT AND PROGNOSIS

The most effective treatment is avoidance of pressure on the carotid sinus. If simple measures such as wearing loose collars do not suffice and the patient is repeatedly symptomatic, permanent pacemaker implantation may be necessary. In the emergency setting, the vagal form of carotid sinus hypersensitivity will respond to atropine and the vasodepressor form will respond to pressors such as aramine or norepinephrine. With the management approaches outlined above, the prognosis is very good.

Stokes-Adams Syndrome and the Sick Sinus Syndrome

The definition of the Stokes-Adams syndrome has broadened so that it includes transient cerebral ischemia in nonanesthetized subjects due to a sudden change in cardiac rate, rhythm, or conduction resulting in reduced cardiac output. This definition excludes the common faint and epilepsy, but technically it includes syncope caused by the sick sinus syndrome.

DIAGNOSIS

Symptoms may vary from slight faintness or giddiness to loss of consciousness, with or without convulsion. In the nonhospital setting, an incorrect diagnosis of primary neurologic disease can be made if the syncopal event is observed without benefit of simultaneous cardiac examination or ECG monitoring. It is not unusual for a nursing home patient to be referred

to an emergency ward with the diagnosis of "seizure disorder." Such a patient may have multiple facial and head contusions from recurrent episodes of paroxysmal syncope. The diagnosis of Stokes-Adams syndrome in such patients can usually be confirmed reliably only when such an episode is observed under ECG monitoring. In contrast to seizures of primary cerebral origin, an aura does not usually precede a Stokes-Adams attack. "Cardiac seizures," if present, usually commence and terminate abruptly. The Stokes-Adams patient may resume a previous conversation or activity without being aware of the pause produced by the period of cerebral ischemia.

Stokes-Adams attacks are characterized by their sudden onset, in contrast to the premonitory light-headedness that usually precedes the common faint. The less frequent the syncopal event is, the most difficult the diagnosis is (Fig. 9.2). If a syncopal episode does not occur during hospitalization, repeated ambulatory Holter monitoring may be necessary in the hope of obtaining an ECG tracing during syncope. In a patient with bifascicular block (right bundle branch block and left anterior hemiblock, *or* complete left bundle branch block, *or* right bundle branch block and left posterior hemiblock) and recurrent syncope that does not occur during ECG monitoring, detailed electrophysiologic testing in a cardiac catheterization lab may be necessary. However, some physicians would proceed with permanent pacemaker placement in such patients without further electrophysiologic study, even though a recently published study suggests that unless a bradydysrhythmia can be documented in patients with bundle branch block, insertion of a permanent pacemaker (even in patients with a prolonged His-Ventricular interval) may not necessarily prolong life.

MANAGEMENT AND PROGNOSIS

In some instances, Stokes-Adams attacks are due to reversible abnormalities such as hypokalemia, hypoxia, or transient myocardial ischemia. Underlying causes of Stokes-Adams attacks should be sought out and treated. Dysrhythmias, both ventricular and supraventricular, can frequently be managed with appropriate pharmacologic agents (Chapter 5). If a patient with Stokes-Adams or sick sinus syndrome experiences recurrent syncope despite correction of reversible abnormalities and antidysrhythmic therapy and if a bradydysrhythmia can be documented, then permanent pacemaker implantation will usually be necessary. Without specific therapy, the prognosis of patients with Stokes-Adams syndrome or sick sinus syndrome due to bradydysrhythmias or ventricular dysrhythmias may be ominous.

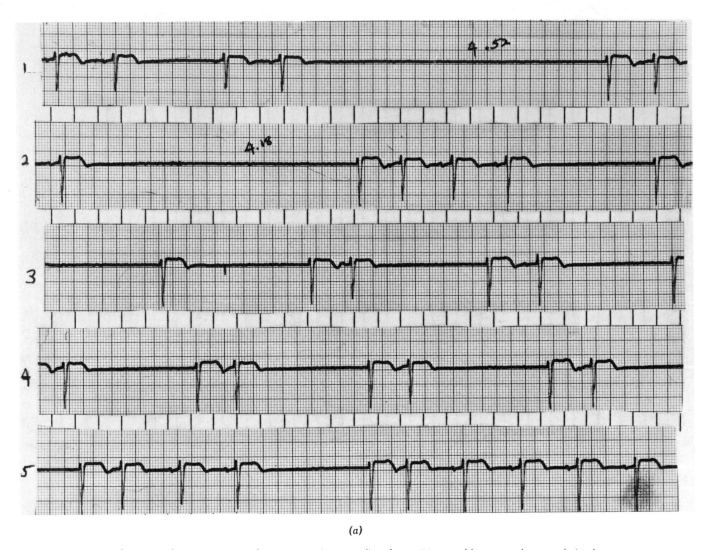

(a)

Figure 9.2 The tracings in panels *a-c* are monitor recordings from a 76-year-old woman who was admitted after a fainting spell. She had no previous history of cardiac disease. On exam, she had pain in her lower back where she fell, and x-ray films confirmed that she had minor fractures of several lower thoracic vertebrae. In the emergency ward, her 12-lead ECG was normal. Her physician did hear an irregular heartbeat and for that reason she was admitted for observation. The tracings show examples of the sick sinus syndrome. This patient underwent permanent pacemaker placement and has had no further symptoms. (*a*) Continuous recording demonstrates frequent sinus pauses, the longest of which is 4.5 seconds. In the third and fourth rows, the sinus pauses are preceded by atrial premature depolarizations. (*b*) Tachycardia is caused by frequent atrial premature depolarizations followed by sinus arrest. (*c*) A supraventricular tachycardia at 136/min followed by bradycardia. (Courtesy of Dr. Walter Kaufmann, Leonard Morse Hospital, Natick, MA.)

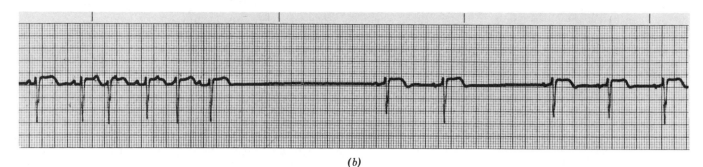

(b)

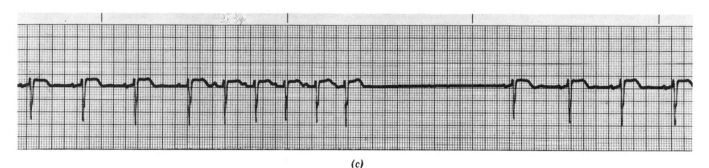

(c)

Figure 9.2 (Continued)

Valvular Aortic Stenosis

Patients with valvular aortic stenosis usually remain asymptomatic until the sixth decade of life. During this long latent period, there is gradually increasing obstruction of left ventricular outflow and increasing pressure overload of the left ventricle. The primary symptoms of aortic stenosis are angina, syncope, and congestive heart failure. After onset of symptoms, median survival is approximately 5 years with angina, 3 years with syncope, and 2 years with heart failure. Atrial fibrillation and the development of pulmonary hypertension and systemic venous hypertension are often preterminal findings.

DIAGNOSIS

The diagnosis of hemodynamically significant aortic stenosis can be suspected by physical examination and confirmed by echocardiography, carotid artery pulse tracing, and cardiac catheterization. M-mode and two-dimensional echocardiography, in addition to carotid artery pulse recording, can be done as noninvasive emergency procedures in the emergency ward. On physical examination, the arterial pulse rises slowly and is small and sustained. Coarse systolic vibrations are felt most readily in the carotid arterial pulse, producing a "carotid shudder." There is a systolic thrill at the right upper sternal border and in the suprasternal notch. There is usually a prominent S_4 and a single S_2. The midsystolic murmur of aortic stenosis is heard best at the base of the heart and has a harsh and rasping quality. The murmur radiates well to the carotids and to the apex, where it frequently has a more musical quality and can be mistaken for mitral regurgitation. The more severe the stenosis is, the longer the duration of the murmur and the later in systole is its peak intensity. More than 80% of patients with severe aortic stenosis meet ECG criteria for left atrial enlargement and left ventricular hypertrophy. On chest roentgenogram, the heart size is usually normal. The left ventricular border and apex often appear rounded. Poststenotic dilatation of the ascending aorta is common. Calcification of the aortic valve can be found either on the plain film or with fluoroscopy. Two-dimensional echocardiography demonstrating marked aortic valve calcification, left ventricular hypertrophy, and poor excursion of the aortic valve leaflets in both long and short axis, in combination with an abnormally delayed carotid artery upstroke documented on a carotid artery pulse tracing are virtually diagnostic. After admission to the hospital, the diagnosis can be confirmed by cardiac catheterization, which reveals a pressure gradient between the left ventricle and proximal aorta. In adults with a normal cardiac output and severe aortic stenosis, this gradient will exceed 50 mm Hg. Catheterization is important to determine whether associated valvular disease is present and, in patients with angina pectoris, to determine the patency of the coronary arteries.

MANAGEMENT AND PROGNOSIS

Almost all patients with severe aortic stenosis should undergo aortic valve replacement. In patients without left ventricular failure, operative mortality is 5–10%. In patients with left ventricular failure, the operative mortality is 10–25%. Even in patients with refractory pulmonary edema or medically non-resuscitatable cardiac arrest due to aortic stenosis, emergency aortic valve replacement can be lifesaving. In such dire circumstances, surgical therapy must at times be undertaken without prior cardiac catheterization since it may offer the only hope for survival.

Hypertrophic Obstructive Cardiomyopathy

The age distribution of hypertrophic obstructive cardiomyopathy (HOCM), also known as IHSS, is bimodal and peaks in the third and seventh decades of life. In elderly patients, HOCM can easily be confused with coronary artery disease or aortic valve disease. The clinical context has a wide spectrum from the asymptomatic patient with asymmetric septal hypertrophy on an echocardiogram that was done because of a family screening program to the unfortunate young athlete whose first manifestation of the disease is sudden death. In patients with symptoms, dyspnea is the most common complaint, but angina, fatigue, and syncope are also frequent. In contrast to its significance in the presence of valvular aortic stenosis, syncope may not be an ominous finding of impending death.

DIAGNOSIS

The diagnosis of HOCM can be suspected on physical examination and confirmed by echocardiography or catheterization. An echocardiogram can be performed in the emergency ward and can establish the diagnosis within minutes. On physical examination, the apical precordial impulse is often displaced laterally, is abnormally forceful, and is enlarged. A prominent presystolic impulse is often present. A systolic thrill is common at the apex or left lower sternal border. There is usually a prominent jugular venous a wave. The carotid pulse usually rises briskly and then declines in midsystole, followed by a secondary rise. There is often a fourth heart sound. The systolic murmur is a harsh crescendo–decrescendo and is best heard between the apex and left lower sternal border. It does not radiate well to the neck. The murmur is often more holosystolic and blowing at the apex and axilla and more mid-systolic and harsher along the left sternal border. The gradient and the murmur will increase with conditions or provocative maneuvers that increase contractility, decrease preload, or decrease afterload (such as Valsalva during strain, standing, amyl nitrate, and exercise). Digitalis, isoproterenol, and nitrates are medications that increase the gradient. Conversely, conditions or maneuvers that decrease contractility, increase preload, or increase afterload (such as squatting and isometric handgrip) will decrease the gradient and the murmur. Phenylephrine and beta blocking agents are medications that decrease the gradient.

The ECG usually shows prominent abnormal Q waves either inferiorly or laterally. M-mode or two-dimensional echocardiograms are usually diagnostic. The prime features are left ventricular hypertrophy, usually preferentially involving the interventricular septum, narrowing of the left ventricular outflow tract, and obstruction to left ventricular outflow (with systolic anterior motion of the mitral valve). Associated echo findings include a small left ventricular cavity, reduced septal motion and thickening during systole, normal or increased motion of the posterior left ventricular wall, reduced rate of mitral valve closure, mitral valve prolapse, and coarse systolic fluttering of the aortic valve. Cardiac catheterization usually reveals a pressure gradient within the body of the left ventricle, which is separated from a subaortic chamber by the thickened septum and the anterior leaflet of the mitral valve that abuts the septum.

MANAGEMENT AND PROGNOSIS

Medical therapy for HOCM traditionally has consisted of beta blockade with propranolol and avoidance of digitalis, nitrates, and β-adrenergic agents. Emergency management necessitates aggressive hydration and withdrawal of potentially deleterious medications. Unfortunately, fewer than one-third of patients treated chronically with beta blockade experience sustained symptomatic improvement. Recently, treatment with verapamil or nifedipine has appeared very promising.

Operative therapy for HOCM usually consists of septal myectomy with a transaortic approach. The operative mortality is 5–10%. Successful operation often yields lasting clinical and hemodynamic improvement and may prevent secondary left ventricular hypertrophy. The procedure is recommended for patients with a resting systolic pressure gradient of more than

50 mm Hg who remain severely symptomatic despite medical therapy.

The prognosis in HOCM is varied. The degree of the gradient does not correspond to the occurrence of sudden death. Younger patients appear more prone to sudden death, especially during strenuous exercise.

Cardiac Tamponade

Acute cardiac tamponade occurs in the setting of acute pericarditis, hemopericardium, and metastatic neoplastic pericardial disease. Chronic cardiac tamponade can be caused by many types of pericarditis, including tuberculous, parasitic, uremic, neoplastic, myxedematous, postirradiation, Dressler's syndrome, postpericardiotomy syndrome, and chylopericardium. Patients with acute cardiac tamponade almost always complain of dyspnea and frequently complain of chest pain that may be pleuritic, dull, or squeezing. Patients with chronic tamponade often complain of weakness, malaise, dyspnea, chest pain, anorexia, and weight loss. If cardiac tamponade causes syncope, the clinical situation is a medical emergency that requires immediate therapy.

DIAGNOSIS

The diagnosis, as discussed in Chapter 20, is suspected by physical examination and echocardiogram and is confirmed by cardiac catheterization. Patients with acute tamponade usually have increased jugular venous pulse (95%), tachycardia (80–90%), pulsus paradoxus more than 10 mm Hg (70–80%), pulse pressure less than 30 mm Hg (50–60%), systolic blood pressure less than 100 mm Hg (40–50%), pericardial friction rub (40–50%), and decreased intensity of the heart sounds (10–40%). The arterial pulse is usually weak and thready. Patients with chronic tamponade have marked jugular venous distension, hepatic enlargement, and ascites. On ECG, low voltage may be seen. However, the most specific ECG finding is electrical alternans. Two-thirds of reported cases of electrical alternans are due to tamponade. Echocardiograms may show a pericardial effusion, dampened pericardial motion, right ventricular compression, a "swinging heart," and marked sudden posterior septal motion in inspiration. Nevertheless, among echocardiographers there is still considerable skepticism as to the reliability of echocardiography in the diagnosis of tamponade. Catheterization usually demonstrates an elevated right atrial pressure, often more than 20 mm Hg. The ventricular diastolic pressures are elevated and equal to each other. As in constrictive pericarditis, in the absence of concurrent cardiac disease or ventricular failure there is equilibration among the right atrial pressure, ventricular diastolic pressures, and the pulmonary capillary wedge pressure. Finally, the existence of low-pressure cardiac tamponade has been well documented.

MANAGEMENT AND PROGNOSIS

The immediate management depends on the clinical urgency of treatment. If a patient with cardiopulmonary arrest is suspected of tamponade, immediate pericardiocentesis (Procedure 20) without any diagnostic tests is warranted. In a patient with gradually increasing dyspnea and possible chronic tamponade whose clinical status is, for example, complicated by chronic lung disease, complete diagnostic workup including cardiac catheterization may be appropriate. If the patient's clinical status is subacute, prudent management would probably include insertion of a central venous pressure line to measure right atrial pressure, aggressive rapid intravenous fluid administration, and an emergency echocardiogram or catheterization. The long-term prognosis depends on the etiology of the tamponade. If pericardial fluid recurs despite pericardiocentesis and catheter drainage, pericardiectomy may be necessary.

Pulmonary Embolism

Pulmonary embolism (PE) is an elusive disease that occurs in many clinical contexts. Some of the more commonly cited predisposing risk factors for PE are bedrest, cancer, cardiomyopathy, chronic lung disease, congestive heart failure, deep venous thrombosis, hip fracture, myocardial infarction, obesity (especially in women), oral contraceptives, pregnancy, sepsis, stroke, and surgery. A review of 132 consecutive cases of acute PE documented by pulmonary angiography indicated that syncope was the initial or predominant clinical feature in 17 (13%).

DIAGNOSIS

Pulmonary embolism is especially difficult to diagnose in the setting of pneumonia, congestive heart failure, or old age. Unfortunately, unless PE is massive and clinically obvious, ECG and radiologic abnormalities are so nonspecific that they are virtually useless as diagnostic aids. Furthermore, the search for a sensitive blood screening test has been disappointing. Any patient suspected clinically of PE should ordinarily undergo ventilation-perfusion lung scanning. In most circumstances, patients with moderate or indeterminate probability lung scanning should undergo pulmonary angiography. The diagnostic features and management of the condition are discussed in Chapters 2–4.

Hypoglycemia

The clinical settings for organic hypoglycemia include (1) overdose of insulin or an oral hypoglycemic agent, (2) an islet cell, insulin-secreting tumor of the pancreas, and (3) depletion of liver glycogen (e.g., after a binge of drinking alcohol). Functional or reactive hypoglycemia may precede diabetes mellitus or accompany peptic ulcer. In this condition, the rise of insulin in response to a carbohydrate meal is delayed, but it then causes an excessive fall in blood glucose to 30–40 mg/100 ml. Hypoglycemia must be profound in order to cause syncope.

DIAGNOSIS

Symptoms and signs of hypoglycemia at about 30 mg/100 ml can include nervousness, hunger, flushed face, sweating, trembling, headache, palpitation, anxiety, malaise, and fatigue. A patient with this degree of hypoglycemia can be confused with someone who appears to stagger and be stuporous from alcohol intoxication. Low levels of plasma glucose can cause confusion, drowsiness, and syncope. Levels of 10 mg/100 ml are associated with deep coma, mydriasis, pale skin, shallow respiration, slow pulse, and hypotonicity of limb musculature. To make the diagnosis of hypoglycemia, it must first and foremost be suspected.

MANAGEMENT AND PROGNOSIS

In a patient suspected of hypoglycemia, blood for glucose and insulin determinations should be drawn quickly and then, immediately afterward, empiric therapy should be administered with 50 ml of 50% glucose solution. The prognosis depends on the underlying etiology of the hypoglycemia, its degree, and the length of time that it persisted. A severe and prolonged episode of hypoglycemia may result in various degrees of impairment of intellectual function or even in protracted coma.

Hyperventilation

The clinical context for hyperventilation, a common cause of syncope, is usually an underlying anxiety state. The symptoms include giddiness, circumoral and extremity paresthesias, and a feeling of suffocation. The signs include dyspnea and tetany. Arterial blood gases will reveal alkalosis and hypocapnia.

Management consists of instructing the patient to rebreathe expired air. This can be accomplished with a rebreathing mask (usually used for oxygen therapy) or, less expensively, with a small paper bag. Simultaneously, attempts should be made to learn about possible precipitants of the hyperventilation attack and to reassure the patient.

Transient Ischemic Attack

Although transient ischemic attacks (TIAs) rarely cause syncope, they should be considered in the differential diagnosis of "light-headedness" or "a spell" or "faintness." The TIAs may last from several seconds to 24 hours. Most last 2–15 minutes; an attack of more than 30 minutes is uncommon. A patient may have a few attacks or several hundred. Between attacks, the neurologic examination may be entirely normal. Postictal paresis (the residuum of a seizure) must be differentiated from a TIA.

DIAGNOSIS

The symptoms and signs of TIA depend upon the area of the brain that is threatened. In the carotid system, attacks may involve either ipsilateral visual disturbance or contralateral sensorimotor disturbance. Usually, initial attacks are ocular and later attacks involve the cerebral hemisphere. In ocular attacks, transient monocular blindness is the usual symptom. During transient monocular blindness, retinal arterioles may show arrest of blood flow or a white plaque, probably representing a carotid arterial embolus. In hemispheric attacks, there is usually transient weakness or numbness of the opposite hand and arm. If such attacks occur in the left hemisphere, transient dysphasia may occur. In the vertebrobasilar system, symptoms can include dizziness, diplopia (vertical or horizontal), dysarthria, bifacial numbness, and weakness or numbness of part or all of one or both sides of the body.

MANAGEMENT AND PROGNOSIS

To prevent acute recurrence of TIA or threatened stroke, heparin has traditionally been the drug of choice. Before anticoagulation, intracranial hemorrhage should be excluded by computed axial tomography. Contraindications to anticoagulant therapy should be sought out and baseline prothrombin time (PT), partial phromboplastin time (PTT), platelet count, and stool guaiac should be obtained.

The Canadian Cooperative Study Group investigated chronic therapy with aspirin, sulfinpyrazone, or placebo in 585 patients with at least one cerebral or retinal ischemic attack in the 3 months before double-blind randomization. Aspirin reduced the risk of stroke or death in men by 48%, but no significant trends were observed for the use of aspirin in women or for sulfinpyrazone in men or women.

It is our practice for all patients with TIA to obtain carotid Doppler and opthalmoplethysmography in order to assess non-invasively possible carotid artery stenosis. The use of two-dimensional cardiac echo to exclude a cardiac source of emboli has a low yield unless the patient has atrial fibrillation or underlying cardiac disease such as prior myocardial infarction with left ventricular aneurysm. In patients with recurrent TIAs who do not respond to medical treatment, carotid angiography should be considered. Such patients should be in generally good medical condition so that if an ulcerated carotid plaque is found, carotid endarterectomy can be undertaken without undue morbidity.

The prognosis of patients with TIAs is highly variable. A stroke may occur after one or two TIA attacks or only after hundreds of attacks. Often, TIAs gradually cease spontaneously. In one study it was found that about 20% of strokes that follow TIAs occur within 1 month of the first attack. About 50% of the strokes occurred within 1 year of the first attack.

CONCLUSION

Syncope is a challenging problem, especially in the emergency ward setting where details of previous medical history and a long-term relationship with the patient are usually lacking. The differentiation of syncope from other conditions such as seizure disorder must first be made. Then the etiology of the syncopal episode must be sought carefully. The emergency ward personnel ideally will act as a team to elicit history pertinent to the syncopal episode. The astute diagnostician will recognize situations for which further emergency evaluation is needed to establish and treat life-threatening conditions such as severe valvular aortic stenosis and cardiac tamponade. Most young, apparently healthy patients will be sent home after a minimal workup. Most older patients, even if apparently healthy, will be admitted for observation (usually with continuous cardiac monitoring). However, generalizations such as these cannot substitute for a sound understanding of the pathophysiology of syncope in addition to experience in dealing with the many clinical settings in which syncope is found.

SUGGESTED READINGS

Adams RD, Victor M: *Principles of Neurology.* New York, McGraw-Hill Book Co, 1981, pp 248–257, 558–563, 732–734.

Alpert JS, Smith R, Carlson J, Ockene IS, Dexter L, Dalen JE: Mortality in patients treated for pulmonary embolism. *J Am Med Assoc* 1976; 236:1477–1480.

Alpert JS, Smith RE, Ockene IS, Ashkenazi J, Dexter L, Dalen JE: Treatment of massive pulmonary embolism: The role of pulmonary embolectomy. *Am Heart J* 1975; 89:413–418.

Antman EM, Cargill V, Grossman W: Low-pressure cardiac tamponade. *Ann Intern Med* 1979; 91:403–406.

Bigger JT Jr: Mechanisms and diagnosis of arrhythmias, in Braunwald E (ed): *Heart Disease.* Philadelphia, WB Saunders Co, 1980, p 680.

Braunwald E: Valvular heart disease, in Braunwald E (ed): *Heart Disease.* Philadelphia, WB Saunders Co, 1980, pp 1095–1165.

Canadian Cooperative Study Group. Randomized trial of aspirin and sulfinpyrazone in threatened stroke. *N Engl J Med* 1978; 299:53–59.

Compton D, Hill PM, Sinclair JD: Weight-lifter's blackout. *Lancet* 1973; 2:1234–1237.

Couch NP, Baldwin SS, Crane C: Mortality and morbidity rates after inferior vena caval clipping. *Surgery* 1975; 77:106–112.

Currier RD, DeJong RN, Bole GG: Pulseless disease, central nervous system manifestations. *Neurology* (NY) 1954; 4:818–830.

Dalen JE, Grossman W: Profiles in pulmonary embolism, in Grossman W (ed): *Cardiac Catheterization and Angiography.* Philadelphia, Lea & Febiger, 1980, pp 336–339.

Darsee JR, Braunwald E: Disease of the pericardium, in Braunwald E (ed): *Heart Disease.* Philadelphia, WB Saunders Co, 1980, pp 1530–1537.

Day SC, Cook EF, Funkenstein H, Goldman L: Evaluation and outcome of emergency room patients with transient loss of consciousness. *Am J Med* 1982; 73:15–23.

DiMarco JP, Ruskin JN: Recurrent unexplained syncope: Use of intra-cardiac electrophysiology. *Primary Cardiol* 1982; 8:21–32.

Dressler W: Effort syncope as an early manifestation of primary pulmonary hypertension. *Am J Med Sci* 1952; 223:131–143.

Dunn MI, Carley JE: Syncope, in Eliot RS, Wolf GL, Forker AD (eds): *Cardiac Emergencies.* Mount Kisco, NY, Futura Publishing Co Inc, 1977, pp 95–118.

Engel GL: Psychologic stress, vasodepressor (vasovagal) syncope, and sudden death. *Ann Intern Med* 1978; 89:403–412.

Glick G, Yu PN: Hemodynamic changes during spontaneous vaso-vagal reactions. *Am J Med* 1963; 34:42–51.

Goldhaber SZ: Pulmonary embolism, in Kloner R (ed): *Synopsis and Manual of Cardiology.* New York, John Wiley & Sons Inc, in press, 1983.

Goldhaber SZ, Hennekens CH, Evans DA, Newton EC, Godleski JJ: Factors associated with the correct antemortem diagnosis of major pulmonary embolism. *Am J Med* 1982; 73:822–826.

Haldane JH: Micturition syncope: Two case reports and a review of the literature. *Can Med Assoc J* 1969; 101:712–713.

Hancock EW: Syncope, in Rubenstein E, Federman D (eds): *Sci Am Medicine*. IV-1 to IV-4, May 1981 (chapter 1).

Jacobson RR, Ross Russell RW: Glossopharyngeal neuralgia with cardiac arrhythmia: A rare but treatable cause of syncope. *Br Med J* 1979; 1:379–380.

Jervell A, Lange-Nielsen F: Congenital deaf mutism, functional heart disease, with prolongation of the QT interval and sudden death. *Am Heart J* 1957; 54:59–68.

Lesser LM, Wenger NK: Carotid sinus syncope. *Heart Lung* 1976; 5:453–456.

Levin B, Posner JB: Swallow syncope: Report of a case and review of the literature. *Neurology (Minneapolis)* 1972; 22:1086–1093.

Longhurst JC: Arterial baroreceptors in health and disease. *Cardiovasc Rev Rep* 1982; 3:271–298.

Lorell BH, Paulus WJ, Grossman W, Wynne J, Cohn PF, Braunwald E: Improved diastolic function and systolic performance in hypertrophic cardiomyopathy after nifedipine. *N Engl J Med* 1980; 303:801–803.

Lown B: Mental stress, arrhythmias and sudden death. *Am J Med* 1982; 72:177–180.

McAnulty JH, Rahimtoola SH, Murphy E, DeMots H, Ritzmann L, Kanarek PE, Kauffman S: Natural history of "high-risk" bundle-branch block. Final report of a prospective study. *N Engl J Med* 1982; 307:137–143.

McIntosh HD, Estes EH, Warren JV: The mechanism of cough syncope. *Am Heart J* 1956; 52:70–82.

MacMurray FG: Stokes-Adams disease: A historical review. *N Engl J Med* 1957; 256:643–650.

Metcalfe J, Ueland K: Maternal cardiovascular adjustments to pregnancy. *Prog Cardiovasc Dis* 1974; 16:363–374.

Moss AF, Davis RJ: Brady-tachy syndrome. *Prog Cardiovasc Dis* 1974; 16:439–454.

Moss AJ, Schwartz PJ: Delayed repolarization (QT or QTU prolongation) and malignant ventricular arrhythmias. *Mod Concepts Cardiovasc Dis* 1982; 51:85–90.

Pathy MS: Defaecation syncope. *Age Ageing* 1978; 7:233–236.

Pomerantz B, O'Rourke RA: The Stokes-Adams syndrome. *Am J Med* 1969; 46:941–960.

Reich P, De Silva RA, Lown B, Murawski BJ: Acute psychological disturbances preceding life-threatening ventricular arrhythmias. *J Am Med Assoc* 1981; 246:233–235.

Rosing DR, Kent KM, Borer JS, Seides SF, Maron BJ, Epstein SE: Verapamil therapy: A new approach to the pharmacologic treatment of hypertrophic cardiomyopathy. I. Hemodynamic effects. *Circulation* 1979; 60:1201–1207.

Rosing DR, Kent KM, Maron BJ, Epstein SE: Verapamil therapy: A new approach to the pharmacologic treatment of hypertrophic cardiomyopathy. II. Effects on exercise capacity and symptomatic status. *Circulation* 1979; 60:1208–1213.

Ross J Jr, Braunwald E: The influence of corrective operations on the natural history of aortic stenosis. *Circulation* 1968; 37 (suppl V):61–67.

Rybak ME, Handin RI: The science and art of using heparin. *J Cardiovasc Med* 1981; 6:265–275.

Sasahara AA, Dalen JE: Should fibrinolytic drugs be used to treat acute pulmonary embolism? *J Cardiovasc Med* 1980; 5:793–814.

Shabetai R, Grossman W: Profiles in constrictive pericarditis, restrictive cardiomyopathy and cardiac tamponade, in Grossman W (ed): *Cardiac Catheterization and Angiography*. Philadelphia, Lea & Febiger, 1980, pp 369–372.

Shy GM, Drager GA: A neurological syndrome associated with orthostatic hypotension: A clinico-pathologic study. *Arch Neurol* 1960; 2:511–527.

Sobel BE, Roberts R: Hypotension and syncope, in Braunwald E (ed): *Heart Disease*. Philadelphia, WB Saunders Co, 1980, pp 952–966.

Thames MD, Alpert JS, Dalen JE: Syncope in patients with pulmonary embolism. *J Am Med Assoc* 1977; 238:2509–2511.

Thomas JT: Hyperactive carotid sinus reflex and carotid sinus syncope. *Mayo Clin Proc* 1969; 44:127–139.

Thomas JE, Schirger A, Fealey RD, Sheps SG: Orthostatic hypotension. *Mayo Clin Proc* 1981; 56:117–125.

Whisnant JP, Matsumoto N, Elveback LR: Transient cerebral ischemic attacks in a community: Rochester, Minnesota, 1955 through 1969. *Mayo Clin Proc* 1973; 48:194–198.

Wynne J, Braunwald E: The cardiomyopathies and myocarditides, in Braunwald E (ed): *Heart Disease*. Philadelphia, WB Saunders Co, 1980, pp 1437–1500.

Ziegler MG: Postural hypotension. *Ann Rev Med* 1980; 31:239–245.

Ziegler MG, Lake CR, Kopin IJ: The sympathetic-nervous-system defect in primary orthostatic hypotension. *N Engl J Med* 1977; 296:293–297.

10
COMA

Dennis M.D. Landis

Chapter 10 outlines an approach to the initial management and diagnostic evaluation of patients presenting to the emergency room in coma. We use the word *coma* to describe a depressed level of awareness from which the individual cannot be roused to a usual level of responsiveness. A comatose patient is unable to perceive or respond adequately to internal and external stimuli; therefore, the physician must protect the patient from aspiration, hypothermia, hypotension, and ventilatory failure. A host of pathologic processes can result in coma, and many of these will lead inexorably to death or to permanent neurologic damage. It is essential to learn as rapidly as possible the nature of the underlying disorder and to institute appropriate therapeutic maneuvers quickly.

DEFINITION AND PATHOPHYSIOLOGY

The words *lethargy, confusion, stupor,* and *coma* describe a range of increasingly severe depression of neurologic function. The confused patient may be alert but is unable to manage the thought processes that subserve perception, memory, and correct language. Stupor is often taken to mean an unconscious state from which the patient may be only transiently aroused to verbalization or fairly appropriate warding responses by noxious stimuli. In coma, there is no evident appropriate response to exogenous or endogenous stimuli, and homeostatic functions are beginning to fail. It is probably unnecessary to label the patient precisely as stuporous or comatose because in a given patient the level of function may fluctuate from moment to moment and because the same pathologic processes will be found to cause a wide range of neurologic dysfunctions.

The normal ability of a patient to perceive exogenous and internal stimuli and to respond appropriately is based on the capacity of the brainstem reticular formation to maintain arousal in the integrating function of the cerebral cortex. Lesions in the upper pons or midbrain interrupt the reticular activating system, and the state of arousal necessary for perception and processing is lost or cannot be sustained. Bilateral damage to the cerebral cortex directly interferes with integrative capabilities and in most clinical situations is also accompanied by an altered level of awareness. Processes that depress both the cerebral cortex and the ascending reticular activating system, such as metabolic derangement or intoxication, may cause both altered arousal function and impaired integrative function.

Transtentorial Herniation

The process that poses the gravest immediate hazard to the patient and that is of utmost concern in the emergency room is transtentorial herniation. This process, which is potentially reversible early in its course, can rapidly lead to death if it is not treated effectively. Transtentorial herniation is basically a pathologic extrusion of brain tissue from one compartment to another within the skull caused by increased pressure and resulting in fatal compression of vital regions. The tentorium is a tough membrane that separates the cerebral hemispheres above from the cerebellum and brainstem below in the tight cavity of the skull. If a space-occupying lesion such as a tumor with its surrounding edema begins to expand within the skull, the intracranial pressure must increase. Early on, there is a decrease in the volume of cerebrospinal fluid and blood as those fluids are pushed out. Continued expansion above the tentorium forces a portion of the brain to herniate through the aperture of the tentorium as the brain mass squeezes from the region of increased pressure toward the single available opening at the foramen magnum, where the spinal cord exits from the skull.

If the mass is in the temporal or parietal lobes, the medial portion of the temporal lobe is the tissue first forced through the tentorium apertures. The herniating temporal lobe directly compresses cranial nerve III (oculomotor nerve), and as a result the ipsilateral pupil dilates and extraocular movements are paralyzed. If the downward pressure continues, the herniating temporal lobe thrusts the brainstem laterally against the unyielding opposite edge of the tentorium; the pyramidal tract is injured and hemiparesis ipsilateral to the herniating tissue results (Figure 10.1). Weakness is bilateral, however, if the expanding lesion has also independently injured the ipsilateral corticospinal system. Unless the distortion and compression of the brainstem are promptly reversed, respiration becomes irregular and then stops as medullary centers are injured. This sequence is sometimes heralded by a dramatic bradycardia or by a widening pulse pressure (Cushing's phenomenon). Coma with a fixed and dilated pupil, ipsilateral hemiparesis, and altered respiratory pattern is a harbinger of imminent death and demands that the increased intracranial pressure be lessened immediately by therapy.

Less frequently, the expanding intracranial lesion is frontal, occipital, or at the vertex and exerts a more symmetric pressure downward so that the diencephalon (the central mass of the

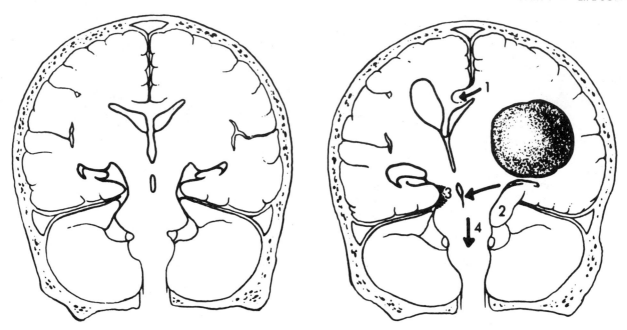

Figure 10.1 Intracranial shifts and transtentorial herniation from supratentorial mass effect. The drawing on the left shows the relationships of the various supratentorial and infratentorial compartments as seen in a coronal section. The drawing on the right illustrates (1) herniation of the cingulate gyrus under the falx, (2) herniation of the temporal lobe past the tentorium, (3) compression of the opposite cerebral peduncle against the unyielding tentorium, producing Kernohan's notch, and (4) downward displacement of the diencephalon and brainstem through the tentorial aperture. (From Plum FJ, Posner JB: Diagnosis of stupor and coma, in *Contemporary Neurology Series* ed 3. Philadelphia, FA Davis Co, 1980. Used by permission.)

cerebrum) rather than the temporal lobe is forced through the tentorial aperture. Distortion of the diencephalon promptly depresses consciousness, and traction on the posterior cerebral arteries and other arteries of the circulation of the midbrain and brainstem will eventually cause patchy ischemia of the midbrain and pons. Such "central" herniation may not be heralded by compression of cranial nerve III and is less easily recognized than herniation of the temporal lobe. An expanding mass below the tentorium, within the posterior fossa that is occupied by the cerebellum and brainstem, can cause herniation of cerebellar tissue either upward through the tentorial aperture or downward through the foramen magnum. In either case compression of the brainstem may be fatal.

In the emergency room the physician initially has to proceed on the assumption that coma and neurologic deficits referrable to the brainstem are due to herniation, and therapy to decrease intracranial pressure must be started immediately. For patients who are actually suffering from brainstem ischemia or hemorrhage, such measures are not harmful although not beneficial.

INITIAL ASSESSMENT

Ideally, evaluation of the patient in coma has the same elements of any diagnostic process: (1) accumulation of a pertinent, detailed history; (2) complete physical examination with special attention to the compromised system; and (3) selection and evaluation of appropriate diagnostic aids.

The temporal sequence of orderly evaluation is inevitably deranged when the physician is dealing with a comatose patient because initial management and sometimes empirical therapy must be instituted before a leisurely history taking or complete examination can be performed. In this section the items of historical data and the pertinent aspects of physical examination will be listed together with some of the reasons for obtaining that information. We have to realize that in actual practice the information will be accumulated as it is possible rather than in tidy sequential fashion. The actual first steps are discussed in the section "Initial Management," below. It is important, however, to acquire all of the information listed in every case as quickly as possible. Occasionally a bit of history or some aspect of physical examination will seem to point to a specific diagnosis, but a thorough evaluation will lead to an entirely different direction. It may be tedious, but it is certainly worthwhile for the physician to gather all of the information possible even though he or she has already formulated a diagnostic impression.

History

Since a comatose patient cannot describe the immediate past, the history must be gleaned from friends, relations, police, ambulance attendants, witnesses, assailants, or old hospital records. Nobody with potential information should be allowed to leave the emergency room until he or she has been adequately questioned. The essential information required in every case includes the rate of onset, probability of trauma, and whether certain predisposing circumstances existed (Table 10.1).

ABRUPT OR INSIDIOUS ONSET

The character of the onset of coma is important. A history of progressing confusion or hemiparesis implicates a slowly expanding mass such as a tumor, an abscess, or a chronic subdural hematoma. In contrast, hypertensive hemorrhage or subarachnoid hemorrhage is associated with the abrupt onset of coma. Occlusive vascular disease in the territory irrigated by

TABLE 10.1 History Immediately Relevant to the Comatose Patient

Abrupt or insidious onset
Recent trauma
Cardiovascular disease (arrhythmia, hypertension)
Metabolic disorders (diabetes, renal insufficiency, Addison's)
Known seizure disorder
Anticoagulation or clotting disorder
Likelihood of intoxication, suicide effort, and so on.

the basilar artery may cause stuttering and waxing and waning deficits that progress by abrupt exacerbations to coma.

RECENT TRAUMA

The likelihood of trauma must be ascertained whenever possible. Massive head trauma sufficient to result in immediate coma or coma emerging in a few hours may have caused an epidural hematoma, one or more subdural hematomas, or intraparenchymal hemorrhage—any of these may require prompt surgical intervention. Major trauma that is followed by immediate coma may also have caused diffuse concussion and contusion that can be accompanied by markedly increased intracranial pressure. Less severe trauma a week or more before the loss of consciousness may have caused a chronic subdural hematoma. Occasionally a history of trauma may be misleading. For example, a patient who has been hemiplegic because of an unsuspected tumor may have fallen many times before finally becoming obtunded. In seeking a history of trauma, we should be impressed only when definite trauma has been observed or when the abrupt onset of coma in the absence of trauma was clearly witnessed. Otherwise we should proceed with the presumption that trauma and its sequelae have not been eliminated as significant factors contributing to the comatose state.

CARDIOVASCULAR DISEASE

Heart or lung disorders are also potentially significant factors in possible etiologies of coma. A history of claudication, for example, often indicates advanced peripheral atheromatous vascular disease, which may be associated with occlusive vascular disease in the basilar or carotid arteries. Severe or longstanding hypertension is almost invariably found to be a concomitant of hypertensive intraparenchymal hemorrhage. A myocardial infarction and arrhythmias related to myocardial vascular disease occasionally produce transient cerebral anoxia severe enough to cause coma. A history of severe pulmonary disease should suggest hypoxia and hypercapnia.

METABOLIC DISORDERS

Any of a number of metabolic disorders, including diabetes, renal insufficiency, and adrenal insufficiency can result in coma. A diabetic, for example, may become comatose from too much or too little insulin. Metastatic carcinoma increases the likelihood of hypercalcemia and eventual coma (see also Table 10.2).

TABLE 10.2 Major Causes of Coma without Focal Deficits

Hypoglycemia
Ketoacidosis/hyperosmolar state
Renal failure
Hepatic failure
Hypo/hypernatremia (can reflect inappropriate antidiuretic hormone syndrome from CNS process)
Hypercapnia
Hypoxia
Adrenal insufficiency
Hypo/hyperthyroidism (hypothyroidism may be betrayed by "hung-up" reflexes)
Hypo/hypercalcemia (hypocalcemia sufficient to cause coma will also cause characteristic ECG changes)
Hyperviscosity (often associated with typical retinal changes)
Hypo/hyperthemia

KNOWN SEIZURE DISORDER

Recurrent seizures may be associated with postictal coma, and the history of a seizure disorder should also be a reminder that drugs such as barbiturates may have been available.

ANTICOAGULATION OF CLOTTING DISORDER

Specific inquiries should be made for diseases or drugs that modify the blood coagulation mechanisms. A patient being treated with warfarin (Coumadin) or suffering from a disorder such as thrombocytopenia is at great risk for intracranial bleeding, with or without notable antecedent trauma. Intracranial bleeding often proceeds to death when hemostasis is compromised; therefore, a history of head trauma in a setting of altered blood coagulation mandates an urgent search for subdural or epidermal hematoma.

LIKELIHOOD OF INTOXICATION OR ATTEMPTED SUICIDE

The direct risks of coma due to intoxication are as life threatening as those caused by a mass lesion, but the patient can be spared potentially dangerous diagnostic maneuvers if a good history is obtained. A brief psychological history may be helpful. A depressed patient may have attempted suicide by taking an overdose of a drug. The availability of psychoactive drugs may be suggested by a history of psychiatric care. Although alcoholics are rarely able to drink themselves into coma, as a group they are vulnerable to trauma, intoxication with meth-

anol or propylene glycol, hypoglycemia, thiamine deficiency, seizures, and hepatic encephalopathy, any of which can result in coma. Intoxication in a drug abuser may be inadvertent.

Physical Examination

Detailed physical examination of a comatose patient is absolutely essential. Often in the confusion of initial management or instituting empirical therapy the physician may be tempted to dispense with portions of an unfamiliar neurologic examination, particularly if the likely etiology for the coma is immediately apparent. Such a relaxed approach, though, will eventually result in disaster. The examination, summarized in Table 10.3 and described in the following section, can be carried out in less than 10 minutes and should be performed as early as possible. The general purpose of the physical examination is to assess the presence and distribution of focal neurologic deficits associated with the altered level of awareness. As outlined in Figures 10.2 and 10.3 and as discussed in the section "Clinical Settings," recognizing specific patterns of neurologic dysfunction together with an understanding of their onset will permit a reasonable choice among the several diagnostic tests and therapeutic maneuvers appropriate to the case. The presence and distribution of neurologic deficits referrable to the brainstem are of critical importance, and special attention must be paid to respiratory pattern, eye movements, oculocephalic or oculovestibular responses, and trigeminal sensory function. Subsequent, repeated neurologic examinations are absolutely necessary to assess the pace and direction of the pathologic process.

TABLE 10.3 Initial Approach to the Comatose Patient

1. Observe the pattern of respiration, and look for spontaneous movement.
2. Stabilize the neck, and inspect for evidence of head trauma.
3. Establish an airway, check pressure and heart rate, draw blood, and inject glucose and thiamine.
4. Look for reaction to visual threat.
5. Look for response to noxious stimuli delivered to each limb, to the chest, and to the face.
6. Test pupillary reaction to light.
7. Fundoscopic exam and inspection of the tympanic membrane.
8. Gag and corneal reflex.
9. Deep tendon reflexes and plantar response.
10. Examine the range of spontaneous eye movements.
11. Test oculocephalic or oculovestibular reflexes.
12. Test for meningeal irritation.

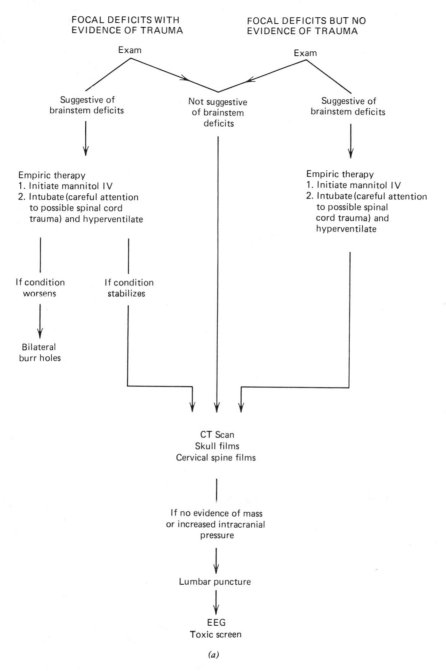

FOCAL DEFICITS WITH
EVIDENCE OF TRAUMA

FOCAL DEFICITS BUT NO
EVIDENCE OF TRAUMA

Exam

Exam

Suggestive of
brainstem deficits

Not suggestive
of brainstem
deficits

Suggestive of
brainstem deficits

Empiric therapy
1. Initiate mannitol IV
2. Intubate (careful attention
   to possible spinal cord
   trauma) and hyperventilate

Empiric therapy
1. Initiate mannitol IV
2. Intubate (careful attention
   to possible spinal
   cord trauma) and
   hyperventilate

If condition
worsens

If condition
stabilizes

Bilateral
burr holes

CT Scan
Skull films
Cervical spine films

If no evidence of mass
or increased intracranial
pressure

Lumbar puncture

EEG
Toxic screen

(a)

Figure 10.2 Sequence of diagnostic tests and initial management when computed tomographic (CT) scanning is available.

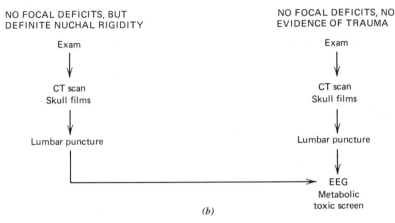

(b)

Figure 10.2 (Continued)

THE FIRST LOOK

While we may be tempted to leap to the bedside and hurry into various manipulations, the very first step should simply be to look carefully for 20–30 seconds. This may be the last opportunity to consider posture, presence or absence of spontaneous movement, respiratory pattern, and evidence of trauma. The patient's posture provides an important index of whether decorticate or decerebrate behavior has emerged (reviewed below). Spontaneous movement may reveal the patient's capacity for volitional movement, whereas focal twitching may provide the only evidence of an ongoing seizure. The presence of vomitus on the clothes or on the face points toward the possibility of aspiration. Periorbital ecchymosis, blood behind the ear (Battle's sign) or in the external auditory meatus, abrasions, and so forth, provide evidence for notable, recent trauma. While inspecting the skin for bruises, we should not overlook hemorrhagic petechiae suggestive of meningococcemia.

The region of brain damage can sometimes be determined by observing the pattern of respiration. Bilateral hemispheric disease or metabolic disorder is often signaled by Cheyne-Stokes respiration, a regular alternation of apnea and hyperpnea with ventilation changing in a smooth crescendo –decrescendo pattern. The length of the cycle and the duration of apnea should be recorded. Many of these patients will demonstrate spontaneous movement at the height of their hyperpneic phase, and their response to external stimuli increases simultaneously. Central neurogenic hyperventilation is rapid, regular, and deep breathing in the absence of hypoxemia and acidosis. This pattern is rare and probably arises from damage between the diencephalon and the middle third of the pons that may reflect compression from transtentorial herniation.

When this pattern is observed arterial blood gasses should be determined to be sure that hypoxemia is not present and to check the arterial pH. If the pH is normal and P_{CO_2} low, an underlying metabolic acidosis is present (for example salicylate intoxication). Apneustic breathing is usually slow, irregularly irregular, and can deteriorate to abrupt apnea. The pattern of ataxic breathing can be encountered in a setting of rapidly expanding posterior fossa masses.

FIRST THERAPY AND CARDIOPULMONARY EXAMINATION

As described below in the section on initial management, a few supportive measures and some empirical therapy must be integrated into the first moments of examination. The exact sequence of maneuvers may vary from patient to patient, but a specific set of tasks must be accomplished in every case. In brief, we must first stabilize the neck to avoid exacerbating any cervical injury. As soon as an airway is assured, the blood pressure, heart rate, heart rhythm, and external evidence of blood loss should be checked to eliminate the specter of hypovolemic shock. Venous blood is drawn for diagnostic studies, intravenous access is established, and glucose and thiamine are injected. Subsequently, we can more carefully review cardiac and pulmonary auscultation and then move promptly to the neurologic examination.

REACTION TO NOISE AND VISUAL THREAT

The patient should be tested for his or her capacity to react to noise and to visual threat. Any response to external stimuli is

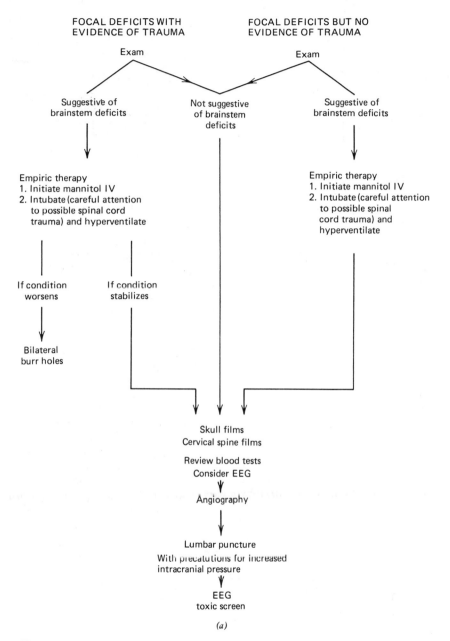

Figure 10.3 Sequence of diagnostic tests and initial management when prompt CT scanning is not available.

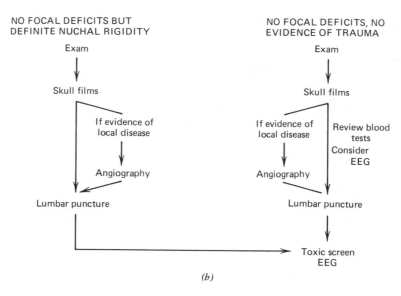

(b)

Figure 10.3 (Continued)

evidence that the pathways subserving the sensory modality are functioning. A patient may not respond to a moderately loud voice, yet a loud clap may elicit a wince; such a reaction indicates that much of the pons is functional.

Reaction to visual threat is gauged by holding open the eyelids and feigning a blow to the eye from the midtemporal visual field; ipsilateral blinking indicates that the retina, optic nerve, contralateral optic radiations and occipital cortex, corticobulbar tracts, and ipsilateral facial motor nucleus and nerve are all working. Caution should be taken to prevent the breeze caused by the threatening movement from stimulating the cornea.

RESPONSE TO PAINFUL STIMULI

Moderately obtunded patients who are not suffering from a structural lesion usually withdraw from a painful pinch on the foot by flexing the knee and hip, and pain inflicted on the fingers often elicits elbow flexion. Such responses, however, may be obliterated by spinal shock or by severe toxic–metabolic insult. Asymmetry of the responsiveness is most often due to an injury somewhere in the corticospinal motor system. A severely noxious stimulus (a pinch just short of laceration) should be applied to the upper extremity or to the sternum; any effort to ward the offending stimulus should be noted, and the laterality of the response should be gauged. A painful stimulus applied to the face, such as compression of the supraorbital with the thumb, sometimes elicits a motor response when

stimuli inflicted elsewhere does not. If response to facial pain is unilateral, other parameters of cranial nerve V (trigeminal) function, especially the corneal response, should be checked to determine whether sensory function has been interrupted.

As we test responses to noxious stimuli, we may observe the emergence of stereotypic decorticate or decerebrate posturing. Decorticate posturing is flexion of the fingers, wrist, and elbow and adduction of the upper arm, rigid extension of the hip and knee, and plantar flexion. When it is observed, the corticospinal tract is probably injured at or rostral to the level of the thalamus. Decerebrate posturing is extension and pronation of the arm with internal rotation at the shoulders, rigid leg extension, and plantar flexion (Figure 10.2). Damage to the rostral half of the pons or to the diencephalon is virtually certain. Decorticate or decerebrate responses may be observed on one or both sides. Although the most troublesome association is with structural disease, either response can develop from toxic–metabolic stress, which usually results in symmetric posturing.

PUPILLARY RESPONSE

Pupillary response to light should be assessed by flashing a bright light into the eye. Normally both pupils constrict, and the stimulated eye usually contracts somewhat more briskly. If both pupils constrict when only one eye is stimulated and stimulation of the other eye elicits no response, the retina or optic nerve of the unresponsive eye is not functioning. Careful fundoscopic examination and inspection for proptosis is necessary in such a setting. When light is flashed into both eyes but only one pupil constricts, the efferent pathway of the unreactive eye may be damaged, possibly because the third cranial nerve is compressed; the oculomotor system should be tested carefully. Parasympathetic fibers originating just rostral to the oculomotor nuclei in the diencephalon and traveling along the third cranial nerve effect pupillary constriction. Sympathetic pathways mediating dilatation of the pupils originate in the hypothalamus and follow a route, most of which is unknown, to synapse in the upper thoracic part of the spinal cord. Sympathetic postganglionic fibers from the superior cervical ganglion follow the carotid artery to the ophthalmic artery and terminate in the iris. Both sympathetic and parasympathetic pathways are tonically active, and much of the brainstem must be intact if they function normally.

Failure of one eye to constrict when stimulated with light is never insignificant. The etiology to be considered most carefully is transtentorial temporal lobe herniation. Bilateral fixed, completely unresponsive pupils that are dilated halfway are usually the result of midbrain lesions involving the oculomotor nuclei. A lesion in the pons that interrupts the sympathetic but not the parasympathetic systems will cause very small but reactive pupils. The abrupt onset of coma with pinpoint reactive pupils is usually a sign of pontine hemorrhage. On the other hand, a lesion affecting only one side of the sympathetic pathways causes Horner's syndrome—pupillary constriction, ptosis, and anhidrosis. The reaction to light is preserved, although at times it is so slight as to require the use of a magnifying glass to detect it. A unilateral Horner's syndrome of recent onset is ominous because it is often associated with the compression of the hypothalamus during an early phase of central or diencephalic transtentorial herniation.

A variety of intoxications can also result in altered pupillary size, but reactivity to light is almost always preserved. An overdose of an opiate (heroin, morphine) or an anticholinesterase (neostigmine, pyridostigmine, or paraquat) can cause pupils to contract; phenothiazines or amphetamines, on the other hand, result in dilatation. A large amount of atropine or scopolamine also causes dilation, but the pupils are unresponsive to light. Glutethimide or a large overdose of barbiturates are associated with midsize pupils that do not respond to light.

FUNDOSCOPIC EXAMINATION AND INSPECTION OF THE TYMPANIC MEMBRANE

Six major fundoscopic findings are of critical importance in establishing the etiology of coma. Papilledema implies that intracranial pressure has been increased for at least 6 hours.

Preretinal (or subhyaloid) hemorrhages, globular accumulations of blood that shift like fluid levels when the position of the head is changed, are due to subarachnoid hemorrhage. Arterial tortuosity and narrowing in association with arteriovenous nicking indicate long-standing hypertension, a frequent concomitant of cerebrovascular disease. Diabetic retinopathy, especially neovascularization, should alert the physician to the possibility of hypoglycemia induced by insulin or by excessive intake of an oral hypoglycemic agent. Occlusion of a central retinal artery or evidence of multiple segmental retinal infarcts may be due to severe carotid atherosclerotic disease. Dilated, sausagelike veins with perivenous hemorrhage occur in hyperviscosity syndromes.

The tympanic membranes should be inspected for three specific entities: rupture of the membrane or blood accumulated behind it from a recent skull fracture; evidence of infection such as may have caused intracerebral abscess or meningitis; old perforations that may interfere with the studies of vestibular caloric responses.

CORNEAL AND GAG REFLEX

The corneal and gag reflexes both give important information about brainstem function. The cornea should be stroked lightly with a cotton wisp. If both eyes blink, the pathways of the sensory root of the fifth cranial nerve to the facial motor nucleus are functional. Blinking of only the unstimulated eye suggests that the facial nucleus of the seventh cranial nerve has been injured on the nonblinking side. No response whatever is a sign of massive brainstem damage or a severe toxic–metabolic insult since the reflex is often preserved even when respirations are low or have been depressed to the point of apnea. The gag reflex, on both the afferent and efferent levels, is mediated principally by the vagus nerve. In contrast to the corneal response, the gag reflex is often lost early from any number of insults. Testing the reflex is useful to determine the likelihood of aspiration. A response on only one side suggests medullary disease; if the response is hypoactive, the corticobulbar tract may be injured.

DEEP TENDON REFLEX AND BABINSKI'S SIGN

The deep tendon reflexes are monosynaptic reflexes at the level of the spinal cord, but the amplitude of the motor response is modulated by the corticospinal tracts. In the initial evaluation of a comatose patient, the symmetry of the deep tendon reflex responses is the key consideration. Unilateral interruption of a corticospinal tract may initially have very little effect on the deep tendon reflexes or it may suppress them; hours or days later, however, the affected reflexes may become relatively hyperactive. We should keep in mind that extremely active, symmetric reflexes may develop in the settings of hypocalcemia or incipient tetany.

If Babinski's sign (extension of the great toe, also described as dorsiflexion of the great toe) is observed in response to firm stroking along the side of the sole from heel to toe, the cortical spinal tract is injured—the normal response is toe flexion. The plantar response is most informative when it occurs on only one side because any one of toxic–metabolic insults may cause bilateral positive Babinski response. Because Babinski's sign may not be demonstrable for hours or days after an acute injury to the corticospinal tract, its absence is rarely informative.

SPONTANEOUS EYE MOVEMENTS

Conjugate lateral gaze is controlled by the cerebral cortex of the frontal lobes in conjunction with the pontine gaze centers near cranial nerve VI nuclei in the pons. Each frontal lobe directs gaze to the opposite side; therefore, a lesion in the right frontal lobe can result in sustained, involuntary, conjugate lateral deviation of the eyes to the right because the left cerebral cortex is functioning unopposed. If damage is limited to the cortex of the frontal lobe, full oculocephalic and oculovestibular responses may be retained (see below). A lesion of the lateral gaze center in the pons prevents gaze to the same side and results in conjugate deviation to the unaffected side; oculocephalic and oculovestibular maneuvers then fail to direct gaze toward the diseased side. Unless a structural injury has occurred, the eyes of an unconscious patient usually are directed straight ahead or are slightly divergent. Roving eye movements, which may be conjugate or disconjugate, indicate that the brainstem is probably intact. Cortical seizure activity can irritate the frontal eye fields and drive gaze away from the abnormally discharging hemisphere, but most often the eyes make episodic movements.

Damage to the rostral pontine tegmentum, usually caused by pontine hemorrhage, may result in a peculiar, characteristic "ocular bobbing." The eyes rest in midposition and intermittently jerk down (and sometimes inward) and then more slowly float back to midposition. The motion was first described as reminiscent of a fishing float as the fish are nibbling.

OCULOCEPHALIC AND OCULOVESTIBULAR REFLEXES

Often the most useful assessment of brainstem function is based on examination of evoked eye movements. The oculocephalic reflexes cause the direction of gaze to be transiently maintained despite passive movement of the patient's head—these reflexes are commonly described as a *doll's eye* or *doll's head* reflex. Normally they are suppressed by voluntary control of gaze, but they can emerge in stupor and coma. The vestibular system and proprioception of head position normally interact with the oculomotor nuclei to produce these reflexes. They must not be tested until fracture or dislocation of the cervical spine has been ruled out; if such an injury is suspected, caloric testing should be substituted for doll's head maneuvers. Testing of oculocephalic or doll's head reflexes is comparatively straightforward. With the patient's nose and eyes pointing straight up, the examiner should briskly rotate the head to aim the nose over the right shoulder. During this passive movement, with intact oculocephalic reflexes, gaze continues to be directed toward the ceiling; thus the right eye adducts toward the nose as a medial rectus contracts (third cranial nerve) and the left eye abducts laterally as the lateral rectus (sixth cranial nerve) contracts. Rotating to the left will test the complementary responses.

Interpretation of the abnormal response can be complicated. Initially we should assume that the afferent portion of the reflex is functioning; abnormal reflexes should then be attributed to failure of the efferent oculomotor system. If abduction seems to be impaired and if the seventh cranial nerve on that side proves to be weak, pontine damage is likely. Failure of adduction in an eye with pupillary dilation suggests that the third cranial nerve itself is being compressed outside the brainstem; the temporal lobe may be herniating. Although isolated failure of adduction may be due to damage in the ipsilateral medial longitudinal fasciculus, it is rarely a result of a pontine lesion causing coma.

The testing of oculovestibular function involves irrigating the ears with warm or cold water. Because almost the same system is evaluated in oculocephalic testing, the procedure is unnecessary if the oculocephalic responses are normal. A maximal response can be elicited when the head is elevated to 30 degrees from supine so the lateral semicircular canal is vertical. However, if injury to the cervical spine is suspected or certain, testing can be performed with the patient supine. After inspecting the tympanic membrane to be sure it is not perforated, we slowly flood the external auditory meatus with ice cold water (50 ml over 30 seconds). The usual response of a moderately obtunded patient is nystagmus with the fast component toward the opposite ear; patients in deeper coma, on the other hand, manifest tonic deviation to the irrigated side within 2–3 minutes. An asymmetric response is most informative. Although a severe toxic—metabolic insult can block all oculomotor responses, it usually does so symmetrically.

A few reservations must always be kept in mind when assessing ocular motility. Because Wernicke's encephalopathy in alcoholics is often accompanied by unpredictable ophthal-moplegia, interpretation of oculocephalics in such patients is nearly impossible. Barbiturate, phenytoin, or glutethimide intoxication also can immobilize the eyes.

TESTING FOR MENINGEAL IRRITATION

When the meninges are irritated by blood or inflammatory exudate, reflexes emerge to keep the spinal column as short as possible and thus minimize traction on the inflamed meninges. Reflex resistence to passive neck flexion between supine and 45 degrees is a common manifestation of that response. Although restricting the test to that range may make it less sensitive in young patients, confusion with the osteoarthritic stiffness of the elderly is avoided. Forced deviation of the neck in the presence of meningeal irritation at times will cause the hip to flex, and the neck may extend if the knee is extended from a flexed position while the hips are flexed.

Diagnostic Aids

Selecting diagnostic aids and deciding about the urgency with which they are obtained require an understanding of the test itself and its relevance to the clinical situation at hand. In this section, we list a set of tests that should be performed in every instance of coma and briefly describe other laboratory or radiologic procedures that may be of use in the evaluation of a patient in coma. The way in which we choose tests is presented in detail in the section "Clinical Settings" below.

The following determinations should be obtained immediately for all comatose patients:

1. Blood tests: arterial blood gases, sodium, potassium, calcium, blood urea nitrogen (BUN), glucose, complete blood count, platelet count, prothrombin time
2. Electrocardiogram (ECG)

The information from these blood tests is essential to evaluating various metabolic and toxic causes of coma (see Table 10.2) and cardiopulmonary status. The electrocardiogram detects acute myocardial infarction or ischemia and may reveal supraventricular arrhythmias attributable to increased intracranial pressure. Blood, urine, and gastric aspirates can be set aside for later toxic screening tests.

Further diagnostic testing usually involves some risk to the patient, either because of the time involved or because of the nature of the tests. Selection of appropriate further tests should involve consideration of the etiologic possibilities in the individual patient and the information generated by each test. It is important to emphasize that selection of diagnostic tests and

the institution of initial management are the responsibilities of physicians in the emergency room. We cannot await the neurologist or neurosurgeon.

COMPUTED TOMOGRAPHY

Computed tomography (CT) is the single most useful test in the evaluation of the comatose patient. This x-ray technique rapidly generates a high-resolution image of x-ray density within the skull and is particularly useful in defining the size and position of ventricles, the presence of intraparenchymal or subarachnoid hemorrage, subdural or epidural hematomas, and the presence of nonbrain masses such as an abscess or tumor. There is essentially no direct risk from this immensely useful examination, but it usually requires that the patient remain supine for 10–30 minutes. Comatose patients should not be allowed to remain unaccompanied during this interval, and it is probably safest for the emergency room physician to be in attendance the entire time. Special precautions should be taken to avoid aspiration. Unfortunately, CT scanning is not available in most emergency rooms, and so the physician is usually forced to rely on the less-powerful combination of skull films and angiography.

SKULL FILMS

Skull films are most often used to look for evidence of fracture. When the pineal is calcified we may also be able to estimate the position of midline brain structures; lateral displacement of the pineal, for example, may provide evidence of mass effect above the tentorium. Infrequently, skull films may reveal focal bone erosion suggestive of a localized mass, clinoid resorption characteristic of sustained increase in intracranial pressure, or calcifications around an arteriovenous malformation or mass. The direct risk is small, but the patient must never be left unattended during this examination.

CEREBRAL ANGIOGRAPHY

Injection of x-ray opaque media into the cerebral vessels, preferably by the femoral route, permits observations of vessel caliber and distribution. This is essentially the only approach to definitive recognition of stenosis, embolic occlusions, aneurysm, and vasospasm. If a CT scan is not available, we can use angiography to detect distortion of vasculature caused by subdural hematomas, mass effect, or hydrocephalus. The risk of the procedure varies with the condition of the patient and the skill of the angiographer, but it is never insignificant. High-pressure injection of contrast media may dislodge an atheroma, causing embolism, or create a traumatic dissection of the arterial wall. For poorly understood reasons, injection of contrast material may precipitate infarction in an ischemic region. Often the chief limitation in this test is that it may take too many hours to arrange.

ELECTROENCEPHALOGRAPHY

Two very significant classes of diagnostic information can be derived from the electroencephalography (EEG) with no direct risk to the patient. Masses such as tumor or abscess may be betrayed by "phase reversal" of brain waves. Seizure activity sufficient to cause a profoundly depressed level of awareness is often evident to the skilled interpreter. In general, brain wave activity is an indicator of cerebral cortex function and may be useful in providing confirmatory evidence of local dysfunction (for example, that resulting from compression by an overlying subdural hematoma). This test is usually done after CT scanning or skull films and angiography.

ECHOENCEPHALOGRAPHY

Echoencephalography is designed to demonstrate the position of the third ventricle (normally in the midline) within the skull by bouncing ultrasound waves from it. While there is no risk, the information is reliable only in very experienced hands and should be used only when a CT scan is unavailable and the position of the pineal gland cannot be seen in the skull films.

LUMBAR PUNCTURE

Lumbar puncture permits analysis of the cerebrospinal fluid and is indispensable in the diagnosis of meningitis. The usual method of lumbar puncture in the lateral decubitus position is described in Procedure 29, and lumbar puncture in the setting of increased intracranial pressure is described below under "Initial Management." In every case, the physician must study the cerebrospinal fluid personally for (1) presence, type, and number of leukocytes; (2) presence and character of microorganisms, especially bacteria; (3) presence of red cells (counting more than one tube); and (4) presence of xanthochromia, a distinctly yellowish discoloration resulting from the breakdown of blood within the subarachnoid space, or pigments leaking from a chronic hematoma.

Lumbar puncture can be mortally dangerous in comatose patients. Removal of fluid from the lumbar sac (and continued drainage of cerebrospinal fluid through the puncture site in the dura) lowers pressure at the end of the neuraxis. If intracranial pressure is increased, particularly if the pressure below the tentorium is increased, skull contents will flow toward the lowered lumbar pressure causing in the worst instant herniation of the cerebellar tonsils and fatal brainstem compression. Whenever possible, the lumbar puncture should be deferred until the presence of an intracranial mass has been ruled out. Methods of dealing with unsuspected raised intracranial pressure discovered during the process of lumbar puncture are discussed in the management section below.

INITIAL MANAGEMENT

General Measures

The following basic measures must be taken in every case:

1. Establish an airway; if at all possible, delay intubation until the neck has been stabilized.
2. Check blood pressure and pulse; institute therapy for hypovolemic shock if clear evidence of blood loss exists.
3. Draw diagnostic studies.
4. Inject glucose and thiamine; glucose is administered as an empiric therapy for the possibility of insulin or drug-induced hypoglycemia and also for the hypoglycemia that occurs in debilitated chronic alcoholics. Thiamine prevents the exacerbation of Wernicke's encephalopathy that can occur in an alcoholic given glucose alone.
5. Establish intravenous access, but do not infuse more than 100 ml/hr until the possibility of cerebral edema is eliminated.
6. Stabilize the neck and inspect for evidence of trauma. Any person unconscious after a major trauma obviously should be protected against cervical subluxation, preferably by a "four-post" collar or simply by sandbags around the head and neck. The same precautions should be taken when the history is even slightly unclear. Appropriate x-ray films should be obtained promptly after the completion of the physical exam because the risk of aspiration is greatest while the patient remains supine. Inspect the scalp minutely for contusion and palpable fracture lines. Blood behind the tympanic membrane is an important sign of temporal bone fracture, and the tympanic membrane may be ruptured by petrous bone or middle fossa fractures. Basilar skull fractures cause ecchymoses behind the ear and over the mastoid. Peculiar periorbital bruises can result from frontal fracture; proptosis can indicate retrobulbar hemorrhage or fracture of the orbit.
7. Monitor the ECG.

8. Place a nasogastric tube to drain gastric contents (set aside an alioquot for toxicologic analysis).

9. Maintain normal body temperature.

Treatment of Increased Intracranial Pressure

INTRAVENOUS MANNITOL

The initial medical therapy for transtentorial herniation, mass effect, and increased intracranial pressure resulting from meningitis or a subarachnoid hemorrhage is aimed at reducing the volume of water in the cranial cavity: Infuse 500 ml of 20% mannitol solution over 30 minutes. More can follow, but first be sure that the patient can make urine. Brain water moves down the resulting osmotic gradient into the vascular space and out of the skull, and it is hoped that intracranial pressure may be reduced sufficiently to arrest or reverse herniation.

HYPERVENTILATION

If respiration is already compromised or if Cushing's signs (bradycardia, widened pulse pressure) are present, the patient should be intubated and hyperventilated to an arterial P_{CO_2} of 20 mm Hg (arterial pH should not exceed 7.55).

DEXAMETHASONE

If the possibility of cerebral edema exists, dexamethasone should be given intravenously as soon as convienient since its effects on cerebral edema will not occur for several hours. A reasonable dose schedule is 10 mg given intravenously to start and 4 mg given intravenously or intramuscularly every 6 hours thereafter.

LUMBAR PUNCTURE IN THE CONTEXT OF INCREASED INTRACRANIAL PRESSURE

When correctly placed, the lumbar puncture needle pokes a hole in the meninges, allowing cerebrospinal fluid to leak around the needle (and draining even more rapidly if the needle is withdrawn from the rent it has created). When intracranial pressure is increased, the leak of cerebrospinal fluid through the needle hole creates a gradient in pressure. The living brain has the consistency of jello and shifts to follow the pressure gradient causing, in the worst instance, herniation of the cerebellar tonsils through the foramen magnum or transtentorial herniation. Both result in acute compression of the brainstem and can end in respiratory or cardiac arrest. Once the needle is in, the disastrous sequence is entrained, and the therapeutic

response must be immediate. The presence of raised intracranial pressure is recognized as the fluid level in the manometer rises past 250 cm H_2O. Stop withdrawing cerebrospinal fluid and *with the needle still in place* have someone else straighten the flexed neck and legs from the usual lateral decubitus position. Recheck the pressure and proceed normally if it has fallen to 180 cm H_2O. If it hovers at 250 cm H_2O, take less than 5 ml of cerebrospinal fluid, withdraw the needle, and arrange to have the patient watched continuously for the next 4 hours. If the pressure remains above 250 cm H_2O, call for an assistant to infuse sufficient intravenous 20% mannitol solution to bring it down to that level before withdrawing the needle. If the cerebrospinal fluid does not provide evidence of subarachnoid hemorrhage or meningitis, presume that a space-occupying lesion is present and that danger from transtentorial herniation remains imminent.

CLINICAL SETTINGS

The orderly sifting of potential etiologies of the coma and selection of appropriate diagnostic tests are facilitated by combining data from the history and physical examination to place the patient in one of several tentative categories:

1. Coma with focal neurologic deficits and evidence of recent trauma
2. Coma with focal neurologic deficits but no history or evidence of trauma
3. Coma with meningeal irritation
4. Coma without focal signs

The value of such an approach is that each category has a set of likely etiologies. A flow chart for selection of diagnostic tests when prompt CT scanning is available is presented in Figure 10.2; alternative approaches that can be used when CT scanning is not possible (but cerebral angiography is) are presented in Figure 10.3. The flow charts are intended to be guides when essentially no useful history is available. They emphasize the necessity of establishing the presence or absence of significant intracranial mass effect before lumbar puncture. In general, proceed to the next step only when the prior test offers no diagnosis and no contraindication.

The urgency with which additional tests are obtained should vary with the particular clinical situation. Whenever transtentorial herniation has occurred or seems imminent, everything to identify the site of a mass lesion must be done immediately so that surgical therapy can be instituted when appropriate. Similarly, when meningitis is a major consideration, steps must be taken to evaluate the possibility of a mass lesion and lumbar puncture must be done as soon as possible. On the other hand, a history and examination characteristic of subarachnoid hemorrhage allows us to arrive at a fairly reliable tentative diagnosis, and confirmation by lumbar puncture could be delayed up to 8 hours while a CT scan is undertaken. Moderate stupor, absence of focal deficits, and a definite history of drug ingestion similarly allow a deliberate pace though eventually the diagnosis of intoxication must be confirmed.

Focal Deficits with Evidence of Trauma

Major trauma followed by immediate loss of consciousness may have caused concussion, brain contusion, and/or intracranial hematomas. A contused brain functions poorly, and the patient may present a bewildering melange of field cuts, pyramidal tract disease, and ophthalmoplegia from brainstem trauma. There is no specific therapeutic response to contusion apart from the usual measures directed against cerebral edema. Unfortunately, it is necessary to be sure that focal deficits have not been caused by more ominous hematomas. Severe head trauma may cause parenchymal hemorrhage, resulting in collections of blood at the frontal poles or temporal lobe tips, epidural hematomas, or acute subdural hematomas, all of which compress and distort the brain and may lead to transtentorial herniation. Epidural hematomas result from bleeding of lacerated arteries outside the meninges. Trauma sufficient to cause an epidural hematoma may often cause immediate loss of consciousness, but occasionally the history is obtained that a child or person under 35 years who has been struck a forceful blow awakes from a transient spell of unconsciousness, walks away, and within 2–4 hours collapses again. The artery, usually a middle meningeal or one of its branches, is lacerated by a temporal or parietal skull fracture and has been bleeding the entire time. Subdural hematoma can be the most difficult of neurologic diagnoses. The bleeding usually comes from torn veins that bridge the space between the dura mater and pia arachnoid. All ages are susceptible, but the combination of brain atrophy and adhesion of the dura to the skull in the elderly makes them particularly vulnerable. Subdurals can accumulate rapidly, creating a clinical picture essentially like that of an epidural bleed and necessitating surgical intervention. A particularly lethal combination can be persistent subdural bleeding in the anticoagulated patient.

DIAGNOSTIC PROCEDURES

The diagnostic procedure of choice in the situation of coma and evidence of trauma is a *CT scan*—without delay. The CT scans precisely define the site and size of intracranial hemorrhage. *Skull films* and *cervical spine films* should also be obtained as soon as possible to detect associated fractures. When CT scanning cannot be done immediately, skull films must be the only screening test. Time is important because some of these hematomas are surgically remediable, and all may lead to permanent deficits over unpredictable, but often short, intervals. If skull films are normal and a CT scan is unavailable, cerebral angiography should be undertaken promptly.

INITIAL TREATMENT

Osmotic Therapy and Hyperventilation

In certain situations following severe head trauma it is prudent to begin empirical therapy for cerebral edema, and it rarely may be necessary to proceed to surgery before completing the list of diagnostic tests. If the traumatized patient presents with or develops signs of brainstem damage, presume that the brainstem deficits reflect herniation and start mannitol infusion and intubation immediately. If clear-cut signs referable to one hemisphere precede decerebration or the development of transtentorial herniation, osmotic therapy and hyperventilation may be insufficient to control the mass effect of an acute subdural or epidural bleed. The failure of osmotic therapy and hyperventilation to arrest neurologic deterioration forces us to the last resort of empirical burr holes to evacuate hematomas.

Burr Holes

The failure of osmotic therapy and hyperventilation to prevent clinical deterioration after recent major head trauma or the emergence of frank transtentorial herniation after the institution of those therapeutic maneuvers are sufficient indications to perform empirical bilateral burr holes to evacuate presumed subdural or epidural hematomas. If the herniation syndrome is accompanied by respiratory arrest or Cushing's signs, the burr holes must be done in the emergency room. This situation is very rare, but it is a true emergency that requires immediate response. If a surgeon cannot be there in 10 minutes, the responsibility for drilling the burr holes falls to the emergency room physician.

If the trauma occurred more than 24 hours before the onset of stupor or coma, the most likely mechanism could be a subdural hematoma. The delayed onset of coma may be attributed to recurrent bleeding or to cerebral edema adjacent to hematoma. In that setting of slow onset, empirical burr holes would probably never be required since initial osmotic therapy and hyperventiltion should be adequate.

ADDITIONAL DIAGNOSTIC MEASURES AS INDICATED

If CT scans or angiography fail to reveal intracranial hemorrhage despite a clear history of trauma, we still have to respect the possibility that the trauma followed a primary intracranial process and is itself comparatively unimportant. As indicated in Figures 10.2 and 10.3, the sequence of lumbar puncture, EEG, and toxic screening allows us to evaluate the possibilities of meningitis, seizure activity, or intoxication.

Coma with Focal Neurologic Deficits but No History or Evidence of Trauma

Coma with focal neurologic deficits but without history or evidence of trauma includes the widest range of etiologic possibilities. The principal diagnoses to be considered initially are the following:

1. Hypertensive hemorrhage
2. Intracranial mass lesion
3. Brainstem ischemia/infarction
4. Hemispheric infarction
5. Encephalitis
6. Unrecognized trauma

Certain classes of hypertensive hemorrhage have characteristic findings and are described in Chapter 30. When the diagnosis of hypertensive hemorrhage seems unlikely on grounds of history and examination of patient, the etiologic possibility of greatest concern remains an intracranial mass with frank or incipient transtentorial herniation.

INITIAL DIAGNOSTIC PROCEDURES AND EMERGENCY TREATMENT

If the examination has disclosed deficits referable to the brainstem, especially if they are asymmetric, we should begin empirical therapy for the presumption of transtentorial herniation. A CT scan and skull film should be obtained as soon as possible; if the CT scan is not immediately available, emergency angiography must be started. If, however, the focal deficits are referable to the cerebral hemisphere, empirical therapy can be deferred unless frank transtentorial herniation emerges. Proceed to CT scan and skull films. If the CT scan is not available and the skull films are nondiagnostic, deliberate before accepting the morbidity of angiography. While, as indicated before, the greatest worry centers on an occult mass, it is possible that the patient is intoxicated, metabolically deranged, or postictal.

DIAGNOSIS IN PRESENCE OF METABOLIC DERANGEMENTS OR POSTICTAL STATE

Metabolic derangements (such as hypercapnia) and intoxications (such as with barbiturates) sufficient to cause coma may sometimes present as obtundation with focal neurologic deficits. The mechanism is not thoroughly understood, but a possible explanation is that certain areas of the brain in some individuals may be predisposed to poor function and may exhibit a disproportionately severe deficit in the setting of a diffuse toxic insult. Such predisposition could result from underlying dysfunction at sites of previous cortical infarctions, healed contusions, seizure foci, or very old subdural hematomas that is usually compensated for. It is important, therefore, to have in hand the result of the several blood analyses obtained at the outset of the investigation so that obvious examples of metabolic dysfunction can be identified. Obtundation and evidence of focal neurologic dysfunction may also be present in the postictal state. The history is usually the critical factor in recognizing this possibility, but gingival hyperplasia or hirsutism in women may also point to chronic phenytoin therapy. A portable EEG, if a reading is available in 4 hours, would be a logical step before angiography.

FURTHER DIAGNOSTIC STEPS AND INITIAL THERAPY IN PRESENCE OF A MASS LESION

Awaiting the results of toxicologic screening before undertaking further diagnostic steps is not safe unless the physician finds compelling evidence of intoxication. If a CT scan has not been done, a mass lesion caused by undisclosed trauma, a tumor, or an abscess are still possibilities. If the metabolic screening tests (and an EEG, if appropriate) do not provide a diagnosis, angiography on an emergency basis may still be necessary. If cerebral angiography reveals only an avascular mass, we still have to deal with the possibilities of brain abscess and encephalitis, and cerebrospinal fluid examination is necessary. It is fair to assume that a mass sufficient to cause coma will also cause transtentorial or cerebellar herniation if a lumbar puncture is performed. The safest approach is to initiate mannitol therapy and hyperventilation and to perform lumbar puncture in an operating room after a neurosurgeon has drilled a burr hole; this precaution facilitates ventricular drainage if it becomes necessary to relieve an acute transtentorial herniation.

Coma with Signs of Meningeal Irritation

Subarachnoid hemorrhage from a berry aneurysm and meningitis are the principle causes of obtundation with evidence of meningeal irritation. *Lumbar puncture* and *examination of the cerebrospinal fluid (CSF)* are the best diagnostic procedures, but they entail some risk. Arterial bleeding from a berry aneurysm causes hemorrhage in the subarachnoid space and can also dissect into brain parenchyma, resulting in a clot that very rarely may predispose to transtentorial herniation after lumbar puncture. Mass effect or a preexisting abscess may also accompany meningitis and similarly pose a small, but real, hazard after lumbar puncture, A *CT scan* should thus be obtained before lumbar puncture if it can be done promptly (often the CT scan alone is sufficient to make a clear diagnosis of subarachnoid hemorrhage). If a CT scan is unavailable, *skull films* should be obtained as a screen for evidence of midline shift or bony changes accompanying abscess. Cerebral angiography is not warranted as a screening examination, but it should be carried out if skull films reveal a mass effect. Lumbar puncture cannot be delayed more than 2 hours in cases of suspected meningitis.

If the CSF is found to be normal, then we have to presume that the impression of nuchal rigidity was incorrect. The subsequent evaluation of possible metabolic disorder, intoxication, or postictal state requires an EEG and toxic screen.

Rarely one will have proceeded to lumbar puncture without a CT scan or angiography under the mistaken impression of nuchal rigidity. If the CSF is acellular (include a Gram stain!) but under high pressure, it is likely that we are faced with a significant mass lesion. Osmotic therapy and hyperventilation must be instituted promptly and angiography done as soon as possible.

Coma without Focal Signs

Metabolic derangement or intoxication is most often the cause of obtundation without focal deficits (see Chapters 27 and 42). The most common etiologies are listed in Table 10.2. Each is associated with a characteristic constellation of findings, and the blood tests obtained at the outset offer clues to them. It is important, however, to keep in mind that mass lesions, meningitis, and subarachnoid hemorrhages are still potential etiologies. If no clear evidence of intoxication is obvious in 2–4 hours, skull films should be obtained after a CT scan. Unless the results contraindicate lumbar puncture, it should be the next test since meningitis is still a possibility: nuchal rigidity depends on reflex mechanisms and may disappear in deep coma. If the CSF is under normal pressure and has normal constituents, the etiology of coma is almost certainly metabolic, intoxication, or postictal phenomena. Then proceed with a screening of urine, blood, and gastric aspirates for toxic substances. On the other hand, if the CSF pressure is greater than 180 cm H_2O, pursue the evaluation of intracranial mass and be wary of a transtentorial herniation.

The myriad toxicologic emergencies are described in Chapters 42 and 43, but clues to several agents will arise in the course of the neurologic examination. Fundoscopic examination provides an unavoidable opportunity to assess the patient's breath. Petroleum distillates, cyanide (burnt almonds), ethanol, paraldehyde—all may be thus revealed. Symmetric ophthalmoplegia without other evidence of brainstem dysfunction may reflect barbiturate or phenytoin intoxication. Pupillary constriction can result from opiate intoxication; the possibility is readily assessed by intravenous administration of naloxone, which should transiently block miosis caused by morphine alkaloids and often awakens the patient.

SUGGESTED READINGS

Fisher CM: The neurological examination of the comatose patient. *Acta Neurol Scand* 1969; 45 (Suppl 36):1–56.

Jennett B, Teasdale G, Braakman R, Minderhoud J, Heiden J, Kurze T: Prognosis of patients with severe head injury. *Neurosurgery* 1979; 4:283–289.

Levy DE, Bates D, Caronna JJ, Cartlidge NEF, Knill-Jones RB, Lapinski RH, Singer BH, Shaw DA, Plum F: Prognosis in nontraumatic coma. *Ann Intern Med* 1981; 94:293–301.

Plum F, Posner J: Diagnosis of stupor and coma, in *Contemporary Neurology Series* ed 3. Philadelphia, FA Davis Co, 1980.

Teasdale G, Jennett B: Assessment of coma and impaired consciousness. A practical scale. *Lancet* 1974; 2:81–84.

11
LIFE-THREATENING ELECTROLYTE ABNORMALITIES

Howard S. Frazier

The purpose of this chapter is to describe the short-term management of the more common life-threatening electrolyte disturbances. Pathogenesis, differential diagnosis, and etiology will be discussed only to the extent that they are important determinants of early therapy for the electrolyte disorder. The focus of the discussion will be on the electrolyte abnormality itself and the therapeutic responses appropriate to the first few hours of hospital care.

To emphasize a manifestation of disease—here an alteration in the concentration of some solute in the serum—rather than cause or mechanism, runs counter to traditional medical teaching, which holds that an understanding of etiology is an essential prerequisite to rational therapeutics. This apparent conflict highlights an important characteristic of the management of medical emergencies. In this context, the crucial judgment concerns the identification of the abnormality that represents the most immediate threat to the patient's life, and the most important response is that directed at the reduction or removal of that threat. With certain exceptions to be mentioned later, the judgment and response do not require the formulation of a unique etiologic diagnosis. If etiology can be proven without prolonging the period of risk, so much the better. The significant requirement, however, is that efforts to establish a precise etiologic diagnosis not delay a response to serious functional abnormalities.

Having begun a therapeutic program directed at the most serious threat, the physician reevaluates the patient and makes a decision as to the next most threatening abnormality. An appropriate program is then instituted to counter this functional problem and the patient again is reevaluated. This iterative process is continued until all of the immediately life-threatening problems are matched by appropriate therapeutic responses. At this point, additional studies aimed at defining etiology are undertaken, and a treatment program is developed that is directed at functional abnormalities to be anticipated over the next few hours or days and at the etiology, if that is possible.

ACID–BASE EMERGENCIES

Normal Physiology

Two sets of mechanisms are responsible for the preservation of normal acid–base status—body buffers and the renal handling of excess acid or alkali. The significance of the buffer system inheres in its capacity to minimize alterations of hydrogen ion concentration, or pH, of body fluids in the face of acute loads of strong acid or alkali. The renal response to acid–base disturbance occurs over a period of hours to days, involves the net excretion of the excess acid or alkali, and restores the buffer system to its normal state. The buffer system temporizes; the kidneys renew. Since we are concerned only with the first few hours of hospital care, the characteristics of the buffer system are crucial, while renal responses have little impact on immediate outcome.

Two features of the buffer system deserve emphasis. First, the major buffer pair of the extracellular fluid (ECF), $HCO_3^- - H_2CO_3$, is the one most accessible to measurement. Although it represents a minority of the total buffering capacity of the body, it has a predictable relationship to other body buffers; hence its state is a useful index of that of the other buffers. Specifically, at commonly encountered levels of metabolic acidosis, one-third of the acid load is buffered by the $HCO_3^- - H_2CO_3$ system and two-thirds by others. The fraction of the acid and alkali load buffered by the former varies with the direction and severity of the disturbance, however, ranging from one-tenth in severe metabolic acidosis to one-half or more in metabolic alkalosis.

Second, the buffering capacity of the $HCO_3^- - H_2CO_3$ pair is substantially enhanced because a precursor of one member of the buffer pair, CO_2, is volatile and its concentration can be controlled independently by changes in alveolar ventilation. The functional significance of this capability can be appreciated when the chemical equation for the reaction of the buffer pair is put in the form described by the Henderson–Hasselbalch equation as follows:

$$pH = pK + \log\frac{[HCO_3^-]}{[H_2CO_3]} \qquad (11.1)$$

where pK = 6.1. The pH can be seen to depend on the ratio of concentrations of the members of the buffer pair rather than on the absolute concentration of either taken alone. Under normal circumstances, the serum bicarbonate concentration, $[HCO_3^-]_s$ is approximately 24 mEq/liter and H_2CO_3 equals 1.2 mmol/liter, yielding a pH of 7.40. The partial pressure of CO_2 in equilibrium with the solution, P_{CO_2}, is determined by the following relation:

$$P_{CO_2} \text{ (in mm Hg)} = \frac{[H_2CO_3^-] \text{ (in mmol/liter)}}{\alpha} \qquad (11.2)$$

where $\alpha = 0.0301$; P_{CO_2} normally is maintained by the activity of the respiratory center and the lungs at 40 mm Hg.

Approach to Acid–Base Disturbances

Management of the patient with an acid–base disturbance requires the formulation of answers to the following three questions:

1. *What is the acid–base disturbance?* Note that its type cannot be inferred from a measurement of [total CO_2]$_s$ alone; [total CO_2]$_s$, the sum of [HCO_3^-]$_s$ and [H_2CO_3]$_s$, yields an unambiguous interpretation only if all other relevant clinical information is available, clear-cut, and correctly interpreted. Since these requirements are rarely met in the emergency room setting, the measurement of two of the three terms of the Henderson–Hasselbalch equation normally is required. The third term can then be obtained from a nomogram. A venous sample drawn without stasis often is sufficient, although an arterial sample may be required at times.

2. *What is the etiology of the disturbance?* Although this question is in apparent contradiction to the principles discussed above, it is an essential preliminary to the next question.

3. *What can the patient contribute to the immediate resolution of the acid–base disturbance?* For example, a patient with a severe attack of asthma may, on occasion, have respiratory acidosis. The fall of pH associated with the increased P_{CO_2} could be reversed, in theory, by the administration of sufficient HCO_3^- to restore the normal ratio of the buffer pair. Knowledge of the etiology of the respiratory acidosis suggests, however, that the achievement of bronchodilatation will increase alveolar ventilation, lower P_{CO_2}, and rapidly restore acid–base status to normal. At the other end of the spectrum, the patient with uremic metabolic acidosis may not be able to respond to any therapy designed to promote acid excretion; correction of the acid–base disturbance requires administration by the physician of an appropriate amount of HCO_3^-.

Metabolic Acidosis

The signs of metabolic acidosis usually are not striking. Kussmaul respirations—deep excursions of normal or even slow rate—are difficult to detect until the serum concentration of bicarbonate, [HCO_3^-]$_s$, has been reduced by the acid load to less than one-half of normal. As pH approaches the lower limit of viability, approximately 7, obtundation and hypotension may supervene.

Blood gases show an abnormally acid pH and, in the presence of normal respiratory compensation, a low P_{CO_2}. Calculation or a nomogram will show [HCO_3^-]$_s$ to be low as well.

Values for other serum electrolytes typically will be available at the same time, and their examination may provide additional information regarding the acid–base disturbance. The usual tests do not identify and quantify a group of organic and inorganic anions normally present in serum. An approximation of the total concentration of these unmeasured anions may be made by calculating the difference between the measured value of [Na^+]$_s$ and the sum of [Cl^-]$_s$ and [HCO_3^-]$_s$. Determined in this way, the anion gap normally has an upper limit of 12 mEq/liter. On the basis of this information, the clinician can distinguish between two major classes of metabolic acidosis: one in which the reduction in [HCO_3^-]$_s$ is associated with an equivalent rise in [Cl^-]$_s$, leaving the anion gap unchanged, and one in which the fall in [HCO_3^-]$_s$ is accompanied by an equivalent rise in the anion gap. Table 11.1 lists the more important members of each class.

Calculation of the anion gap is useful in two respects. First, it narrows the range of diagnostic alternatives and may suggest a previously unsuspected etiology. Second, an elevated anion gap may result from the accumulation of an organic anion that can be metabolized, a process that will regenerate HCO_3^-. A common example is diabetic ketoacidosis. In this situation, replacement of the calculated HCO_3^- deficit while treating the immediate acid–base defect will result in overcorrection of the acidosis because of the metabolism of organic anions to HCO_3^- under the influence of insulin. Forewarned by knowledge of the approximate concentration of metabolic anion, the clinician can make an appropriate reduction in the dose of HCO_3^- to be administered.

A compensatory decrease in P_{CO_2} is an important feature of the normal adaptation to metabolic acidosis. As pointed out in the introductory paragraphs of this section, normal pH could be preserved for any reduced level of [HCO_3^-]$_s$ simply by symmetrical reduction in arterial P_{CO_2} brought about by increased

TABLE 11.1 Major Causes of Metabolic Acidosis

Normal Anion Gap	Increased Anion Gap
Ingestion of ammonium chloride	Diabetic ketoacidosis
Use of carbonic anhydrase inhibitors	Uremic acidosis
Massive loss of pancreatic or small bowel secretions	Lactic acidosis
	Salicylate intoxication
Renal tubular acidosis	Methyl alcohol intoxication
Ureterosigmoidostomy	Ethylene glycol intoxication

alveolar ventilation. In fact, normal people cannot reduce arterial Pco_2 much below 10 mm Hg because further increases in alveolar ventilation result in a rapid increase in CO_2 production due to the increased muscular work of breathing. As a consequence, further respiratory compensation for metabolic acidosis fails when $[HCO_3^-]_s$ is reduced below 6 mEq/liter and pH falls precipitously with further decrements in HCO_3^-.

In patients with cardiac or pulmonary disease, the energy cost of hyperventilation may be 10 times that of a normal person. Such a patient may not be able to lower Pco_2 commensurate with even moderate reductions in $[HCO_3^-]_s$, and blood pH may fall to lethal levels at values of $[HCO_3^-]_s$ that would be of little concern in a normal person. Infusions of $NaHCO_3$ tend to be well tolerated in acidotic patients even in the presence of left ventricular failure. Improvement in myocardial responsiveness to catecholamines and reduction in that component of cardiac output obligated to support the work of breathing usually mitigate the effects on cardiac function of that portion of the sodium load that remains in the ECF.

INITIAL MANAGEMENT

If the etiology and severity of the metabolic acidosis indicate the need for $NaHCO_3$ therapy, a rough calculation of the HCO_3^- deficit can be made by recalling that the apparent volume of distribution of the original acid load approximates three times the volume of ECF. For most patients, a reasonable therapeutic endpoint is a $[total\ CO_2]_s$ of 18 mEq/liter. The total $NaHCO_3$ dose is thus the difference between 18 mEq/liter and the present value of $[HCO_3^-]_s$ times the volume of ECF, about 20% of body weight, times three. Of this amount, from one-third to one-half is given in the first 12 hours, one-third in the second 12 hours, and, after rechecking the serum value, the remainder on the following day. To this schedule must be added an amount of $NaHCO_3$ designed to cover the rate of production of new acid during the treatment period. For most patients, 100 mEq/day will be sufficient, but in some circumstances, spontaneous lactic acidosis for example, 1,000 or more mEq/day may be required.

Finally, as noted previously, when metabolic acidosis is severe, a substantially larger fraction of the acid load is buffered outside of the ECF than is indicated by the calculation shown above. The difference may be as large as a factor of five. This discrepancy serves to emphasize the approximate nature of all such clinical estimates and the importance of monitoring the patient's response to the therapeutic program over intervals as short as an hour or two while it is underway so that appropriate revisions can be undertaken.

Respiratory Acidosis

In addition to the intrinsic risks of low pH mentioned previously, respiratory acidosis inevitably carries with it two additional hazards. The elevated Pco_2 that is responsible for the acidosis begins to depress central nervous system (CNS) function, including that of the respiratory center, at levels in excess of 65–75 mm Hg. Further, 80% of the air we breathe is N_2; 20% is made up of the sum of O_2 and CO_2. Elevations of Pco_2 in the aveoli and the arterial blood necessarily are associated with reductions in Po_2 and the threat of hypoxia for the patient who is breathing room air. Furthermore, treatment of hypoxia by abrupt elevation of Po_2 in the inspired gas poses risks to the patients with chronic ventilatory insufficiency. If the respiratory center has ceased to respond to the elevated Pco_2 and is being driven by hypoxia, substantial elevation of the Po_2 in the inspired gas may remove the latter stimulus, further reduce alveolar ventilation, and result in a precipitous increase in arterial Pco_2, narcosis, and death.

In addition to these considerations, the therapeutic response to respiratory acidosis should be influenced by the chronicity of the problem. If it is acute and severe—as shown by an arterial Pco_2 greater than 60–70 mm Hg or an arterial pH less than 7.2—an endotracheal tube should be inserted and the patient ventilated until the underlying cause can be determined and corrected.

If the condition is known to be chronic, either from the history or the finding of a venous total CO_2 that is elevated in the absence of diuretic therapy, then a trial of controlled low-flow O_2 via Venturi mask is appropriate. For the reasons noted above, the hazards of attempting to increase arterial O_2 content are significant and mandate the continued attendance of the responsible physician or an experienced nurse or respiratory therapist during the first hour or two of treatment. If an improvement in arterial oxygenation is not evident by clinical signs or laboratory studies and the arterial pH remains below 7.25 and the Po_2 below 40 mm Hg, a decision must be made regarding endotracheal intubation. The period of time devoted to a trial of low-flow O_2 by mask will also have been used to conduct a rapid and careful search for reversible causes of acute ventilatory failure—usually infectious—superimposed on chronic insufficiency. Demonstration of a reversible component in the presence of these laboratory values usually can be considered adequate indication for an endotracheal tube and controlled ventilation.

The most difficult judgment concerns those patients with known chronic, severe ventilatory insufficiency who present decompensated without any detectable superimposed acute problem. In such circumstances, the likelihood of eventually weaning the patient from a ventilator is small, and the prospect of a prolonged and uncomfortable death is commensurately large. There remains a spectrum of medical response to this difficult dilemma, and no credible analysis of the issues is sufficiently brief to be appropriate here. Suffice it to say that the thoughtful and skilled primary physician who has anticipated the problem and has outlined the management, and the reasons, he or she feels appropriate for the patient in a prominent place in the record, will earn the respect and admiration of the emergency room physician who next receives the patient.

Although establishment of controlled ventilation solves one acute problem, it creates a new risk for the patient with chronic respiratory acidosis. The normal renal response to an elevation of arterial P_{CO_2} of several days duration is the excretion into the urine of additional acid and the production for the body of additional HCO_3^-. The accumulation of HCO_3^- brings about

an increase in its concentration—a result that raises the pH of ECF back toward normal—and is associated with a reciprocal fall in $[Cl^-]_s$. Under these circumstances, the enthusiastic reduction of arterial P_{CO_2} by controlled ventilation will increase the ratio $HCO_3^-:\alpha P_{CO_2}$ and raise the arterial pH to frankly alkalotic and potentially lethal levels. Since the alveolar and arterial P_{CO_2} is now fixed by the respirator, arterial pH can be normalized only by the renal excretion of HCO_3^-, a response that the kidney can manage with dispatch in the presence of surplus Cl^-. The risk arises because these patients usually are depleted of Cl^- due to antecedent diuretic therapy and often are maximally conserving Na^+ in the glomerular filtrate as well. As a consequence, the adaptive diuresis of HCO_3^- is inhibited and alkalosis persists. From understanding of these mechanisms comes two important guidelines for therapy. First, alveolar ventilation should be increased slowly over several hours, the endpoint being the usual P_{CO_2} for that patient rather than a normal value. Second, throughout this period of change,

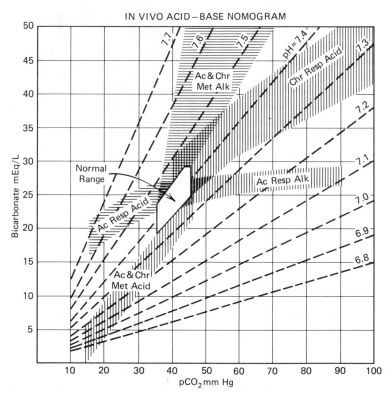

Figure 11.1 Characterization of disturbances of acid–base balance. (Arbus GS: An in vivo acid base nomogram for clinical use *Can Med Assoc J* 1973; 109:291. Reproduced with permission.)

Cl⁻ must be provided, usually with Na^+ and K^+, in amounts at least equal to the desired urinary loss of HCO_3^-.

Mixed Acid–Base Disturbances

The discussion thus far has been based on the assumption of a single primary acid–base disturbance and a coexisting normal respiratory or metabolic response to the primary disorder. Mixed, or complex, disturbances in which there are as many as three primary acid–base disorders are not rare in emergency room practice; their recognition depends upon demonstration of a deviation from the normal compensatory responses to be expected in simple acid–base disturbances. For most of us, recourse to a diagram provides more accurate results than does recollection.

Figure 11.1 is one type of summation of the evidence on normal compensatory responses drawn from studies in humans and laboratory animals. The coordinates are components of the Henderson–Hasselbalch equation (Eq. 11.1), and the shaded regions represent confidence limits for the adaptations expected to occur in vivo in response to a single primary disturbance. An example will be sufficient to demonstrate the use of the figure. Consider a patient whose arterial blood shows a pH of 7.25 and a P_{CO_2} of 70 mm Hg. The coexistence of acidosis and an elevated P_{CO_2} clearly establish the presence of primary respiratory acidosis, but the level of bicarbonate determined by these two values falls outside of the ranges to be expected for either an acute or a chronic process. This observation strongly suggests that if the respiratory acidosis is acute, it is complicated by primary metabolic alkalosis, or, if the respiratory acidosis is chronic, a primary metabolic acidosis is also present. Under these circumstances, the medical history and the presence or absence of an increased concentration of unmeasured anions should permit differentiation between the acute and chronic alternatives and thus allow identification and appropriate management of the second primary acid–base disorder.

ABNORMALITIES OF SERUM POTASSIUM CONCENTRATION

Normal Physiology

An effective therapeutic response to life-threatening disorders of serum potassium concentration, $[K^+]_s$, depends upon an understanding of the normal distribution of the ion among the compartments of the body fluids, of some of the factors that affect this distribution, and of the principal renal mechanisms that are responsible for regulation of $[K^+]_s$.

More than 95% of total K^+ in the body is within cells. Of this amount, the overwhelming majority is in muscles in which its concentration in cellular water may exceed 150 mEq/liter in the presence of a normal concentration of 4.5 mEq/liter in the surrounding ECF. In most tissues, this gradient is maintained by a process of active, or uphill, transport of K^+ and an electric potential difference generated by the active transport of other ionic species that favors the cellular accumulation of K^+. The high intracellular concentration of K^+ is essential to the operation of a variety of cellular metabolic processes and is crucial to the normal function of excitable tissues, including cardiac and skeletal muscle as well as the nervous system.

The distribution of K^+ between cellular and extracellular compartments is dependent on a variety of factors. Since most of the active transport mechanisms are aerobic, a continuous supply of oxygen and metabolic substrate is required to prevent a leak of intracellular K^+ into the ECF. In the presence of otherwise normal metabolism, the acid–base status of the person exerts a strong influence on the distribution of K^+: acidosis results in a loss of the ion from cells into the ECF, while alkalosis favors cellular accumulation with a lowering of $[K^+]_s$.

A number of other factors also play a role in the partition of K^+ between these two major compartments, but it is sufficient for our purposes to mention only one hormonal effect. Insulin favors the entry of extracellular K^+ into both hepatocytes and muscle cells, an effect that is both rapid in onset and, relative to the total amount of K^+ in the ECF, significant in magnitude.

While the distribution of K^+ between intra- and extracellular compartments is not subject to direct control by the kidney, renal mechanisms normally operate to preserve $[K^+]_s$ within narrow limits despite wide variations in the dietary intake of K^+. One important influence on renal excretion of K^+ is the level of circulating aldosterone. Secretion of the hormone is stimulated by low intake of Na^+, as well as by elevation of $[K^+]_s$. Increased levels of aldosterone are associated with increased urinary losses of K^+. Although the relationship is more complex, K^+ excretion also tends to be increased by acidosis.

With these cellular and renal regulatory mechanisms in mind, we will now consider certain features of hyper- and hypokalemia.

Hyperkalemia

The hazards associated with hyperkalemia are the result of changes in the electrical activity of the heart. Although the latter is strongly influenced by the ratio of intracellular to extracellular concentrations of K^+, the concentrations of other ions and metabolites also play a role. In addition, $[K^+]_s$ is not a reliable measure of either cellular concentration or content since, for given values within the cell, the serum level is elevated in acidosis and reduced in alkalosis. It is not surprising, therefore, that fatal episodes compatible with an hyperkalemic etiology have been reported with elevations of $[K^+]_s$ as slight as 2 mEq/liter above the normal upper limit.

Symptoms and signs attributable to hyperkalemia are not uniformly present. They involve little more than muscle weakness or paresthesias and are easily missed in the context of other medical problems. For this reason, the best protection is provided by a high index of clinical suspicion, particularly in patients with anoxia, acidosis, trauma to soft tissues, oliguria, or a history of spironolactone or triamterene ingestion. A value of $[K^+]_s$ in excess of 6 mEq/liter in a properly handled specimen is an indication for immediate procurement of an electrocardiogram to determine if signs of hyperkalemic cardiac toxicity are present.

The threshhold figure for $[K^+]_s$ of 6 mEq/liter requires three qualifications. At normal platelet counts, roughly 0.5 mEq/liter of the measured value of $[K^+]_s$ is contributed by the K^+ released through platelet lysis when the specimen is collected. In the presence of marked thrombocytosis, sufficient K^+ may be re-leased during lysis to elevate normal plasma K^+ levels in vivo above 6 mEq/liter in the serum in vitro. This possibility may be examined by repeating the K^+ determination in the plasma of a specimen collected with heparin. White cells also leak K^+ into serum over time. Marked leukocytosis or inordinate delay in separating serum from cells may also result in a value of $[K^+]_s$ not reflective of the state of the patient. A repeat measurement on a promptly processed specimen will identify this source of potential misinterpretation. Finally, the presence of visible hemoglobin in a serum sample makes the measured $[K^+]_s$ uninterpretable.

Studies in otherwise normal animals demonstrate a progression of electrocardiographic changes as $[K^+]_s$ is raised. In order of increasing severity, these can be summarized as follows:

1. Peaked T waves with normal or shortened QT interval
2. Prolonged PR interval, progressing to absent P waves
3. Prolonged QRS, progressing to ventricular fibrillation or standstill

Electrocardiograms showing manifestations of mild and severe hyperkalemic toxicity are reproduced in Figure 11.2.

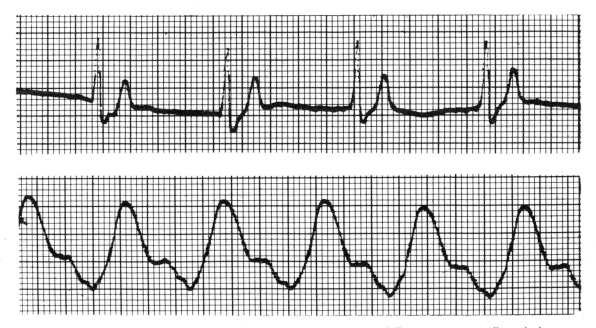

Figure 11.2 The electrocardiogram in hyperkalemia. The upper panel illustrates symmetrically peaked T waves, which is evidence of mild toxicity. The lower panel shows marked prolongation of the QRS complex, which is an indication that toxicity is severe and requires immediate intervention.

Clinical experience emphasizes the importance of two points. First, there is no constant association between an absolute level of $[K^+]_s$ and a particular electrocardiographic manifestation of hyperkalemic toxicity. Second, the rate of progression of cardiac toxicity is highly variable. The therapeutic implications of these facts are apparent. The demonstration, or indeed the suspicion, of cardiac toxicity always establishes the need for close, continuing medical observation and a rapid and careful search for the cause of abnormal regulation of $[K^+]_s$. In addition, it frequently will require therapeutic intervention using one or more of the modalities listed in Table 11.2.

The choice among the alternatives listed in Table 11.2 is conditioned by the severity of hyperkalemic toxicity at the institution of therapy, a judgment as to the rate at which K^+ is entering the ECF, the estimated time interval before normal regulation can be reestablished as a result of etiologically directed therapy, and other patient variables as noted in the last column of Table 11.2.

Hypertonic Na^+ and Ca^{2+} are indicated only if toxicity is far advanced at the time of its discovery. They should be infused under electrocardiographic control and should be viewed as the immediate component of a therapeutic effort that will include other modalities from the list in Table 11.2. Both act to suppress the abnormal electrical effects of elevated $[K^+]_s$ without affecting its concentration significantly.

In the presence of systemic acidosis, the infusion of

TABLE 11.2 Treatment of Hyperkalemia

Therapy[a]	Dose	Onset	Duration	Efficacy
Hypertonic saline	Up to 250 ml of 6% saline IV	Immediate	Short	Poor unless $[Na^+]_s$ is initially low; hazardous in cardiac failure
Calcium gluconate[b]	5–10 ml of 10% solution IV over 2–3 min	Immediate	Short	Relatively good, but hazardous in presence of digitalis
Sodium bicarbonate[b]	2 ampules (90–100 mEq) IV over 5 min; repeat 10 min later if acidosis is severe	Immediate	Short	Poor unless acidosis is present; hazardous in cardiac failure unless acidosis is present
Glucose and insulin	20–30 units of crystalline insulin, half IV and half SC, plus 25 g glucose per/hr IV	15–45 min	4–6 hr	Good
Sorbitol and polystyrene sulfonate resin[c]	Basic mixture: 25 ml of sorbitol + 75 ml of water + 25 g of resin; dose is 25–50 ml orally every 4–6 hours or 100 ml of suspension in enema, retained for 45 min	1 + hr	—	Good
Dialysis	—	30+ min start-up time	—	Good

[a]The first four therapies are temporizing measures that may be instituted while awaiting the effects of either of the last two or the outcome of definitive therapy. The source of K^+ entry into the ECF should be identified and treated if possible.

[b]Solutions containing Ca^{2+} and HCO_3^- for IV administration should not be mixed in the same bottle because $CaCO_3$ will precipitate.

[c]The recommendation is based on the assumption that $[K^+]_s$ is slightly elevated and that K^+ is entering the ECF slowly. In any given situation, the appropriate dose is the amount that is required to achieve the desired effect.

HCO_3^- as isotonic or hypertonic $NaHCO_3$ will lower $[K^+]_s$ by promoting its cellular uptake, an effect that is much less pronounced or predictable in the absence of acidosis. An appropriate initial dose would be two ampules of approximately 50 mEq each infused over 5 minutes, with subsequent doses determined by the severity of the hyperkalemic toxicity and degree of preexisting acidosis.

Elevation of blood glucose and insulin levels will promote the uptake of K^+ into both liver and muscle cells. A dose of 20–30 units of crystalline zinc insulin, one-half given intravenously (IV) and the remainder subcutaneously (SC), coupled with the IV infusion of 25 g glucose per hour, or approximately 500 ml of 5% glucose in water, for a period of 5–6 hours, usually will result in a transient lowering of $[K^+]_s$.

It is important to bear in mind that none of the modes of therapy discussed thus far alters total body K^+, and, except in special circumstances, none should be considered as more than a method for buying sufficient time either to institute definitive therapy or to reduce total body K^+ content. Two methods are available to accomplish the latter. Cationic exchange resins of polystyrene sulfonate may be given either by mouth or by retention enema as a 1:4 suspension in 25% sorbitol. Their binding capacity approximates 1 mEq of K^+ per gram of resin under optimal circumstances with oral administration. In the hyperkalemic emergency, the dose is determined by the estimate of the rate of entrance of K^+ into the ECF, the presence of electrocardiographic abnormalities, and the other therapies to be considered. Doses as high as 50 g of resin in 200 ml of a 25% solution of sorbitol administered as a 45-minute retention enema, repeated hourly, may be required and generally are well tolerated. At these dose levels, the resin may bind sufficient Ca^{2+} to produce symptoms of hypocalcemia, but frequent attempts to elicit Chvostek's sign and, if it becomes positive, the intravenous infusion of small amounts of Ca^{2+} permit easy control of this unusual complication.

The second method for the production of negative K^+ balance is dialysis. Hemodialysis requires access to the circulation and equipment not uniformly available. Although peritoneal dialysis is less efficient with respect to the rate of K^+ removal, it has the advantages of simplicity, short lead time, and no requirement for equipment beyond the commercially available disposable sets.

Hyperkalemia is a relatively common and potentially lethal metabolic disorder with a variety of causes. It usually is readily reversible by the application of an appropriate selection of the methods described above. Unfavorable outcomes are most often the result of failure to appreciate the presence of hyperkalemia or of failure to use the time made available by

these therapies to detect and control the underlying cause of the disorder in K^+ metabolism.

Hypokalemia

The widespread use of potent diuretics has made hypokalemia of mild to moderate severity among the most common of the electrolyte disorders encountered in emergency room or hospital practice. When the disturbance is mild ($[K^+]_s$ more than 2.8 mEq/liter), the patient is asymptomatic or complains only of polyuria resulting from the impact of K^+ depletion on the urinary concentrating mechanism. Except in the digitalized cardiac patient in whom even slight hypokalemia may precipitate serious arrhythmias, the condition is well tolerated in the short run and does not require emergency intervention in the sense in which the term is used here.

More severe hypokalemia results in muscle weakness and occasionally in paresthesia. When $[K^+]_s$ approaches 2 mEq/liter, weakness affecting the respiratory muscles may be sufficient to compromise ventilation.

Additional support for the clinical impression of hypokalemia can be obtained from the electrocardiogram: The T wave will be flattened, the U wave will be apparent and the QU, or apparent QT, interval will be prolonged.

As soon as the presence of hypokalemia is established and before institution of therapy, a urine specimen should be obtained for measurement of urinary K^+ concentration. The result will have no impact on the immediate program of intravenous or oral K^+ replacement, and the latter may be commenced as soon as the urine specimen has been obtained. A value greater than 10 mEq/liter in the face of prolonged hypokalemia points strongly to the kidney as the source of depletion, while a value less than this suggests that excessive losses from the gastrointestinal tract or, rarely, insufficient intake of K^+ are responsible for the hypokalemia. Once K^+ therapy has been started, urinary electrolyte values will become uninterpretable, and an important aid in differential diagnosis will be lost.

Emergency repletion of body stores of potassium and correction of mild or moderate uncomplicated hypokalemia should be undertaken by the oral route if the patient's state permits. If it does not or if the hypokalemia is severe or complicated, intravenous administration of K^+, ordinarily as the Cl^-, should be undertaken. Concentrations greater than 20 mEq/liter are likely to cause local pain when administered into a peripheral vein; the rate of administration should not exceed 40 mEq/hr unless massive, continuing losses or rapid correction of severe acidosis are occurring simultaneously. Under these circumstances the most careful supervision using frequent electrocardiograms and measurements of $[K^+]_s$ is necessary to regulate administration and prevent hyperkalemia. Caution is also appropriate when approaching repletion in the previously severely K^+-depleted patient. The physiologic prerequisites for the brisk normal excretion of excess administered K^+ may not be met, and hyperkalemia can result from continued administration of K^+ at the rates ordered earlier in the course of repletion. As noted earlier, minimizing risk requires frequent monitoring and a readiness to reduce the rate of administration as $[K^+]_s$ approaches normal.

Prior estimation of the absolute amount of K^+ depletion, an imprecise exercise at best, rarely is necessary in the clinical situation since the program of repletion will be governed in any event by the need to avoid hyperkalemic overshoot, on the one hand, and persistent, inadequately treated hypokalemia, on the other.

DISORDERED REGULATION OF THE SOLUTE CONCENTRATION OF BODY FLUIDS

Normal Physiology

The membranes of mammalian cells, with few exceptions, are freely permeable to the water that makes up 50–60% of body weight. As a result, water moves rapidly in response to osmotic gradients, reaching equilibrium when water activity or its equivalent, total solute concentration, is everywhere the same. From this property of cellular membranes, it follows that the total solute concentration of each compartment of body fluids can be regulated by control of any one compartment. In addition, it permits the physician to evaluate total solute concentration, that is, plasma osmolality, P_{osm}, expressed in mosm/kg H_2O, by sampling the plasma or serum.

Changes in P_{osm} from the normal value of approximately 285 mosm/kg H_2O necessarily are related to differences in the rates at which solutes and water enter the body, usually through the gastrointestinal tract, and leave it via the lungs, skin, gastrointestinal tract, and kidney. Ordinarily, P_{osm} is regulated within 1–2% of the normal value by the operation of two mechanisms. The first is the ability of the kidney to excrete water and solute relatively independently of each other. This capacity is expressed in the elaboration of large volumes of urine at a solute concentration one-sixth that of plasma or of small volumes of urine at a fourfold concentration. Because of the continuous loss of water by the insensible route, however, the remarkable versatility of the kidney is not sufficient to defend P_{osm} under conditions in which inadequate amounts of water are being

ingested. The second mechanism, thirst, is the evolutionary response to the requirement for continued ingestion of some minimum amount of water.

Disordered regulation of the solute concentration, then, can be understood as the result of an imbalance between the rates at which solutes and water enter and leave the body fluids. The most common clinical example of pathologic elevation of P_{osm} is the result of failure to ingest sufficient water because of an altered state of consciousness or physical incapacity. Abnormal depression of P_{osm} usually results from a reduced ability of the kidney to elaborate a urine of sufficiently large volume and low concentration to rid the body of solute-free water at the rate it is being ingested. The mechanisms responsible for this restriction of the normal renal capacity to excrete water are discussed in the section on hyponatremia.

Hypernatremia

Elevation of $[Na^+]_s$ in the conscious and otherwise normal patient is associated with thirst. Further elevation to levels above 160–165 mEq/liter in the adult is correlated with depressed consciousness, seizures, and, ultimately, coma. As noted earlier, water deprivation is the primary event in most cases of hypernatremia; acting alone, it produces a symmetrical reduction in the volume of all body fluid compartments, including the ECF. Most of such patients have undergone some loss of salt as well, so that ECF volume is reduced even further. Decreased tissue turgor, tachycardia, and postural hypotension are often observed and may even dominate in the clinical presentation.

TREATMENT

The major hazards, in addition to vascular collapse or altered function of the CNS, are intracranial bleeding related to tearing of vessels coincident with changes in brain volume or cerebral edema related to entry of water into brain tissue during therapeutic lowering of the extracellular hyperosmolarity. The latter risk as well as the commonly associated ECF depletion are the basis for a therapeutic program of gradual correction of the free water deficit using half-normal saline. A rough estimate of the solute-free water required to bring $[Na^+]_s$ down to normal is given by the following formula:

$$\text{Liters of water} = \text{body weight} \times 0.6 \times \frac{\text{observed } [Na^+]_s - \text{normal } [Na^+]_s}{\text{normal } [Na^+]_s} \quad \textbf{(11.3)}$$

When water deprivation and coexisting salt depletion are severe and, as described above, the signs of ECF volume depletion are prominent, it is advantageous to begin treatment with isotonic saline, switching to half-isotonic saline after hemodynamic function has been stabilized. More often, however, initiation of therapy with half-isotonic saline is entirely adequate. Since the deficit of water calculated using Equation 11.3 represents solute-free water, the volume of half-isotonic saline required for correction will be twice this amount. One-half of the total volume can be given on each of the two succeeding days. To this daily ration should be added a volume of glucose and water or half-isotonic saline sufficient to replace the patient's daily insensible losses of water.

Hyperosmolar Hyperglycemic Nonketotic Diabetic Coma

INITIAL THERAPY

Although the solute causing abnormal elevation of serum osmolality is glucose rather than Na^+ and its accompanying anion, the symptoms, signs, and hazards of the hyperosmolar state are those described in the preceding section. One feature deserves additional emphasis, however. The osmotic diuresis associated with severe hyperglycemia during the period before treatment has induced severe salt depletion, and ECF volume is maintained, in part, by the water extracted from cells by the abnormal concentration of glucose in the ECF. If the hyperglycemia is reduced by insulin therapy before ECF volume has been stabilized by saline administration, the patient is at risk for further contraction of ECF volume and vascular collapse. The first priority, therefore, is expansion of the ECF with isotonic saline until blood pressure and urine output are adequate; low-dose insulin therapy may then be begun. Most patients will require less than 200 units of insulin during the first day of treatment; with higher doses blood glucose and, hence, serum osmolality may fall more rapidly than is desirable for the reasons mentioned previously. In addition to glucose concentration, $[K^+]_s$ should be followed closely.

SUBSEQUENT THERAPY

Subsequent therapeutic decisions depend upon an estimation of the *effective* plasma osmolality, P_{osm}, that is, the component of plasma osmolality due to the presence of solutes that penetrate cells slowly. With respect to electrolytes, the quantitative dominance of Na^+ and its anions and the magnitude of osmotic coefficients of univalent electrolytes permit the contribution of the electrolytes to P_{osm} to be calculated simply as $2[Na^+]_s$. The contribution of glucose is estimated, using clinically relevant units, as follows: glucose concentration in mg% ÷ 18. Because urea is a permeant solute, it exerts no differential osmotic force across cell membranes in the steady state and does not enter into the calculation. No other solutes are present in sufficient concentration to require inclusion. Thus, P_{osm} is given simply by the following expression:

$$P_{osm} \text{ (in mosm/kg } H_2O) = 2[Na^+]_s + \frac{\text{glucose in mg\%}}{18} \quad \textbf{(11.4)}$$

If the initial P_{osm} is elevated above the normal value of 285 mosm/kg H_2O and the $[Na^+]_s$ exceeds approximately 130 mEQ/liter, there is a bodily deficit of solute-free water. Achievement of the second priority, reduction of P_{osm} to normal, is accomplished by the infusion of solute-free water in the form of half-isotonic saline with continued administration of insulin as required to bring about gradual reduction of hyperglycemia. For the reasons noted in the previous section, correction of the hyperosmolar state should be made over a period of 2 days. If the state of consciousness worsens during the treatment period, the change may be related to cerebral edema; the rate of correction of the hyperosmolar state should be slowed, and a trial of intravenous hypertonic mannitol or glycerol may be considered. In any event, the rate at which P_{osm} is being lowered should be slowed when the value reaches the range of 320–330 mosm/kg H_2O.

NORMAL OSMOLARITY IN THE PRESENCE OF MARKED HYPERGLYCEMIA

On rare occasions, the initial P_{osm} will be normal or low despite the presence of marked hyperglycemia. Under these circumstances, $[Na^+]_s$ necessarily is low, indicating a surplus of water relative to the amount of Na^+ in the ECF. The osmotic diuresis associated with marked glucosuria consists of urine that is roughly isosmolar with serum and in which glucose is a major solute. Consequently, urinary water losses exceed simultaneous urinary losses of Na^+ and, if there is no intake of solute-free water, osmotic diuresis will tend to elevate $[Na^+]_s$. If examination discloses no significant abnormalities of CNS or cadiovascular function, continued osmotic diuresis from hyperglycemia may be permitted, in this circumstance, to raise $[Na^+]_s$ before insulin therapy is begun. In the presence of signs suggesting either altered function of the CNS or ECF volume depletion, however, hypertonic saline should be administered to raise the level of $[Na^+]_s$ before reduction of the hyperglycemia with insulin.

Hyponatremia

Under all circumstances, the major contribution to P_{osm} is made by the salts of Na^+; in the absence of hyperglycemia, P_{osm} is closely approximated by $2[Na^+]_s$. A patient whose serum is hypoosmolar, therefore, must also be hyponatremic. From the standpoint of emergency management, two types of significance are attached to hyponatremia. First, progressive hyponatremia is associated with confusion, obtundation, seizures, and coma. The level of $[Na^+]_s$ at which symptoms or signs appear is extremely variable: On the one hand, values below 100 mEq/liter may be well tolerated, while on the other hand, a patient with a preexisting convulsive disorder may develop uncontrollable seizure activity at a $[Na^+]_s$ of 120 mEq/liter. It is not the severity of the hyponatremia that determines the degree of emergency, but the severity of the manifestations of hyponatremia in a particular patient and in the context of the underlying disease. Second, the therapeutic response to the finding of hyponatremia and, more important, its life-threatening manifestations, depends upon an understanding of its pathogenesis and the ability to marshal the clinical evidence to distinguish among the three major forms of the electrolyte disorder: hyponatremia associated with reduced volume of ECF, with primary inappropriate release of antidiuretic hormone, and with cardiac disease or severe hypoalbuminemia. The remainder of this section is addressed to the pathophysiology of hyponatremia and its differential diagnosis and management.

PATHOPHYSIOLOGY

If laboratory error, severe hyperglycemia, and marked hyperlipidemia are excluded, the demonstration of hyponatremia indicates a failure of the normal mechanisms that provide for the excretion of the water that is in excess of available solute. The ability of the kidney to generate a sufficient volume of urine whose concentration is more dilute than serum, and thus to elevate the concentration of solute in the body fluids, depends on the fulfillment of three conditions. The first is the delivery of an adequate volume of residual glomerular filtrate containing Na^+ and Cl^- to the distal nephron. Second, the ion pumps in this location must be operational—as they are, for example, in the absence of the loop diuretics furosemide and ethacrynic acid or, to a lesser extent, the thiazide diuretics. Third, release of antidiuretic hormone (ADH) from the posterior pituitary gland must be inhibited. If all three conditions are fulfilled, a large volume of dilute urine will be formed, and hyponatremia either will not develop or, if present, will rapidly be corrected.

HYPONATREMIA ASSOCIATED WITH REDUCED VOLUME OF EXTRACELLULAR FLUID

From the pathogenetic standpoint, three major types of hyponatremia may be distinguished. The first is associated with reduced volume of the ECF. Under ordinary circumstances, reduction in the size of this compartment is reflected in proportionate contraction of one of its components, the vascular space. As a result, glomerular filtration rate (GFR) is compromised and the volume of fluid delivered to the distal nephron is reduced. In addition, ADH, whose release under normal conditions is stimulated by increased P_{osm} and inhibited by reduced P_{osm} of body fluids, is secreted independently of P_{osm} when hemodynamic status is severely compromised. For both reasons, the kidney fails to excrete water in excess of solute and, if water intake is maintained, hyponatremia ensues. The patient's history often will suggest a reason for abnormal loss of salt, and physical examination will reveal decreased tissue turgor, tachycardia, and perhaps a fall in blood pressure on standing. Laboratory studies will demonstrate an elevation of blood area nitrogen (BUN) or creatinine for that patient and, if the kidney is not the route of abnormal salt loss, a urinary concentration of Na^+, $[U_{Na}]$, approaching 0 mEq/liter. Infusion of isotonic saline will restore the volume of ECF, including its intravascular component, enhance GFR and the delivery of volume to the distal nephron, and remove the hemodynamic stimulus for ADH release. Removal of these two constraints on renal regulation of P_{osm} will permit rapid correction of the hyponatremia. Infusion of hypertonic saline is unnecessary and confers increased risk.

HYPONATREMIA ASSOCIATED WITH PRIMARY INAPPROPRIATE RELEASE OF ANTIDIURETIC HORMONE

Hyponatremia of the second type results from the release of ADH or similar material from the posterior pituitary or an ectopic source in the absence of either the normal osmotic stimulus or hemodynamic insufficiency. The syndrome, best characterized as *primary inappropriate ADH release* to distinguish it from *inappropriate release* of hemodynamic etiology, is not rare in general hospital practice. The initial step in the pathogenetic sequence is the expansion of body fluid compartments, including the ECF, due to continued intake of water in the face of renal production of a concentrated urine, the latter obligated by the presence of ADH. If cardiac reserve is normal, expansion of vascular volume results in an increase in GFR and a reduction in aldosterone secretion, both of which are responsible for a diuresis of Na^+ and its anions. The relative retention of water in the face of urinary losses of Na^+ produces hyponatremia.

DIAGNOSIS

In addition to the findings associated with any of the several specific etiologies for the syndrome, the patient demonstrates good tissue turgor and hemodynamic status, an increase of 3–5 kg over baseline weight, no edema in the uncomplicated case, a BUN or creatinine that is lower than the patient's premorbid value, a urine that need not be maximally concentrated, or even more concentrated than plasma, but is more concentrated than expected for the low value of P_{osm}, and a $[U_{Na}]$ that usually exceeds 20 mEq/liter.

It is worth noting that a very similar clinical picture can result from the rapid ingestion of massive amounts of water, a syndrome termed *psychogenic polydipsia*. In the patient with psychogenic polydipsia, however, the rate of urine flow is large and its concentration, appropriately, approaches a physiologic minimum as indicated by a specific gravity close to 1.001.

TREATMENT

At present, there is no clinically available method for inhibiting the release of ADH or its interaction with the renal receptors that initiate the process of urinary concentration. An alternative approach—inhibition of the normal renal response to the hormone—is technically possible. It involves the creation of temporary nephrogenic diabetes insipidus by administration of lithium salts or demeclocycline. Since treatment results in a new, albeit transient disease, and since experience with the regimen is limited, it cannot be considered an established therapeutic option at this time.

Conservative management of the syndrome of primary inappropriate ADH release is directed at restoring renal capacity to conserve Na^+ by reducing the amount of total body water. At a minimum, this requires rigid restriction of water intake so that the combination of renal and insensible losses result in negative water balance. If the manifestations of hyponatremia are not life threatening, no additional therapy is indicated. If the patient's status appears to require more aggressive—and more hazardous—therapy, three major options exist: infusion of hypertonic saline; administration of hypertonic saline concurrently with either ethacrynic acid or furosemide; or dialysis, preferably by the peritoneal route. All three modalities require careful and continuing supervision by the attending physician. Unless he or she is experienced in their use, the latter two options are likely to confer greater risk than the first.

The following principles govern the use of hypertonic saline in this context. First, the therapeutic objective is not the restoration of $[Na^+]_s$ to normal, but its elevation to a level that eliminates the life-threatening manifestations of hyponatremia, such as severe obtundation, convulsions, or coma, in the particular patient. Only rarely will a value greater than 120 mEq/liter be required. Second, because the hypertonic saline is restricted to the ECF, it will generate an osmotic force that will extract water from the cellular compartment, enlarge the ECF volume, and reduce the expected increment in $[Na^+]_s$. In calculating the number of milliequivalents of Na^+ to be administered, assume an apparent volume of distribution equal to total body water, or 0.6 of body weight. Third, there is *no* clinical situation in which administration of hypertonic saline is appropriate that does not also require, at least temporarily, the rigid restriction of water intake.

HYPONATREMIA ASSOCIATED WITH CARDIAC DISEASE OR HYPOALBUMINEMIA

The third type of hyponatremia, and the most common in urban hospital practice, is associated with hemodynamic insufficiency due either to cardiac disease or hypoalbuminemia. The defect in the renal regulation of the solute concentration of body fluids has its origin in the decreased GFR per nephron and hence in the delivery of solute and water to the diluting segment of the distal nephron. If the circulatory insufficiency is severe, release of ADH may further reduce the ability of the kidney to excrete water in excess of solute. In the face of continued intake of water and diminished capacity of the kidney to excrete it, as well as the usual low-salt diet, the patient becomes hyponatremic. The etiology of the hemodynamic insufficiency usually is obvious. Further, the patient commonly is edematous, urinary concentration is inappropriately high for the patient's $[Na^+]_s$ or P_{osm}, the BUN or serum creatinine is likely to be at least slightly elevated, and $[U_{Na}]$ approaches zero.

TREATMENT

From the descriptive standpoint, the fundamental problem is an intake of solute-free water in excess of the ability of the kidney to excrete it. Management of this type of hyponatremia thus depends, first, on anticipating reduced capacity to excrete water in the presence of circulatory insufficiency and, second, on restricting its intake when $[Na^+]_s$ begins to fall below the normal range.

In the presence of established hyponatremia whose manifestations are life threatening, the additional therapeutic options of hypertonic saline, with or without a loop diuretic, and dialysis are all hazardous. If more rapid elevation of $[Na^+]_s$ than can be achieved solely by water restriction is mandatory, peritoneal dialysis in the cardiac patient and hemodialysis in the cirrhotic patient, conducted by experienced personnel, appear to confer the least risk.

Two points merit emphasis. First, prevention of this type of hyponatremia by early restriction of water intake avoids the risks associated with its rapid correction. Second, hyponatremia in this context is an indication of serious disease. Although development of hyponatremia can profitably and easily be prevented, the outcome of the illness is more likely to be affected by the discovery of a treatable cause of the basic disease. An energetic search for constrictive pericarditis, subacute bacterial endocarditis, masked thyrotoxicosis, or other remediable etiology should be a routine part of the prevention or correction of hyponatremia associated with circulatory insufficiency.

THE OLIGURIC PATIENT

Oliguria of recent onset is often associated with life-threatening electrolyte abnormalities at the time the patient is first seen; in the remainder of cases, serious disturbances will develop within hours in the absence of appropriate management. For these reasons, a section on the approach to the oliguric patient is presented here.

Oliguria is usefully but arbitrarily defined as a rate of urine production less than 400 ml/day, or approximately 15 ml/hr. The following discussion proceeds on the assumption that the presence of oliguria has been recognized and that serious electrolyte disturbances already have been addressed as described in previous sections of this chapter.

Evaluation of the patient is directed first at differentiating among the three principal types of etiology of oliguria: prerenal, intrarenal, and postrenal disorders. Within each major category the differential diagnosis need not proceed to a unique etiologic solution since the objective of emergency evaluation is to identify those causes of oliguria that are immediately reversible and will either permit rapid resumption of normal urine flow or halt progressive renal damage. For all other etiologies, emergency management will be based on the presumption of acute and reversible renal failure, and definitive diagnostic studies will be deferred. Using these simplifying principles, manageable descriptions of each of the major etiologic categories may be developed.

Oliguria of prerenal origin is that resulting from renal hypoperfusion. The most important causes are hemorrhage, salt depletion, hypoalbuminemia, sequestration of ECF volume, and circulatory failure due to either intrinsic cardiac disease or the effects of septicemia. The crucial diagnostic feature of prerenal oliguria is its rapid reversal upon amelioration of the cause of renal hypoperfusion.

Intrarenal causes of oliguria include all of the many diseases that can produce acute or chronic renal failure. Emergency evaluation, however, requires only the identification of those conditions that have a potentially modifiable course in the short run. Possibilities include allergic or toxic disorders, hypercalcemia, malignant hypertension, fulminant infection of the kidneys, and arterial or venous occlusion.

Postrenal causes of oliguria are those that cause obstruction at any level of the urinary tract. Anuria, which may be intermittent, is the most suggestive manifestation, and prostatic hypertrophy, tumors, and calculi are the most common causes. It is worth remembering that it is not unusual for patients to have a single functioning kidney. Patency of the lower urinary tract, therefore, does not rule out obstruction as the cause of oligoanuria.

Evaluation

The patient's medical problems are reviewed, with particular emphasis on the mode of onset of the oliguria, fluid balance, trauma, including that due to surgery, infections, exposure to drugs or other nephrotoxins, and historical evidence of hepatic or myocardial disease, nephrolithiasis, or hypercalcemia.

The physical examination is first directed at the discovery of causes of renal hypoperfusion. Evidence for decreased intravascular or ECF volume or cardiac decompensation is carefully sought. The cornea is examined for band keratopathy; the skin is examined for eruptions suggestive of an allergic reaction or vasculitis. The presence or absence of a distended bladder is noted, and pelvic and rectal examinations are performed to seek a potentially obstructing lesion. Finally, foci of infection that may be the source of septicemia are sought.

We have assumed for the purpose of the present discussion that serious electrolyte abnormalities are already under treatment. It should be emphasized at this point, however, that an important component of the physical examination is the search for causes of increased catabolism or accelerated entry of K^+ into the ECF. Ischemic tissue, an abscess, or a large hematoma may require urgent intervention.

If not already available, acquisition of a series of baseline measurements is the next step. These should include an accurate determination of the patient's weight, serum values of Na^+, K^+, CO_2, and BUN or creatinine, and, if clinical suspicion makes it appropriate, Ca^{2+} and arterial pH and PCO_2.

While awaiting these results, the examiner should attempt

to obtain a specimen of urine by spontaneous voiding, if possible, or by urinary catheter if necessary. An aliquot is sent for osmolality, Na$^+$, K$^+$, and BUN or creatinine, and the remainder of the sample is kept for the physician's own analysis.

Next, if the evaluation to this point suggests intravascular or ECF volume depletion, infusion of blood, albumin, or saline as appropriate is begun. In the elderly or in patients with known cardiac disease, insertion of a venous catheter to measure central venous or pulmonary capillary pressure is advantageous. If the clinical evidence fails to suggest fluid depletion as the cause of the oliguria, it frequently will be found useful to test renal function in other ways. A dose of 12.5 g of the osmostic diuretic mannitol or 40–80 mg of furosemide are infused intravenously over 5 minutes. In the subsequent hour an increase in urine output to 40 ml/hr or more suggests that the previous oliguria is of the prerenal type.

If the results of the initial evaluation suggest that urinary obstruction is present, the studies in the preceding paragraph may be omitted and the patient should be sent for x-ray examination. At a minimum, a plain film of the abdomen should be taken to demonstrate the number, size, and position of the kidneys and to determine the presence of calcification overlying the urinary tract. Even in the presence of complete obstruction at or above the trigone, intravenous pyelography with late nephrotomograms may demonstrate the dilated drainage system and establish the presence, and often the general location, of the lesion. If the technique is available, ultrasonography may demonstrate dilatation of the calyces and renal pelvis and obviate the need for injection of dye to establish the presence of obstruction.

While these studies are in progress there is an opportunity to examine the urine specimen obtained earlier. Oliguria of prerenal orgin usually is associated with a specific gravity greater than 1.015, low concentration of protein, a [U$_{Na}$] less that 5 mEq/liter, and a urinary urea nitrogen (UUN) or creatinine concentration more than 12 times that of blood. Oliguria of parenchymal origin is likely to be associated with a specific gravity approximating 1.010, moderate to heavy proteinuria, [U$_{Na}$] greater than 15 mEq/liter, and a ratio of UUN to BUN that is eight or less. A urine sediment that contains large numbers of white cells and bacteria, red cell casts, or renal tubular epithelial cells supports the interpretation of significant parenchymal renal disease. By contrast, urine from a patient with obstructive uropathy is likely to have only slight proteinuria and, depending on the etiology of the obstruction, may show only a few red cells in the sediment. Unfortunately, it is necessary to close this portion of the discussion with the warning that with the exception of the demonstration of obstruction by catheter or pyelography, none of the tests described are absolutely diagnostic. It is the overall weight of the findings, and the risks and benefits to be expected in the particular instance, that will determine the choice of more definitive and hazardous diagnostic procedures.

Treatment

The therapeutic response to oliguria of prerenal origin has been mentioned; the appropriate response to obstruction usually is obvious. Most of the problems arise in the course of managing an episode of parenchymal renal failure. In any case, the patient will have been brought to optimum hemodynamic status by appropriate fluid therapy during the course of initial evaluation. Once it is apparent that the oliguria will not quickly remit, however, further fluid intake must be rigidly restricted to a level comparable to the sum of net insensible losses (about 500 ml/day in the afebrile patient) and all measured fluid losses. If an indwelling urinary catheter is in place, it should now be removed because the risk of infection outweighs the minor advantage to be gained by monitoring hourly urine output. Intake of K$^+$ and protein should be stopped, a program for the provision of 100–200 g glucose per day outlined, and contingency plans made for the management of hyperkalemia, as described in earlier sections of this chapter, of metabolic acidosis, and of the uremic syndrome. The development of a tentative program for the performance of further diagnostic studies and potential treatment completes the phase of emergency management for the patient with oliguria of intrarenal origin.

SUGGESTED READINGS

Cogan MG, Rector FC Jr, Seldin DW: Acid base disorders, in Brenner BM and Rector FC Jr (eds): *The Kidney,* ed 2. Philadelphia, WB Saunders Co, 1981, pp 841–907.

Cohen JJ, Gennari FJ, Harrington JT: Disorders of potassium balance, in Brenner BM and Rector FC Jr (eds): *The Kidney,* ed 2. Philadelphia, WB Saunders Co, 1981, pp 908–939.

Hays RM, Levine SD: Pathophysiology of water metabolism, in Brenner BM and Rector FC Jr (eds): *The Kidney,* ed 2. Philadelphia, WB Saunders Co, 1981, pp 777–840.

Levinsky NG: Fluids and electrolytes, acidosis and alkalosis, in Isselbacher KJ, Adams RD, Braunwald E, Petersdorf RG, Wilson JD (eds): *Harrison's Principles of Internal Medicine,* ed 9. New York, McGraw-Hill Book Co, 1980, pp 415–450.

Valtin H: *Renal Dysfunction.* Boston, Little Brown & Co, 1979.

ACUTE INJURIES

PART II

12

THE CRITICALLY INJURED PATIENT

Harold L. May

There are over 65 million injuries annually in the United States and of these, 105,000 were fatal in 1980, and 10 million were either temporarily or permanently disabling. Accidents are currently the third largest cause of death in the United States, exceeded only by cardiovascular disease and cancer, but they are by far the leading cause of mortality in young people between the ages of 1 and 34. Motor vehicle accidents, which were responsible for 51% of accidental deaths, commonly affect the young, whereas falls, which caused about 13% of accidental deaths, often affect the elderly.

In spite of the facts that one-third of all hospital admissions—approximately 2 million people a year—are the result of accidents, that the cost of trauma to society has been estimated at a staggering $83.5 billion per year, or $228 million per day, and that the evidence that some of these deaths and disabilities could be prevented, it was not until 1961 that a pioneering clinical shock-trauma unit, formed at the University of Maryland, was established. In 1966, the white paper, "Accidental Death and Disability: The Neglected Disease of Modern Society," prepared by the National Academy of Sciences–National Research Council Committees on Shock and Trauma, brought the needs into clear focus. Now that the seriousness of the problem has been recognized, increasing efforts are being made to elucidate the pathophysiology of trauma and to improve the systems for providing care for the critically injured. Such improvement in care requires an understanding of the pathophysiology of the injury and of the body's response to it because it is only with such an understanding of these mechanisms that the physician and the system can respond appropriately.

THE INJURY

Injury occurs only when an energy load that is presented to the body is greater than the body can absorb. Under such circumstances, kinetic energy causes either blunt or penetrating injury; thermal, electrical, chemical, and radiation energy cause other forms of tissue damage and bodily injury, either immediately or over a period of time.

Blunt Injury

INJURING FORCES

*Kinetic Energy, Force,
and Acceleration/Deceleration*

In 1942 attention was first called to the importance of the relationship between stopping distance and the magnitude of injuries suffered in a collision. DeHaven pointed out that the body is far more rugged than formerly believed, reporting survival of individuals after free falls from heights varying from 55 to 146 ft. In each case, survival was possible because, in spite of the violent collision, the victim landed in a variant of the supine or prone position onto a yielding structure such as a roof or soft earth that allowed time for deceleration. Typical of the cases reported was a woman who jumped from a 10-story window, falling 93 ft onto a garden where the earth had been freshly turned, striking the soft earth in a nearly supine position. The stopping distance was 6 in. The magnitude of the energy exchange and the force involved in such a violent impact are expressed primarily in terms of kinetic energy, force, or gravitational units.

An object in motion, whether it is a 2,000-lb automobile, a bullet, or a human body, has kinetic energy represented by the following equation:

$$\text{Kinetic energy} = \frac{\text{mass} \times \text{velocity}^2}{2}$$

The terms kinetic energy and force are often used interchangeably, but they are not the same. *Force* is a push or pull, and weight is the force (pull) exerted by gravity on a given mass. Since weight is the mass of the object multiplied by gravitational acceleration (32.2 ft/sec^2), the *kinetic energy* of a moving object is calculated by the formula,

$$\text{Kinetic energy (ft-lb)} = \frac{\text{weight (lb)} \times \text{velocity}^2 \text{ (ft/sec)}^2}{2 \times 32.2 \text{ ft/sec}^2}$$

(In the metric system, kinetic energy is expressed in joules, weight in kilograms, and velocity in m/sec.) Since the velocity of the 115-lb falling woman at time of impact was 73 ft/sec (50 mph), the kinetic energy of her body when it hit the ground was 9,516 ft-lb.

The dissipation of kinetic energy requires the expenditure of an equal amount of work. Since the amount of work that is required to stop a moving object equals the force that is exerted times the distance over which it acts, the force that is developed at the time of a collision can be calculated by the formula,

231

$$\text{Force} = \frac{\text{kinetic energy}}{\text{stopping distance}}$$

The force generated by (and absorbed by) the 115-lb falling body when it suddenly stopped was 19,090 lb.

Although blunt injury can occur from forces that are applied slowly, it is usually caused by direct impact or by indirect force. These forces of deceleration or acceleration are best understood in terms of gravity (g) units, the factor by which the weight of the body is apparently increased during a sudden velocity change. If the velocity is suddenly reduced to zero by collision, the factor by which the pull of gravity is apparently increased can be calculated by the formula,

$$g = \frac{\text{velocity}^2 \text{ (mph)}}{30 \times \text{ stopping distance (ft)}}$$

The average number of g units during the time of impact of the falling body was 166 g (although the maximum probably reached more than 200 g before the end of the violent deceleration). Survival was possible in the case discussed here because the force of almost 10 tons was distributed throughout the woman's body rather than being concentrated in a small point of impact, and the stopping distance of 6 in., though small, moderated the forces of deceleration.

There are many kinds of force (e.g., gravity, the weight of any object, or atmospheric pressure, the weight of the air that is pressing on a specific area of a surface), but three basic types of force are recognized in terms of their effects on a given mass: tension, compression, and shearing. A tensile force tends to pull apart; a compressive force tends to push together; and a shearing force tends to make part of an object slide over an immediately adjacent part. These forces may act alone or in combination, or they may be coupled in such a way that bending or twisting occurs. In any case, force always causes deformity.

Stress and Strain

Newton's third law of motion—for every action there is always an opposed and equal reaction—helps to explain the difference between externally applied forces and the ones that occur in the body in response to them. Force applied to the human body (or to any body) elicits two responses: stress and strain. Stress is the internal resistance to the deforming effect of an external force. Strain, the reciprocal of stress, is the deformity produced by the applied force. Stress and strain, like force, may be tensile, compressive, or shearing.

Mechanical stress in the body is probably best exemplified by the architecture of the weight-bearing portion of the skeletal system. The trabeculae of the upper femur (Fig. 12.1) are arranged in the familiar pattern of arching, parallel, Gothic-like struts; these lines of stress within this part of the bone are the body's adaptation to the bearing of the weight (force) of the trunk when the person is in an upright position. Similarly, the trabecular pattern of the calcaneus (Fig. 12.2), reflects the stress that makes its weight-bearing function possible. Although stress cannot be seen directly and cannot be measured, it can be computed in terms of the magnitude of the applied force, divided by the cross-sectional area of the distribution of the force. Its units, therefore, are those of pressure: pounds per square inch (psi).

Strain is the deformity produced by a given force; it is measurable by the degree to which a force causes lengthening, compression, or displacement of adjacent tissues in relation to each other. The characteristics of the tissues determine their response. Highly elastic tissue can stretch enormously without breaking in response to an outside force. Even normal bone possesses a small amount of elasticity. The distensibility of organs such as the colon and the bladder make it possible for their walls to be stretched greatly without damage. Most of the

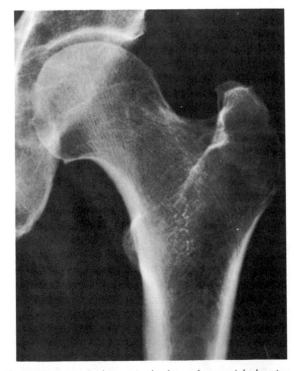

Figure 12.1 Lines of stress in the femur from weight bearing.

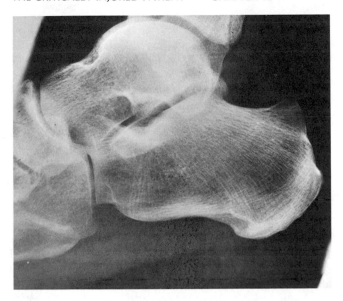

Figure 12.2 Stress lines in the os calcis and other bones of the foot.

TABLE 12.1 Severity of Injury of 57,597 Victims of Rural Automobile Accidents[a]

Severity of Injury	Percent of Injured Occupants
Minor	52.0
Nondangerous	34.5
Dangerous	7.6
Fatal	5.9

SOURCE: Used with permission from Gurdjian ES, Lange WA, Patrick LM, Thomas LM (eds): *Impact Injury and Crash Protection*. Springfield, IL, Charles C. Thomas, Publisher, 1970, p. 15.

[a]From study by Automotive Crash Injury Program of the Cornell Aeronautical Laboratory.

body's structures can stand much greater loads than are required by ordinary activities, but all of the structures have a breaking point and any that is deformed beyond that point will break. Even before that point is reached, however, if some tissues are stretched beyond their normal limits of tolerance they will be injured to some degree (strained) although not broken.

Body Injury

When blunt forces of great magnitude are absorbed by the body, it is not surprising that multiple injuries are frequently the result. The Automotive Crash Injury Program of the Cornell Aeronautical Laboratory, analyzing injury data for 57,597 automobile occupants who were injured in rural automobile accidents, found that 7.6% had serious injuries and 5.9% of them were fatally injured (Table 12.1). As noted in Table 12.2, only 30% of the injuries were limited to one body area; 70% involved at least two body areas and 38% involved more than two. The data from this study and the evidence from many others confirm the observation that multiplicity of injury is a dominant feature for victims injured in automobile accidents. The head was the area that was most often involved, and the lower limbs were more commonly injured than the thorax or the abdomen (Table 12.3). Those injuries that were dangerous or fatal commonly included the head, neck, thorax, and ab-

domen in some combination. On the other hand, less dangerous injuries were generally not multiple and tended to involve the limbs rather than the other parts of the body.

Of 1,286 victims of blunt trauma treated in the Maryland Trauma Institute, 42% had central nervous system (CNS) injuries, 27% had thoracic injuries, 16% had abdominal injuries, and 65% had fractures (Table 12.4). Of those with abdominal injuries, 44% had CNS injuries and 41% had thoracic injury. Of those with thoracic injury, 56% required laparotomy. Simultaneous involvement of the thorax, CNS, and abdomen was present in 6% of the patients.

TABLE 12.2 Number of Body Areas Involved in 57,597 Injured Occupants of Automobile Accidents[a]

Number of Body Areas Involved	Percent of Injured Occupants
One	30.0
Two	32.0
Three	23.4
Four	10.9
Five	3.2
Six	0.5

SOURCE: Used with permission from Gurdjian ES, Lange WA, Patrick LM, Thomas LM (eds): *Impact Injury and Crash Protection*. Springfield, IL, Charles C. Thomas, Publisher, 1970, p. 14.

[a]From study by Automotive Crash Injury Program of the Cornell Aeronautical Laboratory.

TABLE 12.3 Body Areas Involved in 57,597 Injured Occupants of Automobile Accidents

Body Area Involved	Percent of Injured Occupants
Head	70.8
Neck	10.8
Thorax	38.6
Abdomen	17.1
Upper limb	38.9
Lower limb	50.4

SOURCE: Used with permission from Gurdjian ES, Lange WA, Patrick LM, Thomas LM (eds): *Impact Injury and Crash Protection.* Springfield, IL, Charles C. Thomas, Publisher, 1970, p. 14.

[a]From study by Automotive Crash Injury Program of the Cornell Aeronautical Laboratory.

FACTORS INFLUENCING THE BODY'S RESPONSE TO ANY INJURING FORCE

The injuring potential of a force is determined not only by the nature and magnitude of the injuring force but also by the characteristics of the body tissues.

The amount of kinetic energy absorbed by the body tissues is the primary determinant of the magnitude of the injury. Animal experiments have confirmed the common sense observation that a force that seriously injures a small animal may not injure a large one. The magnitude of injuring force is measured against the individual's capacity to withstand it.

The area over which a force is concentrated is an important factor in determining the magnitude of an injury. If a force is distributed over a wide area, the body may be able to absorb it, since the number of pounds of force per square inch is thereby minimized. As the area of distribution becomes smaller, the amount of force that is concentrated over that area in-

TABLE 12.4 Blunt Trauma in 1,286 Victims[a]

Body Area	Number	Percent
CNS	540	42
Thorax	347	27
Abdomen	205	16
Fracture	835	65

SOURCE: Adapted and used with permission from GILL, W and Long, WB: Shock Trauma Manual, Baltimore, Williams and Wilkins Co., 1979, pages 25–27.

[a]Maryland Trauma Institute.

creases, sometimes exceeding the limits of tolerance of the underlying tissues, and injury results. In fact, the smaller the area becomes, the more the injuring force becomes penetrating instead of blunt. A relatively small amount of force can readily penetrate tissues if it is concentrated over a small enough area.

The location of impact of a blunt force helps to determine its injuring potential because of differing responses of body tissues to externally applied forces. Under most circumstances (especially if forces are distributed over a wide area) only a small percentage of the force applied to the experimental animal, and presumably to people in automobile accidents, is actually transmitted directly to vital structures such as the liver because much of the applied energy is absorbed by structures such as the rib cage and the abdominal parietes (Trollope). But relatively small blunt forces may produce severe injuries of solid abdominal viscera when the point of impact is the upper part of the abdomen since fluid-filled, sinusoidal, encapsulated structures such as the liver and spleen transmit applied hydrokinetic energy through their internal architecture to their capsules with bursting force if the pressure is great enough. Much greater force is needed to produce comparatively severe injuries in the lower abdomen because the abdominal parietes can absorb much of the force unless the visceral structures are distended at the time of impact (Mays).

The duration of action also influences the degree of injury. In general, the injury produced by a given force applied over a long period of time is much more severe than if that same force is applied briefly. On the other hand, when compressive force is applied slowly enough, it sometimes allows a turgid organ, such as the liver, to deform to a distorted shape without sustaining injury.

Safety equipment and protective clothing can often prevent or diminish the severity of an injury. It has been estimated that the use of seat belts in automobiles reduces the risk of injury or death by about one-third in the United States and one-fifth in Australia (Haddon). Stapp has noted that most automobile accidents that produce fatal injuries occur at the speed of about 40 mph, as the consequence of delayed braking. Of course, accidents that occur above that speed are more likely to be fatal. As is true of the body in free fall, the critical variable is the stopping distance. If a vehicle that is traveling at a velocity of 40 mph stops in a distance of 2 ft (including the compressing deformation of the front of the vehicle), it is subjected to 26.7 g units. A passenger who is securely strapped in by lap and shoulder belts is subjected to approximately the same g forces. But the unrestrained passenger continues forward at the moment of impact and will not stop until he or she is thrown out of the vehicle or hits the steering wheel, dashboard, windshield, or other obstruction—the second collision. Although the velocity at the time of the second collision is less than that of the automobile at the time of impact, if the structure is unyielding such abrupt crashes are almost always fatal.

Extensive studies in Australia revealed that the use of protective headgear reduced the risk of fatal injuries to motorcyclists to about one-third of the risk without the helmet. Not only does the helmet distribute the impact over a larger area, but it also protects the skull from deformity that would otherwise occur from a direct impact against an unyielding surface. Athletic equipment, such as shoulder pads, offer energy-absorbing protection, and even street clothing (especially heavy clothing) offers some degree of protection. Not surprisingly, leather clothing offers the highest degree of protection to the motorcyclist who is subjected to great shearing forces when thrown off the motorcycle. The tough skin of an animal absorbs shearing forces to which the motorcyclist's skin would otherwise have been subjected.

MECHANISMS OF BODY INJURY

There are three basic mechanisms for the production of blunt injury. It is commonly caused by direct impact to the body surface. Inertial forces, resulting in differential motion of one part of the body in relation to another, may injure by causing shearing and internal collisions of tissues. The force can also be caused by air- or liquid-transmitted blast waves that transmit pressure to large parts of the body or major segments of it. Exposure to a blasting force may involve all three types of force application. Crash injury involves forces of both the first and second type, whereas the acceleration forces encountered in aerospace flight are predominantly of the second type.

Head Injury

A blunt injury to the head may be caused either from a direct or indirect force resulting from a direct blow to the head or from violent acceleration or deceleration of the brain associated with sudden hyperextension or hyperflexion of the neck. In fact, any impact to the head (except very slowly applied compression) involves acceleration or deceleration, whether the head is fixed or free. When deformation (compression, stretching, or shearing) occurs simultaneously or in succession during an impact to the head, the scalp is compressed, thereby absorbing a significant amount of force. The scalp is able to absorb up to 35% of a force so that in certain low-intensity impacts, the scalp and a thick head of hair may be effective in preventing an injury to underlying structures (Gurdjian).

Violent acceleration or deceleration may injure because of differences in the rate of acceleration or deceleration of various parts of the intracranial contents. Cortical veins emptying into the superior sagittal sinus and other veins emptying into the sphenoid sinus may be torn and produce subdural hematomas as a result of such relative movement of the brain in relation to the skull (Fig. 12.3). The base of the skull, which is irregular in the anterior and middle fossae, and the knifelike edge of the lesser wing of the sphenoid and the unbudging sharp border of the tentorium may produce tears and contusions of the brain as it moves in relation to these structures (Fig. 12.4).

Direct impact over the skull may cause a fracture that, in turn, may be responsible for injuring an underlying blood vessel such as the middle meningeal artery (Fig. 12.3), thereby causing an epidural hematoma. If a large force is concentrated over a small area, for example, a blow from a hammer, a depressed fracture may result. The total energy that is required to cause a skull fracture ranges from 33 to 75 ft-lb, which is the amount of energy that is transmitted to the head when it strikes a hard flat surface after a free fall from a height of 5 ft (Gurdjian). Striking the head at 50 mph against a surface that bends or dents 5 or 6 in. may expose it to less force than it may receive when a person slips on the ice. It has been repeatedly noted by Gurdjian and others that 78–80% of patients with linear skull fractures were rendered unconscious. The conclusion is that a linear skull fracture may be taken as an index of severity of a blow, representing an impact effect that is slightly stronger than the impact level that may cause a concussion.

Ordinarily, a combination of forces is involved in producing a head injury. As discussed in Chapters 10 and 15, the intracranial pressure changes that result from a head injury may secondarily produce movement and compression of portions of the brain, which may result in neurologic deficits and threaten life.

Neck Injury

Although the neck is injured much less frequently than the head, blunt injury to it must be suspected whenever the head is injured. Direct force to the anterior part of the neck, such as that caused by the impact of a steering wheel during a collision, may compress and crush the larynx. Commonly, the forces responsible for blunt injury to the neck are indirect. As described in Chapter 16, violent hyperextension or hyperflexion of the neck, associated with violent acceleration or deceleration of the head, may tear the supporting ligaments and protecting muscles and rupture intervertebral discs. If compressive force is great enough, fractures of the vertebrae may result and shear forces may lead to dislocation.

In a comparison of injuries sustained in rear-end collisions with those of front-end and side collisions, significant differ-

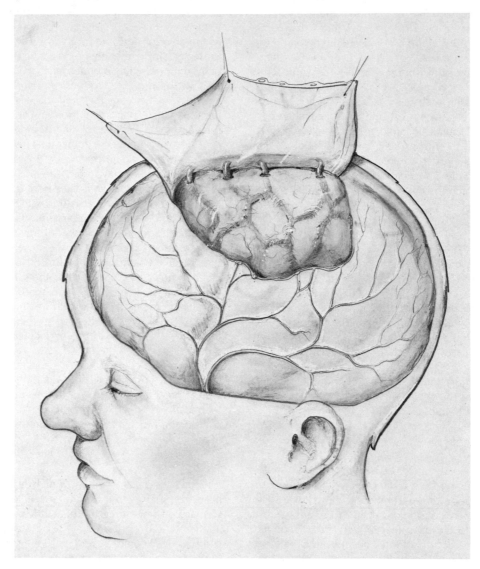

Figure 12.3 The subdural bridging veins between the sagittal sinus and the cortical vessels are shown. These may shear at time of violent deceleration, causing a subdural hematoma. The middle meningeal artery, which runs in the meningeal groove on the inner cortex of the temporal region, may be lacerated by a fracture of the overlying bone, leading to an epidural hematoma.

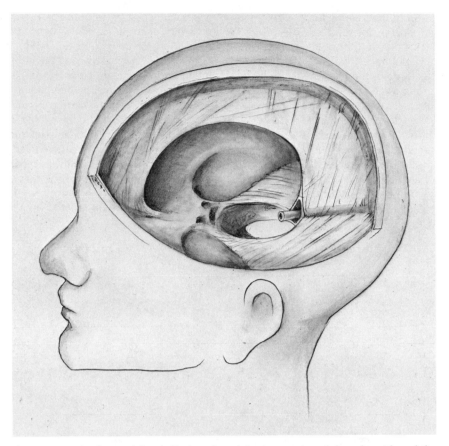

Figure 12.4 The base of the skull, the edge of the lesser wing of the sphenoid, and the unbudging edge of the tentorium are structures against which the decelerating or swelling brain may be injured.

ences were found by MacNab and Hohl. The rear-end collision was generally the most disabling. The explanation is that hyperflexion, caused by front-end collision, has a built in restraint when the chin strikes the chest and, to a lesser extent, the lateral flexion is limited when the head strikes the shoulder. On the other hand, if a rear-end collision is forceful enough, the resulting hyperextension of the neck is stopped only when the head strikes the upper dorsal spine, causing movement well in excess of the range permitted by the anatomical structures.

Chest Injury

Here again, the injuring force may be direct or indirect. Direct impact produces injuries primarily to the chest wall or to in-

trathoracic structures, depending on the force of impact. Indirect forces are partly responsible for injuries to intrathoracic content. Since clothing often provides an effective cushion and protection for the skin, the skin is often unbruised and apparently undamaged in spite of severe underlying soft tissue damage and intrathoracic injury.

Approximately 40% of victims of nonpenetrating thoracic trauma sustain fractures of the ribs, the most common of all chest injuries. Fractures of the ribs are more common in adults than in children because the cartilage in children is more resilient and can absorb an impact without breaking. The ribs of elderly individuals are brittle and can be broken even by minor trauma. The number of ribs fractured, the degree of displacement of rib fragments, and injury to the underlying lung are dependent on the force and direction of the impact and the area of its distribution. If the injuring force is applied over a wide area, especially in the anteroposterior (AP) projection, the ribs tend to buckle outward, breaking in midshaft position without injuring the pulmonary parenchyma (Blair). Direct impact over a limited area of the chest tends to drive the rib fragment inward (in the same way that a similar force may cause a depressed skull fracture) and can cause laceration of the pleura, pulmonary parenchyma, and intercostal vessels, producing pneumothorax, hemothorax, or both.

The sternum is seldom fractured in children and young adults because of the elasticity of the ribs and anterior costal cartilages. It has been demonstrated experimentally that the force of impact can press the sternum backward almost against the spinal column without breaking it. The fact that severe trauma is usually necessary to produce a sternal fracture explains the high incidence of serious associated injuries with such fractures. Blunt direct force readily produces pulmonary contusion or myocardial contusion, and the blunt force may cause sharp intrathoracic damage if ribs are broken and sharp edges are forced backward causing laceration of underlying structures.

Fractures of the first rib are uncommon. Because the first rib is small and protected by the shoulder girdle, fractures of this rib usually occur only if the impact force is tremendous. These fractures, almost always accompanied by fracture of the overlying clavicle, are frequently associated with injuries of the thoracic aorta or major bronchi; they are also associated with an increased incidence of disruption of the neurovascular structures to the upper extremities (Fig. 12.5). The lower two ribs

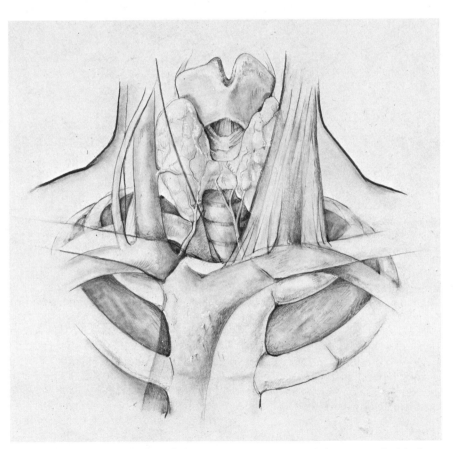

Figure 12.5 The root of the neck showing the relations of the subclavian vessels, which are immediately behind the clavicle, to the first rib, to which they are closely attached. The structures of the brachial plexus, which are immediately lateral to the subclavian artery are not shown.

are mobile and yielding; and therefore they are the least often ones to fracture. Because of the location, lower rib fractures are often associated with injuries to the liver, spleen, and kidneys (Figs. 12.6, 12.7, 12.8, and 12.9). Fractures of the left tenth rib also are sometimes associated with fractures of the spleen.

Myocardial contusion following blunt trauma is usually the result of direct impact of an automobile steering wheel over the precordium, causing compression of the heart between the sternum and the vertebral column. This injury is most commonly associated with multiple rib or sternal fractures.

At the time of direct impact, compression and sudden increase in pressure in an enclosed system may cause further injury. Ordinarily the airway is open, but the open system in the awake and aware subject is converted into a closed box by closure of the glottis at the moment of or just before impact.

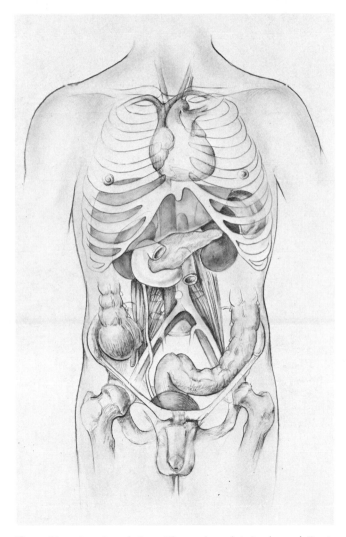

Figure 12.6 Anterior relations. The aortic arch is in close relation to the first rib. The subclavian vessels are more closely applied to the superior margin of the first rib than is shown in the illustration.

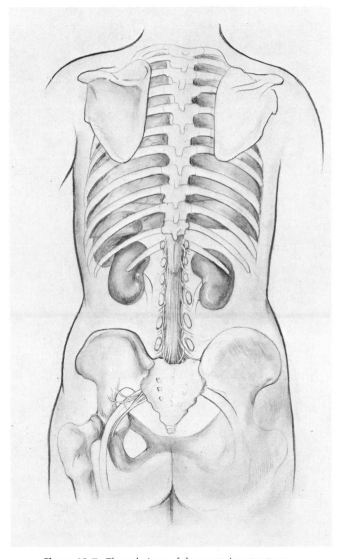

Figure 12.7 The relations of the posterior structures.

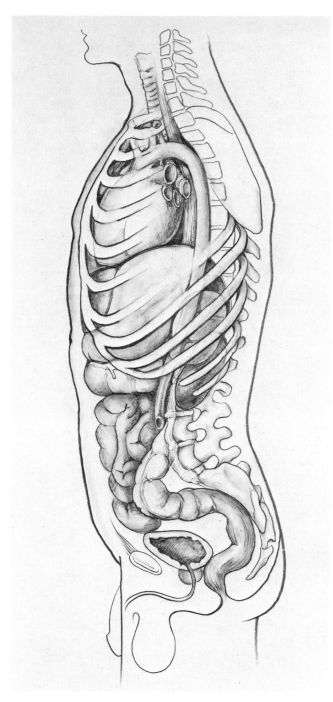

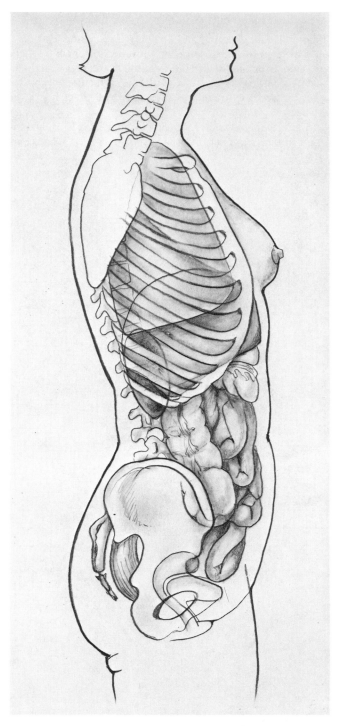

Figure 12.8 The left lateral view of the male showing the relationship of the ligamentum teres to the aorta and pulmonary artery and the relationship of the subclavian vessels to the first rib. Also shown are the relationships of the spleen and the left kidney to the lower left rib.

Figure 12.9 Anatomical relationships from the right lateral aspect in the female.

The increase in pressure may result in bursting phenomena causing mediastinal, pleural, tracheal, bronchial, or intrapulmonary damage. When the force is removed, the distorted thorax springs back, creating an instant of increased negative intrathoracic pressure. It is thought that one possible mechanism for lung contusion may lie in these compressive–decompressive phenomena (Blair).

It has been noted by Blair that mediastinal injuries rarely result from direct impact because the lungs presumably serve as protective cushions, somewhat like plastic air splints while they are momentarily at positive pressure. At time of impact, the sternum is forced posteriorly, displacing and twisting the heart to the left, while the mediastinal contents suddenly decelerate. The decelerating aorta is arrested sharply at points of attachment, such as the ligamentum arteriosum (Fig. 12.10). Although the factors responsible for the tearing or transection of the aorta have not been completely elucidated, it seems clear that an imbalance of forces of deceleration, compression, and restraint are involved. Torsion stress is critical at the base of the heart, and shearing stress is critical at the ligamentum.

The mechanisms for diaphragmatic rupture remains conjectural, but it is believed that it is caused by a tremendously high gradient between intraperitoneal and intrathoracic pressure at the time of injury, if the glottis is not closed when a severe crushing force is applied to the abdomen. At time of impact with the glottis closed, the sudden rise in intrathoracic pressure is usually matched by a rise in intraabdominal pressure. This apparent neutralization of pressures probably accounts for the relative infrequency of diaphragmatic rupture associated with blunt injury to the torso (Blair).

Abdominal Injury

The same blunt force that causes injury to the thoracic contents may also injure abdominal organs, a fact that gives rise to the term *torso injury*. The severity of injury is greatly influenced by the location of the impact. As previously noted, although the turgid liver and spleen are somewhat protected by the rib cage, they are much more easily injured than are the lower abdominal organs. This oft-noted observation is confirmed by the statistics in Tables 12.5 and 12.6, Blaisdell's summary from the literature of the relative incidence of organ injury in blunt and penetrating trauma. The hollow viscera can absorb a considerable amount of transmitted pressure unless they are distended. The small bowel is most commonly injured if a loop

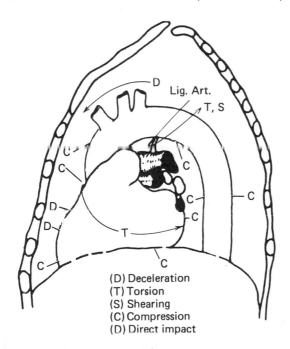

Figure 12.10 Some of the forces involved in injury to the chest. (Used with permission from Blair E, Topulzu C, Deane RS: *Major Blunt Chest Trauma.* Current Problems in Surgery, Chicago, Yearbook Medical Publishers, 1969, p. 9.)

TABLE 12.5 Blunt Trauma: Relative Incidence of Organ Injury

Organ	Percentage
Spleen	25
Liver	15
Retroperitoneal hematoma	13
Kidney	12
Small bowel	9
Bladder	6
Mesentery	5
Large bowel	4
Pancreas	3
Urethra	2
Diaphragm	2
Vascular	2
Stomach	1
Duodenum	1

SOURCE: Used with permission from Blaisdell FW: General Assessment, Resuscitation, and Exploration of Penetrating and Blunt Abdominal Trauma, in Blaisdell FW, Trunkey DD: *Trauma Management, Vol 1—Abdominal Trauma.* New York, Thiene-Stratton, Inc., 1982, p. 13.

TABLE 12.6 Penetrating Trauma: Relative Incidence of Organ Injury

Organ	Percentage
Small bowel	30
Mesentery and omentum	18
Liver	16
Colon	9
Diaphragm	8
Stomach	7
Spleen	6
Kidney	5
Major vascular	4
Pancreas	3
Duodenum	2
Bladder	1
Ureter	1

SOURCE: Used with permission from Blaisdell FW: General Assessment, Resuscitation, and Exploration of Penetrating and Blunt Abdominal Trauma, in Blaisdell FW, Trunkey DD: *Trauma Management, Vol. 1—Abdominal Trauma*. New York, Thiene-Stratton, Inc., 1982, p. 11.

is trapped against the vertebral column and subjected either to a bursting force or a shearing force.

In a report of 307 patients with blunt abdominal injuries, Walt and Griska described the mechanisms of injury as follows:

1. Direct compression with disruption of tissues due to pressure from without, either direct or shearing in nature, seen especially in mid-lying structures caught between the abdominal wall and the vertebral column.
2. Rupture of the hollow viscus due to increased intraluminal pressure which exceeds bursting wall tension, whether or not a closed loop is present.
3. Shearing by torsional forces or relatively fixed and inelastic supporting ligaments, mesenteries, or vessels.
4. Tearing of the diaphragm following sudden marked increase in the pressure of the intra-abdominal cavity.
5. Direct perforation by fragments of fractured bones which form part of the wall of the abdominal cavity, especially the pelvic area.*

---

*Walt AJ, Grifka TJ: Blunt abdominal injury: A review of 307 cases, in Gurdjian ES, Lange WA, Patrick LM, Thomas LM (eds): *Impact Injury and Crash Protection*. Springfield, IL, Charles C Thomas, 1970, pp 101–123.

Associations of injuries included pelvic fractures and rupture of the urinary tract, concomitant hepatic and splenic injuries following steering wheel injuries to the torso, and ruptures of the small bowel and its mesentery with or without lumbar fracture in the "seatbelt syndrome."

Pelvic Fractures

The rigid, strong, bony ring of the pelvis can not be fractured unless great force is applied to it, and bony displacement can occur only if the ring is disrupted in at least two places. Other portions of the pelvis—the obturator rings, sacrum, and coccyx—can be fractured from the application of much less force such as occurs commonly from falls. Although the pelvis can absorb a tremendous amount of force that would otherwise cause injury to underlying soft tissue, once it is broken, it can become the wounding force for underlying pelvic vessels, urethra and bladder, vagina, and rectum and perianal structures. Fractures of the pelvic ring commonly occur from industrial accidents in which crushing forces are applied. In recent years, automobile accidents in which a pedestrian is struck from the side, is thrown sideways in a crashing vehicle, or has the heavy wheels of a vehicle run over the pelvis, have also become a common cause of pelvic fractures.

Penetrating Injury

Classifying all gunshot injuries in the broad category of penetrating wounds is an oversimplification associated with the widely held belief that the seriousness of a bullet wound depends only on the structures that are directly in its path. A stab wound or an injury caused by a low-velocity missile can be rapidly lethal if a vital structure, such as the heart, brain, or a large vessel, is injured. But a wound caused by a high-velocity missile, such as from a hunting or military rifle, can be lethal even if a vital structure has not been penetrated.

The three primary theories that have been used to explain the wounding mechanism of bullets are the kinetic energy, momentum, and power theories. They are expressed as follows:

1. Kinetic energy $= \dfrac{mass \times velocity^2}{2}$

2. Momentum $= mass \times velocity$

3. Power $= mass \times velocity^3$

Most authorities now hold that the kinetic energy theory is most compatible with the experimental observation that the damage inflicted by a penetrating missile primarily depends on the kinetic energy that is absorbed by the tissue. Since the weight of the bullet is usually expressed in grains and approximately 7,000 grains equals 1 lb, the kinetic energy of the bullet at the gun muzzle is approximated by the following expression:

$$\text{Energy (ft-lb)} = \frac{\text{weight (grains)} \times \text{velocity}^2 \text{ (ft/sec)}}{7,000 \text{ (grains/lb)} \times 64.4 \text{ (ft/sec)}^2}$$

$$= \frac{\text{weight (grains)} \times \text{velocity}^2 \text{ (ft/sec)}}{453,600}$$

Before World War I, the emphasis in the development of small arms was upon the mass of the missile in order to maximize the knockdown capability. The U.S. military Colt 45 pistol, which fires a relatively heavy bullet (250 grains, or 16.2 g) at a low velocity (860 ft/sec, or 263 m/sec), was developed for this purpose for use in the Spanish–American War under the assumption that the momentum of the bullet was primarily responsible for its wounding capability. However, the U.S. military M-16 rifle, used in Vietnam, was developed with the recognition of the fact that the velocity of a missile contributes more to its kinetic energy than does its mass. Its bullet is tiny (55 grains, or 3.6 g), but its muzzle velocity is so high (approximately 3,250 ft/sec, or 991 m/sec), that its kinetic energy is 1,218 ft-lb, in contrast to the 410 ft-lb developed by the Colt 45 pistol.

Tables 12.7 and 12.8 indicate the relative contribution of the mass and velocity of a missile to its kinetic energy. By convention, bullet velocity is classified as low if it is under 1,000 ft/sec, medium if it is between 1,000 and 2,000 ft/sec, and high if it is above 2,000 ft/sec. The fact that the bullets of most handguns have low velocity and those of the hunting and military rifles have high velocity explain the vast difference in kinetic energy of these guns. The velocity of all bullets falls off with increasing distance, but the velocity and kinetic energy of handguns fall off so rapidly that the handgun is ordinarily effective only at short ranges (less than 50 yd). The velocity retained by most hunting and military rifles at the range of 300–1,000 yd approximates the velocity of the handgun at close range. Demuth and others have emphasized that the most important determinant of the wounding capability is the impact velocity, and that the kinetic energy absorbed by the victim is a function of the difference between the impact velocity and the velocity that the missile retains after the target has been penetrated. The missile remains within the body only if all of its kinetic energy is absorbed by the body.

Demuth has also observed that the composition and design of a bullet are almost as important as its velocity in determining its wounding capability because they play an important role in determining how much of the kinetic energy of the bullet will be absorbed by the target. The bulk of most bullets consists of a lead alloy. Since lead's melting point is low, it is easily deformed when heated above its melting point. This fact does not limit its use in handguns because their muzzle velocity is so slow that the bullet does not become distorted by frictional heat during its passage through the gun barrel; on the other hand, the portion of a high-velocity rifle bullet that comes in contact with the barrel must be covered with a jacket of metal that has a higher melting point than lead to prevent distortion produced by heat. Geneva Convention rules, established before World War I, required that military bullets must be full jacketed and nonexpanding, but hunting bullets are ordinarily softnosed so that they mushroom after perforating the target, expanding to several times their original caliber and establishing a wide wound tract. Whereas some bullets are designed to expand, others are designed to disintegrate or to tumble once they have penetrated the target. Any of these actions increase their wounding power.

The damaging effect of moving bullets increases with the increase in the specific gravity of the tissues involved (Daniel). This explains the seeming paradox of lung injury that appears to be greater if a bullet strikes the thorax tangentially than if the bullet moves directly through lung tissue. Table 12.9 indicates the specific gravity of a number of tissues. In contrast to the high-velocity bullet that transverses human tissue in a straight line, a low-velocity missile often has its course changed as it encounters tissue of varying density so that its course within the body is not that of a straight line.

Low-velocity missiles inflict penetrating injuries that are similar to those produced by knives or other sharp pointed instruments. Since tissues are pushed aside, the damage that is inflicted is limited to a small radius from the center of the track; morbidity and mortality depend only on the structures that have been penetrated. But when a bullet of similar caliber but high velocity penetrates, the tremendous amount of kinetic energy that is absorbed by the surrounding structures causes momentary acceleration of the tissues in a direction forward and laterally away from the bullet, thereby forming a temporary cavity around the bullet and its track. The cavity, resulting from the expending of an enormous explosive force during the passage of the bullet through the tissues, continues to enlarge to many times the diameter of the bullet after the bullet passes. Since the cavity is initially at subatmospheric pressure, foreign materials and tissue fragments (secondary missiles) may be sucked into it; then within a few milliseconds the cavity begins to collapse under atmospheric pressure. The reforming and collapsing of the cavity continues at rapidly diminishing amplitude until all imparted energy has been dissipated, alternately stretching and compressing the tissues and producing severe damage, sometimes at a great distance from the permanent wound track. The cavity temporarily formed is principly a function of the velocity of the bullet (Demuth).

TABLE 12.7 Representative Ballistic Data for Hunting and Military Rifles

Cartridge	Bullet Weight (grains)	Type	Velocity (ft/sec) Muzzle	100 ft	200 ft	300 ft	Energy (ft-lb) Muzzle	100 ft	200 ft	300 ft
22 Hornet	46	Hollow point	2,690	2,030	1,510	1,150	740	420	235	135
223 M-16 (U.S. 5.56 mm)	55		3,200	2,630	2,120	1,700	1,218	837	541	330
243 Winchester	80	Hollow point	3,450	3,050	2,675	2,330	2,115	1,650	1,270	965
270 Winchester	100	Pointed soft point	3,480	3,070	2,690	2,340	2,690	2,090	1,600	1,216
30-06 Springfield	110	Pointed soft point	3,370	2,830	2,350	1,920	2,770	1,960	1,350	900
30 M-1 U.S.	150		2,970	2,670	2,400	2,130	2,930	2,370	1,920	1,510
300 Winchester Magnum	150	Plastic point Pointed core lok	3,400	3,050	2,730	2,430	3,850	3,100	2,480	1,970
458 Winchester Magnum	510	Soft point	2,130	1,840	1,600	1,400	5,140	3,830	2,900	2,220
460 Weatherby Magnum	500	Full metal jacket	2,700	2,416	2,154	1,912	8,095	6,482	5,153	4,060

Of greater importance in the establishment of the permanent wound tract is the bullet construction. Expanding bullets used for sporting purposes create a permanent track much larger than that produced by a full-jacketed military-type bullet. Demuth observed experimentally that a 0.30 caliber bullet traveling at the speed of 2,900 ft/sec produces chest wound volumes that are approximately 40 times as great with expanding bullets as compared with full-patch military bullets. Figure 12.11 illustrates variations of ballistic effects upon animal tissue.

The wounding capacity of a shotgun differs from that of pistols and rifles. The shot charge consists of a large number of small spheres rather than a single missile. These pellets do not hit the target at the same time; rather, the first pellet may strike a person in one position and the last pellet may strike the victim after he or she has changed from the earlier position.

TABLE 12.8 Representative Ballistic Data for Handguns

Cartridge	Bullet Weight (grains)	Style	Muzzle Velocity (ft/sec)	Muzzle Energy (ft-lb)
22 Rohm	30	Short	965	60
25 Automatic	50	Metal case	810	73
32 Colt	80	Lead	745	100
38 Special	125	Jacket soft point	945	248
38 Automatic	130	Metal case	1040	312
45 Colt	250	Lead	860	410

TABLE 12.9 Relationship of Specific Gravity to Wounding Capacity

Tissue	Specific Gravity	Severity of Wound
Lung	0.4–0.5	Minimum
Fat	0.8	Moderate
Liver	0.01–1.02	Marked
Skin	1.09	Marked
Muscle	1.02–1.04	Marked
Bone	1.11	Extreme

SOURCE: Used with permission from DeMuth, WE: Bullet velocity and design as determinants of wounding capability: an experimental study. *J. Trauma* 6:226, 1966.

The tissue damage depends on the range. At close range, the amount of kinetic energy delivered to the tissues is overpowering (over 2,200 ft-lb). In addition, at close range the wadding that accompanies the shotgun shell is delivered to the wound along with the total mass of shot, adding considerably to the blast effect and driving the foreign body deeply into the body tissues, along with clothing and sometimes other foreign materials (Mays).

The long-range shotgun injury is very different. Mays has noted that at 40 yd approximately 200–300 pellets hit in a circle 30 in. in diameter. As the range from the target increases, fewer pellets will hit it and the kinetic energy at time of impact will decrease so that the seriousness of the injury depends only on the site of injury.

RESPONSE OF THE BODY TO INJURY

If immediate death does not occur at time of injury, the body instantly begins to mobilize a highly organized series of neurohumoral and cellular responses in its effort to meet the energy requirements that will prolong survival. This initial phase, which may not occur if hypovolemia is prevented or is treated promptly, rarely lasts more than 24–36 hours. Conserving blood volume and perfusing vital structures with enough oxygen and energy substrate to maintain life are the highest immediate priorities. The next phase, which is commonly regarded as the period of acute metabolic response to injury, is characterized by increased heat production through catabolism of the tissues and may last for as little as 1 day or as long as 14 days. This phase is followed by an anabolic phase lasting several weeks and characterized by protein synthesis, and then a final phase of convalescence lasting several months, during which energy reserves are replaced. Although the initial stages of these responses may be lifesaving, some of them, if prolonged, become damaging and then fatal if they are not interrupted.

Stimuli and Initial Responses

LOCAL INJURY

The initial stimulus is the injury itself. Depending on the nature of the trauma, some cells are injured or destroyed directly; others begin a rapid or slower process of deterioration because of hypoxia or damage from metabolic products of adjacent damaged cells or from primary or secondary effects of inflammatory cells that are recruited to defend the threatened tissues. Cellular injury releases metabolic products that greatly influence subsequent events.

Arachidonic Acid Metabolites

Perturbation of a cell membrane, even by very slight chemical or mechanical stimulation, can activate the enzyme phospholipase A_2 (or another enzyme) which releases arachidonic acid (eicosatetraenoic acid), a fatty acid that is present in the membrane of all mammalian cells, from the membrane phospholipids and initiates its rapid metabolism to form prostaglandins, thromboxane, and other derivatives. The metabolism may take two major subpathways (Fig. 12.12). The first pathway involves the enzyme, cyclooxygenase, which seems to be present in the membrane of all cells. It leads to the formation of prostaglandins, thromboxane A_2 (TxA_2), and prostacyclin. TxA_2, a very potent vasoconstrictor and inducer of platelet aggregation, is a powerful thrombogenic substance that is formed primarily by platelets, although it may be formed elsewhere to a lesser degree. Prostacyclin, a very potent vasodilator and inhibitor of platelet aggregation, is an important antithrombogenic substance formed primarily by the vascular endothelium of blood vessels (but not found in platelets). As initially described by Moncado and Vane, the generation of prostacyclin appears to be the physiologic mechanism that protects the vessel wall from deposition of platelet aggregates and has led to the suggestion that these substances represent a newly discovered homeostatic mechanism:

> The prostaglandin endoperoxides are precursors of both the proaggregatory vasoconstrictor, thromboxane A_2, formed by platelets and the antiaggregatory vasodilator, prostacyclin$_2$, produced in the vessel walls. Platelets in close contact with the vessel wall (possibly adhering to it) or forced by turbulent blood flow into

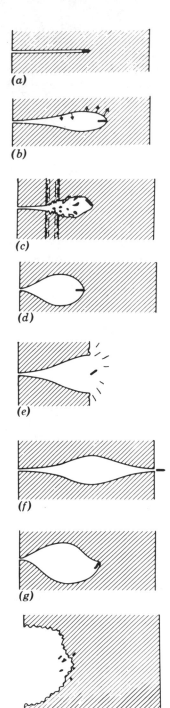

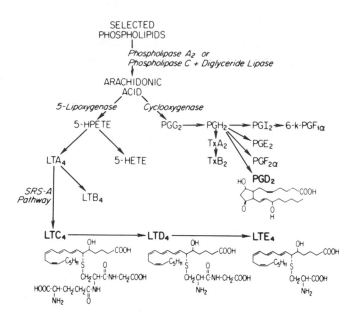

Figure 12.12 Oxidative pathways of arachidonic acid metabolism, emphasizing mast cell–dependent products. (Used with permission from Lewis RA, Austin KF: Mediation of local homeostasis and inflammation by leukotrienes and other mast cell–dependent compounds. *Nature* 293:104, 1981, Macmillan Journals Limited.)

Figure 12.11 Wound ballistics: (a) low velocity, no cavitation, entrance and exit small; (b) higher velocity, formation of cavity, arrows show direction and magnitude of acceleration of tissue; (c) velocity as in (b) but deformation of bullet and creation of secondary missiles upon penetrating bone; (d) very high velocity, large cavity, and small entrance, exit may be small; (e) very high velocity, thin target, large, ragged exit; (f) velocity, caliber, and thickness of tissue such that cavitation occurs deep inside and entrance and exit are small; (g) asymmetric cavitation as bullet begins to deform and tumble; (h) wound predicted for ultra high-velocity, small caliber projectiles now under development, no exit wound, fragmentation of bullet. (Used with permission from Swan KG, Swan RC: *Gunshot Wounds, Pathophysiology and Management.* Littleton, MA, John Wright-PSG, Inc., 1980, p. 9.)

a strong platelet-to-platelet interaction near the wall release prostaglandin endoperoxides that can be used by the endothelial cells to generate prostacyclin. This sequence of events inhibits further platelet aggregation and thus prevents the formation of a thrombus.*

Both of these substances are extremely unstable and are rapidly converted to other substances. Prostacyclin has a half-life of about 3 minutes, whereas TxA_2 has a half-life of only 30 seconds. TxA_2 is converted to the largely but not totally inactive substance thromboxane B_2 (TxB_2); prostacyclin spontaneously decomposes to other metabolites that are stable. Other prostaglandins have been discovered that have potent or weak vasodilator or vasoconstrictor effects, as well as other effects, on platelet aggregation.

Cyclooxygenase, the action of which is inhibited by aspirin, seems to be present in the membranes of all cells, but lipoxygenase has thus far been detected only in platelets, lungs, white blood cells, and recently in tissue mast cells. As depicted in Fig. 12.12, the lipoxygenase pathway leads to the formation of an intermediate 5-hydroperoxyeicosatetraenoic acid (5-HPETE) and 5-monohydroxyeicosatetraenoic acid (5-HETE), as well as leukotriene A_4 (LTA_4). The LTA_4 then enters two different pathways, one yielding leukotriene B_4 (LTB_4) and the other sequentially yielding leukotrienes C_4, D_4, and E_4 (LTC_4, LTD_4, LTE_4). As pointed out by Austin, most slow-reacting substances of anaphylaxis (SRS-A) is a mixture of these last three. LTB_4 is the most potent natural chemotactic factor identified to date, with chemotaxis for eosinophils, neutrophils, and monocytes. The SRS-A is by far the most potent vasoactive and spasmogenic mediator known. On a molar basis, it was found that it was 4,000 times as potent as histamine in compromising airway function in healthy individuals.

Platelet Aggregation and Blood Clotting

When a blood vessel is damaged, its endothelium is disrupted, exposing the underlying layer of collagen. The platelets adhere to the collagen, as well as stick to each other, forming clumps (by the process called *aggregation*) and secreting the contents of their granules (the release reaction). Some of the secreted materials—serotonin, adenosine diphosphate (ADP), calcium, lysosomal enzymes, prostaglandins, TxA_2, and 5-HETE—assist

---

*Reprinted with permission from Moncada S, Vane JR: Arachidonic acid meabolites and the interactions between platelets and blood-vessel walls. *N Engl J Med* 1979; 300:1144.

in producing the local vasoconstriction, and some make the platelets sticky thereby promoting further aggregation of platelets to form a temporary hemostatic plug. Stimulation of the coagulation cascade then causes the formation of fibrin, which consolidates and stabilizes the thrombus. Some of the compounds, such as TxA_2, are strong stimulators of platelet aggregation; others, such as prostacyclin, modulate the response in such a way that when an injury is minor, platelet thrombi form but parts break off to be washed away by circulation. The degree of injury is an important determinant of the size of the thrombus; for the development of a large thrombus, severe damage or physical detachment of the endothelium must occur. Platelet plug formation is especially important in capillary hemostasis, whereas vasoconstriction and fibrin formation seem to be more important for larger vessel hemostasis.

Increase in Vascular Permeability

Inflammation is the normal local reaction of vascularized tissue to injury. Austin notes that the tissue mast cells—the "sentinel" cells of the body—have a distribution that is highly appropriate for sentinels. They are found in cutaneous and mucosal surfaces and around venules—the portals of entry of the body. They contain stored mediators of the inflammatory response—histamine, heparin, and chemotactic factors for eosinophils and neutrophils—and other mediators, including leukotrienes, that are synthesized in response to perturbation of the cellular membranes. These mediators, along with others, participate in a biphasic inflammatory pattern of increased permeability of vessels 20–100 μ in diameter in response to injury. The immediate phase is transient, occurring within minutes after the injury and then disappearing. It is replaced by the delayed phase, which occurs over a 3–6 hour period as the vasopermeability factors induce a reversible opening of the junction between the endothelial cells by producing a contraction of the cells, thereby permitting passage of plasma solutes across the vascular barrier. Depending on the local balance between the vasoconstricting and the vasodilating agents that are secreted or synthesized in response to the injury, there is local vasoconstriction or vasodilatation. The blood flow in the microvascular bed slows because of the increased viscosity of the packed red blood cells associated with loss of fluid from the vessels. These changes permit increased adherence of polymorphonuclear leukocytes to the endothelial lining and their diapedesis into the inflammatory focus. Neutrophils are present in large numbers within 4 hours after injury because of the chemotactic factors generated by blood clotting, injured tissues, complement (especially C5A), bacteria (if present), lymphocytes, and prostaglandins (MacLean).

Blood sequestered in an injured area, together with decreased tissue perfusion brought about by local vascular injury and by edema, leads to local acidosis because of anaerobic energy metabolism of the cells and consequent breakdown of the sodium–potassium pump, allowing sodium to enter the cells and potassium to move from the cells into the interstitial compartment. A disproportionately large rise in interstitial fluid potassium levels during hemorrhagic shock relative to plasma potassium has been found by Shires and others. In some cases, the early movement of sodium into the cells is accompanied by water, leading to swelling of the cells. For cells that are not irreversibly damaged by the initial trauma, the sodium–potassium fluid shifts are reversible early.

PAIN AND EMOTIONAL RESPONSE

In a classic experiment, Egdahl showed that the outpouring of adrenocorticotropic hormone (ACTH) that followed the injury to the hind limb of a dog was eliminated if all nerves to the extremity were divided. This observation confirmed the important fact that the afferent nerves from an injury site play a significant role in mobilizing the body's responses. It is not surprising that paraplegic or quadriplegic patients fail to demonstrate an increase in ACTH following trauma to denervated areas. Pain impulses ascend in the spinothalamic tracts to the thalamus, but because of the association of these pathways to the cortex and limbic system, in the conscious patient, pain commonly evokes strong emotional responses, including fear, anxiety, and possibly anger, which intensify sympathetic outpourings stimulated by the pain. This pain-mediated response occurs before blood volume loss is sufficient to activate the autonomic system. The initial release of norepinephrine may be from the postganglionic sympathetic fibers in the wound. The release of both epinephrine and norepinephrine from the adrenal medulla occurs at a later stage. The local pain is augmented by the local outpouring of prostaglandins, potassium, and histamine. Although the emotional trauma of an injury usually stimulates the endocrine response, it sometimes may also inhibit it. Endorphines, which are released in the central nervous system, may also blunt the sensation of pain and the response of the sympathetic nervous system to the pain.

HYPOVOLEMIA

Although there are many stimuli for the body's neurohumoral response to injury, hypovolemia may be the primary activator (Gann). Loss of up to 10% of the normal blood volume can be readily compensated for by constriction of the capacitance vessels. Since the systemic veins and venules—the capacitance system—normally contain 14 times as much blood as does the capillary bed, loss of up to 10% of circulating blood volume from loss of whole blood or plasma and from sequestration of fluid in the interstitial space can be compensated for by an adjustment in the venous tone, accomplished primarily through an intrinsic mechanism. Further loss of circulating volume is sensed in the low-pressure portion of the circulation by the atrial receptors and by receptors in the great veins and pulmonary vascular system and later by the arterial baroreceptors in the aortic arch and the carotid bodies. As blood volume decreases, the tonic inhibitory influence that these receptors normally maintain over the medullary vasomotor center is reduced. The resulting stimulation of the vasomotor center, the hypothalamus, and the anterior and posterior pituitary gland result in a rapid increase in the secretion of ACTH, vasopressin (antidiuretic hormone, ADH), and growth hormone. Stimulation of the hypothalamus results in enhanced secretion of epinephrine and norepinephrine from the adrenal medulla, of norepinephrine from the autonomic nervous system, of renin from the kidney, and of glucagon from the pancreas.

This mobilization is the body's response to hypovolemia and its attempt to compensate for it initially and to correct it as rapidly as possible by initiating clotting in order to stop blood loss, by repleting blood volume through refilling of capillary beds from the surrounding interstitial spaces, by shunting blood to vital organs, and by minimizing the renal loss of body fluids and sodium.

Plasma Refilling

The body's attempt to restore blood volume occurs in two phases. The first phase depends at least in part on hydrostatic forces. The capillary hydrostatic pressure is reduced because of decreased systemic blood pressure, as well as because of the predominantly sympathetically induced precapillary vasoconstriction. Interstitial fluid, which is essentially protein-free, moves into the capillaries. It was long thought that the hydrostatic pressure differential between the capillaries and the interstitial fluid was the predominant factor in replacement of fluid volume after hemorrhage, but during the past few years the importance of hyperglycemia, first described by Claude Bernard over 100 years ago, to the plasma refilling process has been recognized. Changes in both the capillary hydrostatic pressure and the plasma osmolality (because of hyperglycemia) are equally important in determining the rate of vascular fluid replacement early after relatively severe hemorrhage (i.e., the first 1 or 2 hours) (Friedman and Drucker). Since the fluid that is absorbed into the capillaries is relatively protein-free, the hematocrit and plasma oncotic pressures decrease together as the interstitial fluid pressure decreases during this early phase of plasma refilling (Litwin and Cope). Based on these observations and on other findings, Gann has indicated that a 20–50% restitution of plasma volume occurs in 2–6 hours before an equilibrium is achieved between capillaries and interstitial space, making further restitution of blood volume impossible without the addition of plasma protein.

The second phase of plasma refilling requires movement of plasma protein from the interstitium, either across the capillary membrane or through lymphatic channels. This, in turn, requires an increase in interstitial pressure, which occurs as a result of increased osmolality of the interstitial space; this produces an osmotic gradient between the cells and the surrounding interstitial space and leads to a loss of fluid from the cells to the interstitium. This second phase in the restitution of blood volume, which appears to be critical for cardiovascular stabilization after injury, depends on the metabolic effects of the hormones that are released after injury. Although this response depends critically upon increased concentration of cortisol, preliminary evidence also implicates glucagon, epinephrine, and growth hormone in this response (Gann). In experimental situations these substances have led to full restitution of plasma blood volume over a 24–48 hour period. Although the nonglucose elements responsible for the increased concentration of solute have not been completely identified, the changes in concentration of amino acids, of free fatty acids, and sometimes of lactate are sufficiently large to account for at least a portion of the solute. The antianabolic actions of cortisol and of glucagon, which impede the entry of amino acid into cells, leads to the catabolic effect, a major component of the metabolic response to injury. In one sense, the protein loss, fat mobilization, and hypoglycemia and carbohydrate depletion associated with injury may be viewed as late metabolic consequences of an initial attempt by the body to restore blood volume through this second phase of restitution (Table 12.10). As little as 12% reduction in blood volume, which causes no change in blood pressure, is sufficient to initiate absorption of extracellular fluid.

Shunting of Blood to Vital Areas

The proportion of cardiac output normally available to an individual organ under normal circumstances depends on the perfusion pressure and the degree of smooth muscle tone of the supplying vessels. For most of the body tissues, the pressure–flow relationship is passive: the lower the pressure, the lower the flow. But in the heart, brain, and kidneys, the flow is maintained at an almost normal level, in spite of lowering of blood pressure, until a pressure of 90 mm Hg has been reached. Below this pressure renal blood flow and glomerular filtration decrease to defend blood flow to the brain and heart. When a pressure of about 50 mm Hg is reached the flow to the brain and heart decreases precipitously. This mechanism, autoregulation, is the body's compensation for reduced perfusion pressure to vital organs.

TABLE 12.10 Some Metabolic Effects of Hormones with Generally Increased Secretion in Trauma

	Proteolysis (in muscle)	Gluconeogenesis (in liver & kidney)	Glycolysis Muscle	Glycolysis Adipose tissue	Glycogenolysis Liver	Glycogenolysis Muscle	Lipolysis (adipose tissue, liver, muscle)	Insulin antagonism	Insulin secretion	Plasma sodium	Plasma potassium	Water retention
ACTH-cortisol	+++	+++	0	0	—	0	+++	++	++	+	0	0
Renin-aldosterone		—								+++	00	
Epinephrine norepinephrine	+	++[a]	0	++	+	++	++++[a]	+++	0	+	0	
ADH												++++
Growth hormone	0		0	++			++[a]	++	+++			
Glucagen	+	+++[a]	0		++++[b]		++[a]		++			

SOURCE: Used with permission from Gann DS: Endocrine and metabolic responses to injury, in Schwartz SI (ed): *Principles of Surgery*, ed. 3. New York, McGraw-Hill Book Company, 1979, p. 17.

[a]Only in the presence of the adrenal corticosteroids.

[b]By stimulating catecholamine secretion.

NOTE: Lipolysis stimulates gluconeogenesis; + to + + + + = stimulates or increases; 0 or 00 = antagonizes or decreases.

At the same time that the heart, brain, and kidneys are being protected, the splanchnic region and other parts of the body are being hypoperfused. The following mechanisms for the shock-induced pancreatic hypoperfusion have been noted: passive decrease in vessel lumen diameter in response to a reduced perfusion pressure; vasoconstriction resulting from active increase in sympathetic tone to the splanchnic resistance vessels; release of humoral vasoconstrictor agents such as angiotensin II, TxA_2, and vasopressin; and physical obstruction of the microcirculatory vessels by the formation of microthrombi and platelet aggregation (Lefer). The primary consequence of these events is reduced perfusion to the pancreas and, to a lesser extent, other splanchnic viscera.

Conservation of Renal Water and Salt Loss

Through the action of ADH, aldosterone, renin, and angiotensin, the kidney participates in the body's defense of the blood volume by minimizing the renal loss of sodium and by decreasing (and sometimes stopping) the renal loss of water.

ADH is released from the posterior pituitary in response to decreased blood volume (mediated by the low-pressure receptors in the right and left atria, the great veins, and the pulmonary vessels) or by an increase in plasma osmolality (mediated by the osmoreceptors of the hypothalamus). Pain, anxiety, and other emotions that are aroused from trauma may also stimulate its release. ADH increases the permeability of the cells of the distal tubules and collecting ducts of the kidneys so that water in the tubule enters the hypertonic interstitium. The urine becomes concentrated, and its volume decreases as the body attempts to increase the blood volume and lower the osmolality of body fluids.

Aldosterone, secreted by the adrenal cortex in response to injury, acts also on the distal tubule to increase the reabsorption of sodium with chloride and water and in exchange to excrete potassium and hydrogen. This is an important mechanism since it is the principal one for renal excretion of potassium and acid that build up rapidly in the injured patient. Aldosterone is secreted in response to three factors: angiotensin II, ACTH, and potassium.

The combined action of ADH and aldosterone is extremely effective in preventing renal sodium loss; if sodium is found in the urine of a severely injured patient, it can be assumed that either renal or adrenal failure has occurred. Injured patients continue to produce 800–1,200 mosm of solute per day. Since the normal kidney maximally concentrating in the presence of ADH and aldosterone can excrete 1 mosm/ml of urine,

urine volume after a major injury should be in the range of 800–1,200 ml/day. If urine flow decreases much below 800 ml/day, decreased renal blood flow and glomerular filtration rate or renal failure have occurred.

As previously noted, because of the autoregulation mechanism, the glomerular filtration rate can be maintained almost to a normal level in spite of lowering of systemic blood pressure to about 90 mm Hg. Any fall in blood pressure below that level decreases the ability of the kidneys to excrete waste products while still defending extracellular fluid volume. Renal damage as a result of hypotension does not normally occur until arterial pressure falls below 60 mm Hg and activates the renin–angiotensin system. Then extracellular fluid volume is defended because urine flow stops or decreases to a negligible volume (Wright).

Renin is secreted in the cells of the juxtaglomerular apparatus of the preglomerular afferent arteriole. Its release can be triggered by at least three mechanisms: increased sympathetic stimulation of the juxtaglomerular arterioles, decreased renal arterial perfusion pressure, and decreased delivery of sodium to the macula densa of the distal tubule. The macula densa is a group of modified cells of the distal tubule immediately adjacent to the juxtaglomerular apparatus of the afferent arterioles. The renin acts as an enzyme in the liver to convert angiotensinogen, an α_2-globulin normally found in the plasma, into angiotensin I. Then most of the angiotensin I is converted in the lung or in the plasma to angiotensin II, the most powerful hypertensive agent known. (Its pressure activity is about 200 times that of norepinephrine.) It increases the contractility of the heart and constricts the veins, thereby reducing the capacity of the circulatory system; it also constricts arterioles, thus limiting the excretion of water and sodium by decreasing glomerular filtration. Angiotensin II is an important stimulus for aldosterone secretion by the adrenal cortex, and it also acts to increase the production of ACTH and of ADH from the pituitary gland.

HYPOXIA

Respiratory failure does not occur early in the injured patient unless an injury to the chest has been sustained or an injury to the head, neck, or abdomen has interfered with the mechanics of breathing. During the initial phase of the body's response to injury, the pain and emotional response stimulate the respiratory center, leading to an increased rate and depth of breathing. This hyperventilation response, which occurs even before hypoxia or metabolic acidosis have stimulated the center, produces respiratory alkalosis and, at the same time, increases the work of breathing (discussed below). When hypoxia does occur, it is detected by the chemoreceptors of the medulla and of the carotid and aortic bodies (which are also sensitive to hypercarbia and to acidosis). Chemoreceptor activation stimulates an increased sympathetic output and the increased production of other hormones.

Special Responses

CENTRAL NERVOUS SYSTEM INJURY

The body's response to injury is greatly altered if the CNS itself is injured. In addition to causing immediate or rapid death from damage to vital structures, brain injury may cause pulmonary edema that may occur almost immediately after injury but is more likely to occur as survival time is prolonged. Although the mechanism is not known, it is postulated that an overdischarge of the sympathetic nervous system is sometimes responsible since reversal of pulmonary edema with stellate ganglion block has been described. Head injuries, especially basalar skull fractures, may cause deviation from the normal homeostatic actions of vasopressin. Such inappropriate ADH secretion may involve continued secretion of ADH after the body may have fully compensated for any loss in blood volume, leading to profound dilutional hyponatremia associated with the excretion of a low-volume urine with a high urinary osmolarity. On the other hand, diabetes insipidus, the converse of inappropriate ADH release, leads to polyuria and hypernatremia in some patients. Spinal cord transection not only inhibits the normal ACTH response to injury to a segment below the level of transection, as previously noted, but it also leads to vasodilatation below the level of division, thus impairing the body's compensation for blood loss.

EXTREMES OF ENVIRONMENTAL TEMPERATURE

Environmental temperature in which an injury occurs or to which the victim is subjected after injury can have a profound effect on the body's response to it. Heat and cold by themselves can each produce changes in the output of many hormones, including ACTH, cortisol, aldosterone, ADH, epinephrine, norepinephrine, and thyroxine (Gann). A hot or cold environment produces striking changes in skin circulation, sometimes with associated fluid and electrolyte losses. Fever increases cardiac work and oxygen consumption, which are associated with increased catabolism and water and salt loss.

ANAPHYLAXIS

Of all immunologically active cells, tissue mast cells are the only ones that possess a recognition system that is already in the tissues. The system can recognize "non-self" the moment it enters the organism without the need for recruitment from the blood circulation or from the lymphatics (Austin). The inflammatory reaction, the body's normal response to injury from any outside agent, normally serves a protective function. But in a hypersensitive person, a simple injury such as a bee sting can initiate a devastating response that may cause shock, airway obstruction, coma, and even death. An injuring force that may be trivial for one person may be deadly for another.

Late Consequences

Once some of the body's compensatory defenses that were triggered by the initial injury and resulting shock are set into action, they may lead to a cycle of events that can cause organ failure and eventual death. Whether or not failure of one or more organ systems will occur depends in part on the survival rate of the injury and in part on the severity of shock and the length of time that the body was at risk before the precipitating causes were corrected.

The Fick principle describes the normal interrelationships among cardiac output, oxygen consumption, and arterial venous oxygen content difference. As cardiac output decreases, oxygen consumption in the body's tissues can be maintained only by an increased extraction of oxygen, leading to an increased arterial venous oxygen content difference. Since myocardial oxygen delivery normally requires almost maximal extraction of oxygen, in the presence of a decreased cardiac output the compensatory increased extraction of oxygen is not available to the heart to the same degree that is true of other tissues. On the other hand, the sympathetic discharge with its resultant tachycardia and increase in contractility of the heart achieves a higher cardiac output for a given filling pressure. This requires more work by the heart muscle as the coronaries dilate to increase the blood flow to the heart. An increased fraction of the cardiac output is diverted to the heart itself, and myocardial oxygen consumption increases. As the oxygen supply to the cells decreases and the tissues switch to anaerobic metabolism, the resulting acidosis favorably influences oxygen unloading in the tissues by shifting the oxyhemoglobin dissociation curve, but the oxygen uptake in the lung becomes impaired.

Between 1 and 2% of the total oxygen consumption of the body is normally used for ventilation, but the hyperventilation that occurs after injury (if the injury itself does not prevent it) increases the work of breathing. As ventilatory exchange increases to 15 liters/min, up to five times as much oxygen is required for each additional liter of ventilation, reflecting the increased work of breathing even in patients without chest injuries (Gump). As cardiac output decreases in patients who are in shock, the muscles of respiration receive inadequate circulation, further impairing their efficiency and resulting in a deterioration of ventilatory function. In the low-flow state in which there is maximum extraction of oxygen in the tissues, the low venous oxygen exceeds the oxygen transport capability of the lungs. Cellular adenosine triphosphate (ATP) production in body tissues is severely curtailed in the absence of aerobic metabolism. Ultimately the acidosis decreases the responsiveness of the body to the sympathomimetic agents.

Up to a point, the compensatory splanchnic vasoconstriction that occurs in response to shock serves to divert blood volume to vital organs. As previously discussed, however, the reduced perfusion to the pancreas and, to a lesser extent, other splanchnic viscera, results in acidosis, hypoxia, and ischemia to the pancreas and other viscera. It has been observed that the hypoxia and ischemia are potent stimuli for lysosomal disruption and for activation of zymogenic enzymes, resulting in the release of large amounts of proteolytic enzymes into the cytoplasm of pancreatic acinar cells and in stimulating the production of myocardial depressant factor (MDF) (Fig. 12.13) (Lefer). As one of the toxic factors produced as a result of shock, MDF has a negative inotropic effect on the heart and has other effects that tend to undermine circulatory homeostasis.

Although there is still some controversy about the pulmonary response to pure hemorrhagic shock, it is generally accepted that hemorrhagic shock alone does not seem to produce any significant clinically evident lung injury in humans, but posttraumatic respiratory dysfunction (or posttraumatic respiratory failure) may occur from the superimposition of severe trauma, burns, or sepsis. The lung injury, affecting the distal alveolar–capillary units, seems to be caused, at least in part, by the excessive recruitment and activation of cells that normally participate in the body's response to injury. This condition, which becomes clinically manifest from 24 hours to 7 days after injury, is characterized by increased capillary permeability. A number of humoral agents and vasoactive substances—TxA_2, leukotrienes, and other arachidonic acid metabolites, lysosomal enzymes, histamine, serotonin, and bradykinin—may all be involved in the response. However, since the earliest morphologic change in the lung in this condition is extensive leukostasis, followed rapidly by degranulation of the leukocytes and endothelial cell vacuolization, it has been postulated that although many factors other than granulocytes are probably

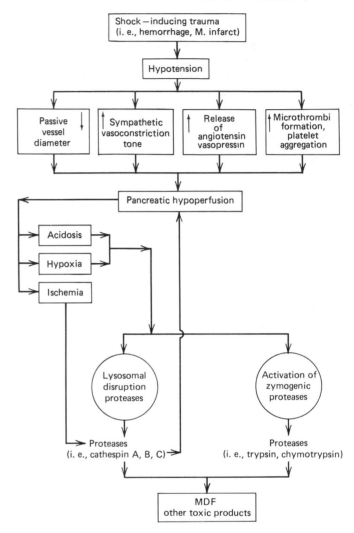

Figure 12.13 Mechanism of the formation of myocardial depressant factor (MDF) from the initial hypotension to the proteolysis. These events occur primarily within the pancreatic acinar cells. (Used with permission from Lefer AM: Vascular Mediators in Ischemia and Shock, in Cowley RA, Trump BF (eds): *Pathophysiology of Shock, Anoxia and Ischemia.* Baltimore, Williams and Wilkins Co, 1982, p. 173.)

important in the genesis of adult respiratory distress syndrome (ARDS), the best hypothesis now appears to be that the contributions of granulocytes and platelets are sequential and aggregation of granulocytes is earlier and perhaps crucial to the triggering of the syndrome (Jacobs). In response to stimulation from activated complement, granulocytes release substances, mainly oxygen radicals such as superoxide anion and hydrogen peroxide, which, in addition to being important microbicides, are also evidently endothelial toxins.

Fluid retention occurs early after injury as a physiologic compensation for hypovolemia. If the low-volume state is not rapidly corrected, however, renal damage occurs secondary to these mechanisms and is sometimes reinforced by toxic injury products in the renal tubules. Most organs are involved to a greater or lesser extent in the process of deterioration that occurs if the compensatory mechanisms mobilized by the body and the therapeutic interventions do not successfully correct the derangements. As discussed in Chapter 13, nutritional deficiency and sepsis with multiple organ system failure may result.

MANAGEMENT OF THE CRITICALLY INJURED PATIENT

Organization

From an analysis of data from San Francisco and Orange County, California, and from Maryland, Trunkey has shown that deaths as a result of trauma tend to have a trimodal distribution. The first peak of deaths occurs within seconds or minutes after the injury. Invariably these deaths are a result of lacerations in the brain, brainstem, upper spinal cord, heart, aorta, or other large vessels (Fig. 12.14). Few patients with such injuries can be

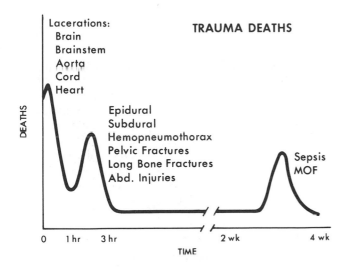

Figure 12.14 The trimodal distribution of deaths from trauma. (This figure was prepared by Donald D. Trunkey, Chief of Surgery of San Francisco General Hospital and used with his kind permission.)

saved. The second death peak occurs within the first 2 hours of injury. These deaths are usually caused by subdural and epidural hematomas, hemopneumothorax, ruptured spleen, lacerations of the liver, fractured femur, or multiple injuries associated with significant blood loss. The third death peak occurs days or weeks after the injury and the deaths are almost always a result of sepsis and multiple organ failure. Many of the deaths that occur in the latter two groups are unavoidable, regardless of the excellence of the care that is given, but some studies have demonstrated that the percentage of preventable deaths related to inadequacies of the trauma-care system ranges from 30–40%. The studies strongly confirm the lessons learned on the battlefield that the most effective way of preventing many of the deaths that would otherwise occur within the first 2 hours after injury is by the adoption of the system, developed in Korea and Vietnam, of transporting patients as quickly as possible to a trauma center in which definitive care for *all* injuries can be given (supporting them with whatever care that is necessary while en route). This means bypassing hospitals where appropriate care cannot be given.

Since almost two-thirds of the 52,600 motor vehicle deaths that occurred in 1980 in the United States were in rural areas and over one-half of all deaths occurred from night accidents, the responsibility for rapid recognition of life-threatening conditions and efficient initiation of appropriate treatment does not rest alone with the trauma teams in trauma centers of large metropolitan hospitals; staffs of hospitals that are being designated in rural areas for initial care of injured patients must also be prepared 24 hours a day, to provide at least initial stabilization before referring the patient to a trauma center. The American College of Surgeons is encouraging the designation of trauma centers—levels I, II, and III—around the country for the care of critically injured patients. The level I trauma center has a trauma team on duty 24 hours a day and the consultation and diagnostic services that may be needed to care for a critically injured patient immediately available. For designation as a level II facility, it is desirable, but not necessary, that a trauma team be available 24 hours a day. But since trauma is a surgical disease, trauma surgeons and appropriate consultants must be available 24 hours a day. The level II center is likely to be a large institution dealing with large numbers of patients presenting with serious trauma in a geographical area lacking a hospital with resources of level I. The level III center, in a community that lacks hospitals of level I or II capability, is one that has made a clear commitment to excellence of trauma care.

The arrival of a critically injured patient in most hospitals should not be a surprise. During the past few years, as emergency medical technicians and paramedical personnel have been trained and ambulance services have been improved, communications systems have been developed that make it possible for ambulance teams to communicate directly with receiving hospitals.

The resuscitation area must always be ready to accept a new patient, whether the area is in the emergency room, the operating room, the intensive care unit, or a special trauma receiving area. In large metropolitan hospitals it is possible to dedicate an area and a team for the resuscitation and initial management of trauma victims. Since so many emergency rooms now function as 24-hour walk-in clinics, which sometimes results in confusion, distractions, and heavy traffic, very few of them are satisfactory sites for the initial management of critically injured patients; unless they are large enough to have a section with its own operating room dedicated to this type of care.

Since surgical procedures such as tube thoracostomy and even laparotomy, thoracotomy, or craniotomy are integral parts of the resuscitation procedure of many critically injured patients, an area within the operating room has been designated in some hospitals as the receiving area for these patients. The operating table is modified to accept the Bucky x-ray unit so that films can be taken before, during, or after any operation that may be necessary. In the operating area everything that is necessary for evaluation, resuscitation, and definitive care is readily available. In some hospitals the intensive care unit is used for the initial evaluation and resuscitation until the operating room can be readied. Wherever the resuscitation area is within the hospital a procedure must be developed and a protocol followed so that trauma victims can be efficiently received and managed.

There is not just one way to organize the team that will care for the critically injured patient in a hospital. The Maryland Trauma Institute has pioneered in developing the model of a trauma team on 24-hour duty in an area used only for the resuscitation and care of injured patients. Such a model can be used, with variations, in large metropolitan hospitals but cannot be used in rural hospitals in which many of the trauma victims have to be taken for initial stabilization. Each hospital that receives a trauma victim must organize its teams according to the experience and availability of the members of its staff.

The key to the organization of a successful team is the team leader. One person must be in charge. That person is usually the most experienced general surgeon of the team, but in some hospitals in which initial care is rendered an orthopedist or generalist, including an emergency room physician, has this leadership responsibility. The leader performs the initial rapid survey, assures the airway if an anesthesiologist is not available, assists in placing intravenous lines if necessary, super-

vises all emergency diagnostic procedures, initiates therapy, calls in appropriate consultants, and decides on priorities for therapy. In some centers the receiving team is responsible for the resuscitation and initial diagnostic procedures but then transfers the responsibility to the appropriate specialists or general surgeons for definitive care. In other centers, the team leader becomes the senior surgeon for that patient throughout hospitalization. In trauma centers an anesthesiologist is a member of the resuscitation team. His or her responsibility is to ensure adequate ventilation and to monitor vital signs, assisting in any additional ways that may be necessary. The other members of the team, whether they be physicians, physician assistants, or nurses, assist in removing the clothing, inserting intravenous lines, instituting any diagnostic and therapeutic measures that are indicated, and monitoring the response to treatment.

In the critically injured patient, especially the victim of blunt trauma, the initial assumption must be made that there are multiple injuries. For this reason, it is dangerous for a specialist to assume responsibility for the care of the victim until those problems that pose an immediate threat to life have been recognized and stabilized. The team leader relies heavily on the judgment of the specialists who are summoned in consultation; the advice of each specialist regarding the necessity for additional diagnostic procedures or operation is carefully considered and priorities are established.

PRIORITIES OF CARE

Since the first priority must be to preserve life, attention must first be given to those derangements that can cause immediate death: ventilatory failure, hemorrhage, and central nervous system injury. Only after therapy has been initiated to correct these problems, the patient's condition has stabilized, and survival seems assured, can attention be given to the second priority—to preserve function. Although preservation of function is an important goal in caring for the critically injured patient, it is not necessary to treat and correct all of the injuries definitively within the first few hours of hospitalization. Sometimes a delay in the repair of extremity injuries or facial lacerations must be accepted while the life-threatening problems are being treated in order to obtain meaningful survival.

Initial Survey

When the critically injured patient is brought into the emergency receiving area, diagnosis and treatment are simultaneous; lifesaving therapy must often be started before a definitive diagnosis has been made. Within the first 2 or 3 minutes after a patient has arrived, the most threatening problems must be identified and life support measures must be initiated.

In some hospitals the patient is put onto a wheeled litter with spine board, if indicated, at the hospital entrance and is transferred immediately to a table in the operating suite, thereby requiring no additional moving before receiving definitive care. In other hospitals the patient is transported on the ambulance litter to the emergency receiving area. In either case, the physician should immediately determine if there are any apparent life-threatening conditions, such as serious hemorrhage or tension pneumothorax, that require immediate correction and should note if the spinal cord is in danger. The extremities should be quickly felt while the neck veins are observed to see if they are distended or collapsed. Distended neck veins in the presence of shock usually indicate a cardiogenic cause such as tension pneumothorax, pericardial tamponade, or myocardial contusion. More commonly, the neck veins are collapsed. This should be interpreted as meaning hypovolemia until proven otherwise.

During these first few seconds, the patient is tentatively categorized as unstable, stable, or potentially unstable. If there is obvious evidence of shock, respiratory distress, altered consciousness, or inability to move the extremities, the patient is considered unstable. The potentially unstable patient is conscious but shows restlessness and/or other signs of sympathetic discharge. He or she is usually a young person who was healthy before the injury, but when decompensation finally occurs, it may be too late to reverse the circulatory collapse unless assessment proceeds immediately and appropriate therapy is initiated quickly. The sense of urgency dominates the evaluation and resuscitation efforts for patients whose vital signs are obviously unstable, but urgent attention must also be given to those patients who are potentially unstable.

The critically injured patient often has the odor of alcohol on the breath. Fifty percent of the trauma admissions to the Maryland Trauma Institute showed alcohol in their blood on arrival, and 25% had over 0.15 mg/100 ml alcohol in their blood (the upper legal limit for driving in Maryland). Since alcohol often masks a serious injury, its presence should not delay the management of the victims.

While the patient is being transferred to the examining table and the clothing is rapidly but carefully and *completely* removed by cutting with large heavy bandage scissors, an abbreviated history is obtained from accompanying ambulance personnel or police. An understanding of the mechanism of injury will help to direct initial attention to areas that pose the most immediate threat to survival. A total evaluation—front and back—of the undressed patient is performed rapidly (within the next 2–5 minutes). This examination is not intended to pinpoint all of the injuries or medical problems but to identify those problems that pose an immediate threat to life. The entire body is scanned. While someone supports the head and neck, the patient is gently turned, by use of the logrolling maneuver, and the back of the head and neck, the back, buttocks, flanks, and posterior thighs are observed and palpated in order to identify obvious injuries. Initial attention, though, must focus on the airway and ventilation, the circulatory system, and the central nervous system.

AIRWAY AND VENTILATION

If the patient is conscious, he or she is asked to take a deep breath. If this can be done without discomfort, most thoracic injuries are ruled out. The bared chest and abdomen are observed, and signs of respiratory difficulty such as stridor or other types of noisy respiration, suprasternal, or intercostal retraction during inspiration and rapid or shallow respiration or abdominal breathing are noted. As previously indicated, soon after the injury the critically injured patient ordinarily hyperventilates, in part in response to the pain and the emotional stimulation; later, hyperventilation is commonly seen as a compensation for the hypoxia and/or the development of metabolic acidosis that results from the inadequate peripheral perfusion. At the same time, a search is made for any external evidence of chest injury (swelling, contusion, deformity, or asymmetry of movement of the chest wall). The chest wall is palpated quickly and gently for tenderness, subcutaneous emphysema, or other obvious evidences of fractured ribs; the position of the trachea is felt, and note is made whether the neck veins are distended or collapsed.

The presence or absence of cyanosis is noted, although it is not a dependable indicator of ventilatory insufficiency. Central cyanosis (observed around the lips and ocular conjunctiva) is not seen unless at least 4–5 g/100 ml of reduced hemoglobin is present in the capillaries and venules of the skin and mucous membrane. If, because of hemodilution from early capillary refilling or early volume replacement with solutions that contain no red cells, the hemoglobin concentration has had time to drop in the critically injured patient who has lost a considerable amount of blood, central cyanosis may not be evident even though a severe ventilatory insufficiency exists. The concentration of reduced hemoglobin is insufficient to produce the cyanosis. Peripheral cyanosis, observed in the extremities of critically injured patients, usually is a reflection of perilously reduced perfusion of the tissues because of major loss of blood volume.

If there is evidence of chest injury or if there is any doubt about the airway and ventilation, a chest film should be obtained as soon as possible and an arterial blood sample should be obtained from the femoral artery and sent for blood gas analysis.

CIRCULATORY SYSTEM

The physician feels the pulse and looks for evidence of shock. A weak, steady pulse should be taken as an indication of hypovolemic shock or obstructive shock from cardiac tamponade. (A very strong pulse usually is a good sign, but the physician must be aware that it may, on the other hand, indicate carbon dioxide retention.) The nature of the pulse is more reliable than the blood pressure as an early sign of shock because it is one of the indicators of sympathetic response. Tachycardia, pallor of the skin and mucous membranes, coolness of the extremities, increased sweating, anxiety, slow capillary filling of the nailbeds, and collapse of the peripheral veins are early signs of sympathetic response. The thready pulse results from a reduction in the pulse pressure and may be a late sign of shock. The diastolic pressure ordinarily is determined by the degree of arteriolar constriction, and the pulse pressure reflects the stroke volume. Because a fall in blood pressure is rapidly compensated by sympathetic responses, a single blood pressure reading is a poor indication of the severity of shock. In a previously healthy individual, the systolic blood pressure may be maintained at normal levels by compensatory responses in spite of blood loss of up to 15% of blood volume.

At the same time, obvious bleeding is controlled by local pressure (see below), and areas of swelling, discoloration, or deformity that may be clues pointing to hidden sources of bleeding are noted. If an antishock garment, pressure dressing, or splint is in place, it must not be disturbed until intravenous lines have been inserted and volume replacement is underway.

CENTRAL NERVOUS SYSTEM

During the initial survey, CNS status must be rapidly assessed. Is the patient conscious? If so, it is certain that pressure coning is not occurring. Is the patient speaking? If he or she is able to speak, the airway must be open. Is the patient moving the extremities spontaneously? Spontaneous movement does not rule out the presence of spinal column injury, but it does indicate that the spinal cord has not been irreparably damaged. Although the presence of a spinal cord injury does not pose an immediate threat to life unless it is located high in the cervical cord, it is important to learn quickly whether or not a spinal column injury is possible or probable in order to protect it from further harm during the resuscitation period. If the patient is conscious and reports discomfort in the neck, at

rest, or during movement or if the patient is unconscious, the neck should be splinted with sandbags until films of the cervical spine can be obtained.

Any disturbance of consciousness should be considered as evidence of head injury until proven otherwise. If the patient is unconscious, the pupils must be quickly observed to be certain that inequality has not developed, an indication that urgent intervention may be necessary. But the examiner must remember that the degree of intracranial trauma cannot be accurately determined in the presence of profound shock.

ABDOMEN AND PELVIS

In any patient who has sustained blunt or penetrating injury to the trunk, the possibility of injury to both the thorax and the abdomen must be clearly in mind since the lower six ribs normally overlie the upper abdomen. If the victim of blunt trauma can take a deep breath without discomfort, it is unlikely that he or she has sustained a chest wall injury. If the comatose patient responds to pain, gentle pressure over the lower ribs usually elicits evidence of pain if ribs are fractured. The contour of the abdomen should be noted, but the examiner must remember that an exsanguinating amount of blood may be contained in the abdomen or retroperitoneum with minimal change in contour of the abdomen. Many guidelines have been established estimating the amount of blood loss associated with typical injuries, but individual variations are so great that their usefulness is sometimes limited. Simple geometric principles can be used to demonstrate the amount of blood loss that can be associated with hidden injuries. Figure 12.15 illustrates a theoretical calculation of the amount of blood loss that could be associated with a 1-cm increase in the radius of the abdomen (Trunkey, Sheldon and Collins).

The abdomen is gently palpated in order to detect any area of increased tone that may indicate an underlying injury. Any penetrating injuries should be observed carefully. (Later, before films are obtained, any penetrating injuries, such as bullet holes, should be marked by radiopaque objects.) Deep palpation may or may not elicit guarding or tenderness (even if blood is present), but the perforation of a viscus should produce signs of peritoneal irritation, the intensity of which depends not only on the presence or absence of associated CNS injury, but also on the viscera that have been penetrated.

The iliac crests and the symphysis pubis should be compressed to detect any obvious evidence of a pelvic fracture. Blood coming from the urethral meatus is diagnostic of urethral injury and presumptive evidence of a fractured pelvis. If the patient can void, a specimen should be obtained promptly and

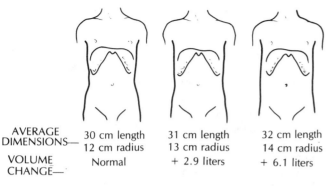

AVERAGE DIMENSIONS—	30 cm length 12 cm radius	31 cm length 13 cm radius	32 cm length 14 cm radius
VOLUME CHANGE—	Normal	+ 2.9 liters	+ 6.1 liters

Figure 12.15 Injured abdomen considered as a cylinder for computational purposes; change in volume corresponds to changes in length and radius. Change in length occurs as raising of the diaphragm and thus remains unapparent to external examination. Exsanguination can occur with minimal change in external appearance. (Used with permission from Trunkey DD, Sheldon GF, Collins JA: The Treatment of Shock, in Zuidema GD, Rutherford MD, Ballinger MD (eds): *The Management of Trauma*. Philadelphia, W.B. Saunders Co, 1979, p. 82.)

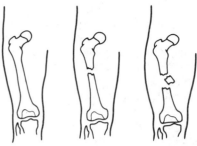

AVERAGE DIMENSIONS	40 cm length 8 cm radius	40 cm length 9 cm radius	40 cm length 10 cm radius
VOLUME CHANGE —	Normal	+ 2.1 liters	+ 4.5 liters

Figure 12.16 Injured thigh considered as a cylinder for computational purposes; change in volume (blood loss) corresponds to changes in radius. (Used with permission from Trunkey DD, Sheldon GF, Collins JA: The Treatment of Shock, in Zuidema GD, Rutherford MD, Ballinger MD (eds): *The Management of Trauma*. Philadelphia, W.B. Saunders Co, 1979, p. 81.)

examined grossly and microscopically for red blood cells. If there is no evidence of fractured pelvis, the bladder should be catheterized gently and the urine should be examined for red blood cells. If there is evidence of pelvic fracture, urethral catheterization should be delayed (see Chapter 21).

Rectal examination should be performed. Fullness in the pelvis is ordinarily diagnostic of pelvic fracture with retroperitoneal hematoma. Blood on the glove usually indicates an injury involving the lower gastrointestinal tract and suggests fecal contamination of the retroperitoneal hematoma.

EXTREMITIES

Obvious fractures with deformity or swelling are readily observed during the quick initial examination. As implied by the theoretical calculations in Figure 12.16, 1 or more liters of blood can be lost in association with a fracture of the femur with relatively modest soft tissue swelling. The primary concerns at the time of the initial survey of extremity injuries are to estimate the amount of blood loss and to minimize such loss and subsequent discomfort.

Resuscitation

Evaluation and resuscitation of the critically injured patient occur simultaneously. Before the initial physical examination has been completed, measures are applied to gain control of the airway and ventilation at the same time that venous access is obtained, blood is drawn for typing and cross-matching and any other urgently needed study, and fluid therapy is initiated.

CONTROL OF AIRWAY AND VENTILATION

Opening the Airway

Any evidence of an inadequate airway must be dealt with immediately by clearing the mouth of foreign material. Solid material that cannot be removed by suction should be cleared manually. Extreme care must be used to position the patient's head to relieve airway obstruction if cervical spine injury has not been completely ruled out. In such a situation, hyperextension of the neck is obviously contraindicated. If the patient appears to be making respiratory efforts but no movement of air can be detected or if the patient is unconscious, the situation will sometimes be corrected if the physician places both hands behind the angles of the mandible and lifts it forward as described in Chapter 1 (Fig. 1.2c). The tongue can sometimes be lifted forward by this maneuver, thereby correcting the obstruction. In the presence of severe facial injury, the tongue will have to be pulled forward, using a towel clip if necessary, if it is causing an airway obstruction.

Endotracheal Intubation

If there is any question about the adequacy of an airway or of ventilation in the critically injured patient, endotracheal intubation should be performed (Procedure 4). Most of the indications for intubation of these patients are obvious: airway obstruction, facial injury or neck injury that may cause airway obstruction, any potentially serious chest injury or significantly depressed consciousness. Patients who are in shock often have no obvious evidence of ventilatory insufficiency; on clinical examination alone it may be very difficult, if not impossible, to detect early respiratory failure in these patients. In the past, the accepted practice was to perform frequent blood gas determinations, especially concentrating on measures of physiologic shunting in the lung and on alveolar–arterial oxygen differences in order to determine whether or not intubation and mechanical ventilation were necessary. It is now recognized that ventilation in patients who are in shock must be maintained at levels greater than normal to compensate for the impaired pulmonary function. Because of their increased work of breathing, all patients are given oxygen (at least by nasal catheter or by face mask); if there is any doubt about adequacy of airway and of ventilatory exchange, the patient should be intubated without delay and ventilatory support should be given. The tube is inserted after the patient has been preoxygenated with a mask at 100% oxygen for 30 seconds. If necessary 100 mg succinylcholine may be used, and the ventilation is then controlled either by using a self-inflating bag or by attaching the endotracheal tube immediately to the volume ventilator (see below). Except in the presence of airway obstruction, intubation can and should be delayed until adequate preparations have been made. Ordinarily, if the airway is not obstructed, even in the presence of ventilatory arrest, a bag and mask or mouth-to-mouth technique of ventilation will provide adequate ventilation until intubation can be performed. Before the intubation is attempted, make sure all necessary preparations have been made; the intubation should then be performed quickly but carefully by the most experienced intubator on the resuscitation team.

In the presence of severe facial injury and in the patient in whom the possibility of cervical spine injury is a real one, a satisfactory method for insertion of an endotracheal tube is to thread the tube over a fiberoptic bronchoscope or laryngoscope and then insert the bronchoscope or laryngoscope through the laryngeal opening, observed under direct vision. This procedure should only be used by one who is familiar with it. Nasotracheal intubation can sometimes be used in the presence of cervical spine injury.

Esophageal Obturator Airway

In increasing numbers, patients are arriving in emergency rooms with esophageal obturator airways in place (Procedure 5). These airways can be inserted by paramedical personnel at the scene of an emergency and by physicians who are not expert in the technique of endotracheal intubation. Although it may be lifesaving when endotracheal intubation is not possible for one reason or another, it is not without risks, especially esophageal perforation, intubation of the trachea, or aspiration of gastric contents into the tracheobronchial tree when the cuff is deflated before the removal of the tube. Based on the increasing numbers of reports of serious complications from its use, the esophageal airway is now considered a dangerous instrument by many. If a patient is admitted with an esophageal airway in place, it should not be removed until a secure airway has been obtained by conventional endotracheal intubation with a cuffed tube. Because of the risk of esophageal perforation, the obturator airway should be left in place for a maximum of only 2 hours.

Cricothyrotomy

In cases of airway obstruction, when for any reason endotracheal intubation is impossible, cricothyrotomy (Procedure 9) should be performed. It is a much easier and safer procedure than a tracheotomy for even the most experienced surgeon to perform under the trying circumstances of resuscitating a critically injured patient. This is especially true in patients with short obese necks. After the airway has been established and the patient's condition has finally stabilized, a semielective tracheotomy can be performed in the operating room under optimal conditions.

Ventilation

Most hospitals that expect to receive multiply injured patients have volume ventilators available in the area in which the critically injured patients are received. The endotracheal tube should be attached to the ventilator immediately in order to provide maximum ventilatory support. If the ventilator is not available in the resuscitation area, satisfactory ventilation can be supplied by a bag with reservoir tail to allow delivery of a high concentration of oxygen (see Fig. 1.9). Respiratory rate may vary from 12 to 20 breaths per minute with tidal volume 1.5–2 times as great as normal. Usually a high inspired oxygen concentration (FiO_2 up to 100%) should be administered while waiting for the results of the initial blood gas determination in order to maintain the arterial PO_2 above 80 mm Hg during the initial resuscitation steps. Maintenance of such a high oxygen concentration poses no clinical problem during the first hour of resuscitation. Problems may arise, however, if such high concentrations are maintained after 1 or 2 hours because of the risk of airway closure that occurs as nitrogen is washed out of poorly ventilated but perfused alveoli. In this case, the rate of oxygen removal by blood exceeds the rate of oxygen entry into the alveoli. As discussed below, in such patients positive end expiratory pressure (PEEP) or continuous positive airway pressure (CPAP) sometimes strikingly improves the arterial oxygenation.

INITIAL MANAGEMENT OF CHEST INJURY

Ordinarily, the emergency medical personnel who transport a victim with an open pneumothorax occlude the opening before the patient is brought to the hospital. Any such emergency measures that have been instituted before admission should be left in place until the patient's condition has stabilized. However, if there is evidence of tension pneumothorax—cyanosis, venous distention, tracheal shift—the occluding dressing should be removed and, if necessary, an 18-gauge needle should be immediately inserted into the second intercostal space of the involved side in the midclavicular line even if there is no available method for applying suction or attaching it to an underwater seal. If the clinical indications are strong enough, this procedure should be carried out even before a roentgenogram is taken.

If there is evidence of flail chest as the cause of ventilatory failure, a member of the team should gently exert counterpressure on the involved portion of the chest wall during expiration to control the paradoxical motion until the endotracheal tube has been inserted and the patient has been placed on a volume respirator. One of the relatively frequent causes of tension pneumothorax is puncture of the lung by a fractured rib when positive pressure ventilation is being applied. For this reason all patients with flail chest who are being treated by positive pressure ventilation should have a chest tube inserted prophylactically (Procedure 19).

If the heart has arrested, closed chest massage must be started. Time should not be wasted in trying to do a difficult intubation during the early stages of this resuscitation. If the chest wall is unstable, if the patient is in extremis, or if the cardiac massage is ineffective for any other reason, the chest must be opened immediately in the left fourth or fifth intercostal space through a long incision from the sternal border toward the midaxillary line. This procedure, performed by a member of the team who is familiar with it, will allow direct access to the heart and if necessary will make it possible to cross clamp the thoracic aorta in order to divert as much blood as possible to the heart and brain.

CONTROL OF CIRCULATION

Control of Hemorrhage

Any significant external bleeding must be controlled at the same time that the airway is being established. It can nearly always be controlled by finger pressure or by pressure bandages. For most critically injured patients who are brought to the hospital by emergency medical technicians, methods of control have been initiated before arrival at the hospital. If control is effective, the pressure should not be released until satisfactory intravenous lines have been established, adequate fluid replacement has been accomplished, more pressing diagnostic and therapeutic procedures have been completed, and the patient is finally taken to an operating room where repair of the injury can be safely performed. Stopping hemorrhage is a first priority; repair of the wound that is responsible for the hemorrhage has a low priority unless the survival of a limb depends on the early restoration of continuity of severed blood vessels.

A severed major artery can usually be better controlled by pressure exerted by one finger than by any other method. This pressure should be maintained until it is time for the definitive repair, at which point a decision can be made by the surgeon whether arterial continuity should be reestablished or whether the vessel should be simply clamped. Diffuse oozing from a soft tissue wound can ordinarily be controlled by a pressure dressing, usually composed of several abdominal pads held in place by an evenly applied pressure bandage that stops the bleeding but allows distal circulation. The pressure dressing should not be applied as a tourniquet but simply as a device for applying even pressure. Some bleeding from deep cavities can be controlled only by a pack, such as a Kerlex roll, inserted with a Kelly clamp. If hemorrhage is uncontrollable by other means, an immediate thoracotomy or laparotomy may have to be performed in the emergency receiving area with cross-clamping of the aorta to control bleeding.

Much has been taught in the past about the application of tourniquets as a means of controlling arterial bleeding. However, frequency of complications—increased bleeding from venous engorgement (caused by too loose an application of the tourniquet) or gangrene (caused by too prolonged an application)—makes it inadvisable to attempt to control bleeding by use of tourniquets, except in the case of traumatic amputation, unless alternative materials are not available or other methods do not adequately control the hemorrhage. The duration of application should always be minimal although the sacrifice of a limb on occasion will be necessary to save a patient's life. Air splints may function as pressure dressings, controlling hemorrhage at the same time they immobilize fractures, if they are carefully applied. Care must be taken to be sure that no part of the extremity protrudes beyond the end of the air splint in order to avoid venous engorgement of the exposed portion of the limb. The splint must not be overdistended and should never function as a tourniquet.

Antishock garments are gaining wide acceptance for the temporary control of pelvic and abdominal bleeding. This three-compartment pressure suit applies pneumatic splinting to the lower half of the body (Procedure 17). Since it can be inflated to 80 mm Hg, it can relatively easily be overinflated if the patient is in shock, although some models incorporate a safety device to prevent this. Its safety and the allowable duration of inflation have not yet been completely determined. If antishock garments have been applied before a patient's arrival in the hospital, the device should not be deflated until intravenous access has been secured, fluid resuscitation is satisfactory, and definitive control is possible.

Intravenous Access

Depending on the severity of the injury, one or more large-bore (at least 15-gauge) catheters must be inserted by members of the team while other members are controlling hemorrhage and obtaining airway access. Peripheral lines should be used for the first catheter and, if necessary, for the second as well. Since the resistance to flow in any tube is directly proportional to its length and inversely proportional to the fourth power of its radius (Poiseuille's law), large-bore, short catheters should be used for early volume replacement. If a large volume of fluid must be infused in a short time, at least two short catheters must be inserted before a central venous line is placed. The site of line placement partly depends on the injuries that are suspected (Figs. 12.17 and 12.18). Veins should be avoided if their central portions are likely to be injured. In patients with severe torso injury, it is usually best to have venous access to at least one vein above and one vein below the diaphragm. Although the saphenous vein at the ankle is not a satisfactory one for long-term use (because of the frequency of the development of phlebitis), it is excellent for initial volume replacement if a cutdown is required since it can be performed very quickly and the largest catheter can be inserted. If necessary, the end of the intravenous tubing can be cut obliquely so that it can easily be slipped into the vein and can be tied in place. The peripheral and central veins are usually collapsed if the patient is in deep hypovolemic shock. The subclavian and internal jugular veins are poor choices for early insertion in these patients because the collapse of the veins makes the insertion of the line more difficult and increases the chance for development of serious complications. In such a situation, the femoral vein can be catheterized percutaneously for initial

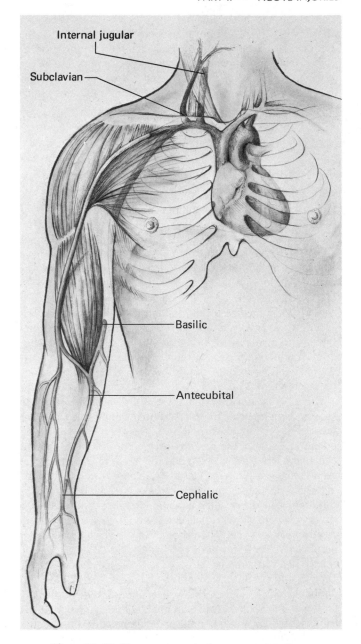

Figure 12.17 Venous access in the upper extremity.

infusion of fluids, and other lines can be inserted after 1,000–1,500 ml of fluid have been given by the femoral route.

The basilic vein, just proximal and anterior to the medial humeral condyle, is an excellent site for cutdown and insertion of the long catheter for central venous pressure monitoring

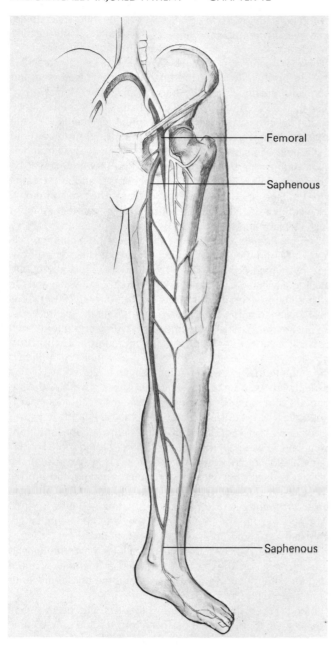

Figure 12.18 Venous access in the lower extremity.

because the catheter can readily be threaded from this position into the central veins. The length of catheter that is required to ensure central location makes this a poor choice for replacement of fluids; its prime use should be for the monitoring of central venous pressure.

Initial Blood Samples

A blood sample should be drawn through one of the catheters and sent to the laboratory for appropriate battery of examinations: blood type and cross-match; hemoglobin and hematocrit, remembering that hemodilution will begin to have an effect on these values within the first hour but the plasma refilling process will only be completed in 24–48 hours; white blood cell count and coagulation profile–prothrombin time (PT), partial thromboplastin time (PTT), platelets, and fibrinogen. Any additional tests that are indicated should be ordered. (An arterial sample should have been sent for blood gas analysis as soon as the patient has been placed on the examining table.)

Administration of Intravenous Fluids

The basic physiologic derangements of shock relate not only to a decrease in peripheral blood flow but also to a decrease in oxygen-carrying capacity of the blood that does reach the tissues, since the hematocrit drops in response to blood loss. Attaining airway control and making sure that ventilation is adequate ensures optimal oxygenation of hemoglobin, but if the patient is in shock, tissue hypoxia will persist in part because of the low-flow state associated with an increased viscosity of the red blood cells and in part because of a tendency of the cells to aggregate. Not only must the intravascular volume be expanded quickly, but the oxygen-carrying capacity of the blood must also be increased in order to reverse the metabolic aberrations that develop very rapidly in the critically injured patient. It is becoming increasingly apparent, though, that the first priority in fluid resuscitation of these patients is restoration of blood volume and flow, because many of the body's responses that rapidly become deleterious, if prolonged, are mediated by hypovolemia, and it is only by the restoration of blood volume that the sluggishness of tissue perfusion that characterizes shock can be reversed. Therapeutic hemodilution results in a decreased viscosity of the blood and the dispersal of aggregated red blood cells so that single file perfusion of red blood cells through the capillaries can be resumed. The second phase of fluid resuscitation requires restoration of red blood cell mass to improve the oxygen-carrying capacity of the blood. The third phase requires the management of any dilutional coagulopathies that may develop during therapy if massive replacement of fluids is required.

It has been repeatedly demonstrated that resuscitation can be satisfactorily attained with hematocrit levels as low as 20%, although 30% hematocrit seems to be a more physiologic level to maintain during the early management of the volume-depleted patient. The following fluids may be used in the restoration of intravascular volume in these patients: crystalloids, colloids, and blood or its fractions.

Crystalloids—lactated Ringer's solution or normal saline solution—are commonly the first fluids that are given. They are isotonic with extracellular fluid, but much of their volume remains in the intravascular space for only a brief period before escaping into the interstitium. It is therefore argued by some that crystalloids rapidly find their way into the third space, whereas colloids are confined to the intravascular space. However, there is evidence that in the patient who is in shock, colloidal solutions may also leak from the pulmonary capillaries, especially if the capillaries are damaged. It seems, therefore, that any fluid may cause interstitial edema if too large a volume is infused. After many years of controversy over the relative merits of colloids versus crystalloids in fluid resuscitation, it is now accepted that crystalloids have a definite important place. As previously discussed, the body itself replenishes plasma proteins by the plasma refill mechanism as interstitial fluid is transferred into the intravascular space, in part through lymphatics, bringing with it albumin from the interstitium. Replenishing of plasma proteins early in fluid resuscitation does not require the infusion of colloid.

Isotonic saline contains 154 mEq each of sodium and chloride, whereas Ringer's lactate solution contains 130 mEq of sodium and 108 mEq of chloride. Because the normal concentration of chloride in the plasma is approximately 100 mEq/liter, saline contains 50 mEq of excess chloride per liter. In the volume-depleted patient with poor renal function, such a burden of excess chloride may result in the development of metabolic acidosis, which would be especially undesirable in the patient in shock who has lactic acidosis.

It is commonly thought that when Ringer's lactate is given to a patient who is in shock it adds to the acid load that is already present. However, the sodium lactate is not lactic acid; it is a metabolic precurser of bicarbonate. When circulation to the liver has been restored, sodium lactate is metabolized to bicarbonate. Since Ringer's lactate contains 4 mEq/liter of potassium, some consider it best to avoid administration of potassium in the first bottle used for resuscitation since renal function is usually unknown at that time. Some recommend that resuscitation begin instead with isotonic saline and continue with Ringer's lactate solution, if and when satisfactory renal function is established (Moss). Two liters of crystalloid solution can be given to the volume-depleted patient while awaiting cross-matched blood.

In patients with mild hemorrhage, not exceeding 20% of blood volume, crystalloid solution alone is adequate to maintain blood volume and homeostasis. In patients with moderate to severe hemorrhage, however, salt solution alone is unable to compensate for the losses. Because of the third-space losses sustained in hemorrhage and severe trauma, Shires recommends that Ringer's lactate be given in addition to blood.

Colloidal solutions contain high molecular weight molecules that do not readily cross the intact capillary membrane and normally remain within the intravascular space for a longer time than do crystalloids. Under ordinary circumstances, they do not have to be used in the initial fluid replacement for the critically injured patient. They should be used in initial fluid replacement in small infants, the elderly, patients with inhalation injuries, and in any other situation in which it will be important to give the fluids to replace losses and at the same time limit the amount of fluid that is given. The two commonly used colloids are albumin and human plasma protein fraction, such as plasmanate.

Normal *human serum albumin* is a sterile preparation of 5% or 25% serum albumin obtained by fractionating blood from healthy human donors. The 5% solution, osmotically equivalent to plasma, is available in 250- and 500-ml vials, and the 25% solution is applied in units of 20, 50, and 100 ml. It is heat treated to minimize the risk of transmitting hepatitis virus. Serum albumin 5% is sometimes used with a crystalloid, such as lactated Ringer's solution, as a plasma substitute. This combination, in a ratio of 250 ml colloid to 1 liter crystalloid, is the solution that is used in some centers to correct a volume deficit while waiting for typed and cross-matched blood. Salt-poor 25% albumin is an extremely expensive solution that is not ordinarily used in the initial resuscitation effort.

Other plasma–protein fractions are sterile aqueous solutions containing 5% human plasma protein in isotonic sodium chloride solution or in some other diluent. They are essentially plasma with fibrinogen and γ-globulin removed and are osmotically equivalent to plasma. Like albumin, they are heat treated to minimize the risk of transmitting hepatitis B virus. Available in 250- and 500-ml vials, they are used interchangeably with 5% albumin as a plasma substitute.

The choice between the use of colloids or crystalloids is usually made on the basis of cost and availability. Colloid solutions are much more expensive, and the crystalloid solutions are usually far more available.

Blood, especially fresh whole blood, would be the ideal replacement for blood that has been lost. It is the only volume expander that can not only replenish the blood volume but can also increase the oxygen-carrying capacity within the circulatory system and provide platelets. In addition, it contains the labile factors—factors V and VIII—which are the hemostatic factors that decay significantly during liquid preservation of blood. But there is not enough fresh blood to meet the need for blood replacement for the most critically injured patients.

Blood loss in these patients is usually replaced by whole blood or packed cells. For elective transfusion, packed cells are more commonly used because the red blood cell mass can thereby be replenished without overloading the circulatory system. In the critically injured patient, however, whole blood is usually a better choice because the viscosity of packed cells precludes their being administered rapidly and also because in the injured patient, early restoration of the blood volume is just as critical as the early increase in oxygen-carrying capacity of the blood. As previously discussed, improvement in the perfusion of blood increases the efficiency of oxygen exchange so remarkably that we should strive for therapeutic hemodilution in the early management of the critically injured patient, aiming to keep the hematocrit at about the level of 30%, a level at which both perfusion and oxygen-carrying capacity are adequate.

The type of blood that is given usually depends on the availability in the blood bank at the time. Citric acid-phosphate-dextrose (CPD) anticoagulant has replaced citric acid-citrate-dextrose (ACD); CPD blood has a lower potassium, higher pH, and higher 2,3-diphosphoglycerate (2,3-DPG) level. Since a reduced 2,3-DPG shifts the oxyhemoglobin dissociation curve to the left, thereby reducing release of oxygen in capillaries, the deficiency of 2,3-DPG had been considered a theoretical disadvantage of administering stored whole blood in the past, but it has never been clinically proved. The patient's body restores 2,3-DPG within a few hours of transfusion of banked blood. Hyperkalemia in stored blood has also been considered a theoretical disadvantage but has seldom presented a problem because much of it is excreted in the patient who is retaining sodium in response to injury.

The need for typing and cross-matching sometimes introduces delays that are unacceptable. In such cases, it is safer to get an uncrossmatched, type specific blood than it is to give "universal donor" O negative blood. If the blood type of the victim is unknown, it is safest to use O negative or O positive packed cells because of the reduced amount of A and B iso-antibodies contained in them.

Currently, approximately 80% of the transfusions that are given in the United States are in the form of packed cells rather than of whole blood. The packed red cells may be diluted with normal saline, single donor plasma, or fresh frozen plasma. Transfusions should always be given through a standard transfusion apparatus that contains a filter that traps particles greater than 170 μ. Without the filter, these particles would be trapped in the pulmonary microvasculature. Normal saline is the only intravenous solution that can safely be used with blood transfusions. Ringer's lactate and other solutions containing calcium may cause clotting of citrated blood.

Hypothermia is a frequent side effect of receiving blood stored at 4°C (39°F). If it is transfused at a rate faster than 100 ml/min, it can lower the body temperature to less than 30°C (86°F). Hypothermia increases the affinity of hemoglobin for oxygen, thereby potentiating the similar effect of 2,3-DPG, and hypothermia impairs the ability of the patient to metabolize metabolic acid and potassium. Ultimately, it produces serious cardiac arrhythmias and death. Multiple transfusions should therefore be administered through warming devices that are designed to warm the blood in the tubing. The warming should not exceed 40°C (104°F) because of the hemolysis of red blood cells that occurs above that temperature.

Autotransfusion is a useful and sometimes lifesaving procedure that makes it possible to reinfuse uncontaminated blood from the chest cavity with a minimum of delay. In the presence of rapid life-threatening bleeding, the 15–20-minute interval required for processing cross-matched blood is not acceptable. Autotransfusion is also especially indicated if there is difficulty in obtaining compatible blood. Patients who lose less than 2,000 ml of blood may have their entire transfusion requirement supplied by autotransfusion. A commercially available system may be used, but the simplest method is to collect the blood from chest tube draining into receptacles containing citrate anticoagulant (CPD), then directly reinfuse this mixture into the recipient. It must be adequately filtered.

Among the potential complications of autotransfusion are disseminated intravascular coagulation caused by the transfusion of activated factors and renal failure resulting from the infusion of large amounts of free hemoglobin. Unless bleeding is especially rapid, blood collected from traumatic hemothoraces is defibrinogenated and does not clot; on the other hand, if blood loss is rapid, defibrinogenation does not occur. Even in the absence of fibrinogen, the shed blood contains normal amounts of factors VIII and IX. Autotransfusion should not be used in patients with crushed chests in which combined thoracic and abdominal injuries and associated rupture of the diaphragm may have occurred. The possibility of bowel rupture, as well as the possibility of contamination of the thoracic contents in the presence of a diaphragmatic injury, present a risk that is unacceptable.

The *prevention or correction of acquired dilutional coagulopathies* is the third phase of fluid resuscitation. It is important in patients who receive massive amounts of fluid and blood and in other patients who receive only a moderate amount of blood but have a complicating medical illness that impairs their coagulation mechanism.

It should be assumed that functioning platelets are absent in any blood that is routinely dispensed from a blood bank since the platelets lose their ability to aggregate in cold storage and their viability is not maintained in preserved blood beyond 72 hours. Additionally, most blood banks that separate blood into its components separate out the platelets. Platelets are rarely required before at least two complete exchanges of blood volume have occurred (10 liters of blood and fluid). The status of the platelets is usually assessed by the Ivy bleeding time, the blood smear, and the platelet count. Platelet transfusion is given to a patient after multiple transfusions if the bleeding time is prolonged (more than 7 minutes) or if there is a severe thrombocytopenia. In some centers, platelet concentrates or "packs" are given whenever 10 units of blood have been administered in less than 1 hour. However, since the hazards of platelet transfusions include hepatitis and sensitization, they should be given only if they are needed.

Fresh frozen plasma contains all of the clotting elements of fresh blood except platelets. The labile factors (factor V and VIII) are the only hemostatic factors that decay significantly in preserved blood. Since the patient who is hemodynamically compensated manufactures factor VIII more rapidly than does the healthy person, the only factor that is deficient in the multiply transfused patient is factor V. Its deficiency does not seem to explain completely the coagulopathy that occurs in the multiply transfused patient. The need for fresh frozen plasma is assessed by the results of PT, PTT, and fibrinogen tests. The PT measures the extrinsic pathway, and the PTT assesses the intrinsic pathway. If either PTT or PT of the patient is abnormal, fresh frozen plasma is indicated; but its effectiveness is not firmly established. Fresh frozen plasma obtained from several donors carries a high risk of hepatitis transmission, but this risk is much less if the fresh frozen plasma is obtained from a single donor. It can cause allergic reactions, and since it contains the normal red blood cell isoantibodies, it must be compatible with the ABO grouping of recipient red cells.

Cryoprecipitate is used most often in the treatment of patients with hemophilia since it contains all of the clotting elements of fresh blood except platelets and is especially rich in factor VIII and fibrinogen. It is occasionally useful in the multiply transfused patient who has prolongation of the PT or the PTT, as well as congestive heart failure or another indication for fluid restriction. A 20 ml unit of cryoprecipitate has the same potency as 200 ml of fresh frozen plasma. If it is indicated, the cryoprecipitate is usually given as a bolus containing 5–10 units.

Because the citrate anticoagulant of the blood binds calcium, it had been customary to give a slow infusion of 14.5 mEq of calcium for every 5 units of blood if that volume of blood was given within a 30-minute period. It is now recognized that calcium is not necessary in this setting. However, since calcium does have an inotropic effect, it is sometimes used as an inotropic agent in the critically injured patient.

Initial Monitoring

Since a patient in shock is either improving or worsening, the patient's response to treatment must be monitored carefully in order to provide guidance for continuing therapy. Sophisticated systems are available that make it possible to monitor the blood volume, peripheral vascular resistance, and parameters such as tissue perfusion, but such equipment is not necessary in the initial care of most critically injured patients. The monitoring that they require initially can be provided by simpler equipment that is readily available in any emergency area.

INITIAL MEASUREMENTS

Pulse and Blood Pressure

For patients who are in shock, the primary concern is blood flow, not blood pressure (recognizing the fact that there is a minimum pressure level that must be maintained in order to assure perfusion of vital organs). The correlation between blood pressure and blood flow is often poor. Since the diastolic pressure is determined by the degree of arteriolar constriction, a rising diastolic pressure is usually associated with poor tissue perfusion. On the other hand, the pulse pressure reflects the stroke volume and is therefore more accurate than the systolic blood pressure as an indicator of blood flow. The strength of the pulse and the arterial pressure provides a good estimation of myocardial adequacy. A normal myocardium cannot maintain a strong pulse in the presence of severe hypovolemia, but a normal blood pressure and a strong pulse indicate that the myocardium is functioning adequately and excludes the diagnosis of cardiogenic shock. A single blood pressure reading is a poor indication of the severity of shock. It must be repeated at frequent intervals during the evaluation and early management of the patient. In the patient who is in profound shock, the blood pressure reading obtained by blood pressure cuff is sometimes false. Accordingly, if there is any doubt, a radial artery catheter should be inserted (Procedure 14), not only to monitor the arterial blood pressure but also to obtain frequent arterial blood gases.

Urinary Output and Solutes

A urinary catheter is inserted and the urine output is recorded every 15 minutes as a guide to the glomerular filtration rate. The urinary output is one of the most sensitive indicators of the adequacy of blood volume; small deficits in blood volume are followed promptly by oliguria before other clinical signs appear. The brain, heart, and lungs all occupy higher levels of priority than the kidneys in their demands on the cardiac output. If the kidneys are making urine, it can be assumed that other vital organs with higher priority on the cardiac output are being adequately perfused unless the arterial supply to these organs is interrupted. The normal 24-hour urine output is approximately 1,700 ml (approximately 70 ml/hr). Oliguria is arbitrarily defined as a urinary output in the range less than 400–500 ml in a 24-hour period (approximately 20 ml/hr).

Early in resuscitation, urine output is measured at least hourly but preferably every 15 minutes. The absolute value is not as important as the trends. The urine output should be maintained at least as high as 40 ml/hr by maintaining adequate fluid replacement. Vasopressors or diuretics should not be used for this purpose in the presence of severe hypovolemia. When the use of these agents is mandatory in order to prevent damage to the kidneys, the urine output can no longer be used as an indicator of the perfusion of vital organs.

The blood–urine urea nitrogen ratio is the most reliable test available for establishing the diagnosis of acute renal failure. The concentration of urine urea is normally 30 times that in the serum, but trauma or other cause of prerenal deviation of water may reduce the ratio to 1:15. A ratio of 1:10 indicates severe kidney damage.

Central Venous Pressure

Overall, the best single guide to the rate and volume of fluid administration during the resuscitation period is the central venous pressure (CVP). It is simple, the results are available immediately, and the determination can be repeated as often as necessary. It is not an indicator of blood volume and it does not necessarily measure the adequacy of the function of the left side of the heart, but it does measure the ability of the right side of the heart to propel blood that is presented to it. Since it measures the myocardial adequacy in relationship to the circulating blood volume, it helps to distinguish cardiogenic shock from hypovolemia and to determine whether the patient will tolerate additional fluid infusion. It is not necessary to know the precise blood volume. It is only necessary to know if the patient can tolerate more fluid or if additional fluid is apt to cause congestive failure and pulmonary edema. Early in the course of treatment, CVP monitoring combined with the urine output monitoring can be used for this determination. When the left side of the heart is incapable of pumping blood normally, pulmonary venous pressure increases before CVP does; monitoring of the pulmonary capillary wedge pressure becomes necessary.

In patients who are in manifest or imminent shock, regardless of cause, the central venous catheter should be inserted during the course of the resuscitation. As previously noted, if the patient is obviously hypovolemic, volume replacement should be well underway before the central venous line is inserted, and it is unwise in those circumstances to use the subclavian or internal jugular route because of the collapse of the central veins in the hypovolemic patient. The basilic route can be approached, either percutaneously or by cutdown and, if necessary, even the inferior vena cava can be approached using the Seldinger technique. It is important that the tip of the catheter be positioned in the superior vena cava 2 or 3 cm above the heart.

Proper interpretation of the venous pressure is as important as careful technique in its measurement. It is of value only in judging the ability of the patient to tolerate fluid replacement and helping to prevent cardiac overloading during therapy. Central venous pressure therefore must never be considered in isolation but should always be used in conjunction with other estimates of cardiac output and peripheral perfusion (see below). If venous pressure is normal or low, the fluid may be administered safely but only if other signs indicate the need. On the other hand, if CVP is high, it does indicate that the patient will not tolerate more fluid. It must always be remembered that CVP may not be elevated in left heart failure, especially in the early stage. CVP monitoring is most useful in preventing excessive transfusion during the rapid administration of fluid to otherwise healthy, young patients. As long as the CPV is not elevated and the chest is clear, fluid can be administered as rapidly as desired with little fear of fluid overload. When CPV increases, the blood volume is approaching the maximum that can be tolerated by the heart, and the rate of administration must be decreased.

Blood Gases

The determination of arterial blood gases is vital in the care of the multiply injured patient. As a guide to therapy, repeat blood gas analysis may be necessary as often as every 10 minutes during the initial phases of resuscitation.

Metabolic acidosis is a relatively late development in injured patients. The arterial pH does not correlate well with the clinical situation soon after injury because respiratory alkalosis rapidly compensates for any metabolic acidosis that is developing soon after injury; this compensation occurs as the venous blood passes through the lungs. As shock deepens, however, the compensatory mechanism is unable to correct for the metabolic acidosis, which becomes profound if circulatory adequacy is not rapidly established.

An adjunct that is extremely useful for some patients and essential for others is the repeated sampling of mixed venous

Po_2. Early in the course of traumatic shock, this is a much more sensitive index of the circulatory status than the arterial pH, since it can be considered an indicator of cardiac output. True value of the mixed venous Po_2 can only be obtained after a Swan-Ganz catheter has been passed centrally, but the early passage of a Swan-Ganz catheter is necessary only in those patients who have antecedent heart disease, or chronic obstructive pulmonary disease or in some patients who require mechanical ventilatory support. A mixed venous Po_2, ordinarily measured in the blood from the pulmonary artery, is normally 40 mm Hg. However, when the cardiac output is reduced and peripheral perfusion is decreased, more oxygen is extracted in the tissues and the mixed venous Po_2 is decreased. A mixed venous Po_2 of 40 or above usually indicates that the circulatory system is meeting the demands that are made upon it; whereas a Po_2 of 25 mm Hg or less usually indicates that the circulatory insufficiency is severe. Although the Po_2 value of blood taken from the central venous catheter gives a somewhat higher value than the true mixed venous Po_2, it is useful as an index because the relationships ordinarily remain the same. Serial measurements are most helpful; a rising value indicates an improving circulatory status, whereas a falling value usually indicates deterioration.

Volume Challenge

After the initial fluids have been rapidly administered, a volume challenge is a useful mechanism for deciding whether additional fluids should be infused or whether they would overload the circulation. There is no uniform procedure for carrying out this test. Crystalloids—sodium chloride or sodium lactate—are commonly infused in volumes up to 200 ml, and the response of the CVP is monitored. However, there is evidence that a colloid—a true volume expander—should be used rather than a crystalloid since the hemodynamic status of the infused crystalloid appears to be too short lived to enable an accurate interpretation of cardiac response to volume stress.

A satisfactory procedure involves infusion of 200 ml of colloid over a 15-minute period. During this period the patient is observed carefully for signs of the development of cardiac failure or pulmonary edema and if necessary is treated appropriately. The CVP and heart rate are measured at 5-minute intervals before, during, and after the completion of the infusion. A CVP that remains persistently low or falls indicates that the circulatory volume is inadequate. If it rises either transiently or steadily but remains within normal range while the heart rate remains steady or decreases, it is an indication that the volume is still inadequate but is in the process of correction. If there is a rise in the CVP and also a rise in the pulse, it must be interpreted as a possible indication of overloading of the circulation, even though the CVP remains within normal range. The literature presents a confusing array of numbers that should be considered the top value for a normal CVP, ranging from 8 cm H_2O to 15 cm H_2O. All clinicians agree that a CVP above 15 cm H_2O should be considered abnormally high under ordinary circumstances. Many advise that a CVP increase to more than 10 cm H_2O represents an imminent overloading of the circulation, and they all agree that the isolated CVP reading can be misleading. It is the trends that must be followed carefully.

CLINICAL STATUS

There is no substitute for repeated clinical evaluation of the circulatory, respiratory, and nervous systems. Monitoring systems yields numbers, but these numbers must be interpreted in the light of the total clinical picture. If rales are heard at both lung bases in spite of a low CVP, the physician must base therapeutic decisions on the rales rather than on the CVP alone. If one pupil suddenly dilates in a patient whose blood gases, urinary output, and CVP are returning to normal, the new physical finding helps to determine the next urgent clinical decision.

URGENT DIAGNOSTIC CONSIDERATIONS

The diagnostic decisions that apply in the care of the multiply-injured patient, especially the victim of blunt trauma, are not usually the same as those that guide in the evaluation of the patient with a single injury. Because of the initial uncertainty about the full extent of injuries and the likelihood that the injuries are serious, urgent questions must be answered quickly. If the patient is in shock, shows no obvious external source of bleeding, and apparently does not have fractures of the extremities, it must be assumed that he or she is bleeding internally, either in the chest, the abdomen, or the retroperitoneum. The bleeding source must be found quickly. A pneumothorax or other correctable intrathoracic problem that prevents adequate ventilation must also be detected early since it is estimated that 10% of victims of high-speed automobile accidents die from unrecognized tension pneumothorax. CNS injury, a frequent cause of death, is commonly associated with other injuries. Since as many as 50–70% of patients cared for in a trauma unit are unconscious upon arrival, urgent diagnostic procedures may be necessary in order to decide whether or not immediate neurosurgical exploration is necessary to save the patient's life.

The only diagnostic procedures that should be performed urgently are those that are necessary to save the patient's life. Only after the preservation of life seems assured should other diagnostic tests be performed. Procedures such as arteriograms to confirm or rule out vascular injury associated with fractures of extremities have no place among the initial diagnostic procedures for the multiply-injured patient. They should not be performed until life-threatening problems have been identified and the patient's condition has been stabilized with adequate therapy. The clinical assessment and splinting of such injuries is all that is necessary during the first few minutes after a patient has arrived.

Chest Injury

CHEST ROENTGENOGRAM

The most important single diagnostic tool for evaluation of a chest injury is the chest roentgenogram. The portable x-ray is perfectly satisfactory as a screening device. In fact, it would be dangerous to send a patient with a possible chest injury to the x-ray suite, which may be far from the resuscitation area, unless the condition is completely stable. Any patient with signs of possible chest injury, such as flail chest, palpable subcutaneous emphysema along the chest wall or neck, tracheal shift, or use of accessory respiratory muscles, and any patient with profound hypotension unexplained by injuries elsewhere in the body should have an early chest film, except in the most extreme emergency situation. The portable film, which requires only a few seconds, should be taken as soon as possible after the airway has been opened, ventilation has been established, intravenous lines have been inserted, and the blood pressure has begun to respond to volume infusion. At the same time the chest film will be used to check the position of the central venous line.

An upright film reveals much more about the chest pathology than does the supine film because it is often impossible to detect the dependent layering of fluid or a collection of air within the injured chest if the patient is in the supine position. Since it is usually very difficult and often impossible or unsafe to take an upright film of a critically injured patient, the head of the examining table can usually be elevated to 45–50 deg for the short time that it takes to obtain the chest film, even if the patient is unconscious. In the patient who is hemodynamically unstable, this position must be held for only a few seconds. It is sometimes possible, and often more satisfactory, if the x-ray tube and film is positioned for an upright film and the patient is held by members of the resuscitation team for a few seconds in order to get an upright film. If this procedure is used, extreme care must be used in moving the patient in order not to cause further injury. If upright or semiupright films cannot be taken, a lateral decubitus film should be obtained in an effort to demonstrate layering of fluid and air.

NEEDLE OR TUBE THORACOSTOMY

Not infrequently, the patient's condition is so unstable that the team cannot wait for a chest film to be taken. If tension pneumothorax is suspected, a large-bore needle (16–18 gauge at least) should be inserted into the second intercostal space anteriorly or into the fourth or fifth intercostal space in the midaxillary line. This maneuver can be lifesaving; it is therapeutic if air is present and diagnostic if blood is present. If the presence of blood is proved by needle aspiration or is strongly suspected, a tube thoracostomy (Procedure 19) can be performed in the fourth or fifth intercostal space in the midaxillary line.

Abdominal Injury

PERITONEAL LAVAGE

Most patients with abdominal injuries survive long enough to receive medical attention if associated injuries are not lethal. Patients with abdominal injuries do have a high mortality, however, because diagnosis is often delayed since the index of suspicion is not high enough and the diagnostic evaluation is not aggressive enough. Clinical findings are useless for the early diagnosis of abdominal injuries in most patients. At the Ramsey Hospital in Minnesota where the technique for peritoneal lavage was developed, the initial clinical impression has been found to be inaccurate in 33–57% of patients with blunt abdominal trauma. In patients with visceral injuries, abdominal signs and symptoms are absent in 16% of patients without head injuries and in 43% of patients with significant head injuries.

Peritoneal lavage (Procedure 24) should be performed early in the evaluation of the patient with a possible abdominal injury, regardless of the clinical findings on abdominal examination (unless the patient is obviously bleeding massively and needs immediate operation or there is another life-threatening contraindication). It should be performed only after the initial resuscitation measures have been initiated and a sufficient volume of fluid has already been given to raise the blood pressure to a safe level.

It is usually best for the lavage to be performed by the surgeon who will be observing the patient or performing the operation if it becomes indicated. Although it is sometimes necessary for a triaging physician to perform the lavage if he or she is faced with the need to refer a multiply-injured patient to a trauma center. Such a decision must be made by the team leader in consultation with the surgeon who will be responsible for the patient.

The minilaparotomy technique is accurate and safe when performed carefully, but great care is necessary in order to avoid iatrogenic bleeding that will vitiate the results of the examination. Recently, a technique that uses a guide wire for the introduction of the lavage catheter has gained wide acceptance. It is easier and quicker to perform than is the minilaparotomy, but the accuracy and safety of the two methods have not yet been compared rigorously.

Interpretation of the lavage findings has not been uniform. Some teams examine the fluid, quantitating the results on the basis of red and white blood cell counts and amylase determinations; others relate the significance of the findings to the ability to read newspaper print through the lavage fluid. The only tap that can be considered to be negative, though, is one that is crystal clear. Any degree of blood tinging of the fluid indicates either poor technique, with contamination of the abdominal cavity with blood from the incision through which the lavage was performed, or intraabdominal pathology. The finding of blood within the abdominal cavity is not, in itself, an indication for operation in all cases. As indicated below, the computed tomographic (CT) scan is being used with increasing frequency in hemodynamically stable patients in whom injury to one of the solid organs of the upper abdomen is suspected. For some of these patients, operation is indicated; for others, the course of watchful waiting is wiser. The indications and techniques for intravenous pyelography and other studies that are useful in the initial evaluation of abdominal and genitourinary injury are discussed in Chapter 21.

Central Nervous System Injury

Monitoring of the clinical signs in a person with a possible CNS injury is the best way to diagnose such an injury and to decide about the follow-up that will be necessary. However, since so many critically injured patients are already unconscious or have associated injuries that require immediate surgery under general anesthesia, the usual markers—level of consciousness, vital signs, pupil size, and response to painful stimuli—may not provide specific enough information to determine whether or not immediate neurosurgical exploration is required. Early CT scan is highly desirable and widely used in delineating intracranial pathology, but a decision about this or any other diagnostic procedure must be made by the neurosurgeon. In the multiply-injured patient, if there is a critical acute head injury with signs of acute deterioration, such as dilating pupil, the patient is taken immediately to the operating

room where bilateral burr holes are placed to explore for epidural or subdural hematoma. In preparation for these burr holes, the patient is intubated and artificially ventilated with ventilation adjusted to obtain a partial pressure of arterial carbon dioxide of 25–30 mm Hg and a partial pressure of arterial oxygen above 100 mm Hg if possible. Mannitol, 1.5–2 g/kg, is given intravenously over a 30-minute period if time permits. If the burr holes do not reveal acute epidural or subdural hematomas, CT scans are performed. The management of acute head injuries is discussed in Chapter 15.

X-ray films of the cervical spine should be obtained at the earliest opportunity to exclude injury to the spinal column in any patient who may have sustained such an injury. The cross-table lateral view of the cervical spine should also include the skull. Acutely, the only finding on a plain skull film that is likely to be helpful would be that of a fracture running across the course of the middle meningial artery, which is evidence that would strongly point to the possibility of a developing epidural hematoma.

Emergency Radiology

In some hospitals, the receiving area in which patients with multiple injuries are initially managed either includes a diagnostic radiology unit or is adjacent to one. Careful radiologic assessment is a vital part of the evaluation and management of the injured patient; such assessment takes place after all conditions that are immediately life-threatening have been ruled out and the clinical condition is stable. However, in the critically injured patient, especially one with multiple injuries, x-ray must be brought to the patient rather than the patient brought to the x-ray department, even if it is adjacent to the resuscitation area. As already described, the portable x-ray film is often the one that will guide the initial clinical decisions. The films that are taken during the first few minutes of the patient's admission should be ordered only to rule out life-threatening conditions. Then, after the condition has stabilized, the ordering of films depends on the organization of care within each hospital and the decisions that are made by the team caring for the patient.

The CT scan is proving to be a valuable addition to the diagnostic tools that can be used in the evaluation of critically injured patients. Under no circumstance should it be used, however, until the patient's condition has stabilized. It can be used to delineate pathology in injuries of the head, maxillofacial region, spine, and abdomen, including the pelvis. In cases of possible spinal cord injury, it can help in detecting whether a fracture is stable or unstable, whether there are bony elements in the canal, and whether there is compression of the cord. In evaluation of abdominal injuries, it is primarily useful in assessment of damage to the solid organs of the upper abdomen, liver, spleen, kidneys, and pancreas. It is not used for most patients with possible abdominal injury, but it is especially useful in evaluating stable patients with possible significant abdominal traumas. It is especially helpful to the surgeon in planning whether or not to explore a patient and in giving an indication of the injuries that have been sustained by the solid organs. The diagnostic radiographic procedures that are used in the evaluation of the critically injured patient are more fully discussed in subsequent chapters.

Preservation of Function

After life-threatening conditions have been identified, effective therapy has been initiated, and the condition of the patient has stabilized, preservation of function becomes a prime concern. A rapid but careful physical examination is performed from head to toe in order to identify injuries that may cause impairment of function if they are inadequately managed. Since the head, neck, and front and back of the torso have been examined already to rule out life-threatening conditions, attention must now be directed to the extremities. The injuries that have been sustained by the musculoskeletal system are for the most part obvious, but secondary impairment that has resulted from injury to adjacent neurovascular structures must be searched for if the condition of the patient makes this evaluation possible. Figures 12.19 and 12.20 indicate some of the sites at which injury to particular neurovascular structures commonly occur. In order to rule out such impairment, it is important to evaluate the circulatory status and the motor and sensory nerve function distal to the point of injury quickly but carefully.

URGENT THERAPY

After adequate ventilation has been ensured, external hemorrhage has been stopped, and infusions have been rapidly given through multiple intravenous sites, a number of additional therapeutic adjuncts should be considered at the same time that monitoring mechanisms are being established and urgent diagnostic procedures are being performed.

Ventilation

POSITIVE END EXPIRATORY PRESSURE
VENTILATION

After volume infusion is well underway and hemodynamic stability has been achieved positive end expiratory pressure (PEEP) on continuous positive airway pressure (CPAP) should be introduced in any patient who has had a blunt injury to the

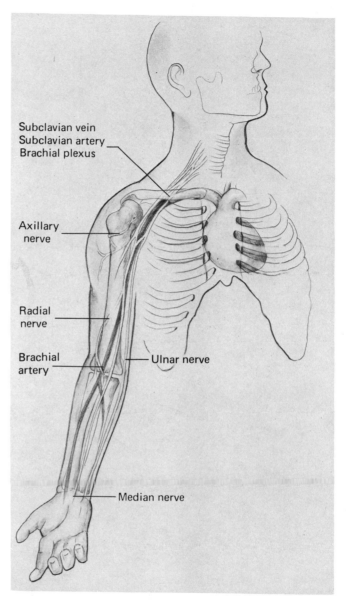

Figure 12.19 Neurovascular structures that may be damaged by fracture or dislocation of overlying bony structures of the upper extremity.

chest, whether or not it has caused a flail chest. Even in the critically injured patient who has not sustained a chest injury, PEEP seems to offer protection from overinfusion of fluid with resulting pulmonary edema, which is a frequent complication of resuscitation. In the press of the efforts to restore blood volume quickly and at the same time carry out the other ur-

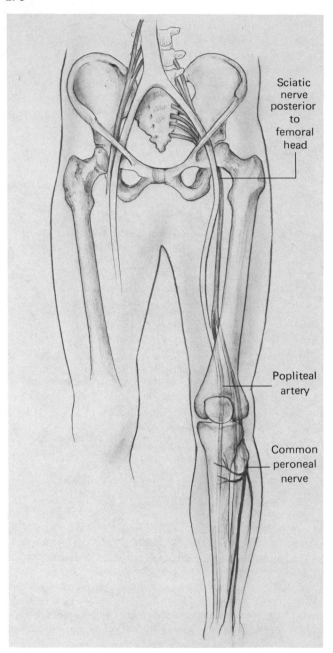

Sciatic
nerve
posterior
to
femoral
head

Popliteal
artery

Common
peroneal
nerve

Figure 12.20 Neurovascular structures that may be damaged from fracture or dislocation of overlying bony structures of the lower extremity.

gently needed diagnostic and therapeutic maneuvers, it is easy to overload the patient with fluids in spite of intensive monitoring. When this situation is recognized, either by the appearance of rales or by a rise in CVP, the rate of infusion is reduced to the point where relative hypovolemia recurs. However, PEEP is able to protect the patient from interstitial edema through such periods when the rate of infusion is being titrated to the patient's needs. In addition, it protects such patients from the microatelectasis that develops. Characteristically, the ratio of dead space to tidal ventilation increases in patients in early shock as the pulmonary blood flow, reduced as it is, is concentrated in the dependent parts of the lungs under the influence of gravity while ventilation is preferentially directed to the upper portions of the lung. In situations in which there is increase in arteriovenous shunting in the lungs, an increase in the concentration of inspired oxygen helps very little; PEEP or CPAP may help a great deal.

Ordinarily, PEEP is introduced at a level 5 cm H_2O. Later the level of PEEP can be modified, increasing it incrementally while the arterial oxygen tension is carefully followed. Eventually the optimal level of PEEP is that which produces the largest increase in arterial oxygen tension without decreasing cardiac output. It is crucial that the level of PEEP not be raised to the point at which it can decrease cardiac output since the resulting lowering of the oxygen delivery to the tissues would defeat the purpose for which it was started. The team should not hesitate to use PEEP in patients with head injuries if it is needed to correct ventilation problems.

High concentrations of oxygen will usually be required during the initial resuscitation efforts in order to maintain arterial P_{O_2} above 80 mm Hg. It may be necessary to give 100% oxygen early, but the oxygen concentration should be reduced to the lowest level that will maintain an arterial P_{O_2} of at least 80 mm Hg as soon as it becomes possible. High concentrations of oxygen do not cause oxygen toxicity in the previously healthy person if they are given for short periods of time, but the risk of toxicity becomes significant if high concentrations are maintained for more than 6 hours. When the oxygen concentration has been reduced to less than 40%, there seems to be relative protection from the subsequent development of pulmonary complications of oxygen therapy.

Circulation

INOTROPIC AGENTS

Inotropic agents are often required in the treatment of shock in critically injured patients. In some patients who are receiving intravenous fluids rapidly, if the urine output remains low in spite of an adequate or high atrial filling pressure (CVP), decreased myocardial contractility must be suspected. In the absence of myocardial contusion or myocardial infarction, an inotropic agent should be given. The most effective of these is digitalis; others that are widely used are isoproterenol, dopamine, and calcium. These agents should only be used after hypovolemia has been corrected, or is being corrected, and the blood pressure, heart rate, and urine flow must be carefully monitored while they are being used.

Digitalis

Digitalis preparations are not necessary and should not be given to patients with a normal heart under most conditions, especially when the patient is under the age of 30. But the critically injured patient who is 18 or 19 years old and has depleted blood volume does not have a normal heart. Its energy stores are depleted; in this circumstance cardiac glycosides are sometimes lifesaving, in part because they restore high-energy phosphate bonds. In some patients they protect, at least partially, against the development of pulmonary edema that sometimes occurs as a result of the myocardial strain associated with factors such as hypoxia, hemodilution, and increasing demands on the heart in spite of depletion of energy reserves.

The disadvantage of the cardiac glycosides in this setting is that they produce a profound splanchnic vasoconstriction, potentiating the preexisting ischemia and enhancing the release of lysosomal enzymes and the myocardial depressant factor, previously discussed. Because of this, their use should probably be limited to patients in whom the presence or the risk of cardiac decompensation is definite.

As discussed in Chapter 6, digoxin is a satisfactory preparation to use since its onset of action is within 15–30 minutes when given parenterally. The dose required to obtain an optimal effect when shock is present may be extremely variable because of changes in acid–base balance, electrolyte abnormalities, and altered cell metabolism, but the usual loading dose for intravenous administration of digoxin is 0.75–1 mg. A commonly used schedule for rapid digitalization is digoxin, 0.5–0.75 mg intravenously immediately, followed by 0.25 mg every 2 hours for two dosages. If necessary, 0.125 mg may be given every 2 hours until there is evidence of digitalis effect (not exceeding 4 doses of 0.125 mg each). An ECG strip must be taken before each dose is given. If there is any change indicating digitalis effect or toxicity—changes in rate, rhythm, or ST segments—no further dosage is given until the maintenance dose is required. It is preferable to dilute the drug in isotonic sodium chloride solution and to make the injection slowly. The facts about previous digitalis medication must be

known, and the dosage must be determined carefully because intravenous use of digitalis is by far the most dangerous. Fatality can occur rapidly if extreme care is not observed in its use.

Isoproterenol

Isoproterenol (Isuprel) is an effective inotropic agent that has a powerful action on all beta receptors and almost no action on alpha receptors. Therefore, its main actions are on the heart, the smooth muscle of the bronchi, the skeletal musculature, and the alimentary tract. When it is used intravenously, cardiac output is raised because venous return to the heart is increased; the contractility of the heart and the heart rate are also increased. Since peripheral vascular resistance is decreased, especially in the skeletal muscle but also in renal and mesenteric vascular beds, the diastolic pressure falls, but the increase in cardiac output is generally enough to maintain or raise the systolic pressure. Renal blood flow is decreased in normotensive subjects but is markedly increased in patients in cardiogenic or septicemic shock. Isoproterenol is an excellent drug to use if the pulse rate is less than 100 beats/min. It should be administered intravenously 1–2 mg in 500 ml D_5W adjusting the rate until the appropriate response is obtained. Unfortunately, its clinical usefulness is often limited because of the presence of tachycardia or the development of tachycardia of over 120 beats/min or arrhythmia when it is used. It must be remembered, too, that in augmenting the cardiac output by increasing the contractility of the heart and the heart rate, isoproterenol also increases the oxygen demand of the myocardium, which, in the profoundly hypovolemic patient, is already ischemic.

Dopamine

Dopamine, the immediate precursor in the synthesis of norepinephrine in the body, is widely used in the treatment of shock. In low doses it stimulates the beta-adrenergic cardiac receptors, resulting in an increase in cardiac contractility, and at the time it stimulates specific dopamine receptors in the mesenteric and renal vascular beds, leading to renal and mesenteric vasodilatation with resulting increase in renal blood flow and urine output and an increase in the arterial blood pressure. Higher doses of dopamine stimulate the alpha-receptors that cause systemic vasoconstriction and reverse the renal vasodilatation seen at lower doses. The dose must therefore be carefully titrated in order that the desired increase in vital organ perfusion will result. The 5-ml ampule containing 40 mg/ml of the drug must be diluted in 250 or 500 ml of an appropriate, nonalkaline, sterile solution (0.9% sodium chloride) to yield a final concentration of 800 or 400 μg/ml. It is given by metered drip infusion at an initial rate of 2.5 μg/kg/min, and the dosage is gradually increased to 10–20 μg/kg or more per minute, if necessary. The urine flow must be monitored frequently because it is the best index of a satisfactory response. Since the action of dopamine is quite brief, the rate of administration can be used effectively to control the intensity of effect. The blood pressure, heart rate, and urine flow should be monitored continuously and the dosage adjusted accordingly. Hypovolemia must be corrected before it is administered, but the prognosis is more favorable when therapy is instituted early, especially before the rate of urine flow has seriously decreased.

Calcium

Calcium is also an inotropic agent. It has long been recognized that there are certain similarities in the effect of calcium and the cardiac glycosides on the cardiac muscle. In fact, it has been postulated that the inotropic action of the cardiac glycosides is mediated by an influx of calcium ions. The inotropic effect of calcium may be rapid and impressive at onset, but it is usually short lived. If hypocalcemia is present, 10 ml of a 10% solution of calcium chloride is given directly intravenously over 2–3 minutes while EGC is monitored continuously for cardiac arrhythmia. Hypercalcemia is potentially lethal; therefore, calcium should always be administered cautiously and the ionized calcium level should be measured periodically, if possible, in such situations.

DIURETICS

Diuretics must sometimes be used in the management of critically injured patients in order to protect renal function. When the urine output is decreased in spite of a CVP that is adequate or increased, it is important to get some indication of cardiac output. This can be measured only after a Swan-Ganz catheter has been passed and the mixed venous P_{O_2} has been measured. If this value is high, the cardiac output probably is adequate. If the urine output is low under these circumstances, it is usually an indication that renal function is decreased and that an osmotic diuretic may be helpful. If the urine specific gravity is above 1.020 or if the urine sodium is below 20 mEq/liter in the presence of oliguria, it usually indicates that the renal blood flow is adequate. If additional fluids cannot be given safely because of an elevated CVP, cardiotonic drugs should be given. If their use does not result in improved urine output, diuretics must be tried.

Mannitol

Mannitol is the osmotic diuretic of choice for critically ill patients if the use of diuretics is indicated. The adult dosage recommended for the promotion of diuresis ranges from 50 to 200 g over a 24-hour period of infusion; the rate is generally adjusted to maintain a urinary output of at least 30–50 ml/hr. In patients with marked oliguria or questionable adequacy of renal function, a test dose of 200 mg/kg (approximately 75 ml of a 20% solution for adult patients) is recommended. The test dose should be infused over 3–5 minutes, and if the first or second dose fails to promote a urinary flow greater than 30-ml/hr for 2–3 hours, the patient's status should be reevaluated before initiation of mannitol therapy. Mannitol infusions should be terminated if the patient develops signs of progressive renal dysfunction, heart failure, or pulmonary congestion.

Mannitol is used extensively to protect patients against the development of acute renal failure, which may occur not only from acutely reduced filtration rates but also from acute changes in tubular permeability. The tubular damage may be caused by a noxious agent, such as myoglobin, that can build up to dangerous concentrations in the tubule, sometimes resulting in actual precipitation. In these situations, mannitol exerts an osmotic effect within the tubular fluid, inhibits water reabsorption, and maintains the rate of urine flow so that the concentration of the noxious agent within the tubular fluid does not reach excessively high levels.

If given in sufficiently large amounts, mannitol raises the serum osmolality, acting as a transient volume expander and improving renal blood flow, while at the same time decreasing cellular swelling. Overloading of the circulation may occur, leading to the development of pulmonary edema. Mannitol must therefore be used with care.

If a Swan-Ganz catheter has not been placed, it is worthwhile to use a volume challenge as an aid in making the decision whether or not mannitol should be used. If in response to a volume challenge of 200 ml of fluid given over a short time the urine flow rate increases, this can be taken as an indication that more volume is needed. If there is no change in urine flow rate in response to the challenge, the assumption must be made that the patient has renal failure, and mannitol should be tried. If there is any suspicion about renal function, it is helpful to give the mannitol early. Often it is given with 2 liters of Ringer's lactate and 1 ampule of sodium bicarbonate to alkalinize the urine.

Furosemide

Furosemide (Lasix) should be given only if there is no response to mannitol or if there is danger that overloading of the circulation will occur from mannitol. Furosemide or other chemical diuretics such as ethacrynic acid should rarely be used in treating patients who are in shock, and they should *never* be given early to patients in shock since they may cause systemic vasodilation as well as redistribution of blood flow within the kidney. In the rare situation in which furosemide is used, it should be used very cautiously; only small intravenous doses such as 10–20 mg, should be given initially unless the patient is in pulmonary edema or there is other evidence of volume overloading, in which case it can be given in 40-mg intravenous boluses.

CORTICOSTEROIDS

The use of massive doses of steroids equivalent to 50–150 mg of hydrocortisone per kilogram of body weight are being used with increasing frequency in the treatment of patients in severe or prolonged shock, although their use is highly controversial. There are conflicting reports about their effectiveness in the management of critically injured patients. Although the mechanism of action of massive doses of steroids is not understood, there is evidence that they may stabilize lysosomal and cell membranes and act as vasodilators. There is controversy as to whether or not pharmacologic doses of cortisone protect the lungs from the hyperpermeable states that characterize post-traumatic pulmonary dysfunction. Jacobs has proved that such doses inhibit the aggregation of leukocytes (which seems to play a central role in initiating the derangements that follow). It is uncertain whether improvement of the cardiac output is a result of a direct inotropic action on the heart or whether it is because of increased venous return to the heart. The hemodynamic actions of massive doses of steroids have not been consistently reproduced, and in any case, more potent agents exist to accomplish these objectives.

There are several techniques for giving massive steroids. Dexamethasone (Decadron), 6 mg/kg, or methylprednisolone, 30 mg/kg, is given intravenously as a bolus over 5–10 minutes followed by another bolus after 4–6 hours or a continuous infusion over 12–24 hours. If the patient improves, infusion or bolus dosage may be repeated. Hydrocortisone may be given in equivalent dosages, 50–150 mg of hydrocortisone per kilogram of body weight.

VASOMOTOR DRUGS

Vasoconstrictors and vasodilators have been of limited value in the treatment of patients in shock. If all of the steps outlined above fail to bring the patient out of shock, the prognosis is usually extremely poor.

Vasopressors, in general, have yielded disappointing results when they have been used to combat shock in critically injured patients. They can only lead to further deterioration if they are given to the hypovolemic patient without first correcting the hypovolemia. They have been used extensively in patients in cardiogenic shock (see Chapter 3), but even in this group of patients, their use has been disappointing. The prime indication for the use of vasopressors in the injured patient is spinal shock in which vasodilation causes a relative hypovolemia because of expansion of the capacity of the vascular system. Inappropriate use of vasopressors for patients in other forms of shock has been caused by the preoccupation with blood pressure as a manifestation of shock. One of the most potent stimuli to evoke a sympathetic response in a patient is blood loss. What the patient with blood loss needs is not a reinforcement of the compensatory sympathetic discharge. The patient needs fluids.

Vasodilators, on the other hand, have proved to be effective adjuncts to therapy for patients who are in some forms of shock. These agents induce vasodilation by inhibiting sympathetic vasoconstriction or by directly relaxing vascular smooth muscle. The protection provided by vasodilators has been attributed to at least three distinct cardiovascular effects: (1) increased cardiac output and total blood flow, particularly in the abdominal viscera; (2) local redistribution of blood flow so that a larger percentage passes through channels that readily exchange metabolites with tissue cells; and (3) reversal of vasoconstriction-induced shift of fluid from the vascular to the interstitial compartment.

Chlorpromazine (Thorazine) has a mildly dilating effect; phentolamine (Regitine) and phenoxybenzamine have a much more pronounced effect. Since the response is unpredictable, the dosage of phentolamine and phenoxybenzamine must be carefully titrated to prevent dangerous hypotension. The blocking agent must be administered slowly, and suitable fluids must be immediately available for use if a sharp drop in blood pressure indicates that replacement has in fact been inadequate. Phenoxybenzamine should not be given unless the CVP has been elevated by fluid administration without an adequate circulatory response.

Care of Wounds and Immobilization of Fractures

After all of the initial measures of resuscitation have been initiated, the fractures should be immobilized and wounds dressed in order to minimize further damage. These procedures can be carried out by one member of the team while other members proceed with urgent diagnostic procedures and complete a careful and complete evaluation of the patient. As described in Chapter 13, antibiotics in high dosages should be initiated early during the resuscitation period if they are indicated, and appropriate protection against tetanus should be given.

Necessary consultations must be obtained whenever they are appropriate, but it is the team leader who must assume responsibility for coordinating the total care. The leader must decide when the time has come for an operation or for further diagnostic studies at a more leisurely pace. If all injuries that threaten life and limb have been ruled out or cared for, the decision must be made about the wisdom of transferring responsibility to another physician and to another area of the hospital. The mechanism of organization of care will vary from one hospital to another, but protocols must be developed and followed. Since attention to detail often determines whether the patient will live or die or whether or not there will be a serious disability, decisions about how the emergency will be managed should be made before the emergency.

SUGGESTED READINGS

Armstrong PW, Buigzie RS: Symposium on hemodynamic monitoring. *Can Med Assoc J* 1979; 121:865–936.

Austin KF: Tissue mast cells in immediate hypersensitivity. *Hosp Pract* 1982; 17:98.

Baker CC, Oppenheimer L, Stephens D et al: Epidemiology of trauma deaths. *Am J Surg* 1980; 140:144–150.

Beisel WR, Wannemacher RW: Metabolic response of the host to infectious disease, in Richards JR, Kinney JM (eds): *Nutritional Aspects of Care in the Critically Ill*. New York, Churchill Livingstone Inc, 1977, pp 135–161.

Blair E, Topuzlu C, Deane RS: *Major Blunt Chest Trauma. Current Problems in Surgery*. Chicago, Year Book Medical Publishers, 1969.

Blaisdell FW: General assessment, resuscitation and exploration of penetrating and blunt abdominal trauma, in Blaisdell FW, Trunkey DD (eds): *Trauma Management. Abdominal Trauma*. New York, Thieme-Stratton Inc, 1982, vol 1, pp 1–18.

Blaisdell FW, Lim RC Jr, Stallone RJ: The mechanism of pulmonary damage following traumatic shock. *Surg Gynecol Obstet* 1970; 130:1.

Blaisdell FW, Schlobohm RM: The respiratory distress syndrome: A review. *Surgery* 1973; 74:251.

Blaisdell FW, Trunkey DD (eds): *Trauma Management. Abdominal Trauma*. New York, Thieme-Stratton Inc, vol 1, 1982.

Boyd DR, Mansberger AR Jr: Serum water and osmolar changes in hemorrhagic shock: An experimental and clinical study. *Am J Surg* 1968; 34:744–749.

Brinkhous KM (ed): *Accident Pathology*. Proceedings of An International Conference, No. FH-11-6595, June 6–8, 1968. National Highway Safety Bureau, 1968.

Chaudry IH, Baue AE: Overview of hemorrhagic shock, in Cowley RA, Trump BF (eds): *Pathophysiology of Shock, Anoxia, and Ischemia*. Baltimore, The Williams & Wilkins Co, 1982, pp 203–219.

Chaudry IH, Clemens MG, Baue AE: Alterations in cell function with ischemia and shock and their correction. *Arch Surg* 1981; 116:1309–1317.

Christou NV, McLean APH, Meakins JL: Host defense in blunt trauma: Interrelationships of kinetics of anergy and depressed neutrophil function, nutritional status and sepsis. *J Trauma* 1980; 20:833–841.

Christou NV, Meakins JL: Neutrophil function in surgical patients: Neutrophil adherence and chemotaxis and cutaneous anergy. *Ann Surg* 1979; 190:557.

Cowley RA, Dunham CM: *Shock Trauma/Critical Care Manual*. Baltimore, University Park Press, 1982.

Cowley RA, Trump BF (eds): *Pathophysiology of Shock, Anoxia, and Ischemia*. Baltimore, The Williams and Wilkins Co, 1982.

Danto LA: Paracentesis and diagnostic peritoneal lavage, in Blaisdell FW, Trunkey DD (eds): *Trauma Management. Abdominal Trauma*. New York, Thieme-Stratton Inc, 1982, vol 1, pp 45–58.

Davis JM, Dineen P: Chemoattractants in trauma, in Dineen P, Hildicksmith G: *The Surgical Wound*. Philadelphia, Lea & Febiger, 1981, pp 26–36.

DeHaven H: Mechanical analysis of survival in falls from heights of fifty to one hundred and fifty feet. *War Med* 1942; 2:586–596.

Demling RH, Flynn JT: Humoral factors and lung injury during shock, trauma, and sepsis, in Cowley RA, Trump BF (eds): *Pathophysiology of Shock, Anoxia, and Ischemia*. Baltimore, The Williams & Wilkins Co, 1982, pp 395–407.

DeMuth WE Jr: Bullet velocity and design as determinants of wounding capability: An experimental study. *J Trauma* 1966; 6:222–232.

DeMuth WE Jr: Bullet velocity as applied to military rifle wounding capacity. *J Trauma* 1969; 9:27–38.

DeMuth WE Jr, Nicholas GG, Mung BL: Buckshot wounds. *J Trauma* 1976; 18:54–57.

DeMuth WE Jr, Smith JM: High-velocity bullet wounds of muscle and bone: The basis of rational early treatment. *J Trauma* 1966; 6:744–755.

Dineen P, Hildick-Smith G: *The Surgical Wound*. Philadelphia, Lea & Febiger, 1981.

Drucker WR, Chadwick CDJ, Gann DS: Transcapillary refill in hemorrhage and shock. *Arch Surg* 1981; 116:1344–1353.

Egdahl RH: Pituitary-adrenal response following trauma to the isolated leg. *Surgery* 1959; 46:9.

Faden AI, Holaday JW: Opiate antagonists: A role in the treatment of hypovolemic shock. *Science* 1979; 205:317–318.

Federle MP: Abdominal trauma: The role and impact of computed tomography. *Invest Radiol* 1981; 16:260–268.

Foley RW, Harris LS, Pilcher DB: Abdominal injuries in automobile accidents: Review of care of fatally injured patients. *J Trauma* 1977; 17:611–615.

Gann DS: Endocrine and metabolic responses to injury, in Schwartz SI (ed): *Principles of Surgery,* ed 3. New York, McGraw-Hill Book Company, 1979, p 1.

Gann DS, Ward DG, Carlson DE: Neural control of ACTH: A homeostatic reflex. *Recent Prog Horm Res* 1978; 34:357.

Gill W, Long WB: *Shock Trauma Manual.* Baltimore, The Williams and Wilkins Co, 1979.

Gilmore KM, Clemmer TP, Orme JF Jr: Commitment to trauma in low-population-density area. *J Trauma* 1981; 21:883–888.

Goodman LS, Gilman A: *The Pharmacological Basis of Therapeutics.* New York, MacMillan Inc, 1980.

Gurdjian ES, Lange WA, Patrick LM, Thomas LM (eds): *Impact Injury and Crash Protection.* Springfield, Illinois, Charles C Thomas Publisher, 1970.

Gurll NJ, Vargish T, Reynolds DG et al: Opiate receptors and endorphins in the pathophysiology of hemorrhagic shock. *Surgery* 1981; 89:364–369.

Haddon W Jr: The prevention of accidents, in Clark DW, MacMahon B (eds): *Preventive Medicine.* Boston, Little Brown & Co, 1967, pp 591–621.

Hardaway RM III: Treatment of severe shock with phenoxybenzamine. *Surg Gynecol Obstet* 1980; 151:725–734.

Hechtman HB, Utsunomiya T, Krausz MM et al: The management of cardiorespiratory failure in surgical patients. *Adv Surg* 1981; 15:123–156.

Hohl, M: Soft tissue injuries of the neck. *Clin Orthopedics and Related Research* 1975; 109: 42–49.

Hunt TK: *Wound Healing and Wound Infection: Theory and Surgical Practice.* New York, Appleton-Century-Crofts, 1980.

Jacob HS, Craddock PR, Hammerschmidt DE et al: Complement-induced granulocyte aggregation. An unsuspected mechanism of disease. *N Engl J Med* 1980; 302:789.

Jennett B, Snoek J, Bond MR et al: Disability after severe head injury. *J Neurol Neurosurg Psychiatry* 1981; 44:285–293.

Kihlberg JK: Multiplicity of injury in automobile accidents, in Gurdjian ES, Lange WA, Patrick LM, Thomas LM (ed): *Impact Injury and Crash Protection.* Springfield, Illinois, Charles C Thomas Publisher, 1970, pp 5–24.

Kulowski J: *Crash Injuries.* Springfield, Illinois, Charles C Thomas Publisher, 1960.

Lefer AM, Properties of cardio-inhibitory factors produced in shock. *Fed Proc* 1978; 37:2734–2740.

Lefer AM: Vascular mediators in ischemia and shock, in Cowley RA, Trump BF (ed): *Pathophysiology of Shock, Anoxia, and Ischemia.* Baltimore, The Williams & Wilkins Co, 1982, pp 165–181.

Lefer AM, Smith EF III: Protective action of prostacyclin in myocardial ischemia and trauma, in Vane JR, Bergstrom S (eds): *Prostacyclin.* New York, Raven Press, 1979, pp 339–347.

Lefer AM, Trachte GJ: Effects of hormones on heart, in Bourne GH (ed): *Hearts and Heart-like Organs.* New York, Academic Press Inc, 1980, pp 1–40.

Lewis RA, Austen KF: Mediation of local homeostasis and inflammation by leukotrienes and other mast-cell dependent compounds. *Nature* 1981; 293:103.

Lloyd JR, Silva Y, Walt AJ, Wilson RF: Trauma in infants and children: Special considerations, in Walt AJ, Wilson RF (ed): *Management of Trauma: Pitfalls and Practice.* Philadelphia, Lea & Febiger, 1975, pp 117–135.

Lowe RJ, Moss GS, Jilek J et al: Crystalloid versus colloid in the etiology of pulmonary failure after trauma. *Crit Care Med* 1979; 7:107.

Mason J, Thurau K: *Physiological Mechanisms Responsible for the Adjustment of Renal Function During Acute Renal Failure.* Sixth International Congress of Nephrology. Stuttgart, Symposium Verlag, 1975, pp 100–105.

Mays ET: *Clinical Evaluation of the Critically Injured.* Springfield, Illinois, Charles C Thomas Publisher, 1975.

McCuskey RS: Microcirculation—basic considerations, in Cowley RA, Trump BF (eds): *Pathophysiology of Shock, Anoxia, and Ischemia.* Baltimore, The Williams & Wilkins Co, 1982, pp 156–164.

Meakins JL, McLean APH, Kelly R et al: Delayed hypersensitivity response and neutrophil chemotaxis: Effects of trauma. *J Trauma* 1978; 18:240–247.

Moncada S, Gryglewski R, Bunting S et al: An enzyme isolated from arteries transforms prostaglandin endoperoxides to an unstable substance that inhibits platelet aggregation. *Nature* 1976; 263:663–665.

Moncada S, Vane JR: Prostacyclin, platelet aggregation, and thrombosis, in deGaetano G, Garattini S (eds): *Platelets: A Multidisciplinary Approach.* New York, Raven Press, 1978, pp 239–258.

Moss GS, Lowe RJ, Jilek J, Levine HD: Colloid or crystalloid in resuscitation of hemorrhagic shock: A controlled clinical trial. *Surgery* 1981; 89:434–438.

Moss G, Staunton C, Stein AA: Cerebral hypoxia as the primary event in the pathogenesis of the "Shock Lung Syndrome." *Surg Forum* 1971; 22:211.

Nahum AM, Gadd CN, Schneider DC et al: Tolerances of superficial soft tissues to injury. *J Trauma* 1972; 12:1044–1052.

Najarian JS, Delaney JP (eds): *Emergency Surgery, Trauma—Shock—Sepsis—Burns.* Chicago, Yearbook Medical Publishers Inc, 1982.

Peitzman AB, Shires GT III, Illner H, Shires GT: The effect of intravenous steroids on alveolar-capillary membrane permeability in pulmonary acid injury. *J Trauma* 1982; 22:347–352.

Peters RM, Hargens AR: Protein vs. electrolytes and all of the starling forces. *Arch Surg* 1981; 116:1293–1298.

Pietra GG, Rüttner JR, Wüst W, Glinz W: The lung after trauma and shock: Fine structure of the alveolar-capillary barrier in 23 autopsies. *J Trauma* 1981; 21:454–462.

Pirkle JC Jr, Gann DS: Restitution of blood volume after hemorrhage: Mathematical description. *Am J Physiol* 1975; 228:821.

Pirkle JC, Gann DS: Restitution of blood volume after hemorrhage: Role of the adrenal cortex. *Am J Physiol* 1976; 230:1683–1687.

Powers SR: Maintenance of renal function following massive trauma. *J Trauma* 1970; 10:554.

Powers SR: Renal response to systemic trauma. *Am J Surg* 1970; 119:603.

Reichard SM, Fletcher JR (eds): *Advances in Shock Research.* Proceedings of the Fourth Annual Conference on Shock. New York, Alan R Liss Inc, 1982, vol 7.

Safar P: Resuscitation in hemorrhagic shock, coma, and cardiac arrest, in Cowley RA, Trump BF (eds): *Pathophysiology of Shock, Anoxia, and Ischemia.* Baltimore, The Williams & Wilkins Co, 1982, pp 411–438.

Sayeed MM: Membrane Na$^+$–K$^+$ transport and ancillary phenomena in circulatory shock, in Cowley RA, Trump BF (eds): *Pathophysiology of Shock, Anoxia, and Ischemia.* Baltimore, The Williams & Wilkins Co, 1982, pp 112–132.

Schumer W: Steroids in the treatment of clinical septic shock. *Ann Surg* 1976; 184:333.

Seelig JM, Becker DP, Miller JD et al: Traumatic acute subdural hematomas: Major mortality reduction in comatose patients treated within four hours. *N Engl J Med* 1981; 304:1511–1518.

Shackford SR, Virgilio RW, Peters RM: Selective use of ventilator therapy in flail chest injury. *J Thorac Cardiovasc Surg* 1981; 881:194–201.

Sheagren JN: Septic shock and corticosteroids. *N Engl J Med* 1981; 305:456–457.

Shires GT: *Care of the Trauma Patient,* ed 2. New York, McGraw-Hill Book Co, 1979.

Shires GT, Cunningham JN, Baker CRF et al: Alterations in cellular membrane function during hemorrhagic shock in primates. *Ann Surg* 1972; 176:288–295.

Shoemaker WC: Pathophysiology, monitoring, and therapy of shock syndromes, in Shoemaker WC, Thompson WL (eds): *Critical Care: State of the Art.* California, Society of Critical Care Medicine, 1980, pp 1–63.

Short BL, Gardner M, Walker RI et al: Indomethacin improves survival in gram-negative sepsis, in Schumer W (ed): *Advances in Shock Research.* New York, Alan R Liss, 1981, pp 27–36.

Stapp JP: Voluntary human tolerance levels, in Gurdjian ES, Lange WA, Patrick LM, Thomas LM (eds): *Impact Injury and Crash Protection.* Springfield, Illinois, Charles C Thomas Publisher, 1970, pp 308–349.

Starling EH: On the absorption of fluids from the connective tissue spaces. *J Physiol (Lond)* 1896; 19:312.

Staub NC: Pulmonary edema due to increased microvascular permeability to fluid and protein. *Circ Res* 1978; 43:143–151.

Swan HJC: The role of hemodynamic monitoring in the management of the critically ill. *Crit Care Med* 1975; 3:83–89.

Thal AP, Brown EB Jr, Hermreck AS, Bell HH: *Shock, A Physiologic Basis for Treatment.* Chicago, Year Book Medical Publishers Inc, 1971.

Thurer RL, Hauer JM: *Autotransfusion and Blood Conservation. Current Problems in Surgery.* Chicago, Year Book Medical Publishers Inc, 1982.

Trunkey DD: The value of trauma centers. *Bull Am College Surgeons* 1982; 67:5.

Trunkey DD, Federle M, Cello J: Special diagnostic procedures, in Blaisdell FW, Trunkey DD (eds): *Trauma Management. Abdominal Trauma.* New York, Thieme-Stratton Inc, 1982, vol 1, pp 19–44.

Trunkey DD, Sheldon GF, Collins JA: The treatment of shock, in Zuidema GD, Rutherford MD, Ballinger MD (eds): *The Management of Trauma.* Philadelphia, WB Saunders Co, 1979.

Virgilio RW, Rice CL, Smith DE et al: Crystalloid versus colloid resuscitation: Is one better? *Surgery* 1979; 85:129.

Walt AJ, Grifka TJ: Blunt abdominal injury: A review of 307 cases, in Gurdjian ES, Lange WA, Patrick LM, Thomas LM (eds): *Impact Injury and Crash Protection.* Springfield, Illinois, Charles C Thomas Publisher, 1970, pp 101–123.

Walt AJ, Wilson RF (eds): *Management of Trauma: Pitfalls and Practice.* Philadelphia, Lea & Febiger, 1975.

Ward PA: The acute inflammatory response and the role of complement, in Dineen P, Hildick-Smith G: *The Surgical Wound.* Philadelphia, Lea & Febiger, 1981, pp 19–25.

Weissman G: *Prostaglandins in Acute Inflammation. Current Concepts.* Upjohn, Kalamazoo, 1980.

Weissman G, Smolen JE, Korchak MM: Release of inflammatory mediators from stimulated neutrophils. *N Engl J Med* 1980; 303:27.

West JG, Trunkey DD, Lim RC: Systems of trauma care: A study of two counties. *Arch Surg* 1979; 114:455–460.

White RJ, Albin MS: Spine and spinal cord injury, in Gurdjian ES, Lange WA, Patrick LM, Thomas LM (eds): *Impact Injury and Crash Protection.* Springfield, Illinois, Charles C Thomas Publisher, 1970, pp 63–83.

Wilkinson AW, Cuthbertson DP (eds): *Metabolism and the Response to Injury.* Bath, England, Pitman Publishing Ltd, 1976.

Wilmore DW: *The Metabolic Management of the Critically Ill.* New York, Plenum Publishing Corp, 1977.

Wright HK, Gann DS, Drucker WR: Maintaining extracellular fluid volume, in Davis JH (ed): *Concepts in Surgery.* New York, McGraw-Hill Book Co, 1965, p 295.

Yurt RW: Role of the mast cell in traumas, in Dineen P, Hildick-Smith G: *The Surgical Wound.* Philadelphia, Lea & Febiger, 1981, pp 37–62.

Zweifach BW: Microvascular aspects of tissue injury, in Zweifach BW, Grant L, McCluskey RT (eds): *The Inflammatory Process,* ed 2. New York, Academic Press Inc, 1973, vol 11.

13
PREVENTION AND TREATMENT OF INFECTION IN THE INJURED PATIENT

John F. Burke

Although there has been a dramatic improvement in the treatment of patients in shock after severe injury, this improvement has been somewhat counterbalanced by an increase in the number of deaths related to infection during the posttrauma weeks. By solving one set of problems a new set has been uncovered. As a result of improved techniques for the management of severe trauma and massive blood loss, patients now live long enough to develop sepsis. If the treatment of the severely injured patient is to be successful, infection must be prevented.

In the overall treatment of the trauma patient it is important to recognize that the patient's own bacterial defenses are the most important in preventing sepsis; a loss of host resistance cannot be replaced by antibiotic therapy that is itself dependent upon some activity on the part of the patient. If tissue resistance against bacterial infection is intact, it provides adequate protection in almost all situations. However, since natural resistance to bacterial invasion varies according to physiologic state and from tissue to tissue, it is imperative that periods of abnormal physiology be promptly recognized and treated.

PREVENTION OF INFECTION

Restoration of Normal Physiology

The rapid and effective use of measures to bring the trauma patient to the state of near normal physiology is the cornerstone on which all other measures must rest. Debridement, accurate repair of vascular occlusion, and the use of antibiotics will accomplish relatively little without the simultaneous resumption of normal physiologic function. In addition to compromising the functions of the brain, heart, and kidney seriously,

low cardiac output and systemic hypoperfusion produce another more subtle but nevertheless potentially lethal effect—sepsis in the bacterially contaminated wound. Although it is recognized that immediate correction of circulatory failure is essential to prevent death, it is not yet widely recognized that immediate reestablishment of adequate circulation is an essential ingredient in the prevention of wound sepsis.

Unfortunately, adequate circulation is at times considered to be clinically achieved with the resumption of urine flow or the recording of a nearly normal central arterial pressure. However, in this situation the peripheral muscle mass and skin may remain seriously underperfused, becoming fertile ground for sepsis in the area of a contaminated wound. Although sepsis may not be manifest for a few days or a week after trauma, the bacterial contamination causing suppuration occurs during or close to the time of injury, and prevention of infection is impossible without adequate circulation to the soft tissue injuries themselves. The circulation must be restored not only centrally but also peripherally. Because vasoconstrictive agents produce peripheral hypoperfusion, their use should be avoided in patients with traumatic shock.

There are other systemic abnormalities that must be corrected before physiologic equilibrium and near normal antibacterial defenses can be expected. Some of these corrective measures must be initiated in the emergency room: Normal respiratory function and adequate gas exchange are vital; and acid–base equilibrium, electrolyte concentration, and hydration are important areas to bring into balance.

Appropriate measures should be taken during hospitalization to correct other systemic abnormalities that cause defects in host resistance. Malnutrition, particularly protein starvation and vitamin deficiencies, seriously compromise the ability to mount a substantial antibacterial effort. The properly functioning immunologic mechanisms form a vital link in the complex chain of defense against bacterial invasion. Agammaglobulinemia or complement defects cause significant weaknesses in bacterial defensive structure. Hormone imbalance, particularly adrenal corticosteroids, has a well-known effect on the inflammatory reaction and in large doses over time decrease the defense against bacterial invasion. Such conditions as Cushing's disease, Addison's disease, diabetes mellitus, and the various leukemias impair the person's ability to deal with bacterial infection.

Preventive Antibiotics in the Management of Traumatic Wounds

Indiscriminate use of antibiotics without careful consideration of the biologic problems presented does not prevent infection but rather exposes the patient needlessly to the risk of allergic reaction, alteration in normal bacterial flora, and the creation of resistant strains of bacteria. The natural antibacterial mechanisms of the patient are the most important factors in preventing infection, and the supplementation of this resistance is only possible during the period immediately after bacterial contamination. For the majority of wounds, the antibacterial mechanisms of the patient, even though compromised, are able to deal effectively with a small amount of bacterial contamination and prevent invasion and infection. Only when the degree of physiologic alteration or bacterial contamination is large enough to present a serious risk of invasive infection should consideration be given to supplementing the host's native resistance with antibacterial therapy during the period of high risk immediately after bacterial contamination. Patients who for a number of reasons have a high probability of post-injury bacterial complications fall into the following three categories:

1. Patients with injuries or preexisting diseases that interfere with the normal function of one or more of the natural mechanisms of host resistance
2. Patients in whom the traumatic injury has produced massive bacterial contamination
3. Patients in whom the extensive nature of the surgical procedure required to repair traumatic defects threatens to overwhelm the host's bacterial defenses

In all three categories increased risk of bacterial sepsis occurs during the well-defined period between onset of trauma and the return of normal physiology. The key period for preventing trauma sepsis is clearly indicated. The dosage schedule must be individually developed to ensure an adequate level of antibiotics in the tissue as soon after trauma and bacterial contamination as possible, as well as throughout the period of decreased host resistance after trauma. Experimental and clinical evidence indicates that the antibiotic substance is most effective if it is circulating in the interstitial space when the contaminating bacteria arrive. Of course, this is not possible for patients who undergo open injury, but the use of accurate debridement and delayed wound closure combined with the early use of preventive antibiotics greatly increases the patient's chances of avoiding posttrauma sepsis. The antibiotic should be delivered intravenously immediately after the establishment of the intravenous line. Appropriate use of antibiotics is discussed in Chapter 28.

Prophylaxis against Tetanus

Although the clinical disease of tetanus is rare today, it is seen sporadically throughout the United States so that its develop-

ment must be considered, and measures to prevent it should be taken routinely after injury. Prophylaxis against tetanus is usually carried out using adsorbed tetanus toxoid in three intramuscular doses of 0.5 ml each (or as instructed on the label of the package because of variation in antigen concentration in various products). The second dose is given 4–6 weeks after the initial dose, and the third is given 6–12 months after the initial dose. A booster dose of 0.5 ml adsorbed tetanus toxoid intramuscularly 10 years after the last dose is indicated. A response to a booster dose may occur for as long as 25 years after active immunization and in many patients may last throughout the patient's life.

For minor clean injuries treated early in a patient who has a clear history of tetanus immunization within the last 10 years, a booster dose may not be required. If there is no immunization or if it is uncertain as to the time of the last booster, 0.5 ml adsorbed tetanus toxoid is indicated. However, when the wound is more serious and there is destruction of tissue and contamination or the wound is old, 0.5 ml adsorbed tetanus toxoid, as well as 250 units of tetanus immune globulin (human) should be given, and penicillin or tetracycline may be considered. In the immunized patient, adsorbed tetanus toxoid should be given as the initial immunization dose for all wounds. Passive immunity should also be given in the case of old wounds except clean minor wounds in which tetanus is most unlikely. The usual recommended dose is 250 units, although larger doses have occasionally been recommended. In severe neglected wounds 500 units of tetanus immune globulin (human) is recommended. In addition to the above schedule, which should be begun immediately, penicillin or tetracycline may be considered. In all wounds strict attention to the wound management including removal of all devitalized tissue and foreign bodies should be carried out.

Management of Contaminated Wounds

Traumatic wounds created in the workaday world are far from free of bacterial contamination. These wounds, having been made under circumstances where asepsis is unknown, are contaminated as they are created. Large numbers of bacteria are present in the wound, and infection is almost sure to follow if the wound is closed primarily without accurate debridement despite the most rigorous aseptic precautions and meticulous surgical technique at the time of closure.

In order to avoid the almost universal development of sepsis, clinical experience has evolved a method of treatment for such wounds that has proven to be effective. Two special steps are often called for in this form of wound care. The first is the debridement of the damaged wound surface in order to be certain that all bacterial contamination, as well as nonviable or marginally viable tissue, is removed. The second principle is the provision of adequate drainage for any possible locus of unrecognized necrosis or extensive bacterial contamination remaining in the wound. Primary closure is therefore often avoided in these cases in order to allow effective drainage of the wound edges, to eliminate the remaining bacteria, and to begin repair with the assurance that devitalized exudate will be removed promptly. Anatomical reconstruction therefore is delayed until the wound edges can be placed together in a "closed" fashion without danger of bacterial inflammation. These procedures are of great practical importance in the rapid rehabilitation of patients who have suffered traumatic wounds. In addition to these procedures, antibiotics are usually added to supplement host resistance during the crucial posttraumatic period as noted above. A close examination of the principles involved will illustrate these points.

DEBRIDEMENT AND IRRIGATION

The debridement of a wound is used to convert a heavily contaminated wound containing devitalized tissue to a viable, sterile one so that primary closure, with its obvious advantages, can be employed. Debridement followed by primary closure is occasionally indicated in patients who present themselves for treatment less than 8 hours after injury. In these cases, if debridement has created a "sterile viable wound," primary healing takes place. However, in many cases following trauma this accurate debridement cannot be relied upon with certainty. Primary closure following debridement, therefore, should only be practiced if the patient is under the constant scrutiny of trained personnel so that developing sepsis, if it occurs, can be managed immediately. It is obvious that where mass casualties are involved primary closure following debridement would be extremely hazardous. As discussed in Chapter 14, irrigation of the wound must usually be combined with debridement in the management of contaminated wounds.

DELAYED PRIMARY CLOSURE

In clinical situations in which a bacteria-free and completely viable wound cannot be obtained through debridement, delayed primary closure is the practice requiring the least deviation from the principles of optimal surgical wound care. The wound at its initial treatment is left open, and textile drainage is used. Daily inspection is important in order to detect developing infection. If none is observed, the wound can be closed on the second to the fourth day. The closure usually may be accomplished in the patient's room, but all of the

adjuncts of aseptic technique must be followed. An example of the wound requiring delayed primary closure is a gunshot wound of the arm suffered 20 hours before treatment. Certainty of the exact extent of blast injury and the extent of bacterial invasion is very difficult at the time of debridement. All obvious necrotic and septic tissue is removed, then the wound is drained using a thin layer of gauze. If no sepsis develops, the patient's wound is primarily closed on the third day.

SECONDARY CLOSURE

Secondary closure is reserved for wounds that manifest obvious superficial or invasive infection at the time they are first encountered or for wounds that develop sepsis during the program leading to delayed primary closure. In these wounds the closure is delayed until a time when granulation tissue has formed (as described in Chapter 14). In general practice this is usually 10 days or longer. Secondary closure following the development of granulations may take two forms. The first is simple closure of the granulating wound, bringing the two granulating surfaces together. The second, and usually the one giving the best functional result, is the excision of the granulating wound together with the indurated scar tissue and the primary closure of the two surfaces. This has been called *excision and primary closure.*

MANAGEMENT OF ESTABLISHED INFECTIONS

The problems of dealing with an already established infection are very different from those of prevention. Here, the general principles of drainage, elevation, heat, and rest are basic. To these classic methods of dealing with bacterial infection, antibiotic therapy has added another specific element that needs to be controlled. The effect of antibiotics on the therapy for bacterial infections is impressive but can be overstated. It is wise to recognize that antibiotics in therapy, as in prevention, are adjuncts to host resistance—they do not replace it. Further, in order to be an effective supplement, the antibiotic used must be effective against the infecting bacteria. It must be used in a concentration that is bacteriocidal or bacteriostatic, and it must be given over a period of days, rather than hours as in the case of prevention. Therefore in the treatment of any infection, it is more important to restore normal physiology than it is merely to prescribe an antibiotic. Allergic and toxic reactions that occasionally occur after administration of all antibiotics must be reduced to a minimum. Therefore a bacterial diagnosis and sensitivity pattern of the isolated bacteria, as well as a careful history, are essential for efficient treatment. Although the press of clinical disease may require the initiation of antibiotic treatment before an exact diagnosis can be established, bacterial smear may provide vital information, and initial careful bacteriologic culture should be carried out in order to allow adjustments to be made when definitive bacteriologic information is available.

Antibiotic treatment has been so prominent in the management of infection that other basic, essential procedures such as surgical drainage and the restoration of normal anatomy in the treatment of certain localized bacterial disease is too often neglected. Thus, it is common to find patients with localized abscesses assigned a prolonged course of antibiotics when simple surgical drainage would solve the problem far more quickly and with less morbidity. Antibiotics in the treatment of bacterial disease must be considered not only as an adjunct to host resistance but also as an adjunct to a surgical procedure in many cases. Surgery may either eliminate the bacterial disease by excision, as in a brain abscess or acute appendicitis, or provide drainage of a closed space infection, allowing effective function of host resistance and healing of the wound.

The clinical manifestation of bacterial infection may be divided into *cellulitis,* representing an active spread of bacteria through the tissue spaces themselves with a resulting intense inflammatory reaction, and *abscess formation,* a localization of infection with the creation of a circumscribed area of necrotic tissue and pus. Bacterial spread through blood or lymphatic vessels (bacteremia and lymphangitis) represent specialized methods of spread of bacteria that are life threatening themselves because of the wide and rapid dissemination of bacteria through these routes. Septicemia denotes multiplication of bacteria within the blood stream, and it is a further progression of bacteremia. These infections are discussed more fully in Chapters 3 and 28.

Tetanus

Tetanus, usually called *lockjaw,* is a clinical syndrome caused by a toxin produced by *Clostridium tetani,* a spore-forming, strictly anaerobic, gram-positive bacillus. The bacteria are widely distributed in nature, being commonly found in the gastrointestinal tract of domestic animals and in soil. Unlike bacterial infections that produce clinical difficulties by direct invasion as well as by intoxication, the tetanus bacillus produces disease by elaborating a toxin that diffuses throughout the tissue. Severe or even lethal tetanus can be caused by minor bacterial growth with little inflammation in the most minor of wounds. Natural tissue resistance to the tetanus bacillus is high, so that under ordinary circumstances contamination of tissue with this bacillus, or its spores, does not result in bacterial growth or invasion. However, if devitalized tissue or foreign bodies are allowed to remain in a wound, anaerobic conditions may be produced and tetanus infection established.

DIAGNOSIS

The incubation period for tetanus is usually 6–10 days after injury, but it may be as long as 20–30 days. Sometimes the first symptom is pain and tingling at the site of innoculation, which is followed by spasticity of nearby muscle groups. More commonly, though, the initial symptoms include stiffness of the jaw and neck, dysphagia, and signs of central nervous system irritation such as irritability. Abdominal pain and spasm occasionally are pronounced enough to suggest a diagnosis of an acute abdominal condition. In the more acute cases, severe spasms of the back muscles produce opisthotonus. Spasms become increasingly frequent and involve increasing numbers of muscle groups. As the condition progresses, spasms of muscles of jaw, face, neck, abdomen, and back often become associated with painful tonic convulsions precipitated by minor stimuli. During convulsions the muscles of respiration and the glottis go into spasm, making it impossible for the patient to breathe effectively. As chest and diaphragm spasms occur the periods of apnea become increasingly long. Not infrequently, urinary obstruction also occurs because of spasm of sphincter muscles.

TREATMENT

The major objectives in the treatment of tetanus are removal of the sources of tetanus toxin production and the neutralization of the circulating toxin already produced. The former is accomplished by thoroughly debriding any traumatic wound by wide excision. Anaerobic conditions must be prevented at all cost; the wound therefore is usually left open after debridement. Circulating tetanus toxin is destroyed by administering tetanus immune globulin (human). The usual dose is 3,000–6,000 units intramuscularly, preferably given proximal to the wound; repeated doses may be necessary. Antibiotics, usually in the form of penicillin, tetracycline, or erythromycin, may be given to prevent further elaboration of the toxin by growth of the tetanus bacillus.

Because the main symptoms of tetanus are muscle spasms, sedation with diazepam and a quiet, dark environment are essential. In severely ill patients with pharyngeal spasm, tracheostomy may be necessary and muscle relaxants may be used to ensure adequate respiration. Nutrition may be maintained with a nasogastric tube, and constant nursing care is required.

Patients being treated for tetanus should have active immunization begun using tetanus toxoid. The clinical disease does not uniformly confirm immunity. Puncture wounds should have special attention because they can easily produce a closed-space infection. The depth of the wound and the narrowness of the opening to the surface prevent efficient cleaning of the wound at the time of injury, and foreign bodies such as dirt, rust, and bits of clothing are not easily removed. In addition, purulent exudate resulting from inflammation in a puncture wound tends to spread in the subdermal region because the external opening of the wound is soon sealed by a protein coagulum and a closed-space infection is produced. For this reason, puncture wounds for the most part should be opened widely in order to ensure adequate cleaning, debridement, and drainage.

Clostridial Myositis (Gas Gangrene)

Clostridial organisms may produce a life-threatening gangrenous infection of muscle that is rapidly progressive and causes extensive life-threatening systemic, as well as local, abnormalities. The infection usually follows open injuries of the extremities, buttocks, or trunk that are associated with devitalized muscle.

DIAGNOSIS

The early diagnosis of gas gangrene, essential if treatment is to be successful, at times may be difficult because the infection often follows treatment of a severe injury, which may obscure early signs of clostridial infection. Pain at the site of the injury is an early symptom of clostridial myositis, which usually appears within the first 24 hours after injury. At this time crepitus may be present in the tissue, but extensive edema may occur in clostridial myositis without gas formation. The patient develops rapidly progressing systemic and local signs; pain is prominent and a striking pallor of the face is common, with weakness, apathy, profuse sweating, prostration, and shortness of breath. The pulse is rapid and feeble, but fever is seldom over 101°F (38.5°C). Other important signs include a thin, watery, brown, foul-smelling discharge, usually containing many bacteria and red blood cells but few white cells, a dusky or bronze appearance of the skin overlying the wound with vesicles filled with dark red fluid, and crepitus and herniation of dark red discolored muscle. Soluble toxins diffusing into the circulation from the involved tissue produce a severe hemolytic anemia and renal, cardiac, and liver damage, as well as septic shock, which may lead to death if treatment does not intervene. Laboratory data include a severe anemia and a relatively low white count, seldom exceeding 15,000 cells per cubic millimeter.

TREATMENT

Treatment includes the immediate surgical exploration of any wound in which the presence of clostridial myositis is suspected. Wide incision and debridement of involved muscle are essentials of effective treatment. Intensive antibiotic therapy should be employed, usually using penicillin intravenously. Supportive therapy is crucial for maintaining fluid and electrolyte balance, as well as for correcting a severe anemia and decreased circulatory volume produced by the infection. Several authors have advised using hyperbaric oxygen treatment of gas gangrene as a method that improves the results of treatment.

SUGGESTED READINGS

Altemeier WA, Burke JF, Pruitt BA Jr., Sandusky WR: *Manual on Control of Infection in Surgical Patients,* by the Committee on Control of Surgical Infections of the Committee on Pre- and Postoperative Care of the American College of Surgeons. Philadelphia, JB Lippincott Co, 1976.

Bernard HR, Cole WR: The prophylaxis of surgical infection: The effect of prophylactic antimicrobial drugs on the incidence of infection following potentially contaminated operations. *Surgery* 1964; 56:151–157.

Boyd RJ, Burke JF, Colton T: A double blind clinical trial of prophylactic antibiotics in hip fracture patients. *J Bone Joint Surg (Am)* 1973; 55A:1251–1259.

Burke JF: Host defects caused by surgical operations. *Symposium on the Infection Prone Hospital Patient.* Boston, Little Brown & Co, 1978, p 175–181.

Burke JF: Preventive antibiotics in surgery. *Postgrad Med* 1975; 58(?):65–69.

Burke JF: The effective period of preventive antibiotic action in experimental incisions and dermal lesions. *Surgery* 1961; 50:1,161–168,184–185.

Burke JF: Wound infection and early inflammation. *Monogr Surg Sci* 1964; 1(4):301–345.

Committee on Trauma of the American College of Surgeons: *A Guide to Prophylaxis Against Tetanus Wound Management*; Chicago, December 1972.

Miles AA: Nonspecific defense reactions in bacterial infection. *Ann NY Acad Sci* 1956; 66:2,353–369.

Miles AA, Miles Ellen M, Burke J: The value and duration of defense reactions of the skin to the primary lodgement of bacteria. *Br J Exp Pathol* 1957; 38:79.

Polk HC Jr, Lopez Mayor JF: Postoperative wound infection. *Surgery* 1969; 66:97–103.

14
MANAGEMENT OF WOUNDS

John B. Mulliken

WOUND HEALING

All fresh wounds—regardless of depth, whether open or closed, with or without loss of tissue—heal with the same biologic mechanism. The process starts with a transient reflex constriction of the local injured vessels and the first signs of *inflammatory response*. Leukocytes adhere to the injured vascular endothelium, particularly in the small venules. Retraction of severed vessels and platelet plugging initiate the hemostatic process. When the injured vessels are sealed, vasoconstriction is followed by vasodilation—and there is increased flow and a concomitant increase in the permeability of the local venules. The endothelial cells appear to swell and "round up," allowing plasma to leak out between the endothelial cell gaps and enter the injured tissues. Macrophages follow the leukocytes into the interstitium. The wound inflammatory phase and tissue edema reach a maximum at 4 hours. The degree of tension set during suture placement and dressing application should be adjusted keeping these phenomena in mind.

The *fibroblastic phase* of wound healing begins during the inflammatory period, as local histiocytes begin to loosen and migrate into the wound along the strands of the recently constructed fibrin network. These activated fibroblasts begin to extrude ground substance and tiny collagen fibrils into the wound within 48 hours after injury. At the same time, there is angiogenesis, budding of nearby capillaries, and growth of new vessels into the healing matrix. This primitive capillary bed is only a microscopic finding in closed wounds that heal per primam. Wounds whose edges remain open become filled with a granular appearing bed *(granulation tissue)*. From the seventh to tenth day, an open wound, providing it is not heavily contaminated with bacteria, begins to close by *contraction*.

Epithelial cells also participate in the healing process. Within 24 hours, there is a loosening, mitosis, and migration of epithelial cells from the wound margins and the surviving dermal appendages. The cells migrate as epithelial sheets, flowing in the direction of cytoplasmic extensions of the cells' free edges. Epithelial migration is guided by the orientation of extracellular ground substance and fibrillar network; this migration stops as the epithelial-free margins touch. Epithelium also grows downward along the dermal puncture wounds caused by sutures. In superficial abrasions, epithelialization—both from the wound edges and adnexal structures—may cover a denuded dermal surface within 72 hours. Topical wound care and dressings should be selected to expedite this process.

Fibroplasia increases apace, yet newly formed collagen fibers contribute very little to the strength of a closed wound during the first week to 10 days postinjury. During this period, only the fibrin network, ground substance, and epidermal continuity bind the wound together. Sutures or tapes provide the mainstays of wound tensile strength during this early period.

By the tenth day, the tensile strength of the healing wound is increasing in a fashion parallel to increasing collagen production. By the second week, net collagen production begins to diminish, whereas wound tensile strength continues to increase. This phenomenon is the result of formation of intra- and intermolecular cross linking between collagen fibrils. A skin wound reaches 20–30% of strength by the second to third week and 60% of strength by the fourth month. Percutaneous sutures should be removed by the seventh day to minimize the chance of suture track scars, leaving buried sutures and maturing collagen to keep the wound secure.

By the third week, the wound has entered its *phase of maturation and remodeling*. The characteristics of the tissue adjacent to the healing wound and external forces, particularly motion, are well-recognized factors that modulate the collagen weave in a scar. Although careful wound management will affect the quality of a scar, the final appearance is primarily determined by the location and extent of the initial wound.

ASSESSMENT

Although a cutaneous wound may be obvious when a patient is first brought into the emergency room, a detailed assessment of the wound should be deferred until the patient has been evaluated for other more serious injuries. Life-saving maneuvers assume first priority. If the wound is bleeding, a pressure dressing should be applied and held in place by elastic gauze or, if necessary, by an assistant's hand. To minimize further contamination, all wounds, however small, should be covered with a dressing a short time after the patient arrives in the emergency unit.

History

Once the patient is stable, careful history should be obtained as to the time, circumstances, and mechanisms of injury (as described in Chapter 12). This information will provide clues as to possible associated injuries beyond the obvious wounds and will give indications about the extent and degree of contamination of the wound. The patient's past medical history should also be taken with attention to any medications or underlying medical conditions (see Chapter 13).

Examination

The protective dressing which has been applied to the wound a short time after the patient was admitted to the emergency room, should now be removed for detailed evaluation of the extent of soft tissue injury. Sterile gloves and mask should always be worn during the examination and treatment of a wound. The number of examinations of the wound should be restricted to minimize the chances for further contamination.

The depth of a *laceration* should be assessed (Fig. 14.1A), keeping in mind the possibility of injury to underlying structures such as nerves, tendons, muscles, or bone. Different anatomical areas contain unique structures that must be evaluated, for example, parotid duct, lacrimal duct, canthal tendon, and seventh cranial nerve in the face (see Chapter 16). Lacerations overlying bones should be probed with a gloved finger to determine whether or not there is a compound fracture. Patients who have small puncture wounds in the head and neck region and thoracoabdominal areas must be managed on the premise that there has been penetration and damage to vital deep structures. A missile wound should be examined for the extent of surrounding tissue damage along its tract and at the site of exit (see Chapter 1).

A *contusion,* usually caused by blunt force, is a disruption of dermal continuity with intact overlying dermis and epidermis. Signs include swelling and ecchymosis resulting from interstitial edema and hemorrhage or hematoma formation with gross extravasation of blood into the subcutaneous space (Fig. 14.1B). Contusion, like a laceration, may be associated with an injury to important underlying structures.

An *abrasion,* caused by a shearing force, is a loss of epidermis and a variable depth of dermis. The depth of an abrasion wound can be assessed by the pattern of bleeding. A deep abrasion occurs at the level of a second-degree burn and exhibits a brisk bleeding pattern from damaged middermal capillaries (Fig. 14.1C). Superficial abrasions bleed very little from injured capillaries in the papillary dermis.

WHO SHOULD MANAGE THE WOUND AND WHERE?

Before wound treatment is initiated, we must decide who should repair the wound and whether or not it should be cared for in

(a)

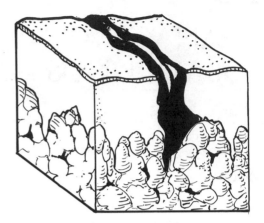

(b)

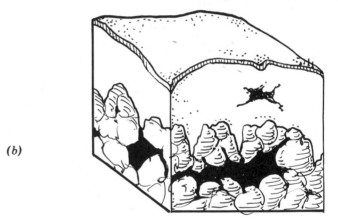

(c)

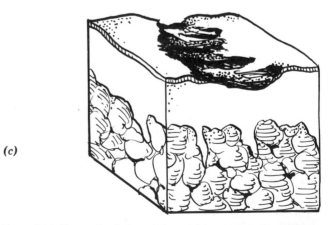

Figure 14.1 Types of soft tissue injury: (a) laceration; (b) contusion; and (c) abrasion.

the emergency room or in the operating room. Important considerations include condition of the patient, type of wound, degree of contamination, possibility of damage to deep structures, and presence of associated injuries.

In general, patients with simple and superficial wounds can usually be managed in the emergency room. This also holds true for children, providing they can be satisfactorily premedicated. Patients with complex wounds, bullet wounds, and wounds where there is damage to underlying nerves, tendons, or bone, require admission to the hospital and surgical consultation. Some avulsion wounds (where there is an actual loss of tissue) can be closed in a linear fashion or with a small split-thickness skin graft by the surgeon in the emergency room; most avulsion wounds are best handled in the main operating theater.

EMERGENCY ROOM MANAGEMENT OF SUPERFICIAL WOUNDS

Tetanus Prophylaxis

Patients with a minor clean wound who give a history of tetanus immunization within the past 10 years do not need tetanus toxoid. However, given a tetanus-prone wound in a patient who has not been immunized in less than 5 years, intramuscular booster injection of 0.5 ml adsorbed tetanus toxoid is indicated. For all wounds in unimmunized patients, toxoid should be given as the initial dose for active immunization. Passive immunization with human tetanus immune globulin (HyperTet) should be considered in neglected wounds that are likely to harbor clostridia (see Chapter 13).

Skin Preparation

Most lacerations of the scalp or beard area are easier to manage if the hair is clipped. The small cut hairs should not be allowed to fall into the wound where they may act as a nidus for infection. Eyebrows should never be shaved.

Antiseptic cleansing of the skin around the wound may be done before or after the wound is anesthetized—usually it is easier for the patient if the anesthetic is injected before vigorous skin preparation. An antiseptic such as 1% povidone–iodine solution should be applied to the skin surface, taking care not to place it in the wound.

Local Anesthesia

Wounds to be repaired in the emergency room require local anesthesia to allow assessment of the wound extent, proper irrigation, debridement, and closure. Lidocaine (Xylocaine), 0.5% or 1% is the most useful agent. The combination solution xylocaine and epinephrine 1:200,000 minimizes troublesome dermal bleeding, decreases the risk of rapid absorption and xylocaine toxicity, and prolongs the anesthetic affect. Epinephrine should not be used in a local anesthetic block of the digits or with infiltration of thin skin flaps with compromised blood supply.

The local anesthetic solution should be injected through a 25- or 30-gauge needle placed through the wound surface to minimize the pain of needle penetration of intact skin. Gloves should be worn by the physician.

Debridement and Irrigation

Clean wounds—those with minimal tissue destruction and foreign body–bacterial contamination—do not require debridement or irrigation. Wounds that are untidy, contain dirt and other foreign material, or present 6 hours or more after injury, are contaminated with bacteria. It is the number of bacteria, rather than the bacterial type, that is the critical determinant of whether or not a wound subsequently becomes infected. The critical level of bacteria is 10^5 organisms per gram of tissue. Below this level, wounds heal; at levels greater than 10^5 bacteria per gram of tissue, wounds often become infected after closure.

Debridement, irrigation, and antibiotics are used to reduce the bacterial level of the contaminated wound (see Chapter 13). All devitalized tissue must be thoroughly excised; for this purpose, a sharp knife is best. Irrigation reduces contamination by dislodging bacteria and foreign material. The oft-used "physiologic saline" solution is acidic and hyperchloric. Buffered Ringer's solution or commercially available balanced salt solutions (e.g., Tis-U-Sol or Physio-Sol) are more physiologic. The pressure of the irrigation is important. A 30-ml syringe fitted with a 19-gauge needle gives 7 psi irrigation pressure. At such a pressure, bacteria or particles are dislodged and not forced into the tissue.

The volume of the irrigation must be enough to dislodge the dirt and lower the concentration of bacteria. Clean wounds require little or no irrigation, whereas bite injuries and other heavily contaminated wounds may require 1 liter or more of irrigation. Irrigation with topical antibacterial agents, such as 1% povidone–iodine solution, should only be considered in the management of wounds heavily contaminated with bacteria.

Suture Selection

Suture selection should be determined by the type of wound, its location, vascularity, viability, and degree of contamination, as well as the physical and biochemical characteristics of available suture materials. *Absorbable sutures* may be indicated for closure of the deep layers of a wound. *Catgut sutures* elicit more inflammatory reaction and potentiate wound sepsis as compared to the newer, synthetic, absorbable sutures such as polyglycolic acid (Dexon) and polyglactin 910 (Vicryl). These sutures remain longer than catgut, although 60–80% of tensile strength is lost after 2 weeks. *Nonabsorbable monofilament sutures* may be used in a buried position in clean wounds, particularly in the fascial layer where it takes considerably more time for tensile strength to approach a normal level. In terms of minimizing the widening of a scar, there is no convincing evidence that nonabsorbable sutures offer any advantage over absorbable sutures in dermal closure. Nonabsorbable braided sutures, particularly silk, should not be used in clean or contaminated wounds.

Whatever monofilament nylon may lack in handling quality, as a percutaneous suture it is far preferable to old-fashioned silk in terms of tissue reactivity. Silk sutures left in place for over a week incite a perisuture inflammatory reaction and miniabscess formation, which are in part responsible for suture track marks. Another cause of suture track marks is leaving the sutures in longer than one week. Monofilament nylon elicits a minimal inflammatory reaction, even with the ingrowth of epithelium along its suture tracks. Braided and coated nylon suture approaches the superior handling quality of silk and possesses many of the desirable qualities of monofilament suture.

Suture Closure of Simple Wounds

Far more important than the character of sutures used is the gentleness and method of placement. The minimum number of absorbable sutures should be used for the task of deep tissue closure. The fascial layer should be approximated with the knots tied above (Fig. 14.2A). Torn dermis retracts because of its elastic fibers. The dermal wound should be definitively sutured; it is the foremost layer for wound strength and aids in apposition of the epidermal edges. A cutting rather than a round (taper) needle is preferred, and the knots in the dermal layer should be inverted (Fig. 14.2B). Make an effort not to include any subcutaneous tissue when placing the dermal (subcuticular) sutures. The buried dermal suture technique is useful for reducing tension, making accurate approximations, and providing immediate tensile strength to the healing wound. If the dermis is very thin (e.g., in an infant or in eyelid tissue), a vertical, buried dermal suture may be difficult to place, and a horizontal suture is useful. A fine skin hook facilitates placement of an everting suture of either type. In very thin tissues,

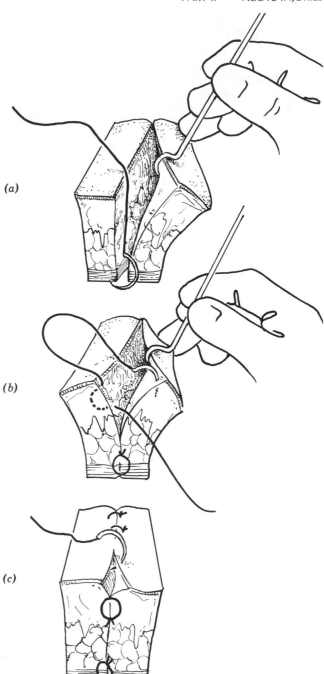

(a)

(b)

(c)

Figure 14.2 Layered wound closure: placement of (a) fascial; (b) dermal; and (c) percutaneous sutures. A skin hook helps to evert the wound edge and is less traumatic than forceps.

particularly in recalcitrant infants, percutaneous sutures alone may have to suffice.

Dermal apposition may be so exact that tape application could then be used for epidermal approximation. However, for fine coaptation, some form of percutaneous suture—usually a fine monofilament nylon—is preferred (Fig. 14.2C). If the edges are already well apposed, a running suture (Fig. 14.3A) can save time and is quite acceptable. Running percutaneous sutures are useful in controlling the brisk bleeding from the edges of a scalp laceration, but this suture technique may compromise the circulation of a more poorly vascularized wound margin in other locations. When interrupted stitches are used, each knot should be placed to one side or the other for "fine adjustment" and to aid in eversion of the wound margins. Also, with the knots to one side, there will be less disruption of epidermis when the sutures are removed (Fig. 14.3B).

When the wound is in lax tissues that are easily approximated, we may choose a running intradermal suture closure with either absorbable suture or monofilament "pull-out" nylon (Fig. 14.3C).

Technical details in suture placement are important at each layer (Fig. 14.4). Sutures should be placed near the cut edge to prevent strangulation of the enclosed tissue. Tissue layers should be approximated without tension. Eversion of the wound edges is important to minimize the formation of a troughlike scar. Eversion is critical in the closure of wounds at margins, such as the eyelids, ears, nasal columella, and alae, to minimize the tendency for late notching. In order to achieve eversion of the wound edge, the needle holder should be held in pronation so that the needle will enter the skin at a 90 deg angle to the surface. At the other wound edge, the needle should enter the cut surface at the corresponding level and emerge equidistant from the edge at a 90 deg angle (Fig. 14.2C). Taking a separate "bite" in each wound edge is preferable to catching both edges with a single thrust to be certain of the angles of entrance and exit. The slight "pouting" of the suture line and ridge affect will smooth out with time.

Adhesive Tape Closure

Adhesive tape closure has been used since the time of the Egyptian Middle Kingdom. Modern Steri-Strips of micropore tape are useful in approximating superficial wounds that have not extended into the subcutaneous layer and for wounds parallel to the "relaxed skin tension lines." Tape closure is particularly useful in dealing with wounds on a flat surface and wounds with thin flaps of tissue where suturing is difficult, particularly in pediatric patients. Sometimes it is difficult to obtain a fine adjustment of epidermal margins and wound edge

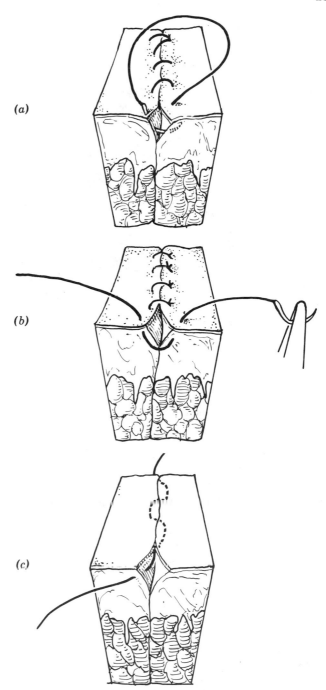

(a)

(b)

(c)

Figure 14.3 Basic skin closure techniques: (a) running percutaneous (continuous); (b) interrupted percutaneous; and (c) running intradermal (subcuticular).

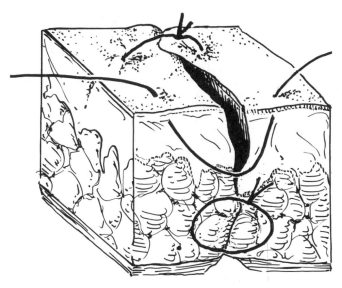

Figure 14.4 Five common errors of suture placement: failure to close fascia; tight suture in subcutaneous layer; improper angle of entry and exit of skin suture causing inversion of wound edges; tightly tied skin suture; and sutures too far from wound edge.

eversion using tape closure. Tape closure alone is unreliable for wounds in areas of motion. The application of tincture of benzoin to the skin improves tape adhesiveness.

Dressing the Wound

Wound management is not complete with placement of the final suture. The dressing should be constructed in a thoughtful manner to aid the healing process. Dressings serve a number of purposes: (1) protection, (2) absorption, (3) immobilization, and (4) compression. A well-conceived and well-fashioned dressing is a reflection of the quality of wound care and character of the physician. If the sutured wound is relatively dry, protection with a layer of transverse or longitudinal Steri-Strips is useful. Any blood or serum that collects underneath micropore tape can be expressed to prevent pooling and maceration. A layer of tincture of benzoin will hold the tape in place until time for suture removal. Tape fixation is aided by epithelial ingrowth into the micropore interstices.

Closed wounds that ooze serosanguinous fluid should not be dressed with tape. Instead, a nonadhering layer of petroleum-impregnated gauze, followed by a layer of absorbent gauze, will keep the wound dry and protected. If it is difficult to affix an absorbent dressing, for example, within the hairline,

the sutured wound may be left open. Repeated application of an antibacterial ointment will minimize crusting and bacterial proliferation around exposed sutures.

So-called pressure or compression dressings are difficult to achieve in practice. Gauze or cotton tends to compact, and experimental studies have shown that pressure over a wound is quickly dissipated. A pad of polyurethane foam may provide gentle pressure to a wound for a period of time. Elastic tape or elastic cloth wraps may also provide several hours of compression; however, these techniques should be used with care in circumferentially dressing an extremity.

CLOSURE OF COMPLEX WOUNDS

The Minimally Contaminated Wound

Once a minimally contaminated wound has been thoroughly debrided and irrigated, it may be closed primarily, particularly in areas where there is excellent blood supply such as the face and scalp. In the closure of such wounds, the number of sutures should be kept to a minimum and often tape closure may tip the balance in favor of primary healing. In an initially contaminated wound, even a single extra suture may mean the difference between subsequent wound sepsis and primary healing. The common practice of closing off "dead space" with sutures in the subcutaneous layer has been demonstrated to potentiate sepsis in experimentally contaminated wounds. The sutures should be absorbable, and the fewest possible knots will minimize the interstices for bacterial growth and total amount of foreign material left in the wound. Antibiotics would ordinarily not be used; however, see Chapter 13 for management of grossly contaminated wounds.

Stellate and Avulsion Wounds

Wounds where there is actual loss of tissue, avulsion wounds, and wounds with ragged and traumatized edges present special problems for closure in the emergency room. If the wound margins are thin, ragged, and traumatized, they should be conservatively trimmed. If a tattered edge is first "scored" with a sharp No.15 blade, the compromised margin can be easily trimmed with fine scissors. This two-step trimming technique is more accurate than sawing the wound edge without prior scoring (Fig. 14.5, above). The beveled wound edge also deserves special consideration before suturing. When there is a sharply angled bevel cut, the edges should be "squared off" before closure using the scoring technique (Fig. 14.5, below).

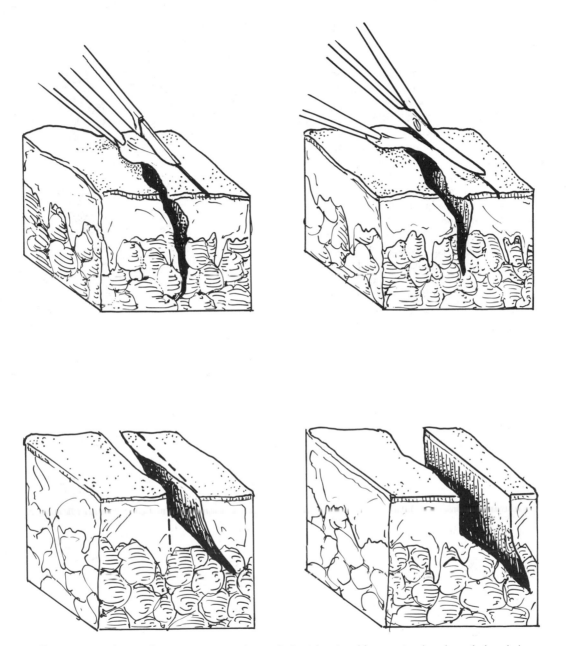

Figure 14.5 Technique for trimming a ragged wound edge (above) and for squaring the edges of a beveled laceration (below).

Every effort should be made to replace the multiple edges of a complicated skin laceration carefully, much like fitting together pieces of a puzzle. The half-buried horizontal mattress suture technique is useful when approximating wound edges of which one is ischemic, for example, the distal end of a triangular flap of tissue (Fig. 14.6). The buried loop of the half-buried mattress should be placed through the dermis of the ischemic wound edge and the knot tied loosely to minimize strangulation of the dermal plexus. It is remarkable how often the pieces of a complicated stellate laceration can be brought together when, initially, there appeared to be actual loss of tissue. However, there can be a true avulsion wound in which the retracted wound edges cannot be apposed, even with tension. At first, the technique of undermining the wound edges in the subdermal plane seems logical. However, undermining is always a double-edged sword. Undermining may allow some relaxation of the closure; however, it also creates more potential dead space and may further compromise the vascularity of the elevated skin edges. Rather than resort to undermining, it is preferable to try to take the tension off the approximated, or near-approximated, skin margins by the proper placement of deep sutures. Most incised and some avulsion wounds can usually be closed by appropriate suture techniques. The emergency room physician should not try to get too fancy in attempting plastic techniques. There is no indication for a Z-plasty flap transposition for the closure of acute wounds.

Major soft tissue avulsion injuries will necessitate expert consultation for possible primary closure with a skin graft or flap tissue. In special cases, particularly those in which consultation is not available, a rational decision could be made to allow a large wound to remain open and to close eventually by contraction. This decision must be based on thorough knowledge of anatomical factors and appreciation of the quality of such healed wounds and possibilities for scar revision. For example, full-thickness wounds of the scalp, extremities, and anterior chest wall should not be allowed to heal by contraction. Nor should contraction be allowed to occur in any wound that lies in a mobile area where the end result would be a contracture. In these cases, split graft or flap coverage is needed. On the other hand, in special cases, deep wounds over the back, posterior neck, abdomen, and buttocks may be allowed to close by contraction with the expectation of minimal scarring and deformity.

CONTUSIONS

Once the possibility of underlying fracture or serious soft tissue injury has been ruled out, little can be done for a contusion except to splint the area (if appropriate) and apply cold packs

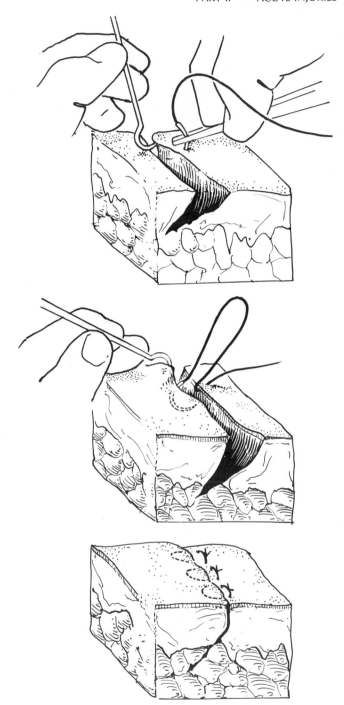

Figure 14.6 Half-buried mattress suture, which is useful if there is vascular compromise of one wound edge. The knot is tied on the more healthy margin.

to minimize edema formation. If there is a large hematoma, consideration should be given to the need for drainage. We must clearly differentiate between interstitial hemorrhage or ecchymosis, which cannot be drained, and true hematoma, which may be drained. Because of the excellent vascularity of scalp tissue, a cephalic hematoma is quite innocuous, notwithstanding the extent and degree of tension in the overlying skin. However, a small hematoma beneath the skin with a poor blood supply, for example, the pretibial region or a compromised flap of tissue, should be promptly evacuated. Red cells are toxic to compromised tissue. In addition, a hematoma is known to be an adjuvant in the presence of bacteria and will thus potentiate wound infection. A contused area without any skin loss may need nothing more than simple immobilization. If incision and drainage are necessary, an appropriate absorbent dressing is indicated.

ABRASIONS

Gross particulate matter in a deep abrasion must be removed. First, the area may be anesthetized, followed by a vigorous scrubbing with a brush or extraction of the foreign matter with fine forceps. If necessary, loupe magnification should be used. If the foreign matter is not removed within a short time after the injury, the particles will become encased in the healing wound with a resultant tattoo. Such a "traumatic tattoo" is near impossible to manage secondarily (see Chapter 17).

The proper dressing for an abrasion requires an understanding of the biology of the healing epidermal wounds. Because an abraded wound usually heals quickly by epidermal migration over the exposed dermis, the dressing should protect the exposed wound surface from desiccation. If the upper dermis is allowed to dry and form a thin layer of dead fibrous tissue, the migrating epithelium from the adnexa and wound edges would then have to produce collagenolytic enzymes to burrow beneath this eschar to find living dermis. This prolongs the time of epithelialization and may cause a thicker scar and more prominent skin pigment changes. If an abrasion wound is not heavily contaminated with bacteria, a petroleum dressing (e.g., Xeroform gauze) will protect the exposed dermis and will allow maximum epithelial migration over its surface. If bacterial contamination is a problem, a topical antibacterial ointment may be used. Above the petroleum gauze layer, another gauze is needed to absorb serosanguinous drainage and minimize crusting. This dressing should be checked every 2–3 days for the possible development of sepsis. If the dressing remains attached to the wound, it should be allowed to separate on its own with the establishment of epidermal continuity.

POSTOPERATIVE CARE AND SUTURE REMOVAL

A sutured wound is effectively closed by the healing process within a few hours, during which dressings provide protection, comfort, and support. Dressings may be continued for these reasons and should be changed as necessary. Dressings applied over wounds that ooze and continue to drain after the closure should be changed more frequently. If the wound was contaminated before debridement and closure, the dressing should be removed after 72 hours so that the wound can be examined for possible infection. The dressing recommended for an abrasion wound should be periodically examined but allowed to separate naturally with epithelialization.

To minimize the formation of suture track scars, percutaneous sutures should be removed by the seventh postoperative

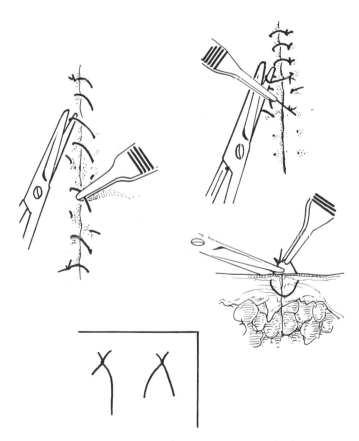

Figure 14.7 To remove a continuous suture, every other loop is cut. With an interrupted closure, each cut suture should be pulled toward the young wound. The cut suture should be checked for unequal tails, signifying removal of the buried portion (inset).

day. Since the face has excellent vascularity and healing abilities, sutures can be removed earlier, that is, 3–5 days. The timing of removal of sutures in other locations depends on the integrity of the dermal closure and the degree of wound motion. For example, sutures usually cannot be removed from hand wounds until after 10–14 days unless dermal closure is secure and prolonged splinting is necessary.

The cut suture should always be pulled out toward the wound. When removing a percutaneous running suture, the exposed portion of a "stitch" should not be pulled into the suture sinus track. When removing interrupted sutures, each should be checked to be certain one end of the loop is longer than the other, indicating that the entire suture has been extracted (Fig. 14.7). A 1-week old wound is still at less than 10% of tensile strength; therefore, Steri-Strips should be applied for another 1–2 weeks for support as well as for protection.

SCAR PROGNOSIS

After the wound is repaired, the patient or relatives will frequently want to know if there will be a scar. It is important to emphasize that there will, indeed, be a scar whenever the dermal layer has been breached. The emergency room physician should prepare the patient regarding the expected degree of scarring.

The factors that determine the scar prognosis are as follows: (1) age of patient, (2) race, (3) type of injury, (4) location of injury, (5) course of wound healing, and (6) psychological reaction to scarring. Lacerations in children under 1 year old and in adults over 60 years old tend to leave fine scars. Patients with dark skin have a tendency to scar pigmentation, hypertrophic scarring, and possible keloid formation. A true *keloid* is defined as a heavy scar that extends beyond the confines of the original wound and that rarely regresses. A *hypertrophic* scar is also heavy, but it does not go beyond the confines of the original wound, and it improves with time.

The important factors in scar prognosis are the type of injury (i.e., the extent of tissue damage and propensity for sepsis) and the location of the injury. Wounds with tissue loss and wounds that become infected will cause prominent scarring. There are regional predispositions to heavy scarring and keloid formation, such as the anterior chest, shoulders, and ear lobules. Lacerations that parallel the relaxed skin tension lines (RSTL) of the face and body tend to close under minimal tension and generally heal with fine scars (Fig. 14.8). Wounds that cross the RSTL or those that cross areas of joint motion (e.g., flexion creases) tend to heal with hypertrophic scars and scar contracture.

The technical aspects of wound management, emphasized

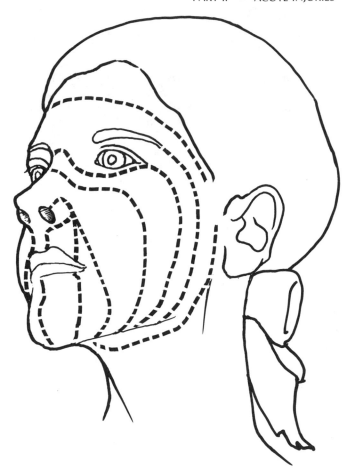

Figure 14.8 Relaxed skin tension lines (RSTL) of the face: In most cases thay follow wrinkle lines. Lacerations parallel to RSTL tend to heal with finer scars than those at right angles to these lines.

in this chapter, are also important in scar prognosis. Wound management is critical so as to minimize the possibility of wound sepsis. Another important determinant in scar prognosis is the perception of the patient. Even in the emergency room, the patient may demonstrate difficulty in accepting a wound and its subsequent scar; early psychiatric support may be necessary.

BITES AND STINGS

Human Bite Wounds

Human bite wounds often have an interesting sociological background. The embarrassed recipient may be reluctant to come to the emergency room. As a result, human bite wounds are frequently seen days after the injury when home remedies have failed and the wound has become infected.

The treatment of human bite injuries depends on the type of wound, the location, and the length of time after the occurrence. Human bites can be of a penetrating or avulsive type or a combination. The hallmarks of successful therapy are copious cleansing of the wound, aggressive debridement of damaged tissue, and removal of foreign material. Given this approach, some human bite wounds of the face could be closed and will heal per primam. Closure should be considered in wounds of the nose, eyelids, ears, or lips. On the other hand, wound sepsis is a frequent occurrence following human bites, particularly in the extremities where the blood supply is not as abundant as in the facial region. Therefore, in general, human bite wounds should be cleansed, debrided, and covered with a dressing—not sutured.

Human saliva is filled with a variety of organisms in the concentration of 10^7 bacteria/ml. They are mostly streptococci, veillonellae, and fusobacteria. Transient flora, present only intermittently, include staphylococci, *Escherichia coli*, *Pseudomonas aeruginosa*, and other coliforms. Notwithstanding the wide variety of microorganisms in contaminating saliva, the most common human bite wound infections occur with streptococci and penicillin-resistant *Staphylococcus aureus*. Therefore, prophylactic antibiotics should be selected with these specific bacteria in mind (see Chapter 28).

Human bite wounds of the extremities are particularly worrisome. The patient frequently will prevaricate regarding the circumstances of the injury. Typical locations are the skin over the metacarpophalangeal joints and fingers. These are usually puncture-type wounds with penetration of the underlying joint space or bone; deep sepsis, tenosynovitis, even osteomyelitis, may result.

Time is an important factor in the management of human bite wounds. Many of these patients come to the physician several days after the injury occurred. At this stage, incision and drainage of loculated pus, dressings, strict immobilization, and elevation of the extremity along with systemic antibiotics are all indicated.

Chemical or thermal cauterization of human bite wounds is no longer considered proper therapy.

Animal Bites

Only serious animal bite wounds and litigious recipients come to an emergency room. All animal bites are reportable by law. They should be considered in the same category as human bites with the added potentially serious problem—rabies.

DOG BITES

There is indeed some truth in the old maxim clean as a hound's tooth. Nevertheless, dog bite wounds must be well irrigated and thoroughly debrided if primary healing is to be expected. The cheek region is a typical location for a dog bite. Although there may appear to be a number of small puncture wounds, on close inspection a large subcutaneous dead space may be found below the skin. This is the result of a shearing pull of the skin away from the underlying aponeurotic fascia. If such a cavity is present, a drain should be placed and brought out through one of the wounds. Occasionally, there will be leakage from a bite wound of the parotid or its duct (see Chapter 17 on facial injuries).

The traumatized edges of dog bite wounds may be trimmed for 1–2 mm by a skilled operator. This will remove damaged tissue and contaminating bacteria. Puncture-type wounds should not be sutured nor should most dog bite wounds of the extremities. However, with proper wound toilette, most bites of the facial area can be closed using a minimum number of sutures and micropore tapes. Antibiotics are routinely given; the bacteria in dogs' saliva are sensitive to penicillin. Tetanus prophylaxis should be given to patients who have had any dog or other animal bite.

Rabies

The rare but potentially most dangerous complication of any dog bite is rabies. Knowledge of the biting animal's health is extremely important. If this is unknown, the treating physician is faced with the decision of whether or not to begin rabies vaccination. Moreover, a rabid dog can be infectious several days before its symptoms appear. Therefore, the best policy is to be certain the animal is confined for observation before initiating antirabies treatment.

If the confined animal appears healthy, treatment need not be initiated unless signs of rabies develop, usually within 5 days after the exposure. If the animal is rabid or the animal has escaped and the signs in the patient suggest rabies, then treatment should be started immediately. There are two methods of treatment—vaccination with duck embryo vaccine and antirabies immune globulin. Duck embryo rabies vaccine produces antibodies by the tenth day; therefore it is useful in cases in which the incubation period is over 3 weeks. For immediate therapy when there is a short incubation period, passive immunity is confirmed using human rabies immune globulin. It is given in a single dose, 20 IU/kg. When feasible, one-half the injection should be infiltrated around the site of injury and the remainder given intramuscularly in the buttocks. The duck embryo vaccine is given in 23 1-ml doses, starting the day that the antirabies serum is given. First, 21 daily doses are given, followed by a 1-ml booster dose at 10 and 21 days after completion of the series. The vaccine should be injected subcutaneously, rotating sites about the trunk and lateral thighs. Therapy may be discontinued if the laboratory examination of the animal is negative. Fortunately, there are only 102 cases of confirmed rabies yearly in the United States.

CAT BITES

Cat bites and scratches often become infected. Because cats clean themselves with their tongues, they harbor large numbers of bacteria in their mouths. Cat wounds should be cleansed, and topical antibacterial ointment should be applied. *Pasteurella multocida,* a small gram-negative rod, is a common pathogen in cat as well as dog bites. It is sensitive to penicillin and tetracycline, and preventive antibiotics should be given to a patient with a deep cat scratch or bite wound.

SNAKE BITES

About 45,000 people are bitten by snakes every year in the United States; however, only 20% of these people are bitten by poisonous snakes. Although there are over 20 species of poisonous snakes in this country, the majority of bites are from pit vipers, so called because of a deep pit lined with heat receptors located between the eye and nostril. The rattlesnake is the most common pit viper and is responsible for the most serious bites. Other members of this species include the cottonmouths (also known as water moccasins) and copperheads. The usually docile coral snake can also bite. They are generally marked with alternating red and black bands, separated by yellow rings. Coral snakes account for only 1% of poisonous snake bites (Fig. 14.9).

Bites from nonvenomous snakes characteristically leave multiple small puncture marks, similar to scratches from a blackberry bush. There is only minimal local swelling and slight discomfort about the injured skin. There are no systemic effects. Nonvenomous snake bites should be cleansed and the patients given tetanous toxoid.

The bite of a poisonous snake results in envenomation in about two-thirds of the cases. There will be a history of instantaneous severe pain in the bitten area. Within a few minutes, the area will become swollen and ecchymotic with bleb formation and rapid appearance of skin necrosis and sloughing of tissue. Viper bites result in the typical double puncture wounds made by the snake's fangs. Coral snake bites produce little or no local tissue changes, and the fang marks look like scratches.

Severe envenomation is signaled by more rapid onset of local signs and systemic symptoms such as nausea, vomiting, thirst, sweating, and fever. More severe effects can also be seen, for example, hypotension, cyanosis, convulsions, even pulmonary failure and circulatory collapse. Coral snake venom is mainly neurotoxic. Systemic effects usually occur within 1–7 hours, but may show up later, evidenced by ptosis, slurred speech, dyspnea, even respiratory arrest (symptoms suggestive of bulbar-type paralysis).

First-aid measures include killing the snake, without damaging identifying marks around the head, and retrieving the snake for identification by a herpetologist. The skin of the victim should be incised longitudinally through the fang marks. Suction is effective for removal of substantial amounts of venom (up to 50%) from the wounds. It should be started after the skin incision and continued for 1 hour. Suction cups are provided in commercial snakebite kits; oral suction can lead to contamination of the wound. Over 90% of snake bites occur in the extremities; in such cases the limb should be immobilized and elevated. A constricting band should be applied proximal to the bite area. This should function to impede superficial venous and lymphatic drainage only; the distal pulse should be monitored.

If the characteristic fang marks and severe local and systemic reactions as described are present, antivenin should be administered. Antivenins are commercially available in horse serum. Reactions to the antivenin serum—anaphylaxis and serum sickness—are frequent. Preliminary testing for sensitivity to serum should be done with the proviso about false-negative reaction to the test. Dosage recommendations vary with the type of snake, severity of the bite, and age and weight of the patient. Two types of antivenin are commercially available: one for rattlesnake and other pit viper bites and another for coral snake bites. The location of antivenin for rare species of poisonous snakes, as well as names and phone numbers of experts on venomous bites, can be obtained from any large city poison center.

Early debridement of the ecchymotic, necrotic, and hemorrhagic tissue surrounding the puncture site can be effective. The important structures such as vessels, nerves, and tendons are spared. The open wound is dressed and covered later with a split-thickness skin graft. Fasciotomy may also be beneficial; a physician familiar with this operative procedure should be summoned.

Snakes harbor tetanus bacilli in their mouths; therefore antitetanus therapy is indicated. Broad-spectrum antibiotics are also empirically given. Some patients may require therapy for hypotension, renal shutdown, and respiratory failure.

Insect Bites

Forty to sixty deaths occur yearly as a result of bites from spiders, bees, wasps, hornets, yellow jackets, ants, and scor-

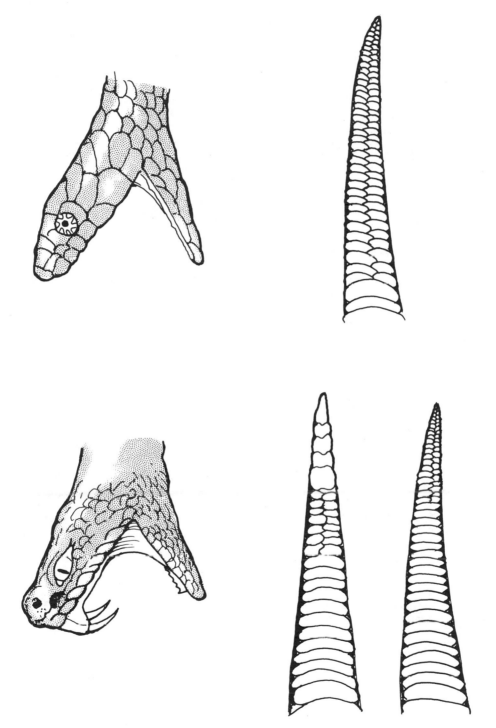

Figure 14.9 Features of poisonous and harmless snakes. (Adapted from Parrish HM, Carr CA, *J Am Med Assoc* 1967; 201:927.)

pions in the United States. Some of these fatalities are due to the poisonous venom per se, while others are due to an anaphylactic response.

HYMENOPTERA

Hypersensitivity to Hymenoptera stings (bees, wasps, hornets, and yellow jackets) accounts for the greatest mortality rate from any venomous animals—30–50 people die each year in the United States from systemic reactions to stings. The common honey bee accounts for more stings and deaths than any other species. It is the only species that leaves its barbed stinger and venom sac in situ as evidence. Therefore its presence makes a positive diagnosis and its absence makes a specific diagnosis difficult.

Treatment of Hymenoptera stings begins with removal of the stinger, taking care not to squeeze the area. The wound should be cleansed with soapy water and ice should be applied. Allergic reactions to Hymenoptera may be immediate (local or generalized, even anaphylaxis) or delayed with serum sicknesslike symptoms. In general, the more rapid the onset of symptoms, the more severe the reaction will be. If there is the slightest manifestation of an allergic response, subcutaneous epinephrine (1:1,000), 0.4–0.5 ml, should be given and the area massaged vigorously to hasten absorption. For severe anaphylaxis, intravenous epinephrine is warranted—0.25 ml in a 0.01% solution—injected slowly and cautiously. For children, the recommended dose is 0.15 ml or 0.01 ml/kg. The patient is watched closely and a repeated dose may be needed in 20–30 minutes. If there are signs of glottal edema or severe hypotension, intravenous therapy, antihistamines, and steroids may be needed.

For future exposure to Hymenoptera, hypersensitive patients should be prescribed a sting kit, including a lymphatic constrictor band, injectible and inhalant forms of epinephrine, an oral antihistamine, and detailed instructions. They should also carry medical identification tags and take reasonable precautions when they are in endemic areas. In addition, Hymenoptera venom extracts are now approved by the Food and Drug Administration (FDA) for hyposensitizing patients who have had severe, life-threatening allergic reactions to Hymenoptera stings.

SPIDER BITES

Brown Recluse Spider

Most spiders are venomous but timid. They seldom bite unless threatened. Typical is the reclusive brown spider, *Loxosceles reclusa*, which can be responsible for a serious bite wound. This arthropod is characterized by the presence of a posteriorly oriented violin-shaped marking on its dorsal cephalothorax. There is very little pain soon after a brown spider bite. The skin forms a central vesicle with surrounding erythema. A few hours later the area becomes indurated and painful, and within 6–12 hours there is evidence of vascular thromboses. Full-thickness necrosis develops.

Local excision of the involved area and delayed skin grafting has given inconsistent results. It is preferable to allow the eschar to separate; topical antibacterials will minimize the chance of secondary bacterial infection. The wound usually heals within 3 weeks; a skin graft may be necessary. An antitoxin may soon be commercially available for brown spider bites.

Black Widow Spider

The black widow spider has a characteristic red-to-yellow ventral hourglass marking. There is immediate pain, followed by redness and swelling near the fang marks of the black widow bite. After one-half hour, spasms may occur in the abdomen and upper truncal muscles. Anxiety, nausea, vomiting, dizziness, headache, dysphagia, ptosis and edema of the eyelids, low-grade fever, and skin rash are common. Black widow spider venom is also responsible for an immediate rise in blood pressure.

Treatment is supportive, including topical cleansing, ice application, aspirin, and analgesics. Mild sedation and bed rest may be indicated. A horse serum antivenin (Lyovac) is available and may be justified, particularly in children. Ten percent calcium gluconate, given intravenously, may be necessary for relief of acute muscle spasms.

Marine Animal Bites and Stings

Emergency rooms near coastal areas will admit patients injured by stingrays, jellyfish, Portuguese man-of-war, sea urchins, and other spiny venomous marine species. Because stinging marine vertebrates such as stingrays and spiny fish (including catfish) possess remarkably similar thermolabile venoms, heat application rather than the usual ice application is the primary mode of therapy. In general, marine venoms are simpler and shorter acting than those of terrestrial animals. Marine animal stings are treated for pain, venom effect, and secondary infection. A tourniquet should be used for extremity bites, and the wound should be inspected for stingers or tentacles. These wounds should be irrigated and debrided. Elevation of the extremity, pain medication, and rest are recommended. Antihistamine and corticosteroids may be of help if the venom effects increase.

SUGGESTED READINGS

Alexander JW, Kaplan JA, Altemeir WA: Role of suture materials in the development of wound infection. *Ann Surg* 1965; 165:192.

Bodvall B, Rais O: Effects of infiltration anaesthesia on the healing of incisions in traumatized and non-traumatized tissues. *Acta Chir Scand* 1962; 123:83.

Borges AF: Scar prognosis of wounds. *Br J Plast Surg* 1960; 13:47.

Brown LL, Shelton HT, Bornside GH, Cohn I Jr: Evaluation of wound irrigation by pulsatile jet and conventional methods. *Ann Surg* 1978; 187:170.

Conolly WB, Hunt TK, Zederfelt B, et al: Clinical comparison of surgical wounds closed by suture and adhesive tapes. *Am J Surg* 1969; 117:318.

Craig PH, Williams JA, Kavis KW, et al: A biologic comparison of polyglactin 910 and polyglycolic acid synthetic absorbable sutures. *Surg Gynecol Obstet* 1975; 141:1.

Crikelair G: Skin suture marks. *Am J Surg* 1958; 96:631.

deHoll D, Rodeheaver GT, Edgerton MT, Edlich RF: Potentation of infection by suture closure of dead space. *Am J Surg* 1974; 127:716.

Edlich RF, Panek PH, Rodeheaver GT, Turnbull VG, Kurtz LD, Edgerton MT: Physical and chemical configuration of sutures in the development of surgical infection. *Ann Surg* 1973; 177:679.

Forrester JC, Zederfelt B, Hayes BH, Hunt TK: Wolff's law in relation to the healing skin wound. *J Trauma* 1970; 10:770.

Gillman T, Penn J: Studies on the repair of cutaneous wounds. *Med Proc* 1956; 2:121 (suppl).

Gross A, Cutright DE, Bhaskar SN: Effectiveness of pulsating water jet lavage in treatment of contaminated crush wounds. *Am J Surg* 1972; 124:373.

Haury B, Rodeheaver G, Vensko JA, Edgerton MT, Edlich RF: Debridement: An essential component of traumatic wound care. *Am J Surg* 1978; 135:238.

Holmlund DEW: Physical properties of surgical suture materials: Stress–strain relationship, stress–relaxation and irreversible elongation. *Ann Surg* 1976; 184:189.

Krizek TJ, Davis JH: The role of the red cell in subcutaneous infection. *J Trauma* 1965; 5:85.

Krizek TJ, Robson MC: Evolution of quantitative bacteriology in wound management. *Am J Surg* 1975; 130:579.

Levenson SM, Geever EF, Crowley LV, Oates JF, Berard CW, Rosen H: The healing of rat skin wounds. *Ann Surg* 1965; 161:293.

Magee C, Haury B, Rodeheaver G, Fox J, Edgerton MT, Edlich RF: A rapid technic for quantitating wound bacterial count. *Am J Surg* 1977; 133:760.

Marshall KA, Edgerton MT, Rodeheaver GT, Magee CM, Edlich RF: Quantitative microbiology: Its application to hand injuries. *Am J Surg* 1976; 131:730.

McGregor IA: *Fundamental Techniques of Plastic Surgery* ed 5. Baltimore, The Williams and Wilkins Co, 1972.

Mulliken JB, Healey NA: Pathogenesis of skin flap necrosis from underlying hematoma. *Plast Reconstr Surg* 1979; 63:540.

Mulliken JB, Healey NA, Glowacki J: Povidone-iodine and tensile strength in wounds in rats. *J Trauma* 1980; 20:323.

Peacock EE Jr, Van Winkle W Jr: *Wound Repair* ed 2. Philadelphia, WB Saunders Co, 1976.

Postelthwait RW, Willigan DA, Ulin AW: Human tissue reactions to sutures. *Ann Surg* 1975; 181:144.

Robson MC, Duke WF, Krizek TJ: Rapid bacterial screening in the treatment of civilian wounds. *J Surg Res* 1973; 14:426.

Rodeheaver GT, Pettry D, Thacker JG, Edgerton MT, Edlich RF: Wound cleansing by high pressure irrigation. *Surg Gynecol Obstet* 1975; 141:357.

Rodeheaver G, Pettry D, Turnbull V, Edgerton MT, Edlich RF: Identification of wound infection potentiating factors in soil. *Am J Surg* 1974; 128:8.

Rovee DT, Miller CA: Epidermal role in the breaking strength of wounds. *Arch Surg* 1968; 96:43.

Schauerhamer RA, Edlich RF, Panek P, et al: Studies in the management of the contaminated wound. VII. Susceptibility of surgical wounds to postoperative surface contamination. *Am J Surg* 1971; 122:74.

Van Winkle W Jr, Hastings JC: Consideration in the choice of suture materials for various tissues. *Surg Gynecol Obstet* 1972; 135:113.

Van Winkle W Jr, Hastings JC, Barker E, et al: Effect of suture materials on healing skin wounds. *Surg Gynecol Obstet* 1975; 140:7.

Wheeler CB, Rodeheaver GT, Thacker JG, Edgerton MT, Edlich RF: Side effects of high pressure irrigation. *Surg Gynecol Obstet* 1976; 143:775.

Bites and Stings

Barclay W R: Emergency treatment of insect-sting allergy. *JAMA* 1978; 240:2735.

Callahan M: Prophylactic antibiotics in common dog bite wounds: a controlled study. *Ann Emerg Med* 1980; 9:410.

Frazier C A: Diagnosis and treatment of insect bites. *Ciba Clinical Symposia* 20 (3) 1968; 75–101.

Glass T G Jr: Early debridement in pit viper bites. *JAMA* 1976; 235:2513.

Guba A M Jr, Mullikan J B, Hoopes J E: The selection of antibiotics for human bites of the hand. *Plast & Reconstr Surg* 1975; 56:538.

Huang T T, Lynch J B, Larson D L, Lewis S R: The use of excisional therapy in the management of snakebite. *Ann Surg* 1974; 179:598.

Hubbard D C: The brown recluse spider and necrotic arachnidism: a current review. *J Ark Med Soc* 1977; 74:126.

Lichtenstein L M, Valentine M D, Sobotka A K: Insect allergy: the state of the art. *J Allergy Clin Immunol* 1979; 64:5.

Malinowski R W, Strate R G, Perry J F, Fischer R P: The management of human bite injuries of the hand. *J Trauma* 1979; 19:655.

Parrish H M, Khan M S: Bites by coral snakes. Report of 11 representative cases. *Am J Med Sci* 1967; 253:561.

Parrish H M, Schwichtenberg A E, Parmentier C J: Clinical features of bites by non-venomous snakes. *South Med J* 1973; 66:1412.

Robinson D A: Dog bites and rabies: an assessment of risk. *Brit Med J* 1976; 1:1066.

Schultz R C, McMaster W C: The treatment of dog bite injuries, especially those of the face. *Plast & Reconstr Surg* 1972; 49:494.

Strickland N E: Snake bites: a review. *J ARK Med Soc* 1976; 73:69.

Thomson H G, Svitek V: Small animal bites: the role of primary closure. *J Trauma* 1973; 13:20.

Tindall J, Harrison C: Pasteurella multocida infections following animal injuries, especially cat bites. *Arch Dermatol* 1972; 105:412.

Watt C H Jr: Poisonous snake bite treatment in the United States. *JAMA* 1978; 240:654.

Wingert W A, Wainschel J: Diagnosis and management of envenomation by poisonous snakes. *South Med J* 1975; 68:1015.

Zook E G, Miller M, Van Beek A L, Wavak P: Successful treatment protocol for canine fang injuries. *J Trauma* 1980; 20:243.

15
HEAD INJURIES

Edwin G. Fischer

Head and neck injuries are a major cause of disability death in Western society, especially among young adults and children. Head injuries occur at an estimated yearly rate of 200 per 100,000, neck injuries at a rate of 5 per 100,000 population. Although a majority of the deaths and vegetative outcomes can be attributed to injury to brain substance occurring at the time of trauma, a significant number are caused by remediable, secondary phenomena, especially intracranial hematomas, and are avoidable when detected and treated promptly. Intracranial hematomas occur in approximately 10% of patients hospitalized for head injury, and the recognition of the hematomas is a major objective in the management of such patients.

The emergency room treatment of head injuries contains many pitfalls. Apparently minor injuries may evolve into neurosurgical emergencies over a short period of time. Cervical spine fractures may be masked by coma or an agitated mental state, and additional neurologic injury may occur if the neck is not properly protected. Depressed skull fractures or basilar fractures with cerebrospinal fluid (CSF) leak may be overlooked. Finally, there are often other accompanying injuries that require a multispecialty approach to the patient's care.

CLINICAL PATHOLOGIC CONSIDERATIONS

Concussion

Transient loss of consciousness frequently follows head trauma and usually lasts several minutes or longer. Retrograde and anterograde amnesia are common. The pathophysiology of these disturbances is not well understood, but dysfunction of medial portions of the temporal lobes and of the reticular activating system of the brainstem has been postulated. If consciousness is not regained promptly after head trauma, the "lucid interval" that is characteristic of acute epidural and subdural hematomas (see below) may be obscured.

Brain Contusion and Laceration

Several mechanisms account for injuries to both brain substance and vessels during trauma: axon stretching and shear strains on brain structures during rotation of the skull; compression of the brain against the skull at the site of impact and distraction in contrecoup locations during deceleration injuries; direct laceration and shock waves in penetrating and missile injuries. The most severe brain injuries appear to occur when the freely movable head is acutely rotated upon impact. Rotational acceleration creates shearing strains within the brain that are disruptive and deforming. Such rotational injuries may affect the cortex alone, especially on the undersurface of the frontal and temporal lobes or, when more severe, the deeper structures of the brain. They may produce diffuse and severe white matter injury accompanied by characteristic injury to the corpus callosum and superior cerebellar peduncle, causing coma, decerebration, and autonomic instability, often erroneously interpreted as a pure brainstem injury and from which a satisfactory recovery is unlikely. Intracerebral hematomas may develop in areas of torn tissue, either as small scattered lesions or as a single, large mass, often in a contrecoup location. They may also occur days or weeks after an injury, in which case a traumatic aneurysm may be responsible. The injured brain may swell either because of vascular engorgement as a result of loss of autoregulation or because of edema, resulting in increased intracranial pressure (see below).

Acute Epidural and Subdural Hematomas

Acute epidural hematomas form between the dura and inner table of the skull usually within minutes or hours of the injury. A torn middle meningeal artery is the most common source of bleeding, but a fracture is not always present. The usual location of acute epidural hematomas is over the temporal lobe. In children, they may occur in the posterior fossa. They are often but not always in the presence of an occipital fracture and are presumably the result of the marked vascularity of a child's dura in the region of the foramen magnum. The clinical syndrome of an acute epidural hematoma in either location is described below (see temporal lobe and cerebellar tonsil herniations). Although they may be rapidly fatal, their prompt evacuation generally leads to complete recovery, especially in young adults and children.

Acute subdural hematomas form within the potential space between the dura and the arachnoid membrane and develop within hours of the injury. They result from tearing of veins that cross from the brain to the dura, especially near the sagittal sinus, or from injury to a cortical artery. They generally extend over the entire convex surface of the hemisphere and cause a clinical picture indistinguishable from that of an epidural hematoma. They may occur after trivial injuries in patients who are on anticoagulant therapy. The mortality rate is high (50–80%), and there is a high incidence of neurologic sequellae, which are thought to be caused by injury to underlying brain substance. *Chronic subdural hematomas,* by contrast, occur more often in the elderly, are often contrecoup in location, are frequently bilateral (10–20%), and have a much better prognosis. Their clinical course may be clinically indistinguishable from that of a tumor, typically occurring over days, weeks, or even months and characterized by progressive headache, lethargy, confusion, and neurologic deficit.

Brain Swelling

Brain swelling may be focal or generalized, may occur in the absence of detectable injury to brain parenchyma, and may be especially severe in children. It generally does not last for more than 4–6 days. Posttraumatic brain edema is caused both by cytotoxic mechanisms in areas of ischemia and direct injury and by vasogenic mechanisms. Expansion of cerebral blood volume also contributes to brain swelling and can occur when autoregulation (which normally restricts flow in the cerebral capillaries during elevation in systemic arterial pressure) is lost and when carbon dioxide is retained causing increased cerebral blood flow. Focal disturbances in cerebral blood flow are thought to account for the transient, posttraumatic neurologic deficits, especially blindness, that are seen in children.

Increased Intracranial Pressure

Any space-occupying lesion can increase intracranial pressure. Although headaches and vomiting may be early symptoms, declining consciousness is the most reliable early sign of increased intracranial pressure. Increased pressure becomes life threatening when cerebral perfusion pressure (the difference between arterial pressure and intracranial pressure, normally 50 mm Hg or greater) becomes compromised. There are only two intracranial mechanisms that can compensate for acute mass lesions: displacement of CSF and reduction of brain vascular volume. These mechanisms have a limited capacity, however, and eventually each unit of added intracranial volume is accompanied by a progressively larger rise in intracranial pressure. Finally, waves of pressure develop, first lasting only a few minutes but then becoming longer (15–20 minutes) and more refractory to treatment (hyperventilation, hyperosmolar agents, barbiturates). Pressure waves are presumably vascular in origin and ultimately result in death from cerebral ischemia or brain herniation.

Temporal Lobe and Cerebellar Tonsillar Herniation

Temporal lobe herniation causes a characteristic clinical syndrome that in the setting of trauma indicates impending death from a usually treatable cause such as an acute epidural, subdural, or intracerebral hematoma. After the initial concussion, there is a variable period and degree of wakefulness. If the concussion is prolonged this "lucid interval" may never be recognized. As intracranial pressure increases, the level of consciousness declines. With expansion of the hematoma, the hemisphere is compressed and the medial portion of the temporal lobe is displaced across the edge of the tentorium and downward (Figs. 15.1 and 15.2). The adjacent oculomotor nerve and cerebral peduncle are compressed (Fig. 15.3) causing dilation of the ipsilateral pupil (the contralateral pupil in approximately 10% of patients) and findings of contralateral pyramidal tract injury (hemiparesis, hyperreflexia, Babinski reflex). As midbrain compression continues, decerebrate posturing develops (opisthotonus, extension, and internal rotation of the upper extremities, extension and plantar flexion in the lower extremities with extension of the big toe), and the eye and motor findings become bilateral. Ischemia and hemorrhage (Duret hemorrhage) develop in the brainstem, brainstem reflexes are lost, and cardiorespiratory arrest ensues. If the entire brainstem is displaced against the opposite tentorial edge thus creating a groove or Kernohan's notch in the cerebral peduncle contralateral to the hematoma, the initial pyramidal findings are on the side ipsilateral to the hematoma.

Herniation of the cerebellar tonsils through the forman magnum, with compression of the medulla, is a feature of posterior fossa hematomas. Although depression of consciousness is generally present before cardiorespiratory arrest occurs, there are no telltale focal neurologic signs as in temporal lobe herniation. Other herniations of less diagnostic importance may also occur such as herniation of the frontal lobe under the falx or compression of the posterior cerebral artery at the edge of the tentorium by the temporal lobe which causes occipital infarction.

Skull Fractures

Although injury to brain parenchyma is generally unrelated to the presence of a fracture, certain skull fractures are important because of other adjacent tissues that may be damaged. A particular vascular structure may have been torn such as the middle meningeal artery, a dural venous sinus, or the vascular dura of the posterior fossa in children. A depressed fracture

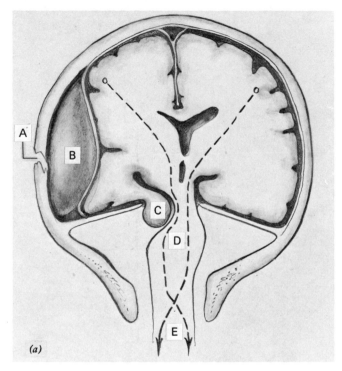

Figure 15.1 Compression of midbrain by temporal lobe herniation. (A) Temporal bone fracture across middle meningeal artery; (B) epidural hematoma; (C) uncus of temporal lobe herniating over edge of tentorium and compressing descending corticospinal tract (D) at level of midbrain, causing contralateral motor defect. Decussation of the coticospinal tract occurs at spinomedullary junction (E).

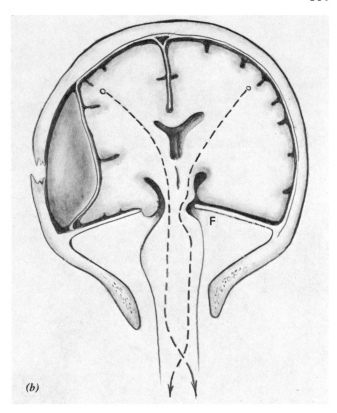

Figure 15.2 Kernohan's Notch (F). Compression of midbrain against opposite tentorial edge resulting in motor deficit on same side as hematoma.

may tamponade an underlying torn vessel and should not be manipulated or disturbed except when the patient is in the operating room.

In infants, because the dura is adherent to the skull at the cranial sutures, skull fractures may be accompanied by tears in the dura, especially if the fracture is diastatic or separated. As the child grows, an expanding cystic deformity may result involving the meninges, the bone, and the underlying brain and resulting in extensive deformity of the skull, seizures, and neurologic deficit.

Depressed skull fractures may tear the underlying dura and brain. It is not known whether seizures are more likely to result if the fracture is not elevated. Nevertheless, fractures depressed more than 1 cm or depressed a distance greater than the thickness of the skull are generally elevated to reduce the risk of posttraumatic epilepsy, especially when the fracture is in the region of the central sulcus.

Fractures are a potential source of meningitis or brain abscess when they are compound or when they occur at the base of the skull, resulting in a communication between the subarachnoid space and the paranasal sinuses or mastoid air cells. Cerebrospinal fluid rhinorrhea or otorrhea may be evident after a basilar skull fracture, or the only clue may be an air–fluid level in the sphenoid sinus seen on an otherwise normal roentgenogram. Fractures of the temporal bone may cause ecchymosis over the mastoid region (Battle's sign) and are occasionally associated with surgically correctable dislocation of the ossicles of the middle ear or transient or permanent injury to the facial nerve.

Fractures of the sphenoid bone often cause periorbital ec-

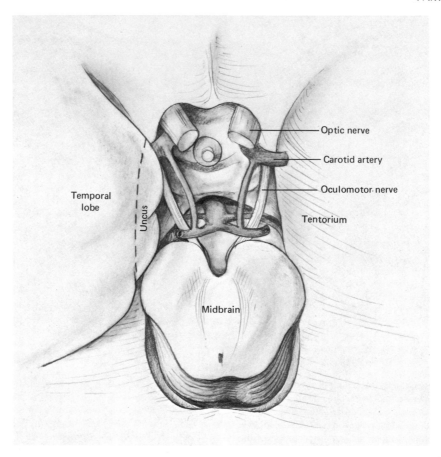

Figure 15.3 Compression of the ipsilateral oculomotor nerve by the uncus of the temporal lobe as it herniates over the edge of the tentorium.

chymosis and edema and can result in a carotid-cavernous fistula when a small branch is torn from the carotid artery within the cavernous sinus. Orbital bruit, conjunctival injection, chemosis, extraocular palsy, and impaired vision may result. Although some fistulas close spontaneously, surgical treatment is frequently required to preserve vision.

Cervical Spine Injuries

Injuries of the cervical spine frequently accompany head injuries, and if the patient is uncooperative or in coma the diagnosis cannot be made clinically. Even when the patient is alert the diagnosis may be difficult to make if there is little neck pain or neurologic deficit. Therefore all patients with head injuries, especially from falls or vehicular accidents, should be suspected of having a cervical spine injury. If they are alert and totally free of neck pain and of signs and symptoms of spinal cord injury, the diagnosis can be excluded. If they are in a coma or uncooperative, the diagnosis is assumed. To prevent further spinal cord injury from occurring in the emergency room or during transport, the neck must be protected from movement and kept in neutral position, even during resuscitative measures that include oral suctioning and endotracheal intubation. (Management of cervical spine injuries is discussed in Chapter 16.)

MANAGEMENT

Initial Resuscitation

A clear airway, adequate ventilation, and adequate blood pressure must be provided, first, as for any patient with trauma. Poor oxygenation or perfusion will result in severe, irreversible brain damage within 3–5 minutes under normothermic conditions. Hypoventilation resulting in hypocarbia will increase cerebral blood flow and may therefore increase cerebral blood volume and intracranial pressure.

The mouth and oral pharynx are suctioned or otherwise cleared of debris. When required, adequate artificial respiration may often be provided with a mask and bag before endotracheal intubation. Assuming that a cervical fracture is present, a second person can stabilize the neck for intubation, suctioning, or turning by applying continuous traction on the head along the axis of the spine while the neck is in a neutral position. When the neck is not being manipulated, it may be stabilized with sandbags, a collar, or other apparatus.

Hypotension is not caused by intracranial bleeding, except in infancy when the cranium is rapidly expandable, and it suggests either external blood loss or bleeding into the chest, abdomen, or extremities. Intravenous catheters are inserted for volume expansion or fluid replacement, but in the absence of hypotension, fluids are given sparingly to avoid brain swelling. Lactated Ringer's solution or glucose and saline are preferable to glucose and water; the recommended rates of administration are 40–60 ml/hr for adults, 1–2 ml/kg/hr for children. Infants who are in shock from blood loss may safely be given a transfusion that is one-half of their blood volume or 3.5% of their body weight.

Blood is drawn for type and cross match, complete blood count, prothrombin time, partial thromboplastin time, platelet count, blood urea nitrogen, creatinine, glucose, and electrolytes, as well as for alcohol and toxic screening when appropriate.

A Foley catheter is inserted to monitor urine output and to prevent bladder distention if hyperosmolar agents are given.

History

When a patient is in coma and has obviously sustained a head injury, the history of neurologic deterioration or of loss of consciousness after a prior lucid interval strongly suggests an evolving intracranial hematoma. An hypoxic or hypotensive episode, drug or alcohol ingestion, seizure disorder, or history of diabetes mellitus may also indicate the etiology of the coma; therefore it is important to learn the circumstances of the injury if at all possible. The presence of other diseases, and especially a history of bleeding disorder, either iatrogenic or metabolic, may be germane to the patient's management.

In less acutely ill patients, a good history may be available from the patients if they do not have amnesia. Any neurologic symptom may be of importance. Headache and vomiting, which are classic symptoms of intracranial hematoma, are common in children. Seizures are also seen frequently in children, especially at the time of or immediately after the accident. When they occur several hours later they may indicate a developing hematoma. After head trauma, transient neurologic deficits, particularly blindness, may occur in children without evidence of other pathology and may be caused by vascular phenomena. Neck pain or limited movement or neurologic symptoms in the extremities of an alert patient indicate possible spinal cord injury.

Examination

In comatose patients, a systematic but rapid assessment is made of both the head injury and of other possible sites of trauma (chest, abdomen, pelvis, extremities). The entire scalp and face are examined for lacerations, puncture wounds, and underlying bony deformity. All lacerations are thoroughly explored for fractures, CSF, or brain tissue. The ears, nose, mouth, and throat are also examined for injury, CSF, and brain tissue.

Scalp wounds should be covered with a sterile, noncompressive dressing. Bleeding from scalp vessels may be controlled with hemostats, but care must be taken not to apply pressure in the presence of an unstable skull fracture or in an area of potentially unprotected brain. Penetrating objects and fragments of depressed bone should be left undisturbed.

A complete neurologic examination may not be feasible, but a systematic examination is done focusing on level of consciousness, pupil equality, and movements of the extremities. The examination is aimed at recognizing evidence of increased intracranial pressure or temporal lobe herniation, spinal cord injury, and gross neurologic deficits. All findings should be recorded, preferably in graphic form, to facilitate recognition of subsequent deterioration or improvement. The mental status or level of consciousness is the best clinical guide to changing intracranial pressure and can be crudely graded by assessing (1) *speech* (oriented, confused, inappropriate, not at all), (2) *eye opening* (spontaneous, to auditory stimuli, to pain, not at all), and (3) *motor response* (appropriate to command, appropriate to painful stimuli, reflex response to painful stimuli, no response to pain). Depressed consciousness and an enlarged pupil on one side usually mean an ipsilateral temporal lobe herniation and is usually accompanied by contralateral corticospinal tract dysfunction: depressed motor response, hyperreflexia, Babinski's reflex, or decerebrate posturing. The pupil enlarges on the side opposite the herniation approximately 10% of the time, and the motor findings are on the same side as the hematoma if a Kernohan's notch exists in the opposite cerebral peduncle. An enlarged pupil does not mean temporal lobe herniation if the patient is fully alert. Spinal cord injury is suggested by bilateral weakness of extremities, intercostal muscle paralysis with abdominal breathing, a sensory level, and bladder distention. The more alert a patient is the more detailed the examination can be for focal deficits of brain or spinal cord function.

Immediate Surgical Treatment

Immediate surgical intervention (burr holes or craniotomy) may be indicated if there is evidence of temporal lobe herniation or rapid neurologic deterioration. There is a direct correlation between poor outcome and delay in treatment of acute traumatic intracranial hematomas. Under these circumstances, other injuries must be managed simultaneously. A computed tomographic (CT) scan of the head, if it does not involve significant delay, is performed to facilitate surgical planning, and lateral x-ray films of the neck are obtained with a portable x-ray machine. If a CT scan does not demonstrate a surgically removable hematoma, the patient is transferred to an intensive care area where intracranial pressure can be monitored and treated. In the absence of a CT scan, diagnostic burr holes, carotid arteriograms, or a ventriculogram may be performed. Placement of *burr holes or twist drill holes* for patients in the emergency room who are thought to be herniating has been advocated by some physicians. It is questionable whether it is worth the delay in moving the patient to the operating room for a procedure of such limited scope. Since the blood of acute epidural and subdural hematomas is usually clotted, it cannot be removed through a burr hole or needle. The most one could hope for would be relief of pressure from an acute subdural hygroma or from a chronic subdural hematoma. Tapping the lateral ventricular through a twist drill hole could relieve acute hydrocephalus caused by a posterior fossa hematoma.

Treatment of Increased Intracranial Pressure

Temporizing measures can be employed to reduce intracranial pressure while preparing the patient for an operation or performing diagnostic tests, but the time they buy is brief. In addition, clinical improvement may mask the diagnostic features of a developing hematoma, and shrinkage of the brain may reduce intracranial tamponade, thereby increasing intracranial bleeding.

Hyperventilation reduces intracranial pressure within minutes by lowering arterial P_{CO_2} (to between 20 and 30 mm Hg) and thereby reducing cerebral blood flow and blood volume in areas of the brain where carbon dioxide responsiveness persists. Intubation and artifical ventilation are required. It is not uncommon for arterial P_{CO_2} to be already low in patients with head injuries because of spontaneous hyperventilation.

Hyperosmolar agents that do not readily cross the blood brain barrier, such as mannitol and urea, selectively dehydrate normal brain and can reduce intracranial pressure over a period of 15–30 minutes. Furosemide may enhance this effect. A Foley catheter must be in place to prevent overdistention of the bladder. Mannitol is the most commonly used agent and has the least rebound effect. The loading dose is 1–2 g/kg by rapid intravenous infusion. Smaller dosages can be repeated every 4–6 hours or as needed in the subsequent management of intracranial pressure. Glycerol is an oral agent and has little rebound effect, which makes it useful for long-term therapy. The initial dose is 1–2 g/kg. The maintenance dosage is 0.5–0.7 g/kg every 3–4 hours.

Steroids are commonly used to treat head injuries even though their effectiveness in reducing traumatic edema or influencing outcome is not proven. Dexamethasone is the most commonly used preparation. The initial dose for adults is 10 mg intravenously (IV), the maintenance dosage is 4–6 mg IV every 6 hours. For children the initial dose is 0.12 mg/kg; the maintenance dosage is 0.06 mg/kg every 6 hours.

Barbiturates, especially high doses of pentobarbitol, may effectively reduce intracranial pressure in some patients with traumatic cerebral edema. The technique is complex and requires continuous monitoring of intracranial and arterial pressure, which makes it impossible to follow the patient's neurologic state and has no role in emergency room management.

Treatment of Patients with Seizures

Seizures at the time of head injury are common in children, and when they occur in the immediate posttraumatic period they may indicate a developing intracranial hematoma. To minimize aspiration and airway obstruction, the patient should be placed on the side, keeping the neck in neutral position if a cervical fracture is a possibility. In adults, 400–600 mg diphenylhydantoin may be given intravenously as a loading dose over a period of 15–20 minutes (cardiovascular collapse may occur at rates greater than 50 mg/min) followed by a maintenance dosage of 300–400 mg/day to keep blood levels within therapeutic range (10–25 mg/ml). When seizures are prolonged or repetitive, intravenous diazepam or phenobarbitol may be more effective. Both drugs suppress respiration significantly, and ventilatory assistance should be available. The dosage of diazapam for adults is 2.5–10 mg, for children 0.25 mg/kg, intravenously over 1–2 minutes and repeated if necessary after 15–20 minutes. The dose of sodium phenobarbitol for adults is 400–800 mg (dissolved in distilled water); for children it is 5–6 mg/kg. Delayed posttraumatic epilepsy occurs in approximately 5% of patients with closed head injuries and in more than 50% of patients with penetrating injuries; it is more common in patients with injuries in the vicinity of the central sulcus. The onset of delayed seizures is generally within the first few months or year but may be much later. Prophylactic anticonvulsants may significantly reduce the incidence of posttraumatic epilepsy.

Radiologic Examination

There is debate about the usefulness of x-ray films in the immediate management of head injuries. The films are frequently normal, and a linear fracture in itself does not require specific treatment. Although not every patient with a head injury needs to have skull films, we cannot be dogmatic about their use.

CERVICAL SPINE FILMS

X-Ray films are essential for evaluating the cervical spine in patients with neck symptoms. The first film should be a lateral one with the patient's neck still supported and in neutral position. Visualization of all seven cervical vertebrae is necessary and frequently requires traction on the arms to pull the shoulders down, or even swimmer's views. If a fracture is not seen in the lateral projection, the collar or other support can be removed with relative safety and additional views taken—an anterior–posterior open mouth view of the odontoid and anterior–posterior and oblique views of the cervical spine. If the base of the skull is included in the brow-up lateral view of the neck, the sphenoid sinus should be inspected for an air–fluid level. High-resolution CT scanners are of great value in defining cervical spine fractures, especially those of the odontoid and the first cervical vertebra.

SKULL FILMS

Examinations of the skull routinely include anterior–posterior, Towne's, and right and left lateral projections. The possibility of an epidural hematoma developing is significantly increased if a linear fracture crosses the groove of the middle meningeal artery, the dural sinuses, or the foramen magnum in children, and alone it would be sufficient reason for admission to the hospital for observation. Roentgenograms are important for the diagnosis of depressed fractures, of occult radiopaque penetrating objects, and of diastatic fractures, which are of special importance in infants. The pineal calcification, if present, should be in the midline. Foreign bodies and abnormal densities of bone should be noted. A localized increase in bone density, or "double density," is seen in depressed fractures that are best demonstrated by tangential projections of the suspicious area. An air–fluid level in the sphenoid sinus or air in the cranial cavity (pneumocephalus) generally indicates a basal fracture, even though the fracture itself is not detectable.

COMPUTED TOMOGRAPHIC SCANNING AND ARTERIOGRAPHY

Because special neuroradiologic studies such as CT and arteriography usually involve delay in treating the patient, they are obtained only as a calculated part of the surgical plan of management. The CT scan has added a new dimension to the management of head injuries. Although arteriography may accurately detect mass effect, subdural and epidural hematomas, and unrelated or unsuspected pathology, such as tumors, aneurysms, and arteriovenous malformations, the technique has been superceded in hospitals where CT scanning is available because CT is quicker, provides more information, and is non-invasive. There may be difficulties in identifying some intracranial hematomas by CT scan. Thin acute subdural hematomas can be obscured by CT scan artifact along the inner table of the skull. Some subdural effusions may be indistinguishable from brain parenchyma because they have the same film density. Lesions that are high on the brain convexity may be missed if high enough cuts are not made. A mass effect will be evident from compression or effacement of the ipsilateral ventricle and a shift of the ventricular system to the opposite side.

Repair of Scalp Lacerations

Lacerations of the scalp associated with skull fractures and tears of the dura may lead to osteomyelitis or brain abscess. Puncture wounds are important for the same reason and may be associated with a foreign body, such as a pencil or stick, that was broken off and retained intracranially. They are easily overlooked, especially if the site of entry is hidden in the orbit, nose, or throat. Because of the vascularity of the scalp, significant blood loss may occur from even small scalp lacerations. In infants and young children, large amounts of blood may collect under the galea, and deformities of the galea when palpated may simulate a depressed skull fracture.

Scalp lacerations must be thoroughly explored. Depressed fractures or lacerations of dura, as evidenced by CSF leak or extruded brain, require debridement and repair in the operating room. Depressed fragments of bone and penetrating objects should be left undisturbed to avoid initiating uncontrollable bleeding. Linear fractures should be noted, but in themselves they do not require special treatment.

The scalp around a laceration should be shaved and prepped with a surgical solution. Troublesome bleeding from wound edges can be controlled with hemostats, self-retaining retractors, or, if there is no skull fracture, direct compression. The wound should be inspected visually and palpated with a gloved finger. Once it has been determined that the skull is intact, the wound should be thoroughly irrigated, foreign material and necrotic tissue should be removed, and the skin edges should be trimmed. The galea and skin should be closed separately, using absorbable suture for the galea and silk or nylon for the skin.

"Stable" and Awake Patients

Most head injuries are minor and patients will not require hospitalization. Approximately 10% of those who are admitted have intracranial hematomas that require surgery. Nevertheless all patients with head injuries require careful examination. It is easy to overlook penetrating wounds, fractures within scalp lacerations, depressed skull fractures, basal skull fractures, CSF leaks, or cervical fractures. A lucid interval may last several hours or even days before deterioration occurs from an intracranial hematoma. It is often desirable to prolong the patient's evaluation in the emergency room so that the clinical course may be observed before making a disposition. In uncertain clinical situations, neurosurgical referral or hospitalization is recommended (see Table 15.1). If the patient is discharged home, it must be with clinical confidence of the physician and to the care of a responsible person who is adequately warned about symptoms and signs of a developing hematoma—persistent headache or vomiting, lethargy or altered mental state, unequal pupils, seizures or any neurologic symptoms. In many hospitals, printed instruction sheets are available for this purpose.

Head Injuries in Infants

Although the basic principles of management of head injuries in older children and adults apply to infants, there are some

TABLE 15.1 Indications for Hospitalization

Firm Indications
  Depressed level of consciousness
  Neurologic deficit
  Increasing headache and vomiting
  Seizures
  CSF otorrhea or rhinorrhea
  Linear skull fracture crossing the groove of the middle meningeal artery, a venous sinus of the dura, or the foramen magnum
  Compound skull fracture
  Depressed skull fracture
  Bleeding disorder (or anticoagulant therapy)
Relative Indications
  Suspected child abuse
  Prolonged loss of consciousness
  Intoxication or illness that may obscure neurologic state
  Adequate observation at home unlikely

important differences. In infants, head injuries commonly result from birth trauma, falls, child abuse, or vehicular accidents. Intracranial pressure can be assessed directly by palpation of the anterior fontanelle if it is open. Because the cranial sutures can be easily separated, allowing the skull to expand, intracranial hematomas in infants may become large enough to result in shock. Subgaleal hematomas may also produce hypotension. When an infant is in shock, half the estimated blood volume (3.5% of body weight) may be rapidly replaced with safety. Maintenance intravenous fluid therapy in infants should be designed to prevent fluid overload to minimize brain swelling and the development of edema. A conservative rate of fluid administration would be 50–60 ml/kg/24 hr. The elevated edge of a subgaleal hematoma in infants may mimic a depressed fracture on palpation. Diastatic (separated) skull fractures in infants and young children may be associated with a tear of the dura through which the arachnoid may protrude. If the tear is not repaired, an expanding, pulsating defect of arachnoid, dura, and bone may form over the next several months. The most frequent head injuries during birth are cephalhematomas, which are treated expectantly, and depressed "ping–pong" fractures, which are easily elevated with an instrument passed through an adjacent burr hole or cranial suture. More rarely, distortions of the skull may result in tearing of the tentorium and bleeding into the tentorium, the posterior fossa, or even the upper brainstem. Large hematomas of this nature are usually fatal, but on rare occasions they may be amenable to surgical removal. Compression or stretch injuries of the facial nerve may occur from the use of obstetric forceps, and these usually disappear. Spinal cord injuries may also occur at birth and are associated with breech presentations and extreme hyperextension of the neck in utero.

CHILD ABUSE

Child abuse is not uncommon in infancy and early childhood and is associated with a significant mortality and reinjury rate when children are returned to their environment without adequate protection. It is required by law to report all suspected cases to the appropriate social agencies and authorities. Such a report is indicated when the head injury is of unknown or implausible etiology or when other injuries of varying age are noted by physical examination or by x-ray films of the ribs and extremities.

CHRONIC SUBDURAL HEMATOMAS IN INFANTS

Chronic subdural hematomas in infants often occur without a history of trauma, without skull fracture, and with nonspecific signs and symptoms, that is, irritability, fever, poor feeding, seizures, enlarging head circumference, bulging anterior fontanelle, and anemia. Rapid deterioration may occur so that the patient presents acutely. The diagnosis is confirmed by bilateral subdural taps, CT scan, or angiography. Serial measurements of head circumference and hematocrit are helpful parameters to follow. The initial treatment consists of daily tapping of the subdural space, removing not more than 15–20 ml from each side at first. If fluid persists for more than 1–2 weeks, alternative therapy may be tried, such as irrigation of the subdural spaces through burr holes, drainage by insertion of a subdural–peritoneal shunt, or, if thick subdural membranes have formed, their removal by craniotomy.

Technique for Subdural Taps

In subdural taps, infants are restrained by wrapping them in a sheet and giving them a pacifier. The head is steadied at the edge of an examining table by an assistant who places one hand over each ear. The entire anterior scalp is shaved to several centimeters behind the coronal sutures. A face mask and sterile gloves are worn. The skin is prepared with povidone-iodine (Betadine), and the field is draped to behind the coronal sutures with a sterile towel held at the ears by an assistant; the anterior scalp and face are left in full view. A skin wheal of 0.5–1 ml of lidocaine hydrochloride (0.5 or 1%) is made over the coronal suture in the midpupillary line. At this site a 1.5-inch 18-gauge lumbar puncture needle is passed through the coronal suture until puncture of the dura is felt. To prevent seesawing of the needle intracranially in case the head moves, one hand always rests against the skull and stabilizes the needle where it penetrates the scalp. The stylet is withdrawn and 15–20 ml is collected in a test tube. Fluid is never aspirated with a syringe. The needle hole in the scalp is closed with a suture, and the procedure is repeated on the opposite side.

SUGGESTED READINGS

Braakman R, Penning L: *Injuries of the Cervical Spine.* Amsterdam, Excerpta Medica, 1971.

Grossman RG: Treatment of patients with intracranial hematomas. *N Engl J Med* 1981; 304:1540–1541.

Jennett B, Teasdale G: *Management of Head Injuries, Contemporary Neurology series.* Philadelphia, FA Davis Co, 1981.

Mealey JJ: *Pediatric Head Injuries.* Springfield, Charles C Thomas, 1968.

Plum F, Posner JB: *Diagnosis of Stupor and Coma.* Philadelphia, FA Davis, 1966.

Walker AE, Caveness WF, Critchley M (eds): *The Late Effects of Head Injury.* Springfield, Charles C Thomas, 1969.

16

SPINAL CORD INJURIES

Robert W. Hussey

The primary protection to the spinal cord is the spinal column; therefore, any injury to the spinal column has the potential of resulting in injury to the spinal cord. If the cord is damaged, the effects are frequently permanent and extremely disabling. Proper initial care and treatment, however, can decrease the likelihood of spinal cord injury. Only 10–20% of spinal fractures result in spinal cord injury, but improper handling can result in damage to the cord, as evidenced by a study of 85 patients with cervical spinal cord injuries at the Massachusetts General Hospital in which eight patients were neurologically worse on admission to the emergency room than they had been at the time of the accident.

The incidence of spinal cord injury is three per 100,000 population per year. The most frequent etiology is motor vehicle accidents, which account for 50% of all spinal cord injuries. This is followed in frequency by falls, sports-related accidents (especially water sports), and gunshot wounds. Initial mortality may be as high as 50%; most occur before the patient arrives at the initial treating hospital and are due to associated injuries. Once the patient is admitted to a hospital, the mortality is 10–20%. After successful initial treatment and rehabilitation, the life expectancy is nearly normal for the patient's age.

The primary goals of emergency management of patients with spine and spinal cord injuries are to prevent or minimize spinal cord damage, to stabilize the injured spine, and to treat the associated life-threatening injuries. At the scene of an accident the main objectives are to recognize a potential spinal cord injury and to manage the patient in such a way as to minimize or prevent injury to the spinal cord. In the emergency department the objectives are to determine the nature of the spine, spinal cord, and associated injuries and to initiate treatment that will meet the primary goals. This immediate stabilization should be carried out as expeditiously as possible so that the patient with a spinal cord injury can be transferred to a spinal cord injury center within hours of injury. These centers, staffed by professionals experienced in treating patients with such injuries, are equipped to offer the comprehensive care and rehabilitation that facilitates recovery and rehabilitation to the fullest extent possible in a reasonable time period and without preventable complications.

MECHANISM OF INJURY AND PATHOPHYSIOLOGY

Mechanism of Injury

Spinal cord injuries are usually caused by forces exerted on the spine indirectly through other parts of the body. The force may result in flexion, extension, rotation, axial loading, or any combination of these motions. Each type of motion tends to produce a characteristic injury pattern at a particular level of the spinal column. This pattern is related to the anatomy of the vertebrae, in particular, the shape and orientation of facet joints and the size and shape of the vertebral body (Figs. 16.1, 16.2). Injuries are more common in an area in which a highly mobile segment joins a less mobile segment, such as the lower cervical spine and the thoracolumbar junction (T-10 to L-1).

Flexion forces in the cervical spine usually produce pure dislocations or fracture dislocations of one or both posterior articulating facets. Although only damaged bones are demonstrated on films the ligaments that support the spine—the posterior longitudinal ligaments, the interspinous ligaments, and the anterior longitudinal ligaments—are often disrupted as well. Extension, on the other hand, is associated with posterior displacement, which frequently reduces spontaneously. If the spine is involved with arthritic process, the spinal cord may be compressed between the buckled ligamentum flavum and the anterior osteophytes. Axial loading tends to produce wedged compression or burst fractures. Compression fractures rarely result in spine instability; however, this type of fracture may compress the spinal cord if bone or disc material is displaced posteriorly.

Pure rotation forces are rare, but rotation combined with any other motion is relatively common. Although any of the forces in isolation may not be injurious, together they may severely damage the spine. Roaf found, for example, that the posterior supporting ligaments are not disrupted in experimental injuries by flexion alone but that slight rotation coupled with flexion does separate the ligaments. Flexion combined with rotation applied to the thoracic spine may result in the slice fracture dislocation.

Pathophysiology

The spinal cord is composed of a central core of gray matter that contains the neuronal cell bodies and a peripheral layer of white matter in which the major ascending and descending

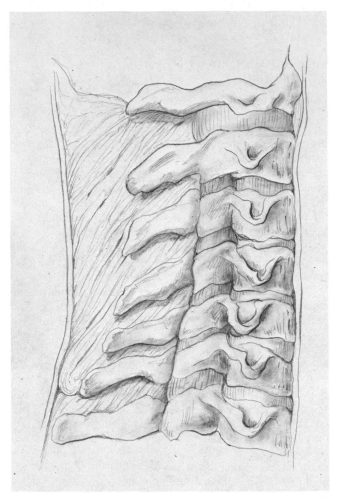

Figure 16.1 Normal cervical spine.

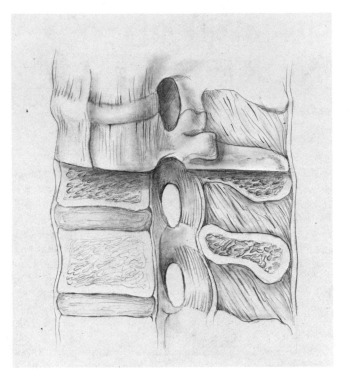

Figure 16.2 Major spinal ligaments.

tracts are located. The major tracts, whose functioning can be determined by routine neurologic examination, are illustrated in Figure 16.3. Blood normally reaches the anterior two-thirds of the spinal cord through the anterior spinal artery and the posterior one-third through the paired posterior spinal arteries. Interconnecting vessels that encircle the spinal cord supply the blood to the periphery of the white matter. Fibers are arranged in a segmental manner, or laminae, within the tracts. The lateral spinothalamic tract and the corticospinal tract are anatomically close to each other and have a common blood supply. If functioning of one tract is impaired, functioning of the other is usually similarly impaired, and the potential of

recovery is the same for both. Impairment and recovery of functioning of these two tracts are, however, unrelated to the impairment and recovery of function of the dorsal column. If there is sparing of pain pathways and preservation of motor function in the lateral tract, the patient has a more favorable prognosis than if only the posterior column is not damaged.

A force strong enough to injure the patient's spinal cord initiates a complex series of biochemical and physical events that may completely destroy the functional tissue of the involved segment within a period of 4–8 hours. When a 400 g/cm force is delivered to the exposed spinal cord of a laboratory animal, pericapsular hemorrhages appear in the gray matter within 15 minutes, coalesce, and expand until they involve all of the gray matter and extend into the white matter. These events are accompanied by a decrease in oxygen saturation and intracellular and extracellular edema. Though the histologic changes evolve over several hours, the effect is an immediate and permanent loss of spinal cord function. On the other hand, if less force is applied, the injury is frequently reversible, even though similar biochemical and physical responses occur (Fig. 16.4). The prognosis is better because only

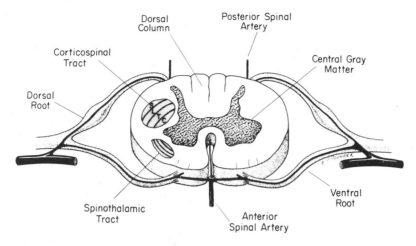

Figure 16.3 Anatomy of the normal spinal cord. The fibers of the sacral distribution are most lateral in position in both the corticospinal and spinothalamic tracts.

a part of the cross section of the cord is affected. The destruction, nevertheless, leaves residual damage in its wake as it recedes.

Spinal cord injuries are classified as follows. If there is no evidence of function distal to the site of injury (i.e., if the patient has no sensation and is totally paralyzed below the level of injury), the injury is *complete*. If no sensation or movement is apparent 12–24 hours after the cord is injured, recovery is extremely unlikely. An *incomplete* injury spares some sensory and motor function below the level of the lesion. Because sparing, which is observed most often in sacral segments, is often slight and can be easily overlooked, the patient should be examined closely in this region. This is important for prognosis and treatment planning since significant recovery is possible in incomplete injuries that are managed properly.

MANAGEMENT AT THE ACCIDENT SITE

Evaluation of the Patient

An evaluation of injuries to the patient's whole body, not just the spine, should begin as soon as the emergency personnel arrive at the site of the accident. The position of the patient and of the parts of the body should be noted, and any external evidence such as bruises, contusions, or lacerations indicating that the spine may have been injured should be sought. Pain in the neck or spine, tenderness of the spine, or paralysis or loss of sensation suggests a spinal injury. In addition, any pa-

tient who sustained a head injury, is unconscious, has fallen from a height, or has had a diving accident should be assumed to have a spinal injury. These patients should be handled as if the spine is so damaged that the cord is threatened. Although the spine should be inspected specifically for deformity, especially abnormal angulation, no attempt should be made to correct the deformity except to position the body in the neutral anatomical position. This can usually be carried out safely, but forceful manipulation should be avoided. Because the forces that produce injuries are often transmitted through the head, shoulders, or pelvic regions, these areas should be examined closely for additional local injury.

The evaluation should include a search for signs of other injuries, such as labored respiration, which may indicate that the airway is obstructed or the chest is injured; external bleeding; limb deformity, which may suggest a fracture; bleeding from the ears, nose, or mouth; and unequal dilation of pupils, which may be a result of head injury. Because injuries below the level of spinal cord injury may be totally asymptomatic and the patient may be completely unaware of them, a thorough search is essential. Life-threatening conditions should be treated immediately but, whenever possible, without moving the patient or the spine excessively. Other conditions that are uncovered may require special handling. If the patient cannot be fully examined before being immobilized and extricated, the examination should be repeated after extrication but before departure for the hospital, if no life-threatening condition is present.

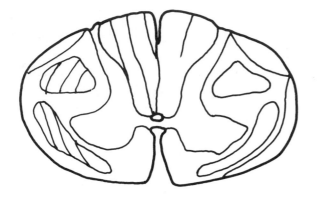

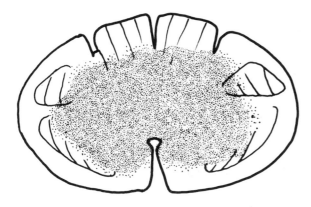

Figure 16.4 Central damage in an incomplete injury.

Immediate Life Support

All injuries to the spinal cord above the tenth thoracic segment (T-10) compromise respiration, which normally requires the coordination of the diaphragm, the intercostals, and the abdominal muscles. The diaphragm is innervated primarily by C-3 and C-4, the intercostal muscles by T-2 through T-8 and the abdominal muscles by T-8 through T-11. Any complete injury above C-3 therefore necessitates application of total respiratory support, and an injury between C-4 and C-5 may also require respiratory assistance. Lack of innervation of the intercostals causes a paradoxical motion of the chest wall when the lower cervical or upper thoracic spine is injured, decreasing the tidal volume and ventilatory capacity. Oxygen should therefore be administered to patients with cervical and upper

thoracic spine injuries. Paralysis of the intercostal and abdominal muscles prevents the patient from producing an effective cough. Suction should be available at all times to keep the pharynx clear of secretions, blood, and vomitus.

History

The personnel at the scene of the accident should elicit as much background information about the accident as possible from witnesses and the patient. Information about how the accident happened, the events that occurred between the time of the accident and the time the emergency personnel first saw the patient, any change in the patient's sensation or ability to move (e.g., was paralysis followed by return of feeling and ability to move, or vice versa?), and the patient's current symptoms (pain and its location or any other abnormal sensation) often provides clues about the type and mechanism of injury. Knowing the mechanism may be useful in deciding how to handle the patient in order to prevent further injury. A good rule of thumb is that the patient should be handled in such a way that he or she is not subjected to the type of motion that seems to have caused the injury. For example, if the injury resulted from flexion, particular attention should be paid in the immobilization to prevent further flexion.

Treatment

IMMOBILIZATION

The entire spine should be immobilized, preferably with a spine board, before the patient is extricated. A short board is appropriate if the patient is sitting in a confined space such as an automobile. One person should maintain firm but gentle longitudinal traction with the patient's head in the neutral position, and another person should place a cervical collar or other immobilizing device (e.g., rolled up towel or newspaper) around the patient's neck. The patient should then be secured to the appropriate board. If a short board was used during extrication, the patient should then be completely immobilized onto the long board before transportation. If the patient is initially found in a nonconfined location, he or she should be immobilized initially on the long spine board. The standard log rolling technique carried out by three to four people is the preferred method. The essential feature of this method is to move the patient as a single unit without bending or twisting the spine.

NEUROLOGIC EXAMINATION

A brief check of motor and sensory functions of any patient who is suspected of having spine injury should be carried out by emergency personnel before transporting the patient. This would involve at least observing the patient's ability to move the hands and feet and checking the patient's ability to feel touch and pain sensation in both feet and both hands. These findings should be documented by the emergency personnel.

Transportation

Patients who are properly immobilized with a spine board can be transported safely in any position. The standard position in which to transport a patient is the supine position. In the event of sudden emesis or excessive collection of fluids or secretions in the pharynx that interferes with a clear airway, the patient, if properly secured to the spine board, can be rapidly turned to the side position or even to a semiprone position in order to allow gravity to help maintain a clear airway.

Transportation from the site of the accident to the nearest treatment facility should be as expeditious as possible, but unless the patient is in critical condition because of nonspine injuries or respiratory involvement, high-speed transfer is unnecessary. Indeed, the inevitable bouncing and jolting may further injure the patient's spine and spinal cord.

MANAGEMENT AT THE INITIAL MEDICAL FACILITY

Resuscitation

Priority is given to stabilizing the vital functions when the patient arrives in the emergency room. An intravenous line with a large-bore needle should be inserted, and treatment for shock and blood loss should be initiated as appropriate. Lesions to the cervical or high thoracic spinal cord result in immediate functional sympathectomy. The patient's signs are altered accordingly: blood pressure 70–90 mm Hg systolic and 50–70 mm Hg diastolic; pulse 50–60 beats/min; and temperature 35–36°C (95–97°F). If the patient is alert and conscious and if the urine output is acceptable, treating these vital signs per se is unnecessary. Bradycardia that is severe enough to cause an arrythmia presents occasionally and can be reversed with atropine, 0.4–0.6 mg. A central venous catheter may be inserted so that the circulation can be monitored. A blood sample is drawn for routine hemogram and chemistries, and arterial blood gases are obtained to determine whether respiration is adequate. Prompt initiation of intermittent positive pressure breathing helps prevent pulmonary complications, which is the most common cause of early morbidity and mortality. If ventilation requires mechanical support, inserting a nasotracheal or an orotracheal tube is preferable to performing a tracheotomy. Extreme caution must be exercised to avoid extending or flexing the neck of a patient who is suspected of having cervical spine injury. Ideally, an anesthesiologist or another physician experienced in inserting endotracheal tubes should perform this procedure. Using a fiberoptic laryngoscope or a bronchoscope with the endotracheal tube passed down over it is a technique that permits difficult intubation without manipulating the patient's neck. A volume respirator should be used if continuous ventilatory support is required.

Evaluation of the Patient

PHYSICAL EXAMINATION

After life-threatening conditions have been stabilized, a thorough examination aimed at finding associated injuries should be begun, but it may have to be conducted in stages as treatment progresses. Above the level of neurologic deficit, the examination should be conducted exactly as it would be if the patient's spine were not injured, Below the level of the spinal cord injury, normal symptoms and signs may be modified or absent: Abdominal pain, tenderness, or reflex guarding, for example, may be absent even if injuries are present with intraperitoneal bleeding. Additional diagnostic procedures such as peritoneal lavage or minilaparotomy to check for abdominal bleeding may therefore be necessary. All body surfaces should be inspected, but unless definite evidence of a life-threatening injury is noted, the patient should not be turned to complete the examination until the skeletal lesion has been defined radiographically and the patient has been immobilized appropriately. This examination should be conducted as rapidly as possible, and ideally the patient should remain immobilized on the spine board until the exact nature of the spine lesion has been defined. Concomitant injuries should be managed in the usual manner and generally have priority for treatment over the spine and spinal cord injuries. Care must be exercised once again throughout this treatment to protect the spine and spinal cord. A fracture below the level of injury should be immobilized using a well-molded splint or bivalve cast, never a solid circular cast. Because the muscles below the level of injury are usually flaccid initially, skeletal traction is not necessary; in fact, it often makes treatment of the spine injury more difficult and may result in complications.

NEUROLOGIC EXAMINATION

The presence of paralysis and the level of completeness of injury can be determined by testing the patient's motor and sensory functioning. Precise recording of the findings on a diagram and marking the level of injury directly on the patient

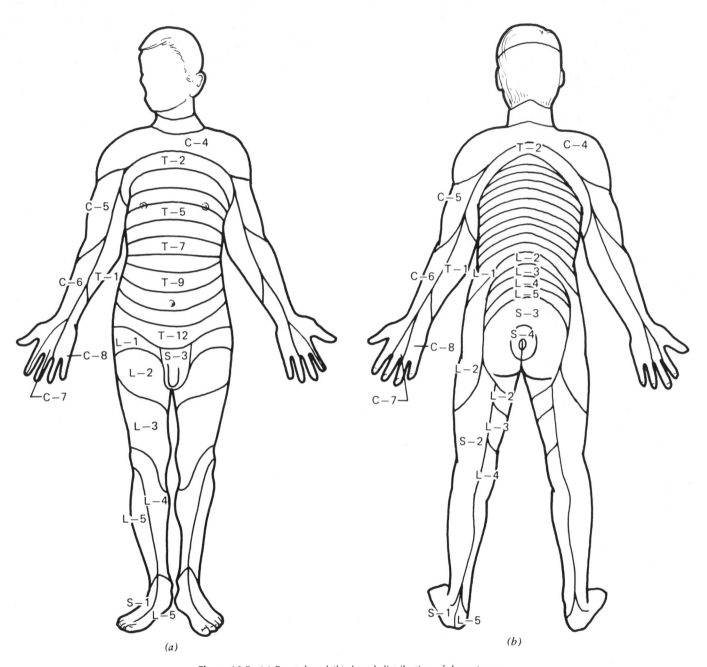

Figure 16.5 (a) Frontal and (b) dorsal distribution of dermatomes.

facilitates frequent assessment. In addition to checking for paralysis by having the patient make purposeful movements with the hands and feet, the physician should observe the patient's sensory response to pinprick, light touch, vibration, and proprioception.

With the patient fully supine with arms extended in the palm-up position, the physician should begin the examination distally and move proximally. The physician should begin in the perianal region, move down the posterior thighs and then proximally along the anterior leg and thigh and up the trunk in the midaxillary line, down the arms, across the palm, and up the preaxial border of the arm (Fig. 16.5). It is preferable to begin this sensory examination distally and move proximally because the level of injury can be identified more easily by going from an area in which sensation is absent. Because the sensory segments from C-5 through T-1 are not represented on the anterior torso, it is preferable to move proximally in the midaxillary to anterior axillary line rather than in the midclavicular line. A precise motor level cannot be defined as rapidly as a sensory level, but certain muscles provide a convenient index to level of injury (Table 16.1). Each muscle is innervated by several spinal cord segments. The segments listed in Table 16.1 are the ones that appear to provide the major innervation to the muscles. Thus, if a muscle has a strength of fair (3 out of

TABLE 16.1 Major Index Muscles for Determining Level of Motor Function

Muscle	Spinal cord segment
Diaphragm	C-3
Sternocleidomastoid	C-4
Deltoid	C-4, C-5
Biceps	C-5
Extensor carpi radialis	C-6
Triceps	C-7
Flexor carpi radialis	C-8
Extensor digitorum communis	C-8
Interossei and lumbricals	T-1
Upper rectus abdominis	T-8
Lower rectus abdominis	T-9, T-10
Quadratus lumborum	T-11
Iliopsoas	T-12, L-1
Adductors of the hip	L-2
Quadriceps femoris	L-3, L-4
Tibialis anterior	L-5
Gastrocnemius	S-1
Gluteus medius and maximus	S-2
Sphincter ani	S-3, S-4

5) or better, the major portion of the segment is probably intact. The representation of segments in the lower extremities is much broader and less precise than it is in the upper extremities.

Any residual sensation or motor function below the level of the lesions signifies that the injury is incomplete. The most common location of sparing, which must be carefully searched for because of its therapeutic and prognostic implications, is the sacral area. The perianal and perineal regions should be tested with pin and light touch, and a rectal examination should be performed to determine whether the patient has any voluntary sphincter response. Sensory response to a pin prick in the sacral segments or motor sparing at any level below the injury has the most favorable prognosis for recovery.

Neurologic deterioration that occurs in an injury that is known to be incomplete is frequently an indication for emergency surgery. The major deep tendon reflexes, the plantar reflexes, and the conus reflexes should be tested. Most patients demonstrate no major deep tendon reflexes below the level of injury, the condition known as spinal shock. The anal wink (contraction of the external sphincter when the skin near the anus is stimulated with a pin) and the bulbocavernosus reflex (contraction of the anal sphincter upon compressing the glans of the penis or clitoris or tugging gently on the Foley catheter) are conus reflexes and frequently are not lost or return a short time after spinal cord injury. The plantar reflex following acute spinal cord injury is extremely variable without regard to the nature of completeness of the injury. This variation is seen in patients with similar lesions and in the same patient at different times after the injury. Reflex testing is important because it occasionally provides evidence that the injury may be incomplete even if no sensory or motor sparing is demonstrated. If hyperactive deep tendon reflex appears soon after injury or if an injury is above the lower thoracic spine and no bulbocavernosus reflex can be elicited, the injury may be incomplete. Such findings do not, however, constitute proof of incompleteness.

RADIOLOGIC EXAMINATION

After neurologic examination is completed, the lesions should be diagnosed radiographically. Lateral views of the entire spine and anterior views of the injured area of the spine are essential. X-ray films of the skull are indicated, particularly if there is any history of unconsciousness, if there is suspicion of head injury or if skull tongs traction is to be applied. In patients with head and cervical spine injuries, in addition, an open mouth view of the atlas and axis should be performed. Figures 16.6–16.9 illustrate the most common types of injury to the cervical and thoracolumbar spines. If x-ray examination reveals that the

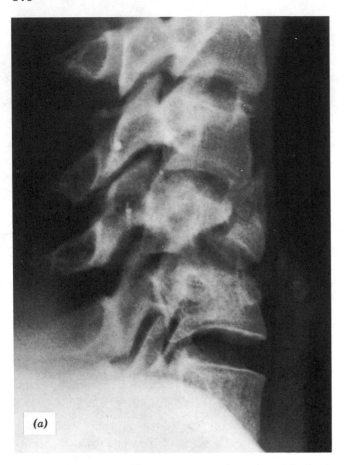

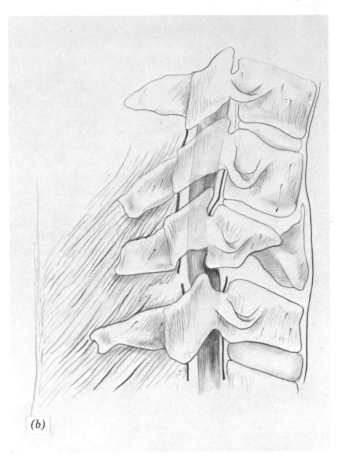

Figure 16.6　(a) Radiograph and (b) drawing of fracture dislocation of the cervical spine.

superior vertebrae is displaced more than one-half the width of the vertebral body below, the patient has sustained a bilateral facet dislocation or a fracture dislocation. A displacement of one-half the width or less of the superior over the inferior vertebral body, on the other hand, suggests that the injury is only a partial dislocation or unilateral facet dislocation. An oblique view of the spine demonstrating the side of the dislocation should be made. This can be accomplished without moving the patient by placing the film flat beneath the patient and angling the x-ray to 50 deg. This view is also of value in identifying injuries to the pedicles or injuries of the lower cervical spine when the lowest vertebrae are obscured on lateral film by the shoulders. Occasionally, x-ray films do not confirm an injury of the cervical spine that is suggested by neurologic

signs. This may result if the entire cervical spine was not visualized, if the injury was caused by extension injury, or if the dislocation spontaneously reduced; occasionally spinal cord injury occurs without demonstrable spine injury. Despite negative initial films, an injury to the spine cannot be ruled out as a possibility and the patient should be treated as if such an injury had occured. Neurologic evidence indicating that the spinal cord is injured between C-6 and T-2 should be confirmed by films of the lower cervical and upper thoracic spine. These areas may be demonstrated radiographically if traction is applied to the patient's arm and shoulders while performing the lateral x-ray. If this method fails, the swimmer's view, taken with one arm over the head and the other at the side, may demonstrate the lesion. Oblique films also can be valuable in

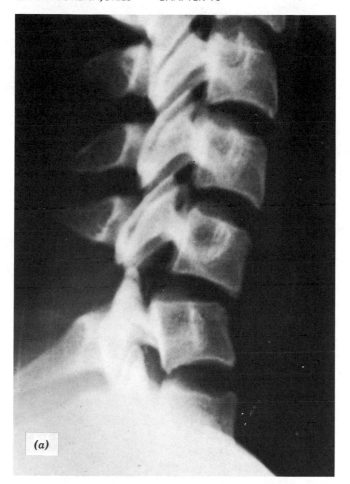 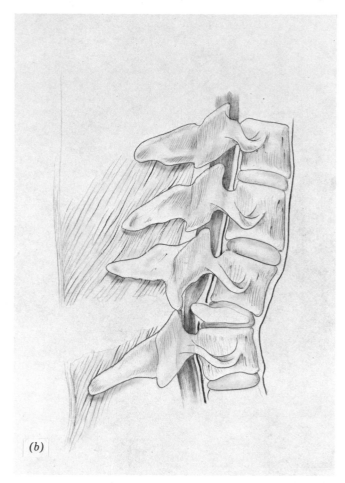

Figure 16.7 (a) Radiograph and (b) drawing of dislocation of the cervical spine with ligament damage.

this situation, as noted above. If these methods fail to demonstrate the lower cervical and upper thoracic spine adequately, tomography may be necessary.

Demonstrating a dislocation that has spontaneously been reduced is also possible. Lateral views should be made while the patient's neck is gently flexed and extended. Although flexion up to 20 deg and extension to 20 deg seem to impose no significant risk, force should not be applied and the motion should be stopped if it causes any additional pain or neurologic symptoms. These views should be obtained only under the supervision of a physician who is experienced in dealing with patients who have had cervical spine injuries. If this expertise

is not available, the patient should be immobilized and transferred to a facility where such physicians are available.

Computerized axial tomography (CAT scan) is rapidly establishing itself as one of the primary emergency means of imaging the injured spine and spinal cord. First and second generation scanners demonstrate well injury to the vertebrae but do not have sufficient resolution to reliably show the spinal cord or nerve roots even with enhancement of contrast material; additionally most of these units are not able to reconstruct sagittal or coronal images. These units can be extremely helpful in evaluating the spine injury, particularly in the area of C-1 and 2, but they do not replace polytomography when

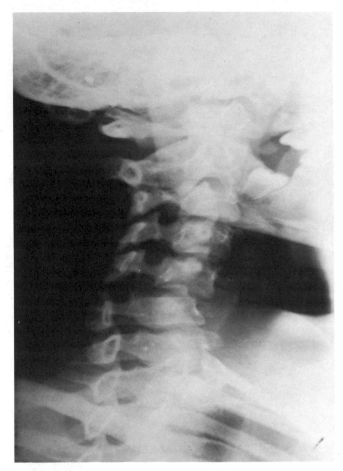

Figure 16.8 Oblique view of a unilateral facet dislocation of the cervical spine.

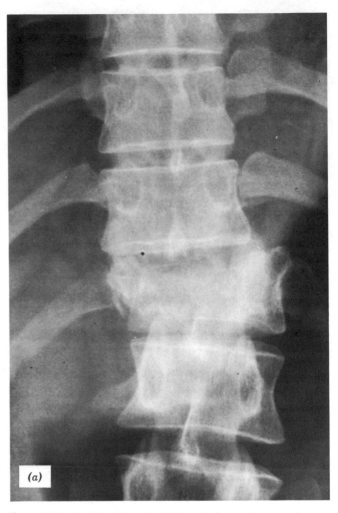

Figure 16.9 (a) AP Radiograph (b) lateral radiograph and (c) drawing of (b). Fracture dislocation of the thoracolumbar spine.

bony detail is required or myelography when it is necessary to determine the status of the spinal cord in the injured area. Third and fourth generation scanners have higher resolution and are capable of producing sagittal and coronal reconstructions and demonstrating the spinal cord. To adequately demonstrate the spinal cord in the cervical and thoracic regions, it is necessary to put metrizamide in the subarachnoid space but this is not needed in the thoracolumbar or lumbar regions. CAT scanning has a definite advantage in studying the acute spine and spinal cord injured patient in that the patient does not need to be turned to positions other than supine to carry out the study, as is the case with tomography or myelography. In hospitals with third and fourth generation scanners, CAT

scan will probably be the next most important radiographic study after plain radiographs, to demonstrate the nature and extent of the spine and spinal cord injury and to guide further treatment, particularly operative intervention.

Treatment

IMMOBILIZATION

A patient with an injured spine should always be immobilized whether or not the spinal cord is injured. Patients with thoracic

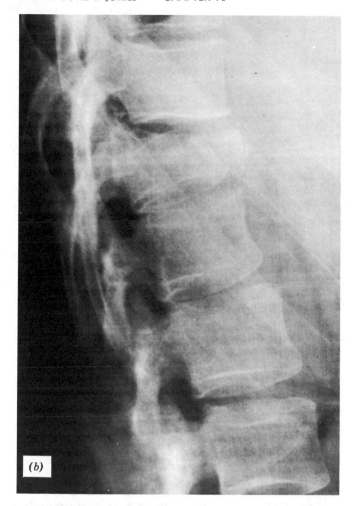

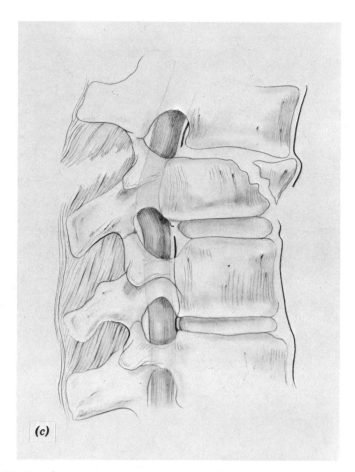

Figure 16.9. (*Continued*)

and lumbar spine injuries are most effectively immobilized in a firm bed with a bed board or in a Striker frame. Patients with cervical spine injuries require traction in addition to postural immobilization. Although head halter traction with a 4.5-kg weight and a cervical collar are acceptable for a short period, skeletal skull traction should be used if traction must be applied for a longer period of time. Several types of cranial tongs (Crutchfield, Cone-Barton, Vinky, Gardner-Wells) are currently available. The choice of device should depend on the physician's experience and of course on what is available in the hospital. The Gardner-Wells tongs have gained wide acceptance. In addition to being simple to use they can be rapidly applied. They require no special instruments or skin incisions

and a spring-loaded device built into them indicates when the proper amount of compressive force has been applied. The Gardner-Wells tongs are inserted 2–4 cm above the helix of the ear below the point of maximum circumference of the skull in neutral axis of the neck. The neutral axis is estimated to be on a line drawn from the tip of the mastoid process through the external auditory meatus (Fig. 16.10). Unless the patient's hair is long, thick, or dirty, the area need not be shaved. The area selected on each side of the head is prepared with an antiseptic solution such as povidone-iodine. Local anesthesia is given to the patient by infiltration by 1 or 2% lidocaine, being certain to infiltrate down to and including the galea and periosteum. The tongs are then placed in the selected position,

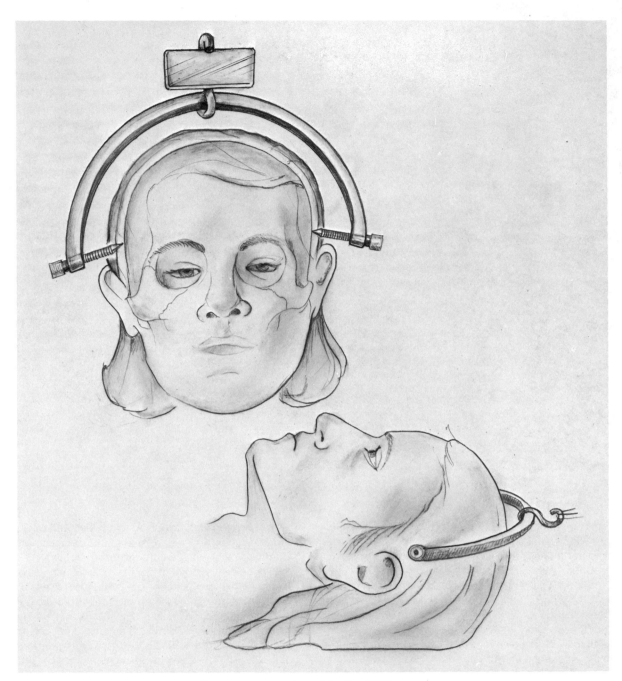

Figure 16.10 Insertion of Gardner-Wells tongs.

and the pins are turned by hand on each side simultaneously until they penetrate the skin and soft tissues and are seated firmly in the outer table of the skull. The pins are tightened until the indicator pin on the spring-loaded side protrudes 1–2 mm. After the axis of the pins and the lock nuts are tightened, the tongs are moved up and down. The following day the pins should be retightened to be sure that the indicator protrudes 1–2 mm. They should not be tightened subsequently.

The patient who presents with symptoms or signs of an injury to the cervical spinal cord should be immobilized with cranial tongs traction whether or not radiographs have demonstrated injury to the cervical spine. This type of immobilization is especially important if a lower cervical or upper thoracic segment has been injured because these parts of the spine are extremely difficult to visualize radiographically and a special technique such as laminography may be required to confirm the diagnosis. Cranial tongs traction is also efficacious if the spinal cord is injured only slightly. Experience indicates that a speedier recovery is effected by such immobilization even if the skeletal injury appears not to be severe enough to cause spine instability.

BLADDER MANAGEMENT

An indwelling Foley catheter should be aseptically placed in the patient's urinary bladder. This enables close monitoring of urine output and prevents bladder distension during this immediate period when it may be necessary to carry out fluid replacement therapy and to give medications intravenously. Intermittent catheterization is the preferred method of long-term bladder drainage to prevent urinary tract infection and retrain the bladder, but it requires careful control of fluid intake and precise technique. An indwelling catheter can be left in place for up to 48 hours without the bladder becoming infected.

MEDICATION

The efficacy of various drugs for reversing or ameliorating the effects of spinal cord injuries has not been proven clinically; however, an initial dose of 10–20 mg dexamethasone intravenously followed by a 4–6-mg dosage intravenously or intramuscularly every 6 hours for 5 days is a generally accepted regimen. Drugs such as plasmin antagonists, sympathetic blocking agents, barbiturates, and narcotic antagonists have been shown in experimental animals to improve the outcome after experimental injury but have not as yet been proven or accepted as therapeutic agents for clinical use.

DECOMPRESSION OF THE GASTROINTESTINAL TRACT

A patient should be given nothing by mouth because ileus usually accompanies any significant spine or spinal cord injury. Nausea, vomiting, or abdominal distension indicates the need for a nasogastric tube either placed on gravity drainage or low suction. Additionally, a nasogastric tube should be inserted before the patient is transported to a secondary or tertiary care facility to reduce the risk of vomiting and aspiration during transportation.

FLUIDS

A crystalloid solution should be administered intravenously; 5% dextrose and water or 5% dextrose and 0.5 normal saline or Ringer's lactate solution are the recommended solutions. These solutions should be given at a rate of not more than 100 ml/hr unless a higher rate is specifically indicated, for example, if there is a large volume of gastric drainage. Blood plasma or colloid solution should be given only if volume replacement is required. The physician must remember that a low blood pressure is normal for a patient with a high spinal cord injury and that patients with spinal cord injuries are extremely sensitive to fluid overload, which is a frequent cause of pulmonary problems as a result of increased secretion and interstitial fluid.

Transfer

Once the patient's condition has been stabilized in the emergency room, plans should be made for transfer to a facility that has the capability for definitive management of spine and spinal cord injuries if such capability is not available at the initial treating facility. Every emergency room should have arrangements and protocols for transferring patients with spinal cord injuries to the nearest spinal cord injury unit or center.

WHIPLASH INJURIES

Soft tissue injuries to the neck present a problem to emergency medical personnel. If patients with a soft tissue or whiplash injury are properly handled at the site of the accident, they should arrive at the emergency room completely immobilized with a collar. Although this procedure may seem to be overtreatment for a benign condition, personnel at an accident site are not equipped to differentiate between a soft tissue injury of the neck and a more serious cervical spine injury. It is the responsibility of the emergency room physician to evaluate the patient and rule out the possibility that a more serious injury has not been sustained and to begin appropriate treatment.

A sudden acceleration that causes the head to move backward rapidly and the neck to hyperextend is the most common way in which whiplash injuries occur. This is frequently experienced in rear end automobile collisions. This type of injury may produce transient cerebral injury and stretch the anterior cervical structures, the esophagus, the neck muscles, and ligaments in the intervertebral disc. These injuries rarely result in a structural instability of the cervical spine or in a spinal cord injury.

Evaluation of the Patient

HISTORY

Two-thirds of patients presenting with soft tissue injuries to the neck have cerebral symptoms (confusion, mental dullness, or mild amnesia), and one-tenth are unconscious for a brief period. Neck ache often followed several hours later by soreness and stiffness in the neck and upper shoulders are the most common symptoms. Patients frequently complain of pain radiating to the occiput and forward to the eyes, the upper scapular regions, or into the arms, but the pains do not follow a nerve root or a peripheral nerve distribution and are not accompanied by objective signs of nerve injury.

PHYSICAL EXAMINATION

The physical examination should include a complete neurologic examination, including state of consciousness, cerebral functioning, cranial nerves, spinal cord function, and peripheral nerve. Except for minor temporary cerebral signs, the findings should be normal if the patient has a soft tissue injury. The neck and upper thoracic spine should be examined for swelling, tenderness, spasm, and restricted mobility. Few if any signs appear in the first hour or two after injury. Spasm and restriction of motion usually do not develop for several hours or even until the day after injury. These symptoms usually subside in 5–7 days. In general, the physical findings are rarely proportional to the symptoms.

X-RAY EXAMINATION

A suspected diagnosis of soft tissue injury should be confirmed by x-ray film to make sure that no bone or major ligament injury has occured. The examination should include anterior–posterior and lateral views of the entire cervical spine as well as odontoid views and oblique or pillar views. If the neurologic and film examinations are negative, lateral views of the flexed and extended neck should be made to rule out significant ligament damage. The patient should flex and extend his or her neck rather than have a technician place the neck at the extremes of the range. An abnormal distance between the spinous processes indicates that the posterior ligaments are torn. Signs of soft tissue injury (i.e., abnormal soft tissue shadows such as widening of the perivertebral space) not just of bone injuries should be looked for on the film. Evidence of preexisting problems such as degenerative disc disease may also be found.

MANAGEMENT

The most important treatment is thorough examination to confirm that the patient has no serious injury. A soft cervical collar, bedrest if spasm is severe, and mild analgesics are usually sufficient to relieve the symptoms. As soon as possible, however, the patient should be weaned from the collar and should begin simple motion exercises in order to resume normal activity. If symptoms and disability persist any longer than 5–7 days, the patient should be referred to a specialist such as a neurosurgeon, orthopedic surgeon, or neurologist for a more specific program.

SELECTED READINGS

Bedbrook GM: Spinal injuries wth teraplegia and paraplegia. *J Bone Joint Surg* 1979; 61-B:267.

Bosch A, Stauffer ES, Nickel VL: Incomplete traumatic quadriplegia; A ten year review. *J Am Med Assoc* 1971; 216:473.

Guttman L: *Spinal Cord Injuries: Comprehensive Management and Research.* Oxford, Blackwell Scientific Publications, 1973.

Harris, JH: *The Radiology of Acute Cervical Spine Trauma.* Baltimore, The Williams & Wilkins Co, 1978.

Holdsworth FW: Fractures, dislocations and fracture-dislocations. *J Bone Joint Surg* 1970; 52-A:1534.

Roaf R: A study of the mechanics of spinal injury. *J Bone Joint Surg* 1960; 42B:810–823.

Stauffer ES, Kauffer H: Fractures and dislocations of the spine, in Rockwood CA, Green DP (eds): *Fractures.* Philadelphia, JB Lippincott Co, 1975, p 817.

17
FACIAL INJURIES

Leonard B. Kaban
Robert M. Goldwyn

People with facial injuries are 2–7% of all patients treated in the emergency rooms of large city hospitals. The most frequent causes of facial injuries among adults are motor vehicle accidents and among infants and children are falls, usually from a bicycle, porch, or steps. Accidents in the home, athletic injuries, fist fights, and animal bites are other frequent causes. Often, intraoral structures alone are injured; trauma to the teeth and dentoalveolar segments are probably the most common injuries in the facial region, especially in children.

Reduction of the speed limit to 55 mph and several recent advances in automobile construction (shatterproof windshields, shoulder seat belts, padded dashboards and roofs, stronger car frames) have helped to decrease the number and severity of facial fractures in the United States. The major soft tissue injuries resulting from shattered glass that in the past so often accompanied facial fractures are less common today.

More than half the drivers involved in fatal car accidents are inebriated. Therefore improvement in automobile safety alone will not eliminate facial injuries. Public education, more effective highway monitoring, and law enforcement directed at offending motorists are equally important efforts to reduce the present number of injuries. The increased use of protective headgear, face masks, and mouth protectors has lowered the incidence of facial trauma in organized amateur and professional sports. However, unprotected amateurs still sustain avoidable skeletal and soft tissue damage.

Facial injuries are often dramatic but they are not life threatening unless associated with airway obstruction, severe blood loss, central nervous system (CNS), chest, or abdominal trauma. These problems must be promptly recognized and treated as the first step in management of the injured patient.

INITIAL ASSESSMENT AND MANAGEMENT

Airway Management

Establishment of a patent airway is the first priority in the treatment of maxillofacial injuries. Airway obstruction may result from intraoral or nasal bleeding; loose teeth, fillings, or den-tures; posterior displacement of the tongue and soft tissues associated with fractures of the mandible or midface; swelling of the intraoral soft tissues; or damage to the larynx and trachea.

Foreign bodies, blood, or clots in the mouth or pharynx must be promptly removed by suctioning, by the fingers, or by an instrument. If the patient is able to sit up, he should be encouraged to clear the airway by coughing. If he is unable to sit up, a semiprone position allows for drainage of the oropharynx and proper positioning of the tongue.

Massive swelling of the floor of the mouth or tongue may interfere with respiration. Even if the airway is not obstructed immediately after the accident, it may become blocked as swelling increases or as a hematoma develops in the floor of the mouth, the submandibular region, or the pharynx. Oroendotracheal intubation is occasionally necessary if soft tissue swelling continues to interfere with respiration or if the patient is unable to tolerate an oral or nasopharyngeal airway; tracheostomy is rarely required today for acute airway obstruction unless oroendotracheal intubation is not possible. The physician must remember that a blow forceful enough to fracture the mandible or midface may also result in an injury to the cervical spine. When there is evidence of cervical spine trauma, the endotracheal tube should be introduced by threading it over a fiberoptic bronchoscope or laryngoscope that is guided carefully into the trachea without hyperextending the neck.

In patients with fractures of the mandible, the tongue may be displaced posteriorly, causing airway obstruction. If the patient is allowed to bend forward or if the tongue is pulled forward with a suture or even a towel clip, his or her life may be saved. If a suspected fracture of the mandibular symphysis is the likely cause of labored respiration, the bone may be stabilized by placing a wire around the teeth adjacent to the fracture site, thus allowing the mandible and tongue to be supported in a forward position.

Control of Bleeding

Patients rarely become hypotensive when they have isolated facial injuries because bleeding is easy to control with external pressure. Clamping or tying of vessels should be avoided except under very controlled circumstances, that is, in the operating room or in a room with good light and suction. Proper light, exposure, and anesthesia are necessary to avoid inadvertent injury to the facial nerve and parotid or submaxillary ducts. Intraoral hemorrhage contributing to airway obstruction can usually be controlled by placing a few sutures or a roll of sterile gauze over the wound and asking the patient to bite down on it. If these measures fail, suction will have to be applied until the bleeding can be controlled. If nasal hemorrhage is brisk, it is most likely associated with injury to branches of the internal maxillary artery. If this is persistent, it will require placement of posterior and anterior nasal packs (see Chapter 32).

Treatment of Shock

Because the face and scalp can bleed massively and yet rarely cause shock, the physician should not assume that persistent hypotension in the patient is caused by a facial injury. The presence of shock mandates a search for serious injury elsewhere; bleeding into the thorax, abdomen, or retroperitoneum is the most likely source for shock-producing hemorrhage. The necessary intravenous lines must be inserted and proper fluid therapy initiated (see Chapter 12).

Identification of Associated Injuries

As soon as conditions that pose an immediate threat to life have been identified and corrective measures have been initiated, a rapid but complete history should be taken and phys-

ical examination should be performed in order to identify associated injuries and to establish priorities of care. Although damage to the face may be the most apparent and anxiety-provoking injury, it may be the least important as far as immediate survival is concerned. It is important that the physician understand the mechanism of injury. How did the trauma occur? What was the impact velocity? Is it likely that there was contamination? How many minutes or hours since the injury? As much information as possible should be obtained from the patient or from witnesses to provide clues to the severity and magnitude of the resulting injury.

Examination of the Face and Oral Cavity

A thorough examination of the face and head, conducted in an orderly manner, must be carried out in order to evaluate the severity and extent of soft tissue injuries and to diagnose facial fractures. Radiography, though a valuable adjunct, is not an acceptable substitute. Since patients with facial injuries

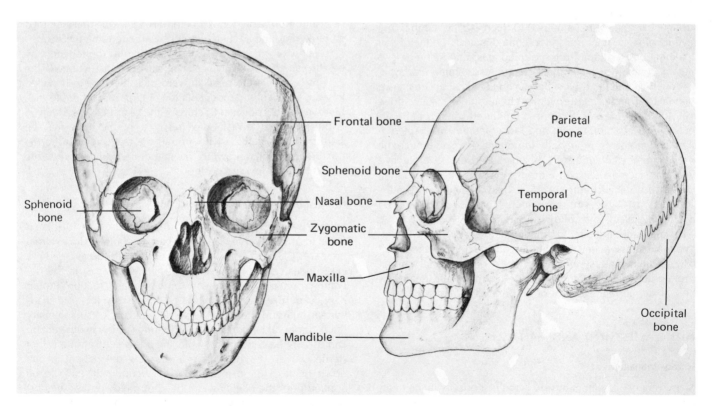

Figure 17.1 Frontal and lateral views of a normal skull.

sometimes become involved in personal injury litigation, it is essential that accurate description of the injury and the method of treatment be recorded carefully. Photographs are most helpful. If a photograph cannot be taken, however, a diagram and careful measurement of lacerations are useful.

Since the face is being examined by inspection, palpation, and x-ray film, it is essential that the examiner have a basic understanding of facial anatomy, especially as it relates to the underlying skeleton, the course of the seventh (motor nerve to the facial muscles) and fifth (sensory) cranial nerves, the parotid glands, and ducts (Figs. 17.1–17.3).

INSPECTION

Soft tissue injuries are usually apparent. The nature, location, and depth of lacerations should be carefully noted. Debris on the face and in wounds and the status of skin edges of any wound must be carefully observed. If the eyelids are closed, they should be separated and the globes should be observed for blunt or sharp injury (see Chapter 18). The mouth should be opened and examined for lacerations and for areas of swelling or discoloration. Missing teeth should be accounted for to rule out aspiration. If the patient is edentulous, dentures should

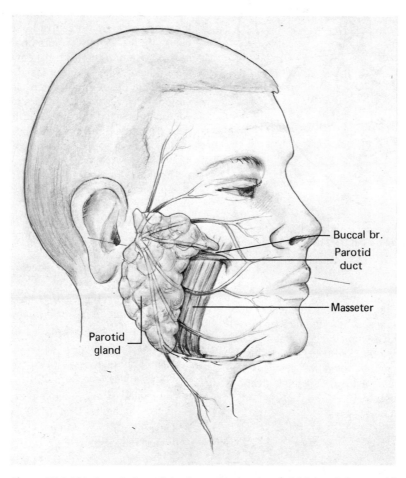

Figure 17.2 This lateral view of the face with the superficial lobe of the parotid gland removed shows the facial nerve, deep lobe of the parotid gland, masseter muscle, and the entrance of the parotid duct into the mouth just anterior to the masseter muscle. Note that the course of the parotid duct follows a line from the tragus of the ear to a point about 1 cm above the commissure of the lip.

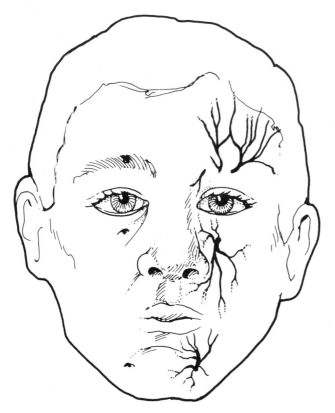

Figure 17.3 Frontal view of the face demonstrating the course of the terminal portions of the first, second, and third divisions of the trigeminal nerve.

be located since they may be helpful in the treatment of maxillary or mandibular fractures. Inspection provides many evidences of facial fractures. Facial asymmetry, ecchymoses, areas of swelling or depression, diplopia, epistaxis, malocclusion, hematomas in the floor of the mouth or the buccal sulcus, and limitation of mandibular movement are among the indications that a fracture is probably present.

PALPATION

The processes of inspection and palpation are not separate. While observing the patient, the examiner also carefully palpates all bony prominences before soft tissue swelling of the face obliterates these landmarks. (Details of the examination are described in the section on specific facial fractures.) When

there has been trauma to the nasofrontal region, nasoethmoidal region, and the orbit, the medial canthi should be carefully evaluated since one or both may be disrupted (Fig. 17.4). One index finger is placed on the medial canthus and the other index finger on the lateral portion of the upper eyelid, which should be stretched laterally. Thus tightened, the intact medial canthus can be palpated. If the medial canthus does not become obviously palpable with this maneuver, disruption of the medial canthal tendon has occurred.

X-RAY FILM EXAMINATION

Radiographic examination is only adjunctive and does not take the place of a well-organized and accurate physical examination. In the seriously injured patient, x-ray films of the face may be deferred until the patient is stable since treatment of facial fractures and even of facial lacerations may need to be delayed. In all cases in which facial fractures may have occurred, however, x-ray films are required to confirm the presence of suspected fractures and to delineate possible unsuspected fractures. Patients with a suspected cervical spine injury should have a lateral x-ray film of the neck before any other x-ray films.

The following are radiographs of the facial bones that are most useful for diagnosis of fractures:

1. Water's view—for fractures of the middle third of the face involving the maxilla, zygomatic bone, and nasal and orbital regions (Fig. 17.5)
2. Posterior–anterior view of facial bones—for frontal and zygomaticofrontal fractures
3. Posterior–anterior view of the mandible—for the body of the mandible from angle to angle (Fig. 17.6)
4. Towne's view—for fractures of the mandibular condyles (Fig. 17.7)
5. Lateral oblique view of the mandible—for fractures of the body, angles, and rami of the mandible (Fig. 17.8)
6. Submental vertex (jug-handle) view—for fractures of the zygomatic arches (Fig. 17.9)
7. Lateral nasal and Water's views—for delineation of nasal bones and septum.

Summary

The emergency room physician should be concerned with the diagnosis of facial injuries and with the early management of

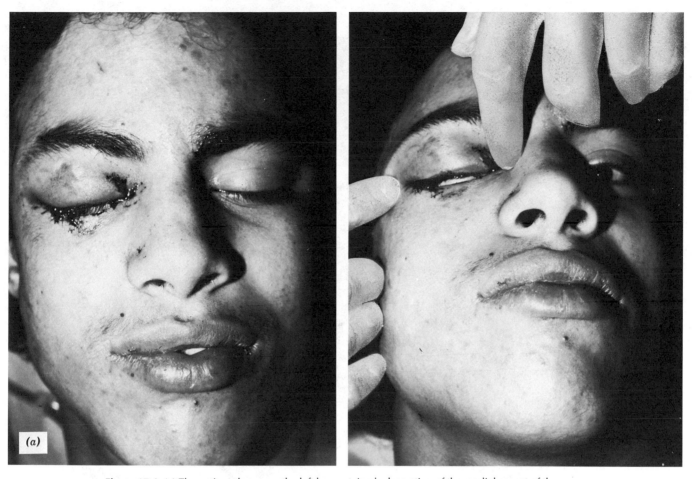

Figure 17.4 (a) The patient shown on the left has sustained a laceration of the medial aspect of the upper eyelid. On the right, examination of the medial canthus is demonstrated.

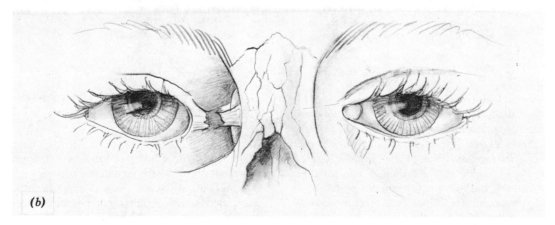

Figure 17.4 (b) This frontal view shows disruption of the medial canthal tendon in association with a nasoethmoidal fracture.

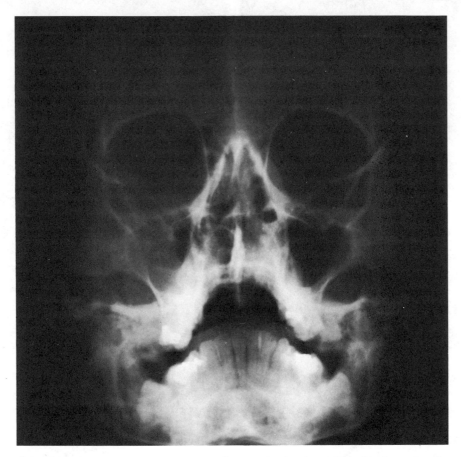

Figure 17.5 Water's view roentgenogram. The Water's view is a standard radiograph to investigate the zygomatic complex, orbits, maxilla, and midface. It shows the orbits, frontal, ethmoid, and maxillary sinuses, as well as the zygomatic complex. This x-ray demonstrtes an opaque maxillary sinus on the right side, indicating fluid in the sinus. The zygomatic bone and orbital rim are intact. The patient has a blow-out fracture of the orbital floor.

potentially life-threatening complications. The diagnosis of facial fractures can usually be made on the basis of history and physical examination; radiographs can be used as an adjunct. If the history is that of a blow of limited force that was directed to a specific area of the face, attention can be primarily focused there. However, in a situation in which there is a potential for multiple facial injuries, the examination should be thorough and systematic. Treatment of specific facial fractures can be delayed, and the patient can be referred to a specialist for definitive care.

EMERGENCY ROOM MANAGEMENT OF SOFT TISSUE INJURIES OF THE FACE

General Considerations

Many soft tissue injuries of the face can be repaired in the emergency room by the emergency room physician. However, if there is extensive soft tissue damage or if there are serious associated injuries, repair should be carried out in the operating room by a specialist. Other injuries that require specialty care include lacerations of the facial nerve, parotid gland or duct, eyelid, canthal tendons, and the lacrimal ducts. If there is full thickness loss of a portion of the ear or if soft tissue injury results in exposure of the cartilagenous framework of the ear or nose, a surgeon who is experienced in the care of such problems should be called.

The general principles of emergency wound care are described in Chapter 14. When repairing facial lacerations, keep in mind the presence of delicate structures in a small area. Tissues should be treated gently, ideally with fine-toothed forceps, small sharp scissors, skin hooks, and small needle holders. Debris and tissue that is obviously dead should be removed; if there is any possibility that tissue is viable, it should be allowed to remain. Since the faces of young patients have little tissue to spare and usually have exceptionally good vascularity, debridement should be reserved for only what is dead or severely contused. The wound must be searched carefully for foreign bodies, and any such material should be removed. If the laceration is deep and could conceivably be associated with a fracture, it is important to make the diagnosis before the wound is closed. The laceration may be used to gain access to the fracture site, and closure may not be necessary in the emergency room.

Fixed facial landmarks, such as the eyebrow line or the vermilion border, should be approximated first. Deep lacerations should be closed in layers in order to eliminate dead space and to prevent a widened, depressed scar. Muscle should

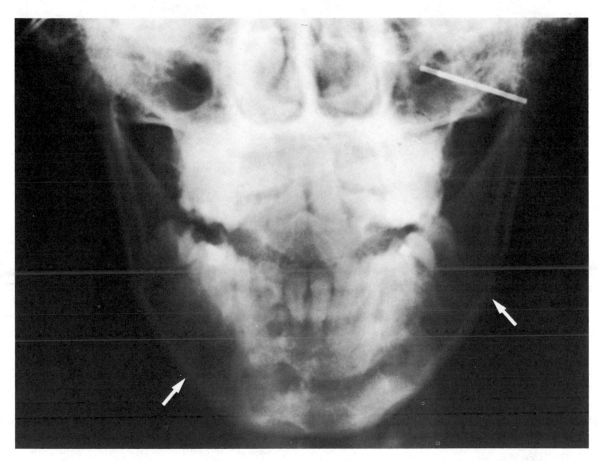

Figure 17.6 Posterior–anterior view of the mandible. This radiograph demonstrates the mandible from angle to angle and shows undisplaced fractures at the left angle and right premolar region (arrows). The radio-opaque structures are hair pins.

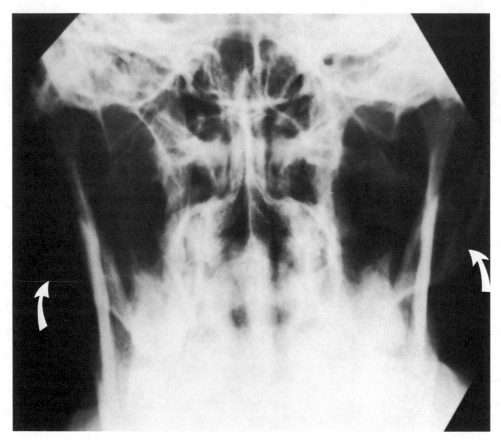

Figure 17.7 The Towne's view radiograph shows the ramus and condyles of the mandible in the medio-lateral plane. In this case, there are no fractures. We can also see the zygomatic arches (arrows).

be approximated with interrupted sutures of absorbable material, either 4-0 polyglycolic acid (Dexon) or chromic catgut. Subcutaneous or dermal sutures should be used so that the skin edges approximate easily without tension; these sutures should be used sparingly. Surgeons differ in their preference, but 4-0 white nylon is acceptable for subcutaneous or subcuticular closure of a clean wound; 6-0 nylon swedged on small cutting needles should be used for skin.

Complicated Lacerations and Other Soft Tissue Injuries

COMPLICATED LACERATIONS

Some facial lacerations are irregular in shape, stellate, or form a flap of tissue. When repairing an irregular laceration, do not anticipate a bad scar by performing a Z- or W-plasty to realign the wound in a more favorable direction with respect to skin tension lines. The scar can be revised months later if necessary. As described in Chapter 14, debridement of ragged edges of lacerations should be as conservative as possible, and every effort should be made to fit fragments together. On the other hand, beveled edges must be carefully trimmed. If a flap has been raised by the laceration, it should not be stitched tightly on all sides or the blood supply to the tip will be compromised. Sometimes Steri-Strips provide better closure than sutures for this type of laceration. If the wound is so small that it can be excised and closed primarily without tension, this method of treatment is very satisfactory. The excision should be in the form of an ellipse with its long axis in the direction of the skin tension line.

AVULSION WOUND

Small losses of tissue can sometimes be corrected by primary excision and closure. However, the defect may be so large that it will require skin graft or local flap. Such a procedure should be performed in an operating room by a specialist.

OLD OR CONTAMINATED WOUNDS

If a soft tissue wound has been open for more than 6 hours, a decision must be made whether or not to close it. With antibiotic therapy, thorough irrigation, and judicious debridement, a tidy, clean wound can be closed even after 24 hours. However, the patient and the physician must be aware that infection is a definite possibility. If in doubt, it is better to leave the wound open and treat it with dressings. In some cases, approximating the wound with Steri-Strips hastens the healing process.

A dog bite produces the most common "dirty wound" in the face. A puncture wound caused by a dog, or any other animal, should not be sutured, but bites that produce a laceration heal best if repaired primarily. Copious irrigation (at least 1,000 ml of normal saline or Ringer's lactated) is a prerequisite to success. The wound should be carefully debrided and penicillin should be given. If the wound is not recent or if the debridement would require sacrifice of a large amount of tissue, the wound should not be sutured, and a surgeon who is experienced in the management of such wounds should be consulted. Careful attention to tetanus prophylaxis is required, and any necessary rabies precautions must be observed (see Chapter 14).

MULTIPLE SMALL CUTS

Multiple small cuts were more common in the days before the shatterproof windshield, but they still occur. They should be

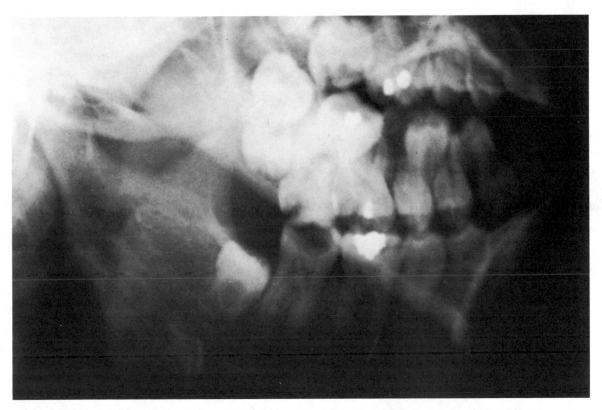

Figure 17.8 The lateral oblique x-ray of the mandible shows the condyle, sigmoid notch, coronoid process, and the body of the mandible in the molar region.

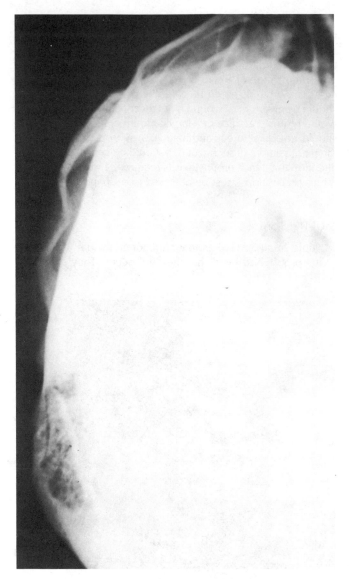

Figure 17.9 The submental vertex or "jug-handle" view illustrates the zygomatic arch and, in this case, shows a classic V-shaped depression of the zygomatic arch.

treated by minimal debridement, thorough irrigation, pressure dressing, and only a few sutures. Too many sutures will cause necrosis of the small flaps. Using magnifying lenses, wounds should be inspected carefully for small pieces of glass or other foreign bodies. An attempt should be made to remove all of the small fragments, but this is sometimes impossible. The patients should be told that glass may work its way out or, if necessary, additional removal may be required in the future. Many patients worry that some of the fragments will work their way into the blood stream. They should be reassured that this will not happen.

TATTOOING

Asphalt, dirt, grease, and gunpowder may enter the dermal and subcutaneous tissues and should be removed within 12 hours by scrubbing with a stiff, sterile hand brush. If foreign material is not removed carefully, it will remain in the tissue as a permanent tattoo. Local anesthesia can be used if the area is small, but general anesthesia is necessary for more extensive injuries. If the material cannot be completely removed by brushing, a No. 11 blade should be used to take the pieces out meticulously under lens magnification. Small amounts of ether or acetone are useful for dissolving grease and paint; the eyes must be carefully protected. If it is not possible to remove all of the debris, the patient should be informed that another operation may be necessary. The treated areas should be covered with an antibiotic ointment dressing.

Postoperative Care

If the patient is well enough to be discharged after soft tissue repair, he or she should be instructed in proper wound care. In general, dressings should be light; abrasion wounds can be left open and covered with antibiotic ointment. Initially, diet should consist of only fluids; soft foods may be added later. Chewing and jaw motion may pull skin against stitches and result in a poor scar. Warm saline intraoral rinses every few hours will help keep intraoral wounds clean.

Any patient with a facial injury should be instructed to return to or to call the emergency room if any of the following symptoms develop: increased pain, fever, nausea, vomiting, headache, diplopia, fainting, weakness, paralysis, slow pulse, or any symptoms suggesting intracranial damage or wound infection. A patient at risk for infection, for example a dog bite victim, should be advised to return in 24–48 hours.

Sutures on the face should be removed after 4 or 5 days; permanent "suture tracks" may result if they are left longer than 7 days. If a patient cannot return to the hospital but is to be checked elsewhere, he or she should be supplied with specific instructions and a summary of the diagnosis and treatment.

Soft Tissue Injuries in Specific Regions

INTRAORAL SOFT TISSUE INJURIES

For generations, it had been taught that intraoral lacerations should never be sutured. However, with the use of prophylactic antibiotics, these lacerations can now be closed. An intraoral wound that is sutured will bleed less and will result in improved soft tissue contour and greater comfort for the patient. For most mucosal and tongue lacerations 4-0 chromic catgut is a satisfactory material. For through-and-through lacerations, the intraoral portion should first be sutured loosely. Then the external portion of the wound may be draped and sutured in layers. The patient should be placed on penicillin or erythromycin prophylaxis (250 mg every 6 hours for 5 days), and the mouth should be rinsed with warm saline frequently in order to maintain optimal oral hygiene.

LIP

Lip lacerations should be repaired in three layers, beginning with mucosa, followed by muscle and then skin (Fig. 17.10). The first skin suture should be in the vermilion border. The mucous membrane, orbicularis, and subcutaneous tissue should be approximated with 4-0 chromic catgut and the skin with 6-0 nylon.

ELECTRICAL BURNS OF THE MOUTH

Electrical burns of the mouth usually occur in children between the ages of 6 months and 3 years. A typical situation is a mother who is interrupted in her ironing and disconnects the appliance plug but leaves the connection to the wall outlet. Her child then places the dangling end in his mouth. Although the contacts are not exposed, electrolytes in the saliva allow completion of the electrical circuit and transmit the current through the local tissues causing considerable destruction.

The oral mucosal burn may appear superficial; however, thrombosis propagates and causes necrosis (Fig. 17.11). Within a few hours, pronounced edema appears, and the injury may extend 2 cm or more beneath the visible edge of trauma. As vacuoles form in the vascular endothelium and intima, the likelihood of late rupture of vessels and hemorrhage increases. Significant bleeding may occur any time within 3 weeks in 25% of patients; therefore hospitalization for 6–21 days of observation is warranted. Although initial treatment is still controversial, most electrical burns are treated conservatively to allow delineation of necrosis and separation of the eschar. Neosporin or bacitracin ointment may be applied to the injured

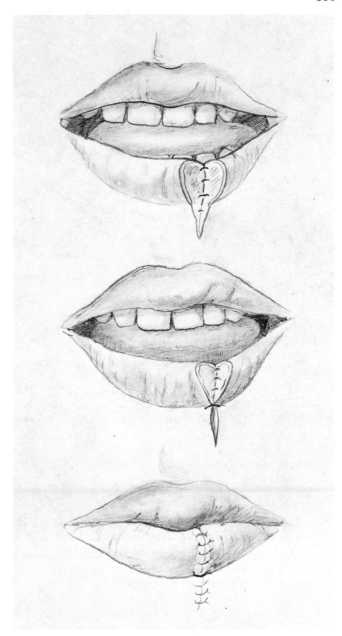

Figure 17.10 The technique of closure of a *through-and-through lip laceration* crossing the vermillion border is illustrated. The vermillion border should be tattooed by needle with methyl blue before anesthesia. Once the mucosal and muscle layers are approximated, skin closure can be started. The first skin sutures should approximate the vermillion border.

NOSE

Full thickness lacerations of the nose must be closed meticulously in layers. To approximate the nasal mucosa, 5-0 absorbable interrupted sutures are used; the knots are placed in the nasal cavity. A continuous subcuticular (intradermal) suture with 4-0 nylon can be used to approximate the skin. Alternatively, 6-0 nylon sutures can be placed in the skin.

EAR LACERATION

The ear has an excellent blood supply that frequently protects it even after severe jagged lacerations and partial avulsions. Flaps survive in spite of what appears to be a very narrow pedicle. For this reason, no part of the ear should be excised during debridement unless it is definitely necrotic. It is essential that hemostasis be precise in order to avoid postrepair hematomas and resultant damage to the underlying cartilage.

Lacerations that involve only the skin can be sutured in the emergency room with 6-0 nylon using a field block around the base of the ear for anesthesia (1% lidocaine with epinephrine 1:200,000). For a simple laceration involving the cartilage, repair should include reapproximation of the cartilage with 5-0 absorbable sutures. If there has been significant full-thickness loss of the ear, if a large area of cartilage is exposed, or if an avulsed segment of the ear has been brought in for reattachment, a surgeon who is experienced in such care should be called. By means of local flaps or storage of the cartilage, the valuable framework of the ear can be preserved to be used for later reconstruction.

HEMATOMA OF THE EXTERNAL EAR

Hematoma of the external ear usually occurs after blunt trauma or a shearing-type injury. The hematoma is subperichondral and is typically fluctuant and purplish in color. Ice packs for 24 hours and oral penicillin, 250 mg 4 times daily for 5 days, are indicated. The patient should be referred to an otolaryngologist or plastic surgeon within 24 hours so that definitive surgical drainage and stenting can be performed.

Careful application of a pressure dressing to an injured ear after it has been repaired is an important factor in the prevention of a seroma or hematoma. A drain between the skin and cartilage may also be used. To create a pressure dressing, moistened pieces of cotton are placed behind the ear and into the convolutions of the auricle. The ear is then covered with fluffed gauze and the head is wrapped with a dressing of gauze and Ace bandage. After 48–72 hours, the ear is inspected.

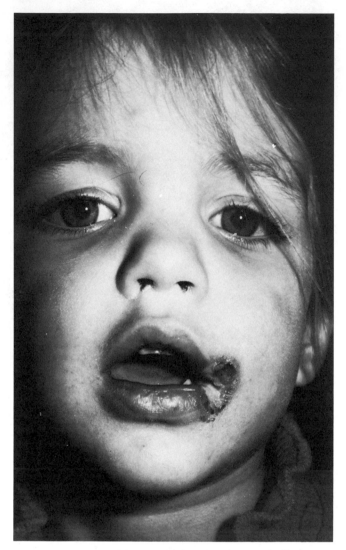

Figure 17.11 Electrical burn of the lip. This photograph illustrates a young girl with an electrical burn in the left labial commissure. This is a typical location of these injuries in children.

area two or three times a day; the patient should be restrained at night to prevent rubbing the burn on the bed coverings, and should be fed with a cleft lip feeder. Whenever possible, a plastic surgeon should be called in immediately because what appears to be a superficial burn may result later in a severe deformity.

EYELID

Any wound of the eyelid mandates a careful examination of the eye to rule out ocular injury (see Chapters 18 and 31). If a laceration involves the tarsal plate of the eyelid at its free edge or the medial aspect of the eyelid, it should be repaired by an ophthalmologist, a plastic surgeon or an experienced general surgeon. Medial injuries of the eyelid are often associated with injuries of the medial canthal ligament and/or the lacrimal duct. These injuries must be recognized and repaired by a specialist. Simple lacerations of the eyelid skin heal well if they are carefully sutured. If a laceration involves the eyebrow, it should be carefully cleaned but the eyebrow should never be shaved. It must be carefully aligned in order to prevent an obvious step deformity. Minimal debridement should be carried out in the region of the eyebrow, even in the presence of complicated lacerations with small flaps. Repair is described in Chapter 18.

FACIAL NERVE INJURY

Every patient with facial injuries should receive careful evaluation of facial nerve function although damage to the facial nerve is rather infrequent because of its position between the lobes of the parotid gland. Occasionally, paresis of the facial nerve or its branches results simply from hematoma formation or from contusion. When in doubt, the physician should refer the patient to a surgeon experienced in the treatment of facial nerve injuries for diagnosis and repair. Branches of the facial nerve that are severed between the stylomastoid foramen and a vertical line dropped from the lateral canthus of the eyelids should be repaired primarily. The terminal nerve branches anterior to that line will usually regenerate satisfactorily if the soft tissues are approximated. A facial nerve repair should be carried out in the operating room within 72 hours.

PAROTID DUCT LACERATION

The parotid duct lies beneath the middle one-third of a line drawn from the tragus of the ear to the midportion of the upper lip (Fig. 17.2). If damage to this duct is suspected because of the location of the laceration, a small polyethylene tube or lacrimal duct probe can be passed into the parotid duct orifice on the buccal mucosa opposite the upper first and second molar teeth. Laceration of the duct is diagnosed by the appearance of the tube in the wound. When possible, the parotid duct should be repaired early; this requires the facilities of the main operating room as well as the skills of a trained specialist.

Failure to recognize a parotid duct laceration may result in a sialocutaneous fistula or a sialocele.

EMERGENCY ROOM MANAGEMENT OF FACIAL FRACTURES

Nasal Fractures

DIAGNOSIS

Nasal fractures, the most common facial fractures in adults and children, may occur as isolated injuries or in combination with fractures of other facial bones. The patient who presents with a history of trauma to the nose should be questioned about the direction and nature of the force that caused the injury and about any possible preexisting nasal deformity or nasal obstruction. Nasal fracture may be indicated by deviation or depression of the bone, ecchymosis, swelling, or nosebleed. A deviated septum, constricted airway, or septal hematoma may be seen on intranasal examination, and subconjunctival hemorrhage or periorbital ecchymosis with edema is common several hours after the injury. One must be careful not to miss a nasal fracture in which the cartilage is telescoped up and under the nasal bone. In this type of injury, the nasolabial angle may be increased and there may be a step deformity at the junction of the septum and nasal bone. The injury site is tender and crepitus is noted on palpation.

Although the standard x-ray films (lateral nasal and Water's view) are necessary for documenting the injury and are possibly desirable for medicolegal reasons, they are not particularly helpful as a diagnostic tool. Delineating the area radiographically is difficult, and because fracture lines do not calcify as they heal, new fractures cannot be distinguished from old ones.

MANAGEMENT

By nasal speculum examination, the emergency room physician must determine whether or not there is a septal hematoma. A specialist should drain a widened and fluctuant septum within several hours. The patient should be started on antibiotics against the normal gram-positive nasal flora. If a hematoma becomes infected, an abscess forms and the septal cartilage becomes necrotic within 24–48 hours, resulting in loss of support of the nasal tip and a saddle-nose deformity.

The results of treatment of nasal fractures are often poor. Since the problem may be a difficult one, even for the experienced physician, it is usually best for these fractures to be treated by surgeons who are experienced in nasal surgery. The emergency room physician should instruct the patient to place iced saline sponges or ice packs over the nose and eyes and to keep the head elevated on several pillows when asleep or resting. This will minimize posttraumatic swelling. The patient should be started on dicloxacillin, 500 mg every 6 hours, or for patients who are penicillin-allergic the same dosage of erythromycin. A decongestant should be started, and the patient should be instructed not to blow his or her nose and not to smoke. The patient should be referred to a surgeon to reduce the fracture in 5–10 days, after the swelling has decreased.

If the nasal fracture is to be reduced in the emergency room, the patient should be supine on the operating table. After he or she has been adequately sedated with an agent such as intravenous diazepam or a combination of diazepam and meperidine HCl (Demerol), the face should be washed with plain soap and water. After the exact nature of the deformity has been determined, topical cocaine (5 or 10%) is used to provide anesthesia and to induce vasoconstriction in the mucous membranes. This is applied by 3-in. rolled cotton pledgets soaked with the agent and thoroughly squeezed out to remove excess solution. Under direct visualization, one pack is placed along the floor of the nose, another along the middle turbinate, and a third along the roof. The external nose is anesthetized by bilateral infraorbital nerve blocks with lidocaine, 1% with 1:100,000 epinephrine and by infiltrating the same agent across the base of the columella and across the glabella region. It is important to wait 15–20 minutes in order to achieve complete anesthesia before the reduction is carried out.

One hand should hold a closed Kelly clamp, covered with a thin piece of rubber tubing, to mobilize and reduce the nasal fracture while the other hand simultaneously molds the nose under direct palpation. Walsham forceps can also be used for this maneuver. If the septum is deviated, an Asch forceps is the best instrument to use to manipulate the nasal bones and septum into position while the fingers of the left hand palpate the bridge of the nose and function as a guide. After careful observation and palpation confirm the fact that the nasal pyramid and the septum are in the midline, nasal packs of petroleum-impregnated gauze should be inserted into the nasal airway to support the fractured bones (without displacing the nasal bones laterally) and to prevent hematomas. A nasal splint made of plaster of paris or a commercially available metal or plastic splint should be placed on the external surface of the nose in order to protect it. The nasal pack should be removed after 48 hours and the splint after 5–7 days. If the septum is injured, the patient should be warned that a nasal deformity may develop gradually over a period of months, and further reconstructive surgery may be necessary.

PROGNOSIS

The prognosis for nasal fractures depends on the severity of injury. In noncomminuted fractures, the prognosis is excellent. After adequate reduction, no further treatment should be necessary. In comminuted fractures and those in which there is a septal hematoma, a varying degree of nasal deformity may occur postreduction and may require further reconstructive surgery.

Maxillary and Midface Fractures

Fractures of the maxilla are less common than those of the mandible. They are often the result of high-speed motor vehicle trauma and, as a consequence, are often associated with skull, central nervous system, chest, or abdominal injury. The most common associated problem involves a dural tear manifested by cerebrospinal fluid rhinorrhea or otorrhea.

Because of the maxilla's relationship to the base of the skull, it is able to absorb and withstand great compressive forces without being fractured. Therefore maxillary injuries rarely occur from a blow to the chin driving the mandible upward into the maxilla. Maxillary and midface injuries most commonly occur from a shearing-type blow delivered from an anterior direction. The patterns of midface fractures were investigated and classified at the turn of the century by Rene Le Fort (Fig. 17.12). The *Le Fort I fracture* is a transverse fracture of the maxilla above the palate and roots of the teeth. The *Le Fort II fracture* is one in which the fractured segment, shaped like a pyramid, contains the nasal bones and the frontal process of the maxilla, as well as the palate, teeth, and lateral walls of the maxillary sinus. The fracture lines usually run through the lacrymal bones and inferior rim of the orbit and extend obliquely and inferiorly along the edge of the maxilla toward the pterygomaxillary fissure. The *Le Fort III fracture* is craniofacial dysjunction. The maxilla, nasal bones, and zygomatic bones will move as a unit from the base of the skull.

DIAGNOSIS

The patient with a midface fracture usually has marked swelling of the upper face with periorbital ecchymosis and edema (Fig. 17.13). In fractures at the Le Fort II level, there may be a significant widening of the inner canthus of the eyes. The patient should be observed in profile for elongation of the middle third of the face and for possible telescoping inward of the nose and midface. A midface fracture may cause the nose to look "cute" or "infantile" when actually the nose has been

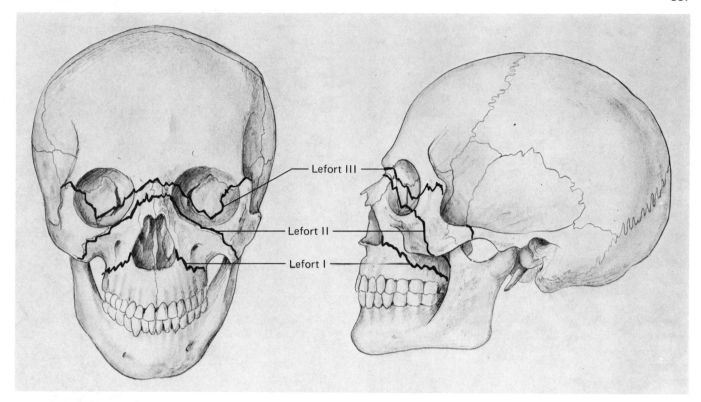

Figure 17.12 Le Fort fracture line. Frontal and lateral views of the skull illustrating the fracture lines of the Le Fort I, II, and III injuries.

foreshortened by the retrodisplacement of the midportion of the face.

Palpation will reveal a mobile segment containing the upper teeth, the palate, and part of the wall of the maxillary sinus (Le Fort I). Using one hand for intraoral palpation while placing the other hand at the frontonasal suture will reveal mobility of the lower maxilla, infraorbital rims, and nasomaxillary complex as one unit. Movement across the frontonasal suture completes the findings at the Le Fort II level (Fig. 17.14A). Using one hand for intraoral palpation while moving the other hand from the frontonasal suture to the frontozygomatic sutures on both sides will reveal movement of the entire midface complex in relation to the cranium in the Le Fort III fracture (Fig. 17.14B).

Sensation should be tested along the distribution of the infraorbital nerve that, in the Le Fort II fracture, may be injured at the infraorbital foramen. The patient's occlusion and the occlusal plane should be observed as described for mandibular fractures, and the patient's subjective evaluation of his or her occlusion should also be determined.

Cerebrospinal fluid rhinorrhea, resulting from damage to the cribriform plate, may accompany a midface fracture and should be suspected if watery fluid drains from the nose or if the patient reports a salty taste in his or her mouth. Cerebrospinal fluid may be suspected if the discharge stiffens a fresh piece of linen on drying. Compared with blood, cerebrospinal fluid contains less protein, uric acid, and sugar but more chloride; the high chloride content is responsible for the salty taste.

The initial x-ray films should consist of a Water's view to evaluate the status of the orbits, orbital rims, and maxillary sinuses (Fig. 17.15). A posterior–anterior view of the skull is very helpful to visualize the frontal sinuses, the supraorbital rims, and the frontozygomatic sutures. In addition, a lateral

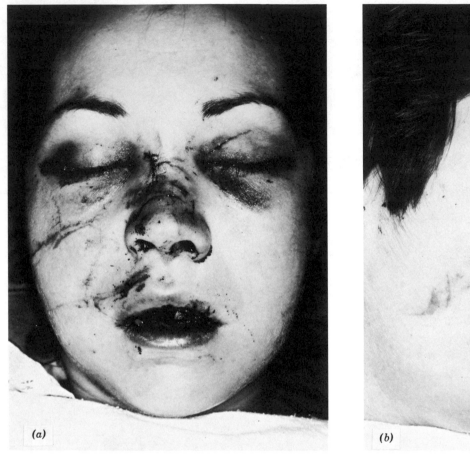
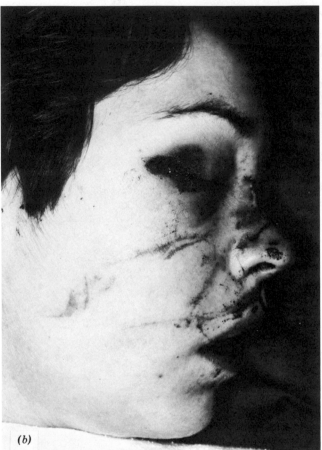

Figure 17.13 Midface fractures. Examination of this patient with a Le Fort III fracture shows bilateral periorbital ecchymosis and edema (the "panda bear" facies) and elongation of the middle one-third of the face.

skull film will illustrate elongation of the midface and tilting of the maxillary occlusal plane.

Although the three patterns of midface fractures described by Le Fort are convenient for classification, variations commonly occur and the fracture should be precisely described. For example, the patient may have a maxillary fracture at the Le Fort III level on one side but a Le Fort I or II level fracture on the other side. In addition, there may be fractures in the midline separating the two sides and there may be severe comminution.

MANAGEMENT

The early treatment of midface and maxillary fractures is similar to that described later in this chapter for mandibular fractures. Oral intake is restricted to clear liquids or is totally stopped. Intravenous penicillin (1,000,000 units) is given every 6 hours, and the patient is placed in a head upright position with ice packs applied to the upper part of the face bilaterally. Close observation is essential for the first 24–48 hours because of the possibility of associated central nervous system or other injuries. The definitive treatment of maxillary fractures requires the same concern for occlusion as described in the treatment of mandibular fractures. In reducing these fractures, we must consider the complex interrelationships among the occlusion, the nasomaxillary complex, orbits, the medial and lateral canthi, and facial aesthetics. For this reason, definitive treatment should be delayed until it can be carried out by an appropriately trained specialist.

PROGNOSIS

The prognosis for midface fractures depends on the severity of the initial injury, that is, the degree of soft tissue damage and the degree of comminution of the bony fragments. There is no question that the best chance for a successful outcome is the first one. It is therefore imperative that a patient with a midface fracture be treated within 5–10 days after injury by a surgeon

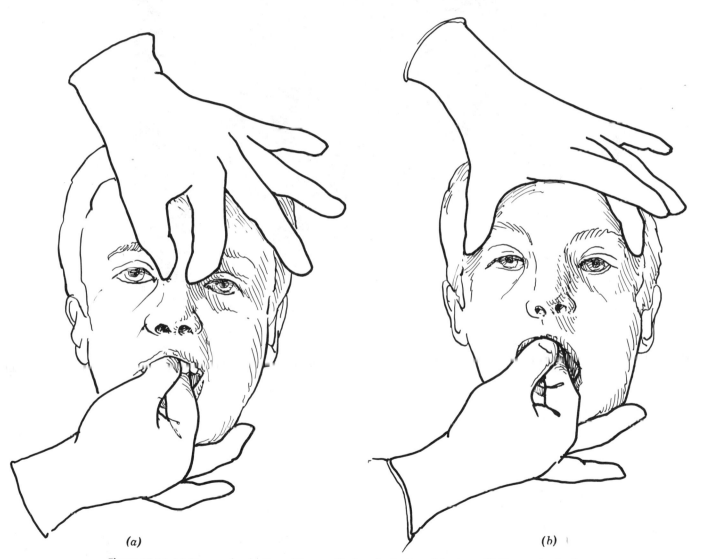

(a)   *(b)*

Figure 17.14 (a) Bimanual palpation of the maxilla for a Le Fort I or II fracture. (b) Bimanual palpation of the midface for a Le Fort III fracture.

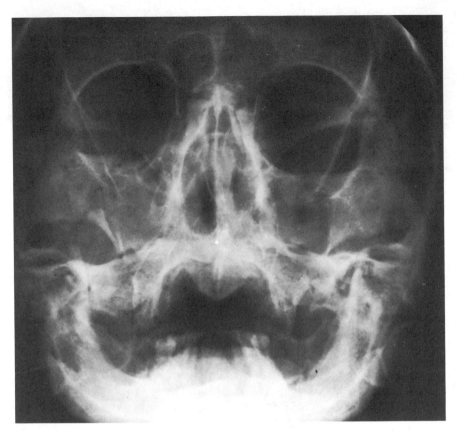

Figure 17.15 Water's view roentgenogram of a patient with a Le Fort III injury demonstrates fractures at the frontozygomatic suture, the infraorbital rims, the nasofrontal suture, and opacification of both maxillary sinuses.

experienced in the treatment of these fractures. If treatment is directed toward reestablishing the correct facial proportions, occlusion, projection of zygomatic bones, and integrity of the orbital floor, then the ultimate outcome will be favorable, even if secondary reconstructive procedures are required.

Inadequate or poor early treatment, resulting in elongation of the middle third of the face, malocclusion, or enophthalmos, is difficult to correct at a later stage.

Zygomatic Complex and Zygomatic Arch Fractures

The zygoma has a thick, long, central portion known as the buttress and four projections that articulate with the maxilla, temporal bone, greater wing of the sphenoid, and frontal bone.

Discontinuity usually occurs at the junction of the zygoma with the other bones. Twenty percent of zygomatic fractures do not result in significant displacement and 10% affect only the zygomatic arch; the other 70% result in depression with or without rotation.

DIAGNOSIS

If the zygomatic complex is fractured, swelling and ecchymosis are seen in the periorbital area, and the malar region appears flat, particularly when observed from above or below (Fig. 17.16). The lateral canthus has an antimongoloid slant (Fig. 17.17)resulting from depression of the lateral portion of the orbital rim; subconjunctival hemorrhage and enophthalmos are present. The zygomaticofrontal, maxillary, and temporal

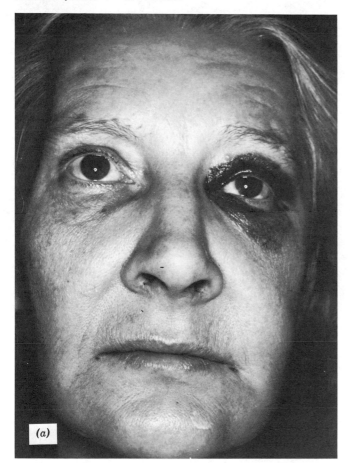

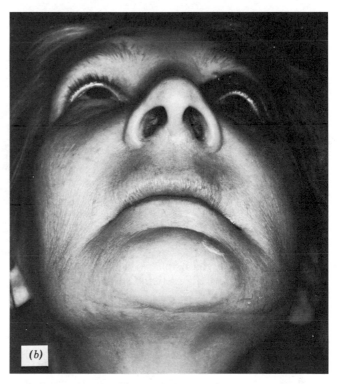

Figure 17.16 (a) Examination of a patient with zygomatic complex fracture reveals periorbital ecchymosis and swelling, antimongoloid slant of the lateral canthus. (b) Examination from below reveals the flatness of the left cheek bone.

sutures are tender, and a separation or step deformity may be appreciated in these areas. The anterior wall of the maxilla is tender on intraoral palpation, and crepitus may be noted; the inferior portion of the zygomatic buttress may be separated or irregular above the posterior maxillary teeth. Neurologic examination often reveals paresthesia or anesthesia in the distribution of the second division of the trigeminal nerve. A test of extraocular muscle function may indicate entrapment of the inferior oblique and inferior rectus muscles in the fracture of the floor of the orbit.

A fracture confined to the *zygomatic arch* may occur as an isolated injury and is most often secondary to a blow directly over the arch. These fractures present with none of the orbital signs and symptoms associated with a fracture of the zygomatic complex. Rather, patients may report pain when they open their jaws and may have only limited motion. The arch fracture causes pain when the mouth is opened because of the relationship of the arch to the coronoid process and temporalis muscle. The zygomatic arch may be ignored because of these symptoms, and x-ray films of the mandible and temporomandibular joint are incorrectly ordered.

When a zygomatic complex fracture is suspected, it can be confirmed radiologically with a Water's or a submental vertex roentgenogram (Figs. 17.18 and 17.9). A submental vertex

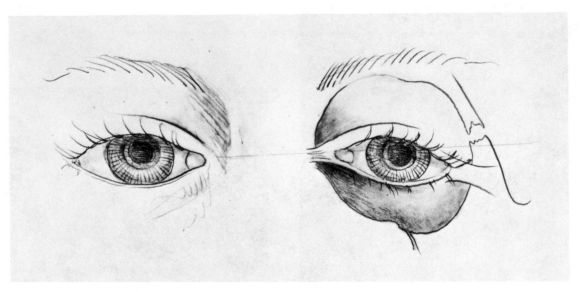

Figure 17.17 Schematic representation of the underlying injury in the patient shown in Figure 17.16.

(jug-handle) view may be helpful in demonstrating the relationship of the zygomatic arch to the coronoid process.

MANAGEMENT

Fractures of the zygomatic bone with significant displacement are usually reduced under general anesthesia. The procedure is performed on a semielective basis after the swelling subsides and the facial aesthetics are evaluated. During the waiting period, the patient is placed on decongestants and antibiotics because of the violated maxillary sinus. The antibiotic of choice is penicillin (250 mg by mouth every 6 hours). Zygomatic arch fractures are treated if the fracture prevents jaw opening or if it produces an aesthetic deformity. These fractures can be treated early, before the onset of maximum swelling, or after 5 days. They are usually reduced by a specialist.

Blow-Out Fractures

The term *blow-out fracture,* coined by Converse and Smith in 1957, refers to a fracture of the orbital floor without a fracture of the orbital rim or zygoma. The term is now used to include isolated fractures of the medial wall of the orbit. The injury is usually caused by a direct blow from a nonpenetrating object larger than the orbital opening (e.g., a fist or tennis ball). The orbital contents are compressed and driven posteriorly into the smaller portion of the orbital cone. The resultant increased

intraorbital pressure causes the weak floor or medial wall to "blow out." Recently, it has been shown that blow-out fractures may also result from an oblique or shearing blow to the zygomatic bone.

DIAGNOSIS

Periorbital ecchymosis, edema, and subconjunctival hemorrhage are seen on examination; chemosis is common. Orbital fat may herniate into the maxillary antrum, resulting in enophthalmos. When the inferior rectus and inferior oblique muscles become entrapped, limitation of ocular movement occurs, particularly in upward gaze (Fig. 17.19). Occasionally, downward gaze is also limited. The presence of diplopia is not necessary for the diagnosis nor is the finding an absolute confirmation of the diagnosis since transient double vision may occur without fracture.

The eye should be examined very carefully for the presence of hyphema, laceration of the globe, retinal tears, or other injuries (see Chapters 18 and 31). In addition, sensation in the distribution of the infraorbital nerve should be tested carefully since paresthesia or anesthesia of this nerve usually occurs (the infraorbital nerve courses along the floor of the orbit before it exits from the infraorbital foramen). Visual acuity should be assessed, and the orbital rim should be carefully palpated in order to detect a separation or fracture.

A Water's view is helpful in the diagnosis of blow-out frac-

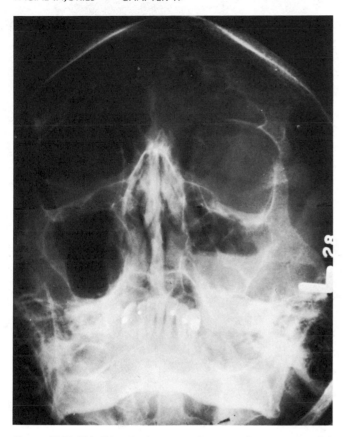

Figure 17.18 This Water's view roentgenogram demonstrates a left zygomatic complex fracture. Note the inward displacement of the frontozygomatic suture, downward displacement of the infraorbital rim, and the air–fluid level in the left maxillary sinus.

tures (Fig. 17.5). Typically, the x-ray film reveals cloudiness and a "hanging drop" of orbital contents in the maxillary sinus. Orbital tomograms in the posteroanterior (PA) and lateral planes are helpful to delineate the size and location of the orbital floor defect.

MANAGEMENT

Whenever a patient sustains trauma to the orbit and/or globe, an ophthalmologist should be called to evaluate these structures and the patient's vision. Once the diagnosis of blow-out fracture is made, the patient is usually observed for several days while the swelling resolves.

Ice packs or iced compresses should be applied to the orbit,

and the patient should be placed on decongestants and antibiotics because of the potential for infection in the violated maxillary sinus. Patients should sleep with their heads elevated and should not blow their noses; if they do, subcutaneous emphysema may increase and further contaminate the traumatized tissue planes. A decision about surgery is made after several days, when enophthalmos, extraocular muscle function, diplopia, and infraorbital nerve paresthesia have been evaluated. Indications for surgical repair are quite controversial; in brief, the decision to operate is usually made on the basis of severe enophthalmos, persistent severe limitation of extraocular muscle movement, and persistent anesthesia or paresthesia (also see Chapter 18).

Mandibular Fractures

Mandibular fractures are the most common facial fractures that require patients to be admitted to the hospital. Because of the great force required to fracture the mandible, associated injuries are frequently found in these patients. Cervical spine injury, particularly, should be ruled out when the mandibular symphysis and condyles are involved (Fig. 17.20).

DIAGNOSIS

In patients with a history of trauma to the mandible resulting in pain, swelling, and difficulty opening their jaws, the most significant finding is the complaint that their bite is changed. Swelling and ecchymosis, contusion, or laceration may mark the site of impact. Gross malocclusion may be visible when the mouth is closed (Fig. 17.21); abnormal interdigitation of the cusps of the teeth or nonalignment of "wear" facets is evidence of a change in bite and thus a fracture. Ecchymosis and hematoma are seen in the floor of the mouth and in the buccal vestibule near the fracture site; the floor of the mouth may be elevated secondary to hematoma or edema, and the gingiva overlying the fracture may be lacerated. Trismus, which prevents the patient from opening the mouth, may make detection of a fracture difficult. Limited opening or deviation on opening may be a result of a fracture in the condylar region, but it may also be a result of a hematoma in the joint space. On palpation, the site of the blow and, if the condyles are involved, the temporomandibular joint region are tender. The teeth in the line of fracture are mobile and tender, and bimanual palpation demonstrates mobility of the mandible across the fracture site (Fig. 17.22). Neurologic examination reveals paresthesia or frank anesthesia in the distribution of the inferior alveolar nerve (the third division of the trigeminal) on the side of the fracture.

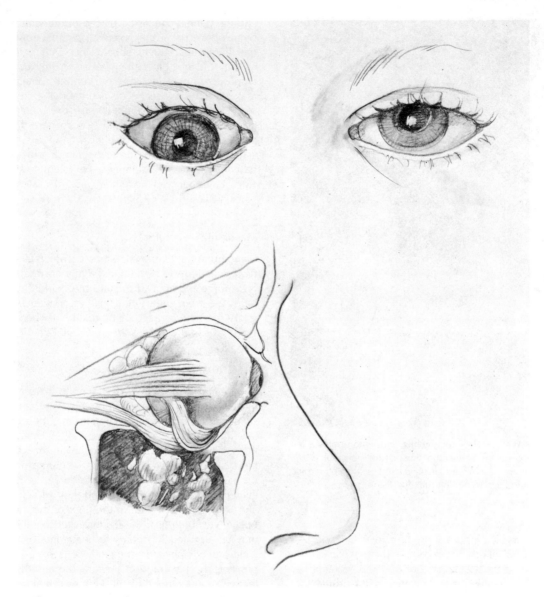

Figure 17.19 Frontal view (top) shows the restriction in upward gaze of the right globe secondary to entrapment of the inferior oblique-inferior rectus muscles. Lateral view (bottom) shows the muscles and periorbital fat herniated down into the maxillary sinus.

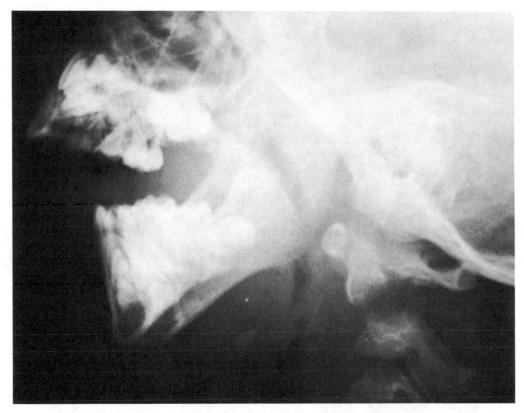

Figure 17.20 This lateral skull and cervical spine radiograph shows an anteriorly displaced odontoid process (C-2) fracture. Note that the mandible is retrognathic and there is an open bite. This is evidence of bilateral subcondylar and mandibular symphysis fractures, although they do not show on this radiograph.

The ramus and subcondylar region, where the bone is thinnest, are the most common sites of mandibular fracture. In fact, two-thirds of all fractures occur within an area bounded by the third molar, the angle, and the condyles. The symphysis, on the other hand, is fractured infrequently because of its thickness. A blow that produces a symphyseal injury drives the mandible posteriorly and superiorly, wedging the condyles against the base of the skull; unilateral or bilateral subcondylar fractures often result. When the symphysis is fractured, the potential for airway obstruction is great, and the patient should be positioned with head elevated and closely observed for respiratory distress.

Fractures in the subcondylar region may be difficult to detect, particularly when trismus prevents movement of the jaw. A swollen, discolored, or lacerated auditory canal may serve as a clue to this injury. When there is a unilateral subcondylar fracture, the jaw will deviate toward the side of fracture on opening because of asymmetric lateral pterygoid muscle action. When the fracture is bilateral, an anterior open bite results from the downward rotation of the body of the mandible by the suprahyoid muscles. Retrusion of the mandible is also common in the presence of bilateral subcondylar fractures.

X-ray films are helpful adjuncts in the diagnosis of mandibular fractures. The standard mandibular views are the posterior–anterior, right and left lateral oblique, and the Towne's view (Figs 17.6, 17.7, 17.8). The posterior–anterior radiograph shows the body from angle to angle. The right and left lateral oblique x-ray films show the ramus of the mandible, condyle,

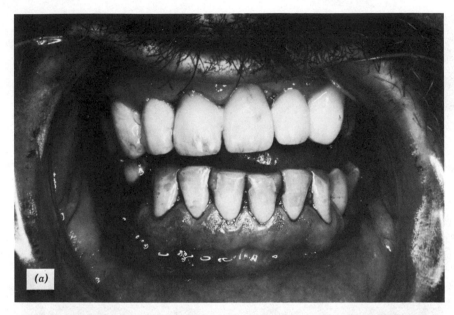

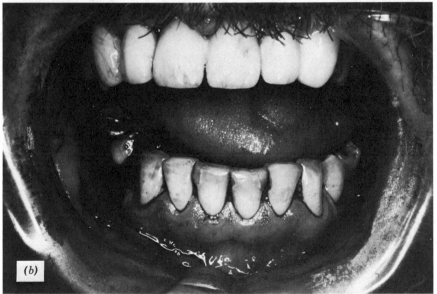

Figure 17.21 This photograph illustrates the intraoral examination in a patient with bilateral mandibular fractures. (a) There is a gross malocclusion with abnormal interdigitation of the teeth and an open bite on one side. (b) The limitation of opening of the jaw (trismus) is shown.

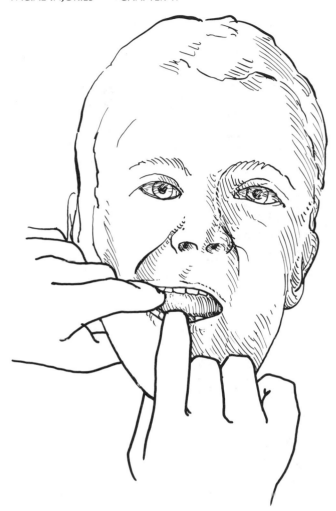

Figure 17.22 Illustration of the bimanual palpation of the mandible.

MANAGEMENT

Oral intake is reduced to clear liquids or is stopped. Moving the jaw in an attempt to chew or swallow food tends to pump bacteria into the fracture sites and into any open intraoral wounds. Since almost all mandibular fractures are compound into the mouth and contaminated by oral flora, antibiotic therapy consisting of 1,000,000 units of penicillin G intravenously every 6 hours is begun. Erythromycin or clindamycin may be used in patients allergic to penicillin. Temporary stabilization with a single wire around the teeth adjacent to the fracture site or with an arch bar should be attempted if a gross malocclusion is present or if there is a fracture of the symphysis of the mandible with collapse of support and respiratory difficulty. This is usually done by an oral surgical specialist. If the fracture is undisplaced and minimally mobile and the patient is having no respiratory difficulty, temporary stabilization is not necessary, and no further treatment need be carried out during the immediate postinjury period. Once the preliminary measures are carried out, the patient is usually referred to a specialist trained in the management of maxillofacial injuries.

The goal of treatment of subcondylar fractures of the mandible is to achieve a mobile, functioning joint and to maintain the height of the mandibular ramus. Immobilization for 4–6 weeks in the presence of a high subcondylar or intraarticular fracture may result in a stiff joint with a fibrous or bony ankylosis. In order to avoid this complication, subcondylar fractures are treated with minimal immobilization. Patients with unilateral subcondylar fractures may be treated with a liquid diet and analgesics alone. They are closely observed and are not immobilized unless a malocclusion develops. Patients with bilateral subcondylar fractures usually require a short period of intermaxillary fixation (2 weeks) and then exercises to maintain function. For patients with isolated subcondylar fractures, the emergency room physician need only to start the patient on a liquid diet and analgesics and to put ice on the area for 24–36 hours followed by heat. The patient should be referred to an oral surgeon for follow-up within 24 hours.

Mandibular fractures in children are often nondisplaced and are treated conservatively with 3 weeks of intermaxillary fixation using arch bars or interdental wiring. Open reduction is avoided because it may damage tooth buds in the body of the mandible. It is especially important for children to be treated and followed-up by an experienced specialist because of potential problems with growth.

Dislocation of the Jaw

The mandible articulates with the base of the skull at the temporomandibular joint (Fig. 17.1). This is an unusual joint in

sigmoid notch, coronoid process, and the molar regions. The Towne's view is an anterior–posterior x-ray film with the head tilted to project the petrous ridges and the mastoid processes away from the condyles. In this x-ray film, the posterior portion of the ramus of the mandible, the condylar neck, and the head of the condyle can be seen. A panoramic x-ray film is very helpful, but many hospitals do not have the machine and the patient must be ambulatory. This view, however, does give the clearest picture of the mandible and is most helpful diagnostically.

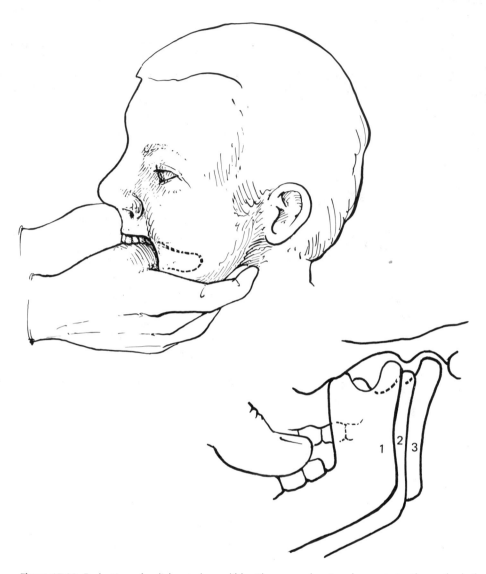

Figure 17.23 Reduction of a dislocated mandible. The upper drawing demonstrates the method of grasping the jaw in order to relocate it. The lower drawing demonstrtes the path taken by the mandible as the bone is pushed inferiorly to clear the articular tubercle. It is then manipulated posteriorly and superiorly back into the glenoid fossa.

that the right and left sides work simultaneously and must be perfectly coordinated. Its anterior aspect is bounded by the articular tubercle of the temporal bone. Initial opening of the jaw occurs on a hinge axis, and there is no anterior translation. Once hinge opening reaches its maximum, however, the mandible translates anteriorly.

Dislocation of the mandible occurs when the condylar head of the mandible moves out of the glenoid fossa anterior to the articular tubercle. It may be caused by a sudden uncontrolled movement such as yawning, laughing with the mouth wide open, coughing, or vomiting. Other etiologic factors commonly seen are trauma, prolonged wide opening of the mouth during induction of general anesthesia, or involuntary movements in patients taking prochlorperazine (Compazine) or other phenothiazines.

DIAGNOSIS

Dislocation of the jaw has occurred when the jaw is locked in the open position. X-Ray films of the mandible are only helpful to rule out fractures when the etiology is trauma. A panoramic x-ray film is most revealing; if this is not available, however, temporomandibular joint views will suffice.

MANAGEMENT

Therapy for a dislocated mandible is directly related to the anatomy and muscle function. With the patient sitting upright in a chair, the physician should stand above and manipulate the mandible into its normal position. Having another person hold the patient's head is often helpful. The mandible which is grasped between the thumb and index finger, is pushed downward until it clears the articular tubercle and is then rotated upward and posteriorly into the glenoid fossa (Fig. 17.23). The jaw should be held in the patient's proper occlusion. If the lateral pterygoid muscles are in spasm, repositioning the jaw may be difficult or impossible without general anesthesia. Once the mandible has been relocated, movement of the jaw should be limited to minimize the chance of recurrent dislocation. A soft diet and muscle relaxant such as diazepam,

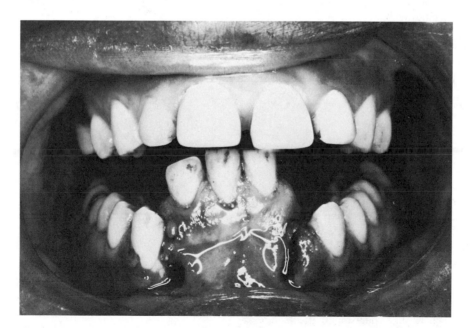

Figure 17.24 Dentoalveolar segment trauma. Intraoral examination reveals a gross malocclusion secondary to fracture and displacement of the mandibular anterior segment with three incisor teeth. The segment was reduced then stabilized with an arch bar wired to the mandibular teeth.

5–10 mg twice a day, are appropriate, and heat therapy is helpful. The patient should be instructed to place a fist under his or her chin to prevent the jaw from opening too wide when he or she yawns, for example. A dislocation that recurs requires immobilization by intermaxillary fixation for 7 days, after which the jaw should be released and allowed to function.

The emergency room physician should attempt to relocate a dislocated jaw as described above without premedication. If this attempt is unsuccessful or if the jaw dislocates again, an oral surgeon should be consulted to treat the patient.

Trauma to the Teeth and Dentoalveolar Segments

Trauma to the teeth and dentoalveolar segments are probably the most common injuries in the facial region. They occur most frequently in children and are the result of a direct blow to the dentoalveolar segments. The most common location is the maxillary anterior region, followed by the mandibular anterior region. The posterior dentoalveolar segments are less commonly involved. These injuries may be associated with fractures of the teeth or jaws and with lacerations of the buccal mucosa, gums, or lips.

Dental injuries consisting of fracture or avulsion of teeth are commonly treated in dental offices, but they may also be seen in patients in emergency rooms. They are usually the result of a fall from a bicycle, steps, or jungle-gym-type apparatus. Other common etiologic factors include athletic injuries or fist fights.

DIAGNOSIS

Dentoalveolar segment injuries are usually quite obvious. The patient complains of a malocclusion and, on physical examination, the teeth and underlying bony segments are out of position and mobile. The overlying gingiva is usually lacerated (Fig. 17.24). A panoramic x-ray film is helpful to document the position of the fractured alveolar segment and to evaluate the status of the teeth within it.

A fracture in a tooth may be superficial, affecting only the enamel (the outer covering of the crown), or it may involve the dentin, pulp, or root (Fig. 17.25). The extent of the fracture is important because it affects the initial symptoms and treatment, as well as the prognosis for the tooth. If only the enamel is involved, the patient is asymptomatic because the enamel does not have nerves. A fracture into the dentin commonly

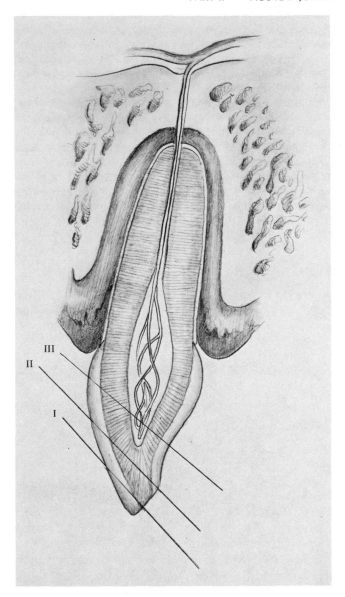

Figure 17.25 A cross section of a maxillary incisor tooth showing levels of fracture that may occur. A class I fracture is into the enamel. A class II fracture is into the dentin. A class III fracture is into the pulp.

causes sensitivity when exposed to changes in or extremes of temperature, to air or to sweets; the pain is much like that associated with dental caries. The yellowish color of the dentin is visible on examination.

Sensitivity when the tooth is percussed or tapped by an instrument is typical when a fracture extends into the pulp, and the pink color of the pulp tissue may be visible. Sensitivity to a thermal, chemical, or physical stimulus and continuous pain are common, and the pulp may bleed.

A fracture of the root can usually be diagnosed by the extreme mobility of the tooth and pain on palpation or percussion. A dental x-ray film is necessary to locate the fracture.

Teeth that are extruded or partially avulsed are visibly malpositioned and mobile. Occlusion may be affected, and the patient is aware of the abnormality of the bite. Because the root of such a tooth may be fractured, x-ray films are necessary. Teeth may also be totally avulsed from their sockets.

MANAGEMENT

Dentoalveolar injuries are treated by reducing the fractured segment and stabilizing it with an arch bar (Figs. 17.26 and 17.27). This procedure should be performed by a dentist or oral surgeon as soon as possible after the injury in order to salvage the teeth and bone. Occasionally, an acrylic splint is fabricated after dental impressions have been taken. The patient is placed on prophylactic penicillin or erythromycin for 5–7 days and should remain on a liquid diet for 3 weeks. The diet may then be advanced and the arch bars removed after 4 weeks. The emergency room physician should manually reduce the segment to make the patient more comfortable and to reduce bleeding, if necessary.

Fractures of the teeth should also be treated by a dentist as soon as possible after the injury. Those involving only the enamel will usually be smoothed off with a dental drill, and x-ray films should be taken to rule out root fractures. If the dentin is involved, the dentist usually places a sedative dressing, such as zinc oxide and eugenol (oil of cloves) over the tooth. When a small amount of pulp is exposed, a covering with calcium hydroxide and a sedative dressing are sufficient in most cases; the calcium hydroxide causes the pulp to regress and stimulates calcification over the opening. If a large pulpal exposure occurs, the nerve is removed by a dentist, and root canal therapy is carried out later.

When a dental root is fractured in the apical third, nothing is done initially, but root canal therapy may be required later. When the root is fractured in the middle or cervical third, however, the tooth is usually removed.

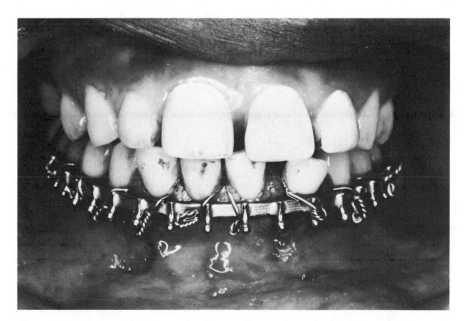

Figure 17.26 Photograph showing the fracture illustrated in Figure 17.24, which has been wired and stabilized into its correct position.

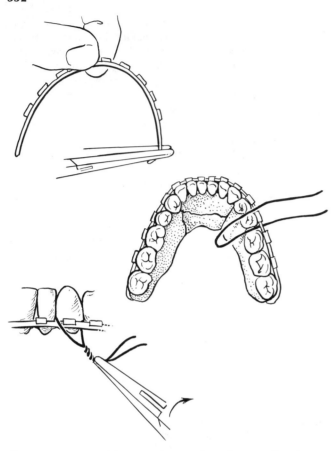

Figure 17.27 Series of drawings showing the technique of bending an arch bar and wiring it into position around the teeth.

Teeth that are displaced or avulsed may be saved. X-Ray films are taken to rule out root fractures, and then the teeth can be manually repositioned into their proper location. The teeth are then fixed and immobilized with an arch bar, interdental wiring, or a composite resin splint to adjacent stable teeth. If a tooth has been totally avulsed from its socket, reimplantation is frequently possible. Therefore, an avulsed tooth should always be brought to the emergency room or to the dentist's office for evaluation. If a dentist is not available, the emergency room physician should clean off the tooth, irrigate and debride the socket, then reimplant the tooth.

Because of contamination of the open socket and hematoma at its apex and because infection almost certainly causes the reimplanted tooth to be lost, the patient should be placed on an antibiotic, penicillin or erythromycin, 1 g per day for 5 days.

SUGGESTED READINGS

Dingman, RO, Natvig P: *Surgery of Facial Fractures.* Philadelphia, WB Saunders Co, 1964.

Kazanjian V, Converse JM: *Surgical Treatment of Facial Injuries.* Baltimore, The Williams & Wilkins Co, 1974.

Mulliken JB, Kaban LB, Murray JE: Management of facial fractures in children. *Clin Plast Surg* 1977; 4:491.

Rowe NL, Killey NC: *Fractures of the Facial Skeleton,* 2nd ed. Baltimore, The Williams & Wilkins Co, 1968.

18
INJURIES TO THE EYE AND ADNEXA

Roger V. Ohanesian

Most traumatic eye injuries may be categorized as blunt, sharp, or chemical. They can range from mild to sight threatening, and the immediate action of the primary care practitioner may determine the ultimate vision of the patient.

Examination of the traumatized eye may be brief or lengthy depending on the extent of injury and the ability of the patient to cooperate. Great care must be taken in this examination, for if the eye is lacerated or even punctured, then manipulation can result in the prolapse of the inner contents of the globe.

If possible, the examination outlined here should be conducted in the following order:

- Visual acuity of each eye
- Penlight examination
- External ocular motions
- Ophthalmoscopy

Of these tests, *visual acuity is the most important test* to determine disorders of the eye, and it should be recorded on *all* patients with ocular emergencies. Acuity of each eye should be recorded using the standard Snellen chart at a 20-ft distance (6 m). Glasses for distance correction should be worn since raw vision scores are useless. If glasses are broken or otherwise not available, pinhole vision should be assessed to determine best visual acuity.

Visual acuity and the remaining tests are basically to compare the injured eye to its mate. Most disorders are monocular, and a difficult diagnosis is made easier by comparison to the nontraumatized eye.

BLUNT TRAUMA

The majority of complaints of blunt trauma are associated with sports injuries, auto accidents and altercations; the order of frequency depends on the locale of the primary care center. Trauma of this nature can affect any part of the eye, from the lids to the optic nerve.

The history after blunt trauma should include the following pertinent information:

- Size of object causing injury
- Place of contact (eye? nose? brow?)
- Decreased vision (immediate? gradual?)

Patients with obvious blunt trauma injuries should be questioned as to the size of the object producing the trauma. A softball may cause facial fractures but rarely injures the globe, which is protected within the orbital recess. In contrast, a golf ball or elbow may cause a blow-out fracture of the orbital floor as well as global injuries.

Patients often consider injuries to the bridge of the nose or the brow as trauma to the eye. It is important to ascertain the point of contact since an indirect blow to the orbit does not cause as severe a visual injury. Immediate decrease of vision indicates vascular compromise or retinal involvement and carries a worse prognosis than gradual decrease in vision, most commonly resulting from corneal edema or hyphema.

Laceration of the Lid and Tear Duct

Laceration of the eyelid commonly accompanies blunt injury to the eye. If the wound is medial then a tear duct laceration should be suspected and is far more ominous than a superficial lid laceration.

DIAGNOSIS

Injuries of the lid should be closely examined with the aid of a penlight. Lid lacerations frequently appear to be little more than abrasions, but upon careful retraction of wound margins, the true extent of the laceration may be seen to involve the tear duct or lid margin (Fig. 18.1). All lid lacerations must be considered to be associated with global injuries until proven otherwise.

MANAGEMENT

Lacerations of the lid margin or tear duct deserve the attention of a specialist; they must be closed layer by layer to prevent disfiguring lid notching or chronic tear problems. Surgery should be performed within 24 hours. A deep wound of the upper lid may sever its levator muscles, causing a resultant ptosis if not adequately repaired.

Blow-Out Fractures

Following blunt injury from a small diameter ball, club, or fist, the eye may be forced posteriorly into the socket, causing a bursting to its surrounding walls, known as a blow-out fracture.

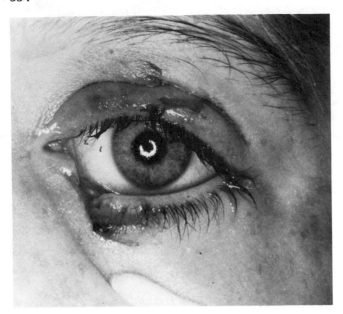

Figure 18.1 Tear duct laceration exposed with lid retraction.

DIAGNOSIS

After blunt injury to the globe, the orbital contents are compressed and may result in fracture of one of the orbital walls. The most common sites to fracture are the medial and/or inferior walls. Inferior wall fractures are associated with much more pathology than the relatively benign medial wall fractures. If the inferior rectus muscle becomes entrapped in the fracture site, vertical eye movements will be limited (Fig. 18.2) and is often associated with pain. Horizontal gaze is usually unaffected after inferior wall blow outs. Reduced tactile sensation of the lower lid, cheek, and alveolar ridge are diagnostic signs of a fracture involving the inferior orbital nerve. X-Ray film evidence, especially in Water's view, frequently demonstrates opacification or soft tissue density within the maxillary sinus of the affected side (Fig. 17.5). This finding should make the primary care practitioner suspicious of the possibility of a fracture of the floor of the orbit.

MANAGEMENT

An ophthalmologist, otolaryngologist, or plastic surgeon should be consulted for patients with blow-out fractures. Usual treatment is hospitalization with systemic antibiotics and surgical repair within 2 weeks. Delay of diagnosis and/or treatment beyond this time increases surgical risks because of increased vascularity of fibrosing tissue. Not all cases of blow-out fracture require surgical repair.

Scleral Rupture

A blow that is strong enough to retroplace the eye may cause the globe instead of the orbital walls to burst. A stronger blow may cause a blow-out fracture as well as a ruptured globe.

DIAGNOSIS

A scleral rupture may be the underlying result of an apparent simple lid injury. The conjunctiva may have evidence of hem-

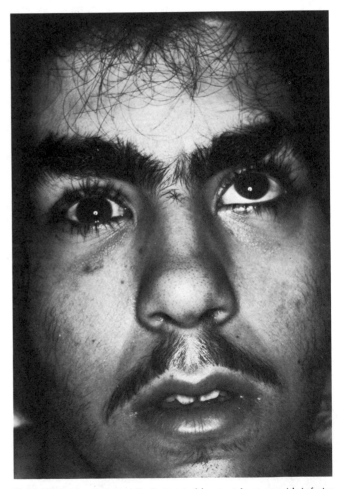

Figure 18.2 Upward gaze limitation in blow-out fracture with inferior rectus muscle entrapment.

orrhage that indicates the site of injury to the globe. This subconjunctival bleeding frequently masks the underlying scleral rupture. A ruptured sclera may also show abnormal pigmentation beyond the circumference of the cornea, representing herniated uveal pigment. This rupture may occur at the site of trauma or at a weak area of the globe. Commonly, the anterior chamber is filled with blood. Wrinkling of the cornea upon slight pressure should arouse suspicions of a ruptured globe. In cases in which this diagnosis is suspected, *no further examination of the globe* should be performed by the primary care physician. Further attempts at examination may cause extrusion of orbital contents through the wound.

MANAGEMENT

An ophthalmologist should be consulted to complete the examination and to repair the wound under general anesthesia in the operating room. Until the ophthalmologist arrives, the patient should be sedated and given appropriate systemic analgesics and a metal shield to prevent rubbing of the eye.

The primary care physician may cause great harm and eventual loss of the eye by inappropriately applying antibiotics to a ruptured globe, since topical ointments are oil based and are intensely reactive to the inner eye.

Corneal Edema

Trauma of a lesser magnitude may cause only corneal injury yet may be intensely painful to the patient.

DIAGNOSIS

Corneal edema may occur after a contusion of the globe by blunt trauma. Alone it may reduce visual acuity to the 20/400 level, but it is often associated with injuries to other ocular structures. Penlight examination reveals a loss of the crisp architecture of the iris when seen through the cloudy cornea.

MANAGEMENT

An ophthalmologist should be called to assist in the management of this disorder since subtle signs of other injuries may escape detection by the primary care practitioner.

Corneal edema, frequently associated with corneal abrasion, may require eye patching for several days to weeks in order for the patient's eyesight to return to clarity. Often a bandage soft contact lens is necessary to reduce pain and allow corneal epithelial ingrowth.

Hyphema

If the blow causes the iris diaphragm to be retroplaced or avulsed, then bleeding into the anterior chamber may occur.

DIAGNOSIS

Blunt trauma often causes a hyphema, blood in the anterior chamber (Fig. 18.3), which is classified as *gross* or *microscopic*. The former is readily diagnosed, but in the latter the blood has not settled and the anterior chamber appears normal to all but slit lamp biomicroscopy.

Both types of hyphema demonstrate a reduction in visual acuity, which, in the microscopic type, may be the *only* evidence of pathology. Visual acuity in the injured eye that is one line worse than in the opposite eye may represent a microscopic hyphema and call for further investigation by an ophthalmologist.

MANAGEMENT

A patient with a hyphema is usually hospitalized, sedated, and the eye is patched. This disease has a potential for rebleeding from the injured iris vessel 4–5 days after the initial trauma. Rebleeding frequently causes the anterior chamber to fill with blood, producing a severe glaucoma that may result in irreversible loss of vision. The prognosis of this potentially grave disease rests entirely upon the primary care physician who must suspect a hyphema in all cases of reduced visual acuity after eye trauma.

Retinal Edema and/or Choroidal Rupture

DIAGNOSIS

Retinal edema may develop after blunt trauma and is a result of a contrecoup injury to the fundus. Pupillary dilation is often necessary to examine the fundus and may be performed by the topical application of 1 drop of tropicamide 1%. Pallor that is clinically obvious by direct ophthalmoscopy is present in the involved retinal tissue. If the macula is involved, vision is reduced to 20/200 or less. A choroidal rupture may also occur in worse cases of blunt trauma. A semicircular white line with adjacent subretinal hemorrhage marks the rupture site, which is often near or through the macula.

MANAGEMENT

Consultation with an opthalmologist is necessary to determine medical treatment. If the edema or rupture does not involve

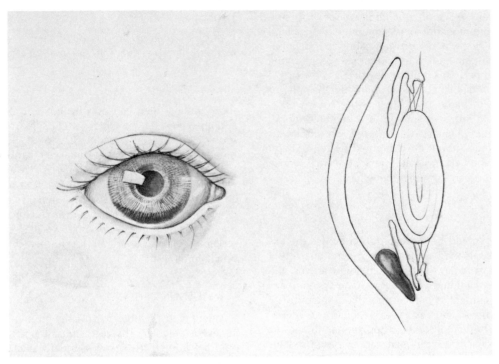

Figure 18.3 Gross hyphema—layered blood in anterior chamber.

the macula, then prognosis for the return of vision is good. If the macula is involved, then prognosis is guarded.

Retinal Detachment

Tears in the peripheral retina followed later by retinal detachment commonly occur after blunt trauma to the eye. Frequently, patients have previously existing retinal holes that develop into detachments after a sudden blow to the eye. The retina should be examined especially at both the site of contact and at the superior nasal quadrant, an area known to have higher incidence of detachments after trauma.

If the central retina is uninvolved, vision will be normal but is in jeopardy since the detachment may continue to progress to the macular region. Once the macula is detached, prognosis for return of normal vision is markedly reduced.

DIAGNOSIS

The primary care physician should be aware that even with a dilated pupil and a direct ophthalmoscope, it is only possible to see to the midperiphery of the eye and that most retinal tears

are beyond the physician's view. Retinal *detachments,* however, can often be seen with the direct ophthalmoscope.
On examination, the vessels overlying the detached retina will be tortuous and out of focus compared to the attached portion (Fig. 31.2*d*). Occasionally, blood will accompany the detachment and make the diagnosis easier. If the retina is greatly detached, it will appear bullous and billowing with eye movements. There will be no vision in the detached portion.

MANAGEMENT

Patients with suspected detachments should be calmed and placed on a flat bed in a supine position until an ophthalmologist can confirm the diagnosis and schedule operative repair. Prognosis is improved if there is early treatment and an uninvolved macula.

SHARP TRAUMA

The vast majority of cases of sharp trauma are associated with industrial accidents. The most important determination in this category is whether the eye has been perforated. Although the globe is extremely resistant to foreign body penetration, sharp trauma is more likely to occur under certain conditions.

The history taken after sharp trauma should include the following pertinent questions:

- What was the immediate preinjury activity? Welding? Grinding? Hammering?
- Were glasses or other eye protectors worn? Are they present? Intact?
- What was the nature of object? Metallic? Steel? Brass? Thorn?

Foreign bodies that penetrate the eye are often the result of high-speed missiles and are frequently metallic. Slivers from a hammered wedge or grinder wheel frequently create hot steel particles that may penetrate the eye, as will shards of glass from shattered spectacles or a thorn from a snapped twig.

In most cases of perforation, patients are unaware of the severity of the injury and consider it of minor consequence. The primary care physician must suspect penetration to all patients who present a history of a propelled foreign body hitting the eye.

Corneal or Scleral Perforation

Despite the severity of the injury, many patients with corneal or scleral perforation present with only a mild foreign body sensation.

DIAGNOSIS

On examination, visual acuity is occasionally normal but is usually reduced by a line or two of the Snellen chart. By penlight examination, the site of entry of a *scleral* wound is often masked by overlying conjunctival hemorrhage. If the *cornea* is perforated, a surface irregularity may be visible at the entry site. Often a brown elevation having a foreign body appearance obscures the wound margins (Fig. 18.4). This is actually a prolapsed iris that has herniated, thereby plugging the wound. This iris prolapse is a diagnostic sign of corneal

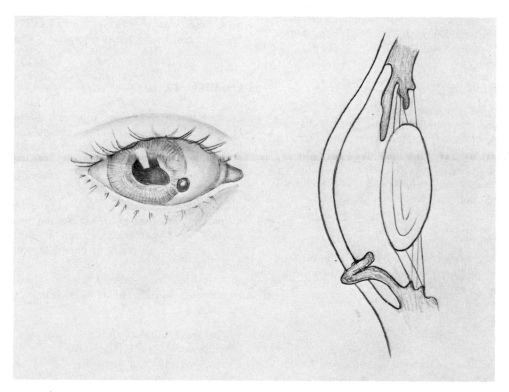

Figure 18.4 Penetrating injury with iris prolapse into the wound resulting in peaked pupil.

perforation, producing an irregular pupil that "points" to the site of the wound. In many cases, the prolapse is small and indistinguishable without the aid of a slit lamp.

MANAGEMENT

Once the diagnosis of corneal or scleral perforation is made, the primary care physician should discontinue the examination. Children and anxious adults are especially prone to squeezing their lids, thus elevating ocular pressure and often eviscerating the entire global contents through a small wound. Surgical repair by an ophthalmologist may be necessary, depending on the size of the perforation and its location. Prognosis should always be guarded because of the grave dangers of infection and latent ocular disease.

Lens Penetration

DIAGNOSIS

When the lens is penetrated by a foreign body, it may rapidly turn opaque. This traumatic cataract may form within 1 hour, become quite dense, and prevent further view of the fundus. Usually the opacity begins at the site of the lens penetration and provides a clue to the position of the foreign body within the eye.

MANAGEMENT AND PROGNOSIS

The lens capsule, once penetrated, usually causes a dense cataract to form. Extraction of this traumatic cataract may be performed at the time of the initial operative repair or may be delayed for months or years.

Prognosis for vision is dependent upon other ocular injuries. After cataract extraction, a contact lens or lens implant is usually necessary for the return of adequate visual acuity.

Posterior Pole Foreign Body

A severe injury from a foreign body is usually quite obvious and results in a profound loss of vision; there is little difficulty in making the diagnosis.

DIAGNOSIS

A foreign body that has come to rest in the posterior pole may be seen as a grey opacity out of focus to the remaining fundus. Intraretinal and choroidal hemorrhage may be seen in the adjacent tissue.

The position of the foreign body and any bleeding should be noted on the patient's chart (e.g., periphery of the 3 o'clock position) since cataract may form so quickly after lens penetration that the first fundus examination may be the only one.

X-Ray films of the orbit, especially Water's view, will identify an intraorbital metallic foreign body in suspicious cases. In unquestionable cases of foreign body penetration, x-ray films should be requested with caution since the added manipulation of transportation and positioning in order to take an x-ray film may cause increased orbital pressure and result in the further prolapse of intraocular contents.

MANAGEMENT

Until the ophthalmologist arrives, the patient should be calmed and given appropriate systemic analgesics, and the eye should be lightly patched with a metal shield. *No topical ointments should be applied* since they are oil based and reactive to intraocular structures and may cause the eventual loss of an eye if applied to a penetrated globe. Prognosis is generally guarded because of the high risk of endophthalmitis, hemorrhage, and detached retina, although with the use of modern microscopic instrumentation for intraocular surgery, many patients who were previously considered hopeless cases have had adequate visual acuity returned.

CHEMICAL TRAUMA

Because of the ubiquitous appearance of toxins in our environment, chemical burns to the eye may occur in the household or in an industrial setting and in people of any age, sex, or race. The emergency care administered during the first few minutes is worth more than the treatment during the first few years.

Chemical burns represent the most dangerous cases in ophthalmology, and their entire course may be determined by the primary care physician. Treatment should be immediate and is the same for all types of chemical trauma, in a word—*irrigation.*

At the time that treatment is being initiated, the history can be obtained and should include pertinent questions such as the following:

- What was the nature of the substance?
  Acid? Alkali? Dry? Liquid form?
- What was any prior treatment?
  How soon after the injury?
  For how long?

Alkaline Burns

Alkaline burns represent the most serious eye emergencies. The degree of damage is determined by the strength of the alkalinity and the time between injury and irrigation. The most common alkaline burns are from lye (NaOH or KOH), lime (CaO), and ammonia (NH_4OH). A pH hydron paper can be used to determine initial alkalinity and can later confirm neutrality. Of importance is whether the chemical was splashed into the eye or propelled from guns, cartridges, or grenades at close range.

DIAGNOSIS

Examination of an eye recently burned by a chemical may reveal surprisingly few positive signs, but this should not deter initiation of complete treatment.

In severe cases, blanching of the conjunctiva and corneal opacities are present before irrigation.

MANAGEMENT AND PROGNOSIS

The hydroxyl radical rapidly infiltrates all layers of the cornea and may appear in the aqueous fluid within 1 minute after injury. It is therefore essential to dilute the alkali with large volumes of *available fluid*. Water *from any source* that can be directed onto the exposed eye should be immediately and copiously used for at least 1 hour. Although the patient's eyelids may be opened manually for instillation of anesthetic drops and initial lavage, a speculum or lid retractor is necessary for long-term irrigation.

Lids and conjunctiva should be examined quickly and carefully for alkaline particles that adhere to the lash margins and mucosal surfaces. A wet cotton-tip swab is used to sweep the fornices and dislodge these particles with surrounding blebs. The pH within these blebs may be 10, although the outer tears are neutral. Seepage from these blebs will cause further corneal damage if the bleb is not ruptured and the particle removed.

Treatment should be 2,000 ml normal saline or irrigating fluid for at least 1 hour. This may be performed or started by the physician and may be continued by an experienced nurse. The order of treatment should be as follows:

1. Instillation of anesthetic drops into each eye (avoid repeated use).
2. Sweep of the under surface of each lid with a wet cotton-tip applicator.
3. Retraction of lids with a speculum.

4. Irrigation for 1 hour with the tip of the tubing directly over the cornea.
5. Evert upper and lower lids, rupture blebs, and remove remaining particles—test fluid within bleb with pH paper to confirm neutrality.
6. Continue irrigation until resumption of neutrality.

The disastrous effect of alkaline burns usually makes the prognosis very poor. The speed and length of treatment become critical determinants of the patient's final vision.

Prognosis is improved if irrigation is performed at the accident site and continued for at least one-half hour. When advising treatment over the phone, care should be taken to require that the patient open his or her eyes during irrigation.

Late corneal transplantation, necessary for badly scarred corneas, is hazardous because of highly vascular host tissue.

Acid Burns

Acid burns, although considered as devastating by the patient, are usually less severe than alkaline burns. A coagulum of precipitated protein prevents the acid radical from infiltrating beyond the first few corneal layers. Exceptions to this relatively benign course are strong acids such as hydrofluoric acid which inflict far more serious corneal damage.

DIAGNOSIS

As with alkaline burns, the patient is often well aware of the particular substance that caused the injury. An exploding automotive battery is a frequent occurrence and may result in an ocular penetrating wound as well as an acid burn.

On examination, the lids and conjunctiva are edematous and erythematous, often with copious tearing. In more severe cases the cornea will lose its transparency due to surface necrosis. Removing the opaque epithelium with a cotton tipped swab reveals an underlying clear cornea

MANAGEMENT

Hydron paper again is helpful, first, in establishing the acidity and, later, following treatment, in confirming neutrality. Irrigation should be performed as in the treatment of alkaline burns, but the consequences of an acid burn are far less damaging. The order and process of treatment should be similar to that listed above. Corneal epithelium may become edematous and slough, causing delayed corneal healing. In most cases, after irrigation the eye may be given antibiotic drops, dilated with homatropine 2% and may be firmly patched with two eye pads. Analgesics and sleeping pills will be necessary to assist patients through the night if they are to be sent home and seen by an ophthalmologist on another day.

Other Toxic Substances

Other toxins of unknown substance can cause irritation to the surface of the eye and, even if not alkaline, can cause severe damage if propelled into the eye.

DIAGNOSIS

Tear gas discharge from an exploding device at close range causes an infiltration of toxin into deeper corneal layers, producing damage as severe as that of an alkaline material. Since particulate matter often accompanies propelled substances, consideration should be given to the possibility of ocular perforation. Examination of the globe as mentioned under sharp trauma should be performed.

Aerosol sprayed toxins such as mace, deodorants, and hair sprays are usually nonalkaline and cause only localized corneal and conjunctival epithelial damage.

Ultraviolet burns from a welder's torch or sunlamp are familiar to most primary care practitioners. The appearance of these unfortunate patients tearing profusely while being led to the examining room by a friend is all too familiar. After 1 drop of anesthetic, however, they are usually relieved to a point where visual acuity and a complete eye examination may be performed without discomfort.

In all of these cases, visual acuity of the affected eye is often slightly reduced. Periorbital and conjunctival edema varies, as do corneal surface changes. Fluorescein staining is often the only way to appreciate minute erosions of the cornea. The remaining examination is usually normal.

MANAGEMENT AND PROGNOSIS

Eyes that have been contacted by a toxin should be managed by irrigation similarly to the treatment mentioned earlier under alkaline burns. Eyelid eversion and sweep with a cotton-tip applicator is necessary to remove concealed particles. Touching the affected tissue with pH paper is helpful to confirm the acid–base balance and postlavage neutrality. These results should be noted on the patient's chart.

In cases in which a toxin was propelled into the eye, an ophthalmologist should be consulted and asked to take over the care of the patient after emergency treatment. People with severely injured eyes often require admission to the hospital for medical or surgical care.

Ultraviolet burns to the cornea are managed differently since irrigation and lid eversion are unnecessary and counterproductive. In these cases and others with extreme photophobia, dilation should be performed with homatropine 2% to prevent intraocular inflammation. Patients should be warned that blurred vision and dilated pupils will persist for a few days.

In milder cases of chemical or ultraviolet burns, ophthalmic antibiotic ointment and eye patching provide sufficient treatment. Two eye patches should be applied to the affected eye; the first patch should be folded to conform to the ocular recess. By this method, a pressure dressing will be created that will allow a greater degree of comfort.

As with other corneal surface injuries, patients may require analgesics and sleeping capsules to assist them through the acute states of their illness.

Prognosis in all but propelled toxins is good. The pain produced is often disproportionate to the long-term effect. People so affected should be reassured that within a few days their vision and pain should be vastly improved. If progressive improvement is not achieved within a few days, patients should be advised to seek follow-up care from an ophthalmologist.

SUGGESTED READINGS

Baylis H et al: Repair of the lacerated canaliculus. *Ophthalmology* 1978; 85:1271–1276.

Bettman J: Medical problems associated with litigation, in *Ophthalmology The Art, The Law and a Bit of Science.* New York, Aesculapius Publishers Inc 1977, pp 96–98.

Bettman J: Medicolegal aspects of ophthalmology. *Int Clin Ophthalmol* 1980; 20 (No 4): 137–139.

Brown S, Tragakis M, Pearce D: Treatment of the alkali-burned cornea. *Am J Ophthalmol* 1972; 74:316–320.

Duke-Elder: *System of Ophthalmology.* St. Louis, CV Mosby, 1972, vol 14, pp 3–356.

Gambos G: *Handbook of Ophthalmologic Emergencies.* Garden City, NY, Medical Examination Publishing Co Inc, 1973.

Grove A: Orbital trauma and computed tomography. *Ophthalmology* 1980; 87:403–411.

Irvine RA: Old and new techniques combined in the management of intraocular foreign bodies. *Ann Ophthalmol* 1981; 13:27–41.

Laigson P, Oconor J (trans): Explosive tear gas injuries to the eye. *Am Acad Ophthalmol Otolaryngology* 1970; 74:811.

Minatoya H: Eye injuries from exploding car batteries. *Arch Ophthalmol* 1978; 96:477–481.

Paton D, Emery J. Injuries of the eyelids and the orbit, in Ballinger W, Rutherford R, Zuidema G (eds): *The Management of Trauma* ed 2. WB Saunders Co, 1973, pp 219–254.

Paton D, Goldberg M: *Management of Ocular Injuries.* Philadelphia, WB Saunders Co, 1976.

Pico G, Boyd B: Lacrimal pathway trauma, in *Highlights of Ophthalmology* ed 25. Panama City, Arcata Press, 1981, Chap 22.

Putterman A, et al: Nonsurgical management of blowout fractures of the orbital floor. *Am J Ophthalmol* 1974; 77:232–239.

Runyan TE: *Concussive and Penetrating Injuries of the Globe and Optic Nerve*. St. Louis, The CV Mosby Co, 1975.

Ryan S, Boyd B: Management of trauma, in *Highlights of Ophthalmology*, ed 25, Panama City, Arcata Press, 1981, chap 2.

Stasior OG, Sorsby A (eds): Blowout fractures, in *Modern Ophthalmology*. London, Butterworth Publishers Inc, 1974, p 990.

Vinger P: Ocular sports injuries. *Int Ophthalmol Clin* 1981; 21(No 4):21–46.

Wergeland, L, Brenner E: Solar retinopathy and foveomacular retinitis. *Ann Ophthalmol* 1973; 12:5–16.

Wilson F: Traumatic hyphema pathogenesis and management. *Ophthalmology* 1980; 87:910–919.

19
NECK INJURIES

Gerald B. Healy
J. Kenneth Koster, Jr.

Major cervical trauma is associated with a significant risk of serious internal injury because of the concentration of important structures within the narrow confines of the neck. Such injuries may be obvious and immediately life threatening, or they may be initially inapparent yet still potentially devastating. In the former situations, the patient must be rapidly and effectively treated; patients in the latter situation must not be overlooked.

Cervical injuries may be either *blunt* or *penetrating;* it should, however, be recognized that in certain cases some overlap will exist. Regardless of the nature of the wounding agent, the initial treatment priorities are the same: assurance of a patent airway and control of exsanguinating hemorrhage.

When stridor or chest wall retraction suggest upper airway obstruction or when obtundation signals the loss of protective reflexes, endotracheal intubation is generally the most effective method of assuring a controlled airway. In cases in which the possibility of cervical spine injury exists, "blind" nasotracheal intubation will allow the least manipulation of the neck. If endotracheal intubation is impossible because of extensive facial trauma or laryngeal disruption, cricothyrotomy affords the most rapid relief of obstruction and is the preferred treatment over emergency tracheotomy.

Hemorrhage from a neck wound should be controlled with direct pressure. Efforts to apply hemostatic clamps blindly to a bleeding vessel in the emergency room without adequate exposure, lighting, and other equipment should be avoided because of the risk of producing further injury.

PENETRATING INJURIES

Most penetrating wounds of the neck result from knife attacks or gunshots. Because of the nature of the deep structures potentially involved in a penetrating cervical wound, immediate surgical consultation should be obtained, and no effort should be made to probe the wound when the patient is in the emergency room. In most medical centers, it is a standard policy that any wound penetrating the platysma is formally explored

when the patient is in the operating room. Wounds at the base of the neck may possibly involve mediastinal structures, and in such cases, the surgeon may rely upon arteriography to exclude the possibility of a major vascular injury.

Vascular Injury

Penetrating injuries to the large arteries of the neck may lead to exsanguination, stroke, arteriovenous fistula, false aneurysm, or an expanding hematoma contained within the fascial planes of the neck. The hematoma may both compress the airway and impede venous return from the head. External bleeding from a penetrating wound should be controlled with direct pressure. The patient should immediately be taken to the operating theater where the neck can be decompressed and the artery either repaired or ligated. Rapid restoration of the intravascular volume to minimize hypotension is especially important in cases of carotid injury because regional cerebral blood supply may be dependent upon collateral flow. Injuries to the large veins of the neck may also produce exsanguination or formation of a compressing hematoma. Moreover, with venous lacerations, air embolism is possible and must be guarded against by immediate compression and ligation.

Visceral Injuries

Penetrating injury to the airway is usually manifest by hemoptysis and subcutaneous emphysema. Signs of obstruction may also be present, and early intubation of the trachea in preparation for repair is indicated. Penetration of the pharynx or esophagus may initially be inapparent or produce only minimal crepitus. Surgical exploration provides the best assurance that such injuries will not be missed.

BLUNT INJURIES

Direct blows to the neck account for most closed cervical injuries, although serious internal damage may also arise from cervical hyperangulation or compression produced by abrupt accelerative–decelerative forces applied to the head or body. Any cervical structure is vulnerable. Direct blows striking the neck from automobile dashboards and steering wheels most frequently injure the upper airway, particularly the larynx. However, blunt trauma can also rupture the esophagus or thrombose or tear the carotid arteries and injure the cervical nerves.

The manifestations of blunt cervical injury are varied and obviously related to the injured structure. Subcutaneous emphysema, variable degrees of airway obstruction, and dysphonia all suggest injury to the larynx or trachea. Esophageal injury may be initially manifest only by subcutaneous emphysema. Arterial injury may produce a hematoma or immediate or delayed signs of cerebral ischemia. In patients with closed head injuries, the risk of injury to the cervical spine is such that anteroposterior and lateral x-ray films showing all of the cervical vertebrae should be routinely obtained with the usual precautions in such cases. Injuries to the cervical spine are discussed in Chapter 16.

Blunt Laryngeal Injury

Blunt laryngeal injury usually occurs when the anterior part of the neck strikes an automobile steering wheel or instrument panel. Concomitant injury of the cervical spine is quite common. Because of its structure and location, the larynx frequently produces very suggestive signs when it is injured. The mucosal lining of the larynx is easily torn, allowing air to enter the surrounding soft tissue rapidly, producing subcutaneous emphysema. By virtue of a relatively exposed position in adults, some of the laryngeal cartilages are quite susceptible to fracture with blunt trauma, often leading to an obvious distortion in the contour of the anterior part of the neck. Thus, distortion of the neck, crepitus, and subcutaneous emphysema in combination with dysphonia, dyspnea, stridor, cough, or hemoptysis should strongly suggest the possibility of a laryngeal injury.

In the absence of signs of airway obstruction that demand immediate intervention, roentgenograms of the neck should be obtained to further define the status of the larynx, trachea, and cervical spine. Manipulation of the neck should be avoided until the possibility of cervical spine injury has been excluded.

Indirect laryngoscopy may be helpful in assessing a suspected laryngeal injury and may be performed without manipulation of the neck. Some assessment of the degree of lar-

yngeal obstruction may often be made with this technique. Manipulation of the larynx with direct laryngoscopy and bronchoscopy should not be undertaken unless the examiner is experienced in evaluating lesions of the upper airway and equipment to intervene surgically is available. Dye studies, such as a laryngograph or barium swallow, add little to the diagnosis and may complicate the situation, especially in patients who have an incompetent larynx.

TREATMENT

Minor injuries to the larynx may result only in edema and hematoma formation. If the airway is not significantly compromised, patients with these minor injuries may be closely observed in an intensive care unit setting. The early administration of large doses of dexamethesone (1 mg/kg to a maximum dose of 30 mg) may limit and even reduce the amount of edema present.

When laryngeal injury is such that stridor, dysphonia, or impending asphyxia are apparent, a cricothyrotomy should be performed as rapidly as is feasible. If the attending physician is not experienced in performing this procedure, an attempt at endotracheal intubation should be made.

SUGGESTED READINGS

Jahrsdoerfer RA, Johns ME, Cantrell RW: Penetrating wounds of the head and neck. *Arch Otolaryngol* 1979; 105:721–725.

LeMay SR: Penetrating wounds of the larynx and cervical trachea. *Arch Otolaryngol* 1971; 94:558–565.

Ogura JH: Management of traumatic injuries of the larynx and trachea including stenosis. *J Laryngol Otol* 1971; 85:1259–1261.

Roon AJ, Christensen N: Evaluation and treatment of penetrating cervical injuries. *J Trauma* 1979; 19:391–397.

20
THORACIC INJURIES

J. Kenneth Koster, Jr.
John H. Sanders, Jr.

Thoracic emergencies are common in a busy hospital's emergency department. Most are related to trauma, and many prove to be relatively minor. All, however, require a constant awareness on the part of attending medical personnel that any chest injury for which there is the potential for significant impairment of cardiorespiratory function may rapidly become life threatening. Such situations demand prompt diagnosis and effective intervention. The key is recognition, for in most cases, once the situation has been properly defined, relatively simple means such as endotracheal intubation, placement of a chest tube, or pericardiocentesis will suffice to meet the immediate demands of the emergency.

INITIAL ASSESSMENT AND MANAGEMENT

In cases of major thoracic trauma, there frequently will be multiple injuries that are not necessarily isolated to the chest. Attention should always first be directed toward those conditions producing immediate compromise of cardiorespiratory function, and the patient evaluation must frequently be conducted in conjunction with initial resuscitative measures. Often the available history is limited since the patient may be agitated or even unconscious. Learning at least the nature of the injuring agent and the circumstances of the injury is useful in allowing some estimate to be made of the possible extent of the patient's injuries.

To avoid distraction by the many simultaneous activities required in instituting care of a seriously injured patient, it is exceedingly important that the physical examination be conducted in an orderly manner by keeping a mental checklist of potential injuries that may complicate a given situation. Such an awareness will make it less likely that serious injuries that may not be immediately obvious, such as an aortic transection or an esophageal perforation, will not be overlooked. Great reliance must be placed upon the intelligent interpretation of physical signs and the chest film.

Assurance of Patent Airway

The initial step in the care of any trauma patient is to provide assurance of a patent airway. Asphyxia from airway obstruction will rapidly produce permanent central nervous system (CNS) injury, rendering other resuscitative measures useless. A rapid assessment of the adequacy of ventilation should be made by observing the rate and quality of the respiratory efforts, noting any stridor or other sign of difficulty. In the obtunded patient, the hypopharynx must be checked and cleared of vomitus, blood, or dislodged dentures. If the degree of obtundation is such that protective reflexes are lost, or if there is any question as to the adequacy of ventilation, *endotracheal intubation* (Procedure 4), using a cuffed tube, should be performed immediately. In the circumstances in which proper equipment is unavailable immediately, the patient's jaw should be pulled forward; and in the absence of a suspected cervical spine injury, the neck should be extended to prevent the base of the tongue from obstructing the pharynx. An oropharyngeal or nasopharyngeal tube will provide a patent pharyngeal airway but will not protect against aspiration. In the unusual circumstance where passage of an endotracheal tube is impossible because of extensive maxillofacial trauma or laryngeal disruption, a *cricothyroidotomy* will provide the most rapid and effective airway (Procedure 9). The cricothyroid membrane, palpable as a subcutaneous indentation immediately inferior to the thyroid cartilage, can be incised with a sharp instrument, allowing placement of the tube directly into the trachea. Later, if there is concern over the potential for cricoid erosion, a standard tracheostomy may be performed electively.

Lower airway obstruction from aspirated material, intrapulmonary bleeding, or mucoid secretions also must not be overlooked once control of the upper airway is assured. In severe blunt chest injuries, intrabronchial accumulations of excessive bronchial secretions and a transudate of red cells and plasma frequently compound the respiratory functional impairment already present because of the edematous, contused lung parenchyma (traumatic wet lung). Vigorous catheter suction of excessive secretions through the endotracheal tube or bronchoscopic lavage with removal of gross clot and other aspirated material are indicated. Bronchoscopy should also be performed in cases in which there is any question of major bronchial obstruction or disruption.

Intravenous Access and Fluid Replacement

When a patent airway has been assured and any immediately obvious life-threatening condition such as a sucking chest wound (see below) or severe external bleeding has been treated, venous access, using large bore catheters, should be established.

This should include a central venous line for critically injured patients. In those cases in which there is an obviously serious intravascular volume deficit, saphenous vein cutdowns in the proximal thigh will allow sterile intravenous tubing to be placed directly into the femoral veins for rapid volume infusion. Lower extremity cutdowns at the ankle or groin should also be used if there is suspicion of disruption of a major intrathoracic venous trunk. Although Ringer's lactate and plasma fractions will suffice for initial volume resuscitation, massive volume infusions obviously include restoration of the red cell mass as well. In critical situations this may be done with O negative blood. Type specific uncross-matched blood should be obtainable about 10 minutes after the blood bank receives a clot and can be administered to bridge the time until fully cross-matched blood is available.

Physical Examination

Once the aforementioned resuscitative measures have been initiated, an orderly physical examination is performed, and an early chest film with the patient as upright as possible is obtained. This film should be obtained at the earliest opportunity in the emergency department. Vital signs and, particularly, any upward or downward trends should be closely observed. The examination should begin with the thorax and neck with the patient fully unclothed. The neck should be examined for tracheal deviation and the fullness of the external jugular veins. A quick check of each hemithorax for breath sounds should be followed by a careful inspection of the chest wall for symmetry and any paradoxical motion. When penetrating trauma is involved, entrance and exit wounds must be carefully noted. The chest wall should be palpated for fracture or any areas of instability. Percussion may suggest either a large pneumothorax or a collection of pleural fluid. Auscultation of the heart may demonstrate a number of important signs, including the diminution of the heart sounds because of intrapericardial blood, a possible new murmur, or even the characteristic crunch of mediastinal air.

Special Studies

If there is suspicion of a major intrathoracic injury, early thoracic surgical consultation should be obtained. Special studies such as aortography should be undertaken only after such consultation. In any event patients with potential major chest injuries should never be sent to the x-ray film department without being accompanied by a person qualified to assess any change in status reliably.

BLUNT THORACIC TRAUMA

Most blunt chest injuries are seen in victims of automobile accidents, although some of these injuries result from falls, contact sports, physical assaults, and the like.

Awareness of the potential intrathoracic injuries possible in a given situation is a large factor in the recognition of the injuries. With blunt chest injuries, the force of impact and decelerative stress dictate the pattern and extent of injury. Massive pulmonary contusion, cardiac trauma, and disruptions of the great vessels, tracheobronchial tree, or diaphragm are more likely to be seen in victims of vehicular accidents that involve motorcycles, pedestrians, or high-speed automobiles. "Simple" rib fractures are not infrequently complicated by pneumothorax, hemothorax, or pulmonary contusion, and the likelihood of these complications is greatly increased if the fractures are multiple. Intraabdominal injuries must be considered when there are fractures involving the lower rib cage. Because of the relatively protected position of the ribs, a fracture of the uppermost ribs, particularly the first two ribs, indicates that the chest has received very severe trauma. There is a very high probability of multiple system injuries when there are such fractures.

Chest Wall Injury

CONTUSIONS

Contusions of the chest wall, although painful, are usually not serious in themselves. When uncomplicated, chest wall contusions require only analgesics and a heating pad. However, they should alert us to the possibility of intrathoracic injury even in the absence of rib fractures. This is especially true in young people who have relatively flexible rib cages that often can sustain a heavy blow without fracture.

SUBCUTANEOUS EMPHYSEMA

Subcutaneous emphysema, a condition usually not significant in itself, is an indication that air has dissected along deeper fascial planes into the subcutaneous tissue. In patients with major blunt trauma, it may be a marker of bronchial injury, but much more commonly, air enters these facial planes from a pneumothorax in which there is some disruption of the mediastinal or parietal pleura. Less frequently, air reaches the subcutaneous tissue through the mediastinum by way of retrograde dissection along the bronchial tree from a small bronchopulmonary air leak without a pneumothorax. Treatment is directed at controlling the source of the air leak, and this usually involves reexpansion of the pneumothorax with a chest tube. In the absence of pneumothorax or bronchial injury, the patient's condition is usually self-limiting. Direct measures such as using needle aspiration or skin incisions to decompress the subcutaneous emphysema should rarely be necessary.

RIB FRACTURES

Rib fractures are usually related to external trauma, although they are occasionally seen in osteoporotic persons following the stress of coughing. Because a considerable amount of force is usually required to produce a rib fracture, we must be alert to the frequent occurrence of associated injuries such as pneumothorax, hemothorax, and pulmonary contusion.

Diagnosis

The injured area is usually quite painful, and the patient tends to voluntarily splint the affected side. Pain is intensified by breathing, coughing, or moving. There is usually marked point tenderness over the fracture site, and, occasionally, crepitus or grating of the fractured bone can be palpated. Rib detail x-ray films may be obtained specifically to demonstrate the fracture, although certain fractures, especially those located anterolaterally, may be difficult to identify on film. A standard chest film should always be taken to assure that there is no intrapleural air or fluid.

Management

In the absence of underlying injuries, the primary treatment goal of an isolated rib fracture is the relief of pain. Strapping the chest with tape or an elastic rib belt is only variably effective in pain relief and potentially can produce atelectasis by limiting chest wall excursion. Pain relief is most effective with an *intercostal nerve block* (Fig. 20.1). This is best performed by infiltrating several milliliters of a long-acting anesthetic, such as bupivacaine, at the inferior margin of the ribs posteriorly several interspaces above and below the fracture site. This can be repeated several times if necessary, and oral analgesics can be used in combination. In the elderly or in patients with obstructive airway disease, the pain and muscular splinting associated with rib fractures may further diminish already compromised functional lung volumes and lead to atelectasis and retention of secretions. Hospital admission for these patients

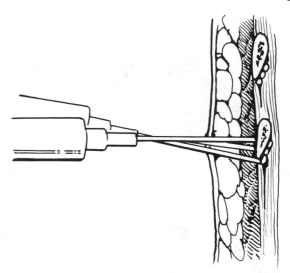

Figure 20.1 Intercostal nerve block. A 22-gauge needle is used to infiltrate the tissues at the inferior margin of the rib with a long-acting local anesthetic such as bupivacaine (Marcaine).

is warranted to ensure that adequate pain relief and proper pulmonary toilet are maintained.

FLAIL CHEST

Multiple rib fractures secondary to major blunt chest injury may render a significant portion of the chest wall unstable and allow it to move paradoxically inward with inspiration and outward with expiration (Fig. 20.2). Such instability, which is called a *flail chest,* may greatly compromise respiratory mechanics by impairing the ability of the thoracic bellows to generate negative inspiratory pressures.

Diagnosis

The chest wall instability that results from such fractures is not always immediately apparent because of muscular splinting, and it may become manifest only upon repeated examinations over several hours as muscular fatigue allows chest wall mobility. Instability should be anticipated and specifically examined for whenever a patient has fractures of three or more ribs, especially if there are anterior and posterior fractures. A sternal fracture of costochondral cartilaginous disruption in association with rib fractures may also produce a flail chest. Underlying pulmonary injury, particularly pulmonary contu-

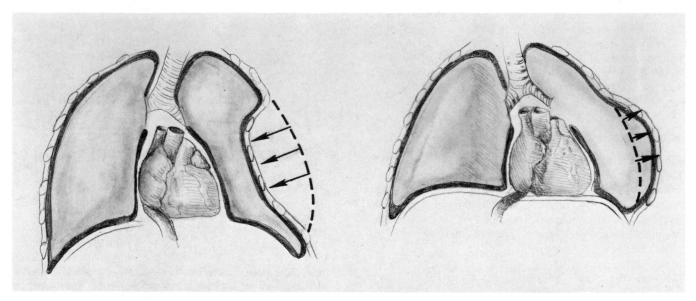

Figure 20.2 Flail chest. Instability of a chest wall section during respiratory effort destroys the effectiveness of the thoracic bellows, thereby limiting the generation of negative intrathoracic pressure with inspiration.

sion, very frequently complicates a flail chest. Hypoventilation, secondary to the unstable chest wall, may, in combination with the alveolar edema of the contused lung, rapidly precipitate severe respiratory insufficiency.

Management

Initial therapy is directed toward stabilization of the flail segment of the chest wall. Several approaches may be used to do this, including immobilization of the unstable segment with either compression or external traction, tracheal intubation and positive pressure ventilation, or surgical fixation. In acute emergencies, the most direct method is the application of pressure over the unstable segment using either the hand or some heavy object such as a sandbag. This should be considered only as a temporary maneuver until the patient can undergo endotracheal intubation and positive pressure ventilation. Once the patient has been placed on the ventilator, a chest tube should be inserted on the injured side even in the absence of an obvious pneumothorax because the lung frequently will be injured by bony spicules, and any air leak from an injured lung will rapidly create a tension pneumothorax with positive pressure ventilation. A decision regarding definitive therapy relative to long-term mechanical ventilation versus early surgical fixation of the flail segment can be deferred until after the patient has been well stabilized and the possibility of other significant intrathoracic injuries, such as myocardial contusion or aortic transection, has been ruled out.

STERNAL FRACTURE

Fractures of the sternum occur much less frequently than rib fractures, but they are not rare. In certain cases they may be caused by hyperflexion, but they usually result from a direct blow to the anterior chest. Sternal fractures represent a significant injury; because of the great force required to fracture the sternum, there is a high likelihood of associated major intrathoracic injury. The possibility of myocardial contusion, a thoracic aortic tear, pulmonary contusion, and other injuries of this magnitude requires that the patient be admitted to the hospital and investigated.

Diagnosis

A nondisplaced sternal fracture is usually marked by local tenderness and possibly some crepitus. Pain is variable but often significant and exacerbated with any effort to breathe or move. The best radiographic demonstration of the fracture is on the lateral chest film.

Management

In most cases the pain from sternal fractures can be controlled with analgesics or injections of local anesthetic agents into the fracture site. Operative reduction and fixation are necessary only if the fracture is severely displaced or unstable and is undertaken only after the treatment of other more pressing injuries has been effected.

Pulmonary Contusion

Pulmonary contusion frequently complicates significant non-penetrating chest trauma. It is often a serious injury that is occasionally overlooked initially in the rush of caring for a victim of multiple trauma. Although the mechanism of pulmonary contusion has not been completely elucidated, it appears that transmission of an abrupt compressive–decompressive wave across the lung parenchyma from a strong force that has distorted the chest wall will produce alveolar and interstitial edema and hemorrhage. This transudation of fluid, in combination with a reflex increase in bronchial mucous secretion, impedes local gas exchange and produces broncheolar obstruction and atelectasis. Alterations in pulmonary blood flow worsen hypoxemia. The patient's clinical presentation depends in great part upon the extent of pulmonary parenchymal injury. When the area of contusion is relatively localized, it may be manifest only by a small patchy infiltrate on an x-ray film with the patient exhibiting little or no sign of respiratory functional impairment. However, pulmonary contusions that initially may appear to be only of moderate severity may significantly worsen in their clinical manifestations over the first few hours after the injury occurred.

Diagnosis

Patients who have lesser degrees of contusion may be asymptomatic or only slightly dyspneic and tachypneic when they are first examined. Scattered rales may be heard over the area of injury, and the patient often will be coughing mucoid or even blood-tinged material. The chest film will usually show an infiltrate that tends to be patchy, irregular, and streaky. With milder injuries, the Pa_{O_2} is normal or only slightly depressed whereas the Pa_{CO_2} may be low because of tachypnea. In situations of more severe contusions, the degree of obvious respiratory difficulty is greater, and in the worst injuries the patient may be severely dyspneic or cyanotic and may be coughing frothy, bloody fluid upon arrival in the emergency department. Such patients show significant arterial desaturation, usually with some degree of metabolic acidosis, and in

the most severe injuries, there may be an ominous elevation of the Pa_{CO_2}.

Respiratory function frequently deteriorates over the initial period after injury. Patients who at first have signs of only mild respiratory difficulty may become desperately ill within several hours. Careful monitoring and repeated observation are necessary. Radiographic findings do not necessarily correlate well with and often lag behind changes in the patient's clinical status. Serial blood gas determinations are the only accurate measures of the severity of a pulmonary contusion and its response to treatment.

Management

It cannot be overemphasized that therapy for pulmonary contusions is most effective when begun as early as possible after injury. Good bronchial toilet should be maintained through vigorous physical therapy for the chest, nasotracheal suctioning, and, if required, therapeutic bronchoscopy. Intercostal nerve blocks will help alleviate chest wall pain, as well as aid coughing and lessen the requirement for narcotic analgesia. For patients with milder degrees of contusion, supplemental oxygen should be given by mask or nasal catheter to maintain the Pa_{O_2} at normal levels. For patients with more serious injuries, manifest by significant arterial desaturation at the time of admission ($Pa_{O_2} < 70$ mm Hg on nasal oxygen), there should be early institution of respiratory support through mechanical ventilation. Positive end expiratory pressure should be added if the Pa_{O_2} cannot be maintained at greater than 60 mm Hg with an Fi_{O_2} of 50%. In all cases, intravenous fluid overload should be avoided since there is evidence that large infusions of crystalloid solutions worsen the wet lung pattern of injury. Intravascular volume deficits in patients with possible pulmonary contusions should be replaced with colloid-containing fluids such as plasma fractions of whole blood. Salt-poor albumin should be given to increase plasma oncotic pressure to minimize fluid transudation into the lung. Diuretics should also be given to minimize excess intrapulmonary fluid. Early institution of broad-spectrum antibiotics may minimize the chance of a superimposed bacterial pneumonia in the obstructed and traumatized pulmonary segments. (Bacterial sensitivities from periodic cultures of the tracheobronchial aspirates may indicate a need for a special antimicrobial agent.) Steroids may be beneficial in lessening capillary membrane permeability and enhancing lysosomal membrane stability. If steroids are used, they should be reserved for the more severe injuries, and they should be given early and in pharmacologic doses.

Although much of the care for patients with a pulmonary contusion occurs after they have left the emergency ward, the final outcome is often very heavily influenced by the adequacy of the early treatment they have received.

Pneumothorax

Normally, the lung is held fully expanded against the chest wall, and there is negative pressure within the potential space between the opposed smooth visceral and parietal pleural surfaces. Disruption of the seal between these surfaces by the entry of air into the pleural space from either a leak from the lung (closed pneumothorax) or through a chest wall defect (open pneumothorax) will allow collapse of the lung to a variable degree.

CLOSED PNEUMOTHORAX

Spontaneous closed pneumothoraces are relatively common. Most occur in otherwise healthy young adults and are the result of a rupture of a small subpleural pulmonary bleb. Rupture of such blebs often appears to be unrelated to any particular exertion since many people have the onset of symptoms in the course of normal activity or when at rest.

Diagnosis

Variable sudden sharp chest pain and some degree of dyspnea usually mark the onset of a spontaneous pneumothorax. Dyspnea is related both to the extent of lung collapse and to any preexisting pulmonary disease. Healthy people may experience little sense of breathlessness with total collapse of one lung, whereas other people with extensive pulmonary parenchymal disease may be quite dyspneic with even a relatively small pneumothorax. Physical signs vary with the size of the pneumothorax and may be limited to only a slight diminution of breath sounds on the affected side. With larger pneumothoraces there may be ipsilateral hyperresonance. The chest radiograph confirms the diagnosis and allows an estimate of the degree of lung collapse.

Management

In the absence of complicating factors, treatment of a patient with a closed pneumothorax can be generally individualized along the following lines: An asymptomatic small pneumothorax of less than 20–25% in an otherwise healthy patient can be safely observed in most instances. A somewhat larger pneumothorax can often be managed with simple aspiration (Procedure 18) using an Intracath with an attached three-way

stopcock placed through the second intercostal space anteriorly, especially if the time span from the onset of symptoms along with the finding of an incompletely collapsed lung suggest that the initial air leak may have sealed. If an x-ray film taken after aspiration of air from the pleural space demonstrates virtual full expansion of the lung, it is reasonable to assume that there is no further pulmonary air leak, and a reliable patient may be released and instructed to return in 24 hours for a follow-up chest film (or earlier should any symptoms supervene). In those cases in which the degree of pulmonary collapse is significantly greater than 50%, in which aspiration has been ineffective, or in which an ongoing air leak is otherwise suspected, closed tube thoracostomy is necessary (Procedure 19). A chest tube is also advisable when the pneumothorax results from a small pulmonary laceration incurred with thoracentesis or placement of a central venous line. In the absence of significant pleural fluid, a 24 F chest tube in the second intercostal space at the midclavicular line is generally satisfactory. For women a better cosmetic result may be obtained through placement immediately posterior to the lateral margin of the pectoralis muscle and up through the third intercostal space. The chest tube is connected to an underwater seal system, and approximately 20 cm of suction is applied to facilitate lung reexpansion.

TENSION PNEUMOTHORAX

In certain circumstances the tissue around an air leak from the lung or (uncommonly) through the chest wall will, by acting as a one-way valve, allow air to enter the pleural space during inspiration but not to escape during expiration. Such progressive accumulation of intrapleural air under pressure will produce marked collapse of the ipsilateral lung and a contralateral shift of the mediastinum, producing some compression of the contralateral lung (Fig. 20.3). As the accumulation of intrapleural air under pressure increases, systemic venous return to the heart is impeded by increasing positive intrapleural pressure and mediastinal angulation. If this process continues unchecked, progressive hypoxemia and a falling cardiac output will lead to marked dyspnea, tachycardia, cyanosis, and vascular collapse. A tension pneumothorax may arise from rupture of a pulmonary bleb, a missile wound, or a lung laceration of virtually any size. A tension pneumothorax may complicate any condition in which there is a pulmonary air leak into the pleural space and will invariably do so when the patient is on positive pressure ventilation. Respirator patients, especially those requiring high inspiratory pressures or positive end-expiratory pressures (PEEP), are particularly at risk of developing a spon-

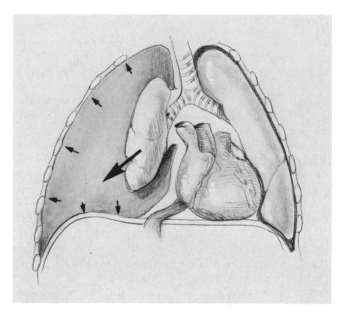

Figure 20.3 Tension pneumothorax. Progressive one-way air leak of air into the pleural space increases the intrathoracic pressures, angulating and compressing the great veins in the mediastinum thus hindering venous return to the heart.

taneous tension pneumothorax through rupture of a bleb, and the possibility should always be considered if there is sudden unexplained deterioration of a patient on a ventilator.

Diagnosis

Physical signs in patients with tension pneumothorax are usually more striking than those observed in patients with a simple closed pneumothorax—diminished or absent breath sounds, hyperresonance over the involved hemithorax, tracheal shift away from the affected side, and, in alert patients, some degree of dyspnea. Although an x-ray film will confirm the diagnosis, if the patient is symptomatic and a tension pneumothorax is suspected, we should proceed with decompression of the pleural space on the basis of the physical findings alone.

Management

Immediate placement of a chest tube in the second anterior interspace is indicated. In cases in which the patient is severely symptomatic, simply placing an 18-gauge needle through a high anterior interspace will convert the tension pneumothorax to a simple pneumothorax and will allow more leisurely placement of the chest tube.

Tracheobronchial Injury

Blunt tracheobronchial injuries are not frequent, but they may present difficult management problems. The usual bronchial injury consists of an incomplete circumferential disruption of the cartilaginous portion of the mainstem bronchus, whereas the less frequent intrathoracic tracheal injuries are usually longitudinal tears near the carina. Tracheobronchial injuries result from severe trauma, usually from high-speed vehicular accidents, and frequently there are associated injuries in other areas.

Diagnosis

Several clinical presentations are possible. Hemoptysis may be caused by bronchial arterial injury, and occasionally it is severe. A complete transection of the bronchus may produce total obstruction at the point of injury with distal atelectasis. However, the much more commonly observed partial bronchial separations are usually marked by large air leaks, either into the mediastinum or into the pleural cavity. If the mediastinal pleura remains intact, air tends to dissect soft tissues of the chest and neck, producing subcutaneous emphysema that may reach remarkable proportions. If the airway tear freely communicates with the pleural space, the resultant pneumothorax is complicated by a continuing large air leak. A tension pneumothorax may result if the pleura overlying the bronchial tear acts as a one-way valve permitting only an outward air leak into the pleural cavity. In certain instances, the peribronchial tissue will maintain continuity of the airway despite even a complete tear of the bronchial wall, and the injury may pass undetected unless healing results in late bronchial stenosis.

Management

The possibility of a tracheobronchial injury particularly should be considered in patients who, following closed thoracic trauma, have hemoptysis, who develop mediastinal and subcutaneous emphysema, or who have a large or a persistent air leak following evacuation of a pneumothorax with a chest tube. In such patients bronchoscopy is indicated at some point to allow identification of any bronchial injury. The timing of this, in part, depends upon the extent of the patient's associated injuries. Operative repair of large or irregular bronchial tears is advisable, and in circumstances in which the air leak after chest tube placement is so large as to compromise ventilation severely, immediate thoracotomy is necessary.

Blunt Cardiovascular Injury

Major blunt chest trauma may produce a variety of severe cardiovascular injuries either through decelerative stresses or by direct compressive forces. The spectrum of potential injury is broad, including, in part, myocardial contusion and rupture, cardiac valvular disruption, pericardial tamponade, and tears of the intrathoracic great vessels. Of these, myocardial contusion and aortic disruption are by far the most frequent. Initial physical findings may be surprisingly subtle and few, especially in view of the severity of the intrathoracic pathology. In addition, for an otherwise traumatized patient, they may be relatively nonspecific, such as hypotension and tachycardia. An awareness of potential cardiovascular injuries in a given setting in conjunction with a careful and orderly evaluation of the patient is necessary in order to avoid overlooking significant lesions.

MYOCARDIAL CONTUSION

In any patient with severe blunt chest trauma, the potential for cardiac injury and, particularly, myocardial contusion, should be considered. The signs associated with myocardial contusion may be few and transient and easily overlooked in the process of caring for other more obvious injuries. Whereas fractures of the sternum or several ribs should particularly alert us to the possibility of myocardial contusion, serious intrapericardial injuries may exist with no evidence of chest wall bony fracture or cartilaginous disruption. The heart is most subject to contusion from an anterior blow of the type that causes it to be abruptly decelerated against and compressed by a posteriorly displaced sternum and anterior chest wall (steering wheel injury). However, because the heart's suspension within the pericardial sac allows it mobility, it may be forcefully driven against the spine posteriorly or sternum anteriorly in any situation in which abrupt decelerative forces are applied to the chest.

The myocardial pathologic lesion can range from scattered petechiae to intramyocardial hematoma and local cellular necrosis. In the absence of associated injury, the clinical manifestations of a myocardial contusion appear to depend upon the extent and location of the myocardial damage. The majority of myocardial contusions do not result in gross functional cardiac impairment. In a few instances, necrosis is so severe as to result in delayed cardiac rupture or late aneurysm formation.

Diagnosis

Although it is possible that patients may have no cardiac symptoms, many will complain of precordial pain that is similar to that experienced in pericarditis or myocardial infarction. Clinical evidence of congestive heart failure is uncommon, although experimental studies have demonstrated that contusion can produce some loss of cardiac functional reserve. The physical signs of uncomplicated contusion are few, the most common one being sinus tachycardia. The diagnosis is most strongly supported by electrocardiographic changes consistent with focal pericarditis or myocardial infarction. Such changes may not be immediately present, and in certain instances they take up to 48 hours or, rarely, longer to develop. They also do not tend to persist as long as the changes observed in typical myocardial infarctions. Myocardial radionuclide scanning and creatine phosphokinase–myocardial fraction (CPK–MB) determinations may be useful in establishing a diagnosis of myocardial contusion, although experience in this context still is not great. The prognosis for myocardial contusion is usually that of complete recovery.

Management

Treatment of myocardial contusions consists of 1 week of bed rest followed by several weeks of restricted activity. Because cardiac arrhythmias represent the most commonly observed complication of myocardial contusion, patients should have continuous electrocardiographic monitoring during the initial days of observation. Although ectopic atrial and ventricular beats are most common, virtually all arrhythmias, including heart block, ventricular tachycardia, and ventricular fibrillation have been observed. Standard antiarrhythmic therapy is indicated. In the unusual circumstance after blunt trauma in which hypotension is felt to be cardiac related, pericardial tamponade should be excluded and inotropic support instituted, monitoring the left atrial filling pressures with a Swan-Ganz catheter.

Nonurgent surgical procedures requiring general anesthesia should be delayed in patients with myocardial contusion during the initial weeks of myocardial healing.

OTHER BLUNT CARDIAC INJURIES

Nonpenetrating cardiac injuries other than myocardial contusion are much less common. Hemopericardium from epicardial bleeding following blunt trauma is not rare, but it is usually limited and only infrequently produces pericardial tamponade. Tears or detachments of the aortic valve leaflets may produce acute insufficiency. Similarly, disruption of the papillary–chordal attachments of the atrioventricular valves may render them incompetent. Interventricular septal rupture, either acutely or following softening of a severe contusion, may produce a ventricular septal defect. Coronary arterial injury is also possible with nonpenetrating trauma, although apparently it is rare.

NONPENETRATING VASCULAR INJURIES

Blunt trauma, usually resulting from vehicular accidents, may injure any of the intrathoracic great vessels. The aorta is by far the most frequently involved. Of the less commonly injured vessels, the innominate and subclavian arteries are particularly vulnerable to avulsion or tears in their more proximal segments. The typical aortic injury is a relatively sharp tear that is generally transverse or spiral. Occasionally, the injury may consist of several closely grouped tears. Autopsy studies of victims of automobile accidents have shown that blunt aortic injuries may involve any segment, but in the group of patients who survive to reach emergency care, the great majority of aortic tears are in the proximal descending aorta immediately distal to the origin of the left subclavian artery. The frequent localization of aortic disruptions at the isthmus suggests that the mechanism of injury may be related to decelerative stresses at this junction of the more mobile transverse arch and the relatively fixed descending aorta (Fig. 20.4a). Initial survival with aortic tears is permitted only when the tear is not completely transmural and the adventitia and loose periaortic tissue contain the hematoma for an unpredictable period. Should the aortic injury pass unrecognized, the chances are overwhelmingly great that the resulting false aneurysm will progress to rupture with exsanguination during the first few days or weeks after the accident.

Diagnosis

The clinical presentation of blunt aortic injuries is varied. Frequently, there are coexisting severe injuries in other areas that also require assessment and treatment. It is surprising, especially considering the magnitude of the internal derangement, that specific physical findings with aortic rupture may be quite subtle or even nonexistent. For this reason the potential for an aortic tear should be considered for *any* patient who has sustained high-speed decelerative trauma. The suspicion of aortic injury may be heightened if there is evidence of severe trauma to the thorax, such as fractures of the sternum or upper ribs, but it should be remembered that a significant percentage of

aortic disruptions occurs with no external evidence of chest injury. Similarly, the physical findings that have been associated with aortic disruption—upper extremity hypertension, posterior thoracic systolic bruit, and diminution of distal pulses resulting from partial aortic obstruction by the periaortic hematoma at the site of injury—are more frequently absent than present.

The chest radiograph often provides the first evidence suggestive of traumatic aortic disruption. Several radiographic signs have been correlated with aortic injury, although none is diagnostic or even specific for aortic rupture; these are superior mediastinal widening, tracheal deviation to the right, inferior displacement of the left main stem bronchus, obliteration of the sharp outline of the descending aorta or aortic knob, opacification of the clear region between the aorta and pulmonary artery, and left pleural effusion (Fig. 20.4b). In a small percentage of cases, the initial chest radiograph may be normal.

Management

Angiography is the only means of providing a definitive preoperative diagnosis of traumatic disruption of the aorta or of any other great vessel. For this reason angiography should be used in any case in which there is a reasonable suspicion of this possibility. Most aortic disruptions are demonstrable on the aortogram as contained pseudoaneurysms immediately distal to the origin of the left subclavian artery. If the diagnosis of aortic rupture or other major vascular injury is confirmed, an operation should follow immediately.

PENETRATING CHEST TRAUMA

Most penetrating chest wounds are produced by knives or low-velocity gunshot wounds. Many result only in a hemopneumothorax and are definitely treated with a closed tube thoracostomy. Wounds of the heart, aorta, and great vessels may be partially tamponaded by the pericardium, surrounding tissue, or accumulation of clot, allowing an initial period of survival. Bleeding from the lung and chest wall is often self-limiting. Plotting the course of the bullet between the entrance wound and point of lodgement or exit wound allows some estimate to be made of what structures may have been injured, although the missile path is not invariably straight. Possible penetration of the diaphragm must also be considered, especially when the wound is at the level of or below the midchest.

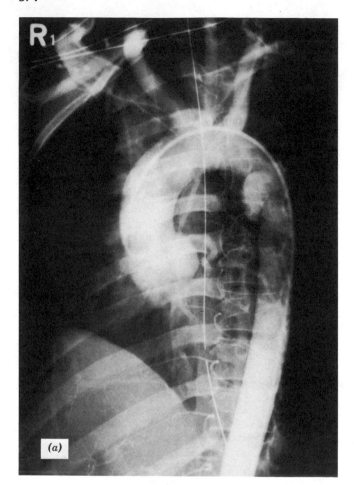

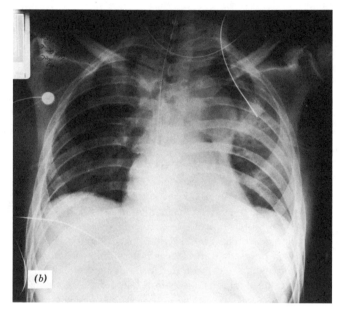

Figure 20.4 (a) Traumatic disruption of the thoracic aorta. Note hematoma surrounding aortic knob, inferior displacement of left mainstem bronchus, and left apical hemothorax. (b) Thoracic aortogram showing disruption of the thoracic aorta distal to the left subclavian artery with false aneurysm formation.

Open Pneumothorax

An open pneumothorax resulting from penetrating trauma represents a serious thoracic injury. In general, the severity of the clinical problem is a function of the size of the chest wall defect. This is not absolute since even a small stab wound that causes no other intrathoracic injury may produce a tension pneumothorax in the course of lacerating the lung. An open pneumothorax becomes especially critical in cases in which the chest wall defect is large enough to allow free communication of the pleural space with the outside atmosphere (sucking chest wound). Severe respiratory insufficiency may rapidly result. Intrapleural pressure on the side of the injury becomes atmospheric, and respiratory excursions of the chest move air in and out through the defect, diminishing the tidal volume passing through the glottis into the lungs (Fig. 20.5). Moreover, as air is drawn into the pleural space with inspiration, the mediastinum shifts toward the uninjured lung in which there is still some negative intrapleural pressure and returns with expiration (mediastinal flutter). This back and forth movement of the mediastinum tends to move increasingly stagnant air in a to-and-fro manner from the aerated to the partially collapsed lung, further diminishing the effective tidal volume.

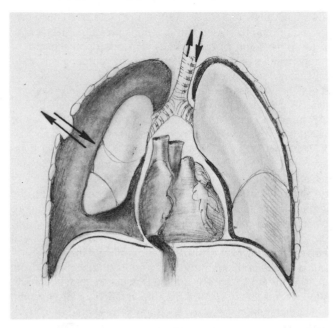

Figure 20.5 Open pneumothorax. Airflow through the chest wall defect into the pleural space with inspiration minimizes development of intrathoracic negative pressure. Tracheal airflow into the lungs is greatly limited by the lack of an inspiratory negative pressure gradient.

Management

Therapy is directed at immediate occlusion of the chest wall defect. This is usually done with a pack of sterile plain or petrolatum gauze. However, if no sterile materials are readily available, a clean wadded cloth held in place is quite adequate. It is best to occlude the defect at the end expiration in order to evacuate as much air as possible from the pleural cavity. Closure of the sucking wound stabilizes the situation and allows placement of the chest tube at a point away from the wound to reexpand the lung fully. When the patient has been otherwise stabilized, debridement and closure of the chest wound should be undertaken in the operating room.

Hemothorax

Hemothorax frequently complicates both blunt and penetrating thoracic trauma. Excluding blunt rupture of the aorta, larger collections of pleural blood generally follow penetrating trauma. Because the source of bleeding may be the chest wall, the lung, or the heart and great vessels, it is difficult to categorize treatment of hemothorax rigidly as an isolated entity. Bleeding

from the lung and chest wall veins is often self-limited, whereas that from the heart and arteries requires operative control.

Diagnosis

On physical examination, intrapleural blood is characterized by a variable area of overlying dullness to percussion and diminished or absent breath sounds. In cases of larger hemothoraces, there may be mediastinal shift and tracheal deviation away from the involved hemothorax. A chest film provides the best estimate of the amount of intrapleural blood. The chest film should be obtained when the patient is positioned as upright as possible because several hundred milliliters of blood layered posteriorly may produce only a faint haziness on a supine film.

Management

Generally, once detected, any significant collection of pleural blood should be evacuated in coordination with other resuscitative measures, including intravascular volume replacement. In the usual trauma setting, closed tube thoracostomy is preferable, although thoracentesis may be considered if the hemothorax is small (200–300 ml) and there is no associated pneumothorax or other injury. Satisfactory drainage may usually be obtained with chest tube placement through the fifth intercostal space in the midaxillary line. This represents a safe compromise in the emergency situation between the more dependent drainage of placing the tube somewhat more inferiorly and posteriorly and the risk of diaphragmatic injury. The initial volume of blood obtained from the chest or the rate of continued bleeding provides indication for conservative therapy or for the necessity to proceed with exploratory thoracotomy. If chest tube placement is followed by the immediate drainage of 800–1,000 ml of blood, immediate thoracotomy should be undertaken because of the great likelihood of a major intrathoracic injury that will not stop bleeding spontaneously. Similarly, in the hours subsequent to initial tube placement, an operation for surgical control of bleeding should be performed if the drainage exceeds 300 ml for any 1 hour or if the bleeding does not appear to be diminishing after the first 3–4 hours. The patient with a hemothorax who remains in shock after vigorous resuscitative measures should be transferred to the operating room for immediate thoracotomy.

Patients brought into the emergency ward in extremis following penetrating chest wounds should have endotracheal intubation immediately followed by a left anterolateral thoracotomy through the fifth interspace. Although such an approach is aggressive, it also offers the only small hope of saving a patient who would otherwise die from the injury. Pericardial tamponade may be relieved by the direct evacuation of blood and clot, and effective open-chest cardiac massage may be instituted. Massive bleeding from tears or gunshot wounds in the heart and great vessels may possibly be temporarily controlled with application of direct pressure, application of vascular clamps, or suture while intravascular volume is being replaced.

Pericardial Tamponade

The limited space between the heart and the surrounding, relatively inelastic, pericardium is normally occupied by only a few milliliters of serous fluid. A chronic slow increase in the volume of fluid within the pericardial space up to several hundred milliliters can be accommodated by a gradual stretching of the pericardium with minimal hemodynamic consequence. However, the capacity of the pericardium to adapt to rapid accumulations of intrapericardial fluid by stretching is limited. When fluid accumulates at a rate or to a volume that exceeds the capacity of the pericardium to enlarge, intrapericardial pressure will increase and impede diastolic filling of the heart. When inflow is limited, cardiac output progressively falls, and the atrial and central venous pressure will rise. The severity of the derangement depends upon the degree of intrapericardial pressure elevation. Pericardial tamponade may be severe and life threatening, or it may be mild and, although hemodynamically demonstrable, not necessarily clinically significant in terms of requiring pericardial drainage.

Pericardial tamponade may complicate virtually any pathologic process that produces an intrapericardial fluid accumulation. This includes effusions associated with the full spectrum of infectious pericarditis, malignancy, autoimmune disease, uremia, and other metabolic disorders. In certain cases, tamponade is the first manifestation of previously unrecognized pericardial disease. Intrapericardial hemorrhage from blunt and, especially, penetrating chest trauma may produce tamponade. In cases of penetrating wounds of the heart, tamponade occasionally may in a sense be initially lifesaving by preventing immediate exsanguination into the chest, thereby allowing a short period of survival during which the patient may reach medical care.

Diagnosis

The clinical signs of pericardial tamponade may be subtle or dramatic. Sustained tachycardia indicates compensation for a diminished stroke volume. The signs of arterial hypotension and an elevated central venous pressure indicate a falling cardiac output and increased cardiac filling pressure. The rapidity of the progression of these signs depends upon the rate of intrapericardial pressure rise. If the onset of tamponade is gradual enough, signs of compensatory adrenergic activity such as peripheral vasoconstriction and cool, clammy skin may precede a significant fall in the blood pressure. Neck vein distension from the elevated central venous pressure (CVP) may or may not be observable depending upon neck anatomy and the degree of intravascular volume depletion, and a direct measurement of the CVP should be obtained for any patient suspected of having pericardial tamponade unless the urgency of the situation does not allow it. In normal circumstances, the systolic blood pressure diminishes slightly with inspiration. When this inspiratory fall in pressure exceeds 10 mm Hg, it is termed *pulsus paradoxus* and is highly suggestive of pericardial tamponade. However, pulsus paradoxus is not invariably present with pericardial tamponade, and its absence should not argue against the diagnosis if there is evidence to the contrary. Although the heart sounds may be muffled or distant with pericardial fluid collections, such a finding should be considered as being quite relative and equally dependent upon other factors such as chest wall thickness and the amount of overlying lung tissue.

The chest film may demonstrate an enlarged globular pericardium with chronic effusions. In acute tamponade following trauma, however, the pericardial silhouette is often relatively normal. When the situation allows, echocardiography is the most reliable means of confirming the presence of pericardial fluid.

Management

In situations in which pericardial tamponade from hemopericardium is diagnosed or even suspected following thoracic trauma, immediate pericardiocentesis (Procedure 20) is indicated. Evacuation of even a small quantity of blood may be marked by a significant hemodynamic improvement. Although controversy exists as to the subsequent management of these patients after initial pericardiocentesis, many thoracic surgeons feel that early thoracotomy before reaccumulation should be undertaken for definitive control of the bleeding point and certain evacuation of intrapericardial blood clot, rather than relying upon repeated pericardial aspiration.

In contrast, when pericardial tamponade complicates the various forms of effusive pericarditis, repeated pericardiocentesis may be more useful, and surgery may be reserved for those cases in which there is refractory reaccumulation or a considerable risk of late constriction.

ESOPHAGEAL INJURIES

Esophageal perforations, particularly those that occur within the intrathoracic segment, represent extremely serious injuries. The entry of saliva containing anaerobic mouth organisms into the visceral spaces of the neck and mediastinum or into the pleural cavity produces a rapidly progressing infection in areas in which there are few barriers to extensive spread. Any delay in the recognition and treatment of such injuries seriously jeopardizes the potential for favorable outcome.

Most esophageal perforations result from penetration of the esophageal wall from within, either by a swallowed foreign body such as a pin or small bone or from an endoscopic accident. Instrumental perforation usually occurs proximal to a stricture or tumor or at a point of natural esophageal narrowing such as the inferior constriction or at the diaphragmatic hiatus. Whereas the esophagus may be injured by external penetrating trauma, this is not a frequent occurrence because of its relatively deep and central position. Blunt injury to the esophagus has been reported, but it is rare. Spontaneous esophageal rupture from retching, while not common, occurs more frequently than is perhaps generally recognized, and the diagnosis is often made only after a significant delay.

The clinical manifestations of esophageal perforation depend upon the site of injury and the degree of periesophageal contamination with digestive juices. Cervical perforations are characterized by early pain from swallowing followed by progressive cervical tenderness and crepitation to deep palpation. Intrathoracic perforations are usually accompanied by variable substernal pain and, especially with pleural contamination, some degree of dyspnea. Early physical signs are limited when there are intrathoracic perforations. Cervical crepitation may develop as gas dissects superiorly through the mediastinum.

Auscultation may demonstrate a "mediastinal crunch" of air within the soft tissues. Fever and tachycardia usually develop within a few hours.

Radiographic studies are very useful in confirming the diagnosis of esophageal disruption. When cervical perforation is suspected, early anteroposterior and lateral films will usually demonstrate air within the soft tissues of the neck. X-Ray films taken later may show a periesophageal fluid collection, edema of the prevertebral tissues, and even superior mediastinal widening. When there are intrathoracic perforations, mediastinal widening, pleural effusions, and mediastinal air may be visible on the plane film, but they are inconstant early findings, and contrast studies with water-soluble medium should be obtained any time there is a suspicion of an esophageal injury.

When the diagnosis of an esophageal perforation is suspected, early surgical consultation should be obtained to expedite any necessary surgical drainage and repair.

SUGGESTED READINGS

Glenn WWL, Ziebow AA, Lindskog GE: *Thoracic and Cardiovascular Surgery with Related Pathology.* New York, Appleton-Century-Crofts, 1975, chap IV, pp 85–116.

Johnson J, MacVaugh H III, Waldhausen JA: *Surgery of the Chest,* ed 4. Chicago, Year Book Medical Publishers Inc, 1973.

Kirsch MM, Sloan H: *Blunt Chest Trauma: General Principles of Management.* Boston, Little Brown & Co, 1977.

Naclerio EA: *Chest Injuries.* New York, Grune & Stratton Inc, 1971.

Symbas PN: *Trauma to the Heart and Great Vessels.* New York, Grune & Stratton Inc, 1978.

Zuidema GD, Rutherford RB, Ballinger WF II: *The Management of Trauma,* Philadelphia, WB Saunders Co, 1979.

21
ABDOMINAL AND GENITOURINARY INJURIES

Robert T. Osteen
Frederick W. Ackroyd
Gary P. Kearney

Before the twentieth century, an abdominal injury was a mortal wound. Not until exploratory laparotomy and repair of damaged organs became possible and safe did a person with an injury of the abdominal viscera survive—except by good fortune.

Physicians and surgeons in civilian practice see fewer major penetrating injuries than do military surgeons in wartime. What physicians in civilian emergency rooms witness is a sad byproduct of our high-speed society: the blunt trauma of automobile accidents. Urban violence contributes to the casualty list, but the family automobile is the major culprit. In a recent review of civilian experience, 67% of patients with abdominal injuries had sustained blunt trauma from automobiles, farm equipment, or athletic injuries; 17% had been stabbed; and 14% had been shot.

As in other fields of medicine, prevention is more desirable than treatment. The Roman legionnaires in Gaul, the crusaders at Tyre, and, most recently, the United States servicemen in Vietnam all wore body armor. Unfortunately, the knife fighter in the street and the victim of the ubiquitous "unknown assailant" are not so well protected. Even though automobile manufacturers are gradually devoting attention to safety features, many of these devices have their own innate problems. For example, the use of seat belts often trades neurologic trauma for abdominal injuries. Finally, patients in the hospital are not always safe from abdominal injury. The increasingly effective and aggressive diagnostic use of endoscopes, needle biopsies, and vascular catheters are accompanied by a small but disturbing number of injuries.

INITIAL ASSESSMENT AND MANAGEMENT

The arrival of a patient with abdominal injuries in the emergency room is usually accompanied by clamor and confusion proportional to the severity of the injuries. The physician on duty must transform this disorderly scene into an efficient task force in order to provide the appropriate sequence of diagnostic and therapeutic maneuvers. A quiet room without unnecessary chatter is essential.

As early as possible, an assessment should be made of the staff and specialists available to provide the care required for an injured patient. Any time that there is a patient with severe abdominal trauma, a surgeon and possibly a urologist should be called. A patient with pelvic trauma invariably requires that the emergency room physician consult with an orthopedist, a urologist, and a general surgeon. Many hospitals have a disaster plan that can be activated when emergency facilities become overloaded. A train wreck or other large-scale accident is not the only circumstance in which the plan should be implemented. Indeed, the facilities of the hospital can become saturated by the victims of a two-car collision.

It is impossible to separate completely the multiple features of resuscitation and diagnosis. Initial management of the patient with abdominal trauma may combine resuscitative and diagnostic measures. For example, the response to fluid therapy is an important indicator of intraabdominal bleeding. It may not be possible to make the diagnosis of an injury to a specific organ. Diagnoses tend to be more generic, such as "ruptured viscus" or "continuing intraabdominal hemorrhage." Central to the process of diagnosis and treatment is the decision of whether there is or is not a need for laparotomy.

Immediate Measures

The patient must be completely undressed. Unless the patient is awake and cooperative, the clothing should be cut away to minimize the chance of displacing an unsuspected fracture or vertebral injury. An unconscious patient should be viewed with a high index of suspicion for abdominal and spinal cord injuries.

Combative, intoxicated patients present a problem. Although they may have serious abdominal injuries, definitive evaluation may have to be delayed until they are calmed; minimal light and noise and the sedative effects of the alcohol may help to achieve this. During this period, however, their vital signs should be monitored if they will cooperate. The urge to use drugs to tranquilize such patients must be avoided.

The lighting in the examining room should be adequate to assess the patient's true color. The patient's level of consciousness and breathing characteristics can be determined at a glance. If breathing is impaired, patency of the airway must be ensured and, if necessary, ventilatory support provided. The stability of the patient's chest can be tested by gentle compression of the sternum and the lateral thoracic walls.

If there is a possibility of cervical spine injury, rotation of the head must be prevented by sandbags until roentgenograms can be obtained. In the unconscious patient, the cervical spine should be palpated for alignment.

Blood pressure and pulse should be determined, blood should be drawn for laboratory studies, and intravenous fluids should be started through one to three large-bore catheters. Because the vascular systems of young people are extremely unresponsive to blood loss, blood pressure and pulse may not change until a massive amount of blood has been lost. In these patients, however, tachypnea or dyspnea may be an early sign of hypovolemia.

Except in patients who have major pelvic trauma, a bladder catheter should be inserted to ensure that volume replacement is adequate to maintain a good flow of urine. The urine specimen obtained by catheterization should be examined for blood. If a conscious patient with pelvic trauma is unable to void voluntarily, urethral injury is likely and catheterization should be delayed until the integrity of the urethra has been confirmed. In the unconscious patient with pelvic trauma or in any patient with gross blood at the urethral meatus, a retrograde urethrogram should be performed before catheterization. Whenever there is a question of urethral injury, a urologist should be consulted before an attempt is made at bladder catheterization.

Details of the accident or assault should be obtained from the patient and any available witnesses. The patient's position when shot may give some indication of the course of the bullet. A small penknife is less likely to penetrate the peritoneal cavity than is a long butcher knife or a stiletto. With an eye toward the patient's subsequent course, a few routine questions should be asked. A history of allergies, immunizations, and medications should be obtained. The time of the patient's last meal should be established since this may influence the anesthesiologist's technique of intubation if the patient needs an operation. If cranial trauma can be ruled out by history, a clouded sensorium may be an early indication of cerebral hypoperfusion secondary to internal blood loss.

A complete physical examination must be performed. All information, including pertinent negative findings, should be recorded in detail. Because the process of diagnosis may take many days and involve many people who will not have seen the patient immediately after the accident, the initial examiner's observations are crucial in order to evaluate changes in the patient's condition. The physician must bear in mind that surgical exploration may be necessary at any time from the moment that the patient is first seen. Evidence of peritoneal irritation or bleeding signals the need for surgery. Such physical findings, which often appear within several hours, include gradually disappearing bowel sounds, systemic evidence of infection, or abdominal tenderness. Particularly in the setting of blunt trauma, the signs of intraabdominal injury may evolve slowly, and examination of the abdomen should be repeated frequently by the same examiner.

Laboratory Tests and Diagnostic Studies

In most civilian emergency wards, the patient is seen soon after the injury and before fluid shifts have diluted the hematocrit, before peritonitis has raised the white blood count, before amylase has been absorbed from the peritoneal surface, and before massive fluid replacement has diluted the serum sodium. Although the initial tests have little diagnostic value, they do provide baseline levels against which later results can be compared to evaluate changes in the patient's condition. Normal values should never be used to support an attitude of complacency toward the patient who demonstrates clinical evidence of abdominal injury. After an episode of major blood loss, dilution of the remaining red cell mass begins immediately, but the hematocrit may not be significantly lowered for several hours. The process of hemodilution continues for approximately 3 days after a single episode of bleeding. A rising serum amylase may suggest injury to the pancreas or duodenum. An early leukocytosis should not be interpreted as anything more specific than evidence of major trauma.

Blood in the urine is a major indicator of urinary tract trauma. Gross or microscopic hematuria should be pursued with appropriate radiologic studies, including cystography and intravenous urography.

An electrocardiogram (ECG) should be performed to establish the baseline condition of the patient's heart. There is no electrocardiographic finding, including myocardial infarction, that would contraindicate a laparotomy in a patient who has evidence of significant intraabdominal trauma.

ROENTGENOGRAMS

In general, plain roentgenograms of the abdomen are of little diagnostic value for assessing abdominal trauma. Some subtle signs of organ damage or intraperitoneal bleeding may be seen, but they must be interpreted in light of the evidence from the physical examination. Chest films should always be ordered to check for a pneumothorax and to look for free air under the diaphragm. Radiographic views of the urinary tract can be extremely helpful and should be used to investigate any degree of hematuria.

Roentgenographic studies should not be attempted until the patient is resuscitated. At that time, and in consultation with the involved specialist and the radiologist, the appropriate studies can be ordered. Some particularly well-equipped emergency rooms have x-ray facilities in their resuscitation rooms. In too many hospitals, the patient must be moved from the brilliantly lighted, well-staffed, and well-equipped emergency room to a small, dim x-ray cubicle where only the x-ray technician is in attendance. If intraabdominal bleeding continues, the recently resuscitated patient can slide back into shock. In the radiology department, vital signs of the patient should be monitored as frequently as they were in the emergency room, and a person skilled in the diagnosis of hypovolemia should be present. A physician qualified to make decisions regarding transfusion and the need for immediate laparotomy should be available. Adequate support and observation must be provided while adequate x-ray studies are performed. The use of portable x-ray equipment in the emergency room is a compromise in the evaluation of abdominal trauma. The quality of a portable x-ray film is never as good as one taken by regular x-ray equipment.

Computerized Body Tomographs

Computerized body tomography (CBT) provides an excellent noninvasive technique for accurately assessing, simultaneously, injuries of the head, neck, thorax, abdomen, pelvis, and extremities. The patient need not be moved from one position, and the study can be serially repeated as necessary. The Body Scanner provides images of the liver, spleen, kidneys, bladder, bowel, and bony skeleton. These views demonstrate findings characteristic of organ disruption, subcapsular hematoma, and bleeding, permitting rapid assessment of multisystem trauma patients. Pancreatic injuries are well demonstrated, and the addition of intravenous contrast media outlines the abdominal vasculature. This technique is valuable in evaluating patients with blunt trauma, and a negative scan may permit a more cautious, nonoperative approach, rather than emergency operation. The CBT scans can be interpreted with confidence, and decisions in management may often be made without multiple additional tests, since CBT is, in many cases, the most sensitive and specific for the various conditions.

Urography

Intravenous urography is mandatory for the management of patients with hematuria. Many surgeons order intravenous urograms to help with the evaluation of gunshot wounds of the abdomen without hematuria. One milliliter of 60% iodide radiopaque material, diatrizoate meglumine and diatrizoate sodium (Renografin 60) per pound of body weight, not to exceed 150 ml, is injected as a bolus. More complicated studies of the urinary tract are ordered in consultation with the urologist.

Nephrotomography, if available, may help to delineate the renal outline and the integrity of the renal cortex. The early or "nephrogram phase" gives the best view of the renal outline and indicates the homogeneity of the renal vascular supply. The collecting systems are generally seen on the 5-minute film. The 15- and 30-minute films are most useful for establishing the integrity of the collecting system and for detecting extravasation. Injecting the patient with the contrast material in the emergency room before transporting the patient to the x-ray department may save time; however, such irregular studies may cause the loss of information that is gained from the standard timing sequence. Selective renal arteriography should be performed to rule out major vascular injury if the kidney fails to show up on the intravenous urogram. Retrograde pyelography is only indicated for the definition of ureteral injuries that are suspected by extravasation of contrast on the standard intravenous urogram. Even bullets of low velocity can be expected to traverse the peritoneal cavity and produce a hematoma in the posterior retroperitoneum. It may be difficult during the laparotomy to tell whether a transected ureter lies within such a hematoma. The surgeon may order an intravenous urogram to prove that the urinary tracts are normal and thereby avoid opening a retroperitoneal hematoma.

Cystography

Potential injuries of the urinary bladder should be investigated by the urologist with gravity retrograde cystography before intravenous pyelography. After catheterization, gravity cystography is carried out with half-strength contrast (Renografin 60 mixed half and half with sterile saline or full-strength Cystografin). The bladder is filled until the patient complains of pressure or, in the unconscious patient, until the flow stops. If the initial x-ray films show no extravasation, an additional 20 ml of contrast is instilled with a syringe to show minor leaks that may have been missed without the additional pressure (stress cystogram). Anterior and posterior views are obtained, and additional views are made if indicated. The most important view of this study is the postevacuation film.

If there is evidence of urethral injury, a catheter should *not* be inserted until the integrity of the urethra is confirmed by voluntary voiding after the bladder is filled in antegrade fashion from the intravenous urogram or by retrograde urethrography. If the bladder is in a normal anatomical position and the patient is able to void voluntarily, integrity of the urethra can be assumed. If retrograde urethrography is needed to confirm a urethral injury, the study is performed by injecting 10 ml Renografin 60 or Hypaque into the urethra through a No. 10 or No. 12 Foley catheter, the tip of which has been inserted into the urethra and the balloon inflated to 3 ml of saline using a careful sterile technique.

Arteriography

Selective arteriography is a highly refined, elegant technique for demonstrating injuries to specific vessels. Diagnostic arteriography is appropriately ordered by a surgeon for a stable patient with suspected occult blood loss. Selective arteriography may also be helpful when a kidney fails to opacify on intravenous urography or for the diagnosis and treatment of bleeding from pelvic fractures. When arteriography is performed to control bleeding from a pelvic fracture, the other abdominal organs can be examined at the same time. A pelvic fracture often confuses the diagnosis of intraperitoneal bleeding, and an arteriogram that demonstrates a normal liver and spleen is evidence against the need for laparotomy.

Radionuclide Scans

The liver–spleen scan can demonstrate defects in the distribution of isotope caused by subcapsular or parenchymal hematomas. A hematoma may produce pain without significant blood loss or evidence of generalized, peritoneal irritation. In such circumstances, a scan may be ordered by the surgeon to confirm the diagnosis.

Ultrasound

Although ultrasound can show free fluid in the peritoneal cavity and blood around the liver or spleen, there is little use for diagnostic ultrasonography in the routine evaluation of abdominal trauma. In certain circumstances, ultrasonography may lead to a paracentesis or some other study that would result in a surgeon performing a laparotomy, but it is unlikely that ultrasonography would yield data so compelling that laparotomy would be performed on the basis of that information alone. The interpretation of an ultrasonic examination is frequently complicated by the increased amounts of intralumenal gas caused by a paralytic ileus.

PERITONEAL LAVAGE

Since the introduction of peritoneal lavage by Root in 1965, it has largely replaced other aspiration methods for the diagnosis of intraperitoneal hemorrhage. It is a simple test that can be performed in the emergency room to establish or rule out bleeding in the stable patient with suspected intraabdominal

injuries or in the comatose patient whose signs and symptoms of abdominal injuries are blunted by neurologic trauma. The test can be performed either by the primary emergency room physician or by a surgical consultant. A catheter is introduced into the peritoneal cavity either with a trocar or by exposure and direct incision of the peritoneum (Procedure 24). One liter of saline or balanced salt solution is infused and drained. If the lavage fluid contains gross blood, bile, or intestinal contents, a significant injury has occurred. Lavage should not be performed before obtaining chest and abdomen films since the small amount of air introduced with the catheter will be seen as free air on the films, confusing the diagnosis of bowel injury. Peritoneal lavage is unnecessary when laparotomy is indicated for other reasons, such as free air on the roentgenograms or an unstable blood pressure.

Peritoneal lavage is an extremely sensitive test. When lavage fluid is stained pink but is not grossly bloody, the correlation with important injuries is less good. If the fluid is so turbid that newsprint cannot be read through it or if the red blood cell count is greater than 100,000 cells per cubic millimeter, it is likely that significant bleeding has occurred. The incidence of false-negative lavages is very low—approximately 4%. The red blood cell content of the lavage fluid yields the most important information. The white blood cell count does not correlate well with intestinal injuries, and injuries of the pancreas that may increase the amylase content of the lavage fluid are almost invariably associated with bleeding into the peritoneal cavity.

Although peritoneal lavage has made a major contribution to the diagnosis of intraabdominal injury, some caution is advised. The extreme sensitivity of the test can yield a large number of false-positive examinations unless the criteria for the amount of blood necessary to make an examination positive are rigidly followed. Significant retroperitoneal injury to the duodenum, pancreas, or kidney may occur without intraabdominal bleeding. Care must be taken when introducing the catheter into the abdomen if the patient has had previous surgery because of the possibility of injuring bowel that is stuck to the abdominal wall.

The four-quadrant tap, an older technique for the diagnosis of hemoperitoneum, is a paracentesis performed at several different sites in the flank (Procedure 25). The needle is inserted lateral to the rectus sheath to avoid damage to the epigastric vessels. Blood from a visceral injury will form a pool in the paracolic gutters where it can be aspirated. When the volume of free blood is small, the more sensitive lavage technique will have fewer false-negative examinations than will the four-quadrant paracentesis. Since the four-quadrant tap takes less time than peritoneal lavage, there may be occasions when the faster technique would be appropriate in order to establish the fact that there has been major bleeding into the peritoneal cavity.

BLUNT INJURIES

The definitive evaluation and management of abdominal injuries differs depending upon the wounding agent. There are two major divisions of injuries—blunt trauma and penetrating wounds. *Blunt trauma* presents a difficult diagnostic problem in that a blow to the abdominal wall may not produce significant visceral injury. Furthermore, bleeding into or irritation of the peritoneum may be insufficient to produce symptoms until many hours after the accident. Patients who have sustained blunt abdominal trauma may be asymptomatic at first even though they have significant injuries. Indeed, many patients initially deny that they are injured, though a short time later they gradually begin to perceive the severity of their injuries. Injury to solid organs such as the liver or spleen are more likely to cause rapid blood loss and early appearance of the signs of hypovolemia. Injury to the hollow gastrointestinal tract may cause symptoms of peritonitis initially, and hypovolemic symptoms may develop later.

Assessment of Blunt Trauma

HISTORY

An estimation of the potential for significant visceral injury can be made from the history of the accident. The faster the automobile was traveling or the greater the distance of the fall, the more likely a severe injury has occurred. The history of a sharp blow to the left flank will focus the examiner's attention on the spleen and kidney. Cross-lap seat belts have been associated with mesenteric tears, small bowel lacerations, and rupture of the gravid uterus. The accident victim who is unconscious for any period of time should be a suspect for abdominal as well as intercranial injuries simply because of the force involved. Even an asymptomatic patient who has sustained a major impact should be admitted to the hospital for 24 hours of observation.

PHYSICAL EXAMINATION FOR BLUNT TRAUMA

The best single approach for the evaluation of blunt abdominal trauma is a series of careful physical examinations. Close observation and monitoring of vital signs are essential. The initial physical examination is performed in the emergency room by the emergency room physician.

After immediate measures are taken to provide an adequate airway and to stabilize the patient, a complete physical examination is performed. The abdomen, flanks, and back should be inspected for abrasions and discoloration. Bluish discoloration of the flanks may indicate bleeding into the retroperitoneum. Similar discoloration arising from the pelvic area or perineum may result from a pelvic fracture. Abrasions or contusions of the lower abdominal wall may be caused by a seat belt. The lower part of the rib cage is inspected for ecchymoses and is palpated for crepitance. Fractured ribs are not diagnostic of abdominal trauma, but they do indicate that major trauma has occurred. A blow that is forceful enough to fracture the lower left ribs could also rupture the spleen or kidney by direct puncture, crushing against the vertebral column, or shearing (see Fig. 12.8).

The examination of the abdomen for tenderness must be done so gently that pain from a fractured rib or vertebra does not interfere with the evaluation of peritoneal irritation. Light percussion is a better test for rebound tenderness than is the sudden release of pressure after deep, bimanual palpation. Concurrent spinal cord injury will eliminate abdominal muscle tone and blunt the perception of pain, making the evaluation of peritoneal irritation difficult. Patients with spinal cord injuries will feel abdominal discomfort relayed through the autonomic nervous system, but sensations from the peritoneum that has somatic innervation may be obliterated. X-Ray film studies, selected on the basis of clinical evidence, are helpful when the patient's condition permits. Peritoneal lavage plays a valuable role in the evaluation of comatose patients or stable patients with suggestive but not conclusive evidence of intraperitoneal injury.

Injury to the abdominal wall with bleeding from epigastric vessels may produce a tender abdomen associated with a visible and palpable mass in the abdominal wall. Guarding and tenderness should not be ascribed to a rectus hematoma unless a mass is present. If the abdominal wall is the source of the patient's discomfort, tensing the abdominal muscles will increase pain; but if the pain is from an intraabdominal injury, tensing the abdominal muscles will lessen it.

The physician should listen for bowel sounds. Because bowel sounds may persist for a while after the intestine has ruptured and because ileus is common after chest trauma, even when the abdominal contents have not been injured, the presence or absence of bowel sounds initially is not diagnostic. However, the gradual disappearance of sounds is suggestive of intraabdominal injury.

A rectal examination should be performed in men, and rectal and pelvic examinations should be performed in women. Blood in the rectum indicates damage to the colon or rectum.

Pelvic fractures may be suspected when gentle pressure on the iliac crests or symphysis pubis causes pain. One leg may occasionally be noticeably shorter than the other. Pelvic fractures may be associated with injuries to the rectum, bladder, or male urethra. The short female urethra is rarely injured. Trauma to the bladder causes hematuria that is not usually associated with frank bleeding from the urethral meatus. Blood at the tip of the urethral meatus is a sign of urethral injury and a contraindication to catheterization until the continuity of the urethra has been confirmed. The urethra may rupture on either side of the urogenital diaphragm. Anterior rupture of the urethra typically causes extravasation of blood and urine through Buck's fascia into the superficial tissues of the perineum, scrotum, penis, and anterior abdominal wall with swelling and discoloration of those structures. Rupture of the posterior urethra (on the bladder side of the urogenital diaphragm) is associated with less obvious physical findings because the extravasation of blood and urine is into the retroperitoneum and tissues surrounding the bladder. The hematoma from a posterior urethral rupture may be palpated on rectal examination as a fullness that obliterates the normal feel of the prostate (Fig. 21.1). If the posterior part of the urethra is completely transected and there is rupture of the puboprostatic ligaments, the prostate is no longer fixed in its normal position and cannot be palpated. In young men who normally have a small, barely palpable prostate, the absence of a palpable prostate is not a reliable sign.

Although the initial physical examination is performed in the emergency room by the emergency physician, consultation with a general surgeon should be sought when the signs and symptoms indicate intraabdominal injury or when the magnitude of the force or the nature of the accident was such that the patient should be admitted for observation even though he or she lacks significant evidence of visceral injury. In the unstable patient, exploratory laparotomy is carried out when there is evidence of continued blood loss with persistent or recurrent signs of hypovolemia despite vigorous fluid administration. In the stable patient, exploratory laparotomy is performed if there are signs of peritoneal irritation, intraperitoneal bleeding diagnosed by peritoneal lavage, and roentgenogram evidence of rupture of a hollow viscus.

Clinical Settings

Although the need for laparotomy rests on evidence of continued occult blood loss and/or signs of peritoneal irritation, there are some differences in the presentation of various injuries. It is not always possible to make a diagnosis of specific organ injury preoperatively, but an understanding of the special considerations relating to specific organs is helpful.

SPLEEN

The spleen is the organ most susceptible to injury by blunt trauma. The spleen can be crushed by a force that deforms the left side of the lower part of the rib cage, or the spleen's ligamentous attachments can be torn by rapid deceleration.

Diagnosis

Deep left-sided abdominal pain with coughing and pain in an epaulet pattern distributed over the left shoulder are characteristic of spleen injuries. Subcapsular hematomas may cause pain without significant blood loss. A liver–spleen scan is indicated in the stable patient who has epigastric pain if the diagnosis of subcapsular hematoma is suspected.

Management

Because the spleen plays a major role in the immune response of children, many pediatric surgeons try to avoid removing demonstrably ruptured spleens in children who are hemodynamically stable. In adults the immune function seems to be less important, and a ruptured spleen is generally considered to be an indication for splenectomy. In some instances, it is possible to repair a minimally damaged spleen. It is not clear what action should be taken when a subcapsular hematoma can be demonstrated by a radionuclide scan, but there is no compelling reason for an immediate operation. A subcapsular hematoma may progress to a delayed rupture days or months after the original injury, but no data are available to estimate that risk. At the present time, conservative, expectant treatment seems to be advisable for the asymptomatic patient.

Prognosis

Patients who have isolated ruptures of the spleen have an excellent prognosis. If an operation is performed before the secondary problems of hypervolemia complicate the situation, the patient should survive.

LIVER

Trauma to the liver may be as inconsequential as a minor self-limiting laceration or as severe as exsanguinating hemorrhage from major vessels.

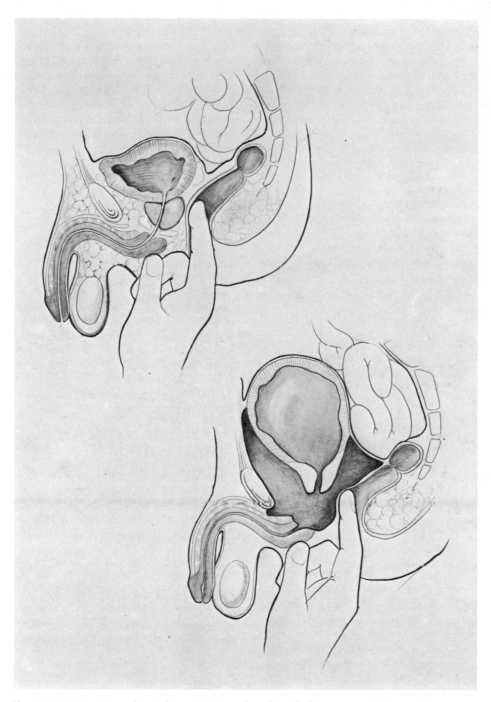

Figure 21.1 Top—Normal rectal examination when the palpable prostate is in normal position. Bottom—when there is urethral disruption, the prostate is not palpable and spongy consistency is present because of retroperitoneal hematoma.

Diagnosis

Injuries to the liver frequently result from a direct crushing force to the right upper quadrant of the chest with fractures of the ninth to the twelfth ribs on the right (see Figs. 12.7, 12.8) or laceration of the diaphragm. Right upper-quadrant pain and evidence of intraabdominal bleeding are the signs of liver injury. Like the spleen, the liver can contain a subcapsular hematoma.

Management

When the liver has ruptured, laparotomy is necessary to control bleeding and to debride devitalized parenchyma. Small cracks in the liver capsule can be treated by simple drainage. Controlling bleeding from tears in the liver parenchyma and the hepatic veins where they join the inferior vena cava may be difficult.

Prognosis

Patients who have small injuries with all nonviable tissue removed have an excellent prognosis. Patients who have more complex injuries that require debridement of large portions of the liver and are associated with trauma to other organs have a higher mortality rate.

DUODENUM AND PANCREAS

The duodenum and pancreas are usually damaged when forces crush them against the rigid vertebral column. Death is common unless the injury is treated promptly.

Diagnosis

Establishing the diagnosis of duodenal or pancreatic injury may be difficult. Because the organs are retroperitoneal, the usual signs of intraperitoneal bleeding may be absent. If there is evidence of retroperitoneal air on the abdominal X-ray films or an elevated serum amylase, the patient should undergo an upper gastrointestinal series with water-soluble contrast material. Elevation of the serum amylase may indicate pancreatic trauma, but the amylase may be normal if only the duodenum is ruptured. Signs and symptoms, when they do appear, may be delayed for 12–24 hours, and peritoneal lavage may be negative.

Management

A pancreaticoduodenectomy is necessary for the treatment of major injuries to the pancreas and/or duodenum. The hematoma that occasionally develops in the duodenum from an injury that is less than transmural may show up as a gastric outlet obstruction several days after the accident as bowel sounds return and oral alimentation resumes. Only nasogastric suction and supportive care are required to treat a patient with a hematoma.

Prognosis

The high mortality rate associated with pancreaticoduodenal injuries is in part a result of massive trauma involving other systems, especially the brain, and of delays in diagnosis.

SMALL AND LARGE INTESTINES

Trauma may perforate the bowel or shear it from the mesenteric vessels. Perforation usually results from a direct crushing force that pinches the bowel against the vertebral column or from high pressures that develop suddenly within an air-filled loop and cause a blowout. The colon may be punctured by a spicule of bone from a pelvic fracture. Shearing injuries are produced by decelerating forces and are frequently associated with wearing seat belts.

Diagnosis

Perforation of the bowel is usually detectable early. Signs of peritoneal irritation are manifested soon after the accident, and free intraperitoneal air is seen on x-ray films. Perforation from the ischemic bowel that has been sheared from the mesenteric vessels may not occur for several days.

Management

Surgery is always necessary for intestinal rupture. If the pelvis is fractured and laceration of the rectum is even suspected, a colostomy is necessary to divert the fecal stream because the contamination of a pelvic hematoma is frequently fatal.

Prognosis

Patients who have isolated injuries of the small intestine or colon have a good prognosis. The prognosis is more guarded when intestinal injury is associated with trauma to other systems.

KIDNEY

The muscles of the back posteriorly and the abdominal viscera anteriorly protect the kidney from injury. Nevertheless, direct trauma to the kidney can result in contusion or laceration, and rapid deceleration can cause an arterial intimal tear with subsequent thrombosis. Rarely can blunt trauma cause complete disruption of the ureteropelvic junction.

Diagnosis

When a patient is admitted with hematuria, the emergency room physician should be alerted to the possibility of renal injury. Most often, gross blood in the urine is associated with major damage, whereas minor contusion tends to produce only microscopic hematuria that clears rapidly. Tenderness in the areas of the lower ribs, upper lumbar vertebrae, flank, or abdomen may reflect hemorrhage or extravasation of urine. When renal damage is suspected, a urologist should be consulted and intravenous urography should be obtained. If the kidney fails to opacify, the urologist will order aortography and selective renal arteriography to determine whether a major vascular injury is present and to define the extent of damage to the kidney. Selective studies of the other aortic branches are useful to rule out other major visceral injuries, particularly to the spleen. Cystoscopy and retrograde pyelography are rarely indicated.

Management

The management of patients with blunt renal trauma depends upon the degree of renal injury and the presence or absence of injuries to other abdominal viscera. Surgery is reserved for patients who have persistent or life-threatening bleeding. If arteriography demonstrates that the main renal vessels have been disrupted, revascularization or nephrectomy is necessary. A few patients with gross hematuria and x-ray film abnormalities eventually require surgical intervention if their clinical status deteriorates. Patients who have gross hematuria with normal intravenous urographic findings require bed rest in the hospital until their urine is clear. Monitoring with frequent blood pressure determinations, hematocrits, and physical examinations is essential because the hematoma, if present, may expand. When hematuria is microscopic, the physical examination is unremarkable, and excretory urogram is normal, the patient can be released from the hospital and followed-up as an outpatient until the hematuria resolves.

Prognosis

Patients who have renal trauma that does not require an operation for control of bleeding have an excellent prognosis. If an operation is required, the prognosis is more guarded because the patients sustained more forceful blows and other systems are likely to be injured.

URINARY BLADDER

Injuries to the urinary bladder are frequently associated with injuries to the bony pelvis. However, if the bladder is distended at the time of direct blunt trauma or deceleration, rupture is possible. Rupture of the renal pelvis may also occur in this circumstance. Most bladder perforations are extraperitoneal. When the bladder wall has been penetrated by a fragment of pelvic bone or when an empty bladder is injured, vessels commonly bleed into the retroperitoneum. Intraperitoneal bleeding is associated with injuries from a direct blow, such as from a kick or seat belt, when the bladder is distended.

Diagnosis

Hematuria, difficulty voiding, and pelvic discomfort are the most common findings when the bladder is ruptured. The diagnosis of a bladder injury may be missed if intravenous urography is the only urologic study. If a ruptured bladder is suspected, the appropriate test is a gravity retrograde cystogram.

Management

The accepted management for a ruptured bladder usually includes surgical repair and drainage, but some selected stable patients with an extraperitoneal bladder rupture and no urinary infection have been managed by simple catheter drainage without formal, operative closure of the bladder.

Prognosis

Patients who have bladder injuries only usually recover quickly. The mortality rate is much higher and the hospital stay longer when the bladder injury is associated with a pelvic fracture.

PELVIC FRACTURE

Pelvic fracture adds a new, complicating dimension to the problem of abdominal trauma. A powerful force is required to break the stout ring of pelvic bones in an adult. The vascular supply to the bones themselves is disrupted, and the adjacent large vessels to the extremities and pelvic viscera are torn resulting in massive retroperitoneal blood loss. Despite the major blood loss, surgical intervention is rarely indicated. When the peritoneum is allowed to remain intact, it will tamponade the bleeding.

Diagnosis

Pelvic fracture should be suspected when compression of the iliac limbs, pressure on the symphysis pubic, or rotation of the hip causes pain. The fracture can sometimes be palpated on rectal or vaginal examination. The diagnosis is confirmed by x-ray films. A pelvic hematoma complicates the diagnosis of injuries to extrapelvic organs. Blood from the hematoma inevitably seeps through small tears in the peritoneum and can be found, in varying quantities, free within the peritoneal cavity. Peritoneal lavage is of limited usefulness in this setting. Pain from a pelvic injury and reflex ileus obscure the physical findings. If arteriography is indicated for the diagnosis and control of pelvic bleeding, the celiac axis and mesenteric vessels can be studied at the same time. The contrast will give an adequate intravenous urogram if follow-up films are timed appropriately.

Management

Direct surgical attack on the hematoma releases the tamponading affects of the peritoneum, may contaminate the hematoma, and is rarely successful in locating a single bleeding source. Ligation of the internal iliac arteries is rarely helpful because the blood supply to the pelvis is so diffuse. Arteriography is the most successful technique for the control of pelvic bleeding. Balloon tamponade and clot embolization are two of the techniques that have been used effectively for control of bleeding.

Prognosis

Major pelvic injuries require a massive force and are frequently associated with other injuries. Patients are often in the hospital for 1–2 months after a pelvic fracture.

MALE URETHRA

The male urethra can be injured directly from blows such as straddle injuries or indirectly in association with a pelvic fracture.

Diagnosis

Urethral bleeding, as opposed to hematuria, is an important sign of urethral injury. Injury to the anterior urethra, distal to the urogenital diaphragm, produces obvious perineal swelling and discoloration. If the posterior urethra is completely transected, there is usually no urinary extravasation because the bladder neck remains competent. An incomplete urethral injury can be converted to a complete transection, and infection can be introduced by ill-advised catheterization. X-Ray films to confirm the diagnosis of posterior urethral injury have been discussed in the cystography section.

Management

Injuries of the anterior urethra may be handled with simple catheter drainage alone. In more extensive cases, surgical repair of the damaged urethra may be necessary. Disruption of the posterior urethra may be treated with extraperitoneal cystotomy for urinary diversion at the time of an exploratory laparotomy. A secondary repair of the urethra can be performed at a later date after the pelvic fracture has stabilized.

Prognosis

Because of modern management techniques, the prognosis for a patient with a functional urogenital system is excellent. Stricture at the site of urethral injury remains a common concern.

MALE GENITALIA

The scrotal sac and penis can contain large quantities of extravasated blood. Relief of pain and prevention of additional bleeding by immobilization, elevation, ice packs, and narcotics are important. In situations in which the testicles cannot be palpated and in which there is any question of injury to the testes, surgical exploration is necessary to determine whether the tunica albuginea has been ruptured with extravasation of intracapsular contents.

UTERUS

The normal uterus is a tough, mobile organ that is rarely injured by blunt trauma. Direct blows to the more vulnerable, extremely vascular, gravid uterus can rupture that organ and produce life-threatening intraperitoneal hemorrhage. The presence of fetal heart sounds is good evidence for the integrity of the gravid uterus. The fallopian tubes and normal ovaries are rarely damaged by blunt trauma.

PENETRATING INJURIES

Gunshot Wound

The prevalent use of handguns is distressing but persistent. The severity of a gunshot wound depends upon the energy expended by the bullet as it passes through the tissue. The expended energy is related to the velocity, weight of the missile, and the tendency of the missile to deform. Soft-nose bullets become deformed and expend all of their energy before exiting, whereas steel-jacketed bullets may pass easily through the tissues giving up less energy and causing less injury. The velocity of the bullet is inversely related to the distance from the gun. The bullet's weight generally increases with increasing caliber. Shotguns present a different problem in that the pellet pattern is tightly grouped at short range but rapidly widens, and the energy rapidly decreases as the distance from the gun increases. Whereas shotgun wounds inflicted at close range are devastating, shotgun wounds from 55 m away may be trivial at the edge of the pattern. In addition to the pellets, shotgun wounds may contain the paper or plastic wadding. At close range, shotgun wounds may cause a major tissue loss from the abdominal wall resulting in external blood loss as well as evisceration of abdominal contents. Bullets are sterilized by the heat generated in passage through the weapon and the air, and they need not be retrieved from a patient simply because they are foreign bodies.

Assessment

Initially, it is safest to assume that a bullet wound of the trunk may have injured anything in the abdominal or thoracic cavities. The physician's priorities are for airway maintenance, ventilatory stability, and blood volume support. From knowledge of the caliber of the weapon, the position of the patient, and the distance from the weapon, inferences can be made regarding the extent of injury.

Bullet wounds of the lower part of the chest are difficult to evaluate. During expiration, the dome of the diaphragm may rise as high as the fourth interspace and bullets that enter the chest may penetrate the peritoneal cavity through the diaphragm. When the patient is stable, the entrance and exit wounds can be marked with radiopaque markers for comparison with the level of the diaphragm on inspiratory and expiratory chest films. Peritoneal lavage may be helpful to establish the diagnosis of peritoneal penetration in the patient who has been shot in the lower part of the chest. The consulting surgeon may perform a peritoneal lavage either in the operating room if the patient is undergoing thoracotomy or in the emergency room if the chest injury is not severe enough to require a thoracotomy.

The other major preoperative diagnostic problem is whether the kidneys and ureter have been damaged in the retroperitoneum. Injuries to the bladder are usually apparent when the abdomen is explored. It is preferable not to explore the retroperitoneum; consequently, preoperative knowledge that the urinary tract is uninjured may obviate the need to explore that area. In the stable patient with adequate renal perfusion, an intravenous urogram may be ordered by the consultant in order to simplify the operation.

Since injuries to the colon are likely, patients should be advised of the possibility of a temporary colostomy.

Management and Prognosis

All patients who are shot in the abdomen should have an exploratory laparotomy. Intraoperative management consists of inspection and repair of all damaged organs.

Patients who survive long enough to reach the operating room will usually survive the injury. The mortality rate for intraabdominal injuries from gunshot wounds is about 12%. Death is usually caused by blood loss in patients who never reach the operating room or are in refractory shock from major vessel injury when they do reach the operating room.

Stab Wounds of the Abdomen

Many stab wounds do not penetrate the peritoneal cavity, and many wounds that do penetrate the peritoneum do not injure the abdominal contents. Except for gaping wounds with protruding intestines or omentum, the size and characteristics of the entrance wound give no information regarding possible visceral injury. The length of the weapon and the force with which it was wielded determine the potential for injury.

Assessment

The physical examination of patients with stab wounds is confusing because there is always some tenderness and rigidity around the entrance site whether there is peritoneal irritation or not. Tenderness at a distance from a stab wound may indicate intraperitoneal bleeding or irritation of the peritoneum by bowel content. Tests for rebound tenderness must take into account the local discomfort around the entrance wound.

Management

Assessment and management are inextricably blended. The problem is to identify visceral injury, and a laparotomy is frequently the primary diagnostic procedure. In contrast to the established general opinion favoring universal exploration for gunshot wounds of the abdomen, many centers are now favoring a conservative "wait and see" policy regarding stab wounds of the abdomen. In 1960 the policy of selective laparotomy was given impetus by Shafton who reported that, in the absence of definite clinical criteria of visceral injury, there was a high incidence of negative explorations for abdominal stab wounds. Maynard and Oropeza argued in favor of mandatory laparotomy. They found visceral injuries in some patients in their series during their operations despite the lack of physical signs. Since a patient with unrecognized visceral injury may be harmed by a delay in treatment, we recommend exploratory laparotomy if peritoneal penetration has occurred. Unfortunately, the diagnosis of peritoneal penetration is not always easy. The surgeon may employ peritoneal lavage, wound exploration, sinography, minilaparotomy, and peritoneoscopy to improve the diagnosis of abdominal wall penetration.

Wound exploration carried out in the emergency room by the emergency room physician under local anesthesia is the simplest technique for the evaluation of a deep stab wound penetration. Those patients who have only superficial wounds without fascial penetration can usually be identified by wound exploration. When fascial penetration is confirmed, the patient should be taken to the operating room so that possible peritoneal penetration can be investigated under general anesthesia by wound exploration, peritoneoscopy, or laparotomy. Under local anesthesia, it may be difficult to trace the knife tract beneath the fascia through a wound obscured by hematoma, active bleeding, muscle edema, and muscle spasm.

A minilaparotomy performed in the operating room involves a small incision near the entrance wound. The incision can be extended for general exploration if penetration of the peritoneum is found. Peritoneoscopy is similar to minilaparotomy but is slightly less traumatic and calls for a peritoneoscope instead of a small incision. Peritoneoscopy is less useful, more difficult, and carries a greater risk if a patient has had previous abdominal surgery. Minilaparotomy and peritoneoscopy are not intended to rule out retroperitoneal injuries from wounds in the flank or back. The only purpose of these techniques is to confirm whether the anterior peritoneum has been penetrated. If peritoneoscopy is negative, the patient may be discharged from the hospital after recovery from anesthesia; if minilaparotomy is negative the patient may be discharged in 24–48 hours. If penetration of the peritoneum is confirmed by wound exploration, minilaparotomy, or peritoneoscopy or if damage to retroperitoneal organs from a wound in the flank or back is suspected, then exploratory laparotomy is necessary. Stab wounds of the lower chest may enter the peritoneum through the diaphragm. Damage to intraperitoneal organs and intraabdominal bleeding can be detected by peritoneal lavage.

A sinogram of the wound tract can be performed by injecting contrast material under pressure into a catheter that has been sealed into the wound by a tight, purse-string suture. Entry of contrast material into the peritoneal cavity as demonstrated by plain x-ray film or fluoroscopy is proof of penetration of the abdominal wall. Although this simple technique can be performed by an emergency room physician and a positive test is definitive evidence for peritoneal penetration, sinography has an unacceptable incidence of false-negative results and is not recommended. False-negative results are caused by muscle spasm, obliquity of the tract, and difficulty in obtaining a tight seal at the skin.

Iatrogenic Injuries

COLONOSCOPY

Perforation of the colon, most frequently at the rectosigmoid and the junction of the sigmoid and descending colon, has been reported as a complication of 0.4–1% of colonoscopies. The bowel wall may be penetrated when the base of a polyp is coagulated and the polyp is severed from the bowel wall with a snare. A diverticulum may be blown out by excessive insufflation. Most perforations are treated with exploratory laparotomy and closure of the perforation. Occasionally, however, a colostomy is necessary. Because most perforations are small and the bowel has been cleansed in preparation for the study, surgery may not be necessary for all patients for whom free air is seen on abdominal x-ray film following colonoscopy. Indeed, isolated case reports suggest that some asymptomatic patients who have free air seen on routine abdominal x-ray films after colonoscopy may be treated nonsurgically. Which patient should be treated in this manner is not clear. If laparotomy is postponed until an asymptomatic patient develops symptoms, the surgeon may lose the opportunity to close the colon primarily and be forced to perform a colostomy. In that case, the overall morbidity of the complication would be increased. Until better guidelines are available for selecting patients to be managed without surgery, laparotomy and closure of perforated bowel appears to be the safest course of action.

GASTROSCOPY

Fiberoptic gastroscopy also carries a small risk of perforation. Some patients with free air in the peritoneal cavity after fiberoptic gastroscopy fail to demonstrate extravasation when radiologic studies are made with a water-soluble contrast medium, and no perforation is found in some patients who undergo laparotomy. Because the stomach is empty during endoscopy and because gastric juice is sterile, small perforations of the stomach can frequently be managed with nasogastric suction and antibiotics. However, if an endoscope is passed through a tear in the stomach, laparotomy to close such a large perforation is advisable.

NEEDLE BIOPSIES OR CHOLANGIOGRAPHY

Needle biopsies of the liver or kidneys may cause intraperitoneal bleeding that should be treated with transfusion and observation. If the transfusion requirement exceeds 3 units, laparotomy is indicated. Percutaneous cholangiography carries the added risk of bile leakage from penetration of distended biliary radicles.

SUGGESTED READINGS

Blaisdell FN, Trunkey DD: *Trauma Management*. New York, Thieme-Stratton, 1982, vol 1.

Clark SS, Prudencio RF: Lower urinary tract injuries associated with pelvic fractures. Diagnosis and management. *Surg Clin North Am* 1972; 52:183.

Davis JJ, Cohn I, Nance FC: Diagnosis and management of blunt abdominal trauma. *Ann Surg* 1976; 183:672.

Ecker MD, Goldstein M, Hoexter B et al: Benign pneumoperitoneum after fiberoptic colonoscopy. *Gastroenterology* 1977; 73:226.

Federle MP, Goldberg HI, Kaiser JA, et al: Evaluation of abdominal trauma by computed tomography. *Radiology* 1981; 138:637–644.

Lucas CE: The role of peritoneal lavage for penetrating abdominal wounds. *J Trauma* 1977; 17:649.

Maynard A de L, Oropeza G: Mandatory operation for penetrating wounds of the abdomen. *Am J Surg* 1968; 115:307.

Parvin S, Smith DE, Asher WN, Virgilio RW: Effectiveness of peritoneal lavage in blunt trauma. *Ann Surg* 1975; 181:255.

Root HD, Hauser CW, McKinley CR et al: Diagnostic peritoneal lavage. *Surgery* 1965; 57:633.

Shafton GW: Indications for operation in abdominal trauma. *Am J Surg* 1960; 99:657.

22
MUSCULOSKELETAL INJURIES

Roger H. Emerson, Jr.
St. George T. Aufranc

The emergency room physician will be called upon to evaluate a wide spectrum of musculoskeletal injuries occurring in young athletes on the school playing field, in the elderly in nursing homes, or in people with multiple injuries from motor vehicle or industrial accidents. Whereas the ultimate treatment for these injuries can be complex, requiring specialized skills and knowledge, the initial management follows basic principles and can significantly affect the patient's ultimate outcome.

Some extremity injuries are obvious, but many, including the most severe, can be overlooked. Frequently, deformity, swelling, pain, and local skin changes will be a clue to the presence of injury. This is especially true of injuries in the arm and leg. Injuries to the spine, pelvis, hip, and shoulder, on the other hand, are often unaccompanied by these signs because of the soft tissues covering these deep structures. Accordingly, injuries to these areas are frequently missed. In addition, if the patient is unable to cooperate and provide information, the evaluating emergency room physician must suspect injuries based upon the circumstances of the trauma. Each bone should be palpated and all joints put through a range of motion. All unconscious patients with trauma should have an x-ray film of the pelvis, hips, and entire spine taken.

There is a tendency for the busy emergency room physician to rely too heavily on radiographic evaluation. Needless to say x-ray films are an important aid to diagnosis but "normal x-ray films" should not lull the practitioner into a false sense of security. Ligamentous injuries and neurovascular compromise (e.g., a compartment syndrome) will not be apparent on radiographs but will be evident upon a quick but thorough physical examination. At the same time, x-ray films that reveal bony damage cause the practitioner to focus on these very obvious abnormalities and possibly miss the associated soft tissue injuries. This is most common in patients with pelvic fractures who have a mortality rate of up to 40% as a result of the associated soft tissue pathology.

In the case of fractures, the soft tissues are extremely important because they are the source of vascular supply needed for fracture healing as well as for providing a barrier to infection. The state of the soft tissues at the time of the injury should be noted and documented. Frequently the associated soft tissue injuries will manifest themselves during the first few hours after an injury. For example, skin necrosis, vascular thrombosis, or compartment syndrome from a crushing injury are usually not present at the initial evaluation. The amount of swelling, the absence of pulses, and the coloration of the skin noted on the initial report will help greatly in determining the next stage of management. The soft tissue injury that is present is based on the circumstances of the injury, especially the amount of energy imparted to the extremity, as well as the age of the patient and the time elapsed since the injury.

INITIAL ASSESSMENT OF THE IMPAIRED EXTREMITY

The examination of patients with musculoskeletal injuries must be methodical and organized in order to prevent oversights and to be efficient. The emergency room physician should assume that the patient is seriously injured with life and limb threatening injuries and then should proceed to establish that such injuries do not, in fact, exist. The methods of resuscitation of the musculoskeletally injured patient do not differ from those methods discussed in Chapter 11. Needless to say, the patient's airway, circulatory status, and vital signs take precedence over injuries of the extremities. For example, an extremity can remain ischemic for up to 6 hours without irreversible damage. This does not mean, however, that the extremity can be completely ignored during the care of higher priority items. Extremities with deformity or false motion should be prevented from possible further injuries as a result of unprotected movements or falls. The use of adhesive tape, pillows, and sandbags is sufficient to accomplish this. The use of such measures can be delegated to others while the physician tends to the higher priority areas.

After the initial resuscitation of the polytrauma victim, the current thrust in care is to manage the extremity and skeletal injuries concurrently with head, chest, and abdominal injuries.

History

A clear and chronological history is unquestionably important. The physician should assume that the patient may lapse into unconsciousness at any minute; therefore, during the first few moments of the interview, the physician should establish the presence of allergies, the use of medications, and the presence of other medical ailments. Once this has been accomplished, the details of the injury can be obtained. The physician should not assume anything since many patients present with injuries or fractures that have taken place days before, and they may or may not have received some form of treatment of which the physician should be aware.

The magnitude of the trauma involved should be known. If the patient cannot provide this information, the examining physician should discuss the details of the accident with the emergency personnel who were involved in transporting the patient to the hospital. The possibility of associated injury is increased when the patient has been involved in a high-speed collision or in a fall from a great height. A trivial injury resulting in a major fracture should be a clue to an underlying pathologic disorder. People frequently fall from causes other than clumsiness or accidents. Witnesses or paramedical personnel may be able to provide details of traumatic events that may suggest unsuspected head injury, seizure disorder, or a cardiac event, for example. The patient's preinjury status should be established soon after an injury. This is especially true, for example, in the case of elderly patients who may not have been ambulatory before their hip fractures. Such knowledge will influence treatment and will help predict functional outcome.

Examination

Examination of the musculoskeletal system does not take long. In the situation of a patient with multiple injuries, the patient's clothes should be entirely removed to permit adequate access and accurate observations.

The examination should follow the format outlined in Table 22.1. The first part of the examination should be the observation of the skin and the assessment of deformity. After this, each bone of the area and each joint should be palpated and each joint should be put through a range of motion. (Muscular strength testing, if appropriate, should follow, depending on the status of the corresponding bones and joints.) The vascular status should be established next, followed by the assessment of sensation. Further neurologic testing would depend upon the clinical situation.

The examiner should be able to see asymmetry by comparing

TABLE 22.1 Outline of Musculoskeletal Examination

1. Observation; skin changes, deformity, swelling
2. Palpation of bones and joints; crepitation, effusions, defects
3. Range of motion of joints
4. Motor strength
5. Vascular assessment
6. Sensory assessment

one side to the other. Areas of abrasions or ecchymoses should lead the examiner to suspect underlying pathology. For example, when there are abrasions on the forehead, a cervical spine injury should be ruled out, and when there are significant abrasions on the knee, the possibility of a dislocation of the hip or patellar fracture should be considered. Each bone should be palpated, looking for tenderness or a defect, malalignment, false motion, or crepitation. The examiner should start at the top of the cervical spine, feeling each spinous process. The clavicles should then be palpated from the sternal attachment to the acromioclavicular joints. The thoracic and lumbar spine should be palpated, followed by bimanual compression of the iliac crests and palpation of the pubic rami. The long bones, starting with the humerus, radius, and ulna, followed by the femur, tibia, and fibula, should be palpated. Next, each joint should be put through a range of motion, actively by the patients if possible, but assisted by the examiner if need be. Clearly, an emergency lateral radiograph of the cervical spine should be obtained before permitting a patient to move his or her neck if there is suspicion of a cervical spine injury from the palpation or history.

Many methods of measuring range of motion exist, and all are satisfactory as long as the examiner is consistent throughout the examination. The American Academy of Orthopedic Surgery has established a standardized range of motion format based on the zero extended position. According to this method, the extended anatomical position is 0 deg of motion. Joint motion is described as flexion, extension, abduction, adduction, internal rotation, or external rotation, depending on the joint in question. Figure 22.1 is an example of the zero extended position method applied to the elbow joint. See the suggested readings at the end of this chapter for a more detailed discussion.

The motor examination should test for active motor function. Stroking the foot and observing a motion of the toes do not rule out a spinal cord injury. The evaluating physician must have the patient perform the functions actively, thereby establishing that the normal motor pathways from the cerebral cortex through the spinal cord and peripheral nerve to the muscle are functioning. Since motor strength in an extremity is dependent on many variables, including the health of the joints, ligaments, bones, and nerves, it is not a helpful parameter in assessing acute situations in detail.

The circulatory status of the extremities should be examined next. The presence or absence of peripheral pulses and the state of capillary filling should be recorded on the patient's chart. This is especially important before any manipulation of an injured extremity in order to ascertain if that manipulation caused a change in the vascular status. Frequently a Doppler

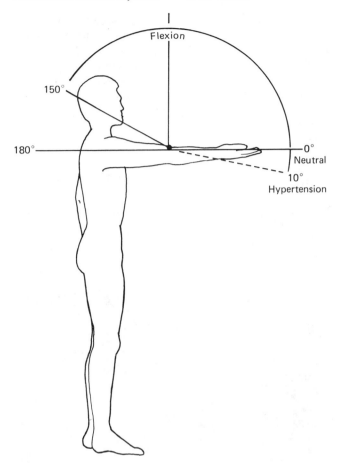

Figure 22.1 The zero extended position of measuring joint range of motion as adopted by the American Academy of Orthopedic Surgery. Note that hyperextension refers to extension beyond the usual range of motion for that joint. A wrist joint would have both flexion and extension from zero, whereas the elbow, hip, and knee normally do not extend beyond the neutral position and therefore further extension is referred to as hyperextension.

unit is required to "hear" pulses in swollen extremities. The presence of normal pulses to palpation does not rule out a compartment syndrome. A pulse volume recording, if available, is another method of objectively assessing the circulation in an extremity.

Testing for sensation can vary from the crude to the elegant, but it is of major importance to ascertain whether or not what the patient feels is normal for that patient. Testing by light touch is a sufficient screening examination of the sensory system. If its appreciation is diminished or absent, a more detailed sensory examination is indicated. The use of a pin prick for sensory testing is a poor choice since it can be felt in the presence of rather major neurologic injuries. Besides leading the examiner astray, it is an unpleasant test for the patient.

Associated Injuries

There are a number of orthopedic injuries that are frequently accompanied by other injuries. The association is so common that if one such injury is present, the other must be ruled out in every case (Table 22.2). When the patient is unconscious, the presence of a cervical spine fracture, pelvic fracture, or hip dislocation cannot be assumed to be absent. Clavicle fractures may injure the brachial plexus and vessels. Fractures of the distal half of the clavicle are frequently associated with acromioclavicular derangements. Shoulder pain with unremarkable anterior–posterior x-ray films may represent a posterior dislocation. Scapular fractures are generally from high-energy injuries, and it is necessary to look for the presence of a first rib fracture and pneumothorax. With mid- and distal humerus fractures, the status of the radial nerve should be routinely tested for and documented on the patient's chart. Supracondylar fractures of the humerus are frequently accompanied by vascular injuries to the brachial artery. When there

TABLE 22.2 Commonly Associated Injuries

What Is Found	What to look for
Unconscious patient	Spine, pelvis fractures
	Hip dislocation
Clavicle fractures	Vascular, neurologic injury
	Acromioclavicular injury
Shoulder pain	Posterior dislocation
Scapular fractures	First rib fractures
	Pneumothorax
Mid-, distal humerus fractures	Radial nerve injury
Supracondylar fractures humerus	Brachial artery injury
	Compartment syndrome forearm
Ulnar shaft fracture	Radial head dislocation
Elbow pain	Radial head fracture
Wrist pain	Scaphoid fracture
Patellar fracture	Dislocated hip
Dislocated hip	Sciatic nerve injury
Knee ligament disruption	Popliteal artery injury
Heel pain	Os calis fracture
	L-1 or L-2 compression fracture
Foot pain	Midfoot dislocation
Excessive pain, normal pulses	Compartment syndrome

are ulnar shaft fractures, look for dislocation of the radial head. The more proximal the ulnar fracture, the more likely there is radial head dislocation. Elbow pain with an unremarkable x-ray film usually indicates a radial head fracture. Wrist pain with a normal x-ray film is indicative of a navicular fracture until such a fracture is ruled out 10 days later with subsequent x-ray films. (The patient's wrist should be immobilized with a thumb-spica cast or splint until the second set of x-ray films.) A patellar or femoral fracture is frequently accompanied by a dislocated hip, especially if the injury was sustained when the patient was in the sitting position. In all patients with dislocated hips, the status of the sciatic nerve should be documented. Ligamentous disruptions of the knee place the popliteal artery in jeopardy. All dislocations of the knee should be evaluated with a femoral arteriogram. Heel pain may be indicative of an os calcis fracture and is frequently accompanied by compression fractures of the first and second lumbar vertebrae. Lower lumbar pain or thigh pain in an elderly patient with trauma can be exclusively from a compression fracture of the twelfth thoracic vertebra. Foot pain with swelling but without gross deformity can be a result of a Lisfranc's dislocation of the tarsal and metatarsal bones of the foot. This condition can be subtle on an x-ray film, and comparison views of the other foot may be necessary. In an extremity, excessive pain associated with swelling despite normal pulses can represent a compartment syndrome. Measurement of the individual compartment pressures is diagnostic.

Radiographic Evaluation

The above examination of the patient should take place before ordering or sending any patient with multiple injuries to the radiology suite. A thorough examination will allow the physician to order the appropriate x-ray films and will prevent a potentially unstable patient from spending time away from resuscitative equipment and trained personnel. If the examination reveals a cervical spine injury, portable x-ray films before any manipulations of the patient should be obtained. After the patient's vital signs have been stabilized, there is no excuse for poor quality films that hinder an accurate diagnosis. Two views of each injured extremity are needed at 90 deg angles to each other. There are few circumstances in which such views cannot be obtained. In general, the emergency room physician should order the routine views and leave stress films, arthrograms, tomography, and computed tomographic (CT) scanning to the discretion of the physician who assumes the care of the injured patient. There are, however, special views with which every emergency room physician should be familiar.

The proximal humerus is difficult to assess with standard anterior–posterior and lateral views because the thorax obscures shoulder detail on the lateral view. Two oblique views at 90 deg angles to each other eliminate this problem, the first oblique view being a true anterior–posterior of the scapula, and the second being a tangential view of the scapula. Using these views, fractures of the humeral neck and proximal shaft, as well as dislocations of the shoulder joint and fractures of the scapula, can be diagnosed (Figs. 22.2 and 22.3). These x-ray films are easily obtained when the patient is in a sitting position in a sling.

Pelvic fractures should be assessed with three views: a true anterior–posterior view, an inlet view, and an outlet view. These can be obtained with the patient supine by simply tilting the x-ray beam.

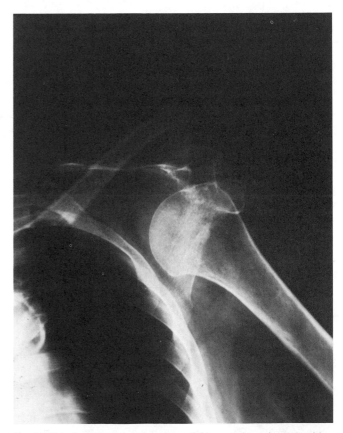

Figure 22.2 Anterior–posterior view of the scapula and proximal humerus with an anterior dislocation of the glenohumeral joint.

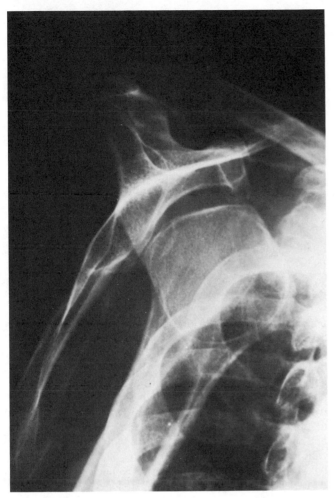

Figure 22.3 Lateral view of the scapula and proximal humerus fracture showing the humeral head anterior to the glenoid process and beneath the corocoid process. This view reliably indicates the presence of a glenohumeral dislocation and the x-ray film is taken without discomfort to the patient.

X-Ray films of fractures of long bones should include both the joints above and below the fracture, ideally, on the same film or, at the very least, on a subsequent x-ray film. X-Ray films of carpal bones and feet can be confusing, especially to the nonspecialist, and comparison views of the other side are helpful. The same is true for children with epiphysial fractures. Such comparison views should not be ordered routinely, but the practitioner should have no hesitancy in ordering them on an individual basis.

No patient with any type of injury should be sent to the radiology suite without appropriate splinting. See the discussion below for techniques in splinting.

FILM INTERPRETATION

There are several important points to remember when interpreting extremity x-ray films. Always look at the soft tissues before looking at the bony outlines. The bleeding that accompanies a fracture produces soft tissue swelling, which can either obliterate or deform the overlying muscle planes that are easily seen on x-ray films. A slightly impacted fracture or a completely undisplaced one may not be visible at all when we look at the bony contours on the film, but the resulting effusion distends the capsule so that the swollen borders on the x-ray film may be the only clues to the underlying injury. Interestingly, both blood and muscle have the same water density on x-ray films so that their shadows are undistinguishable. There are, however, fat pads in the areas of joints, especially in the elbow. An intraarticular effusion elevates these structures, producing a more lucent area in the vicinity of the fracture.

After the soft tissues have been evaluated, the bones themselves should be studied. The contour of each bone should be followed completely. The examiner's eye should focus along the outer margin of each bone and follow this line until the starting point is reached again. In the adult, this contour is unbroken and smooth. The fracture line at the cortical surface presents as a lucent interruption of the smooth contour. For the most part, such lucencies can be traced completely through one side of the bone to the other. As a matter of caution it is important to remember that such fracture lines may be confused with the nutrient vessel to the bone. In the case of the vessel, however, the lucency has an oblique course and a rounded starting point and does not traverse the entire width of the bone involved. Always correlate the area of injury as indicated by the physical examination and the findings on the x-ray films.

In children the bony contour is interrupted by the epiphyseal plate, which appears as a lucent line completely detaching the epiphysis from the metaphysis. It is easy to see therefore that if a fracture existed across the epiphyseal plate and was undisplaced, it could go undetected by x-ray film. Accordingly, nondisplaced epiphyseal fractures are a clinical, not radiographic, diagnosis. In general, the practitioner should have a low threshold for treatment for any injury that may represent a fracture but for which x-ray film confirmation is lacking. Reexamination at a later date will reveal the true nature of the injury.

Description of an Injury

The description of an orthopedic injury, namely a fracture, should be in simple and understandable language. In order to communicate all of the important information reliably, the practitioner should adopt an organized format that can be used to describe a series of injuries. The American Academy of Orthopedic Surgeons has suggested a standardized method of measuring and recording joint motion. The extended anatomical position of an extremity is defined as 0 deg, and all motions are measured from this defined zero starting position. Thus, the degrees of motion of a joint are added in the direction the joint moves from the zero starting position (Fig. 22.1). Deformities are described from the reference point of the distal in relation to the proximal positions.

The following features should be described for any orthopedic injury (see also Table 22.3):

1. Location (shaft, juxta-, or intraarticular)
2. Closed/open, skin condition
3. Simple/comminuted
4. Displaced/nondisplaced
5. Neurovascular status

In general, long bones are divided into thirds, namely, the proximal, middle, and distal thirds. A fracture line adjacent to a joint, but not entering, is referred to as a juxtaarticular fracture. If a fracture line enters a joint, it should be described as being intraarticular.

A fracture is either *closed* or *open*. In a closed fracture, there is no break in the skin. In an open fracture, the skin is broken either right over the fracture site or near it and communicates with the fracture site. When the bone is sticking out of the wound, the fracture is obviously open. An open fracture may go unrecognized, however, when the arm or leg looks fairly straight and there is a small laceration some centimeters away from the actual fracture site. Frequently these lacerations communicate with the fracture site itself. There are three grades of open fracture: A grade I fracture is a wound less than 1 cm long that is a result of an underlying sharp fracture fragment piercing the skin from within. These wounds are clean and have a low incidence of infection. A grade II open fracture is a larger laceration up to 5 cm long, without contamination or crush. A grade III open fracture involves a large laceration with associated crushing and contamination. There is frequently a segmental fracture. A traumatic amputation is considered a grade III open fracture.

A fracture is either *simple* or *comminuted*. A simple fracture means that the bone is broken in only two pieces. If the bone has been splintered into any more than two pieces, the patient has a comminuted fracture.

Fractures are either *displaced* or *nondisplaced*. An undisplaced fracture has no deformity. There is accordingly very little disruption of the blood supply to the bone and these fractures heal relatively quickly with a high rate of union. When there is deformity present, a displaced fracture exists. The features of displacement that must be described are (1) the length, (2) the alignment or angulation, (3) the opposition of the fragments, and (4) the rotation (Table 22.4).

The fracture fragments can be *distracted* or *foreshortened*; the latter is called *overriding* or *bayonet opposition*. Such foreshortening leads to shortening that may be tolerated in the upper extremity but not in the lower extremity. At the same time the rate of union is much diminished by opposition of less than 50% of the diameter of the fractured end in most bones. Whereas most deformities are clear and easily discernable on the x-ray film, rotational fractures deserve a special note. In general, rotational malalignment must be determined by looking at the extremity itself. There are, however, hints as to rotational asymmetry on the x-ray film since most bones are not perfectly cylindrical. Accordingly, malrotated fragments will have different widths on the x-ray film. Again, it should be emphasized that according to convention, a deformity is described as the distal fragment in relation to the proximal fragment.

Finally, the condition of the skin and the *neurovascular status* of the injured extremity should be described. Even when there are no actual cuts or breaks in the skin, there are frequently abrasions or contusions. This is important to recognize since some fractures that may require surgery will have to be treated on an emergency basis if there are abrasions over the intended operative site. The abraded area will rapidly colonize bacteria

---

TABLE 22.3 Fracture Description

1. Location; diaphyseal, metaphyseal, juxta, or intraarticular
2. Closed/open, skin condition
3. Comminution
4. Displacement
5. Neurovascular status

TABLE 22.4 Features of Fracture Displacement

1. Length
2. Alignment or angulation
3. Opposition of fragments
4. Rotation

and make a delay in surgery of a few days less attractive or even contraindicated because of the added risk of infection. Very contused skin or a massively swollen extremity will lead to problems in the healing of the skin, and, accordingly, surgery would not be performed at that point, all other things being equal.

INITIAL MANAGEMENT OF THE INJURED EXTREMITY

Initial Handling

The injured extremity, especially as a result of a fracture or a crush, must be handled carefully. The patient will not have normal muscular control of the arm or leg because of reflex inhibition of the controlling musculature or because of direct injury to the nerves or muscles themselves. The extremity is at risk of further injury due to uncontrolled movements because of the presence of sharp bony fracture fragments. Increased bleeding, pain, and increased contamination at the wounded area will result from inadequate protection.

The examiner should handle the injured extremity with good control to prevent deformity. This will usually require an assistant to lift and hold the patient while the examiner removes the clothing and dressings and assesses the limb. If large open wounds are present, especially over the fractures, the examiner should use sterile gloves and a face mask and should not probe the wounds. Such introduction of objects into a wound will only increase contamination and bleeding, and there is very little benefit in terms of additional clinical information. These wounds should be covered with a sterile dressing soaked in povidone–iodine and should not be inspected further until the patient is in the operating room.

As long as the vascular status of the limb is satisfactory, deformity should not be corrected before radiographic evaluation. An exception to this rule is the situation of a bony fragment impinging tightly on the skin. This will produce ischemic damage to the skin, if not actually cause laceration of the skin, thereby creating an open fracture.

Immobilization

The injured extremity should be splinted at all times. The best method varies with the location of the injury. Generally speaking, the splint must provide adequate immobilization and, if possible, must permit safe and comfortable transferring of the patient to and from stretchers and x-ray tables.

Fractures of the femur are best immobilized by means of Buck's traction, further supported with sandbagging to prevent rotation. Other extremity injuries can be immobilized adequately with splints. There are several types of commercially available splints for the elbow, wrist, hand, knee, and ankle. Although these splints work well, there are many patients who do not fit the available sizes, and a prefabricated splint may not sufficiently accommodate their particular deformities.

The simplest and most efficient splinting material is plaster of paris, which is readily available in all hospital emergency areas. Splints can be made to any size, width, or thickness depending upon the clinical situation. Splints for the upper extremities need not be as thick as those for the lower extremities, and splints for stronger, heavier people need to be stronger than those for thinner, less-muscled people. Five or six layers of plaster are sufficient for the upper extremities, whereas twice as many layers are required for the lower extremities. The opposite uninjured extremity can be used as a template to measure the length of the splint needed. For most hand and wrist injuries, 3-inch plaster is sufficient, for elbow injuries, 4-inch plaster is sufficient, and for the lower extremities 5- or 6-inch plaster is adequate. Three or four layers of cast padding are prepared in the shape of the splint. The plaster is dipped into lukewarm water and placed onto the previously cut cast padding after the excess water is removed. One more layer of cast padding is placed on top of the plaster, and the splint is then held up to the injured extremity and positioned there by an assistant while the physician secures the splint to the extremity with a circular gauze dressing or an elasticized dressing. If an elastic dressing is used, care must be taken to prevent excessive tightening of the dressing as a result of the elastic. Adhesive tape around the edges of the splint and across the layers of circular dressing helps to prevent the dressing from loosening.

There are three commonly used splints for the hand. They are the ulna gutter splint, which incorporates the ring and little fingers, wrist, and forearm (Fig. 22.4); the usual wrist splint, which can be placed on the volar or dorsal side of the wrist and can be extended to the metacarpophalangeal joints or to the tips of the fingers, depending on the clinical situation (Fig. 22.5); and the radial gutter splint, which incorporates the thumb, first metacarpophalangeal joint, hand, and wrist (Fig. 22.6). If a hand splint is designed to immobilize the wrist, the splint should stop just proximal to the distal palmar crease to permit full metacarpophalangeal joint flexion. If the fingers are included in the splint, they must be held with metacarpophalangeal joint flexion of 70 deg and interphalangeal extension of 30 deg. The tips of the fingers should be visible for vascular inspection. If the thumb is immobilized, it should be held in an abducted position from the palm.

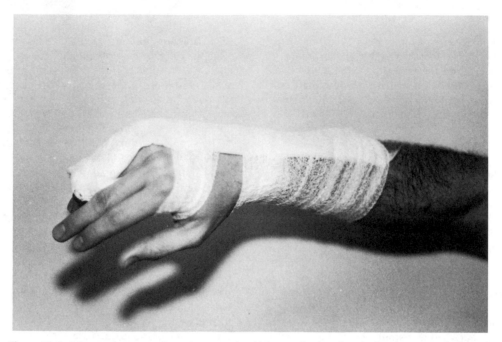

Figure 22.4 Ulna and gutter splint. The wrist should be gently dorsiflexed, the metacarpophalangeal joint flexed 70 deg, and the interphalangeal joints flexed 30 deg. Adequate padding must be placed over the dorsum of the metacarpophalangeal joints.

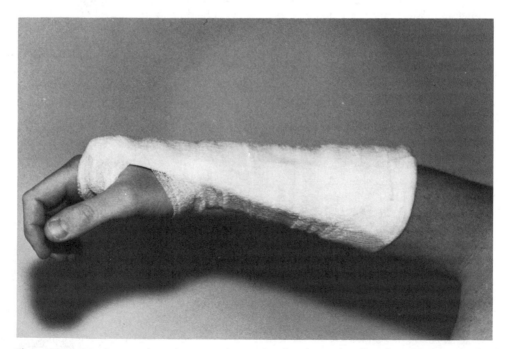

Figure 22.5 Dorsal wrist splint. The wrist splint can be placed on either the volar side or dorsal side of the wrist. It is more likely to interfere with finger motion when placed on the volar side.

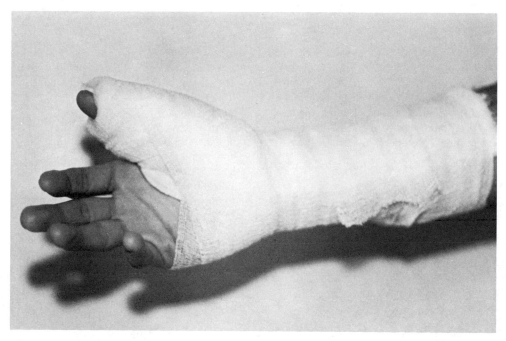

Figure 22.6 Radial gutter splint. The splint starts at the tip of the thumb and crosses the joints of the thumb and wrist immobilizing both the thumb and the wrist. It is especially good for tendonitis conditions across the wrist.

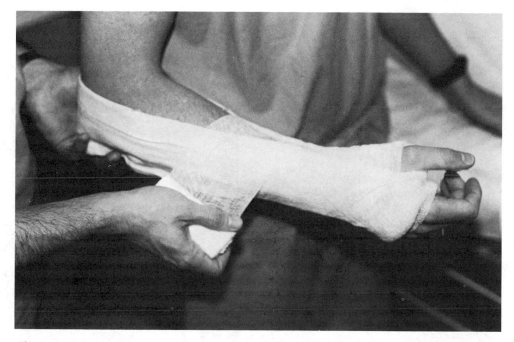

Figure 22.7 Sugar-tong forearm splint. This splint immobilizes the wrist and forearm and prevents rotation at the elbow. It is especially appropriate for a nondisplaced Colles' fracture.

401

There are two splints commonly used near the elbow. The first is the sugar-tong splint (Fig. 22.7), which also immobilizes the wrist. It is designed especially for forearm injuries in which rotation of the forearm needs to be controlled. An example of such an injury is a Colles' fracture of the distal radius. The other splint is the posterior splint, which can include the hand if need be. If the hand is uninjured, however, the splint should start at the wrist and progress posteriorly up the back of the arm to the axilla.

The humerus is best splinted by means of medial and lateral splints or coaptation splints in which the arm is supported with a cuff around the wrist suspended from the neck (Fig. 22.8). The weight of the arm will help align the fracture (Fig. 22.9). If there is no fracture motion, a regular sling is sufficient to support the arm.

Lower extremity splints need to be thicker and stronger in design. The best way to immobilize the knee is with medial and lateral splints (Fig. 22.10). A simple posterior splint on the knee frequently is not sufficiently strong to give good immobilization. The other commonly used splint in the lower extremity is the posterior ankle splint. This splint is made stronger by triangulating it with plaster slabs that connect the proximal splint with the distal splint across the medial or lateral aspect of the ankle joint or by combining the posterior plaster slab with a U-shaped stirrup splint (Fig. 22.11).

Once the splint has been put into position the splint and extremity should be held until the plaster has set. This is especially true for the ankle, which has a tendency to fall into an equinus or plantar flexed position if not held in the neutral position, and for the fingers, which tend to drift into excessive metacarpophalangeal joint extension.

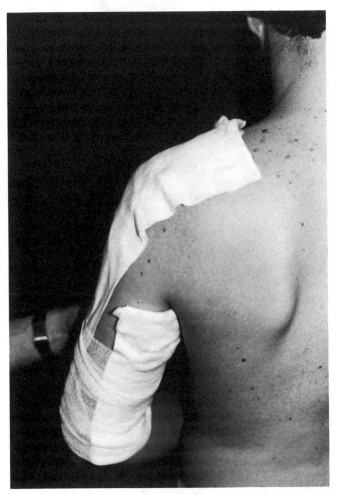

Figure 22.8 Coaptation arm splints. These are lateral and medial splints that start across the shoulder laterally and extend to the elbow with a medial splint from the axilla to the elbow. It is especially appropriate for a humeral fracture.

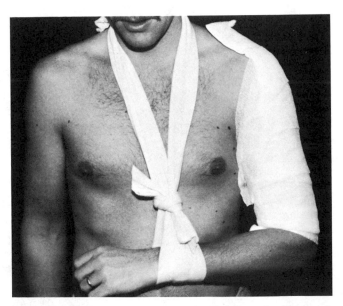

Figure 22.9 Coaptation splints combined with collar and cuff to permit the weight of the arm to provide traction.

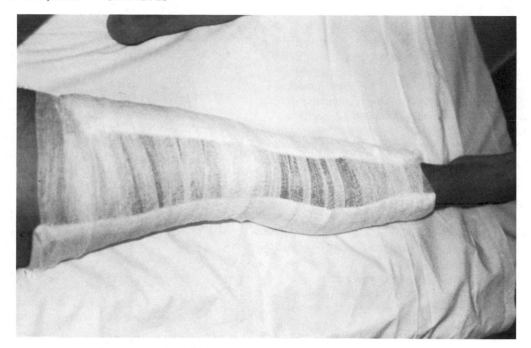

Figure 22.10 Medial and lateral knee splints. These splints start above the malleoli and progress to the proximal thigh. Placement of a skin adhesive helps prevent these splints from becoming malpositioned. The knee should not be immobilized in hyperextension.

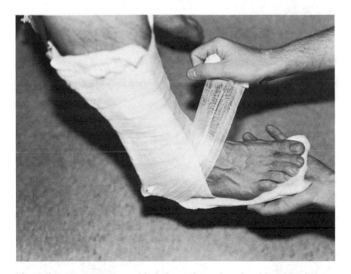

Figure 22.11 Posterior ankle splint. This splint should start at the toes and progress up the back of the calf to the popliteal space. No interference with knee flexion should occur.

SPECIFIC INJURIES

Forearm Injuries

Upper extremity injuries are generally the result of a fall on an outstretched arm. The specific injury, whether to the shoulder, elbow, forearm, wrist, or hand, depends upon the positioning of the extremity at the time of the fall.

As a rule the older the patient the more osteopenic the bone and the more trivial the trauma leading to the injury. From a similar fall, a young child will tend to fracture both bones of the forearm, a young adult will sustain a carpal bone fracture, and an elderly patient will sustain a Colles', or distal radius, fracture. Similarly, a young adult will dislocate a shoulder whereas an older patient with a more osteopenic humerus will sustain a proximal humerus fracture. Since children have open epiphyses and the mechanical strength of the joint ligaments exceeds that of the cartilaginous growth plate, they do not sustain ligamentous injuries to joints, but rather sustain epiphyseal fractures.

COLLES' FRACTURE

Colles' fracture is one of the most frequent upper extremity injuries that the emergency room practitioner will see. Most patients who sustain this fracture are elderly with markedly osteopenic bone. The younger patient who sustains a Colles' fracture tends to have been involved in a high-energy injury that is usually motor-vehicle related. Although the x-ray films of older and younger patients may be identical, younger patients will have more stiffness of the wrist and a higher incidence of neurovascular compromise as a result of the amount of energy dissipated in the trauma.

Diagnosis

The Colles' fracture is a distal radius fracture within 2.5 cm of the articular surface. It is frequently accompanied by a fracture of the tip of the ulna—the styloid process. The distal fragment is dorsally displaced in relation to the proximal fragment (Figs. 22.12 and 22.13). The fracture commonly occurs when someone falls on an outstretched hand and bends the wrist backward, resulting in a typical deformity that makes the hand look like a dinner fork when viewed from the side. Even in this deformed position, the forearm and hand may safely be splinted and the patient may be sent for an x-ray film. The patient's arm should be routinely elevated while the patient is waiting for the x-ray film to be taken.

SMITH'S FRACTURE

Smith's fracture is the reverse of Colles' fracture; it is the result of the wrist having been bent toward the palm and the distal fragment volarly displaced with respect to the proximal fragment. Accordingly, the deformity is the reverse of that seen with the Colles' fracture.

Diagnosis

Generally speaking, the differential between Colles' fracture and Smith's fracture requires an x-ray film. The hand should be splinted in the position of the deformity pending x-ray films.

Initial Therapy

A person with a nondisplaced distal radius fracture can safely be treated by the primary emergency room physician. Initially, these fractures are best treated with a splint to avoid any neurovascular compromise from the swelling within a circular dressing. A sugar tong or long arm splint that starts below the metacarpophalangeal joints, permitting full motion of the fin-

gers and immobilizing the elbow, is sufficient. The patient with a nondisplaced fracture should have repeat x-ray films in 1 week to document the continued satisfactory alignment of the fracture. If the fracture reduction has been lost, it is a simple matter to perform a rereduction at that time. A short arm cast applied after 1 week will usually suffice with nondisplaced fractures, and it should be left on for a period of 3 weeks, followed by a rehabilitation program for the wrist and fingers.

The primary physician should not attempt to treat a displaced Colles' or Smith's fracture. The fracture should be splinted

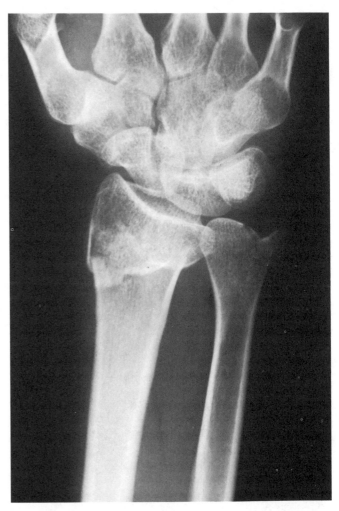

Figure 22.12 Anterior–posterior radiograph of a Colles' fracture. Note the displacement of the ulnar styloid process and the shortening of the radius relative to the ulna.

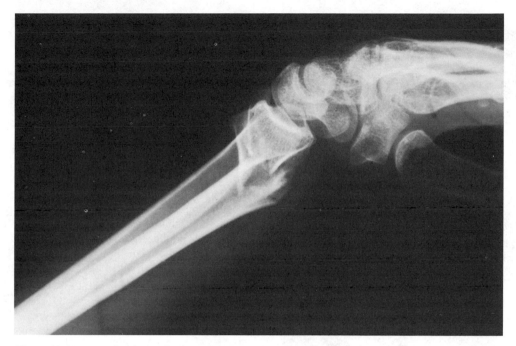

Figure 22.13 Lateral radiograph of a Colles' fracture with dorsal angulation of a distal fragment relative to the proximal fragment.

while the patient is awaiting care by a specialist. The timing of the reduction will depend upon the amount of swelling and the neurovascular status of the hand. Most of the patient's displaced fractures can be managed with an immediate reduction under either a general or regional anesthetic, followed by immobilization in a long arm cast or splint. There is a tendency for treating these fractures with external fixation, thus allowing more anatomical reduction, eliminating the need for a long arm cast, and permitting use of the fingers and elbow and thereby avoiding stiffness of these joints. If external fixation is used, reduction should be delayed 4–5 days.

At the time of discharge from the emergency ward, the patient should be carefully instructed in elevation of the injured arm at home. Such elevation is best accomplished by having the patient's arm rest on one or two pillows that are placed on the lap while sitting or on the chest while lying down. Ice should be applied intermittently to the fractured area, and there should be adequate protection from thermal injury. The patient should be instructed to fully extend and fully flex all of the joints of the fingers several times a day to diminish the swelling and subsequent stiffness. Medication for a discharged patient should be only mild analgesics such as codeine since a well-

immobilized fracture that has been elevated should not be uncomfortable. If there is pain, it may be the first sign of neurovascular compromise and should be brought to the attention of the caring physician.

Prognosis

There is a high incidence of stiffness of the hand and wrist in distal radius fractures because of the proximity of the hand and wrist joints to the fracture, as well as the immobilization required in fracture management. In general, patients do not regain full return of motion of the wrist, but most patients do regain functional activity of the hand. There is no excuse for stiffness of the elbow or shoulder, but care must be taken to prevent this complication.

RADIUS AND ULNAR SHAFT FRACTURES

Radius and ulnar shaft fractures are most frequently the result of falls onto the arm but they can also be caused by a direct blow to the forearm. Either the radius or the ulnar shaft may of the distal radial–ulnar joint, and fractures of the ulna, especially proximally, frequently result in a dislocation of the radial–humeral joint.

Initial Therapy

Radius and ulnar shaft fractures are best treated by a specialist. Most patients with these fractures require admission to the hospital. The function of the forearm, especially rotation, depends upon the anatomical·configuration of the forearm bones. Accordingly, the criteria for a satisfactory reduction is quite strict and usually nothing short of anatomical alignment is satisfactory. This is especially true for adults, whereas some angular deformity may be tolerated in young children. Most fractures in children can be managed closed, whereas most fractures in adults require open reduction and internal fixation. The primary physician should splint the arm in the position in which it lies and should note the neurovascular status. The elbow and wrist should be immobilized to control the rotational forces across the fracture site. Nondisplaced forearm fractures can safely be immobilized in a long arm splint, and the patient can be discharged from the hospital and referred to a specialist for ongoing care. The patient must be carefully instructed in the signs of neurovascular compromise. Follow-up of patients with these injuries should be within 1 week, especially in children, since healing can proceed quickly, making a second reduction difficult.

Prognosis

The incidence of union of radius and ulnar shaft fractures is high. The one exception is the isolated ulnar shaft fracture, which is notorious for delayed union. Most forearm fractures heal with some loss of rotational motion. Loss of pronation is better tolerated than loss of supination because of the inability of the shoulder to compensate for supination.

Elbow Injuries

Fractures near the elbow are a result of both direct falls onto the elbow and falls on the outstretched arm with forces transferred through the elbow joint. X-Ray films of the elbow, especially in children, can be confusing because of the multiple ossification centers. Comparison views of the opposite elbow will often help clarify the situation, but they should not be ordered as a routine. The physical examination is helpful since there are very distinct anatomical landmarks that can be easily palpated (Fig. 22.16). The olecranon, which is the point of the elbow, is the easiest to feel and the most familiar. The medial

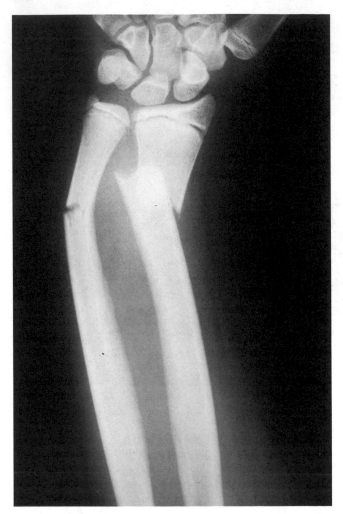

Figure 22.14 Anterior–posterior radiograph of a distal ulnar and radial shaft fracture with displacement.

be fractured individually with the other bone intact, or they may be fractured together (Figs. 22.14 and 22.15).

Diagnosis

Radius and ulnar shaft fractures are frequently characterized by marked deformity. The wrist and elbow should be carefully examined at all times, looking for disruptions of these joints. X-Ray films of both the wrist and elbow should be taken along with x-ray films of the forearm bones themselves. Fractures of the distal third of the radius frequently result in a dislocation

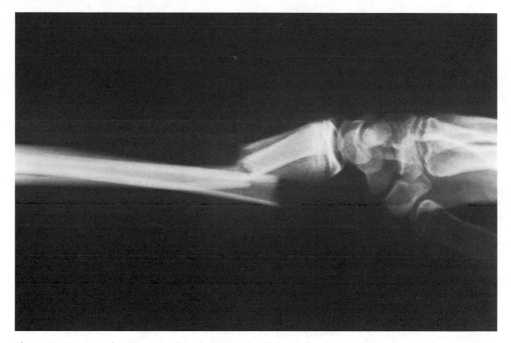

Figure 22.15 Lateral radiograph of displaced distal radial and ulnar fracture. The open epiphyses indicate a pediatric patient.

and lateral epicondyles can be easily felt even in the presence of considerable swelling, and the motion of the radial head may be felt on the outside of the elbow when the forearm is pronated and supinated (Figs. 22.17, 22.18, and 22.19). The points of the epicondyles and the olecranon of the flexed elbow form an equilateral triangle (Fig. 22.20). Tenderness over these bony prominences, especially the radial head, or deformity in this area suggests a fracture. If there is tenderness present in a fairly localized area, a questionable finding on the x-ray film will take on more meaning. A careful examiner can detect an effusion in the elbow, which is palpable posterior to the radial head on the outside of the elbow.

The elbow is subject to several overuse syndromes. These are caused by repetitive microtrauma, resulting in painful injury, rather than the acute catastrophic injury represented by a fracture. These overuse entities are olecranon bursitis, medial and lateral epicondylitis, and osteochondritis of the elbow.

OLECRANON BURSITIS

Olecranon bursitis presents in middle-aged adults who give a history of performing a new repetitive activity involving flexion and extension of the elbow or leaning onto the flexed elbow.

Diagnosis

The olecranon bursa is located over the point of the elbow—the olecranon. A localized mass results when the olecranon bursa, a well-defined sac overlying the olecranon, is distended with blood or synovial fluid. X-Ray films should be taken to rule out an underlying fracture, but usually none is present. There is frequently a redness of the skin over the bursa, which is more pink than that seen with a cellulitis. There should be no axillary adenopathy, and the patient should be afebrile, which further helps to differentiate nonseptic from septic bursitis.

Initial Therapy

Treatment should be a bulky soft dressing and an arm sling. The swelling will usually disappear over the next week or so. Although it is tempting to aspirate the fluid with a needle, the fluid will rapidly reaccumulate, and this area is subject to easy infection. Oral antiinflammatory medications are also helpful in management.

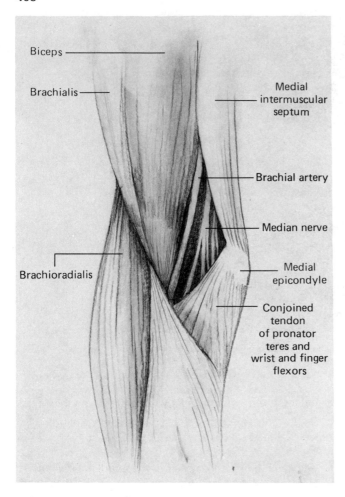

Biceps

Brachialis

Medial
intermuscular
septum

Brachial artery

Median nerve

Medial
epicondyle

Brachioradialis

Conjoined
tendon
of pronator
teres and
wrist and finger
flexors

Figure 22.16 Anterior aspect of the elbow joint showing the prominent medial epicondyle of the humerus and the relationships of the anterior muscles.

Prognosis

Olecranon bursitis, on occasion, is slow to resolve, and aspiration and installation of steroid preparation is indicated if the bursitis is chronic. On rare occasions excision of the bursa is required. The patient who is subject to recurrent olecranon bursitis needs additional protection during use of the elbow.

EPICONDYLITIS

Diagnosis

Epicondylitis is on the medial and lateral aspect of the elbow and is also known as tennis elbow. More commonly, it is found on the outside of the elbow. It represents a tendonitis of the insertion of the extensors and flexors onto the epicondyles of the humerus. They again represent an overuse type of injury. In addition to patients who participate in racquet sports, patients who perform hammering activities and rotatory activities with the forearm are also at risk.

Initial Therapy

Patients present with localized tenderness and frequently pain upon flexion or extension of the elbow. The x-ray films are normal. There is no neurologic involvement of the forearm. Treatment using a bulky dressing and a sling and orally administered antiinflammatory agents is the first line of management. Later steroid injections and physical therapy with ultrasound may be needed.

Prognosis

Epicondylitis can be chronic and shorten the athletic career of serious athletes. When conservative measures are not successful, surgical treatment may be indicated.

OSTEOCHONDRITIS OF THE ELBOW

Osteochondritis of the elbow involves a traumatic fracture of the osteochondral surface of the elbow, usually the capitellum—that part of the humerus that articulates with the radial head. It is most frequently found in little league pitchers.

Diagnosis

The presenting history is one of insidious onset of elbow pain after performing a repetitive activity with the elbow, especially throwing a ball. X-Ray films will show the injury to the articular surface.

Initial Therapy

If there has been no displacement of the osteochondral fragments, simple rest with a sling followed by avoidance of heavy use of the arm may permit healing of the fracture. If there has been displacement of the osteochondral fragment, surgical excision followed by physical therapy to the elbow may be needed.

Prognosis

The outcome for osteochondritis is generally good, but the patient's full return to vigorous use of the arm for athletic

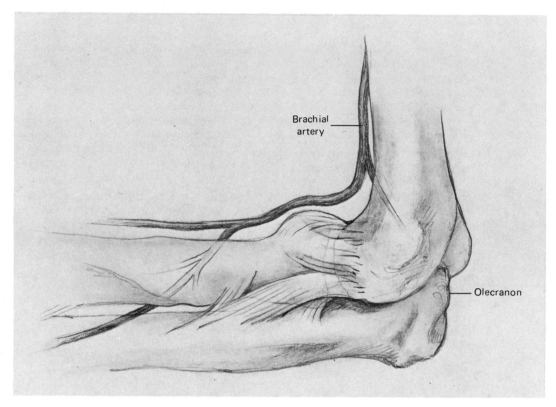

Figure 22.17 Lateral view of the elbow joint showing the relationship of the brachial artery to the anterior elbow joint. Note that a fracture of the distal humerus at this point would easily injure the brachial artery (See Fig. 22.25).

purposes may not be possible. If healing does occur the person's return to athletic competition should be carefully supervised and progressive in order to avoid reinjury.

OLECRANON FRACTURE

Olecranon fracture is an avulsion type of fracture as a result of the pull of the triceps or of the humerus acting as a wedge splitting the olecranon (Fig. 22.21).

Diagnosis

Anterior–posterior and lateral x-ray films of the elbow are sufficient to make the diagnosis of an olecranon fracture. The ulnar nerve passes medial to the olecranon, and the ulnar nerve function in the hand should be routinely checked when these fractures occur.

Initial Therapy

All olecranon fractures are intraarticular. A displaced fracture should be reduced operatively and fixed in an anatomical position. While waiting for reduction, the arm should be splinted in near full extension to relax the triceps and prevent further displacement. Nondisplaced fractures should be splinted in a 90 deg position of elbow flexion with a posterior splint and sling. In a few days x-ray films should be taken again to rule out late displacement.

Prognosis

The advantage of internal fixation of olecranon fractures is that earlier motion of the elbow can be allowed and, generally speaking, better elbow function results. Patients with these fractures routinely lose the last 30 deg of full extension. It is for this reason that a small olecranon fragment that involves

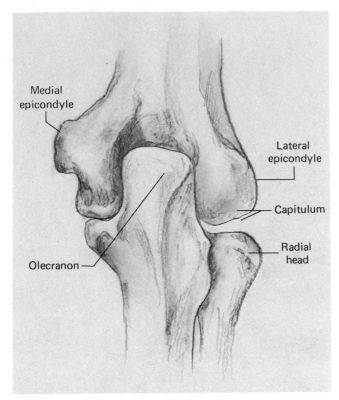

Figure 22.18 Posterior view of the elbow joint in elbow extension, showing the bony landmarks.

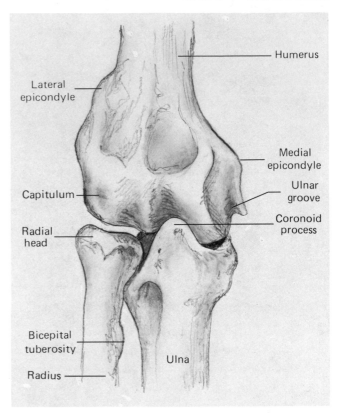

Figure 22.19 Anterior view of the elbow joint in elbow extension, showing the significant bony landmarks.

less than 50% of the olecranon surface area, in an older patient, will be treated with excision and advancement of the triceps into the proximal ulnar shaft. Whether to fix internally or to excise an olecranon fragment is a decision made on a case-by-case basis.

RADIAL HEAD FRACTURES

Radial head fractures are the most common fractures near the elbow and should be suspected in any patient with a history of a fall and subsequent elbow pain (Figs. 22.22 and 22.23). Frequently the x-ray films are normal and the diagnosis is a clinical one based on tenderness over the radial head. Radiographic evidence of an intraarticular effusion strongly suggests a nondisplaced radial head fracture. The fracture line may not be apparent, but the radial head should be tender in this situation.

Diagnosis

Patients with radial head fractures present with their elbows held flexed at 90 deg and with inability to rotate or flex and extend their elbows. Anterior–posterior and lateral x-ray films should be taken. The wrist joint should be palpated, looking for tenderness suggestive of an associated fracture of the distal radius or navicular. Any wrist tenderness deserves an x-ray film.

Initial Therapy

The nondisplaced fracture should be placed in a sling. If the patient is very uncomfortable a posterior splint will add a measure of comfort. Even if the patient's elbow is in the splint, the patient should be instructed to rotate the forearm frequently into supination and pronation.

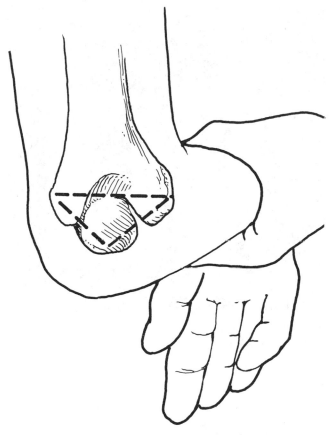

Figure 22.20 Posterior view of the elbow in full flexion, showing the relationship between the olecranon and the epicondyles of the humerus. Note the equilateral triangle formed by the bony landmarks at the apices.

An undisplaced radial head fracture can be treated by the primary physician in the emergency room. Any displaced radial head fracture, no matter how trivial, should be cared for by an orthopedic surgeon. The geometry of the radial–humeral joint is such that any malalignment of the articular surfaces will prevent normal rotation. Injection of a local anesthetic intraarticularly after aspiration of the hemarthrosis will permit comfortable rotation into supination and pronation. This will frequently mold the joint surfaces into alignment, permitting normal rotation after healing. Inability to obtain full rotation generally is an indication for radial head excision or open reduction and internal fixation of the fracture.

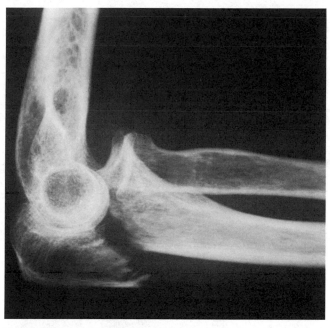

Figure 22.21 Lateral radiograph showing a fracture of the olecranon with associated dislocation of the radial head. All fractures of the forearm can be associated with either dislocation or subluxation of the radial head at the elbow.

Prognosis

Nondisplaced fractures heal quite well with the full return of function and motion of the arm. Displaced or comminuted radial head fractures have a bad prognosis with loss of rotation and frequently loss of elbow extension. If the rotational loss is severe, excision of the comminuted fragments and radial head proximal to the annular ligament should be done. For optimal results, it is important to perform the surgery within the first few days.

FRACTURES OF THE CORONOID PROCESS OF THE ULNA

A fracture of the coronoid process of the ulna is a common fracture that is of the avulsion type and is a result of the pull of the brachialis.

Diagnosis

The patient presents with a history of minor trauma, and x-ray films reveal a small avulsion off the tip of the coronoid process.

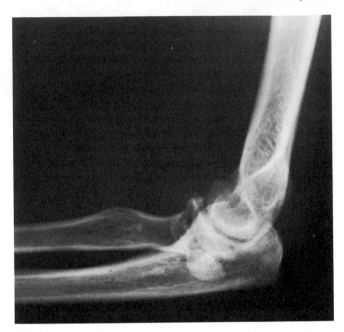

Figure 22.23 Lateral radiograph of a comminuted radial head fracture. Note the displaced fracture fragments in the joint.

ELBOW DISLOCATIONS

Elbow dislocations are frequently the result of simple falls, but they are also seen in patients involved in motor-vehicle and sporting accidents (Fig. 22.24).

Diagnosis

Although there are several types of elbow dislocations, the most common is a posterior dislocation of the ulna on the humerus. It is especially important to assess the neurovascular status in these injuries because of a high incidence of brachial artery injury. X-Ray films will reveal the type of dislocation, as well as presence of any fracture fragments.

Initial Therapy

Elbow dislocations are reduced by direct traction. The patient should be manipulated by a specialist unless the emergency room practitioner has experience. A general anesthetic is frequently required, especially if the dislocation occurred more than 24 hours ago. Once the joint is relocated, a careful assessment of the stability of the joint needs to be made; this situation is unlike that of the shoulder. Younger people's joints

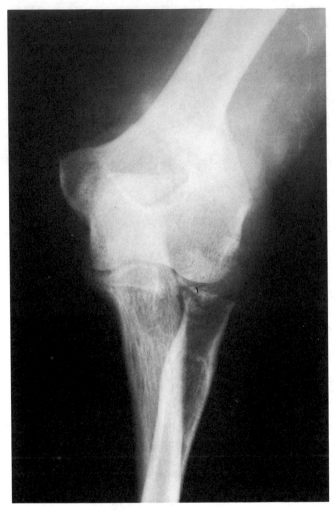

Figure 22.22 Anterior–posterior radiograph showing a complete radial head fracture with the fracture line across the radial neck.

Initial Therapy

These fractures can all be treated with a posterior splint and sling.

Prognosis

These fractures frequently result in loss of extension of the arm. The patient should be advised of this eventuality as soon as possible.

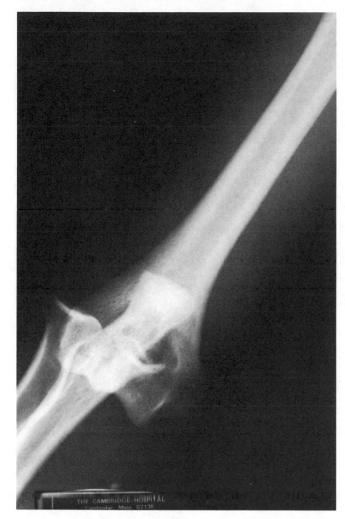

Figure 22.24 Anterior–posterior radiograph of a dislocated elbow. Elbow dislocations are associated with a high incidence of neurovascular compromise, and the fractures heal with considerable loss of joint movement.

should be held in a posterior splint for 2 weeks, after which the range of motion therapy should be started. Older patients need their joints to be held for only 1 week before physical therapy is initiated.

Prognosis

As with other elbow injuries, there is a high incidence of loss of motion, especially extension, after elbow dislocations. Fre-

quently there will be heterotopic ossification in the elbow capsule.

EPICONDYLAR FRACTURES OF THE HUMERUS

An epicondylar fracture of the humerus is a common fracture in patients in the pediatric age group, and because of the number of ossification centers in the elbow, radiographic diagnosis is made very difficult. All epicondylar fractures should be evaluated by a specialist, no matter how trivial.

Diagnosis

The major flexors of the wrist originate from the medial epicondyle, whereas the extensors come from the lateral epicondyle. When either of these epicondyles is fractured, these muscles keep the fracture displaced, and a reduction can rarely be maintained without surgery and internal fixation. An x-ray film interpretation of fractures near the elbow is treacherous, and a comparison view of the uninjured elbow is particularly helpful. Children's elbows are largely cartilagenous, making the fracture diagnosis difficult by x-ray film. A seemingly minimally displaced fracture can have a large displaced intraarticular component.

Initial Therapy

The primary care physician should splint the elbow with a long posterior plaster splint and a sling and then notify the orthopedic surgeon. The neurovascular status should be determined and noted on the patient's chart.

Prognosis

When there is anatomical restoration of the joint, epicondylar fractures heal well, although there can be loss of full elbow motion. Malunion, however, causes a significant decrease in elbow function with marked restriction of motion and progressive deformity in the young child.

INTERCONDYLAR FRACTURES OF THE ELBOW

Intercondylar fractures of the elbow occur after a fall on the flexed elbow, and are especially common during the winter months. The olecranon acts as a wedge by splitting the medial and lateral condyles.

Diagnosis

The elbow is markedly swollen and there is a great deal of bleeding, so much so that a tense and swollen elbow can compromise the circulation to the forearm and hand. In such cases, the neurovascular examination of the hand should be performed every few minutes during the initial management in order to assess any changing status in circulation, sensation, or motor function. Patients with these fractures should lay on a stretcher with their arms supported on a pillow that is placed across their chests. Ice should be applied to the area in order to minimize the ongoing swelling. The interpretation of x-ray films of these fractures is frequently difficult because of the marked distortion of the anatomy.

Initial Therapy

Patients who have intercondylar fractures of their elbows need to be admitted to the hospital. Their ultimate treatment involves either internal fixation of the fracture fragments or traction. The primary physician should place the injured arm in a well-padded long posterior splint and should make sure that ice is constantly applied to the arm and that the arm is elevated. Frequent neurovascular checks need to be ordered; therefore, the splint should not prevent easy access to the hand.

Prognosis

The final result in patients with these fractures depends on the restoration of the elbow's articular surface. Rarely is full motion restored.

SUPRACONDYLAR FRACTURES OF THE HUMERUS

Supracondylar fractures of the humerus occur just above the condyles of the elbow. They are most frequently seen in children (Fig. 22.25).

Diagnosis

These fractures are particularly dangerous because of the high incidence of neurovascular compromise that can occur with an intact pulse. The most frequently seen fracture pattern is posterior angulation of the distal fragment in relation to the proximal fragment, causing the brachial artery to be stretched across the proximal fracture fragment of the humerus (see Fig. 22.17). Even without actual arterial occlusion there is an in-

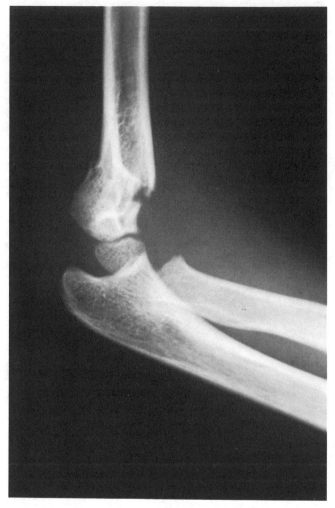

Figure 22.25 A lateral radiograph of a posteriorly angulated supracondylar fracture in a pediatric patient. Comparison with Figure 22.17 will show why the brachial artery is jeopardized by this type of fracture.

creased pressure within the forearm because of the swelling and ongoing bleeding from the fractured bones, and the distortion of the anatomy at the fracture site obstructs venous return. Surgical decompression of the fracture site, exploration of the brachial artery, or fasciotomy of the forearm may be necessary. Vascular compromise from these fractures represents a true surgical emergency. If not recognized, the high tissue pressure results in a necrosis of the forearm muscles, scarring, and contractures that profoundly impair hand function. This is called Volkmann's contracture. Increasing pain in spite of adequate immobilization is the first sign of ischemic injury. Pain with passive extension of the fingers is another sign of early vascular compromise.

Initial Therapy

The primary physician should splint these fractures in the position in which they present using a well-padded posterior splint. Again, the orthopedic surgeon will usually treat these fractures either with a closed reduction and a limited form of internal fixation or with traction. Simple fractures can be treated with a cast. Patients who have sustained such fractures should be admitted to the hospital.

Prognosis

These are treacherous fractures to treat, and there is an alarming incidence of angular malalignment of the elbow and injury to the epiphyseal growth centers of the elbow necessitating a later corrective osteotomy to provide an optimal result.

Arm Injuries

HUMERAL SHAFT FRACTURES

Humeral shaft fractures, again, are the result of falls on the arm, but they also result from direct trauma to the arm, frequently producing midshaft fractures (Fig. 22.26). The humerus is a much larger bone than is generally believed. When it is broken, there may be substantial bleeding from the fractured ends, resulting in an alarmingly swollen arm.

Diagnosis

The physician making the initial evaluation should pay close attention to the status of the radial nerve. Midshaft long oblique and distal third oblique fractures of the humerus are the most notorious for radial nerve injury. The radial nerve may be damaged at the time of the fracture or at the time of treatment. In cases of distal one-third fractures, the nerve may become entrapped within the fracture site since it lies closely approximated to the shaft of the humerus as it winds around the bone (Fig. 22.27). The radial nerve provides for dorsiflexion of the interphalangeal and metacarpophalangeal joints of the hand as well as the wrist. The dorsal sensory branch of the radial

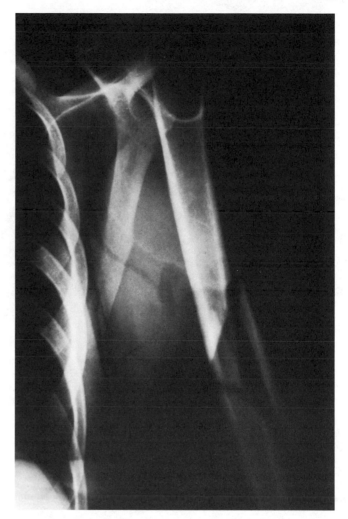

Figure 22.26 Anterior–posterior radiograph of the humerus showing an oblique midshaft fracture line with a single large comminuted fragment. The status of the radial nerve should be checked in all such fractures.

nerve supplies sensation over the dorsum of the thumb and the first web space.

Initial Therapy

The treatment by the primary physician should include adequate splinting. Usually a sling with a swath against the patient's chest wall is sufficient. Plaster splints over the humerus

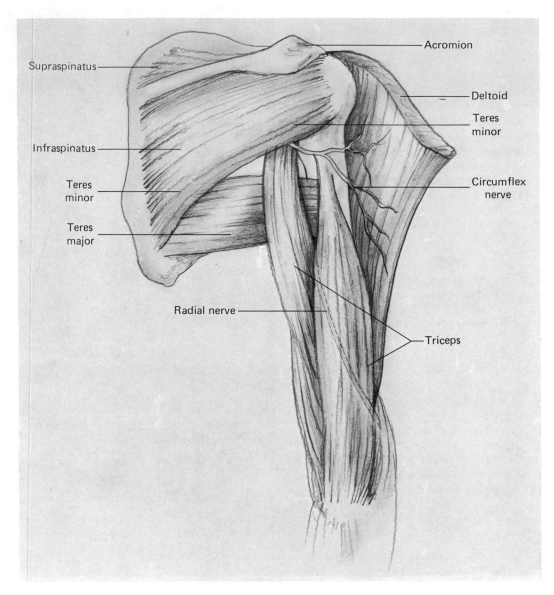

Figure 22.27 Posterior aspect of the shoulder and arm showing the musculature of the rotator cuff as well as the extensors of the elbow. Note the position of the circumflex nerve which is frequently injured in anterior shoulder dislocations, as well as the position of the radial nerve as it winds along the posterior shaft of the humerus.

incorporated into the swath will add to the patient's comfort. All rings should be removed from the fingers since swelling can be anticipated. When these fractures are displaced, they should be treated by an orthopedic surgeon. The modalities of treatment include, in most cases, a closed reduction followed by coaptation splints, or possibly a so-called hanging cast, which provides continuous traction by virtue of gravity aided by the weight of the cast. Most of these fractures can be managed in such a closed fashion. If angulation cannot be prevented, then surgical internal fixation is necessary.

Prognosis

In general, these fractures heal quite well, and there is a very low incidence of nonunion. There is, generally speaking, little in the way of stiffness of the elbow or shoulder. From 8 to 12 weeks are required for useful return of arm function.

Shoulder Injuries

Fractures and dislocations near the shoulder are an extremely common musculoskeletal injury. Except in young people, such fractures routinely result in restricted motion of the shoulder joint. The shoulder is a very unconstrained joint and, for its stability and motion, depends on the gliding of the soft tissue layers (Fig. 22.28). Swelling and bleeding with the resulting fibrosis will lead to restriction of shoulder motion. Careful and supervised physical therapy for these injuries is of paramount importance.

The shoulder joint is also subject to overuse injuries from repetitive microtrauma.

BURSITIS OF THE SHOULDER

Bursitis of the shoulder is extremely painful and most commonly seen in patients who are in their 40s and 50s. There is

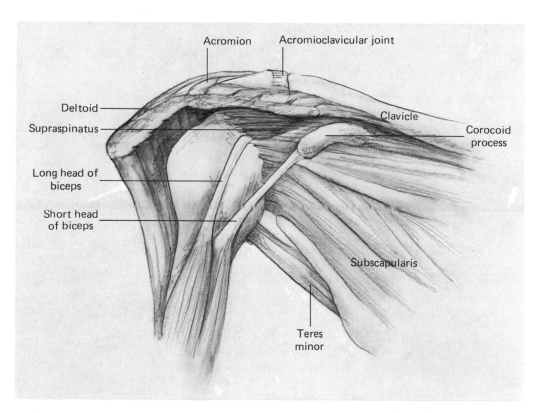

Figure 22.28 Anterior view of the shoulder showing the muscles of the rotator cuff, the anterior flexor of the elbow. Note the great dependence of the shoulder on the investing soft tissues in order to provide stability and motion.

usually a history of some new or unusual activity such as raking leaves or some other type of repetitive activity that has caused overuse of the shoulder.

Diagnosis

The patient presents to the emergency ward with severe pain in the shoulder. There is exquisite tenderness just off the end of the acromion at the point of the shoulder. Shoulder motion is extremely limited because of the pain. Patients who can still move their shoulders have a painful arc of motion that is usually most painful in abduction and external rotation. The patients give a history of not being able to sleep at night. The level of pain appears out of proportion to the pain seen with seemingly more severe injuries. X-ray films of the shoulder may reveal the presence of a calcific density in the rotator cuff region, but the film may also be enitirely within normal limits. The patient will frequently give a history of having had similar episodes of shoulder pain in the past.

Initial Therapy

For patients who can still move their shoulders fairly well, much relief can be provided by the use of a sling, ice, adequate

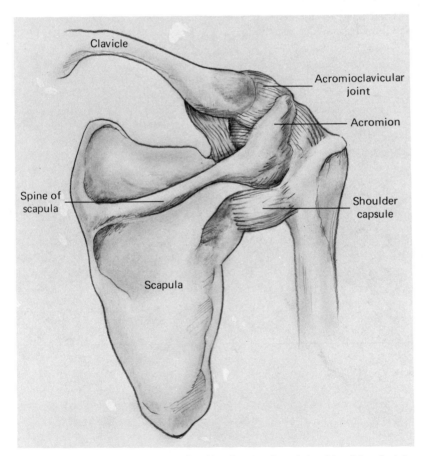

Figure 22.29 Posterior view of the shoulder showing the relationship of the clavicle to the acromion and proximal humerus. The simplest way of injecting the subdeltoid bursa is to place a needle under the posterior acromion that would deposit the antiinflammatory medication in the bursa layer between the deltoid fibers and the fibers of the rotator cuff.

narcotic analgesics, and antiinflammatory medications. For patients who are in more obvious distress and have little motion of their shoulders, injections with a combination of local anesthetics and a steroid are necessary. Injections in this area require a sterile technique and a knowledge of the underlying anatomy (see Fig. 22.28).

The simplest and most reliable method for injecting the acutely painful shoulder is to approach the subdeltoid bursa posteriorly at the posterior edge of the acromion (Figs. 22.29 and 22.30). The area should be prepared and the needle introduced such that it just passes beneath the acromion into the bursa. The entire bursa should then be distended with a large volume of solution; a good combination is a 10-ml solution comprised

of 5 ml of a long-acting local anesthetic such as bupivacaine 0.5%, 4 ml of a short-acting anesthetic such as lidocaine (Xylocaine) 1%, and 1 ml of steroid solution such as 8 mg dexamethasone. After the injection, the area should be gently massaged and the arm gently rotated to disperse the medication. If this is properly done, the relief is dramatic and the shoulder motion improves considerably if not completely. If there are calcific deposits in the rotator cuff, the injection techniques may vary. If these deposits are large enough, they can be irrigated out under appropriate anesthesia (local) using large bore needles. This latter technique is complex and should be done by an orthopedic specialist. When the patient is discharged from the emergency room he or she should have ad-

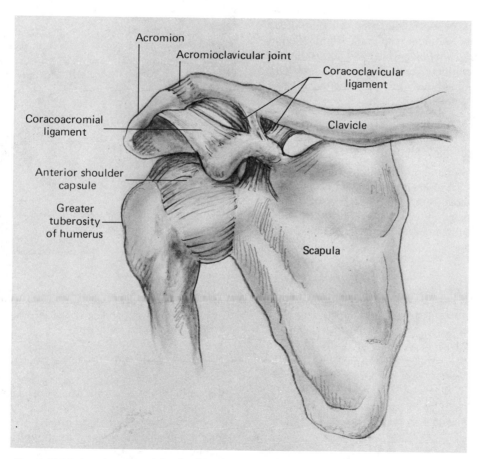

Figure 22.30 Anterior view of the shoulder showing the bony structures as well as the capsule of the acromioclavicular joint and the coracoclavicular ligaments.

equate pain medication since the pain may intensify after the local anesthetic wears off and before the time the cortisone preparation starts to take affect.

Prognosis

In most patients who have episodes of acute shoulder bursitis, these are isolated events that are over within 5–7 days. There is another group of patients, however, who tend to develop recurrent episodes of shoulder bursitis and these patients need to be studied for the presence of small rotator cuff tears or hypertrophy of the anterior edge of the acromion that would account for the recurrent symptoms. A third group of patients, is a group, who after one or several episodes, will develop an adhesive capsulitis of the shoulder with marked restriction in motion, called the *frozen shoulder*. This condition is difficult to treat and may lead to a permanent impairment in range of motion in the shoulder, although most patients have some return of shoulder motion after 1–2 years.

FRACTURES OF THE PROXIMAL HUMERUS

Fractures of the proximal humerus are most commonly seen in elderly patients who fall on their outstretched hands. Most of these fractures are stable injuries in which the shaft of the humerus has been impacted into the humeral head with minimal displacement of the fracture fragments (Fig. 22.31).

Diagnosis

X-Ray films of the shoulder are difficult to obtain unless we use the two views described earlier in this chapter, which are in fact an anterior–posterior of the scapular and a tangental view of the scapular (see Figs. 22.2 and 23.3). These films can be obtained when the patient is sitting with his or her arm resting in a sling. They provide two views that permit the practitioner to determine the presence of a dislocation of the humeral head from the glenoid.

Initial Therapy

Patients who have fractures of the proximal humerus should be placed in a sling. The impacted fractures need no other care unless the patient is quite uncomfortable, in which case a swath across the chest wall for a day or two is sufficient. When the arm is swathed against the chest wall, an absorbent pad should be placed in the axilla to protect the skin from

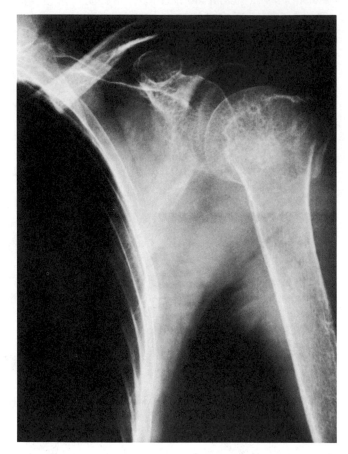

Figure 22.31 Minimally displaced proximal humerus fracture. There are three fracture fragments—the articular surface, the shaft of the humerus, and the greater tuburosity fragment. Early treatment consists of immobilization with a sling combined with a swath if needed, followed by early range of motion.

masceration. If the x-ray film shows displacement of the fracture, multiple fragments, or malalignment of the proximal humerus, whereby the articular surface of the humerus is not aimed at the glenoid, then the fracture requires a reduction maneuver (Fig. 22.32). This can be accomplished by closed reduction in most cases and treated with a sling or collar and cuff. The primary care physician can easily manage the impacted fractures, and an orthopedic surgeon can follow up the patient within 7–10 days. Patients who have displaced fractures should be managed by an orthopedic surgeon from the start.

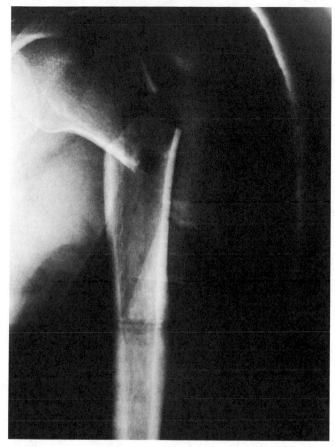

Figure 22.32 Anterior–posterior radiograph of a low humeral neck fracture with unacceptable angulation. This fracture requires a reduction maneuver.

Prognosis

There is a high incidence, as mentioned above, of loss of motion at the shoulder with these fractures. The patient should be advised of this possibility at the outset. Healing of the fracture requires 6 weeks, but improvement in shoulder motion will occur over a 12-week period.

SHOULDER DISLOCATIONS

Dislocations of the glenohumeral joint (Figs. 22.2 and 22.3), are extremely common injuries. They are especially seen in young athletes. Dislocation in patients under age 20 is a serious injury in that the incidence of recurrent dislocations and the ultimate need for surgery is quite high. Patients who have dislocations after age 20 tend to do much better in terms of stability (fewer recurrent dislocations), but they are more plagued with restriction of shoulder motion.

Diagnosis

Patients arrive at the hospital in extreme distress, holding their injured arms by their sides in an attempt to prevent any motion. There may be a history of previous dislocations. Before a frank dislocation, many patients will experience recurrent subluxations. They will describe a sense of the shoulder popping out but popping right back in again without medical intervention. Observation of the dislocated shoulder will reveal a fullness anteriorly with an anterior dislocation and a fullness posteriorly with a posterior dislocation. In heavy-muscled people this is not a reliable physical sign, however. Although the examiner should pay attention to the distal pulses, sensation, and motor function, these injuries tend to cause a brachial plexes traction injury especially involving the axillary nerve and producing a proximal deficit (Fig. 22.33). The axillary nerve supplies the deltoid muscle as well as a patch of cutaneous sensation over the deltoid itself (see Fig. 22.27). Checking for sensation over the deltoid is sufficient to assess this nerve. The status of the axillary nerve must be noted before reduction of the shoulder. X-Ray films should be obtained as soon as possible because of the extreme pain the patient experiences. If there is an axillary nerve injury, it is an orthopedic emergency and should have the highest priority. X-Ray films should always be obtained before reduction to rule out the possibility of a fracture or fracture dislocation.

Initial Therapy

The primary physician who has experience at reducing shoulders can accomplish a reduction in the situation of a routine anterior dislocation that has been out for only a few hours. This is especially true in the case of a recurrent dislocation. After 6 hours and in some patients with first dislocations there can be marked muscle spasm, and the reduction of the dislocation is frequently quite difficult and may even require a general anesthetic.

The reduction of a dislocated shoulder should take place under adequate analgesic usually supplemented with some mild muscle relaxants, such as diazepam, using only gentle maneuvers regardless of the type of reduction technique used. The simplest and most effective maneuver is one whereby the elbow is extended and the arm is held adducted against the chest wall. The patient's chest is stabilized with a sheet held firmly by an assistant.

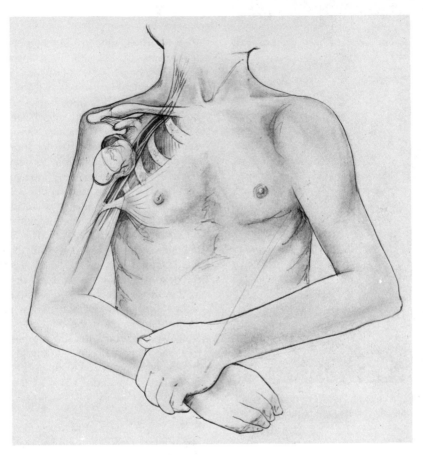

Figure 22.33 Anterior shoulder dislocation. Note the prominence of the acromion at the point of the shoulder. Also note the position of the brachial plexus between the dislocated humeral head and the anterior chest wall. The status of the brachial plexus, especially the axillary nerve, must be assessed with all anterior dislocations. The axillary nerve (see Fig. 22.27) provides innervation to the deltoid as well as a patch of sensation below the point of the shoulder.

The practitioner then provides gentle axial traction with one hand while the arm is gently elevated over the patient's head. At 90 deg of elevation, the humerus will usually relocate. The opposite hand can help push the humeral head into position. This maneuver relaxes all of the structures in spasm, namely, the anterior deltoid, subscapularis, and pectoralis, major and minor, which are holding the humeral head in the unreduced position.

After reduction, a shoulder immobilizer should be used or a sling and swath should be applied such that the arm is held in internal rotation against the chest wall. If the patient is under 20 years of age and this is the first dislocation, then the arm should be immobilized for at least a 3-week period, followed by a careful mobilization with avoidance of any external rotation for a full 6 weeks. The older patient needs to be immobilized for 1–2 weeks and then is allowed to regain motion. Patients with these injuries should be followed up by an orthopedic surgeon and seen within 7–10 days.

Posterior shoulder dislocations are quite rare and frequently misdiagnosed. They should be cared for by a specialist.

If a dislocation is associated with a fracture of the proximal humerus, the problem becomes more difficult since there is now no "handle" to hold on to in order to manipulate the humeral head back into the joint. These injuries need to be cared for by an orthopedic surgeon since they may require a general anesthetic and frequently require open surgery.

Prognosis

There is a high incidence of complications with these injuries. The younger patients, especially those under 20 years old, are at risk of instability, namely recurrent dislocations that can limit sports activities and at times, even routine activities of daily living. The older patient will develop stiffness near the shoulder, although full functional return is the rule. Axillary nerve injuries generally heal after 6 weeks. A rotator cuff tear may also be present. See discussion below.

GLENOID AND SCAPULAR INJURIES

Occasionally there will be a small chip fracture off the glenoid (the socket of the shoulder joint that is part of the scapula), and this usually represents an avulsion injury or an injury associated with a partial dislocation of the head of the humerus. It should be treated in much the same way as a dislocation by using a sling for support, giving analgesics, and arranging for appropriate follow-up by the orthopedist. If the fragment does not have a sharp edge and looks rounded off, then in all likelihood it represents an old injury.

Scapular fractures are unusual and generally represent a high-energy trauma. Fracture of the first rib, pneumothoraces, and mediastinal injuries should be looked for in every instance. The fractures themselves rarely displace because of the muscular support of the fragments. They are treated similarly to glenoid injuries. Patients should be followed-up by an orthopedist in order to monitor their analgesic requirements and to supervise the mobilization of their shoulders.

ACROMIOCLAVICULAR INJURIES

Acromioclavicular shoulder injuries are generally the result of a fall on the lateral aspect of the shoulder such as occurs on the playing field or in a fall off of a motorcycle or bicycle.

Diagnosis

Acromioclavicular injuries are commonly referred to as a *shoulder separation* (see Fig. 22.30). The patient has local tenderness over the acromioclavicular joint and hesitates to move the shoulder, although movement can be accomplished if properly supported. There is a notable swelling or bump that looks like a step off of the distal end of the clavicle. X-Ray films may need to be taken of both shoulders for comparison; the patient should stand and allow the arms to be resting unsupported when films are taken. The weight of the arm will demonstrate the magnitude of the true separation. Additional weight is usually not required. The articulation between the distal end of the clavicle and the acromion should be carefully inspected, looking for translation up or down between these two structures. If the patient supports the arm when the x-ray film is being taken, the true degree of separation will be minimized.

There are three degrees of acromioclavicular joint separations. They represent increasing degrees of disruption of the structures surrounding the joint (see Fig. 22.30). A first-degree separation involves a partial tear of the capsule of the acromioclavicular joint. These injuries are painful, but no visible separation of the joint is seen on x-ray films or physical examination. A second-degree acromioclavicular separation is a complete capsule tear such that there is a physical separation of the distal end of the clavicle and the acromion that is noticeable both on physical examination and x-ray film. Third-degree acromioclavicular separations are the most severe, including not only complete capsular disruption but also complete disruption of the conoid and trapezoid ligaments that attach the clavicle to the coracoid process of the scapular. There is a significant deformity present in the third-degree acromioclavicular separation, and, accordingly, it is frequently mistaken for a clavicular fracture.

Initial Therapy

In general, acromioclavicular joint disruptions are best managed conservatively. There is controversy over the value of surgery to repair the major disruptions since the long-term results of conservative management are so excellent. The cosmetic deformity present is rarely of functional significance and may eventually be treated by excision of the distal end of the clavicle, beveled to provide an acceptable cosmetic result. Early repairs of these injuries using various metallic devices, wires, or fascial slings are frought with technical difficulties, breakage of the implant, and stretching out of the soft tissue repairs. A well-padded sling, analgesics, and early application of cold to the injured part will provide excellent early relief for these injuries. Whereas patients with first- and second-degree shoulder separations may be referred to be seen within 1 week, it is equally appropriate to call the orthopedic surgeon if there is a possible third-degree or major acromioclavicular separation.

Prognosis

Grade I separations uniformly do very well. From 10 to 15% of the grade II and grade III injuries may cause some pain with time over the acromioclavicular joint because of chronic subluxation of the joint. This pain is generally experienced with elevation of the arm above 100 deg. The injury is well treated by distal clavicle resection.

ROTATOR CUFF RUPTURE

The rotator cuff is a group of muscles coming from the scapula and inserting on the proximal humerus, the subscapularis, supraspinatus, infraspinatus, and teres minor. Their exact roles in shoulder motion is controversial, but it is generally held that they are necessary for complete shoulder motion. They help depress the humeral head thus permitting clearance of the greater tuberosity under the coracoacromial arch during shoulder elevation.

People in their 50s and 60s will frequently have degenerative changes in their rotator cuff, and relatively minor trauma— usually a fall—resulting in a resisted abduction by the shoulder can rupture the rotator cuff.

Diagnosis

Patients who have rotator cuff tears present with pain and a history of trauma. The routine shoulder x-ray film is normal. These injuries distinguish themselves from others by a profound weakness of the shoulder that is out of proportion to the extent of injury. The involved arm can be elevated to 90 deg passively, but the patient is totally unable to maintain that position.

Initial Therapy

When the patient is in the emergency room, the shoulder should be checked for fractures and neurovascular injury. A sling and adequate analgesics should be prescribed. The patient should be referred to a specialist for follow-up after 1–2 weeks.

Prognosis

Many patients with rotator cuff tears regain satisfactory strength and motion, but they will have difficulty performing activities requiring elevation of the shoulder. There is usually audible, but frequently painless, crepitation in the shoulder. If adequate strength does not return, then a shoulder arthrogram will be necessary to establish the diagnosis. If the arthrogram is performed too late—after more than 6 weeks—the tears may be difficult to demonstrate arthrographically. Larger tears are amenable to surgical repair.

CLAVICLE FRACTURES

Clavicle fractures are extremely common shoulder injuries that usually occur after falls onto the shoulder (see Fig. 22.30).

Diagnosis

The patient presents with an acutely painful shoulder that requires support of the arm on the side of the affected clavicle. There may or may not be significant deformity present. X-Ray films will show the type of fracture (Fig. 22.34). The most common fractures are in the middle one-third of the clavicle. The brachial plexus and subclavian artery pass beneath the clavicle, and the neurovascular examination of the affected arm should be carefully checked. The sternoclavicular joint, as well as the acromioclavicular joint, should be examined clinically to detect any changes in these joints as a result of the fracture.

Initial Therapy

Simple clavicle fractures that are nondisplaced without disruption of the sternoclavicular or acromioclavicular joint can easily be treated by the primary physician. A simple sling, analgesics, and ice applied to the fracture site will suffice. Patients should be instructed that it will take several days before they will be comfortable and up to 3 weeks before they will tolerate an unsupported arm. The patients may feel more comfortable sitting in a chair and may require several pillows to maintain a somewhat sitting position. For the midshaft fractures a figure-eight-type dressing or splint may provide some comfort by immobilizing the shoulder. For adults, in particular, and especially if they have fractures with gross displacement and overriding of the fragments, the figure-eight splint is not helpful. These patients do better with a shoulder cast, which immobilizes the entire hemithorax and arm. Displaced fractures and fractures involving the distal tip of the clavicle with disruptions at the acromioclavicular joint should be treated by an orthopedic surgeon.

Prognosis

Most fractures of the clavicle go on to union within 6 weeks for adults and 3 weeks for children. As long as the acromioclavicular joint is undisturbed, the ultimate shoulder function is quite good. On occasion, a large callus formed at the site

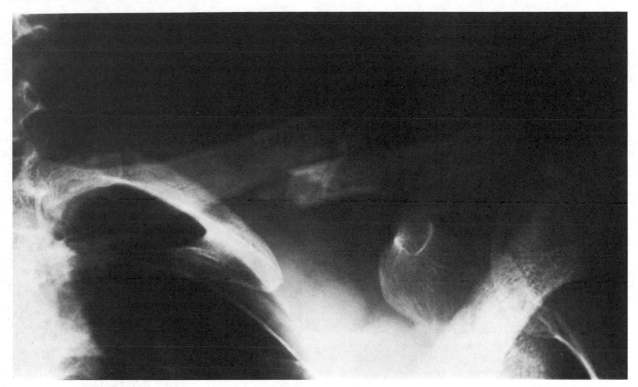

Figure 22.34 Anterior–posterior radiograph of a midshaft clavicular fracture. Note the overriding of the fracture fragments. It is not necessary to restore the clavicle fully to length for satisfactory shoulder function. Excessive overriding, however, should be avoided. The brachial plexus and subclavian artery pass beneath the clavicle, and, accordingly, assessment of these structures should be carried out on all clavicular fractures.

of the clavicular fracture will cause a thoracic outlet compression syndrome.

Thigh Injuries

As with upper extremity injuries, the type of lower extremity injury sustained is determined by the age of the patient and the circumstances of the injury. For example, from the same injury the young athlete will sustain a knee ligament disruption, whereas the older patient will incur a tibial plateau fracture because of the changing strengths of the tissues with age.

There are more open fractures with lower extremity trauma, and bone union tends to be slower. Lower extremity joints are weight bearing, giving increased significance to intraarticular fractures in this area. Accordingly, treatment must be aimed at maintaining joint congruity to help prevent posttraumatic degenerative arthritis. Most lower extremity intraarticular frac-

tures will require an open reduction and, usually, internal fixation.

HIP FRACTURES

Hip fractures are extremely common injuries; there are 200,000 hip fractures per year in the United States, predominantly in women in their 70s and 80s.

Diagnosis

The history reveals that the patient has usually fallen because of a misstep. On occasion, the patient will accurately describe feeling the hip break and falling because of it. The patient's history should be checked for high blood pressure, stroke, cardiac problems, seizure disorder, and any medications that may have contributed to the fall itself.

The physical examination usually shows that the patient has a shortened leg, which is externally rotated and painful to any motion. The amount of swelling present is an indication of the blood loss, which can amount to several units. The circulation sensation and motor function should be ascertained.

Initial Therapy

The leg should be splinted with sandbags, and 5 lb of Buck's traction should be applied to the leg with the weights suspended over the end of the hospital stretcher. These patients should not go to the x-ray film department without some immobilization or traction. There are several types of Buck's traction available. A foam boot that straps to the leg is commonly used and is quite satisfactory. Several layers of cast padding and adhesive moleskin straps held in place with a loose ace bandage is also satisfactory. Two people are needed to apply the traction properly: one person to internally rotate the leg gently and hold it and an assistant to apply the traction straps. When the leg is relatively internally rotated, the fracture surfaces are usually partially reduced, which will lessen the bleeding and provide more comfort for the patient.

By and large, these patients have a number of associated medical problems that may be either known or unknown to them. In most cases the treatment of choice is surgery, and, accordingly, the patient should undergo a complete medical evaluation. In the emergency room the patient should have a chest film, a cardiogram, and blood typing and crossmatching for 2 units of blood. The usual panel of preoperative laboratory determinations should be sent.

Prognosis

There are two main categories of fractures: femoral neck fractures and intertrochanteric fractures. These behave quite differently and are seen in different types of patients. The femoral neck fracture is intracapsular and does not lead to major blood loss since the fracture hematoma is contained within the joint capsule (Fig. 22.35). However, because of the local anatomy, these fractures interrupt the blood supply to the femoral head and therefore may lead to osteonecrosis of the femoral head. Nonunion is common. The orthopedic surgeon must decide whether or not to attempt to save the patient's femoral head. The surgeon will reduce the fracture hoping that union will occur with a normal femoral head. In the elderly, resection of the femoral head and insertion of a prosthesis is frequently resorted to since this provides adequate function when the patient is not a vigorous ambulator.

Intertrochanteric fractures occur in more elderly patients and

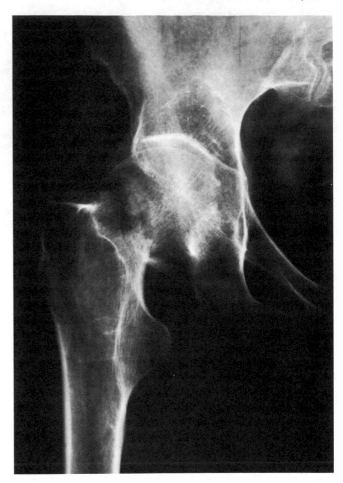

Figure 22.35 Anterior–posterior radiograph of a displaced femoral neck fracture. This is an intraarticular fracture that may have significantly disrupted the blood supply to the femoral head.

present with more deformity (Fig. 22.36). The leg is quite shortened and externally rotated. The patient can easily loose 2–3 units of blood in the thigh within the first few hours of the injury. These fractures do not interrupt the blood supply to the femoral head. The rate of union is high.

DISLOCATIONS OF THE HIP

Dislocations of the hip occur from high-energy trauma, usually a motor-vehicle accident. Classically, the patient is sitting with hip and knee flexion. A blow is sustained on the knee, which forces the femoral head out of the acetabulum posteriorly.

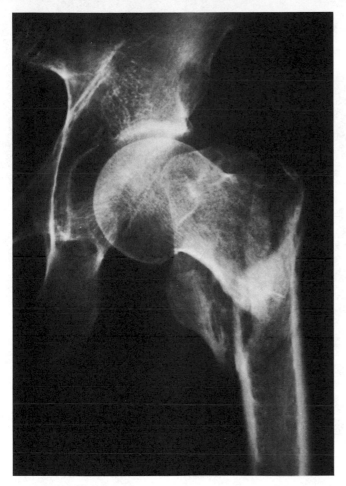

Figure 22.36 Anterior–posterior radiograph of an intertrochanteric fracture. Note the displacement of the lesser tuburosity. Such disruption of the medial femoral neck renders this fracture unstable.

Initial Therapy

The reduction of the fracture itself requires an orthopedic surgeon. It frequently must be done under a general anesthetic. The primary care physician should provide support for the injured side with sandbags and pillows but should make no attempt to correct the deformity. The function of the primary physician in an emergency room is to make certain that no associated injuries are overlooked and to obtain appropriate x-ray films and other medical studies preparing the patient for anesthesia.

Prognosis

A dislocated hip is a devasting injury for the hip joint. If there is no fracture of the acetabulum and the hip is reduced within 6 hours, the prognosis is quite good. The longer the time the hip is out of the acetabulum, the poorer is the prognosis. After 24 hours of dislocation there are no satisfactory results. Sciatic nerve injury, when present, usually resolves after a reduction such that most people regain protective sensation on the bottom of their foot but frequently retain a foot drop.

FEMORAL SHAFT FRACTURES

Femoral shaft fractures are associated with high-energy injuries and frequently with associated trauma in other organ systems (Fig. 22.37). They tend to be more common in young people.

Diagnosis

Femoral shaft fractures are alarming-looking injuries associated with a great deal of soft tissue damage, blood loss, and deformity. We must not lose site of the basics of resuscitation and volume replacement while making sure there is an intact neurocirculatory system distal to the injury. The closer the fracture site is to the knee, the more the popliteal artery is in jeopardy.

Diagnosis

The dislocations can be anterior as well as medial, involving a fracture of the medial wall of the acetabulum. Assessment of sciatic nerve function and distal pulses should be routinely done because there is a high incidence of sciatic palsy in these injuries. There may be other associated injuries, such as a patellar fracture and femoral fractures on the same side, as well as injuries to other organ systems commensurate with the level of trauma sustained.

Initial Therapy

Most of these patients arrive with a splint applied by the ambulance crew. Usually this is a Thomas splint with a traction apparatus attached to the ankle. Buck's traction, 5 lb with medial and lateral thigh splints, is also satisfactory. For distal femoral fractures just above the knee, medial and lateral splints alone are sufficient. The patient should not be sent to the x-ray department unless splinted appropriately. Blood routinely should be typed and crossmatched for these patients.

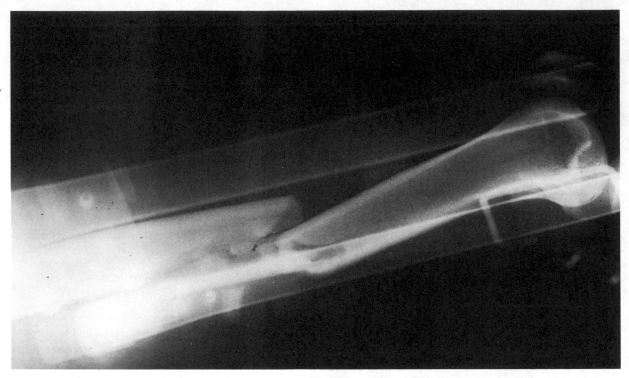

Figure 22.37 Lateral radiograph of a minimally comminuted transverse midshaft femur fracture. Reduction of this fracture would require both correction of the angular malalignment as well as the bony apposition and regaining of the femoral length.

Treatment varies depending on the age of the patient and circumstances causing the fractures. In general, all femoral fractures in pediatric patients are treated with traction followed by a cast. Most fractures in adults are treated with internal fixation using either an intramedullary rod or a plate. No matter what the ultimate form of therapy, the initial therapy for the first 3–7 days is the same, namely, insertion of an upper tibial or distal femoral Steinmann pin for skeletal traction. It is by this means that the fracture is pulled out to length and held immobile, while the soft tissue swelling and hemmorhage subsides. The pin insertion should be done by an orthopedic surgeon.

Prognosis

Femoral fractures have a low incidence of nonunion. It is quite difficult to maintain equality of leg lengths with these injuries, especially if there is comminution at the fracture site. These long bone fractures are the most frequent fractures associated with posttraumatic pulmonary insufficiency or fat emboli syndrome.

SUPRACONDYLAR FRACTURES

Supracondylar fractures are seen in older people and are frequently a result of rather innocent falls.

Diagnosis

Supracondylar fractures occur above the knee joint and unless undisplaced or perfectly impacted the fragments may be angulated by the pull of the gastrocnemius muscles on the distal fragment. The sharp edges of the fracture fragments can easily jeopardize the neurovascular structures at the back of the knee. These fractures are frequently intraarticular, and this must be looked for carefully.

Initial Therapy

If there is no neurovascular compromise, supracondylar fractures can be splinted in the position of deformity with medial and lateral plaster splints, and the patient can be sent to the x-ray department. Frequently, there is a large amount of blood lost with these fractures as with other femoral shaft fractures, so that blood should be typed and crossmatched in the blood bank. Initial therapy involves skeletal traction. Most patients are treated operatively with internal fixation using a plate or intramedullary rods.

Prognosis

Because of the proximity of the knee joint to the fracture, there is uniformly a loss of knee motion with these fractures. Most patients will obtain 100% of knee flexion.

Knee Injuries

Knee injuries compromise a large group of musculoskeletal injuries, which include fractures on the one hand and soft tissue injuries on the other. Patients frequently get these injuries from sports activities as well as motor-vehicle accidents. Ligamentous injuries are more common in younger patients, and fractures are more common in older patients.

MENISCOLIGAMENTOUS INJURY

Diagnosis

The difficult part about the knee examination is the interpretation of the findings from the physical examination, not the physical findings themselves. Specifically, it is the soft tissue injuries that give rise to difficulty. These soft tissues are the

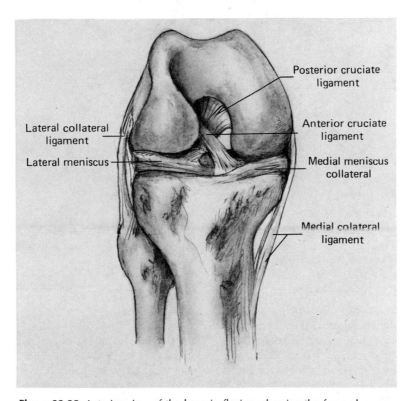

Figure 22.38 Anterior view of the knee in flexion, showing the femoral groove for articulation of the patella as well as the cruciate ligaments, menisci, and collateral ligaments. Note that the medial collateral ligament inserts onto the shaft of the tibia well below the joint line.

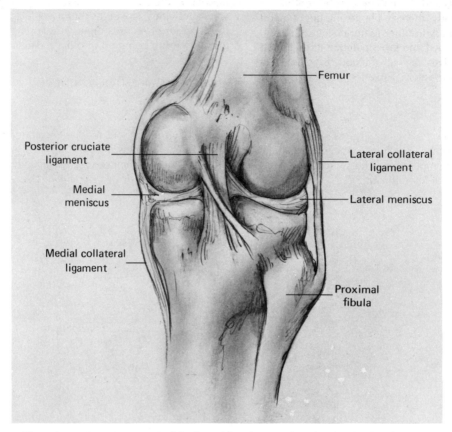

Figure 22.39 Posterior aspect of the knee joint showing the posterior cruciate ligaments and posterior menisci. Note that the medial collateral ligament inserts onto the back of the medial meniscus whereas the lateral collateral ligament does not.

collateral and cruciate ligaments, the capsular structures about the knee joint, the tendons and their expansions as they cross and intermesh with the capsular structures of the knee joint, and finally the medial and lateral menisci (Figs. 22.38 and 22.39). Even in expert hands, the correlation between the clinical findings and the actual pathology seen at surgery is low. When arthrography and arthroscopy are performed, the accuracy of preoperative diagnosis rises dramatically. These tests are rather specialized and are not helpful in the emergency room setting. The emergency room practitioner should develop a systematic knee evaluation that permits the physician to categorize whether a ligamentous, meniscal or bony injury has occurred and therefore to refer the patient appropriately for treatment.

History

The important points to obtain in the history are the presence of prior injury and the mechanism of the current injury in question. Usually the patient can distinguish a twist injury from a direct blow, whether the leg was bent to one side or the other, and if the leg was hyperflexed or hyperextended. Accordingly, the practitioner can then determine the structures at risk in any of these injuries, both on the tension and the compression sides of the joint. Frequently the patient will hear a pop, which is indicative of a cruciate rupture, usually the anterior cruciate, or will feel something tear in the knee, which is usually more suggestive of a meniscal injury. Whether or not the knee is locked, that is, unable to flex or extend from a bent position, should be ilicited. True locking of the knee means that there is mechanical inability to straighten the knee out completely, even if pain were ignored. Most patients describe what they think is locking of the knee when it seems they cannot move it because of pain; they go on, however, to describe being able subsequently to "work it out" over a short period of time. This history is suggestive of hamstring spasm rather than true mechanical locking. Usually a displaced loose body or displaced meniscus tear that interposes itself between joint surfaces causes true mechanical locking, which unlocks with a distinct sensation either heard or felt by the patient. When there are chronic injuries, the presence of buckling or giving way should be determined. This is a nonspecific complaint that either could be a result of intraarticular pathology or of instability of the extensor mechanism of the knee. If the patient gives a history of the knee coming out of place transiently, this is suggestive of a partial dislocation or subluxation of the patella.

Physical Examination

The components of the knee examination are listed and discussed below:

1. Deformity
2. Range of motion
3. Measurements
4. Effusion
5. Tenderness
6. Ligaments
7. Extensor mechanism
8. Other tests
9. Film evaluation

DEFORMITY.   If the patient is able to stand or walk, the examiner should look for the presence of knocked-knees (genu valgum) or bowlegs (genu varum). The presence of a flexion deformity or hyperextension should also be noted. The presence of a limp should be looked for. Deformities at the knee are usually more accentuated when standing than when sitting or lying down.

RANGE OF MOTION.   When the patient is supine, the range of motion is measured. Full extension is designated as 0 deg flexion. Normal knee flexion would be up to 140 deg. Hyperextension is listed in negative degrees from full extension to no extension. Crepitation, indicative of a loss of smoothness of the articulating surfaces, should be examined for while flexing and extending the knee.

MEASUREMENTS.   The circumference of the thigh and calf at an equal distance above the joint line or the patella should be measured, looking for evidence of thigh and calf atrophy or swelling.

EFFUSION.   The presence of a joint effusion should be noted on the record. The examiner should ask the patient over what period of time the swelling in the knee developed. Tense swelling that develops over 1–2 hours represents a hemarthrosis. A swelling that comes on over a 24-hour period represents a transudation into the knee joint. In general, a hemarthrosis is indicative of torn tissue, usually the anterior cruciate ligament or a peripheral meniscus tear. The menisci themselves are avascular, but a peripheral tear will cause bleeding. Detection of an effusion is important as a solid piece of evidence that something is distinctly wrong. In addition to mechanical derangements, an effusion is present with inflammatory diseases such as gout, rheumatoid arthritis, and osteoarthritis, as well as infection. In general, if patients give a distinct history of trauma to the knee and have an acute effusion, they have torn intraarticular tissue; if there is no effusion, the injury is frequently a ligamentous injury or represents an injury to the patella or extensor mechanism of the knee.

A joint filled with fluid will not easily flex or extend fully unless the capsule has been chronically stretched out enough to accommodate increased pressure. The skin lines on the front of the knee are stretched out, and the usually distinct margins about the joint, especially the patella, are blurred. Excess fluid in the joint may be manually ballotted from one side to the other by first putting compression on one side to squeeze out the joint fluid, releasing it, and quickly pushing on the opposite side, looking for a slow fluid wave that is visible as it comes across to the "emptied side." Another means of determining a knee effusion is to squeeze the fluid gently from the suprapatellar pouch underneath the patella and then ballot the patella against the top of the femur. A distinct "tap" is felt when the fluid separates the surfaces and the patella is pushed through this fluid layer and strikes the femoral groove. In a normal joint, the fluid coats the surfaces but does not physically separate the patella from the femur.

LIGAMENTS.   Ligamentous integrity of the knee should be determined by several maneuvers. In full extension the ability to displace the knee medially or laterally relative to the femur should be determined. This should then be repeated at 30 deg of flexion. Lateral or medial instability in extension indicates disruption of the posterior capsule and/or posterior cruciate ligaments. At 30 deg of flexion the posterior structures are relaxed, and this test will indicate injury to the medial collateral and lateral collateral ligament structures. Next, the knee should be flexed at 90 deg and a drawer maneuver performed with care to note the state of relaxation of the hamstrings. A drawer maneuver should also be performed with the knee at 30 deg of flexion. An anterior drawer sign, especially in extension, indicates anterior cruciate ligament insufficiency. At 90 deg of flexion a posterior drawer sign or posterior sag are suggestive of posterior cruciate insufficiency. The foot should be in neutral position when performing these tests.

There are several other tests for ligamentous injury to the knee; see the suggested readings at the end of this chapter for a more lengthy discussion of ligamentous evaluation.

The menisci are C-shaped structures on the medial and lateral sides of the joint (see Figs. 22.38 and 22.39). Their function is to distribute the weight bearing of the relatively curved femoral surfaces onto the relatively flat tibial surfaces. They also guide the femoral condyles during flexion of the knee. The usual mechanism for tearing of one of these structures is an uncontrolled flexion maneuver when the meniscus is unable to be retracted out from under the articular surface, is trapped between the femur and tibia, and is subsequently torn from its attachment on the knee capsule. The presence of ligamentous instability, especially anterior cruciate instability, permits this uncontrolled motion to happen more frequently. The patient who gives a history of a twist injury to the knee and presents with an effusion and joint line tenderness has a meniscal tear until proven otherwise. Frequently, there is locking of the knee and a history of giving way. The best test during the physical examination to see if there is meniscal tear is to flex the knee fully and then internally or externally rotate the foot. Flexion increases the pressure on the menisci and therefore elicits pain. Internally or externally rotating the foot will further increase the stress. After fully flexing the knee and rotating the foot, extending the knee may elicit a "klunk"—the McMurray test—suggesting that a torn portion of the meniscus has been caught under the femoral condyle and subsequently relocates as the knee is extended. Before any meniscal excision, careful documentation of the state of the menisci with arthrography or arthroscopy, should be performed. In general, meniscal tears should be observed for 4–6 weeks to determine the mechanical affect on the knee. Surgery is indicated only if there is chronic effusion, pain, and knee instability.

EXTENSOR MECHANISM.   The patella and quadriceps make up the extensor mechanism of the knee. This is a large source of pathology, especially in young women. When the knee is in full extension, the examiner should translocate the patella medially and laterally, looking for pain. The medial and lateral facets of the articular surface can be palpated with the patella displaced laterally or medially. The presence of subpatellar crepitation should be noted as the knee is placed through a range of motion. The presence of crepitation suggests chondromalacia of the articular surface. There does not need to be disruption of the smoothness of the articular surface, however, to have patellar pain. Chronic subluxation and maltracking of the patella are frequent sources of pain in young people and are dynamic problems that are difficult to elicit during static testing. Arthroscopy has been especially helpful in evaluating the extensor mechanism.

FILM EVALUATION.   Four views of the knee are needed in order to fully evaluate the knee radiographically. These views are an anterior–posterior, lateral, and tangential of the patella at a 40 deg angle of knee flexion and "tunnel view," which views the interchondylar area of the femur. Any bone disruption in the knee, no matter how small, can be significant since it represents an intraarticular fracture.

Initial Therapy

The appropriate therapy depends on the diagnosis. The comfort of the patient should also be taken into account. Any patient with a significant effusion should not be permitted to bear full weight on that knee. Accordingly, crutches and a touch-down, weight-bearing gait should be prescribed for the patient. An effusion will also be diminished and the patient will be more comfortable with a compressive dressing on the knee. In general, it is not necessary to immobilize the knee fully but simply to put on a bulky dressing that will partially immobilize the knee. This is called a Jones dressing. It is easily made by applying a skin adhesive, followed by several layers of cast padding, loose gauze, or cotton to the knee, building up a moderate amount of bulk, although not tight, followed by an elastic bandage. In order to be effective for the knee, this dressing must go from the supramalleolar area up to the thigh. Suspected meniscus tears or cruciate injuries are also adequately treated in the above fashion. Any significant ligamentous instability or intraarticular fractures of the knee should be treated by a specialist. In such instances, when the patient is in the emergency room, the knee should be placed in plaster splints medially and laterally on the leg. These splints should go from the thigh to the ankle.

Prognosis

Minor knee ligament sprains heal well after 3–6 weeks without residual instability. A more major knee ligament injury with some instability heals with residual laxity after 6 weeks. The laxity is slight and usually of no clinical significance as long as there has been good muscular rehabilitation of the leg. Severe knee ligament injuries, complete disruptions, will heal with marked instability and, as a rule, are best treated with operative repair within the first week after injury.

PREPATELLAR BURSITIS

Chronic irritation of the knee, such as repetitive kneeling, will frequently cause a swelling and redness over the top of the patella. This is often well circumscribed and may be confused with intraarticular swelling. The treatment is local measures, such as heat, as well as oral antiinflammatory medications. The differential diagnosis is between an aseptic and a septic process.

PATELLAR TENDONITIS

Patellar tendonitis is also known as "jumpers knee." It is the result of a patella tendon injury, usually a resisted extension of the knee such as occurs with repetitive kicking or jumping. There is local tenderness, usually over the distal pole of the patella, and pain with resisted extension of the knee. The treatment is avoidance of injury and local antiinflammatory measures. If the patient is extremely uncomfortable a Jones dressing or splints can be applied.

PES ANSERINUS BURSITIS

Pes anserinus bursitis occurs underneath the pes tendons as they come around the medial side of the tibia, four finger breadths below the joint line. It is frequently seen in older patients after a new activity involving repetitive flexion and extension of the knee. It can be confused with a meniscus injury because of the tenderness adjacent to the joint line. There should not be a joint effusion, and the true joint line should be comfortable to palpation. Treatment includes local antiinflammatory injection, avoidance of the precipitating activity, and local measures.

LATERAL KNEE TENDONITIS

There are two structures on the lateral side of the knee that cause pain and, frequently, snapping. These include the ili-
otibial tract and the popliteus tendon. Clinically, these two entities are difficult to differentiate. The history is usually that of a repetitive activity, such as running, and the onset of lateral pain. There may be a snapping or crepitation over these lateral structures with range of motion of the knee. Treatment includes antiinflammatory medications and avoidance of the activity that precipitated the inflammation.

Leg Injuries

FRACTURES OF THE TIBIA AND FIBULA

Fractures of the tibia and fibula are extremely common and represent a wide spectrum of injury, from simple closed non-displaced tibial fractures to the grade III open fracture with significant bony, soft tissue, and neurovascular compromise. The injuries that occur during sporting events and from simple falls tend to be easily managed with few complications, whereas injuries from motor-vehicle accidents and falls from a height may appear radiographically and clinically the same, but they have a high incidence of neurovascular compromise, especially compartment syndromes. The healing time of these injuries is proportional to the degree of energy dissipated in producing the injury.

Diagnosis

At presentation, all fractures of the tibia and fibula should be splinted before sending the patient for x-ray films. Frequently, splinting has been done by the emergency personnel at the site of the injury. The physical examination should include careful testing of the pulses, sensation, and motor function with particular attention to peroneal nerve function. If the patient can extend the big toe or ankle and has normal sensation to light touch on the dorsum of the foot, especially in the web space between the first and the second toe, this nerve is intact. Careful inspection of the skin over the pretibial area is required to rule out small puncture wounds that may represent open fractures. Anterior–posterior and lateral x-ray films of the tibia, which include both the knee and the ankle on the same film to permit determination of fracture alignment, should be ordered. No patient should be x-rayed without a splint on the fracture. The newer air splints are particularly suited to tibial fractures (Fig. 22.40). Another excellent splint for the tibia is a pillow folded around the leg and held with adhesive tape.

Initial Therapy

By and large, all tibial and fibular fractures should be treated by a specialist. The isolated fibular fracture is an exception

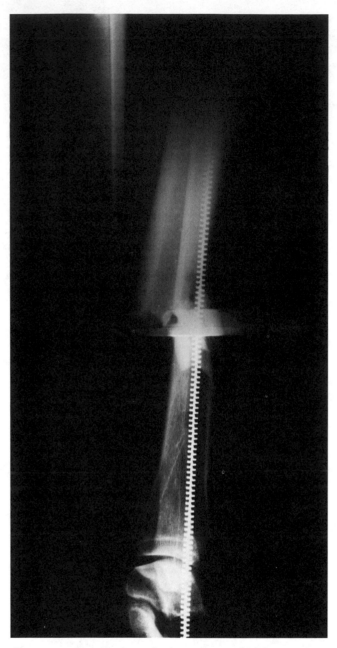

Figure 22.40 Lateral radiograph of a transverse tibial fracture. Note the loss of apposition of the fracture fragments. The fractured extremity has been x-rayed through an air-filled splint.

since it is not a weight-bearing structure. Midshaft transverse fibular fractures are common injuries and do not disturb the stability of the leg. The primary physician can easily treat these. There is bleeding associated with these injuries, and compartment syndromes of the anterior and lateral compartment are a distinct possibility. Consequently, the physician must carefully inform the patient of the signs and symptoms of a compartment syndrome, and the patient should be carefully instructed in strict elevation of the leg. Only mild analgesics should be provided so as to not mask neurovascular compromise. The leg should be immobilized in a well-padded splint that goes from the upper calf to the toes, and the patient should be placed on crutches. Follow-up should be arranged for within 7–10 days. Another common fibular fracture is the proximal fibular neck fracture at the level of the knee joint. The peroneal nerve should be checked. This fracture is also easily treated by the primary physician. The patient is made more comfortable by a splint that immobilizes the knee, as well as the foot. Again, elevation and neurovascular observation should be routine.

All nondisplaced tibial fractures are potentially treacherous in that a compartment syndrome can develop. Nondisplaced fractures may also displace significantly, thus complicating their care and prolonging their healing time. Accordingly, all nondisplaced fractures need to be appropriately immobilized with splints or a cast. Patients with all but the most benign tibial fractures should be admitted to the hospital for 24 hours of observation and instructions on how to walk with crutches, and application of a cast.

The tibial plateau fracture is an intraarticular knee injury and, unless nondisplaced, requires specialized care. Treatment may be surgical. Generally speaking, all patients with these fractures should be admitted to the hospital.

The displaced tibial plateau fracture requires the care of a specialist. The reduction criteria are quite strict. The emergency practitioner should be sure the injured leg is splinted with immobilization of the knee and foot.

Prognosis

The average healing time for tibial fractures is 14–20 weeks, depending on the age of the patient and the energy imparted by the injury. Frequently patients develop stiffness of the ankle, especially if the fracture line is in the distal third of the tibial shaft. Tibial fractures have a 10% incidence of a nonunion. Many patients will experience a small amount of shortening—up to 1 cm is acceptable—during the healing of these fractures.

Ankle Injuries

Injuries to the ankle are the most common joint injuries. Again, as with other joints there is a wide spectrum of injury from the most simple ligamentous sprain to the most complex intraarticular fractures.

LIGAMENTOUS INJURY

Diagnosis

There is very little subcutaneous tissue over the ankle joint. Accordingly, ligamentous injuries do not tolerate prolonged deformity or swelling without compromise of the skin. Accordingly extreme care needs to be taken in the initial management of ankle injuries.

All emergency room practitioners will see a great number of ankle sprains. There is an unfortunate temptation to treat the patients automatically, depending upon the x-ray film evaluation: fractured, call the orthopedist; no fracture, ace bandage, ice, crutches, pain medication, and a return appointment. Although this may suffice for many sprains, it should be recognized that the sprained ankle has a wide range of anatomical damage, and appropriate treatment depends on many factors including the life-style and age of the patient. The minor tears will heal independent of treatment, whereas major tears will need at least plaster mobilization and some may even require surgery. The undertreated severely sprained ankle may become chronically uncomfortable with possible instability. Anatomically, tears of ankle ligaments extend not only across the major portion of the ligament complex but also include the joint capsule.

The most common ligaments sprained in the ankle are the lateral ones, especially the anterior talofibular ligament (Fig. 22.41).

It is important to know exactly how the injury happened, that is, whether the foot twisted in or out and how severe the actual trauma was. The history of past injuries should be elicited. Many "chip fractures" seen on x-ray films are merely residual calcifications in the capsules or ligaments in joints subjected to repeated injuries. The time since the injury is important to note since massive swelling will accompany even a minor ankle sprain if the ankle has not been elevated. Many patients will mistakenly apply heat or hot compresses to an ankle fracture and present with fantastically swollen ankles.

The physical examination should test for the presence of good distal capillary filling and peripheral pulses. A thorough neurologic examination of the foot should be done. The patient is more comfortable if the ankle examination is performed when the knee is flexed which relaxes the calf muscles. The palpation part of the ankle examination should start at the knee joint since fractures of the proximal fibula can accompany ankle sprains. At the same time, avulsions of the muscles of the lateral or anterior compartment may also accompany ankle sprains, and these should be noted. The examiner should start by feeling away from the site of the swelling and pain, gently compressing first one malleous and then the other all along the bony prominences. Tenderness here may be a clue to a fracture, although in a severe sprain, the bone itself may be tender even with a negative x-ray film. The tenderness probably represents a partial tearing or stripping off of the periosteal covering of the bone, which results in hemorrhage under it. Next, the examiner should palpate across the front of the ankle joint to each side of the extensor tendons. This area represents the capsule of the ankle joint, which is directly under the examining fingers. Exquisite tenderness here is a clue to further extension of the "sprain." An experienced examiner can frequently palpate the defects in the ligaments or capsules. The area feels "hollow" in spite of the swelling present on the surface, and the sensation is "mushy," as if there were a lack of substance under the examining fingers. Next, the practitioner should examine the opposite ankle to determine what ligamentous "give" exists for the patient. The practitioner should then return to examining the injured side and should first gently stress the ligamentous complex that appears not to be involved, followed by the ligamentous complex under suspicion. This is performed by cupping the heel in one hand and gently rocking the ankle from side to side to see if it comes to a stop or if it suddenly gives way. If the side of the ankle seems to drop away, then it is likely that the tear is complete. If, when stressed, the ankle does not open up and has a real end point similar to the other ankle when it is similarly stressed, then it is likely that there is only a partial ligamentous disruption. The use of a locally instilled anesthetic may permit a better examination. This decision is best left to the orthopedic surgeon.

Initial Therapy

Ankle sprains can be treated initially by the primary physician without difficulty. Ankle fractures, however, should be referred directly to the orthopedic surgeon for consideration. A severe ankle sprain should also be brought to the orthopedist's attention so that he or she can plan on-going therapy. If the patient can fully move the ankle joint, has minimal swelling, and has only moderate tenderness over one spot, the routine of an elastic bandage, crutches, ice, elevation, and progressive return to full activities is sufficient. No orthopedic follow-up is necessary if the patient is ambulating comfortably by the end

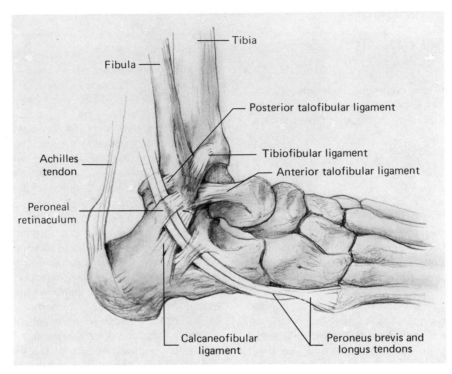

Figure 22.41 Lateral view of the ankle showing the anterior talofibular, calcaneofibular and posterior talofibular ligaments. Note the peroneal tendons crossing behind the fibula inserting on the lateral border of the foot.

of 1 week. The elastic wrap goes from the tips of the toes, includes the heel, and extends to the top of the calf in order to provide adequate compression and to prevent edema above or below the dressing. Put on a 4-inch bandage from the toes to just above the malleoli, then overlap it with a 6-inch bandage that goes from the heel to the top of the calf. A more effective compression dressing for moderately swollen ankles is achieved by using a layer of gauze or cotton pads about the swollen area, holding them in place with cast padding or a gauze bandage, and then covering this with the elastic bandages.

For the severely sprained ankle, the patient will require more immobilization for comfort. This is most easily accomplished with a plaster splint included in the dressing. A simple posterior splint if sufficiently thick, will suffice; however, a second stir-rup splint will markedly strengthen the splint (see Fig. 22.11). The patient will need crutches and should be instructed in a touch-down, weight-bearing gait.

The practitioner should be specific in instructions for home care. The leg should be elevated on one or two pillows so that it is above the level of the heart. The patient is permitted to get up to go to the bathroom and to eat meals but for little else for the first 48 hours. Ice should be applied over the swollen areas by using crushed ice in a plastic bag with sufficient protection from cold injury for the skin. The ice should be applied for 15-20 minutes every 2 hours for the first day depending upon the amount of discomfort and the degree of swelling. The patient should ambulate with crutches, placing as much weight on the foot as is tolerated as long as there is no pain. Gradually, the amount of weight bearing is progressed until the patient can easily walk without a limp. During the first 48 hours, adequate analgesic medication should be taken on a regular basis. The patient should start moving the ankle up and down as soon as possible to prevent the joint from getting too stiff and to aid in pumping the calf to prevent venous stasis.

The patient should have a return appointment to see a specialist if there is a severe sprain or if the patient cannot comfortably ambulate at the end of 1 week.

Prognosis

Ankle sprains are the most common joint injury, and most heal well without joint instability or chronic discomfort.

ANKLE FRACTURES

Ankle fractures are common and important since the ankle is a crucial weight-bearing joint. The shape of the ankle is that of a mortise: it is made up of the articulating surface of the tibia and the medial malleolus, as well as the distal fibula laterally. The talus serves as the tendon that fits into the ankle mortise. Needless to say, disruption of this arrangement would lead to incongruity and degenerative arthritis of the joint. All ankle fractures should be cared for by a specialist because the criteria for reduction are quite strict and even nondisplaced ankle fractures can lose their alignment and require later reduction.

Diagnosis

Frequently ankle fractures cannot be differentiated from ankle sprains by gross inspection. Careful palpation of the soft tissues and bony landmarks will often reveal crepitation or true bony tenderness, rather than ligamentous tenderness, suggesting the presence of the fracture. The most important diagnostic tool, however, is the x-ray film, which will reveal the type of bony disruption. Three views are necessary: an anterior–posterior view, a lateral view, and a 20 deg internal rotation oblique view, which is referred to as the *mortise view* since it reveals the bony arch surrounding the talus (Fig. 22.42). The neurovascular status of the foot should be assessed and the ankle splinted before sending the patient for an x-ray film.

Initial Therapy

If the ankle presents with gross deformity, the practitioner should realign the foot grossly to prevent ischemic damage to the overlying skin as well as to the distal structures. If the practitioner is concerned about the type of injury, a quick x-ray film in the emergency area, before performing the realignment, can be obtained.

All ankle fractures need immobilization. For the nondisplaced single malleolus fracture, a stout splint is sufficient, followed by nonweight-bearing gait with the patient on crutches and strict elevation of the injured extremity until a cast is applied. If there is injury to both the medial and lateral aspects of the ankle, whether bony or ligamentous, a long leg cast is required. If there is incongruity of the weight-bearing surface

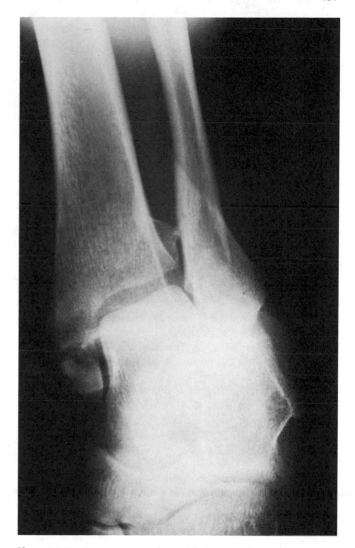

Figure 22.42 A mortise view of an ankle fracture. There is a transverse fracture of the medial malleolus at the level of the plafond of the tibia, as well as an oblique angulated fracture of the fibula.

of the ankle or incongruity of the ankle mortise, a reduction is required. This is best done within the first few hours of the injury. The criteria for reduction are quite strict, and open reduction and internal fixation of the fracture fragments should be accomplished if the closed reduction does not produce a near anatomical result. The orthopedic specialist should be involved in caring for all ankle fractures except the most minor.

Prognosis

Injuries to weight-bearing joints are always potentially serious, and this is also true of the ankle. The more severe the injury, the more impairment the patient will experience. For practical purposes, all ankle fractures result in some loss of motion, but the patient usually retains a functional range.

Foot Injuries

Foot injuries are caused by direct trauma, such as a crush, and indirect trauma, such as occurs in a twist injury. The bones around the foot have interconnecting capsules and ligaments that weave about in a complex fashion, usually preventing complete dislocation of the individual bones except in rare circumstances. Like the ankle, there is very little subcutaneous tissue about the foot, so deformity and swelling are poorly tolerated.

DIAGNOSIS

The bones of the foot are quite superficial, and therefore careful physical evaluation will permit accurate anatomical diagnosis of underlying damaged structures. The examiner should look for the point of maximum tenderness, noting any swelling that can be localized and making note of the ecchymotic area that reflects underlying bleeding. The distal circulation, sensation, and motor function should be assessed. The area of maximum tenderness should be carefully scrutinized on the x-ray film.

The examination of the foot should start with the hind foot and progress to the toes. The heel should be cradled in both palms and rocked from side to side to appreciate subtalar motion. Next, by supporting the heel and holding it stationary, the rest of the foot may be brought from side to side and slightly twisted in order to determine motion and discomfort in the midtarsal joints. The first and fifth metatarsals are easily moved about and palpated throughout their length. The other metatarsals and cuneiforms can similarly be palpated. The balls of the feet represent the metatarsal heads, which are palpable on the soles of the foot. All of the toes are quite easy to inspect visually.

Occasionally, a patient will present with a "lump" of the medial midfoot. This frequently represents an accessory navicular attention having become tender or swollen because of local injury or an excessive pull of the posterior tibial tendon. On the x-ray film there is what looks like an isolated extra bone that has smooth rounded edges and that is also present on the other foot (if it has been x-rayed also). Treatment consists of reassurance and referral for follow-up. Fractures of the talus,

calcaneus, navicular, and cuboid bones deserve a call to the orthopedic surgeon for advice and require follow-up treatment. The examiner should be aware that many small excessory bones reside in the foot and are not fractures. The excessory navicular mentioned above is the largest of these. There are common bones along the back of the talus and the lower surface of the cuboid bone. Frequently, there are "chips" seen on a lateral

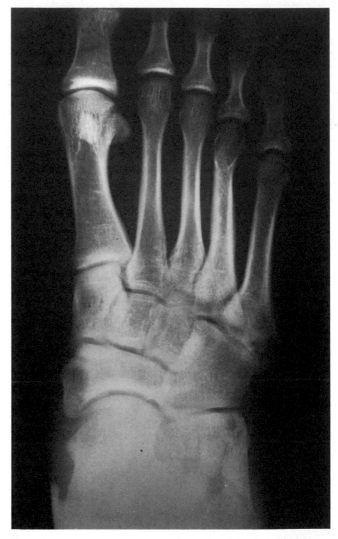

Figure 22.43 Anterior–posterior radiograph of the foot showing an avulsion fracture of the proximal fifth metatarsal. These heal well in 3–6 weeks. Occasionally treatment consists of a cast, but if the patient is sufficiently comfortable, a soft dressing and crutches are sufficient.

film of the ankle or foot that look like multiple bony flecks on the anterior ankle capsule and reflect calcification because of repeated injury and are not acute fractures. True "chip" fractures are avulsion fractures that have sharp jagged edges, and often the examiner can see the defect in the bone from where they come. Tenderness near these avulsion fractures is quite local. A common avulsion fracture is seen at the base of the fifth metatarsal (Fig. 22.43) since the peroneus braevis inserts at this point and actually pulls the bone off when it is suddenly put on stretch.

INITIAL THERAPY

All foot injuries should be elevated at the time of presentation in the emergency room. Severe injuries of the foot, especially crush injuries, require that the patient be supine and the leg maximally elevated above the level of the patient's heart. Such injuries are insufficiently elevated if the patient is in a wheelchair and the injured leg is extended on the leg rest.

Nondisplaced fractures of the foot are best treated by ap-plying a bulky compressure dressing and providing the patient with crutches for a supported gait. If the patient is quite uncomfortable, a posterior plaster splint will better immobilize the foot. In general, circular casts are not indicated during the first few days after an injury. As with other injuries about the foot, fracture of the toes are best treated conservatively. The x-ray film alignment of these fractures is not significant. The visual appearance of the toe is the most important feature predictive of a satisfactory outcome. The toe should have a normal appearance so that it would fit comfortably in a shoe. No bony projections can be directed at the plantar surface that would disrupt comfortable weight bearing. Toe fractures that are quite comminuted or involve one of the interphalangeal joints will heal with some stiffness. This should be mentioned to the patient but is usually of no functional significance.

Fractured toes are best treated by immobilizing the injured toe to the adjacent toe by strapping the toes with tape. The web space should be protected with a layer of gauze to prevent masceration of the skin. The patient should be advised to take an old sneaker and cut out the toe area to fashion a comfortable

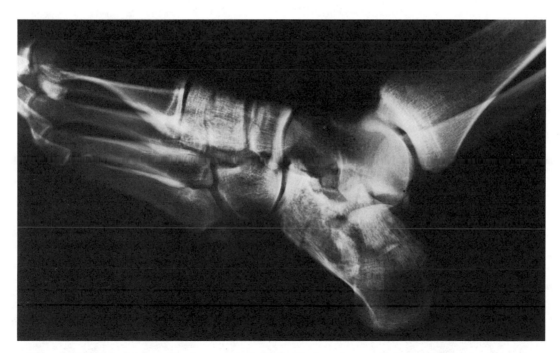

Figure 22.44 Lateral radiograph of a comminuted intraarticular calcaneus fracture. Note the complete disruption of the normal architecture of the subtalar joints. There is an incidental nonunion of a fifth metatarsal fracture that was entirely asymptomatic. There is a high incidence of lumbar spine compression fractures associated with severe calcaneus fractures.

walking shoe. Patients with these fractures should be referred to an orthopedist for follow-up. In general, they are best treated with early weight bearing and early motion. If the patient is uncomfortable, a short leg walking cast may be used.

PROGNOSIS

Fractures of the phalanges, metatarsals, and tarsals have a good prognosis. Nonunions are extremely rare. Fractures of the talus and os calcis, on the other hand, are serious injuries. Talus fractures frequently result in avascular necrosis and chronic ankle pain. Os calcis fractures that are intraarticular result in permanent subtalar stiffness and/or pain. On occasion, arthrodesis of the subtalar joint or the use of an ankle–foot arthrosis to control motion is necessary for comfort.

Lumbar spine compression fractures are frequently associated with calcaneus fractures. Calcaneus fractures deserve special mention (Fig. 22.44). The heel skin is firmly applied to the bone such that swelling is poorly tolerated. As a result, all people with calcaneus fractures should be admitted to the hospital. The functional loss from these fractures is usually significant, especially if the subtalar joint has been injured. All patients with calcaneus fractures should be managed by a specialist.

SUGGESTED READINGS

American Academy of Orthopedic Surgeons: Joint Motion—Method of Measuring and Reading. Chicago, 1965.

Bateman JE: *The Shoulder and Neck.* Philadelphia, WB Saunders Co, 1972.

Charnley J: *The Closed Treatment of Common Fractures.* London, Churchill-Livingston, 1974.

Edmonson AS, Crenshaw AH: *Campbells' Operative Orthopedics.* St. Louis, The CV Mosby Co, 1980.

Helfet AJ (ed): *Disorders of the Knee.* Philadelphia, JB Lippincott Co, 1974.

Heppenstall RB (ed): *Fracture Treatment and Healing.* Philadelphia, WB Saunders Co, 1980.

Hoppenfeld S: *Physical Examination of the Spine and Extremities.* New York, Appleton-Century-Crofts, 1976.

Iverson LD, Clawson DK: *Manual of Acute Orthopedic Therapeutics.* Boston, Little Brown & Co, 1977.

Mann RA (ed): *DuVries, Surgery of the Foot.* St. Louis, The CV Mosby Co, 1978.

Post M (ed): *The Shoulder, Surgical and Non-Surgical Management.* Philadelphia, Lea & Febiger, 1978.

Sharrad WJW: *Pediatric Orthopedics and Fractures.* London, Blackwell Scientific Publications, 1979.

Turek SL: *Orthopedics.* Philadelphia, JB Lippincott Co, 1977.

23

HAND INJURIES AND OTHER ACUTE DISORDERS OF THE HAND

Paul Feldon
Edward A. Nalebuff

The outcome of an injury to the hand is often determined by the care provided in the emergency room. Hand injuries are common, comprising over 30% of all industrial accidents. Seventy-five percent of the injuries that result in permanent partial disability involve the hand. Optimal initial care of hand injuries can minimize the physical and emotional handicaps as well as the loss of productivity that results from these injuries. The ability to make an accurate diagnosis, that is, to determine what can be treated by the primary physician in the emergency room and what should be referred to a specialist, is the key to providing optimal care.

EVALUATION OF THE PATIENT

First aid for patients with injured hands should be provided before a detailed history and physical examination are undertaken. Watches, bracelets, and, especially, rings should be removed immediately so that they will not become tourniquets as swelling occurs. Open wounds and massive injuries of the hand should be wrapped in a dry, sterile bandage while the patient is waiting for clinical or x-ray examination. The hand should *not* be immersed in a pan of water to soak.

History

The mechanism, time, place, and other circumstances of the injury must be determined. A snap or pop at the time of injury suggests a ligament disruption or a fracture. Prolonged copious bleeding from a finger wound suggests neurovascular bundle division. Injuries from glass may result in damage to deep structures that are not apparent from the superficial wound or

may result in fragments of glass being retained in the soft tissue. Hands that are caught in machines may sustain a combination of lacerations, crush, and thermal injuries, depending on the type of machine and nature of the moving parts. The exact nature of the substance in chemical burns will affect the choice of treatment. The age, occupation, avocations, hand dominence, and general health of the patient should be recorded. The patient should specifically be asked about the use of daily medications, the status of tetanus immunization, and oral intake before and after the injury. The patient should be asked about old hand injuries or any preexisting disability of the hand.

If a patient presents with unexplained swelling and tenderness consistent with infection but no obvious source of contamination, the patient should be asked about puncture wounds or insect bites or possible medical conditions, such as gout, that can imitate infection.

Physical Examination

Proper diagnosis of the injured hand requires a knowledge of the functional anatomy of the hand—the locations and functions of the muscles that control it, the skeletal framework, and the major and "minor" nerves that supply the hand. It is perfectly acceptable, even advisable, to use an anatomical atlas to refresh one's memory. Potentially dangerous exploration or probing of open wounds should not be undertaken in the emergency room to establish a diagnosis; the diagnosis should be made by clinical and x-ray examination. A systematic examination should be carried out with the following questions in mind:

1. What is the extent and nature of the skin wound?
2. Has a neurovascular bundle been injured?
3. Is there tendon damage?
4. Is there bone, joint, or ligament damage?

In general, assume that all longitudinal structures crossing the site of an open wound are divided and that swollen joints have unstable ligament disruptions or dislocations until proven otherwise.

The stance of the hand is important for quickly discovering major tendon and joint injuries. The normal posture of the fingers in relation to each other and to the palm is familiar and can be checked by comparing the injured hand against the noninjured hand or the examiner's hand. The fingers normally lie in sequence with each joint in slight flexion (Fig. 23.1). Loss of continuity of one or more tendons or an alteration in skeletal alignment, changes this stance. Gentle palpation of the hand will reveal areas of local tenderness, skeletal irregularity, or joint instability. An alteration in skin moisture sug-

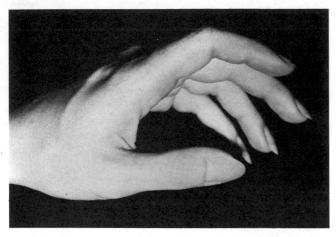

Figure 23.1 When the hand is at rest, the fingers lie in slight flexion. Note the normal "cascade" of progressive flexion from the index to the small fingers.

gests damage to the sensory nerves in the affected area. The skin loss, the amount of tissue crushed, and the presence of cleanly incised wounds, ragged lacerations, or combinations of these will determine where and how the injuries must be handled. The amount of bacterial contamination that has occurred should be estimated and, if indicated, cultures should be obtained. Occasionally, the amount of dirt present obscures the nature of the wound and preliminary cleansing must be done. Soap and water usually are best for cleansing the skin adjacent to the wound, although occasionally degreasing agents such as ether or a solution of hydrogen peroxide to remove coagulated blood may be required. The wound itself should be cleansed only by irrigation with a physiologic solution such as Ringer's solution or normal saline in amounts sufficient to remove superficial contaminants and foreign material from the wound (usually 1–2 liters).

EXAMINATION OF TENDONS

A loss of tendon function following upper extremity injury may be secondary to transection of the tendon, rupture of the tendon, or paralysis of the muscle unit. Tendon transection must be suspected in any open wound of the hand. Complete division of the tendon must be differentiated from partial or incomplete transection. A laceration in the appropriate anatomical area, pain from active or passive motion of the finger, and tenderness over the tendon, without loss of the normal finger posture or active motion suggest a partial tendon laceration. These must be treated to prevent subsequent rupture or ad-

herence. Open wounds should not be probed in an attempt to detect tendon damage. Rather, a careful detailed examination should be done.

Flexor tendon ruptures can occur and must be suspected when tendon function is suddenly lost in the absence of an open wound. The flexor digitorum profundus tendon of the ring finger is not uncommonly avulsed from its distal attachment in football players holding on during a tackle. This may occur either with or without an avulsion fracture of the distal phalanx. Any sudden extension force applied to the hand during grip can cause tendon rupture, although significant force is required.

A tendon's function also may be lost if the nerve innervating its muscle belly is damaged. Thus both the integrity of the tendon and the integrity of the nerve supplying the musculotendinous unit must be determined.

Flexor Tendons

Each finger has two flexor tendons; the *flexor digitorum superficialis,* which inserts on the middle phalanx and flexes the proximal interphalangeal joint, and the *flexor digitorum profundus,* which inserts on the distal phalanx and flexes both the distal and proximal interphalangeal joints (Fig. 23.2). The thumb has one extrinsic flexor tendon—the flexor pollicis longus—which inserts on the distal phalanx and flexes the interphalangeal joint (and metacarpophalangeal joint). Division of one or more of these tendons will alter the posture or stance of the finger with respect to the other fingers and will result in the inability to flex the digit fully. The tendons are tested by asking the patient to make a fist. The tips of all of the fingers should touch the distal palm crease. The thumb tendon is tested by asking the patient to touch the head of the fifth metacarpal with the tip of the thumb. The inability to flex a finger actively at the proximal interphalangeal (PIP) joint suggests division of both the superficial and deep flexor tendons (Fig. 23.3). The diagnosis of damage to a single flexor tendon in the finger is more difficult since the remaining tendon has considerable functional capacity and the posture of the digit may be altered only slightly. Thus, each deep and superficial tendon must be tested individually.

The profundus tendon is tested by stabilizing the PIP joint in extension and asking the patient to flex the tip of the finger (Fig. 23.4). The profundus is the only tendon that can flex the distal interphalangeal (DIP) joint, and the absence of this function is diagnostic. Each finger and the thumb are tested in sequence. Isolated injuries of the sublimis (superficial) tendon are more difficult to detect since the profundus tendon is ca-

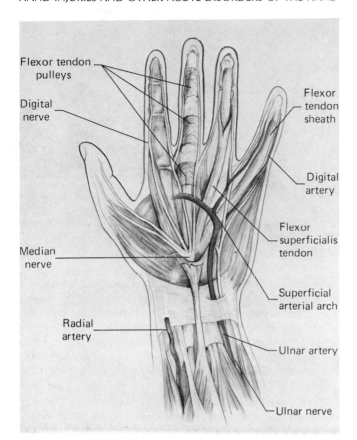

Figure 23.2 The flexor aspect of the hand. The locations of the digital nerves and arteries are illustrated in the index and small fingers; the flexor tendon and sheath and pulley mechanism are shown in the long finger; and the superficial and deep flexor tendons are illustrated in the ring finger.

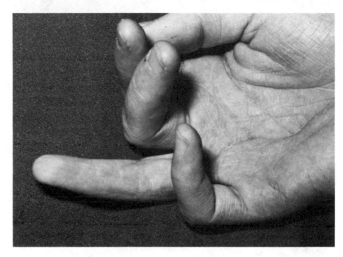

Figure 23.3 Stance of the ring finger when both superficial and deep flexor tendons are cut.

Extensor Tendons

Extension of the fingers is the result of a complex structure composed of interlacing fibers from the extrinsic extensor tendons (extensor digitorum communis, extensor indicis proprius, and extensor digiti quinti) and from the intrinsic muscles (interossei and lumbricals) (Fig. 23.6). The long or extrinsic extensor tendons are responsible for extension of the metacarpophalangeal (MP) joints, whereas the intrinsic tendons combined with the extrinsic tendons act to extend the interphalangeal (IP) joints. The combination of the extrinsic extensor tendons and the intrinsic tendons is called the *extensor mechanism*. The ability to extend the fingers fully at all joint levels suggests that there is no interruption in the continuity of this mechanism. However, a lag in extension of the MP joint suggests an injury of the extrinsic extensor tendons. The extrinsic extensor tendon should be tested against resistance because of the juncturae that interlink the extensor digitorum communis tendons at the midmetacarpal level and that can provide weak extension in the case of a divided tendon. A lag in extension of the PIP or DIP joints suggests an injury of the extensor mechanism distal to the MP joints. Closed as well as open injuries on the dorsal aspect of the digit may damage the extensor mechanism and result in finger deformity (see section on closed tendon injuries). The extensor pollicis longus tendon should be tested by palpation of the tendon at wrist level during active extension since the interphalangeal joint may be extended by intrinsic muscles and division of the extensor pollicis

pable of flexing the digit fully by itself. Therefore the posture of the finger may not be changed, and full active motion may be present in spite of damage to this tendon. Testing the sublimis tendon requires that the profundus tendon action be eliminated. This is done by holding all of the fingers not being tested in extension (Fig. 23.5). This limits profundus tendon action in the finger being tested because of the interdigitation of the profundus muscle bellies in the forearm. Any motion of the PIP joint now is the result of sublimis tendon action alone. The exception to this will occur in a patient with an independent profundus tendon in the index finger. Since this usually is present bilaterally, the injured side should be tested.

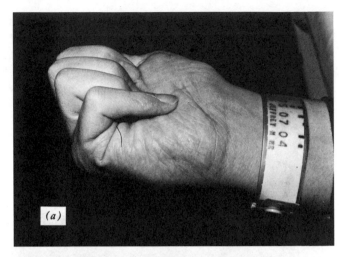

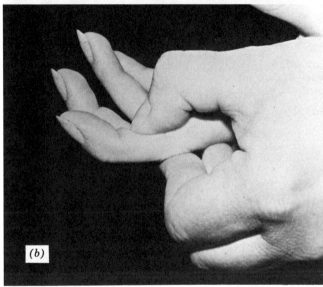

Figure 23.4 (a) The appearance of the hand during maximum active finger flexion with a complete division of the deep flexor tendon to the small finger. Note the absence of flexion of the DIP joint. (b) Method for testing for deep flexor tendon function. The PIP joint is held in extension and the patient is asked to flex the DIP joint actively.

longus may cause the posture of the thumb to reflect only incomplete extension of the MP joint.

NERVE EXAMINATION

Nerve function should be assessed before the use of any form of local anesthetic. Sensory function can be evaluated quickly

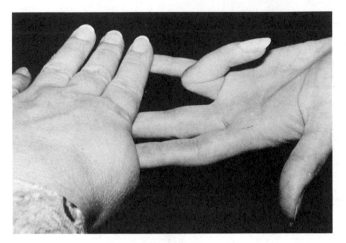

Figure 23.5 Test for superficial flexor tendon function. All fingers except that one being tested are held in extension to eliminate the effect of the deep flexor tendon. If the superficial flexor tendon is intact, the finger can be flexed actively at the PIP joint.

by testing both sides of each digit using light touch, either by the examiner's finger or with a wisp of cotton, and comparing the patient's report of subjective sensation to that on the adjacent or contralateral (noninjured) fingers. Sharp pins are not necessary to test sensibility and can cause discomfort when nerve function is intact. In children this discomfort will make the frightened child uncooperative. We should not ask, "Do you feel this?" but rather, "Does this feel the same as the other side (or finger)?" Sympathetic dennervation at the time of sensory nerve damage results in cessation of sweating. Therefore areas of dryness on the volar surfaces of the digits are very suggestive of nerve damage. The pattern of dryness may help determine which nerves have been injured when the clinical examination is difficult (such as with a child or an unconscious patient) or when nerve damage proximal to the digit is suspected. Injuries proximal to the digits require that the function of the three major nerves supplying the hand be tested (Fig. 23.7).

Median Nerve

The median nerve in the hand provides sensibility to the volar surfaces of the thumb, index, long, and one-half of the ring fingers, as well as to the dorsal surfaces of these fingers distal to the MP joints. It innervates the thenar muscles (opponens, abductor pollicis, and one-half of the flexor pollicis brevis) and the lumbricals of the index and long fingers.

To test for the thenar muscle function, have the patient place

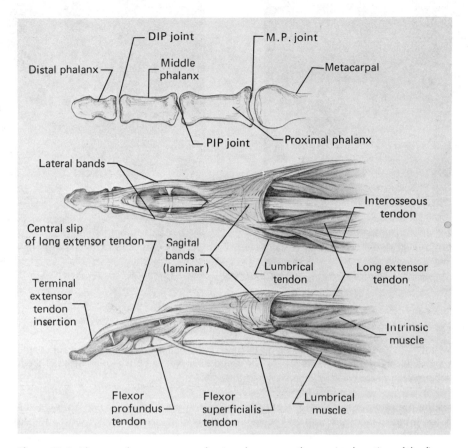

Figure 23.6 The complex extensor mechanism drapes over the proximal portion of the finger and is composed of interlacing fibers with contributions from the long extensor tendon that terminates in the central slip inserting at the base of the middle phalanx and from the interosseous and lumbrical tendons that terminate in the lateral bands.

the hand palm up on a flat surface. Then ask the patient to point the thumb to the ceiling. The ability to perform this maneuver confirms function of the opponens and abductor pollicis brevis muscles. Contraction of these muscles can be palpated adjacent to the thumb metacarpal during the test. Only an intact opponens and abductor pollicis brevis will abduct the first metacarpal bone away from the plane of the palm and rotate the pulp of the thumb to oppose that of the small finger. However, one must observe carefully during thenar muscle testing. An intact ulnar nerve will allow a patient with a divided median nerve to bring the tip of the thumb toward the small finger. However, in this case, the patient will "oppose" the tip of the thumb and small finger by flexing both

digits, rather than by bringing the thumb away from the palm to meet the small finger in space (Fig. 23.8). Rarely, all of the thenar musculature is innervated by the ulnar nerve. If present, this anomaly may confuse the physical examination.

Ulnar Nerve

The ulnar nerve provides sensibility to the volar surfaces of the ulnar half of the palm, the ulnar half of the ring finger, and to the entire volar surface of the small finger. The dorsal branch of the ulnar nerve arises 3–5 cm proximal to the wrist flexor crease and innervates the dorsal skin on the ulnar half of the hand and on the ring and small fingers. The motor portion of

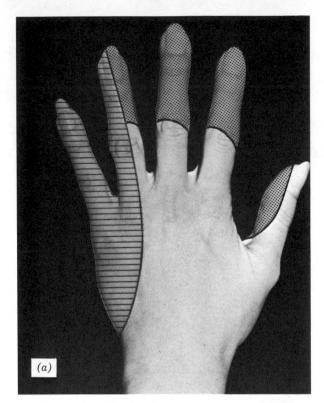
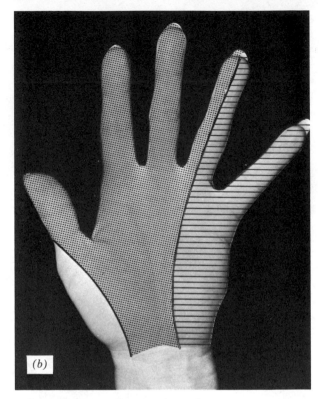

Figure 23.7 (a) The sensory innervation on the dorsum of the hand is a combination of contributions from radial, ulnar, and median nerves. (b) The sensory innervation on the volar aspect of the hand is divided between median and ulnar nerves.

the ulnar nerve innervates the hypothenar muscles, the dorsal and volar interossei, and the lumbricals of the ring and small fingers, half of the flexor pollicis brevis, and the adductor pollicis muscle. In the forearm, it innervates the profundi to the ring and small fingers and the flexor carpi ulnaris muscles.

Damage to the ulnar nerve may result in a "claw" deformity of the ring and small fingers, which is manifested by hyperextension of the MP joints and incomplete extension of the IP joints (Fig. 23.9). Weakness of abduction and adduction of the fingers (spreading and closing the fingers) and flexion of the IP joint of the thumb during pinch are also indicative of ulnar motor nerve damage (Fig. 23.10).

Radial Nerve

The sensory branch of the radial nerve provides sensibility to the radial aspect of the dorsum of the hand. Transection of branches of the sensory portion of this nerve may cause exquisitely sensitive subcutaneous neuromas and/or painful dy-

sesthesias. The radial nerve provides three major motor functions distal to the elbow: wrist extension, MP joint extension, and thumb extension and abduction.

Tests for radial nerve motor function should include active wrist extension, MP joint extension, and active firing of the extensor pollicis longus (demonstrated by palpation of the tendon rather than interphalangeal joint extension for the reason discussed previously). Do not assume that the ability to extend the PIP and DIP joints of the fingers implies an intact radial nerve since this function is shared with the median and ulnar nerves and remains present in the absence of radial nerve function.

EXAMINATION OF THE SKELETAL SYSTEM

Deformities, tenderness, and areas of soft tissue swelling signal skeletal injury. X-ray films confirm the diagnosis and provide information about the nature and location of the fracture or dislocation.

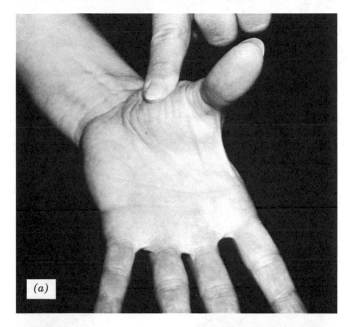

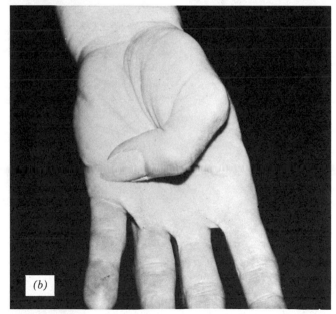

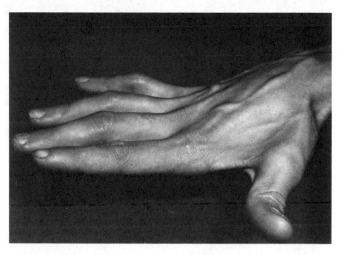

Figure 23.9 Claw deformity of the fingers with hyperextension of the MP joints and incomplete extension of the PIP joints.

Joint Examination

Injured joints will be swollen and tender. Localization of tenderness to the dorsal, volar, or lateral sides can aid diagnosis of the structures injured and can be facilitated by the use of a small blunt object (such as the eraser of a pencil) for palpation. Joints should be stressed gently in the anteroposterior (AP) and

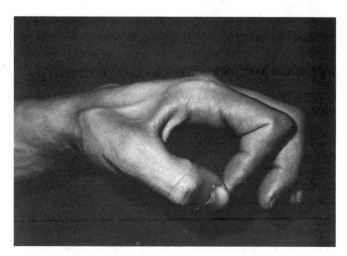

Figure 23.8 (a) The thenar musculature innervated by the median nerve is tested by asking the patient to point the thumb toward the ceiling with the dorsum of the hand resting on a flat surface. Active firing of the median nerve innervated thenar muscles can be palpated during this maneuver. (b) "False" test of the median nerve controlled thenar musculature. This motion can be accomplished using only the ulnar nerve innervated thenar muscles to flex the thumb.

Figure 23.10 Test of pinch strength demonstrating flexion deformity of the IP joint of the thumb (Froment's sign) as the result of weak ulnar nerve innervated intrinsic hand muscles following damage to the ulnar nerve. Note atrophy of the first dorsal interosseous muscle (see Fig. 23.26b).

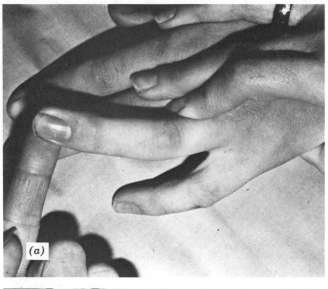

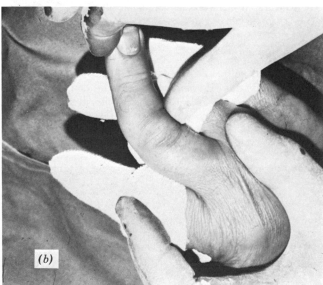

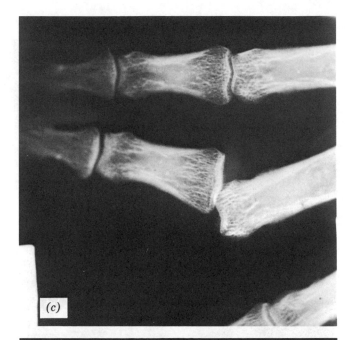

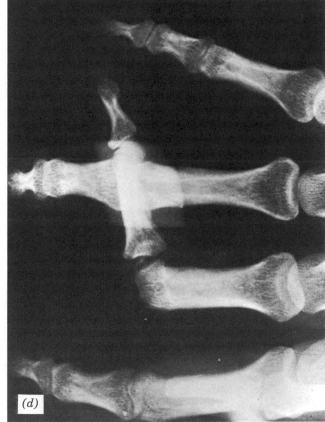

Figure 23.11 (a) Moderate instability of the PIP joint collateral liga-ment demonstrated by a stress test. (b) Gross instability of the PIP joint collateral ligament when stress tested. Stress roentgenograms show (c) partial and (d) complete collateral ligament instability.

lateral planes to detect gross instability. Occasionally, examination under local anesthesia is warranted. The most common joint injuries involve partial damage to the ligamentous supporting structures of the joint—the volar plate and collateral ligaments.

Collateral ligament injury occurs as the result of lateral stress. If the collateral ligament has been damaged, there will be tenderness over the involved structure on the side of the joint. If the ligament has been stretched severely or avulsed, some instability of the joint in the lateral plane may result. This can be detected by gentle stress testing as described above. The amount of instability should be compared to the same joint in an uninjured finger since people may normally be "loose jointed" or "tight jointed" (Fig. 23.11).

The volar plate supports the volar aspect of the joint. This fibrocartilaginous structure may be injured by hyperextension stress (catching a ball or falling with the fingers extended). Tenderness is most marked on the volar capsule of the joint, and the joint may be held flexed because of pain.

Complete dislocation of a joint is usually evident and most commonly is lateral or dorsal. Complete dislocations are most common at the IP joints of the fingers and at the MP joint of the thumb. Carpometacarpal joint dislocations occur but often are overlooked since they may present with minimal deformity and only slight or moderate swelling over the joints. These dislocations can be missed on routine film views, and oblique views may be required.

X-RAY EXAMINATION

X-ray examination should be obtained before attempts at reduction. A digit with compromised circulation is the exception to this. Posteroanterior (PA) and lateral views of the fingers and thumb should be obtained. Lateral views are facilitated by using the "fan" position of the hand with progressive flexion from the index to the small fingers or by placing cardboard cassettes between the fingers. Oblique views of the metacarpal bones are helpful (Fig. 23.12).

Although x-ray findings usually are straightforward, pitfalls are possible. Multiple views may be necessary to detect carpal injuries. Fractures of the carpal scaphoid may not appear on the initial films and may become apparent only after bone resorption at the fracture site has occurred. Epiphyseal lines must be recognized as such. Nutrient vessels penetrating the cortex are occasionally mistaken for hairline fractures. Avulsion or chip fractures are indications of complete ligament avulsion and alert the examiner to the need for careful evaluation of a specific joint. If there is a question regarding the significance of a radiograph, a comparison view of the uninjured part can be obtained. Communication with the techni-

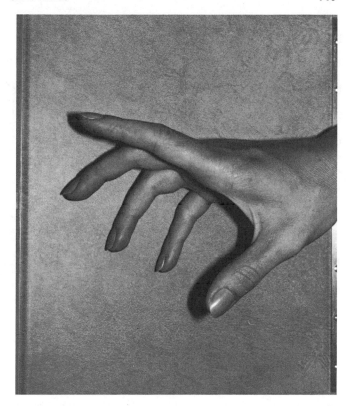

Figure 23.12 Hand placement on a film cassette for obtaining a "fan" lateral view of the hand.

cians and radiologist will enhance the information obtained from the radiographs.

MANAGEMENT

Massive Hand Injuries

Severe, mutilating injuries of the hand involving multiple fracture, skin or bone loss, and damage to neurovascular structures and tendons will require care by an experienced surgeon. In the emergency room, the wound should be cultured, dressed with a dry sterile dressing and roller bandage, and, if necessary, a plaster splint. The hand consultant and the operating room team are notified, and the patient is admitted to the hospital. An intravenous line should be started and a broad-spectrum antibiotic (such as a cephalosporin) begun. Tetanus antitoxin and/or toxoid should be given. If bleeding is profuse, blood should be typed and cross matched. X-ray films should be obtained, through the dressing if necessary. The appropriate laboratory studies required before general anesthesia should be obtained to minimize delay in transporting the patient from the emergency room to the operating room.

Uncomplicated Hand Injuries

OPEN WOUNDS

Commonly, the emergency room physician is the primary physician in the treatment of minor hand injuries. The care of superficial hand lacerations is similar to that of lacerations elsewhere on the body.

The wound should be cleansed of blood and foreign material as described earlier in this section (see section on skin examination). If an open or puncture wound of the hand has occurred, tetanus toxoid and/or human immune globulin should be administered according to the guidelines set forth in Chapter 13 after the status of the patient's tetanus immunization has been determined.

Skin Closure

The decision to close an open wound of the hand and the type of closure to be used depends on the extent and nature of the wound and the extent of damage to structures underlying the skin. If the wound is a sharp laceration without division of underlying structures or excessive skin damage or loss, primary closure can be performed in the emergency room. In most hand or finger lacerations, a single layer closure of the skin with 5-0 nylon is all that is required. Layered closures rarely are indicated. The use of vertical mattress sutures will prevent overlapping of the skin edges in the palm and the inversion of skin edges in loose dorsal skin. In children, the use of 5-0 or 6-0 plain gut suture for skin closure will obviate the need for suture removal after the wound has healed.

Hand wounds generally heal with minimal scarring, particularly if there is no tension on the wound. Wounds with the potential for retained foreign material, such as glass injuries, should be x-rayed, using soft tissue technique, before closure. Ragged lacerations have variable degrees of contamination, as well as damage to circulation in the skin. These will require careful debridement and closure, perhaps by combination of primary suture, skin graft, and local flap coverage. Slicing or avulsion wounds that result in flaps (especially distally based flaps) must be evaluated carefully for viability of the flap, rather than sutured primarily as a matter of course. Although the arterial blood supply of these flaps may be sufficient, venous drainage may not be, and flap necrosis can result. If significant crushing of tissue has occurred or if there is considerable soft tissue swelling without skin loss, the wound should be left open rather than closed under tension. In these cases, a bulky sterile dressing can be applied and secondary closure done in 5–7 days.

SPECIAL WOUNDS

There is very little extra skin in the hand. If the hand injury has resulted in skin loss, it is not advisable to bring the skin edges together under excessive tension. Skin loss can be treated either by allowing the wound to heal secondarily by granulation or by adding skin in the form of a graft or flap. Allowing the wound to granulate is acceptable only for small areas of skin loss (up to 5 mm in diameter) or for small wounds in children. Skin grafts can be either split or full thickness.

Skin Grafts

Split thickness grafts are indicated most commonly and are the simplest method to obtain closure of hand wounds. They may be used to provide a physiologic cover in severe wounds, even though revision or replacement with more suitable skin may be required later. Small grafts often can be applied by the emergency room physician. These grafts can be taken free hand with a sterile surgical blade or with a dermatome. Portable, battery-operated dermatomes are now commonly available in emergency rooms and allow even a neophyte to harvest a good graft. Larger grafts will require the expertise of a specialist.

The donor site of a split thickness skin graft leaves a scar that is noticeable and occasionally unsightly, particularly if the graft is thick. For this reason, the donor site must be chosen with care. The forearm, although convenient, should not be used since the scar in this area is often the source of patient discontent. Ideally, the donor site should be from an area covered by a bathing suit. Usually, the upper thigh or buttocks is suitable. The grafts may be sutured in place or held with Steri-Strips. A gentle pressure dressing and immobilization are essential since a hematoma under the graft will elevate the graft from its base and shear stress on the graft will disrupt capillary ingrowth.

Full thickness grafts are indicated less frequently in emergency situations. If there is any doubt about the ability of the full thickness graft to survive, it is preferable to apply a split thickness graft. If the area of skin loss uncovers bone or a joint, an alternative method of skin closure is required. Free grafts, split or full thickness, will not survive over joint surfaces, cortical bone, or bare nerve or tendon. Coverage by a flap will be necessary. This is best done by an experienced surgeon.

Tourniquet

The debridement and repair of hand injuries in a bloodless field is essential, whether done in the emergency room or in the operating room. The emergency room physician who treats hand injuries should be familiar with the use of a tourniquet and should not hesitate to use an appropriate tourniquet when indicated. If bleeding has stopped or is minimal, a tourniquet is not necessary. If bleeding is profuse, a tourniquet should be used. The use of a rubber band or Penrose drain applied to the base of the finger is dangerous. The pressure applied with these is uncontrolled, and damage to the delicate neurovascular structures at the base of the finger is possible. The use of a blood pressure cuff applied to the upper part of the arm also is risky. These instruments were not designed to maintain sustained pressures in the range of 250–300 mm Hg. Pressure usually is lost slowly, and the tourniquet changes from an arterial to a venous tourniquet. This not only allows arterial bleeding in the field, but also increases venous congestion and edema and is worse than no tourniquet at all. Only modern pneumatic tourniquets designed for use in the upper extremity should be used. The upper part of the arm is padded with two to three layers of circumferentially wrapped 4-in. cast padding, and the tourniquet is applied snugly around the arm. Tourniquet pressure should be maintained in the range of 250–300 mm Hg (depending upon arm size) in adults and 200 mm Hg in children. Before application of the tourniquet, blood is expressed from the hand and arm with an elastic rubber bandage. Most patients can tolerate 15–20 minutes of tourniquet pressure with minimal discomfort.

Nerve Injuries

Lacerations of digital nerves in the fingers are not uncommon, but they are frequently missed because of inadequate examination at the time the finger wound is closed in the emergency room. Prompt recognition will allow a considered decision regarding primary, delayed primary, or secondary repair of the nerve by the appropriate consultant. In addition, patient discontent will be avoided if the correct diagnosis is made at the time of the initial visit rather than days or weeks later.

Management

Nerve repair should not be attempted in the emergency room. Optimal results from digital nerve repair require fine suture material (8-0 to 10-0), magnification, and an experienced operating room team. As with flexor tendons, it may be advisable to close clean wounds with underlying nerve damage and refer the patient to an experienced surgeon for definitive care.

Damage to major nerves at the wrist level requires the same surgical techniques described for digital nerves. The care of mixed motor and sensory nerves (the median and ulnar nerves) is even more difficult because of the necessity of accurately aligning and matching major fascicular groups (motor to motor and sensory to sensory). This so-called grouped fascicular repair of mixed nerves requires high-power magnification.

Damage to the superficial radial nerve on the dorsal radial aspect of the wrist deserves special mention. This nerve supplies sensibility to the dorsal and radial aspect of the hand. Its integrity is not critical to the function of the hand. However, damage to this nerve or its terminal branches may result in either an exquisitely painful neuroma or a chronic pain syndrome (causalgia or reflex sympathetic dystrophy) that may either be limited or cause dysfunction of the entire upper extremity. For this reason, we recommend that acute laceration of this nerve be repaired primarily in an attempt to minimize both symptomatic neuromata and/or minor or major causalgia. Injuries on the dorsum of the hand and wrist require a high index of suspicion combined with routine sensory examination of the dorsal and radial aspect of the hand.

Tendon Injuries

CLOSED TENDON INJURIES

Closed injuries of the extensor mechanism are common and result in characteristic deformities that make the diagnosis straightforward. The common levels of injury are at the DIP and PIP joint levels.

Mallet Deformity

A mallet deformity results from avulsion of the terminal portion of the extensor tendon from the distal phalanx, either with or without a flake of bone. The patient is unable to extend the DIP joint actively. If x-ray reveals a large fragment of displaced bone and/or volar subluxation of the distal phalanx, the injury should be considered a fracture–dislocation and the patient should be referred for treatment. Most injuries, however, result in only a small avulsion fracture or a pure tendon avulsion. These can be treated by splinting the distal joint in full extension with a volar or dorsal metal splint (Fig. 23.13). It is not necessary to splint the PIP joint. However, these injuries require splinting for prolonged periods—8–10 weeks—and premature discontinuation of splinting may result in recurrence of the deformity. Even after the full course of treatment, splinting should not be discontinued abruptly but should be weaned

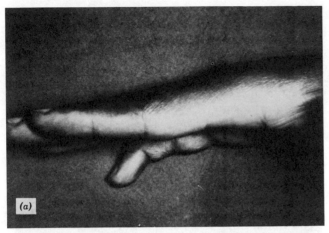

(a)

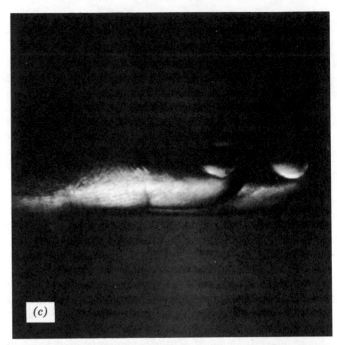

(c)

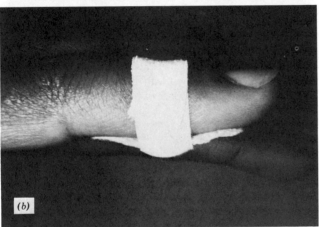

(b)

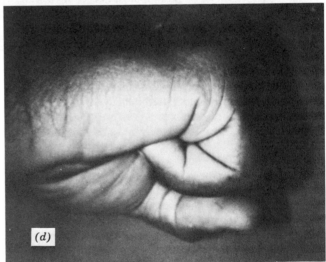

(d)

Figure 23.13 (a) Mallet deformity of the small finger with inability to extend the DIP joint. (b) Volar splint used to keep the DIP joint in extension. (c) Active extension of the DIP joint after 8 weeks of splinting. (d) Active flexion of the DIP joint after splint has been discontinued.

over a 2-week period. The patient will need to change the splint daily to prevent maceration of the dorsal skin and should be instructed to keep the DIP joint extended when doing this. Even when the patient is not seen for several weeks after the initial injury, these deformities sometimes can be improved by splinting. Treatment may be started by the emergency room physician, and the patient may be referred to the appropriate consultant for follow-up. Occasionally, a swan neck deformity of the fingers (hyperextension of the PIP joint combined with extensor lag of the DIP joint) may occur after mallet injuries secondary to extensor mechanism imbalance in people with lax volar plates. In open mallet injuries, the tendon may be repaired, as will be described later, but prolonged splinting is still necessary.

Boutonnière Deformity

A laceration or a closed injury of the "central slip" of the extensor mechanism overlying the PIP joint (Fig. 23.6) may result in a deformity of the finger characterized by flexion of the PIP joint and hyperextension of the DIP joint (the boutonnière). Recognition of this injury is important since inadequate initial treatment may lead to progressive deformities that are very difficult to treat secondarily. Again, a high index of suspicion may be necessary with injuries on the dorsal aspect of the PIP joint since the deformity may be very subtle or even absent initially but progresses as the PIP joint is flexed repeatedly. Closed injuries should be splinted with the PIP in full extension and the DIP joint left free (Fig. 23.14). Active flexion of the distal joint will preserve balance between the central slip and the lateral band portions of the extensor mechanism. Splinting of the PIP joint in full extension is continued for at least 4 weeks, after which active, but protected, flexion is started. The patient should be referred for follow-up observation and care.

Closed Flexor Tendon Injuries

Rupture of the flexor digitorum profundus in young athletes has been described previously (see section on examination of tendons). Early recognition of these injuries allows recovery and repair of the avulsed tendon. Delayed recognition, even for several days, often precludes definitive repair because of retraction and scarring of the tendon. The complaint of inability to flex the distal joint actively and an appropriate clinical history should be heeded.

OPEN TENDON INJURIES

Open tendon injuries may occur with apparently superficial skin wounds as well as with extensive open injuries to the hand. Therefore, careful examination of tendon function of every patient who has an open wound in the hand and/or fingers should be undertaken.

Extensor Tendons

Laceration of the extensor tendons may occur either proximal or distal to the juncturae tendinae—the cross connections be-

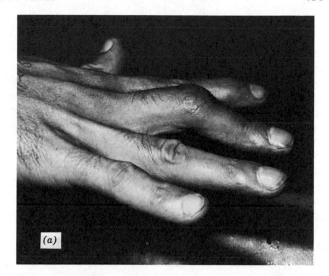

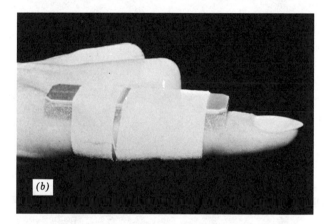

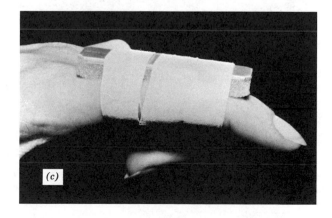

Figure 23.14   (a) Boutonnière deformity (flexion deformity of the PIP joint and hyperextension of the DIP joint) as a result of damage to the extensor mechanism overlying the PIP joint. (b) Method of splinting closed injuries of the extensor mechanism that have resulted in a boutonnière deformity. The PIP joint is held in full extension. (c) The splint should allow flexion of the DIP joint. This motion is encouraged to prevent adherence of the extensor mechanism.

tween the extensor digitorum communis tendons at the level of the necks of the metacarpal bones (Fig. 23.15). Lacerations proximal to these interconnections will allow the tendon to retract and preclude repair in the emergency room since extensive exposure may be necessary to retrieve the tendon. However, if a laceration of the extensor tendon has occurred distal to the interconnections, the tendon will not retract and repair can be carried out primarily by the emergency room physician. The ends of the tendon should be approximated with either one or more simple interrupted sutures or with a horizontal mattress suture using nonabsorbable material such as 4-0 nylon. The affected joint is splinted in extension. The type of suture material used is not important as long as it is *not silk*. Recently, 4-0 Dexon or Vicryl have been used with satisfactory results. Postrepair immobilization *is* important to prevent the repair from pulling apart if the finger flexes.

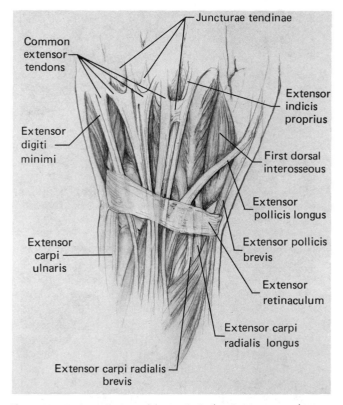

Figure 23.15 Arrangement of the extrinsic (long) extensor tendons on the dorsum of the hand. Note the junctura that interconnect the extensor tendons just proximal to the MP joints.

Flexor Tendons

Since there are two flexor tendons in each finger (Fig. 23.2), the problems of treating flexor tendon injuries differ completely from those of treating extensor tendon injuries. From the distal palm to the midportion of the middle phalanx, these tendons are surrounded by the so-called fibroosseous tunnel, which is a tight tunnel composed of bone and volar plate tissue on one side and the flexor tendon sheath with its pulley mechanism on the other side. Surgery within this delicate area is difficult, and even skilled surgeons may find that the results of tendon repair may be compromised because of adhesions, joint stiffness and limited active motion. Although flexor tendon lacerations distal and proximal to the fibroosseous tunnel are easier to repair and the prognosis for good postoperative tendon function is better, all tendon surgery on the flexor aspect of the hand should be performed in a completely equipped operating room by a surgeon experienced in flexor tendon surgery. If in doubt, it is wiser to close the skin of a tidy wound and refer the patient rather than to attempt primary repair under suboptimal conditions.

Fractures

Because bones of the hand are small, the consequences of injury to them often is minimized. However, improper treatment of finger and hand fractures can result in prolonged morbidity, and frequently the resulting malunion and stiffness is amenable only to surgical treatment.

Precise rotatory alignment of phalangeal and metacarpal fractures is necessary to prevent overlap of the fingers during flexion (Fig. 23.16). Even a small residual rotatory displacement can interfere significantly with hand function. Fractures that appear stable and nondisplaced on x-ray and even on cursory clinical examination may have significant rotatory displacement.

Rotary alignment is tested by flexing the finger into the palm and noting proper alignment of each finger with the next. Although fingernail alignment and/or alignment of the fingers with the pulps pointing toward the carpal scaphoid bone are useful guides, the final check can be done only with the fingers in nearly full flexion. Angular deformity is easier to detect, both clinically and by radiograph.

Fracture healing may result in adherence of the tendon to the bone because of the proximity of the extensor and flexor tendons of the fingers to the phalanges. This will limit tendon excursion and thus finger motion. Prolonged immobilization compounds the problems of tendon adherence and may cause joint stiffness as well. Therefore early motion is necessary when

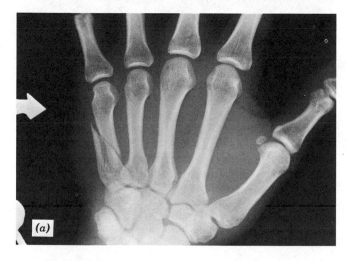

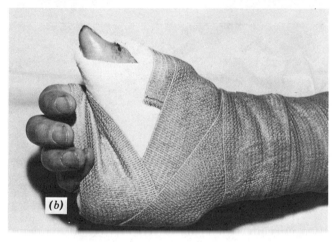

Figure 23.16 (a) Spiral fracture through the midshaft of the fifth metacarpal bone with rotatory malalignment. (b) Overlap of the small and ring fingers during flexion as the result of rotatory malalignment.

dealing with patients who have finger and hand fractures. The adage of 6 weeks of immobilization for a fracture does not apply in the hand; its use will complicate and prolong rehabilitation of the hand. Follow-up care for patients with even simple fractures is necessary to obtain satisfactory functional recovery.

The treatment of fractures of the small bones of the hand is simplified by classifying them as stable, unstable, and intraarticular.

STABLE FRACTURES

Stable fractures usually involve linear "cracks" of the shaft of a phalanx or metacarpal or fractures of the distal phalanx after a crush injury. They are stable either because there is not tendon pull across the fracture site to displace the fracture or because the periosteum and soft tissue surrounding the fracture are intact and are sufficient to counteract any forces tending to displace the fracture. They do not require reduction. *Any fracture that is displaced enough to require reduction should be considered unstable and treated as described in the following section.*

Stable fractures cause no deformity of the hand other than soft tissue swelling. Films of these fractures show minimal, if any, displacement. The treatment of these fractures consists of a brief period of immobilization until the acute pain and swelling subside, followed by early active motion of the adjacent joints. These fractures are "clinically" united before the x-ray film demonstrates complete bone healing. Complications of this group of fractures are most often the result of prolonged immobilization. Molded plaster or metal splints are used, and as little of the hand as possible is immobilized. The metacarpophalangeal joints should be splinted in flexion to keep collateral ligaments at their maximum length and thereby prevent extension contractures. The fingers should *not* be immobilized with the interphalangeal joints in full extension. Thus the use of straight splints such as tongue blades is precluded. Cotton or a gauze sponge is placed between adjacent fingers that are splinted together to prevent skin maceration. Follow-up films within the first week are mandatory to ensure that no change in alignment has occurred. Immobilization for 10–21 days is necessary before the splint is removed and an exercise program to regain motion is started. Full use of the hand should be restricted for a total of 4–6 weeks.

Crush fractures of the distal phalanx are common. However, these fractures are stable and are treated as soft tissue injuries rather than as fractures. Reduction is not required, and a protective splint with immobilization of the DIP joint for 2–3 weeks is all that is necessary. The frequent subungual hematoma that occurs after this injury should be treated as described later to provide relief from pain.

UNSTABLE FRACTURES

Unstable fractures require immobilization to prevent displacement or maintain reduction. Closed reduction under adequate anesthesia should be attempted. However, if satisfactory position of the fracture cannot be obtained or if position is lost either immediately or within the first week, open reduction

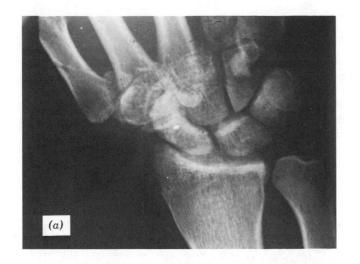

(a)

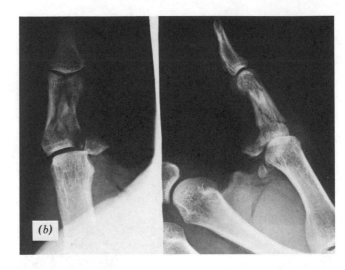

(b)

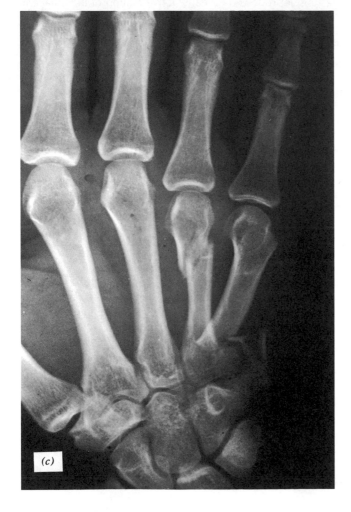

(c)

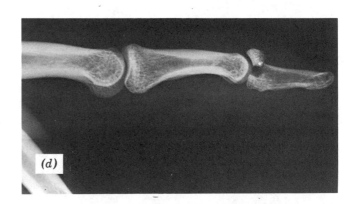

(d)

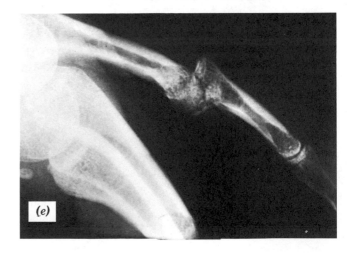

(e)

with internal fixation may be indicated. The stability achieved by open reduction and internal fixation will allow earlier motion and reduce the risk of tendon adherence and joint stiffness. If any question remains after initial care of a hand fracture, the patient should be referred for appropriate consultation and follow-up. Traction in the treatment of hand fractures is mentioned only to condemn its use.

Common unstable fractures include displaced and angulated fractures of the shafts of the metacarpals and of the proximal and middle phalanges, supracondylar fractures through the neck of the middle phalanx, fracture–dislocations of the PIP joint, and fracture dislocations of the thumb carpometacarpal joint (Bennett's fracture) or of the carpometacarpal joint of the small finger ("baby" Bennett's fracture) (Fig. 23.17).

INTRAARTICULAR FRACTURES

Intraarticular fractures are difficult to treat and require experienced judgment for decisions regarding operative versus nonoperative treatment. Several fracture–dislocations usually require percutaneous wire fixation or open reduction and internal fixation. Bennett's fractures (fracture–dislocation of the base of the thumb metacarpal), "baby" Bennett's fractures (fracture–dislocation of the base of the fifth metacarpal), and those mallet fingers that are the result of the avulsion of a significant portion of the dorsal articular surface of the distal phalanx and/or result in volar subluxation of the DIP joint fall into this category, and those patients should be referred.

OPEN FRACTURES

Open fractures, which are those fractures that communicate with an external skin wound, require surgical debridement, and patients should be referred to the appropriate consultant whether the fractures are stable, unstable, or intraarticular.

Figure 23.17 Examples of unstable fractures of the hand. (a) Fracture–dislocation of the carpometacarpal joint of the thumb (Bennett's fracture). (b) Intraarticular fracture of the metacarpal joint of the thumb. (c) Fracture–dislocation of the carpometacarpal joint of the small finger ("baby" Bennett's fracture). (d) Mallet fracture avulsion of the insertion of the extensor tendon from the distal phalanx with a displaced intraarticular fracture of the dorsal lip of the distal phalanx. (e) Fracture–dislocation of the PIP joint.

Minimally displaced fractures of the neck of the fifth metacarpal associated with either tooth marks or a cut on the dorsal skin overlying the bone should be considered and treated as a human bite (see section on human bites).

Carpal Injuries

The carpus consists of eight small bones arranged in two horizontal rows and linked to one another by their contours and a complex set of dorsal, volar, and interosseous ligaments. Carpal bones bear tremendous stress during both direct and indirect trauma and thus are easily injured. The nature of the injury, the bone involved, and bony versus ligamentous injury depends on many factors including the age of the patient and the position of the wrist and forearm at the time of the injury. Most carpal injuries occur after a fall on the outstretched hand or a twisting injury, for example, when a tightly gripped steering wheel is suddenly twisted as the vehicle's wheels strike an obstruction or pot hole or when the torque of a power drill motor rotates the hand and wrist when the bit binds. High-energy injuries such as falls from ladders and other heights as well as motorcycle injuries cause more significant fractures, ligamentous injuries, or fracture–dislocations of the wrist.

Carpal injuries may appear trivial initially if they present with minimal swelling and deformity, moderate pain, and subtle changes on routine x-ray examination. Therefore, a high index of suspicion is necessary so that carpal injuries may be detected and treated at the onset—rather than when the sequelae of these injuries (nonunions, collapse deformities, and posttraumatic arthritis) have occurred.

Carpal scaphoid bone fractures are the most common carpal fractures and typically occur in young men (14–40 years of age) after a fall on the outstretched hand. Clinically, these patients present with tenderness to palpation in the "anatomical snuff box" (the triangular hollow area at the base of the thumb outlined by the outcropping tendons of the thumb) (Fig. 23.18). The waist of the scaphoid bone lies directly beneath this area and thus can be palpated through the overlying soft tissue. Films may or may not show a fracture line through the bone. As described previously, if the fracture remains undisplaced, the fracture line may not be detected for 2–4 weeks until bony resorption on either side of the fracture has occurred. For this reason, a wrist with a scaphoid fracture suspected by clinical examination but not confirmed by films should be immobilized and the patient referred for follow-up evaluation. Failure to do so may increase the already significant tendency of the scaphoid bone not to heal.

Even if a scaphoid fracture is not present, other serious ligamentous injuries with subtle clinical and x-ray findings may

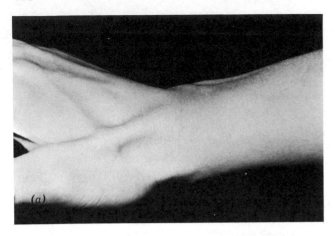

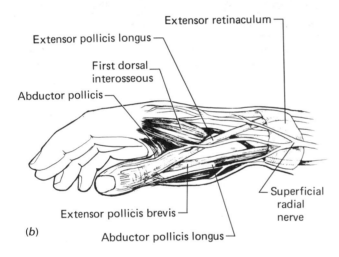

Extensor retinaculum

Extensor pollicis longus

First dorsal interosseous

Abductor pollicis

Superficial radial nerve

Extensor pollicis brevis

(b)

Abductor pollicis longus

Figure 23.18 (a) The radial aspect of the hand showing the extensor pollicis longus and brevis tendons, the abductor pollicis longus tendons, and the "anatomical snuffbox". (b) Drawing of the anatomy of the tendons described, as well as the location of the superficial branch of the radial nerve and its divisions. The extensor tendon compartments are numbered.

be present. These include rotatory subluxation of the scaphoid bone, which produces a decrease in the normal height of the scaphoid bone and a gap greater than 2 mm between the scaphoid and lunate bones on the PA film; injuries of the ligaments stabilizing the lunate, triquetrum, and hamate bones;

and damage to the triangular fibrocartilage, the junction of the distal ulna, and the carpus. Carpal avulsion fractures represent ligamentous injuries that may or may not be significant (Fig. 23.19). Therefore, any wrist injury about which the emergency room physician is not entirely sure should be splinted and reevaluated in several days or the patient should be referred to the appropriate specialist for evaluation.

Dislocations and fracture dislocations of the wrist require immediate care. The emergency room physician should suspect these injuries on the basis of the history alone, for example, a fall from a height or a motorcycle injury. Films of the wrist with these injuries may be difficult to interpret or may show subtle findings, but in any case they will not look normal when compared to that of an uninjured wrist. A lunate dislocation may be accompanied by paresthesias and numbness in the median nerve distribution since the volarly dislocated bone impinges the median nerve within the carpal tunnel. Lateral roentgenograms will show the dislocation clearly. Lateral films usually are the most important views of the wrist and the emergency room x-ray examination is not complete without them.

Joint Injuries

COLLATERAL LIGAMENTS

Collateral ligament injuries result from forceful lateral stress applied to the extended digit. The radial aspect of the PIP joint is injured more frequently than the ulnar side. In the thumb, the ulnar collateral ligament is at risk and is injured more frequently than the radial side ligament, resulting in the so-called "gamekeeper's thumb." The thumb MP joint should be tested for stability in both flexion and extension (Fig. 23.20). If there is more than 45 deg of instability in flexion, operative repair of the ligament is indicated. Acute repair of these ligaments is much more satisfactory than secondary reconstruction.

X-ray examination is important and will confirm suspected ligament injuries with small avulsion fractures. Both AP and lateral stress should be applied gently to the injured joint. A complete tear will allow the joint to open easily. Pain during this maneuver is suggestive of a stretched ligament, and digital block anesthesia may be required to determine the degree of joint laxity. Joint laxity varies from person to person, and the degree of laxity found in the injured digit should be compared to that in a noninjured digit. Stress films of both the injured and the noninjured joint may be helpful. If the joint is stable to lateral stress or opens only minimally, the injury is, at most,

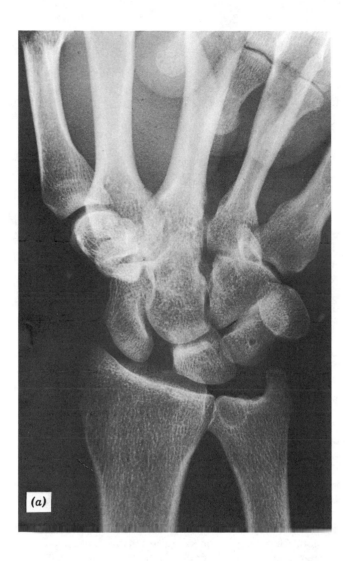

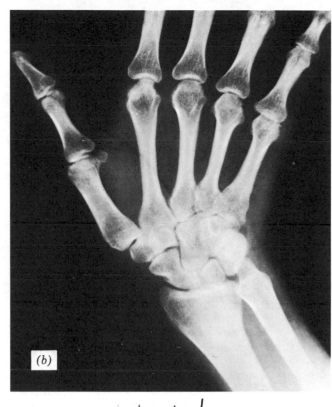

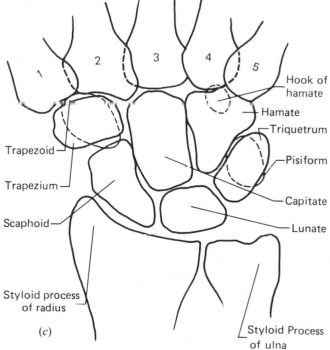

Figure 23.19 (a) PA roentgenogram of the wrist showing a wide gap between the scaphoid and lunate bones indicating severe ligamentous damage and scapholunate dissociation. (b) PA roentgenogram of the normal wrist. (c) Nomenclature and positions of carpal bones.

459

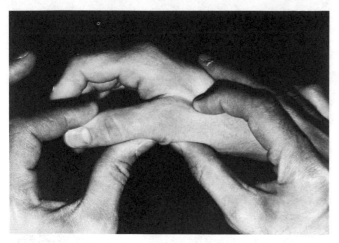

Figure 23.20 Method of testing the stability of the ulnar side collateral ligament of the thumb metacarpophalangeal joint. Comparison of laxity on the injured and noninjured sides should be made.

a partial tear and nonoperative treatment is indicated (Fig. 23.11).

The finger with an incomplete collateral ligament injury can be immobilized with a padded volar aluminum splint positioned in slight flexion for 10 days. Gentle, gradual joint motion is begun after this period, although the joint can be protected from lateral stress by "buddy" tapping the finger to the adjacent digit for an additional 10 days. Full function is not regained for 4–6 weeks, and some residual enlargement of the joint may persist permanently. If the joint is unstable to lateral stress, a complete tear is present and surgical treatment is required. Nonoperative treatment of complete collateral ligament tears often is followed by permanent joint laxity, instability, and chronic synovitis. The late sequelae of these injuries can be degenerative arthritis and stiffness. If there is any question of significant joint injury, the joint should be splinted and the patient referred.

DISLOCATIONS

Dislocations of a joint represent the end stage in soft tissue injury. They usually are either dorsal or lateral, and damage to the volar plate and collateral ligaments is assumed. Dislocations can be classified as either simple or complex. *Simple dislocations* can be reduced by closed methods, whereas *complex dislocations* have interposed soft tissue structures that prevent reduction except by open methods. Dislocations in the fingers occur most often at the IP joints. Dislocations of the thumb usually occur at the MP joint. Dislocations of the MP

joints of the fingers can occur, but are rare. Carpometacarpal joint dislocations can occur but are often overlooked because of the subtle clinical findings. These are most common at the fourth and fifth carpometacarpal joints.

PIP Joint Dislocations

Interphalangeal joint dislocation, when seen early (before swelling and muscle spasm occur) can usualy be reduced by gentle traction and manipulation. When traction is applied, the deformity is increased slightly to release trapped soft tissues. The joint is then flexed to accomplish the reduction. Occasionally, these can be reduced without anesthesia, although a digital block is preferable. Multiple attempts to reduce the joint should be avoided, and brute strength should not be used. The emergency room physician should attempt a closed reduction once. A dislocation that cannot be reduced closed will require open reduction. If reduction is accomplished in the emergency room, the joint should be stress tested and carried through a complete range of motion. Joint laxity or incomplete motion signal a more serious injury. Stable PIP dislocations are immobilized in slight flexion for 14 days, after which gentle motion is started. As with other ligament injuries, full function will not be regained for 4–6 weeks.

The *DIP joint dislocations* are frequently unstable after reduction, and the joint may sublux if the reduction is not maintained with a small Kirschner wire for several weeks. Patients with joints that are unstable after reduction should be referred to the appropriate specialist. Open joint dislocations are less frequent, but when they occur they require immediate surgical care.

Metacarpophalangeal joint dislocations usually reduce easily, but occasionally they are complex and require open reduction. Closed reduction of these joints is performed in a manner similar to that described for the MP joint of the thumb. Persistent volar dislocations of the MP joints of the fingers can cause pressure on the digital nerves resulting in a neuropraxia.

Metacarpophalangeal joint dislocation of the thumb is a relatively common injury resulting from a hyperextension force that tears the volar plate and allows the metacarpal head to herniate through the capsule. These often are complex dislocations and cannot be reduced by closed methods. One attempt to reduce this dislocation closed is justified. If this fails, the patient should be referred for open reduction.

Dislocations of the carpometacarpal (CM) joint of the thumb without fracture can occur—usually with hyperextension stress. If treated early by closed reduction and immobilization in abduction, healing can occur with satisfactory stability. Occasionally there is disruption of the deep ulnar ligament of the carpometacarpal joint. In these cases, chronic laxity with subluxation of the CM joint can result and ligament reconstruction is required.

Dislocations of the carpometacarpal joints of the fingers are usually the result of significant trauma. Recognition of this injury is important since soft tissue swelling may obscure the deformity. X-ray findings tend to be overlooked, but careful review of the PA films show a loss of normal joint space and a lateral or oblique view will show the dorsally displaced metacarpal. Localized tenderness over the CM joints is the clue to injury, and comparison films may be very helpful. These dislocations are deceptive in that they are easily reduced (when treated early) but are very difficult to maintain in the reduced position. Patients with these injuries should be referred for temporary Kirschner wire fixation.

Volar Plate Injuries

A hyperextension stress applied to the joint of a digit can damage the volar plate. A complete dorsal dislocation usually results in a tear of the volar plate. However, tears can occur without joint dislocation. These are more difficult to diagnose. A tiny avulsion fracture on the volar aspect of the joint seen in the lateral view may be present. In most volar plate injuries, the stability of the joint is maintained. The joint should be splinted in slight flexion while the plate heals. Healing with some laxity of the ligament is desirable so that a fixed flexion contracture does not occur. On the other hand, complete instability or marked laxity of the volar plate may result in hyperextension of the joint and/or a swan-neck deformity.

Nail Injuries

The fingernail provides support for the volar skin and pulp of the finger and is important during pinch and other fine hand functions. Injuries to the nail are often overlooked, either because the damage is considered to be minimal or because of other associated and more serious appearing injuries of the hand. However, damage to the nail bed may permanently affect nail growth and result in deformity of the nail plate and/or fingertip.

NAIL PLATE AVULSION

Partial avulsion of the nail plate without damage to the underlying bed should be treated by trimming and replacing the nail into its normal position. It may be held in place with a dressing. The damaged nail will gradually be replaced by a new nail. In complete nail avulsions, the nail should not be replaced, but the bed should be protected from a nonadherent dressing (petrolatum, Xeroform, etc.). A firm membrane will

form over the nail bed in a 1–2 weeks. When this has occurred, the nonadherent dressing can be removed. The skin fold (eponychial fold) surrounding the nail margin must be preserved if the nail is completely avulsed. This is done by packing petrolatum or other nonadherent gauze between the skin fold and the bed. The raw nail bed is quite sensitive and anesthesia by digital block may be necessary to perform this procedure. Failure to preserve this space may result in a deformed nail. Patients who have lost a nail plate should be told that new nail growth occurs very slowly and that 4–5 months is required before a completely new nail is present.

NAIL BED INJURY

Lacerations of the nail bed should be repaired carefully and accurately, using closely spaced 6-0 or 7-0 absorbable sutures after the damaged nail plate is removed (Fig. 23.21). Loss of nail bed tissue should be covered by a split thickness skin graft. These procedures will prevent or minimize subsequent nail plate deformities.

Injury loss of the germinal matrix or nail root will result in complete or partial arrest of nail plate gowth. Because the amount of damage to this germinal tissue cannot be determined clinically, the patient should be advised of this possibility. Reconstructive procedures may be required in the future if the amount of nail deformity is unacceptable either functionally or cosmetically.

SUBUNGUAL HEMATOMA

Subungual hematomas occur after blunt trauma and crush injuries, either with or without fractures of the distal phalanx. These are painful and should be drained to provide relief. A hole in the central portion of the nail plate can best be made using a No. 18-gauge needle. This can be drilled through the nail plate without the need for excessive (and painful) pressure on the nail. Some emergency rooms have a battery-operated instrument that provides an electrically heated filament that will burn a hole in the nail quickly and painlessly (Fig. 23.22).

SUBUNGUAL SPLINTER

Subungual splinters are also painful. The splinter should be removed using a splinter forcep or fine straight hemostat or a No. 20 needle or No. 11 scalpel blade under digital block anesthesia. Attempts to remove the splinter without anesthesia will not be tolerated by the patient. Occasionally a small portion of the nail may have to be removed so that the splinter can be retrieved.

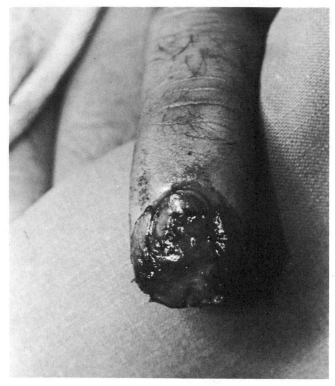

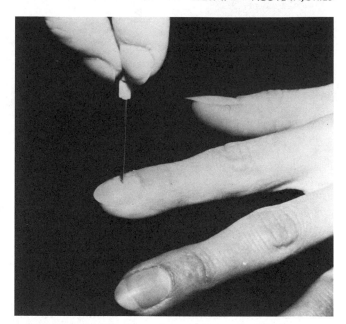

Figure 23.22 Subungual hematoma decompressed by drilling through the nail plate with a No. 18 needle. The point of a No. 11 scalpel blade also can be used.

Figure 23.21 Laceration of the nail bed repaired with fine absorbable sutures (5-0 or 6-0 gut). The eponychial fold is packed open with petrolatum impregnated gauze and a nonadhering dressing is applied to the nail bed.

Fingertip Injuries

Fingertip injuries with pulp damage or loss occur frequently. Small areas of skin or pulp loss (particularly in children) can be cleansed, dressed, and allowed to granulate. Larger areas of pulp loss or partial amputation of the tip will require coverage by skin grafts or local flaps. In these cases, exposed bone should be trimmed with a rongeur. Flap procedures are best done in the operating room by surgeons familiar with these techniques. However, most fingertip amputations can be debrided and covered with a split thickness skin graft in the emergency room. Reconstruction can be done secondarily, if necessary. Many such injuries covered by split thickness skin grafts result in functional digits because of the tendency for the graft bed to shrink and draw normal pulp skin in from the edges of the wound (Fig. 23.23). Bone directly under a split thickness skin graft or large areas of insensate skin will not be functional and will require revision.

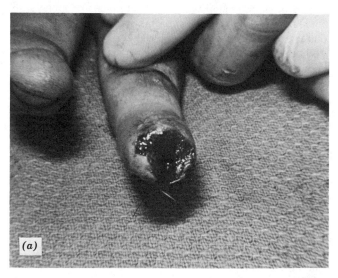

(a)

Figure 23.23 (a) Finger-tip injury with loss of soft tissue from the distal portion of the pulp. (b) Split thickness skin graft from the lateral thigh applied to the area of tissue loss and sutured in place. (c) Stent dressing tied over graft for compression. (d) After healing, there has been contraction of the bed to which the graft was applied resulting in satisfactory appearance and function of the distal pulp without the need for revision. (e) Normal nail plate growth and appearance after healing.

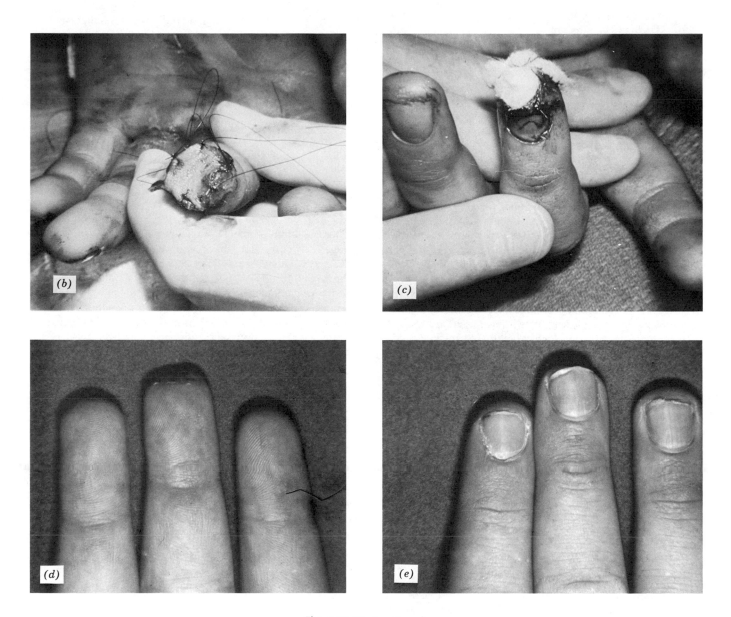

Figure 23.23 (continued)

Amputations

Partial or complete amputations of the hand or digits must be evaluated in the light of recent advances in microsurgical techniques and the possibility of revascularization or replantation of the injured parts. Massively traumatized, crushed, or severely contaminated injuries usually are not suitable for these procedures. Cleanly amputated parts or those with mild crushing may be preserved and transported with the patient for evaluation by a microsurgical team, even though relatively long periods of time may elapse between the initial injury and the definitive surgery.

Parts considered appropriate for replantation should be transported as follows: After arrangements have been made with the nearest replantation team, the part should be washed carefully with normal saline, wrapped in a sterile dressing moistened with normal saline, placed into a plastic bag, and then placed into an ice chest filled with regular ice. Freezing of the tissue must be avoided; thus direct contact of the part with ice or the use of dry ice is precluded (Fig. 23.24).

Amputations that are not suitable for replantation or partial amputations that are not suitable for revascularization should be closed in the operating room under controlled conditions. Occasionally, the cleanly amputated finger may be closed in the emergency room using local skin or split thickness skin grafts. The patient should be referred for follow-up care or revision, if necessary.

Burns

The depth and extent of a burn wound determines what treatment is necessary. The extent of the burn is determined by the nature of the injury; a flash or flame burn will involve more of the hand than a burn produced by contact with a hot object. The depth of a burn often is difficult to ascertain and may vary within the same wound. Burn wounds can be classified as partial or total thickness. In a *partial thickness burn* (first or second degree), some dermal elements remain viable and reepitheliazation is possible if the wound is kept clean and sterile. In these injuries, the skin appears erythematous but blanches with pressure. Sensibility is present and the wound is painful. Blisters or raw weeping surfaces may be present. In a *total thickness burn* (third degree), there is destruction of all dermal elements, and wound debridement and skin replacement are necessary. Areas of total burn appear blanched, grey, or charred. Sensibility over the wound is absent, and the wound is painless. The skin on the dorsal surface of the hand is thin, and total thickness burns with damage to the underlying extensor tendons are common. In contrast, the palmar skin is thicker and more often burn injuries in this area are only partial.

Small areas of burn with partial skin loss can be treated in the emergency room with a topical dressing such as silver sulfadiazine (Silvadene) or mafenide acetate (Sulfamylon), a sterile dressing, elevation, and careful follow-up. Debridement and skin grafting may be required during the recovery period. Burn blisters should be opened and debrided under sterile conditions to prevent secondary bacterial contamination.

A small contact burn with total skin damage but without damage to underlying structures can often be excised and closed primarily in the emergency room. However, if any questions of the extent of damage remains or if extensive damage is present, the patient should be referred to a specialist. Hospitalization under these circumstances is advisable to minimize hand dysfunction as a result of tissue loss or scar formation.

CHEMICAL BURNS

Chemical burns (contact with acid or alkali agents) are treated initially by copious irrigation with water to dilute and remove the agent. Dilute neutralizing agents can be used (with care) for irrigation; dilute acetic acid is used for alkali burns and sodium bicarbonate solution is used for acid burns. Alkali burns require copious and prolonged irrigation since these chemical agents are difficult to remove from the skin. Hydrofluoric acid burns are very serious and must be neutralized by injecting the wound area with 10% calcium gluconate. If there is any question that hydrofluoric acid was the agent involved, the place of work should be contacted and detailed information should be obtained from a knowledgeable source.

ELECTRICAL BURNS

Although high-voltage electrical burns may cause only a small area of superficial tissue damage, extensive deep tissue damage may be present. For this reason, the injury may be far worse than it appears initially. Vascular damage may be widespread, resulting in thrombosis, ischemia, and ultimately tissue death. Because the extent of high-voltage electrical burns will only become apparent after several days, patients with these injuries should be hospitalized and observed. Low-voltage burns to small areas are not as serious and may be cared for as thermal burns.

Frostbite

Prolonged cold exposure in temperatures below freezing will cause ice crystal formation in dermal cells. Fingers are particularly prone to this injury. The resultant cell damage or death turns the affected skin white or grayish. The initial treatment for the frostbitten part is rapid rewarming to body temperature

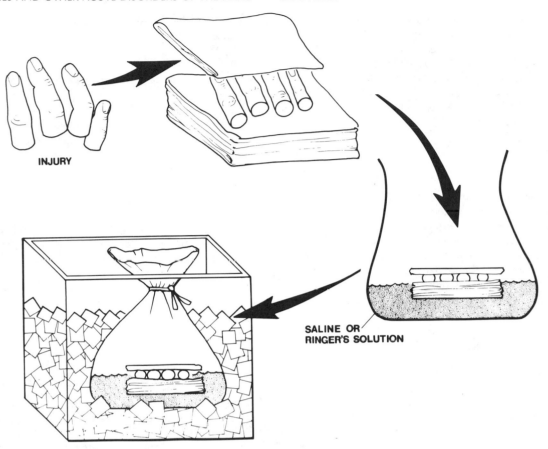

Figure 23.24 Amputated fingers to be transported for possible replantation are placed between stacks of sterile 4-by-4 inch gauze and immersed in a plastic bag filled with sterile saline or Ringer's solution. The bag is placed in a container filled with ice. (Used with permission from Daniel RK, Terris JK: *Reconstructive Microsurgery*. Boston, Little Brown and Company, 1977, p. 130.)

by immersion in water heated to 42°C (107.6°F). Debridement should not be done until the affected areas are allowed to demarcate. In contrast to high-voltage electrical injuries, the damage often is more superficial than the initial appearance indicates. Patients with minor areas of frostbite should be referred for follow-up care after rewarming and application of a sterile bulky dressing. Patients with major frostbite injuries should be hospitalized.

The fingers of children are at risk from subclinical damage to the epiphyses from cold exposure. Although no clinical signs or symptoms may be present initially, the subsequent growth impairment of the fingers becomes manifest near the end of the growth spurt at puberty. Parent education about the danger of prolonged unprotected cold exposure will minimize these injuries.

Bites

ANIMAL BITES

Animal bites on the hand are particularly dangerous because of the potential for deep closed space infections, joint infections, and tendon sheath infections. After aerobic and anaerobic cultures are obtained (if possible), these wounds should be washed thoroughly with soap and water or hydrogen peroxide. Ragged skin edges should be debrided. Primary closure usually is not indicated. The wound should be dressed and treated open. Antibiotics should be given prophylactically. Penicillin is the drug of choice because of its efficiency against *Paturella multocida,* a common infection-producing bacteria found in the mouths of dogs and cats. Follow-up care is advised so that infections of the bone, joints, or tendon sheaths can be detected early.

HUMAN BITES

Human bites may occur either as the result of altercations or, occasionally, during the emergency care of patients having seizures, dental procedures, cardiac arrest, and so forth. Most commonly, the "bite" is an open wound over the dorsal aspect of the fingers or hand from a tooth as a clenched fist strikes an opponent. Because of the virulent nature of the flora in the human mouth, these wounds must be treated as potentially serious infections. The wounds should be washed, debrided if necessary, and dressed open. Broad-spectrum antibiotics such as penicillin, ampicillin, cephalosporin, or lincomycin should be started after the wound is cultured. The patient should be made aware of the serious nature of the injury and the necessity for frequent follow-up examination. Unreliable patients should be hospitalized for observation. Established infections from human bites are limb threatening and will require hospitalization, intravenous antibiotics, and surgical drainage and debridement.

Injection Injuries

Small puncture wounds on the tips of the fingers caused by high-pressure grease guns, paint spray guns, or broken hydraulic lines may initially appear innocuous to both the patient and the emergency room physican. However, the fluids carried by these devices are injected deep into the tissues under very high pressure and are forced along the tissue planes of least resistance, sometimes all the way from the fingertip into the forearm. These fluids cause an extensive chemical inflammatory reaction with subsequent tissue necrosis. Hydraulic fluid is hot and will cause thermal as well as chemical damage. Several hours after the injury, the injured finger and hand will begin to swell and become severely painful.

Patients with these injuries will require emergency surgical exploration, decompression, and debridement of the involved finger and hand far beyond the point of penetration. Failure to do this may result in such extensive tissue necrosis that amputation may be required.

Infections of the Hand

ACUTE PARONYCHIA

Acute paronychia is an infection of the skin fold surrounding the nail plate. It is manifest by reddened and swollen tissue adjacent to the nail on the dorsal aspect of the finger. Early cases can be treated by oral antibiotics and soaks. If the infection is established or if the treatment described above fails, surgical drainage is necessary. This is accomplished by passing a scapel blade between the skin fold and the nail plate at the point of maximum swelling or erythema (Fig. 23.25). Occasionally a portion of the nail plate must be removed to drain the infection adequately. This is done under digital block anesthesia by passing a straight sharp pointed scissor blade longitudinally along the lateral one fourth of the base of the nail on the affected side between the nail bed and the nail plate. Occasionally both edges of the nail plate must be removed. The patient is then instructed in dressing changes and soaks two to three times daily until all symptoms have resolved. Antibiotics are usually not necessary once the infection has been drained.

SUBUNGUAL ABSCESS

Subungual abscess is the collection of pus under the nail plate as the result of the volar extension of an acute paronychia. The diagnosis is suspected when the fingertip appears inflamed and the fingernail is opaque, discolored, or lifted away from its bed. The treatment of subungual abscess requires removal of the base of the nail plate under digital block anesthesia. The distal portion of the nail may be left in place. A 7–10-day course of oral antibiotics (dicloxacillin or cephalosporins) are given, and the patient is instructed in daily dressing changes as described above.

FELON

A felon is an infection of the pulp tissue of the finger, usually as the result of a puncture wound. The septae of the pulp form closed spaces, which, when infected, cause the pulp to become swollen, tender, erythematous, and acutely painful. These infections require prompt surgical drainage. This may be done under digital block anesthesia. A straight incision is made 3 mm volar to and parallel with the nail plate on each side of the fingertip. A hemostat is passed from side to side to open the pulp space, and a slip of Penrose drain or Silastic sheeting is passed through the open space and left protruding through each skin incision (Fig. 23.26). The finger is dressed and oral

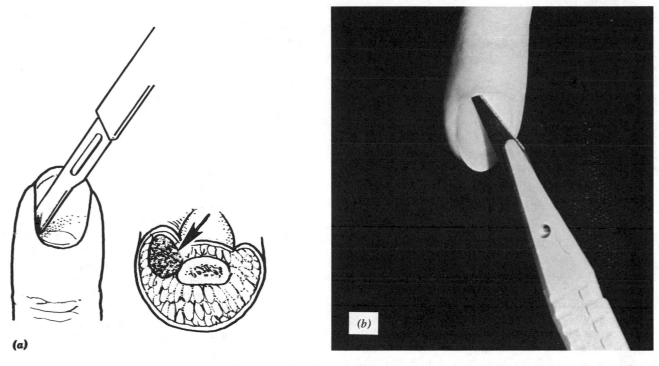

Figure 23.25. (a) Diagram of the method used to drain a collection of pus beneath the nail fold (paronychia). (b) Scalpel blade is inserted beneath the fold parallel to the nail plate.

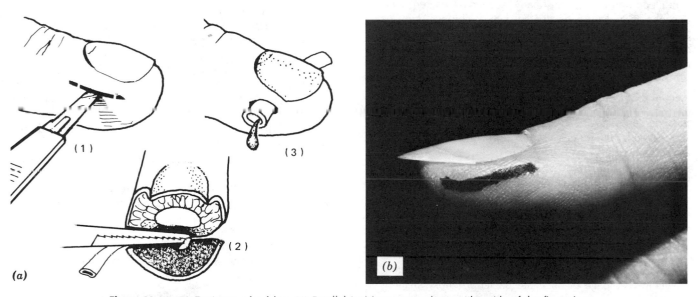

Figure 23.26 (a) Drainage of a felon. (1) Parallel incisions are made on either side of the finger just volar to the nail plate. (2) A hemostat is inserted through the incisions and spread to open the septa of the finger pulp. (3) A through-and-through drain is inserted. (b) Incision used to drain a felon. The "fishmouth" incision should not be used.

antibiotics are prescribed. The drain can be removed in 3–5 days, and the patient should be instructed in dressing changes. A "fishmouth" incision should not be used. If the abscess is pointing at one location on the surface of the pulp or has broken through the pulp, drainage may be accomplished by incising directly over the area. Necrotic skin and pulp should be removed and the wound dressed open and allowed to granulate. Untreated or advanced cases of felon may result in osteomyelitis of the distal phalanx. Films should be taken if there is any question of bone involvement. Unless the emergency room physician is familiar with the surgical drainage of felons, patients with this condition are best referred to a consultant.

HERPES SIMPLEX

Herpes simplex infection of the finger (herpetic whitlow) may be mistaken for a paronychia or felon with erythema and tenderness of the fingertip. However, small vesicles containing clear or turbid fluid usually are present on the surface of the inflamed areas. The occupation of the patient is the diagnostic clue since these infections occur most often in dentists, dental hygienists, phyicians, and nurses whose fingers are exposed to contamination by saliva or other secretions or excretions containing herpesvirus. The condition is self-limited and will resolve spontaneously in 2–3 weeks if the affected finger is kept clean and dry. Occasionally, secondary bacterial infection occurs and must be treated with antibiotics. However, attempts to incise and drain fingers affected with herpes is contraindicated. This will delay healing and may increase the risk of bacterial infection.

DEEP INFECTIONS OF THE HAND

Bacterial tenosynovitis, web space infections, subepithelial abscesses (collar button abscesses), and palmar space infections are serious infections of the hand. They present with painful swelling and erythema over the affected part. Palmar space infections may present with marked dorsal swelling because the dorsal skin and soft tissues are more distensible. Tenosynovitis presents as a swollen, erythematous finger with tenderness over the tendon sheath and pain with active and passive motion of the finger.

Surgical drainage of established infections in these areas is necessary in order to prevent serious functional impairment of the hand. Drainage of an acute bacterial tenosynovitis is a surgical emergency since the increased pressure in the closed tendon sheath from pus accumulation compromises the vascular supply of the tendon and may result in tendon necrosis. These procedures should be done in the operating room under controlled conditions. Attempts to drain these infections in the emergency room by inexperienced personnel may damage underlying structures. The use of improper incisions may cause excessive scarring or joint contractures. Early or incipient infections can be treated by antibiotics, immobilization and elevation, and frequent follow-up vistis.

Hand Dressings

Minor wounds will require a minimal dressing, for example, bandages or tubular gauze. However, more extensive injuries can best be dressed using a bulky compression dressing, usually with a volar or dorsal plaster splint to immobilize the wrist and to protect and position the fingers. This dressing is multifunctional. It will diminish pain by limiting motion of the hand and wrist, it will limit edema by applying gentle compression, and it will protect the injury site. The dressing can be used for temporary immobilization of massive hand injuries or for injuries that require transport of the patient to another facility. It can be used along with multiple fracture or with infections with edema, as well as after surgical repair of injuries.

The "safe" position of the hand places the MP joint 90 deg of flexion and the interphalangeal joints in slight flexion. The thumb is abducted to preserve the first web space. This position will diminish the possibility of joint contractures by keeping collateral ligaments in their positions of maximal length. The positioning of the hand, fingers, and wrist can be modified for specific purposes or injuries.

Open wounds should be covered with a nonadhering dressing. The bulky dressing is applied by placing a single layer of 4-by-8 inch gauze between each finger and multiple layers in the first web space. Gauze is placed in the palm to provide bulk. The first layers are held in place with roller gauze. Excessive pressure should not be used in applying the roller dressing. However, gentle compression is advantageous if applied with care. A padded plaster splint made of 10-to-12 thicknesses of 4 inch plaster is applied either volarly or dorsally. This should immobilize the fingers in the desired position and should extend far enough down the forearm to immobilize the wrist, usually in slight dorsiflexion (Fig. 23.27).

Post–Emergency Room Instructions for Patients with Hand Injuries

Hand elevation is important in minimizing both pain and swelling. In general, a sling will position the hand below the level of the heart and thus will not provide optimum venous drainage. The patient should be instructed to keep the hand at eye

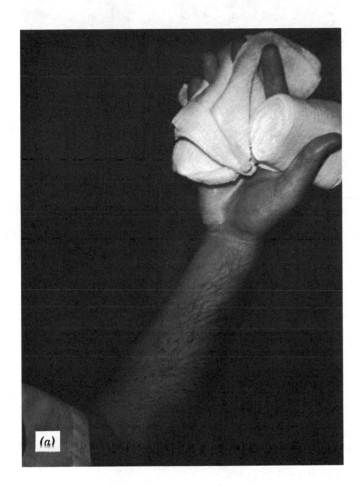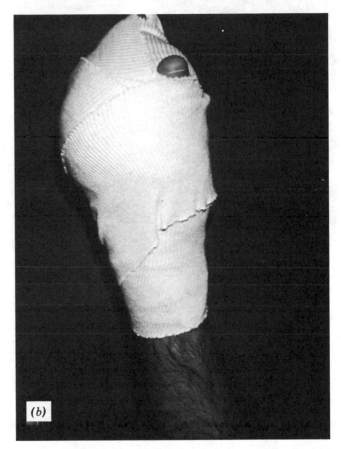

Figure 23.27 Bulky compression hand dressing with a dorsal plaster splint. (a) Sterile gauze dressings are placed between each finger to prevent skin maceration. The first web space is maintained by placing the thumb in abduction and extension (opposition). (b) The initial dressing is held in place with bias-cut stockinette or a roller bandage. (c) A dorsal plaster splint is applied from the tips of the fingers to the proximal forearm and held in place with bias-cut stockinette or a loosely wrapped elastic bandage. The wrist usually is held in slight dorsiflexion. (d) Completed dressing with fingertips exposed for inspection of color and sensibility.

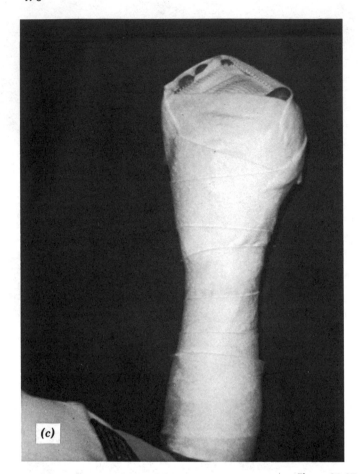

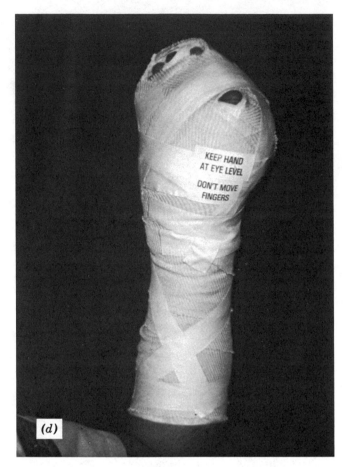

KEEP HAND
AT EYE LEVEL

DON'T MOVE
FINGERS

Figure 23.27 (continued)

level. Usually the patient's arm muscles are sufficient to maintain this position while the patient is ambulatory, although occasionally a modified sling can be applied. When the patient is at home or in bed, pillows may be used to support the forearm and hand. The elbow and shoulder should be moved through their ranges of motion (unless other associated injuries or casts or dressings preclude this) several times a day to prevent stiffness. This is particularly important in older patients.

The patient should be advised to call the physician or return to the hospital if progressive loss of sensation in the fingers occurs, if pain is uncontrolled by minor analgesics, or if a fever, erythema, swelling, or other signs of infection develops.

At least one follow-up visit is necessary for most injuries to ensure that healing is proceeding satisfactorily and that hand motion and function have been regained.

THE PAINFUL HAND

Several painful, but not necessarily traumatic, conditions of the hand may present to the emergency room physician. Recognition of these will allow a diagnosis to be made and reassurance and/or symptomatic care provided. The patient can be referred to the appropriate consultant unless urgent care is indicated.

Nerve Compression

CARPAL TUNNEL SYNDROME

Compression of the median nerve as it passes through the carpal canal (a tunnel formed by the carpal bones and the thick transverse carpal ligament—Fig. 23.2) may occur either acutely as the result of swelling associated with hand, wrist, or forearm trauma or chronically with no apparent underlying cause. It may occur temporarily during pregnancy as the result of swelling secondary to fluid retention or in association with tenosynovitis of the flexor tendons as the result of rheumatoid arthritis or other systemic conditions. It is commonly referred to as *carpal tunnel syndrome.*

The predominant symptoms of carpal tunnel syndrome are paresthesias and numbness in the distribution of the median nerve in the hand associated with pain and discomfort in the hand and forearm at night. These symptoms may be worse after vigorous use of the hand or after driving. The discomfort may be described as aching pain that radiates to the palm, wrist, or forearm. It frequently awakens the patient at night and may be partially relieved by shaking or wringing the hand, immersion in hot or cold water, or changing the position of the wrist. Patients may complain that they frequently drop objects and are "clumsy" or have difficulty in handling or picking up small objects.

Physical examination may reveal either no objective changes in the hand or a combination of signs including impaired sensibility in the median nerve distribution, diminished or absent sweating with resultant dry skin in this distribution, tenderness to percussion over the volar aspect of the wrist, increased numbness or paresthesias when the wrist is held in acute flexion (Phalen's test), and, in advanced cases, atrophy of the thenar musculature.

The treatment of this chronic condition in the emergency room is explanation and reassurance, as well as a plaster or commercial splint to maintain the wrist in a slightly dorsiflexed position. The patient should be referred to a consultant for follow-up and, if necessary, definitive care.

ACUTE COMPRESSION

Acute compression of the median nerve may occur after injuries to the hand, wrist, or forearm that result in swelling or after the application of dressings or rigid casts to the upper extremity following trauma. In these cases, the dressing should be split or removed immediately. Casts should be bivalved with a cast cutter or "univalved" by removing a longitudinal strip 1 cm wide from one surface of the cast. The cast padding is split to the level of the skin, and the edges of the cast are spread apart. The patient's primary treating physician should be notified. Although mild nerve compression may be relieved by the procedures described above combined with elevation of the extremity, occasionally surgical decompression of the nerve on an urgent basis is required.

Compression neuropathy of the median and ulnar nerves may occur after severe closed injuries such as crush injuries by rollers, heavy machinery, or washing machine wringers or by prolonged compression of the upper extremity by the pa-

tient's body during periods of unconsciousness (usually resulting from intoxication by drugs or alcohol). These injuries cause soft tissue damage that results in marked swelling and thereby compression of the neurovascular structures in the closed facial compartments of the forearm and ischemia of nerves and muscles. Occasionally, compression syndromes of the forearm result from acute hemorrhage in patients with a coagulopathy or who are taking anticoagulant medication for other conditions. These closed compartment compression syndromes are surgical emergencies and require urgent decompression by extensive fasciotomy to avoid permanent damage to the nerves and muscles and a deformed functionless extremity (Volkmann's ischemic contracture).

Stenosing Tenosynovitis

TRIGGER FINGER

Patients who present with painful motion of a finger or thumb associated with tenderness over the proximal portion of the digit or distal portion of the palm and with snapping or locking of the digit during active motion may have stenosing tenosynovitis or "trigger finger." The symptoms may be referred to the proximal interphalangeal joint. The condition is caused by impingement of the flexor tendon on the proximal portion of the tendon sheath (first annular pulley) as the tendon glides in the sheath (Fig. 23.2). It occurs most commonly in women and results from thickening of the flexor tendon, either from repetitive trauma, infiltration of the tendon by rheumatoid synovium, or occasionally from a partially lacerated or otherwise damaged tendon.

Temporary immobilization and antiinflammatory medication may give relief in very early or mild cases. Steroid injection into the tendon sheath can be used in moderately severe cases, although care must be taken so that no additional damage is done to the flexor tendon by the needle tip. Advanced cases will require surgical release of the proximal portion of the tendon sheath.

DE QUERVAIN'S DISEASE

Stenosing tenosynovitis may also occur on the radial aspect of the wrist as the tendons of the first dorsal compartment (the extensor pollicis brevis and the abductor pollicis longus) pass through a tight tendon sheath (Fig. 23.18). Stenosing tenosynovitis of the first dorsal compartment is known as de Quervain's disease and again occurs most commonly in women. It is the result of chronic inflammation of the tendon sheath and can occur with repetitive use of the thumb or as the result of direct trauma. Patients present with pain and tenderness localized to the area of the radial styloid bone or with pain radiating along the radial aspect of the thumb, hand, and forearm. These symptoms are worse during use of the thumb and hand, especially during grasp and pinch.

Physical examination reveals maximum tenderness to palpation over the radial styloid of the radius and along the first dorsal compartment of the wrist. There may be mild swelling in this area. Abduction and extension of the thumb against resistance results in pain. Passive forced flexion of the thumb with concomitant ulnar deviation of the wrist results in pain (Finklestein's test).

Mild cases may respond to splinting, antiinflammatory drugs, or the local injection of a steroid solution. The splint should be of the thumb spica type to immobilize both the wrist and the thumb. Advanced or persistent cases require surgical decompression of the first dorsal compartment.

Reflex Sympathetic Dystrophy

Reflex sympathetic dystrophy, also known as *causalgia,* is a pain syndrome that occurs most often in the upper extremity and is thought to be related to a disorder of the autonomic nervous system that results in excessive and prolonged sympathetic response to painful stimulation. The syndrome was originally described following major injuries to peripheral nerves, but it is now known to occur in varying degrees in response to painful trauma of any type in susceptible individuals. Even minor injuries such as superficial cuts, contusions, and bites or fractures or surgical procedures may elicit the syndrome. In addition to the severe pain described above, the patient may complain of severe dysethesias of the involved area. These may be so severe as to preclude contact of the area by anything, including air currents, clothing, bed sheets, or an examiner's hand. The joints of the involved parts are held motionless, and attempts to move these joints actively or passively result in severe pain. There may be mild erythema, swelling, or stiffness and even deformity in addition to the pain. However, the patient may have few, if any, of the objective signs described above. Patients affected with reflex sympathetic dystrophy often have a history of multiple return visits to the emergency room because of pain for which no reason can be found. They are often mislabeled as neurotic personalities or drug abusers if the correct reason for their complaints is not recognized.

The care of reflex sympathetic dystrophy is difficult and requires the expertise of an experienced consultant. The basis for proper treatment is early recognition. Sympathetic blockade to relieve pain and carefully supervised active hand exercise are the cornerstones of the treatment program. Failure of diagnosis or treatment results in a chronic pain syndrome ac-

companied by stiffness and deformity of the extremity that is very refractory to any mode of treatment.

ANESTHESIA

Local infiltration anesthesia and local block anesthesia are used for the control of pain in the emergency room. Occasionally peripheral nerve blocks are necessary and can be administered in the emergency room. However, extensive wound repair or the incision and drainage of infections requires more complete and prolonged anesthesia that can be provided only by intravenous regional, axillary block, or general anesthesia. These procedures are best reserved for use in the operating room where experienced help is available for patient monitoring.

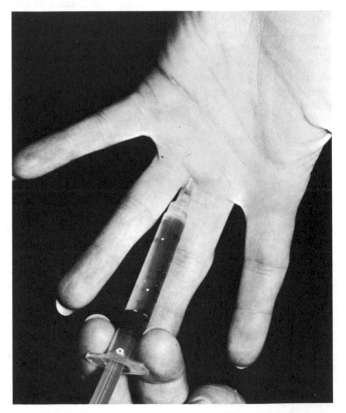

Figure 23.28 The technique of performing a metacarpal block for digital anesthesia A three-eighth-gauge needle is inserted to its hub through the skin of the web space and 2–3 ml of lidocaine are injected.

Local Infiltration

A solution of 1% lidocaine (without epinephrine) infiltrated into subcutaneous tissue provides satisfactory anesthesia for the suture of lacerations of the palm or the dorsum of the hand. Insertion of a small gauge needle (25, 26, or 30 gauge) through the wound edge rather than through the intact skin minimizes discomfort associated with the procedure. Local lidocaine infiltration is useful in obtaining small skin grafts from donor sites in the arm, groin, or thigh. The injection of large volumes of solution into a digit should be avoided because of the possibility of compression of the neurovascular bundle within the closed space of the digit.

Digital Block

If extensive anesthesia of a digit is required, a digital (metacarpal) block should be performed. The digital block is performed in the distal palm rather than within the digit. Two milliliters of lidocaine (without epinephrine) are injected into the web space between the fingers through the thin dorsal skin with a 25-gauge needle (Fig. 23.28). Two separate injections are required since both the ulnar side and radial side digital nerves for each finger must be blocked to obtain complete anesthesia. The use of epinephrine in the fingers is avoided because of the risk of vascular compromise of the digit from the constriction of terminal vessels.

Peripheral Nerve Block

If multiple fingers must be anesthetized, peripheral nerve block may be more satisfactory than multiple digital blocks. Two percent lidocaine should be used since lower concentrations often are not effective in blocking large-diameter nerves. The median, ulnar, and radial nerves may be blocked at the wrist (Fig. 23.29).

The *median nerve* lies directly beneath the deep fascia beneath the palmaris longus tendon. A 25-gauge needle is inserted through the skin directly overlying the tendon and advanced through the fascia. If this results in paresthesias, the tip of the needle should be withdrawn slightly before injecting 1 ml of plain lidocaine. This technique usually, but not always, provides satisfactory anesthesia in the thumb, index, and long fingers. If anesthesia is incomplete, it can be supplemented using the digital block technique described previously.

The *ulnar nerve* can be blocked at either the wrist or the elbow to provide anesthesia of the ring and small fingers. The ulnar nerve lies just beneath and parallel to the flexor carpi ulnaris tendon. The tissue adjacent to the nerve is infiltrated as described above, using the palpable flexor carpi ulnaris as

the landmark. The nerve also can be blocked at the elbow where it is palpable in its groove in the medial epicondyle.

The *sensory branch of the radial nerve* divides into several small branches at the wrist. These can be blocked by the subcutaneous infiltration of 1% lidocaine in the region of the radial styloid. However, a median nerve block must be done to provide complete anesthesia of the digits supplied by this nerve.

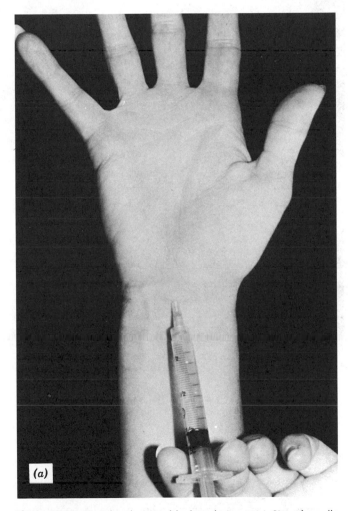

(a)

Figure 23.29 Peripheral nerve block technique. (a) Site of needle insertion for median nerve block at the wrist. (b) Site of injection for ulnar nerve block at the wrist. (c) Site of needle insertion for radial nerve block at the wrist. Note the proximal injection to block the main branch of the superficial nerve as well as its branches (see Fig. 23.18).

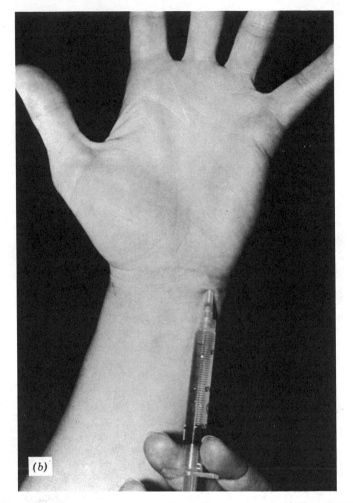

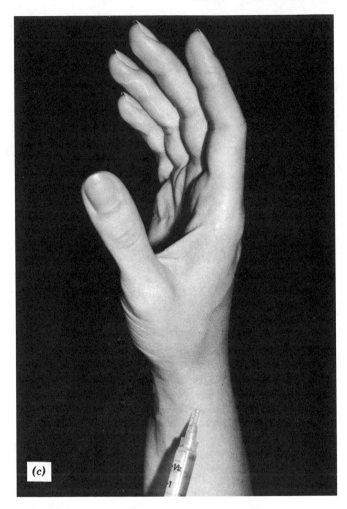

Figure 23.29 (continued)

SPECIAL PROCEDURES

Removal of Fishhooks

The skin surrounding the fishhook should be cleansed. Anesthesia is obtained either with local infiltration or digital block. The hook is then grasped with a plier or needle holder and advanced until the barb end protrudes through the skin at a point separate from that of the entrance wound. The barb is cut off with a wire cutter and the remainder of the hook backed out of the wound. If the hook is too deeply imbedded or is imbedded in an area adjacent to vital structures, such as the neurovascular bundle, surgical excision of the hook may be required. Prophylactic antibiotics are used because of the contaminated nature of the wound.

Removal of Rings

If finger swelling is minimal and there is no damage to the digit, a ring often can be removed by lubricating the finger with a solution of detergent and water and sliding the ring distally with a twisting motion. If finger swelling is moderate and the method described above does not work, the finger can be wrapped tightly with one-fourth inch wide umbilical tape to compress the soft tissues from distal to proximal. The tape is pulled beneath the ring with a small curved hemostat. The tape then is unwound from proximal to distal, sliding the ring with it.

If there is vascular compromise or an open wound, or if time is of the essence, or if excessive swelling precludes the use of other methods, the ring should be cut with a commercially available ring cutter and removed.

SUGGESTED READINGS

Flatt AE: *The Care of Minor Hand Injuries,* 4th ed. St. Louis, CV Mosby Co, 1979.

Lister G: *The Hand: Diagnosis and Indications.* Edinburgh, Churchill Livingstone, 1977.

Mittelbach HR: *The Injured Hand.* New York, Springer Verlag, 1979.

Romanes GJ: *Cunningham's Manual of Practical Anatomy,* 14th ed. London, Oxford University Press, 1976.

Weeks, PM, Wray RC: *Management of Ācute Hand Injuries—A Biological Approach,* 2nd ed. St. Louis, CV Mosby Co, 1978.

24
PARTIALLY OR TOTALLY SEVERED PARTS

Joseph Upton

Recent technological improvements in instrumentation, in operating microscopes, and especially in the mass production of microsutures have transformed small vessel (0.5–2 mm) surgery into a clinical reality. Although applications of microsurgery have been developed in virtually all surgical subspecialities, the most dramatic and widespread is the reattachment of severed parts. Initial assessment and management of patients requiring this procedure is the first critical step in a successful replant* effort.

Microsurgery is surgery performed under high-powered magnification that in the clinical setting involves loupe magnification or operating microscopes. A *revascularization* procedure restores arterial and venous flow to a partially severed part, which if left alone would not remain viable. *Replantation* is the reattachment of a totally severed part. Revascularization of partially severed extremities outnumbers replantation efforts 5:1.

THE REPLANTATION TEAM

Teamwork is critical. Each member of the team must make a major personal commitment, and the hospital must make a significant institutional commitment. In the United States, most microsurgery has become regionalized in large cities and major academic centers. There are, however, many smaller community hospitals where these procedures are also performed. Because most amputations involve limbs, the management is usually within the orthopedic or plastic surgical hand service of the hospital. Busy general surgical trauma services may also become involved with extremity and other amputations. The team must be available 24 hours a day and staffed with enough trained people to handle whatever emergency presents. The leaders must be experienced surgeons in the management of major trauma and in all aspects of acute and reconstructive hand surgery. The decision of these individuals to reattach or revascularize salvageable parts to preserve function will require great flexibility, experience, and frequently innovation. In order to have the necessary expensive and delicate microinstruments and microscopes, the properly equipped operating rooms, recovery rooms, and rehabilitation centers, and the trained nursing personnel the hospital must make a major commitment to microsurgery. Operating suites and individual surgical services must be ready to delay or reschedule elective cases in order to accommodate these often lengthy procedures. Enough physicians must be trained and coordinated into units to avoid frustration and fatigue. Older, more experienced surgeons who may not be enthusiastic about working all night must nevertheless be on the team. Their input will undoubtedly improve the care of the patients.

CARE OF THE PATIENT

Initial Assessment

The patient usually arrives on the emergency ward with a towel or handkerchief wrapped around the injured extremity. Profuse bleeding in the palm or digit can always be controlled with direct pressure and elevation. The same is true for the scalp, facial and perineal regions. Blind clamping of vessels will often inflict unnecessary damage to adjacent nerves. Careful ligation of major vessels in the forearm or upper arm may be necessary to avoid severe hemorrhage and hypovolemia. Large vessel hemorrhage for proximal limb amputations may require several tourniquets. The initial estimation of blood loss is notoriously inadequate.

Multiple trauma patients must be carefully assessed for associated injuries. Sometimes the extremity amputation may be a low-priority injury. More often, preoccupation with the amputation may cause the examining physician to overlook a ruptured spleen, a pneumothorax, or other potentially life-threatening injuries.

Initial resuscitation should include placement of intravenous lines, monitoring of vital signs, and a careful physical examination, regardless of the extent of the injury or level of amputation.

The decision to reattach or revascularize a severed part should be made by the surgical team. Emergency room staff personnel must refrain from promising the patient too much (or too little) before the condition of the patient and amputated part has been thoroughly evaluated.

---

*The terms *replant* and *reimplant* are inaccurate because nothing was really planted initially. They are, however, colloquial terms that are commonly used.

477

History

An accurate and complete history will pay tremendous dividends for the surgeon responsible for making the decision regarding the feasibility of a reattachment effort. During the past decade, a great deal of controversy has existed around the indications for replantation, much of which will undoubtedly be refined over the next 10–15 years. Currently, experts in the field differ, and absolute guidelines cannot be established. Many factors should be considered in the decision. The ultimate goal is to restore as much function as possible without jeopardizing uninjured parts of the limb. The following items should be included in the history of all patients:

1. Associated injuries
2. Age
3. Level of amputation
4. Digit involved
5. Mechanism of injury
6. Hand dominance
7. Occupation
8. Past medical history
9. Psychological and intellectual status
10. Socioeconomic factors

ASSOCIATED INJURIES

Closed- and open-head trauma and major cardiopulmonary injuries often negate the feasibility of limb reattachment efforts. In addition, other small fractures, contusions, adhesions, dislocations, and other less dramatic injuries are often missed and may become the source of the patient's primary long-term disability.

AGE

Younger patients achieve much better long-term results, probably secondary to superior sensory return and motor function. Every effort should be made to reattach major parts that have been amputated in children.

LEVEL OF AMPUTATION

Very proximal amputations in the upper arm or midforearm contain a significant amount of muscle tissue that is quite susceptible to warm ischemia. Major parts that have been amputated are considered to be poor candidates for reattachment when muscle ischemia time has exceeded 6 hours. In addition, avulsion–traction amputations involving the brachial plexus

achieve poor secondary motor and sensory recovery. Amputations at the level of the proximal phalanx pose difficult challenges in terms of flexor tendon function. In contrast, distal amputations at or beyond the level of proximal interphalangeal joints may do remarkably well after reattachment. The level of amputation correlates well with the feasibility of reattachment efforts.

DIGIT INVOLVED

The mobile thumb is essential to all functioning hands and should be reattached if at all possible. Most present controversy surrounds the isolated border digit amputation of the index or fifth finger. Often, reattached border digits are subsequently amputated at the request of the patient because the reattached finger has been "functionally neglected." Stiffness in any of the ulnar three fingers will significantly limit strength because of the common origin of the profundus tendons.

MECHANISM OF INJURY

A detailed description of the circumstances surrounding the injury may be very helpful initially in determining the need for bone shortening or vein grafting. The type of injury probably correlates best with the ultimate prognosis of a successful reattachment effort. Injuries have been classified into the following four categories, each with a different prognosis:

Sharp, Guillotine Injuries

Sharp injuries are usually civilian amputations from knives, glass, meat cleavers, industrial cutting machines, or band saws. Minimal debridement is required for structures that are minimally traumatized. Prognosis is usually excellent, especially in digital amputations beyond the level of the proximal phalanx.

Localized Crush Injuries

Accidents involving industrial presses, farm machinery, saws, and slammed doors are often the cause of localized crush injuries. More extensive debridement, shortening of the digit, and intercalated vein grafts are necessary. The prognosis is not very favorable.

Avulsion Injuries

Avulsion injuries, which are often combined with crush injuries, are the most difficult to manage. Degloving amputations, ski rope amputations, rip saw injuries, and many pediatric amputations fall into this category. Children often instinctively withdraw a hand, finger, or foot that has become caught within a door or elevator. Small vessels and nerves have been stretched over long segments and must be carefully evaluated under magnification and often replaced with autogenous nerves or vein grafts. Although viability can be predictably restored with vein grafts, sensory return is often poor with these injuries. Avulsion of digital arteries may often result in "red streaks" along the midlateral border of the digits, which is a grave prognostic sign. The prognosis for upper arm and forearm amputations is poor because of prolonged ischemia time and frequent postoperative vascular thrombosis.

Diffuse Crush and/or Explosion Injuries

Bomb blasts, firecracker accidents, vehicular accidents, and severe industrial crush accidents predominate. The tissue damage often exceeds the initial evaluation. Multiple-level injuries are often found. Initial revascularization attempts may result in thrombosis and tissue demarcation after 3–4 days as injured tissue becomes more edematous and congested. Although the prognosis is guarded, these patients should always be evaluated, if possible and practical. Portions of the traumatized and/or amputated part may be salvageable and useful as part of a primary reconstruction procedure, for example, to reattach an amputated but nontraumatized fifth finger to the index position to function as an index finger.

HAND DOMINANCE

Indications for reattachment become much more critical in bilateral injuries and in injuries to the dominant hand, especially the thumb. In bilateral injuries, priority should be given to the dominant hand.

OCCUPATION

The functional demands of the patient are important. The thumb is critical to all functioning hands, and in most evaluation scales it accounts for 40–50% of total hand function. The demands of a left index finger of a concert violinist requiring precision pinch may vary tremendously from that of a manual worker requiring power grip and grasp. Careful individualization of each patient and his or her functional needs becomes quite important.

PAST MEDICAL HISTORY

Besides obtaining careful tetanus immunization and allergy history, a thorough review of systems regarding cardiac, pul-

monary, and peripheral vascular systems is important in adults. In children with sickle cell disease (not sickle cell trait), the use of a pneumatic tourniquet is contraindicated. Children with a personal history or family history of malignant hyperthermia should be anesthetized with analeptic techniques. Patients with a history of collagen vascular disorders as well as many other medical problems may be poor candidates for prolonged surgery and subsequent immobilization and extensive rehabilitation. History of bleeding problems should always be obtained when the use of anticoagulants is anticipated.

PSYCHOLOGICAL AND INTELLECTUAL STATUS

It may be unwise to reattach an isolated digit (not a thumb) on the hand of a manual laborer, farmer, or other worker who needs to return to work immediately. The psychiatrically unstable patient, specifically schizophrenics, are often poor candidates for cooperation in postoperative rehabilitation. Mental retardation is not a contraindication for these procedures, but considerable ancillary services must be available to help the patient through the difficult postoperative rehabilitation. Although patients with self-inflicted amputations are often poor candidates for reattachment efforts, they must be considered individually since a portion of the amputated part may be useful to provide a well-padded amputation stump.

CARE OF THE AMPUTATED PART

Once the patient has arrived in the emergency room, the amputated part should be located and labeled. If the part has not been obtained, attempts should be made to retrieve it. Asking a scuba diver to search the bottom of a lake or pool or a mechanic to dismantle a machine or car may not be an unreasonable request when the amputated part has a favorable chance for reattachment. Once located, debris should be gently washed away with cold water or isotonic saline. Prolonged irrigation should be avoided. Small remaining skin or soft tissue bridges should not be incised from partially severed extremities. Often subcutaneous veins and arteries are present that will help sustain flow. An x-ray film of both the injured extremity and the amputated part should be obtained.

The amputated part should then be wrapped in a sponge moistened in a physiologic solution, placed in a plastic bag, and inserted into an *ice bath* at 2–4°C. Direct placement on ice cubes will not afford as homogeneous cooling as the ice bath. Dry ice will crystallize and destroy cells. The fluid within any container in the hospital should be checked to avoid inadvertent placement into formalin. The ice bath should then be transported in a cooler along with the patient. Eventual survival of the reattached part is greatly dependent upon the ischemia time and the anoxic tissue damage. Immediate cooling is essential. Muscle tissue is the most sensitive and undergoes irreversible damage after 6 hours of ischemia time at room temperature (20–25°C). Fingers and thumbs contain no muscle tissue and have survived 20–30 hours of cold anoxia.

FAVORABILITY FOR REATTACHMENT

Recent publicity given to this dramatic type of reattachment surgery has both educated the public and created often unrealistic expectations. Each individual case must be carefully evaluated with the preceding criteria in mind. Special consideration must be given to the prognosis for sensory return, which correlates best with the ultimate functional result. Favorability for reattachment is difficult to summarize, but general guidelines are listed below.

If possible, all of the following should be reattached:

1. Mid- or distal forearm amputations with low ischemia time
2. Wrist amputations
3. Transmetacarpal or hemihand amputations
4. Major thumb amputations, including those distal to the interphalangeal joint
5. Multiple digit amputations
6. Major amputations in a child
7. Scalp amputations

The following cases should be carefully evaluated on an individual basis:

1. Proximal forearm, elbow, and upper arm amputations
2. Isolated digital amputations, especially border digits (index and small fingers) excluding the thumb
3. Ring avulsion injuries at all levels
4. Any amputation in elderly patients (over 60 years of age), patients with history of collagen disease, peripheral vascular disease, or any chronic illness
5. Amputations with prolonged ischemia time
6. Amputations with excessive contamination of tissues
7. All avulsion injuries
8. Pediatric lower limb amputations with good prognosis for sensory recovery.

Do not consider the following under ordinary circumstances:

1. Gross mangle, explosion, or crush injuries at any level
2. Toe amputations

3. Self-inflicted penis amputations at any level
4. Multiple-level amputations
5. Patients with significant life-threatening associated injuries

TRANSPORTATION OF THE PATIENT

After communicating with the replant team, the following specific instructions regarding transfer should be given:

1. Stop hemorrhage with elevation, pressure dressing, and/or vessel ligature if necessary.
2. Intravenous line to control hypovolemia and to administer antibiotics.
3. Monitor vital signs.
4. Provide adequate analgesia.
5. Patient should be accompanied by a qualified ambulance attendant, especially if intravenous fluids are being infused.

SUMMARY OF MANAGEMENT

1. Resuscitate the patient, evaluate associated injuries, tetanus prophylaxis.
2. Obtain accurate history, including type of injury, level of amputation, ischemia time, condition and location of amputated part.
3. Contact replantation team and gain more specific instructions regarding transfer.
4. Care for the amputated part: wash debris, put in sterile wrap, insert in plastic bag and place within ice bath.
5. Transfer patient.
6. Notify receiving team of exact estimated time of arrival.

SUGGESTED READINGS

Biemer E, Duspiva W, Herndl E, Stock W, Ramatschi P: Early experiences in organizing and running a replantation service. *Br J Plast Surg* 1978; 31:9.

Lister GD, Kleinert HE: Replantation, in Grabb WC, Smith JW (eds): *Plastic Surgery*, ed 3. Boston, Little Brown & Co, 1979, p 697.

Manktelow RT: What are indications for digital replantation? *Ann Plast Surg* 1978; 1:336.

O'Brien B McC: *Microvascular Reconstructive Surgery*. Edinburgh, Churchill-Livingstone, 1977.

25
THERMAL INJURY

Nicholas O'Connor

Burns are a common form of trauma in the United States, ranging from sunburns to catastrophic life-threatening injuries. There are approximately 2,000,000 burn patients annually; about 100,000 require hospitalization. Burn injuries are a major cause of death especially in children under 15 years of age. Most severe burn injuries occur in or around the home. In fact, fires are the leading cause of accidental death in homes.

The major source of burn injuries in most patients are flames from stoves, flammable liquids, fires, and explosions. In children under 3 years of age the most common cause of burns is scalding. Curious children who reach up and pull down cooking pans from the stove or knock over containers of hot liquid such as coffee pots frequently suffer scald burns. In children ages 3–14, flame burns resulting from clothing catching fire are the most common. Because girl's clothing tends to be more flammable than boy's clothing, these burns are more common in girls and tend to be more serious in their depth and extent. The rest of the burns in this age group occur from house fires. In people aged 15–60, industrial or work-related accidents account for the largest number of burns. Chemical and electrical burns are relatively rare and are usually the result of industrial accidents.

In people over the age of 60, burns occur in those who are somehow susceptible to being burned. Alcohol and drug overdose in this age group are common factors relating to burn susceptibility. Other factors such as loss of consciousness from cardiac arrhythmias, cerebral arteriosclerosis, and epilepsy also make this population more susceptible to injury. Finally, generalized debility in aged people frequently prevents them from escaping from the source of the fire. Burns suffered by this group of susceptible individuals tend to be very large; there is a high mortality rate.

CLASSIFICATION OF BURNS

In thermal burns, the depth of the surface injury is dependent on the temperature and caloric content of the thermal source, the length of exposure, and the area of exposure. These relationships have been well worked out in scald burns with hot water. For example, full-thickness burns producing epidermal necrosis can be caused by 1 second of exposure to water at 70°C. It requires 5 seconds of exposure to produce the same effect with water at 60°C temperature.

The skin consists of two main layers (Fig. 25.1); the surface epithelium, or epidermis, and the subjacent connective tissue layer, the corium or dermis. Beneath the dermis is a looser connective tissue layer, the superficial fascia or hypodermis, which in many places is transformed into subcutaneous fatty tissue. The epidermis varies from 0.07 to 0.12 mm in thickness on most parts of the body, although on the palms and the palmar surfaces of the fingers it may be up to 1 mm thick and on the soles and toes it may be 2–6 mm thick. The dermal appendages of the skin, hair follicles, sebaceous glands, and sweat glands extend down to the deeper layers of the dermis and occasionally project into the subcutaneous layer. These appendages are important in that the cells lining them can proliferate to form an epidermal layer in the healing of burns.

Depth of Burn

Burns can be classified into four categories according to their depth, namely, first, second, third, and fourth-degree burns. A *first-degree burn* involves only the epidermis. It is characterized by redness and pain that appear sometime after the initial injury. The most common cause of first-degree burns is excessive exposure to sunlight. An instantaneous exposure to more intense heat may also cause a first-degree burn. First-degree burns imply only a very superficial injury to the skin and usually subside over a 1–2-day period. Healing takes place in about 3–7 days and is characterized by some peeling of the outer layer of epidermis. A first-degree burn covering large areas of the body may cause the patient to feel somewhat ill and to have a slightly elevated temperature.

The *second-degree burn* is a deeper injury and involves all of the epidermis and some part of the dermis. A very deep second-degree burn will destroy not only the epidermis but much more of the dermis leaving only some portions of the skin appendages intact. Redness, pain, blisters, and peeling skin characterize second-degree burns. A deep second-degree burn may closely resemble a third-degree burn with a leathery brown appearance to the skin. The length of time required for a second-degree burn to heal depends on the depth to which the dermis has been destroyed and ranges from 10 to 30 days. If not cared for properly, a deep second-degree burn can easily be converted into full-thickness third-degree burn because of infection.

Whereas first- and second-degree burns are partial-thickness injuries of the skin, a *third-degree burn* is a full-thickness injury destroying the epidermis and dermis down to the subcutaneous fat layer. This destruction includes the skin appendages so that

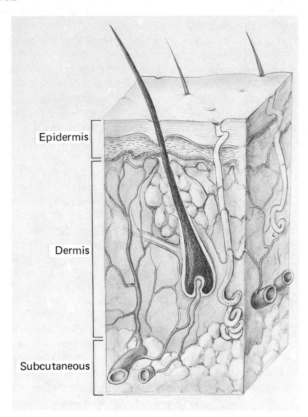

Figure 25.1 A cross section of skin showing the epidermis and the projection of the epidermal appendages deep into the dermis.

Epidermis

Dermis

Subcutaneous

no regeneration of the epithelium in a third-degree burn area is possible. A full-thickness burn can be leathery brown in appearance, have a white marblelike appearance, or be black. Occasionally thrombosed blood vessels can be seen through the burned skin, especially when it has a marblelike appearance. Full-thickness burns are seldom painful because the pain-sensitive nerve endings are destroyed. Patients with these burns correspondingly have little sensation on neurologic testing.

A large amount of edema in the injured area is common to both second- and third-degree burns and develops over the first 12 hours after injury. Deep second- and third-degree burns over the course of days will form a thick eschar that consists of a coagulum of the dead skin layers.

Fourth-degree burns occur when the injury extends through the subcutaneous tissue to involve deeper structures—fascia, muscle, tendon, blood vessels, cartilage, and bone. Such deep injuries usually occur in the extremities, the nose, or the ears and result in permanent loss of tissue. The injured area will

be hard, dry, and black, and there will be very little accumulation of edema.

Extent of Burn

The extent of the burn is expressed as a percentage of the body surface area that is injured. The usual method to determine how much of the body surface is burned in adults is the *rule of nines*. The body is divided into areas, each representing 9% or multiples of 9% of the total body surface: The head and neck equal 9%, the anterior trunk equals 2 × 9, or 18%, the posterior trunk equals 18%, each upper extremity equals 9%, each lower extremity equals 2 × 9, or 18%, the perineum equals 1%. In children under 2 years old, the rule of nines is modified as follows: The head and neck equal 18%, each upper extremity equals 9%, the front of the trunk equals 18%, the back of the trunk equals 18%, each lower extremity equals 1.5 × 9, or 13.5% (Fig. 25.2).

Types of Burn Injuries

A classification of burn injuries can be made on the basis of the extent of body surface area (BSA) involved and the depth of the injury (Table 25.1). Second-degree burns covering less than 15% BSA in adults or less than 10% BSA in children and third-degree burns covering less than 2% BSA in adults or children are classified as *minor burn injuries*.

Second-degree burns covering 15–25% BSA in adults or 10–20% BSA in children and third-degree burns covering less than 10% BSA in adults or children are classified as *moderate burn injuries*. Burns of specific areas such as hands, feet, eyes, ears, face, or perineum are classified as moderate.

Second-degree burns covering more than 25% BSA in adults or more than 20% BSA in children and third-degree burns covering more than 10% BSA in adults or children are classified as *major burn injuries*. Electrical burns, burns associated with traumatic or inhalation injuries, or burns in patients with preexisting diseases are also classified as major.

Nature of Burn Injuries

A thermal insult severe enough to cause a second- or third-degree burn destroys three of the most important protective functions of the skin: (1) a barrier to water evaporation, (2) a sensitive regulation of body core temperature, and (3) a defense against microbial invasion. Heat necrosis of the epidermis leads to an immediate loss of the complex lipids in the epidermis that provide a barrier to water evaporation. As a result, water freely evaporates through the burn eschar resulting in large

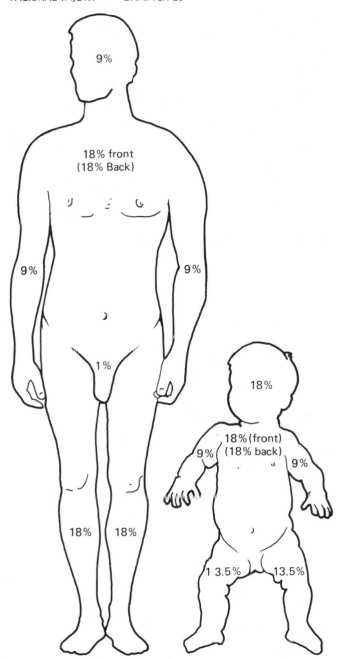

9%

**18% front
(18% Back)**

9%   **9%**

1%

18%   **18%**

18%

**18% (front)
(18% back)**

9%   **9%**

13.5%   **13.5%**

Figure 25.2 The rule of nines to calculate the percentage of body surface area involved with the burning injury is shown for adults and for children under 12 months of age.

TABLE 25.1 Classification of Burn Injuries

Major Burn Injury
   Second-degree burn > 25% BSA—Adults
   Second-degree burn > 20% BSA—Children
   Third-degree burn > 10% BSA—Adults and children
   All burns involving hands, face, eyes, ears, feet, and perineum
   All patients with inhalation injury, electric injury, burn injury complicated by other major trauma
   Poor risk patients with burns

Moderate Uncomplicated Burn Injury
   Second-degree burn 15–25% BSA—Adults
   Second-degree burn 10–20% BSA—Children
   Third-degree burn > 10% BSA—Adults and Children
   Excludes those with burns involving eyes, ears, face, hands, feet and perineum; electric injury; inhalation injury; burn injury complicated by other major trauma; burns in poor risk patients

Minor Burn Injury
   Second-degree burn < 15% BSA—Adults
   Second-degree burn < 10% BSA—Children
   Third-degree burn < 2% BSA—Adults and Children
   Excludes those with burns involving eyes, ears, face, hands, feet, and perineum; electric injury; inhalation injury; burn injury complicated by other major trauma; burns in poor risk patients

losses (as high as 2,000–3,000 ml in very large burns) from the body until the burn wound heals or skin is grafted onto the area.

The evaporation of large amounts of water causes the patient to lose an increased number of calories or amount of heat. The body normally regulates heat loss by altering both the blood flow to the skin and the amount of sweat produced. In burn patients these mechanisms are seriously interfered with so that they can no longer regulate heat loss from their skin surfaces. When this loss of regulation is accompanied by a large increase in evaporation of water, the patient can be in serious danger of dropping the core body temperature. This problem is more common in burns covering more than 50% of the body surface and in burns in very old or very young patients.

The loss of integrity of the epidermis causes the protection against bacterial invasion of the underlying tissues and the blood stream to be lost in these patients as well. The burn wound presents a large vulnerable interface to the external environment. Very quickly burn wounds become colonized by bacteria, which, if they are allowed to proliferate, will become invasive causing severe local damage and systemic septicemia. The most common cause of death of hospitalized burn patients is therefore from infection.

Finally the thermal input damages the extensive network of capillaries in the dermal and subdermal plexus. The thermally injured capillaries are no longer an effective semipermeable membrane, and large amounts of plasma leak out into the injured area creating burn wound edema. There is also thought to be a large release of histamine that further contributes to the "leakiness" of the capillaries in distant unburned areas, as well as the injured area. This injury to the capillaries heals in 24–36 hours so the plasma loss stops by that time. Until healing occurs, however, a large amount of edema, as much as 10% of preburn body weight, accumulates. Further, the huge loss of plasma from the vascular space leads to burn shock if the patient is allowed to go untreated.

Inhalation Injuries

Injury to the respiratory tract is one of the most dangerous and frequent complications of burn injuries and is the leading cause of death in fire victims. In the United States, over one-half of the 12,000 people who die annually from fires die from an inhalation injury. There are three kinds of inhalation injuries: carbon monoxide poisoning, upper airway damage, and pulmonary parenchymal injury.

CARBON MONOXIDE POISONING

Carbon monoxide poisoning, the most common single cause of death in burn victims, is quite separate in its pathophysiology from upper airway or pulmonary injuries. Carbon monoxide is a colorless, odorless, tasteless, nonirritating gas that is liberated from incomplete combustion of carbon compounds. Carbon monoxide combines with hemoglobin to form carboxyhemoglobin. The affinity of hemoglobin for carbon monoxide is 200 times greater than for oxygen, and therefore even a small amount of carbon monoxide in the atmosphere successfully competes with oxygen for the binding sites of hemoglobin. The resultant carboxyhemoglobin, besides rendering the patient functionally anemic, shifts the oxyhemoglobin dissociation curve to the left making the patient even more hypoxic. Death is a result of hypoxia, hypoventilation, hypercapnea, and acidosis.

UPPER AIRWAY DAMAGE

Upper airway and laryngeal edema are produced by the inhalation of hot gases and the irritating chemicals in smoke. The tissue damage caused by these agents leads to upper airway edema and laryngeal spasm and edema usually within 3–6 hours after injury. Increasing hoarseness, inability to swallow secretions, and an increased respiratory rate are signs of impending upper airway obstruction.

PULMONARY PARENCHYMAL INJURIES

Pulmonary parenchymal injury should be suspected in patients caught in a fire that occurred in a closed space or a fire associated with copious smoke production and if other victims of the same fire also have inhalation injury. The same irritating chemicals (aldehydes and nitrates in wood smoke, cyanides and phosgene in smoke from synthetic materials) that cause airway damage are toxic to the pulmonary parenchyma and may lead to necrotizing bronchiolitis, intraalveolar edema, and hyaline membrane formation. These parenchymal changes interfere with gas exchange so that the patient becomes hypoxic and pulmonary infiltrates become visible on x-ray examination within 48 hours. Further, the injured lung is much more susceptible to bacterial invasion and subsequent pneumonia.

INITIAL ASSESSMENT AND MANAGEMENT

Immediate Care and Transportation

The first person to arrive at the scene of a burn accident should remove the victim from further danger of being burned. If the patient is in a burning house, he or she should be removed as quickly as possible from the house or from the source of fire. If the patient's clothing is on fire, the fire should be put out quickly, usually by smothering the burning clothing with a wet blanket. If no wet blanket is available, a dry blanket or overcoat will serve. Burning or smoldering clothing should be removed immediately from the patient; it may be necessary to cut the clothing away with scissors. If any cloth sticks to the burn, it should be left alone until the patient reaches a treatment center. Once the patient is removed from the source of the fire and the burning clothing has been removed, the patient should be placed in a reclining position and should be evaluated for other injuries. If possible, the burned area should be covered with a clean sheet, and a blanket should be placed over the sheet to keep the patient warm. Rings, bracelets, and any constricting clothing should be removed from the patient even if they are on areas of the body that are not burned.

Most patients are able to perform a moderate amount of activity for several hours after they have been burned. If there are no other injuries, patients may be capable of transporting themselves to whatever vehicle is waiting to take them to a treatment center. The patient should be taken to the center quickly, but great rush is usually unnecessary unless there is a respiratory problem. No stimulants or liquids should be given by mouth, and the burn surface should not be covered by butter or any greasy medicated ointments. If time permits, it may be important to find out what caused the burn. Also, if the burn is large or serious, the emergency department of the hospital should be notified that the patient is coming.

Initial Hospital Assessment and Management

All patients with moderate or major burns should be taken to the emergency room of the nearest general hospital. Patients with moderate burns can be taken care of in general hospitals, but those with major burns should be transferred to hospitals with burn facilities after receiving initial care in the emergency room. Emergency room care of patients with major burns should consist of the orderly execution of several routine procedures: obtain a history, rapidly assess pulmonary function, assess injuries other than the burn, estimate the extent and depth of the burn, draw blood samples for laboratory determinations, insert intravenous catheters, and place a nasogastric tube and an indwelling bladder catheter. Tetanus immunization should be instituted and the patient's fluid therapy planned.

ASSESSMENT

The history should include when, where, and how the accident happened. Information should be obtained concerning the status of the patient's health before the injury with particular references to prior history of pulmonary, cardiac, or renal disease. The patient's height, preburn weight, and prior drug history should be obtained.

On examination, the presence of face or neck burns, singed nasal hairs, inflamed or swollen posterior pharyngeal mucosa, and edema of the glottis suggest potential airway difficulty. Patients with such difficulties should be considered for immediate endotracheal intubation. If the airway edema has progressed too far, intubation may be impossible and tracheostomy will be necessary. Humidified air should be provided through the tube.

Carbon monoxide poisoning is suggested by any of the signs associated with inhalation injury but can be confirmed by determining the level of carboxyhemoglobin in an arterial or venous blood sample. A blood carboxyhemoglobin level greater than 15% suggests mild carbon monoxide poisoning. A level greater than 25% suggests serious poisoning especially if the injury occurred more than 1 hour before testing. Patients with mild poisoning are treated with face mask oxygen. Patients with serious poisoning are intubated and placed on a ventilator

with 100% oxygen. The 100% oxygen is continued until the carboxyhemoglobin level is below 10%.

Soot particles in the sputum and an elevated blood carboxyhemoglobin concentration indicate possible pulmonary injury. The injury produces the pathophysiologic changes seen with bronchopneumonia. The changes are not usually manifest for 12–24 hours. Then the patient may develop an increased respiratory rate, auscultatory signs or bronchospasm, a chest film appearance compatible with congestion and edema or bronchopneumonia, and a falling arterial P_{O_2}. The chest film signs may lag behind the clinical signs. Early fiberoptic bronchoscopic examination is helpful in determining the extent of the damage of the lower airways. Patients with this injury are treated for its complications, namely, hypoxemia and infection. Steroids and prophylactic antibiotics are not recommended.

Associated Injuries

Patients who received burns from explosions, motor-vehicle accidents, or burning buildings may have associated skeletal injuries or blunt injuries of the chest and abdomen. Electrical burns are notorious for having a relatively innocent-looking surface injury accompanied by very serious injury to other organ systems. In the initial evaluation of burns, therefore, in addition to characterizing the depth and extent of the burn injury itself, it is critical to assess injuries to other areas. The history of the injury itself is the single most important clue to detecting trauma to organs other than the skin.

Criteria for Admission

Determining the extent and depth of the injury is essential in burn therapy, particularly in deciding whether or not the patient needs to be admitted to the hospital. No criteria for admission should be strictly adhered to; however, the following guidelines for whom to admit may be helpful: (1) children under the age of 10 and adults over the age of 65 with second- or third-degree burns covering 10% or more BSA; (2) children and adults between the ages of 10 and 65 with second- or third-degree burns covering 20% or more BSA; (3) those of all ages with deep second- or third-degree burns of the face, perineum, hands, or feet; (4) those of all ages with minor burns but with other associated severe injuries.

Fluid Therapy for Moderate and Major Burns

Minor burns do not require any special form of intravenous fluid therapy. However, second- and third-degree burns covering more than 20% BSA require resuscitation with large amounts of fluid. These large volumes of fluid are necessary to replace the losses of plasma and extracellular fluid to the burn edema. There is also a corresponding loss of sodium to intracellular fluid spaces and a large increase in the evaporative loss of water through the burned skin. These large fluid losses, unless adequately replaced, lead to two major hazards—burn shock and renal failure.

There are many fluid resuscitation formulas or budgets, all of which are designed to maintain circulating plasma volume, blood pressure, and urine output. Several of these formulas are outlined in Tables 25.2 and 25.3, and one of them is discussed in greater detail below.

To deliver such large volumes of fluid to these patients usually requires the insertion of two large bore venous catheters, one of which is a central venous line. As a rule no catheters or cutdowns should be inserted in the lower extremities since there is a high incidence of thrombophlebitis associated with such lines in burn patients. Generally the lines are placed in the upper extremities, and the central line is frequently placed in the internal jugular or subclavian veins. If possible the lines should be placed through unburned skin; however, it is frequently necessary to insert lines or to do cutdowns through burned skin. These lines should be placed and the fluid therapy initiated a short time after the patient reaches the emergency room.

Patients must be monitored carefully during the first 48 hours of their fluid resuscitation. Their vital signs and intake and output should be recorded hourly. Blood pressure should be maintained within the normal range for the individual patient, and the hourly urine output should be maintained between 50 and 100 ml/hr. Central venous pressure will provide a rough guide to adequacy of volume replacement but is not as important

as the above two measures. Daily weights and total fluid balance are useful guides over the long course.

The Brooke formula meets the patient's fluid requirements with lactated Ringer's solution and a plasma–protein solution. The amount of lactated Ringer's solution is calculated at 1.5 ml per kilogram body weight per percent burn; one-half the amount is given in the first 8 hours, one-fourth in the second 8 hours, and one-fourth in the third 8 hours. The plasma is calculated at 0.5 ml/kg/% burn during the first 24 hours. During the second 24 hours, from one-half to three-fourths of the first 24-hours requirement of both fluids is given. This formula represents a guide to the requirements of the patient. The hourly input of fluid is modified by changes in hourly urine output.

Many patients with large deep burns or electrical burns will have considerable amounts of hemoglobin or myoglobin in their urine. These pigments stain the urine a wine color. Both of these large pigmented protein molecules easily precipitate in the renal tubules causing acute renal failure. Therefore in patients with large amounts of pigmented protein in their urine, it is necessary to maintain a urine output of over 100 ml/hr, and since these proteins precipitate more easily in an acid urine, it is helpful to alkalinize the urine with bicarbonate. It may be necessary to give mannitol (10 g/hr), an osmotic diuretic, to augment urine volume. The hemolysis of red blood cells seen with thermal injury is occasionally severe and increased by associated diffuse intravascular coagulation and may necessitate transfusions with whole blood.

Gastrointestinal Complications

Major burns have a high incidence of stress gastritis with multiple tiny erosions and petechial hemorrhages in gastric mucosa. This gastritis may lead to gastric dilation or hemorrhage

TABLE 25.2 Formulas for Estimating Fluid Needs of Burned Adults

	First 24 Hr			Second 24 Hr		
	Electrolyte	Colloid	Glucose in Water	Electrolyte	Colloid	Glucose in Water
Baxter	4 ml/kg/% burn				20, 50, 60% of calculated plasma volume	2,000 ml
Brigham	100 ml/hr	7.5% of body weight	2,000 ml	100 ml/hr	2.5% of body weight	2,000 ml
Brooke	1.5 ml/kg/% burn	0.5 ml/kg/% burn	2,000 ml	½ to ¾ of first 24-hr requirement	½ to ¾ of first 24-hr requirement	

TABLE 25.3 Formulas for Estimating Fluid Needs of Burned Children

| | First 24 Hr | | | |
	Electrolyte	Colloid	Glucose in Water	Second 24 Hr
Brooke	3 ml/kg/% burn	—	—	Both budgets call for glucose in water ad lib to maintain urine output
Brigham	3 ml/kg/% burn	0.3 ml/kg/% burn	—	

as soon as 2 hours after the burn injury occurred. To avoid these two serious complications, patients with major burns should have nasogastric tubes inserted, and they should be placed on suction while in the emergency room. Antacids are instilled down the tube every 4 hours for the first 48 hours. After this period of time, if the patient is able to eat, the tube is removed; if the patient is unable to eat, the tube is used for tube feedings.

Wound Care

After initial assessment is complete and respiratory and fluid therapy have been instituted, all patients, while still in the emergency room, should have their burn surfaces gently cleansed with a mild antiseptic solution such as half-strength povidone-iodine (Betadine). Any loose dead skin should be removed; however, blisters are usually left intact. Topical agents may then be applied to the burn surface. Most commonly, a light coating of silver sulfadiazine is applied to the burn surface, and the surface is wrapped in sterile gauze or covered with a sterile sheet. Hand burns are splinted in a position suitable for function and are elevated to reduce the accumulation of edema.

The burn eschar in circumferential burns of an extremity may so constrict a limb such that with the accumulation of edema under the eschar, the circulation in the limb is compromised. The circulation in hands and feet should be checked frequently in such patients by feeling for arterial pulsations, observing capillary refill, and checking arterial pulse and flow with Doppler recorders. Escharotomies are frequently necessary to prevent ischemic damage, and indications should be reassessed every few hours. A circumferential burn of the thorax associated with a thick eschar can seriously limit respiratory motion and increase the work of breathing. The patient is completely relieved with escharotomies, and these should be carried out before ventilation is compromised. It will usually become apparent whether escharotomies are necessary 6–12 hours after the injury. Escharotomies are a precise surgical

procedure and should be carried out only by experienced surgeons.

Electrical Burns

Electrical burns are frequently very deceptive and have a high incidence of associated skeletal injury. The surface component of an electrical burn may be very small and involve only the point of entry and exit of the current. The passage of the current through nerves, blood vessels, and muscle may cause extensive damage to these structures. A careful neurologic examination should be carried out to detect not only damage to the peripheral nerves but injury to the spinal cord as well. Since spinal cord injury seen with electrical burns may be progressive, the patient should be repetitively examined. Damage to small arteries can be assessed by examination of the arterial system and is usually easily recognized. Myonecrosis leads to myoglobinemia and myoglobinuria as an immediate hazard and loss of muscle function as a long-term problem.

The electrical current can pass through the heart damaging the myocardium and leading to an infarct. With or without an infarct the patient may develop malignant arrhythmias and should have careful electrocardiographic monitoring. All patients who receive electrical burns, even if the burns appear to be minor, should be admitted to the hospital for observation.

Treatment of Minor Burns

With small burns, immediate relief of pain can be accomplished by applying a cold treatment. A wet towel wrapped around ice cubes applied to the area or placing the burned area under running cold water will be effective especially if the treatment is applied within the first 30 minutes from the time of injury. Cold should be applied to minor burns only.

After applying the cold treatment for 5–10 minutes, the wound should be gently cleansed with mild soap and water or with half-strength Betadine. Devitalized or dead skin is debrided, but blisters are generally left intact. Minor burns are usually more comfortable if treated with a soft gauze or dressing. To prevent the dressing from adhering to the burn, the wound first may be covered with silver sulfadiazine cream or Betadine ointment or covered with petroleum gauze or adaptic and then covered with soft dry gauze. Such dressings should be changed every day in the clinic or at home by a visiting nurse. Tetanus prophylaxis should be carried out according to the usual regimens.

COLD INJURY

There are basically two kinds of cold injuries—hypothermia and cold-induced tissue injury. There are three categories of the latter, namely, frostbite, trench foot, and immersion. Hypothermia may be associated with tissue injury and vice versa.

Hypothermia

Accidental hypothermia, whether from exposure to cold air or cold water, simply reflects an imbalance between the heat produced by the body and the heat lost from it. By adjusting rates of heat production and heat loss, we maintain a stable core body temperature range for optimal enzyme functioning. For example, for each 1°C of temperature drop there is about a 10% decrease in biochemical activity. The normal core body temperature is in a narrow range of 36.4–37.5°C. Heat may be convected, conducted, radiated, or released by evaporation from the body surface. Control of the environment and the use of protective clothing is our major defense against heat loss. The physiologic adjustments to protect ourselves from loss of body heat include exercise, shivering, basal thermogenesis under the control of the hypothalmus, and peripheral vasoconstriction. For example, shivering can increase the basal metabolic rate four or five times the normal rate.

There are basically three types of accidental hypothermia: acute, subacute, and chronic. A person who is plunged into cold water that causes his or her core body temperature to drop swiftly experiences acute immersion hypothermia. A person who, for example, is lost in a sparsely populated area or is incapacitated for some reason and much of the night lies exposed to snow or rain in cold weather with insufficient clothing or shelter to maintain body core temperature suffers from subacute hypothermia. Chronic hypothermia in which the cooling occurs over several days is more frequent in a person who, as a result of drugs, disease, or failure of the body's temperature-regulating mechanism, perhaps combined with age, experiences a slow but nonetheless potentially lethal cooling over a period of days.

This may occur without the person ever leaving his or her living quarters if the room temperatures are lower than the person can safely tolerate. Patients with chronic hypothermia almost always have some other serious disease.

Accidental hypothermia is defined as the pathologic state occurring after core body temperature is reduced below 35°C as a result of accidental cold stress. If there is continuing stress the condition may be progressive and fatal unless body temperature is restored and the concomitant metabolic aberrations are corrected. The diagnosis is made by taking a rectal temperature with a low-reading thermometer. Axillary and oral temperatures are misleading. If the body temperature is below 35°C shivering and vasoconstriction become very intense, and the patient loses manual dexterity but is still relatively well oriented. At this stage, the hypothermia is easily reversible. If the body temperature is below 32°C, the hypothermia becomes severe; shivering is replaced by marked muscular rigidity and stiff movement. The patient is obtunded and is progressing to full stupor. The blood pressure may not be detectable at this time, but a strong carotid or femoral pulse can be palpated. Breathing becomes shallow and irregular and the heart rate begins to slow. If the body temperature is below 27°C, the hypothermia is profound, and the patient experiences deep coma and rigidity. Pulmonary edema can occur, and there is great risk of ventricular arrhythmia.

The most devastating effect of hypothermia occurs when the core temperature drops below 24°C. Below this temperature, ventribular fibrillation generally will occur, and as the core temperature falls below 20°C asystole will occur. If the hypothermia has been acute there may be only relatively mild associated acidosis. If the hypothermia has been chronic a more serious acidosis may accompany cardiac arrest.

TREATMENT

As soon as hypothermia is recognized, wherever the patient may be, action must be taken to prevent further cooling in the patient. Wet clothing must be removed and the patient placed in a dry blanket. Rewarming should begin as soon as possible but only in hospital facilities where medical resources are available to deal with any resulting complications. This is especially true for patients with severe and profound hypothermia. Patients with mild hypothermia can have heat from external sources, such as from the bodies of warm companions, applied, can be given hot drinks, and can be encouraged to do some isometric exercises.

In rewarming patients with severe or profound hypothermia, it is important, if possible, to warm the core of the body before the shell. If the shell or periphery of the body is warmed first by immersing the patient in warm water, peripheral vasodilation occurs. As the cool blood returns centrally, the core body temperature will drop further, and rewarming shock will occur when the supercooled heart cannot return the amount of blood that the rewarmed skin demands. The most effective way of rewarming the patient's core is to use peritoneal dialysis or lavage. This is carried out by inserting a peritoneal dialysis catheter and using isotonic peritoneal dialysate that is heated by a blood-warming coil to 35–37°C. Two liters of the dialysate are exchanged every 20–30 minutes in order to raise the rectal temperature above 30°C as soon as possible to obviate the danger of refractory ventricular fibrillation. At the same time, an endotracheal tube should be inserted to protect the airway since vomiting may ensue with central rewarming. Once the rectal temperature exceeds 30°C, a hypothermia pad or warm water bath can be used to raise the temperature more slowly. The patient will require an infusion of saline to support blood pressure as the periphery becomes rewarmed. Furthermore, any associated acidosis should be corrected carefully; over-correction with resultant alkalosis should be avoided. Although the prognosis for survival is poor with core temperatures below 25°C, there are many case reports of patients with profound hypothermia and cardiac arrest who have been successfully treated using prolonged cardiopulmonary resuscitation and rewarming.

Cold-Induced Tissue Injuries

FROSTBITE

Except in rare instances frostbite is restricted to the extremities of the body or to areas such as the chin, cheeks, nose, and ears. The severity of the injury is influenced by the intensity of the initial exposure and the length of time before adequate circulation can be restored.

The type and duration of contact are the two most important factors in determining the extent of frostbite injury (Table 25.4). For example, touching cold wood is not nearly as dangerous as coming into direct contact with metal, particularly if the hands are wet or even damp, because metal is an excellent thermal conductor. Air itself is a very poor thermal conductor.

TABLE 25.4 Types of Cold-Induced Tissue Injuries

Type of Contact	Duration of Contact	Temperature
Frostbite	Minutes to 16 hours	−60−+7°C
Trench foot	2 hours to 14 days	−7−+10°C
Immersion foot	12 hours to 7 days	−4−+16°C

Cold air alone is not nearly as dangerous as a combination of wind and cold. Hence, the chilling effect of 20°F(−6.7°C) combined with a 45 mph wind is identical to that of −40°F(−40°C) temperature with no wind.

The susceptibility to injury is influenced by training, geographical, background, and cold adaptation. During the Korean War, black soldiers had six times greater incidence of frostbite than white soldiers, and southern whites had almost a two times greater incidence than northern whites. Furthermore, general physical condition influences susceptibility; for example, injured soldiers were much more susceptible to frostbite no matter what their initial injury was.

Two types of reaction occur when tissue comes in contact with cold. First, the superficial tissue at the site of contact actually freezes to a depth that is dependent on the degree of cold and the duration of contact. When this freezing occurs ice crystals grow between cells, and if the source of cold is not removed, these crystals continue to grow, dehydrating and severely damaging the adjacent cells. Intense freezing causes crystals to form within the cells damaging the cells immediately.

Second, arteriolar vasoconstriction occurs in the tissue adjacent to the frozen layer thereby rapidly reducing the blood flow in this zone. When there is arteriolar constriction, shunts occur that allow blood to bypass the affected capillary bed, and if the source of cold is not removed, the whole area begins to freeze.

Diagnosis

The following is a retrospective classification designed by the United States Army during the Korean War. This classification divides frostbite injury into four degrees of seriousness: (1) erythema and swelling with no blister formation, (2) erythema and swelling with blisters, (3) full-thickness injury with gangrene and no loss of part, (4) complete necrosis with loss of part.

This classification is useful in reporting frostbite injuries, but a more useful classification is to divide frostbite injuries into superficial or deep, determined before the injured part has been thawed. *Superficial frostbite* involves only the skin or the tissues immediately beneath it. The frozen part is white and firm on the exterior but soft and resilient below the surface when depressed gently and firmly. After rewarming, the frostbitten area will first become numb, mottled blue, or purple and will then swell, sting, and burn for some time. In more severe cases, blisters will occur beneath the epidermis after 24–36 hours. These blisters slowly dry up and become hard and black after about 2 weeks. General swelling of the injured area will occur and subside in the same period of time. After the swelling disappears, the skin will peel and remain red, tender, and extremely sensitive to even mild cold, and the area may perspire abnormally for a long time.

In *deep unthawed frostbite,* a much more serious injury, the injured part is hard and solid and cannot be depressed at all. The damage not only involves the skin and subcutaneous tissues, but also goes deep into the tissue beneath (even including bone) and is usually accompanied by the formation of huge blisters. These blisters may take from 3 days to 1 week to develop. Swelling of the entire hand or foot will take place and last for 1 month or more. After rewarming, blue, violet, or gray discoloration takes place, and throbbing pains may occur and last for up to 8 weeks. The blisters eventually dry up, blacken, and slough off leaving an exceptionally sensitive red, thin layer of new skin that will take months to return to normal. In extreme cases of deep frostbite the area, with thawing, turns a lifeless gray and remains cold. If blisters and swelling occur, they will appear along the line of demarcation between the acutely frostbitten area and the remainder of the limb. In 1 or 2 weeks after the injury the tissue becomes black, dry and shriveled right up to the beginning of healthy tissue, and eventually the injured tissue will fall off. If this dead tissue becomes infected it will become wet, soft, and inflamed, causing the remainder of the limb to become painful and swollen and increasing the eventual loss of tissue.

It is noteworthy that tendons and bone are resistant to frostbite, whereas nerves, muscles, and particularly blood vessels are highly susceptible.

Treatment

The first and most important principle in treating frostbite is rapid rewarming of the injured part. This can be done by inserting the injured part into either a large bucket or bathtub filled with water that is carefully kept at a temperature between 37 and 40°C. A thermometer should be used to keep a check on the temperature of the water. Rewarming by immersion in 37–40°C water usually takes only 20 minutes; rewarming for a longer period of time is not thought to be helpful. Using water at higher temperatures than those mentioned can be harmful. Rewarming is painful, and if the patient's condition is otherwise good, he or she may be given pain medication. After the injured part is warmed, it should be carefully covered with sterile bandages to minimize any friction or trauma to the injured part. It is critically important to protect the injured tissue at this stage. A frozen part should never be rubbed before, during, or after rewarming.

Other measures that can be used are much the same as those used for a patient with a burn injury. That is, the patient should be given tetanus toxoid, should be placed on penicillin for several days, and can be given intravenous fluids if necessary. The administration of low molecular weight dextran to help improve circulation to the injured part and heparin to prevent further thrombosis of small vessels in the injured area is sometimes carried out and largely depends on the circumstances of the patient. Once the patient is admitted to the hospital, the use of alpha-blocking drugs and sympathectomy may be considered. Finally, one should never debride or amputate any tissue because it is very difficult at first to determine eventual viability in a cold-injured extremity. The prognosis in most cases of frostbite is excellent.

TRENCH FOOT AND IMMERSION FOOT

Trench foot and immersion foot are the subacute and chronic variations of frostbite. The eventual tissue injury can be as severe as with frostbite, and therefore these injuries should be cared for in the same way. Trench foot and immersion foot are rare in civilian life.

SUGGESTED READINGS

Baxter CR: Fluid volume and electrolyte changes of the early postburn period. *Clin Plast Surg* 1974; 1:693.

Boswick JA: Symposium on burns. *Surg Clin North Am* 1978; 58.

Moore FD: The body-weight burn budget. *Surg Clin North Am* 1970; 50:1249.

Renler JB: Pathophysiology, clinical settings and management. *Ann Intern Med* 1978; 89:519.

Towne WD, Geiss WP, Yones HO et al: Intractable ventricular fibrillation associated with profound accidental hypothermia. *N Engl J Med* 1972; 287:1135.

Washburn B: Frostbite. *N Engl J Med* 1962; 266:974.

Zikria BA, Budd DC, Flock F, Ferrer JM: What is clinical smoke poisoning? *Ann Surg* 1975; 181:151.

26
RADIATION INJURY

David E. Drum
Carol B. Jankowski

Accidental injuries involving radiation are rare. Radiation exposure, skin or wound contamination, and inhalation or ingestion may occur alone or in combination as a consequence of a number of mishaps during the following activities: (1) transportation of radioactive materials, (2) use of radioisotopes or radiation sources in medical research or treatment, (3) commercial use of radiation sources for radiography, (4) operation of radiation-producing machines such as accelerators or cyclotrons, (5) noncombat military operations, and (6) operation of research or commercial nuclear reactors. The Joint Commission on Accreditation of Hospitals, which recognizes these potential sources of radiation accidents, requires all hospital emergency rooms to have a written procedure for treating patients exposed to or contaminated by radioactivity. Because the initial emergency care of such victims and precautions for the personnel present at the accident site may be critical, it is essential that every health care provider be familiar with the principles of handling such problems.

CLINICOPATHOLOGIC CONSIDERATIONS

Physical Biology of Radiation Injury

RADIATION DEFINITIONS

Radiation is energy in the form of particles or electromagnetic waves. *Alpha* and *beta particles* are charged emissions from the nuclei of radioactive atoms; *neutrons* are uncharged particles of the same origin. *Gamma rays,* also known as photons and physically identical to x-rays, are a kind of high-energy nonparticulate radiation of the electromagnetic spectrum. *Radioisotopes* are unstable forms of elements that emit radiation. Each isotope has a characteristic rate of decay described by its half-life, a unique array of radioactive emissions, and physiologic properties defined by its elemental nature.

The quantity of any radioisotope is measured in *curies* (Ci), a unit representing 3.7×10^{10} radioactive disintegrations per second. Radiation exposure is quantified in terms of the *roentgen* (R), a measure of ionization produced in air. The *rad* is a measure of absorbed dose determined by the nature of the radiation and by the characteristics of the tissue being irradiated. The *rem* (roentgen equivalent-man) is a special unit of absorbed dose used to indicate the biologic consequences of a given absorbed dose. For most beta, gamma, and x-rays of low energy, the rem is used as if it were equivalent to the rad.*

Because radiation cannot be identified by any of our senses, instruments such as Geiger-Müller counters are necessary for detecting the presence of radiation and are calibrated either in counts per minute (cpm) or milliroentgens per hour (mR/hr). The film badge or thermoluminescent dosimeter (TLD) worn by radiation workers registers cumulative radiation exposure in milliroentgens. Other dosimeters often worn by radiation workers or emergency personnel working with radioactivity include pen dosimeters, which allow an immediate readout of cumulative exposure, and ring badges, which more accurately reflect finger exposures.

PATHOGENESIS OF RADIATION INJURIES

The biologic consequences of radiation depend somewhat on the type of radiation involved. Charged particles of low energy interact with tissues very rapidly and deposit most of their energy in the skin; generally they are not dangerous unless their parent isotopes gain entrance into the body by inhalation or ingestion. For example, alpha particles emitted by heavy transuranic isotopes such as uranium 238, have a maximum range of less than 1 mm in tissue and will not penetrate even the outer layers of skin. The smaller beta particles are attenuated within several millimeters of tissue. Tritium (H3), the best known beta emitter, is the isotope most commonly used in research and is the most abundant component of low-level radioactive waste.

Neutrons are an extremely dangerous form of radiation and are usually generated either in a reactor or by high-energy x-ray machines or linear accelerators. They cause exposure damage only, never contamination, and hence do not require precautions in the emergency room.

Gamma rays and machine-produced x-rays, are highly penetrating, reach all parts of the body with increasingly hazardous effects as the exposure increases, and are the most common source of accidental overexposures. Many radioisotopes emit mixed radiation; for example, iodine 131 decay produces both gamma and beta emissions.

The direct cellular effect of radiation is to ionize or dissociate

---

*The following new universal units are now supplanting all of those mentioned above: 1 becquerel (Bq) = second^{-1} $\simeq$ 2.7×10^{-11} Ci; 1 gray (Gy) = 100 rad; 1 sievert (Sv) = 100 rem.

water molecules to form reactive radical species with unpaired electrons. These then destroy parts of protein side chains or DNA molecules, disrupting normal cell function. Thus, tissues most susceptible to radiation are those that depend on rapid turnover of nucleic acids and on proper control functions within the cells, that is, the bone marrow, the gastrointestinal (GI) epithelium, and the developing gametes. One other important consequence of radiation injury is deposition of heat in the tissues. At low doses this is dissipated through normal homeostatic mechanisms, much as is the heat of the sun. At high doses heat accompanying radiation can produce cellular damage resulting in swelling of cells and enhanced permeability of small blood vessels.

Types of Radiation Injury

Radiation injury may result from two circumstances: (1) accidental *exposure* to a large radioactive source or radiation field or (2) *contamination,* either internally or externally, caused by the presence of radioactive gas, liquid, or particulate material within or on the body. The distinctions must be clear because management differs markedly.

WHOLE BODY EXPOSURES

Perennially, the most frequent radiation accidents have been the overexposure of industrial workers to unshielded radioactive sources (cobalt 60, cesium 137, iridium 192). These accidents have occurred at industries using sealed radioisotope sources for radiography or sterilization. Within seconds or minutes, depending on the level of radioactivity, the workers may receive a whole body dose requiring definitive medical treatment. An approximate estimate of absorbed dose can usually be made by the industrial health physicist at the scene and by quick processing of the victim's dosimeter. More rarely, explosions at weapons research or reprocessing facilities have caused fatal exposures along with equally fatal blast and thermal injuries.

LOCAL EXPOSURES

Overexposures to extremities, especially hands, are not uncommon, are usually not disabling, and are probably frequently unreported. They arise from carelessness during industrial radiography (shipbuilding and metal fabrication), x-ray diffraction work, power plant maintenance, and handling of accelerator target materials. Generally no other significant injuries accompany localized radiation overexposures.

INTERNAL CONTAMINATION

Radioactive material may gain entrance to the body by way of inhalation (e.g., during a fire or explosion), ingestion (i.e, oral intake of accidental, therapeutic, or suicidal origin), and absorption from an open wound, a burn, or a puncture wound. Internal contamination should elicit prompt therapeutic measures to prevent permanent deposition within a critical organ.

EXTERNAL CONTAMINATION

External contamination denotes the presence of radioactive material on the body or clothes of the victim, or in a wound, or complicating a burn. There may be embedded radioactive fragments or particles emitting considerable radiation. The entire outer body may be contaminated, or only a single extremity may be involved. Surface contamination is generally of less medical significance to the patient than acute exposure or ingestion, but it is necessary to conduct appropriate decontamination procedures for the following reasons: (1) to prevent further radiation and internal contamination of the patient, (2) to minimize exposures of attending staff, (3) to prevent spread of radioactive materials elsewhere, and (4) to document, by sampling, the nature and location of radioisotopes contributing to surface contamination.

Accidental contact of the skin with radioactive material in liquid commonly occurs during laboratory and maintenance work in hospitals, universities, and many industries. Serious contamination would be anticipated only in situations of an explosion, valve leakage, apparatus breakage, fall into a contaminated area, or container rupture. Transportation accidents involving trucks carrying medical isotopes or contaminated ion-exchange resins from nuclear power plants offer a potential contamination hazard.

PLANNING AND ORGANIZING MANAGEMENT

Whole Body Exposures

Because patients whose injury is simply overexposure to radiation are not in any way radioactive, initial management can be accomplished within the framework of general emergency room practice. If the radiation dose is estimated to be greater than 150–200 rem, plans should be made to provide a sterile environment with concomitant support systems for the patient. This may require that the patient be transferred to a medical center equipped with reverse isolation units.

Internal Contamination

Patients who have ingested or inhaled radioactive material also may be treated in the emergency room without special precautions if there is no possibility of external contamination. Someone familiar with radiation survey instruments should be available in case such measurements are necessary. The gamma cameras located in all nuclear medicine departments should be used to identify the internal location of significant contaminants.

A whole body counter may be useful for detecting very minimal quantities of radioisotopes, but its use could be delayed several days. Moreover, the presence of *any* external or intraluminal gastrointestinal contamination would interfere with interpretation of data from whole body counting.

External Contamination

Managing patients with surface contamination is quite different from managing those with exposures or internal contamination alone. It requires coordination of several health care disciplines and careful preparation of the treatment area. Preparation and logistical responsibilities generally are assigned to the nursing service. In an emergency, the physician may have to fulfill or delegate many roles; these roles ideally may be segregated as follows: (1) medical—to direct the patient's management; (2) radiology—to interpret radiation measurements and to ensure staff protection (A health physicist or radiology technologist who is familiar with survey meters could serve as monitoring technician. Many firemen and police personnel have been trained to use survey meters, although they may be unfamiliar with the interpretation of the measurements.); (3) nursing—to give direct patient care and provide overall logistical support; (4) maintenance—to set up and isolate an emergency treatment area and to assist with the final cleanup after completion of the emergency; (5) security—to restrict public access to the accident site or to the emergency room during the initial excitement; (6) public relations—to provide the news media with accurate information concerning the casualty.

Once the patient is medically stable, either local officials or hospital administrators may request assistance, if needed, from their state departments of public health or from the Regional Coordinating Office for Radiological Emergency Assistance of the U.S. Department of Energy. Consultation is also available by phone directly from the Radiation Emergency Treatment Center at Oak Ridge, Tennessee. If the injury occurs offsite, (e.g., a highway accident), emergency medical care would take priority, and the area should be immediately secured until

radiation surveys establish the presence or absence of area contamination.

Because most medical personnel are unfamiliar with the procedures of dealing with contaminated radiation casualties, it is essential that a written procedure manual delineating detailed job descriptions be available. Periodic drills involving scenarios with contamination should be conducted by health centers or emergency teams who may conceivably attend accident victims.

RADIATION EMERGENCY TREATMENT AREA

It is preferable to use a treatment area or room remote from other patients as the radiation emergency treatment area (REA), but there should be ready access to emergency equipment and supplies. A marked buffer zone should be designated adjacent to the REA to permit the receipt of needed supplies and discharge of samples and contaminated materials. Ideally, such an area designed as part of an emergency department would have a separate negative pressure air circulation to filter particulates selectively and thereby prevent spread of airborne contaminants. Control of access to the area is necessary to prevent interference by or contamination of nonessential people. Warm running water is essential for decontaminating the patient.

NOTIFICATION OF THE ACCIDENT

When possible, it is important to ascertain from the accident site personnel whether contamination is present, what isotopes were involved, and whether there was major whole body exposure. When the nature of the accident is unknown, preparations must be made to deal with the presence of surface radioactivity. If radioiodine is a suspected contaminant, such as in any nuclear power plant accident or in a thyroid laboratory accident, all attending personnel should take potassium iodide (KI) solution in advance. For unannounced or undefined radiation casualties, it is advisable to keep the victim in the ambulance or at the accident site, depending upon his or her medical status, until the area and personnel are adequately protected. If medical attention must be given or if contamination is discovered after admission to the hospital, any area through which the victim has passed must be considered contaminated.

PREPARATION OF THE RADIATION EMERGENCY AREA

The focus of area preparation is the provision for strict containment of all radioactive materials and the assembly of essential emergency supplies. Ideally the floor or topsoil of the area should be covered to prevent contamination, and plastic bags should be available in which to put clothing and rags or towels. Used wash water may be collected from the stretcher top pan in large plastic containers for later radionuclide analysis and disposal. Radiation survey meters, with probes covered by plastic wrap to prevent contamination, should be available and operational in order that frequent radiation surveys can be made.

Details of protective measures by the medical staff should be modified only by the radiation specialist on site. Personnel in direct contact with the victim will need protective clothing, such as double gowns, plastic aprons, head and shoe coverings, masks, and double gloves. Although this clothing does not protect against penetrating radiation, it does prevent skin and airway contamination. All personnel should use film or TLD badges, and those with close contact should wear ring badges and pen dosimeters if anticipated surface radiation is greater than 50 mR/hr.

EVALUATION AND INITIAL TREATMENT

General Considerations

In a radiation emergency there are four medical objectives; in order of priority they are as follows: (1) to establish adequate airway, respiratory, and circulatory functions; (2) to minimize any internal contamination that may increase the patient's later risk of leukemia or other cancer; (3) to minimize spread of unsealed radioisotopic contamination; and (4) to evaluate and treat the acute radiation syndrome.

Immediate care for the seriously injured patient should follow standard medical practice; secondary consideration should be for the patient's surface radiation levels. It would be rare that sufficient surface contamination would be present so as to preclude life-saving emergency care.

If surface contamination is present, ambulatory patients may remove it by taking a shower and washing with soap and water after sampling of the skin surface is completed. A large pan with controlled drainage fitted on top of a mobile stretcher should be used for the more seriously injured victim who must be washed down while injuries are being treated. After decontamination, the question arises of whether the washings should be contained or should be discharged into the sanitary sewer system. There are no statutory limits to sewer disposal of contaminated washings *from a patient* in a general hospital. In addition, radioisotopes disposed of in such a manner may be integrated theoretically over an entire year's volume of sewer water output. Hence, it would be extremely unlikely that in-

stitutional disposal limits for even occupational activities would ever be exceeded.

STABILIZATION

The first action when dealing with any radiation accident is to ensure that the patient is medically stable, that is, circulation is intact, airway is open, and immediately life-threatening conditions are corrected (Fig. 26.1). While major life-support measures are being initiated, a quick report outlining the injuries and nature of radiation exposure and contamination may be elicited from accompanying attendants or police officers. It should be determined if the level of radioactivity is sufficient to be hazardous to attending staff; it is highly unlikely that surface contamination would emit enough radiation to present an immediate health hazard. Only a metal fragment or foreign body (e.g., cobalt 60) could be so highly radioactive as to require immediate removal. Priority for treating injuries before decontamination depends on the judgment of the emergency physician in consultation with available radiation experts.

Reassurance of the victim, an essential step, is especially important because the victim may not understand the need for extraordinary precautions and may be deeply concerned about the consequences of the exposure depite the absence of any symptoms. Radiation is not perceived by the human senses; even fatal whole body exposures may have no early specific physical findings. Extreme exposures (>500 R) to extremities may cause later erythema.

RADIATION SURVEYING AND SAMPLING OF THE CONTAMINATED CASUALTY

Initially, the entire body is surveyed in detail in order to determine the extent and location of radioactivity. A probe should be passed *slowly* over the surface, and at the same distance, approximately 3–5 cm, from the skin. Readings should be recorded on a body chart analogous to a burn diagram. Most contamination will be removed when the victim's outer clothes and shoes are removed and are placed in plastic bags. Swab samples are then taken from all body orifices, those skin areas exhibiting excess radiation measurements, and any wounds. Clippings of hair, paper tissues into which the nose is blown, and samples of clothing and metal accessories such as a ring or watch are useful sources for identifying the specific contaminating radionuclide and whether neutrons were involved in the exposure. These samples are also important because alpha and low-energy beta particles may not be detected by conventional survey equipment. Samples should be labeled

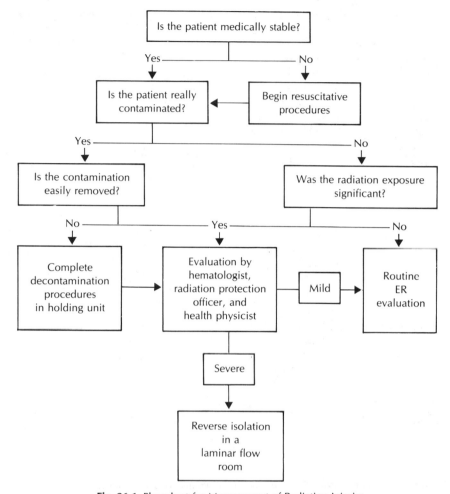

Fig. 26.1 Flowchart for Management of Radiation Injuries.

according to their sites of origin, placed in glass or plastic containers and identified as radioactive for later analysis. The identifying number for each sample should be written on the patient's body chart to identify the origin of the samples. Most general hospitals have laboratory radioisotope counters capable of detecting the presence (not the specific type) of gamma-emitting isotopes.

DECONTAMINATION

Careful and prolonged washing of body surfaces should eliminate all but a trace of contamination. It is essential that contaminated wash water not be internalized by mouth or other orifices. Irrigation of the eyes should be done so as to avoid ingestion.

If there is a serious open wound or burn, the area should be considered contaminated until sampling proves otherwise. The wound should be decontaminated before the rest of the body by irrigation and débridement such as would be appropriate in any case. When the area is clean it should be temporarily sealed off by plastic wrap to avoid recontamination while washing off other areas. Further removal of radioactivity is accomplished by washing the body surface with any mild detergent in lukewarm water. Soft brushes or 4 × 4's can be used on the skin; care must be taken not to abrade the skin, which would allow the radioactive material to enter the body.

Irrigation of nose and ears with water should follow general procedures, and care should be taken to save all washings for analysis. Hair may require several washings and even trimming. Frequent surveys will rapidly determine the progress in removing contaminants. If residual radioactivity (i.e., more than twice true background cpm or 0.02 mR/hr) remains on the surface after several minutes of washing, the area may be covered with plastic wrap and labeled as slightly radioactive. Final decontamination may be conducted later with reducing, oxidizing, or chelating agents, depending upon the nature of the contaminating radioisotope and advice from radiation medical specialists.

PERSONNEL MONITORING AND GENERAL CLEANUP

Once the patient is finally decontaminated and monitoring shows little more than background radiation levels, the patient may be transferred without precautions to an area for definitive care of any injuries. Strictest conformance to measures for containment of residual radioactivity in the REA must be followed. The attending staff should be carefully surveyed for radioactivity before and after degowning. All supplies, linens, and equipment that have been in close proximity of the patient should be secured in plastic bags that are surveyed and clearly marked as potentially radioactive. These materials should be removed to the radioactive waste disposal room of the hospital or picked up by government or industry representatives.

MINIMIZING RADIATION EXPOSURE TO ATTENDING PERSONNEL

Many procedures for handling a patient with contaminated radiation are no different from those for handling a patient suspected of hepatitis or meningococcemia. It is the presence of radioactivity that uniquely distinguishes this care. Its hazard, albeit minor in the short run, is continuous and cannot be neutralized. Throughout the care of such a victim an underlying legitimate concern of staff is that of personal radiation exposure. However, it is most unlikely that any accident victim would ever exhibit surface radiation levels sufficient to cause emergency personnel to receive exposures greater than statutory limits for nonoccupationally exposed workers.

For patients who are extensively contaminated or who have a highly radioactive fragment, *mimimizing time* of exposure and *maximizing distance* from the patient are extremely effective protective measures. Because most significant contaminants emit medium-energy gamma rays, lead aprons are *not* effective protective measures.

TABLE 26.1 Working Time Limits for 125 mR Exposure at a Distance of 1.5 Ft

Survey Meter Reading[a]		
cpm	mR/hr	Time Personnel May Work (hr)
30,000	10	12.5
75,000	25	5
300,000	100	1.25

[a]The relationship of counts per minute (cpm) and milliroentgens per hour (mR/hr) varies according to the nature of the radiation source and the calibration of the survey meter.

As shown in Table 26.1, the radiation survey information given by the survey meter is a useful approximate guide to the time that attending personnel may be permitted to work safely near the patient. Needless to say, an offscale survey meter reading should *always* be interpreted as "Danger—High Radiation Field—Move Away" until proven otherwise.

Clinical Settings

WHOLE BODY EXPOSURES

The acute affects of radiation exposure on the body should rarely ever contribute to symptoms or treatment needs in the early minutes after an exposure. Treatment of the victim's other injuries, if present, should predominate. Exposures below 100 R rarely cause any physiologic symptoms, but the victim may be extremely upset by the situation. His acute anxiety may be mistakenly interpreted as a symptom of more severe overexposure; therefore, it is important to get a calculated estimate of exposure dose. If the exposure is significant (> 50–100 R), then evaluation by a hematologist or other health physics professional is warranted to decide whether and when appropriate supportive measures should be instituted.

Exposures in the range of 200–400 R will generally produce early signs of the acute radiation syndrome, including nausea, vomiting, and fever. A baseline complete blood cell count (CBC) should be drawn as soon as possible. The absolute lymphocyte count is the most practical and effective biologic dosimeter of the radiation exposure and indicator of prognosis. A lymphocyte count less than 1,500 within 48 hours indicates a significant exposure; after severe exposures, the lymphocyte count may dip beneath 500, indicating a poor prognosis. Significant radiation exposures may require subsequent reverse isolation in a special facility, such as a laminar airflow room, designed to minimize infection.

At exposures over 1,200 R to the whole body, prognosis is poor and survival may not be expected even with the best treatment. Such an exposure should be evident very early by central nervous system damage manifest as lethargy, somnolence, ataxia, and seizures, which obviously complicates the differential diagnosis.

LOCAL EXPOSURES

Regional exposures, such as that restricted to a hand, are the most common single form of radiation accidents; they never constitute a therapeutic emergency. Redness, swelling, and blistering indicate very severe injury; slow ischemic necrosis will proceed for months. Local exposures of less severity (< 500 R) may not exhibit any topical changes at first, but the patient should be followed-up for some time.

Initial treatment of patients with local exposures is nonspecific and identical to that of patients with burns of similar severity.

The patient should be counseled in regard to the need for long-term follow-up. Progressive friability and necrosis requiring amputation may develop months after hand or foot exposures over 1,000 R.

INTERNAL CONTAMINATION

Table 26.2 summarizes the likely sources for the most common isotopes implicated in internal contamination. It should be emphasized that deliberate therapeutic (e.g., iodine 131 for thyroid cancer) and diagnostic (e.g., technetium 99m for bone scans) internal contamination are commonplace in medical practice. The biologic hazards of internalization become significant with those radioisotopes that have long half-lives and that emit beta and/or alpha particles. Pulmonary deposition may be anticipated during a fire if respiratory protective devices are not available or properly used.

If a victim accidentally inhales or swallows radioactive gas,

TABLE 26.2 Sources and Treatment of Internal Contamination

Radionuclide				Recommended Treatment	
Class	Example	Likely Accident Sources		Alert Patient	Unconscious/ Airway Injury
Iodines	Iodine 131	Hospital; transport; reactor; laboratory		SS KI, 10 drops	$NaClO_4$, 200 mg IV
Tritium	Hydrogen 3	Reactor coolant; laboratories		Water diuresis	Water diuresis
Noble gas	Xenon 133	Hospital; reactor		Air ventilation	Air ventilation
Diagnostic	Technetium 99m	Hospital; transport		Water diuresis	Water diuresis
Fission products	Cesium 137	Reactor coolant or deionizers		Emesis, purgatives, Bio-Rex 40,[1] 10 g every 4 hr p.o.	Lavage, purgatives; Bio-Rex 40, 10 g every 4 hr
	Strontium 90	Reactor coolant or deionizers		Emesis; purgatives; Gaviscon,[2] 40 ml every 2 hr	Lavage, purgatives; Gaviscon, 40 ml every 2 hr
Corrosion products	Manganese 54	Reactor coolant or deionizers		Emesis; purgatives	Lavage; purgatives
	Cobalt 60	Reactor coolant or deionizers		Emesis; purgatives	Lavage, purgatives
Uranium	Uranium 238	Metallurgical laboratories; mines		$NaHCO_3$, 45 mEq IV every 4 hr	Same as for an alert patient
Transuranics	Plutonium 239	Reprocessing plants; weapons accident		Zn-DTPA, 1 g IV in 500 ml 5% D/W in 30 min	Same as for an alert patient
	Americium 241	Reprocessing plants; weapons accident		Zn-DTPA, 1 g IV in 500 ml 5% D/W in 30 min	Same as for an alert patient

[1] A strong cation exchange resin.

[2] An aluminum hydroxide-magnesium carbonate antacid containing sorbitol, sodium alginate, and edetate sodium.

fluid, or particulate matter (as in a fire), it is essential that procedures be initiated *immediately* to eliminate the radio-active material from the body. Therapy is dependent upon the particular radioisotope involved (Table 26.2). A careful history may elicit the isotopes involved; research laboratories primarily use tritium (H3), carbon 14, and iodine isotopes. A truck delivering medical diagnostic isotopes may contain technetium 99m, molybdenum 99, gallium 67, and thallium 201. Metallurgical industries use depleted uranium, a flammable heavy metal that emits low energy x-rays.

Treatment generally involves water diuresis, emesis or lavage, purgation, or administration of a specific blocking or chelating agent. For example, if radioiodine is a suspected contaminant, saturated solution of potassium iodide, 10 drops in liquid, is administered orally as soon as possible. For patients who are unconscious or have head injuries, sodium perchlorate (200 mg intravenously) is effective for blocking any uptake of radioiodine by the thyroid gland.

Most inhaled particulates are coughed up and reach the gastrointestinal tract. For this reason, much of the treatment effort is aimed at emptying the stomach or intestines and preventing absorption (see Chapter 42).

Patients with internal contamination alone do not emit sufficient radiation to require attending medical personnel to use protective measures. All body waste fluids and serial blood samples should be handled with gloves, labeled as radioactive, and saved for later analysis to help determine the quantity of material internalized. Contaminated wounds must be irrigated thoroughly with a surgical detergent, and only repeated sampling and analysis can determine when the wound is completely decontaminated. Puncture wounds that deposit long-lived alpha emitters, such as americium 241, may require excision to remove the radioactive source.

SUMMARY

Emergency management of accident victims with skin areas contaminated by radioactive material is based on goals of minimizing further injury to the patient, containment of contaminating nuclides, and provision of a safe environment for attending personnel. The procedures are guided by use of radiation survey meters, and prior written plans periodically tested in drills are essential for effective action.

Radiation injuries caused by accidental exposures or internal contamination require medical treatment appropriate to the severity of exposure and specific isotopes involved and do not require special efforts to protect the medical staff. No radiation injury ever preempts immediate airway and circulatory support. The consultative services of radiation medical specialists are available and should be planned for in advance.

SUGGESTED READINGS

Adelstein SJ, Dealy JB: Hematological responses to human body irradiation. *Am J Roentgenol* 1965; 93:927–934.

Andrews GA: Hematologic data for estimating injury in radiation accidents. Prepared for International Workshop on Recent Advances in Medical Management in Radiation Accidents, Washington, D.C. September 17–19, 1973.

Hübner KF, Fry SA: *The Medical Basis for Radiation Accident Preparedness.* New York, Elsevier North-Holland Inc, 1980.

International Atomic Energy Agency: *Manual on Early Medical Treatment of Possible Radiation Injury,* Safety Series 47. Vienna, IAEA, 1978.

International Commission on Radiological Protection: *The Principles and General Procedures for Handling Emergency and Accidental Exposures of Workers,* Publication 28. Elmsford, NY, Pergamon Press, 1978.

Karas SJ, Stanbury JB: Fatal radiation syndrome from an accidental nuclear excursion. *N Engl J Med* 1965; 272:755–761.

Leonard RB, Ricks RC: Emergency department radiation accident protocol. *Ann Emerg Med* 1980; 9:462–470.

Lincoln TA: Importance of initial management of persons internally contaminated with radionuclides. *Am Ind Hyg Assoc J* 1976; 37:16–21.

Lushbaugh CC, Hübner KF, Ricks RC: Medical aspects of nuclear radiation emergencies. *Emergency* 1978; 10:32–35.

Mettler FA, Rocco FG, Junkins RL: The role of EMTs in radiation accidents. *Emerg Med Serv* 1977; 6:22–25.

National Council on Radiation Protection and Measurements: *Management of Persons Accidentally Contaminated with Radionuclides,* Report No 65. Washington, D.C. NCRP, 1980.

Steidley KD, Seik GS, Oullete R: Another Co-60 hot cell accident. *Health Phys* 1979; 36:437–441.

OTHER ACUTE DISORDERS

PART III

27

ENDOCRINE AND METABOLIC EMERGENCIES

Lee A. Witters

The most common emergencies in endocrinology and metabolism are crises in diabetes mellitus, alcoholic ketoacidosis, lactic acidosis, hypercalcemia, and adrenal insufficiency. Other less common emergencies are referenced in the selected readings at the end of this chapter.

CRISES IN DIABETES MELLITUS

Diabetic Ketoacidosis

Diabetic ketoacidosis (DKA) may occur in three groups of patients. Most commonly, it is seen in patients with known insulin-dependent diabetes, either juvenile or adult onset. The second group consists of patients with known mild diabetes who develop DKA in association with an intercurrent stressful illness. The third group consists of undiagnosed diabetics for whom DKA may be the initial presentation of the disease. In fact, 50% of juvenile-onset diabetics present initially with DKA.

PATHOPHYSIOLOGY

Diabetic ketoacidosis may be thought of as a syndrome of insulin deficiency that metabolically mimics accelerated starvation. But other hormonal abnormalities, especially hyperglucagonemia, increased activity of the sympathetic nervous system through catecholamines, and increased cortisol secretion, are also associated with its evolution. The consequences of these hormonal changes are shown in Figure 27.1. Two major metabolic derangements—hyperglycemia and ketosis—lead to the clinical evolution of DKA.

Hyperglycemia results from a decrease in glucose uptake in the absence of insulin by muscle and adipose tissue and from an increase in hepatic gluconeogenesis, even if hyperglycemia is present. The major consequence of this sustained hyperglycemia is hypertonic dehydration. Osmotic diuresis as a result of glucosuria leads to a loss of water that exceeds the losses of sodium and potassium, and the attendant increase in serum osmolality causes cellular water to be depleted. Prolonged diuresis eventually results in a reduction of extracellular fluid volume, which in turn leads to a decrease in the glomerular filtration rate. A patient who weighs 70 kg, for example, suffers renal losses of 5–8 liters of water, 350–600 mEq of sodium, and 200–400 mEq of potassium.

Ketosis, the second metabolic derangement in DKA, results from increases in the blood levels of acetoacetic acid, β-hydroxybutyric acid, and acetone. Without insulin and with increased levels of glucagon, catecholamines, and cortisol, lipolysis in adipose tissue is unrestrained and, as a consequence, the level of circulating free fatty acids increases. These fatty acids reach the liver, where because of the hormonal milieu present in DKA they are preferentially converted to ketones, which are liberated into the plasma. The ketonemia is further heightened by a decrease in the peripheral use of ketones, principally by muscle. If elevated levels of acetoacetic acid and β-hydroxybutyric acid are sustained, serum bicarbonate is depleted and metabolic acidosis results. Ketonuria, by its obligate cation excretion, contributes to the loss of electrolytes.

DIAGNOSIS

The symptoms of DKA are generally nonspecific and thus should not be the basis of the definitive diagnosis. The usual syndrome evolves over 2–4 days. The "polys" (polyuria and polydipsia) may predominate, and vision may be blurred. The patient may have lost weight before the first episode of DKA. Gastrointestinal complaints, especially nausea and vomiting, are common. Any diabetic who experiences significant nausea and vomiting requires special attention; the disruption of oral intake of food and fluid may necessitate intravenous therapy and possibly hospitalization, even if full-blown DKA is not yet present. Abdominal pain mimicking a variety of acute intraabdominal illnesses is occasionally present, especially in children, and changes in mental status, from mild depression of consciousness to frank coma, may occur.

A physical examination likewise usually uncovers only nonspecific signs. Dehydration, signaled by loss of skin turgor and absence of axillary sweat, is common. If fluid and electrolyte losses have been extreme, hypotension and tachycardia may be noted, but the skin is, nevertheless, warm, flushed, and dry. Hyperventilation (Kussmaul respirations), suggestive though it is, is not a definitive sign since it may accompany any form of metabolic acidosis or cardiopulmonary disease. The absence of hyperventilation, however, may portend severe metabolic acidosis (pH < 7). The odor of acetone on the breath, if detected, may be very helpful in diagnosing DKA. Alteration

501

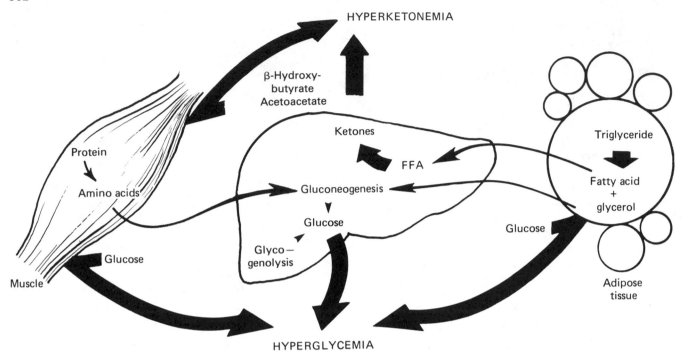

Figure 27.1 Pathogenesis of hyperglycemia and hyperketonemia in diabetic ketoacidosis. Hyperglycemia and hyperketonemia are the two cardinal manifestations of DKA. *Hyperglycemia* results from exaggerated glucose output from the liver through accelerated glycogenolysis and gluconeogenesis (principally from amino acids and lactate derived from muscle and from glycerol derived from adipose tissue) and from diminished peripheral glucose utilization (muscle and adipose tissue) in the absence of insulin. *Hyperketonemia* results from enhanced lipolysis of adipose tissue to fatty acid, preferential conversion of free fatty acids to ketones (β-hydroxybutyrate, acetoacetate) in the liver and diminished peripheral utilization of ketones (muscle).

in mental status is not unusual, but frank coma and focal neurologic signs are rare. This is in contrast to hyperosmolar nonketotic coma, in which these neurologic changes occur frequently, and their appearance should suggest a diagnosis other than DKA. Temperature elevation hardly ever occurs in patients with uncomplicated DKA, so a fever should be regarded as evidence of infection until proven otherwise.

During the initial evaluation of the patient, the physician should keep in mind the *precipitating causes* of DKA, which are frequently not considered in the enthusiasm of treating this metabolic catastrophe. The mortality from DKA in most of the large studies that have been reported ranges from 5–15%. However, most deaths are due to a concurrent illness; mortality from ketoacidosis alone is only about 1%. Failure to follow a prescribed regimen of insulin therapy may precipitate the syndrome in an insulin-dependent diabetic. Increases in the in-

sulin requirement are necessary to maintain normoglycemia and prevent ketosis during infection, severe illness (acute myocardial infarction, stroke, pancreatitis), surgery, and pregnancy. Infection, which may be occult or seemingly trivial, must always be diligently sought. Certain drugs that influence carbohydrate metabolism, such as potassium-depleting diuretics (thiazides, loop diuretics), corticosteroids, diazoxide, and phenytoin, may precipitate DKA. A rare cause is immunologic insulin resistance; a clue to this disorder is a history of a recently escalating insulin requirement to levels of 200 units/day or more.

LABORATORY EVALUATION

Because clinical signs and symptoms of DKA are nonspecific and nondiagnostic, laboratory testing is essential. The diagnosis should be DKA if *significant ketonemia* is demonstrated in the presence of anion-gap metabolic acidosis. Though hyperglycemia is common, blood sugar level alone is insufficient for making a diagnosis. Venous blood should be drawn; levels of blood sugar, electrolytes, ketones, and blood urea nitrogen (BUN) should be measured, and a complete blood count (CBC) should be obtained. Arterial blood gases and pH should be determined from an arterial blood sample.

The blood sugar level in patients with DKA usually ranges from 400 to 800 mg/dl or higher, with an average of about 600 mg/dl. However, so-called euglycemic DKA has been reported for several patients. Most of these patients have been known insulin-dependent diabetics who continued to take insulin throughout the development of DKA, often with a disruption of oral intake. The blood sugar level in some patients is only minimally elevated, yet in others it is normal or hypoglycemic, even when ketoacidosis has been significant.

Because significant ketonemia is the sine qua non of DKA diagnosis, ketonemia should be tested for by checking the patients nitroprusside reaction (Acetest). Several tablets should be pulverized, each in a separate pile on a piece of filter paper. Serum or plasma obtained from the patient should then be serially diluted in several tubes with normal saline (1:1, 1:2, 1:4, etc.), and 1 or 2 drops applied to the powder. The endpoint should be the dilution that yields the last 4 + reaction (lavender or deep purple); the reaction should not be titered to the smallest observable change. *If a 4 + reaction is present in undiluted serum, DKA with significant ketonemia is virtually certain.* Alcoholic ketoacidosis, which is discussed later in this chapter, may, however, cause an important false-positive reaction. On the other hand, a false-negative reaction may result if DKA and lactic acidosis are present concurrently. In this situation, the measurement of serum ketones by the nitroprusside reaction may be artifactually low because the ratio of β-hydroxybutyric acid to acetoacetic acid is increased. Acetoacetic acid and acetone—but not β-hydroxybutyric acid—are measured by the nitroprusside reaction; if the equilibrium between acetoacetic acid and β-hydroxybutyric acid has shifted in the direction of the latter, as it does when lactic acidosis is present, the measurement of serum ketones by this reaction is spuriously low and the diagnosis of ketoacidosis is masked. Any diabetic who presents with what appears to be lactic acidosis should be suspected of having concurrent ketoacidosis.

Anion-gap metabolic acidosis can be tested for by analyzing serum electrolytes and arterial blood gases. If acidosis is confirmed, it is the anion-gap variety if the concentration of Na^+ plus K^+ is 16 mEq/liter greater than the concentration of Cl^- plus HCO_3^-. The differential diagnosis of anion-gap metabolic acidosis that must be entertained includes not only diabetic ketoacidosis, but alcoholic ketoacidosis, lactic acidosis, uremia, and a variety of toxic ingestions including methanol, ethylene glycol, and paraldehyde.

Other features of laboratory testing are important too. The concentration of sodium in serum may be high, normal, or low. The serum level of potassium is usually normal or slightly elevated; fewer than 5% of patients present with hypokalemia. Regardless of the serum potassium concentration, total body potassium has been depleted, and the condition may be especially severe in patients with initial hypokalemia. Urine tests for sugar and "acetone" are of no value in diagnosing DKA.

THERAPY

There is no fixed therapy for the disorder throughout its course; continuous reevaluation of patient response and laboratory parameters are mandatory during critical care monitoring. A scheme for treating DKA is presented in Table 27.1, which outlines the five therapeutic decisions that must be made repeatedly during the three phases of DKA.

Insulin

The first decision that has to be made is the dosage and route of administration of insulin. Regular crystalline insulin should be used throughout the first two phases until the ketonemia and the acidosis are corrected. In the past, dosage and route of administration were usually chosen empirically. During the initial phase of treatment, these traditional regimens used 50–200 units/dose, given entirely intravenously or divided between intravenous and subcutaneous routes. The advantage of the divided dose is that it achieves an immediate effect that is long lasting; if the intravenous route is used exclusively, insulin must be administered every hour to maintain a therapeutic effect. These large doses were based in part on the premise that severe insulin resistance accompanies DKA. Recent studies using so-called low-dose administration, by an intramuscular or a continuous intravenous infusion route, have demonstrated, however, that such severe resistance is uncommon. It now appears that blood sugar decreases at a fixed rate of 75–125 mg/dl/hr regardless of dosage. More critical than dosage is achieving and maintaining a level of circulating insulin that is adequate to reverse the metabolic abnormalities; this level can usually be achieved by using a low-dose regimen.

Two low-dose regimens have been advocated. The *intramuscular regimen* consists of an initial injection of 10–20 units by intravenous bolus followed by intramuscular dosages of 5–10 units every hour. The equivalent pediatric dosage is 0.25 unit/kg of body weight by intravenous bolus followed by 0.1

TABLE 27.1 Treatment of Diabetic Ketoacidosis

	Phase I	Phase II	Phase III
Insulin	Regular Insulin Traditional regimens 50–200 units/dose Give half IV, half SC q2hr *or* Give all IV q1hr (especially if hypotensive) Low-dose regimens IM: 10–20 units IV initially; then 5–10 units IM q1hr IV: Loading dose: 10–20 units by IV bolus; continuous infusion at 6–8 units/hr (30–40 units in 250 ml saline at 50 ml/hr)	Regular insulin Amount variable (10–25 units) given subcutaneously every 3–4 hr dependent on blood and urine sugar If low-dose regimen used, give SC dose with last IM dose or 1 hr before infusion discontinued	Intermediate-acting insulin (NPH, lente) supplemented by short-acting insulin (regular, semilente) as necessary by blood and urine tests
$H_2O + Na^+$	Normal saline initially 1 liter first hr; then half-normal saline 1 liter q2–3hr	Half-normal saline	Continue orally as necessary
K^+	Do not give until urine output established; then 20–40 mEq/hr as KCl Vigorous early replacement necessary if initial hypokalemia, bicarbonate administration, or digitalis toxicity	Continue at 20–40 mEq/hr IV Must continue to monitor serum K^+, ECG, urine output	Continue orally as necessary
Bicarbonate	Generally not necessary; if shock or very severe acidosis present, may give 1–2 ampules of sodium bicarbonate to raise pH to range of 7.1	No	No
Glucose	None, unless initial blood sugar less than 250 mg/dl	When blood sugar reaches 250–300 mg/dl, begin as 5% dextrose in IV fluids	Establish regular intervals or oral intake; if not able to take orally, IV route must be continued

unit/kg intramuscularly every hour. The initial dose avoids the occasional poor response to the first intramuscular injection. On occasion, the initial intravenous bolus must be repeated if the blood sugar has not decreased at the expected rate within the first 2 hours. The intramuscular route has the advantage of being easy to administer; however, this method probably should not be used if the patient is severely hypotensive, since the intramuscular depot may not be readily absorbed.

The *continuous intravenous infusion regimen* is initiated by a loading intravenous bolus of 10–20 units. Thereafter, administration must be regulated by a continuous-infusion apparatus. Though insulin adheres to the glass bottle and infusion tubing, adding albumin to the insulin solution is probably not necessary if a reasonably concentrated solution (30–40 units of regular insulin in 250 ml of normal saline, given at a rate of 50 ml/hr), which will deliver insulin at 6–8 units/hr, is used.

A disadvantage of the infusion technique is the need to maintain a patent intravenous line and to carefully control the drip rate.

The time of response to either low-dose regimen does not differ substantially from that of the traditional regimens. Blood sugar generally reaches a level of 250 mg/dl in 5–7 hours, and ketoacidosis is corrected in 10–13 hours.

The regimen to follow should be decided upon after weighing the advantages and disadvantages of each. We believe that although the two types of regimens are equally effective in correcting hyperglycemia and ketosis, the low-dose regimens are preferable for treating patients with DKA. They represent the application of sound pathophysiologic principles to the disorder and deciding on the insulin dosage empirically is not necessary. Furthermore, there is evidence that the low-dose regimens are less frequently attended by hypoglycemia and hypokalemia during the later stages of treatment. Nevertheless, no difference in mortality has been demonstrated for patients treated by the traditional regimen and those treated by a low-dose regimen. Regardless of the insulin protocol used, however, the patient's response to therapy must be monitored and the insulin dosage, route, or frequency of administration changed if a therapeutic response is not evident.

Intravenous Fluids

The second decision is the choice of intravenous fluids. A reasonable program is that of infusing 1 liter of normal saline in the first hour in order to expand the extracellular fluid (ECF) volume, followed by half-normal saline at the rate of 1 liter every 2–3 hours (recall that the total water deficit ranges from 5 to 8 liters). Plasma expanders, such as albumin, are occasionally necessary in treating severely hypotensive patients.

Potassium

The third decision is whether to give potassium. Though most patients have normal or slightly elevated serum potassium levels, all have significant total body potassium depletion. Potassium should not be given until urine output is established, but vigorous early treatment is necessary if the patient is initially hypokalemic, if bicarbonate is given, or if an electrocardiogram (ECG) clearly indicates digitalis intoxication. Replacement may be begun at a dosage of 20–40 mEq/hr; close monitoring of serum potassium is essential and dosages must be adjusted as necessary.

Sodium Bicarbonate

The fourth decision is whether to give sodium bicarbonate. Administering sodium bicarbonate to patients with DKA is usually unnecessary; in fact, it may lower the serum level of potassium even further. If the patient is in shock from severe acidosis (pH < 7), sodium bicarbonate may be given—but only until the pH nears 7.1—in order to prevent the life-threatening cardiovascular effects of acidosis. Repeated administration should be avoided. Large doses of sodium bicarbonate intended to return the pH to the normal range rapidly may lead to paradoxical acidosis in the cerebrospinal fluid (CSF).

Glucose

The fifth decision is whether to give glucose. Glucose should not be added to the intravenous fluids when severe hyperglycemia is present. When the patient's blood sugar level reaches 250–300 mg/dl, the fluids should be switched to half-normal saline and 5% dextrose. If the blood sugar level initially is in this range or below, fluid therapy should be begun with solutions containing 5% dextrose.

Phosphate

Some physicians recommend the addition of phosphate replacement during therapy for DKA. This recommendation is based on the frequent finding of hypophosphatemia associated with a depression of erythrocyte 2,3-diphosphoglycerate (2,3-DPG) levels, which theoretically may impair tissue oxygenation. However, despite these observations, recent studies suggest that phosphate repletion neither alters the course of therapy nor affects its ultimate outcome. Indeed, there have been reported cases of hypocalcemia with tetany resulting from phosphate administration. Thus, we would recommend that routine phosphate administration be avoided.

Course of Management

As the patient is improving, the five decisions must be repeated continually. Blood should be tested for blood sugar, electrolytes, and arterial blood gases determined every 2–3 hours. After ketonemia and acidosis have been corrected, insulin administration should be changed to the subcutaneous route to achieve more prolonged action (phase II). Subcutaneous dosages can be given every 3–4 hours; dosages are variable, but 15–25 units/dosage, depending on the blood sugar level, is reasonable. Half-normal saline and potassium replacement should be continued; when the blood sugar level reaches 250–300 mg/dl, intravenous glucose infusion should be begun by changing to a fluid of 5% dextrose in half-normal saline. Preventing hypoglycemia is important.

In phase III, after the DKA has been corrected, an effective insulin dosage must be continued. An intermediate-acting insulin (NPH, lente) should be given to smooth control; it should be supplemented with a short-acting insulin (regular, semilente) administered at regular intervals, as determined by urine and blood tests.

Patients with DKA should be treated with an intensive care approach. A central venous pressure (CVP) line may be helpful while volume is being replaced, especially if the patient's cardiac reserve is impaired. Respiratory function should be monitored; patients with antecedent chronic pulmonary disease may experience respiratory failure as a result of sustained metabolic acidosis. A nasogastric tube aids in the management of the gastric atony commonly seen in patients with DKA; in the obtunded patient, an endotracheal tube must be inserted before gastric intubation. Bladder catheterization should be avoided in the diabetic and used only if the patient is unconscious or unable to void. A metabolic flowsheet detailing vital signs, laboratory parameters, and therapy used throughout the patient's course is mandatory during management. A careful search for precipitating causes is absolutely essential.

Complications of DKA sometime arise. The patient may be in shock on admission. Vigorous correction of volume depletion, acidosis, and hypokalemia is necessary, but other causes of shock should not be ruled out immediately. Irreversible coma is seen but rarely; its pathogenesis is unclear. Complications during the course of therapy are largely iatrogenic; hypoglycemia and hypokalemia can be avoided by careful monitoring and judicious application of therapy. Secondary coma occurs occasionally, and cerebral edema is uncommon.

Hyperosmolar Nonketotic Coma

Hyperosmolar nonketotic coma (HNKC), in contrast with diabetic ketoacidosis, generally occurs in middle-aged or elderly patients. These patients usually suffer from mild or previously undiagnosed diabetes; only rarely does an insulin-dependent diabetic present with HNKC.

PATHOPHYSIOLOGY

Hyperglycemia arises in HNKC by mechanisms similar to those responsible for DKA. However, hyperglycemia accompanied by hyperosmolarity is more severe and results in a greater loss of fluid and electrolytes. Osmotic diuresis is more sustained and leads to severe intracellular and extracellular volume depletion. Glomerular filtration rate falls, and severe azotemia is common. Large amounts of body water (up to 25%), sodium, and potassium may be lost.

Ketonemia is not a feature of HNKC, but the reason is unclear. Some observers have attributed the absence of ketones to lower levels of free fatty acids; others have suggested lower levels of circulating cortisol and growth hormone as the mechanism. Though ketonemia is not present, mild metabolic acidosis is common in HNKC. Acidosis probably results from several factors, including prerenal azotemia and possibly mild lactic acidosis secondary to hypotension.

Patient mortality also distinguishes HNKC from DKA. Most studies report a mortality rate of 40–60% for HNKC, in contrast with 5–15% for DKA. The reasons for the higher mortality rate include more severe fluid and electrolyte losses because of the prolonged development of the syndrome, concomitant serious underlying illnesses, and the fact that the patient population affected is older. The delay in diagnosing HNKC in patients who present with apparent neurologic illness also contributes to the higher mortality rate. Vigilance and awareness in diagnosing the syndrome are therefore essential.

DIAGNOSIS

The symptoms of HNKC are nonspecific. Classically, there is a history of a prodrome of increasing polydipsia and polyuria, which is generally more prolonged in HNKC than in DKA. The neurologic features are among the cardinal manifestations of HNKC. Disturbances in mentation, from drowsiness to confusion, stupor, and frank coma, are the rule. A history of seizures, either focal or generalized, may be elicited. The most common presentation is an apparent neurologic catastrophe, such as a stroke, which the physician must be alert to diagnose.

During the initial evaluation of the patient, the physician must keep in mind the common precipitating factors. Drugs, particularly potassium-depleting diuretics, may be implicated; corticosteroids, phenytoin, and diazoxide have all been associated with HNKC. Intercurrent illness (including infection, particularly gram-negative infections such as pneumonia and pyelonephritis) is not unusual. Myocardial infarction, pancreatitis, or gastrointestinal hemorrhage may precipitate the syndrome. Patients subject to increased glucose intake (e.g., through peritoneal dialysis or hyperalimentation) may develop HNKC. If the patient has experienced fluid loss during the evolution of the syndrome and has had limited access to water (e.g., a debilitated nursing home patient or a patient with severe burns), the syndrome may be accentuated. A careful search for such underlying causes is absolutely essential since they contribute significantly to the high mortality rate from HNKC.

LABORATORY EVALUATION

When the blood sugar level is greater than 600 mg/dl, the serum osmolarity is greater than 350 mosm/liter, and ketones measure less than 4+ in undiluted serum, HNKC is present. The blood sugar level of HNKC patients averages 1,000 mg/dl, but values higher than 3,000 mg/dl have been reported. The Dextrostix test may assist in rapidly estimating a very high blood sugar level. Serum osmolality should be determined by the method of freezing point depression; if facilities for this procedure are not readily available, the following formula yields a reasonably accurate estimation of osmolality:

$$\text{Serum osmolality (mosm/liter)} = 2(Na^+ + K^+) + \frac{\text{Blood sugar}}{18} + \frac{\text{BUN}}{2.8}$$

The serum level of sodium is generally normal to high, though hyponatremia is sometimes present early in the illness. Potassium concentration is normal or slightly elevated. Despite the serum values of sodium and potassium, their total body levels are significantly depleted. Sodium bicarbonate concentration, reflecting metabolic acidosis, may be slightly low. Renal function, determined by BUN and creatinine measurements, is invariably diminished (initially BUN is usually between 60 and 90 mg/dl). This diminution of renal function is in large part secondary to severe dehydration; however, once HNKC is corrected, many patients have a chronic mild reduction in creatinine clearance. The hematocrit may be spuriously elevated or deceptively normal, but it may fall when therapy begins.

THERAPY

Many of the therapeutic principles detailed in the section on DKA apply to patients with HNKC as well. Critical care monitoring and close attention to detail are absolutely essential.

Insulin therapy has been largely empirical in the past. Whereas some patients have required small doses of insulin, others have seemed to need large ones. These observations should be reinterpreted in light of recent data on low-dose insulin regimens. Low-dose regimens, administered according to the methods detailed in the section on DKA, have been successful in treating patients with HNKC and are certainly acceptable choices of therapy, by either the intramuscular or the continuous intravenous infusion route. More traditional regimens, using 50–100 units of insulin intravenously as a bolus as an initial dose, have been used; subsequent dosages, generally 25–50 units, based on the response of the blood sugar level, have been given every 1–2 hours. A rapid lowering of blood sugar level, accompanied by a rapid decline in serum osmolality, has been associated with transient hypotension as well as with an exacerbation of cerebral symptoms; both effects appear to be mediated by rapid intracellular shifts of water. When the patient's blood sugar level reaches 250–300 mg/dl, glucose should be given intravenously and the fluids and insulin dosages repeated; careful attention should also be given to blood and urine sugar levels.

Fluid and electrolyte therapy is equally important in managing HNKC. Fluid and electrolyte losses are more severe in patients with HNKC than in those with DKA; water loss, averaging 9–12 liters, represents up to 20% of total body weight. In the presence of severe hyperosmolality, the logical choice would appear to be hypotonic fluid, such as half-normal saline. However, ECF volume, already depleted, must be monitored; if insulin therapy corrects hyperglycemia rapidly by translocating glucose into cells, ECF water follows and the result is

further ECF depletion. If the patient shows any evidence of hypotension or vascular collapse, normal saline (1–2 liters) should be given rapidly to correct the circulatory instability; plasma expanders such as albumin may also be administered. After initial therapy with normal saline, half-normal saline may be administered to correct 50% of the estimated water deficit in the first 12 hours. If severe hypernatremia supervenes during this period, 5% dextrose in water (D_5W) may be necessary. Correcting the total deficit in 24–36 hours is the goal, but supplying adequate replacement, 4–5 liters, in the first 12-hour period should be the primary concern.

Potassium replacement is necessary because total body potassium has been depleted. Once a good urine output is established, potassium may be given in the form of potassium chloride, 20–40 mEq/hr, in the intravenous fluids. Again critical care monitoring is essential. It cannot be overstressed that an important part of the treatment of HNKC is the search for a precipitating cause, which so often is the reason for death; infection should be of paramount concern. Chest films, urinalysis, urine cultures, and blood cultures should be obtained routinely for all patients.

After recovery from HNKC, patients should be monitored by urine and blood sugar tests every 4–6 hours. The use of an intermediate-acting insulin supplemented, as necessary, with short-acting insulin is recommended.

Hypoglycemia

Hypoglycemia should be suspected in every comatose patient and in every patient with an acutely altered mental status. Rapid diagnosis and treatment are crucial and may be lifesaving.

DIAGNOSIS

The neurologic manifestations of hypoglycemia are protean, ranging from mild confusion to belligerence to lethargy, stupor, and coma. Focal neurologic signs that mimic stroke syndromes and seizures may be present. Suspicion should be especially high for four groups of patients: insulin-treated diabetics, diabetics on oral agents, patients with acute or chronic ethanolism (with or without liver disease), and patients with apparent adrenal insufficiency.

Hypoglycemia can usually be easily diagnosed by the Dextrostix test; but a blood sample should be taken when this test is made—before therapy—and sent to the laboratory to confirm the diagnosis. Because the treatment of hypoglycemia can be lifesaving for a comatose patient and is not harmful if hypoglycemia is not present, it should be initiated immediately after blood is drawn and not be postponed until the results of the blood test are available. A single ampule of 50% dextrose (50 ml) should be given as an intravenous bolus.

THERAPY

The response to treatment is generally immediate; failure to respond if hypoglycemia has been documented implies either that the hypoglycemia is not of recent onset and has resulted in severe neurologic damage or that the cause of coma is not the hypoglycemia but another condition. Thiamine should be administered simultaneously with glucose to alcoholics who have hypoglycemia. Repeated dosages of 50% glucose or a continuous intravenous infusion of $D_{10}W$ may occasionally be necessary. Patients who present with hypoglycemia should be observed carefully after initial treatment. Unless overinsulinization is implicated as the cause of coma, patients with hypoglycemia should be admitted to the hospital for further evaluation. This is especially true for diabetics taking sulfonylureas, in which hypoglycemia may be protracted or recurrent over several days.

ALCOHOLIC KETOACIDOSIS

The syndrome of alcoholic ketoacidosis, though not a crisis as is diabetes mellitus, deserves mention because it is common and can be confused with diabetic ketoacidosis. Alcoholic ketoacidosis, which usually occurs in nondiabetic patients, tends to be triggered by binge drinking in those who typically have histories of heavy chronic ethanol intake. Binge drinking is often accompanied by little or no food intake and by vomiting. Consequently, ethanol intake may have been discontinued, so ethanol may not be detected in a blood sample. Abdominal pain is often present, and acute pancreatitis is sometimes observed. Physical findings are nonspecific and include tachypnea, the odor of acetone on the breath, and abdominal tenderness. Signs of gross volume depletion are generally absent. Alcoholic ketoacidosis has been reported more frequently in women than in men.

LABORATORY EVALUATION AND DIAGNOSIS

The patient's blood sugar level during alcoholic ketoacidosis may be low, normal, or slightly elevated. The nitroprusside test generally reveals a low-to-moderate level of ketones in undiluted serum because of the preponderance of β-hydroxybutyrate. A reaction of 4+ in such serum, though rare, has been observed and is responsible for the confusion of alcoholic

ketoacidosis with diabetic ketoacidosis. Serum electrolytes reflect an anion-gap metabolic acidosis, generally of a mild degree. Arterial pH usually ranges between 7.20 and 7.25. The key to diagnosis of alcoholic ketoacidosis is correlating the history with the appropriate laboratory studies.

THERAPY

The treatment of alcoholic ketoacidosis is accomplished with intravenous normal saline rehydration, small amounts of sodium bicarbonate, and intravenous glucose as necessary. Insulin is not required to reverse the metabolic abnormalities; therefore, the distinction between diabetic ketoacidosis and alcoholic ketoacidosis is important. A concomitant lactic acidosis may be present, but because it is usually mild or moderate, it does not require independent therapy. The amount of sodium bicarbonate required is usually low—about 133 mEq on the average. Thiamine should be given with glucose replacement.

LACTIC ACIDOSIS

PATHOPHYSIOLOGY

Lactic acid is the end product of the anaerobic metabolism of glucose. It is formed from pyruvic acid by the action of lactic acid dehydrogenase (LDH) in the presence of reduced nicotinamide adenine dinucleotide (NADH):

$$\underset{\text{Pyruvic acid}}{CH_3\overset{\overset{\textstyle O}{\|}}{C}-COOH} + NADH \underset{}{\overset{LDH}{\rightleftharpoons}} \underset{\text{Lactic acid}}{CH_3-\overset{\overset{\textstyle OH}{|}}{C}-COOH} + NAD$$

Excessive amounts of lactic acid are produced when the catabolism of pyruvic acid through other pathways, particularly the tricarboxylic acid cycle, is inhibited. The most common causes of this inhibition are insufficient oxygenation of tissues and metabolic or respiratory alkalosis. A decreased removal rate of plasma lactic acid may also be responsible, particularly during acute ethanolism.

The syndromes producing lactic acidosis may be divided into two categories. One category includes the following conditions that result in insufficient tissue oxygenation:

1. *Cardiovascular insufficiency.* Shock from any cause accompanied by decreased tissue perfusion is the most common

cause of lactic acidosis. Cardiopulmonary bypass also produces this syndrome.

2. *Acute hypoxemia.* Lactic acidosis is well recognized as a complication of acute respiratory failure and pulmonary edema. It is not a feature of chronic hypoxemia.

3. *Severe anemia.*

4. *Exercise.* Prolonged muscular exertion leads to an "oxygen debt" and may produce a transient lactic acidosis, which quickly reverts when the person stops exercising. Status epilepticus with continuous muscular exertion may lead to persistent lactic acidosis.

The other category of syndromes that produces lactic acidosis comprises a variety of states, including the following:

1. *Diabetes mellitus.* Diabetics have an increased propensity to develop lactic acidosis. The diagnosis may be difficult because uremia or ketoacidosis, either of which can also produce an anion-gap metabolic acidosis, may be present. The diagnosis of concomitant lactic acidosis and ketoacidosis may be especially difficult because the measurement of serum ketones by the nitroprusside reaction may be artifactually low because of an increase in the ratio of β-hydroxybutyric acid to acetoacetic acid. The nitroprusside test measures only acetoacetic acid and acetone; if the equilibrium between acetoacetic acid and β-hydroxybutyric acid is shifted in the direction of the latter, as it is when concomitant lactic acidosis is present, the measurement of serum ketones is spuriously low and thus masks the diagnosis of ketoacidosis. All diabetics who present with apparent lactic acidosis should be suspected of having concurrent ketoacidosis until the possibility is disproved.

2. *Phenformin therapy.* Phenformin may produce lactic acidosis, most commonly in adult-onset diabetics with diminished renal or hepatic function. Phenformin increases the rate of lactic acid production in all treated diabetics, and its use should be discouraged in the presence of renal or hepatic dysfunction. In fact, phenformin has been withdrawn from general use by the Food and Drug Administration because of its association with lactic acidosis.

3. *Acute ethanolism.* Ingestion of excessive amounts of ethanol may produce lactic acidosis by decreasing the rate of lactic acid clearance. The simultaneous use of alcohol and phenformin thus synergistically raises the plasma lactic acid level; alcohol should therefore be abstained from during phenformin treatment.

4. *Malignancy.* Lactic acidosis, both acute and chronic, may occur if a patient has acute leukemia or a lymphoproliferative disorder.

5. *Congenital.* Rare causes of chronic lactic acidosis include glycogen storage disease type I and enzymatic defects in pyruvate metabolism.

6. *Idiopathic.* A small group of patients presenting with rapid-onset metabolic acidosis prove to have developed spontaneous acute lactic acidosis for no apparent reason. This syndrome presents precipitously; hyperventilation progresses to coma, which is usually fatal.

DIAGNOSIS AND LABORATORY EVALUATION

Lactic acidosis must be diagnosed in the laboratory. States of *hyperlacticacidemia* must be carefully distinguished from the syndromes of *lactic acidosis*. There are at least three common clinically important circumstances in which the accumulation of lactic acid does not produce a primary metabolic acidosis: hyperventilation (developing spontaneously or during respiratory support), metabolic alkalosis, and infusion of large amounts of glucose intravenously, as may be seen in patients with hyperalimentation. Thus, the first criterion for establishing a diagnosis of lactic acidosis is to demonstrate that a metabolic acidosis is present. Second, this metabolic acidosis must be the anion-gap type; if the sum of the Na^+ and K^+ concentrations minus the Cl^- and HCO_3^- concentrations exceeds 16 mEq/liter, an anion-gap metabolic acidosis is present. Third, other causes of such an anion-gap acidosis (including uremic acidosis, diabetic or alcoholic ketoacidosis, and ingestion of salicylate, methanol, ethylene glycol, or paraldehyde) must be ruled out. Fourth, if the preceding three criteria are satisfied and if the plasma lactic acid concentration approaches the estimated anion gap, the diagnosis is confirmed. If, however, the lactic acid concentration, though elevated, is far less than the anion gap, a mixed metabolic acidosis should be suspected.

Lactic acid should be measured in arterial blood; venous blood should be drawn without a tourniquet. Normal lactate levels range from 0.6 to 1.8 mEq/liter. Measuring pyruvate simultaneously is not necessary.

THERAPY

The treatment of lactic acidosis is in part dependent on the etiology. The cardinal rule, therefore, is to treat the underlying disorder appropriately. Additional therapy should be aimed at correcting cardiovascular insufficiency to maintain adequate tissue perfusion and oxygenation, and sodium bicarbonate should be administered to correct the acidosis. Massive amounts of sodium bicarbonate may be necessary; it is extremely important to monitor arterial pH since lactic acidosis is commonly associated with fluctuations in pH. Hemodialysis has likewise been of equivocal benefit, but it should be considered for treating lactic acidosis associated with phenformin use and renal insufficiency.

HYPERCALCEMIA

DIAGNOSIS

Severe hypercalcemia is life threatening. Its pathogenesis is complex and multifactorial as any standard textbook of endocrinology makes plain. The diagnosis is often not entertained as a possibility because the signs and symptoms of the illness are nonspecific and because the serum calcium level is not routinely measured in an emergency setting. A history of certain diseases, however, should raise the index of suspicion during the evaluation. The causes of severe hypercalcemia are listed in Table 27.2.

The symptoms of hypercalcemia, which are generally nonspecific, include malaise and fatigue. Gastrointestinal complaints (anorexia, nausea, vomiting, constipation, and a metallic taste in the mouth) may predominate. Polydipsia and polyuria may be present. Neurologic symptoms are frequent; disorders of mentation range from mild lethargy to coma. Muscle weakness is a common complaint. Bone pain may suggest metastatic malignancy or myeloma but may result from primary hyperparathyroidism.

The physical examination is likewise not usually helpful. The patient is often dehydrated. Palpable masses or local bone tenderness should suggest possible malignancy. Band keratopathy, if detected, is a helpful sign, since it suggests chronicity of the hypercalcemia, usually accompanied by renal dysfunction. Such limbic calcifications or a history of renal nephrolithiasis favors a diagnosis of primary hyperparathyroidism, vitamin D intoxication, or milk-alkali syndrome, rather than malignancy. Hepatosplenomegaly or lymphadenopathy, on the other hand, suggests malignancy or sarcoidosis.

LABORATORY EVALUATION

Measurement of the serum calcium is obviously the sine qua non of diagnosis. Hypercalcemia should be regarded as potentially life threatening if the level exceeds 14 mg/dl. Serum phosphorous should also be measured; if the level is low, primary hyperparathyroidism may be the cause but other conditions are sometimes responsible.

Serum electrolytes may reflect hypertonic dehydration from

TABLE 27.2 Causes of Severe Hypercalcemia[a]

Disease	Likely Setting
Frequent causes	
Malignancy	Carcinoma (especially breast, renal, lung), either metastatic to bone or by production of PTH-like substance
	Multiple myeloma
Vitamin D intoxication	Chronic vitamin D therapy for treatment of chronic renal failure or hypoparathyroidism
	Megavitamin use
Sarcoidosis	
Primary hyperparathyroidism	Common cause of hypercalcemia, but infrequent cause of severe hypercalcemia
Milk-alkali syndrome	Peptic ulcer disease treated with high doses of antacid
Infrequent causes	
Thyrotoxicosis	
Adrenal insufficiency	
Vitamin A intoxication	
Idiopathic hypercalcemia in infants	
Immobilization	Bone disease (Paget's disease)
Renal failure	Chronic hemodialysis or transplantation

[a]Causes listed are not necessarily in order of frequency with which any degree of hypercalcemia occurs, but are according to how commonly severe life-threatening hypercalcemia may be present.

hypercalcemia; water loss greater than sodium loss results in hypernatremia. A metabolic alkalosis that elevates the sodium bicarbonate level and decreases the chloride level may be present, particularly if there has been prolonged vomiting. Mild hyperchloremic metabolic acidosis frequently accompanies primary hyperparathyroidism but is not diagnostically useful. Renal function is variably altered; the dehydration may lead to prerenal azotemia with the BUN elevated disproportionately to creatinine. If the hypercalcemia has been more chronic, such tests may reflect underlying renal damage. Despite plasma hyperosmolarity the urine is usually isosmotic because in all states of hypercalcemia the concentrating ability of the kidneys is diminished.

An ECG may reveal a shortened QT interval; but if such a change is not noted, hypercalcemia should still not be ruled out as a possible diagnosis. Digitalis intoxication may result from an elevated level of serum calcium.

Serum calcium may be reduced in several ways. The commonly used therapies are aimed at promoting Ca^{2+} excretion, decreasing the rate of bone resorption or increasing the rate of Ca^{2+} deposition. Attempting to decrease the rate of gastrointestinal Ca^{2+} absorption, though successful for some forms of chronic hypercalcemia, should not be relied on for patients with life-threatening hypercalcemia. Treating the underlying disorder is paramount.

Promoting calcium excretion, the most reliable method, is also the most rapid means of reducing serum Ca^{2+}. Sodium diuresis with its attendant calciuria is effective in most patients. The diuresis is achieved by the intravenous infusion of normal saline in combination with furosemide or ethacrynic acid. The goal of therapy is to maintain a diuresis of 200–500 ml/hr; therefore, the rate of fluid administration and the dosage of diuretic should be dictated by the rate of diuresis. The patients are generally volume depleted, and normal saline is generally begun at a rate of 200 ml/hr, which should be adjusted as necessary to achieve the correct rate of diuresis. Such a diuresis also leads to significant losses of potassium and magnesium, which must be replaced in amounts that match the urine losses. The diuretic is given to maintain the diuresis and to prevent the overexpansion of ECF volume. A reasonable starting dose is 40 mg of furosemide or 50 mg of ethacrynic acid intravenously; the dosage should be repeated at intervals of 2–4 hours as necessary in conjunction with the normal saline to maintain the sodium diuresis. Thiazides must be avoided since they may elevate the serum calcium level. Any evidence of underlying cardiopulmonary disease indicates that the diuresis should be initiated with the diuretic alone; once urine output is established, intravenous saline can be initiated and increased slowly from 50 to 200 ml/hr over a period of 1–2 hours. Absolutely

critical to the care of the patient is frequent monitoring of the response to therapy by accurately measuring the rate of diuresis, the serum levels of electrolytes and calcium, and the tolerance of the rate of saline infusion.

Caution must be exercised when treating patients with congestive heart failure or severe impairment of renal function. Therapy must be undertaken in an intensive care setting. Intravenous sodium sulfate, generally not available, is a satisfactory alternative to normal saline if the diuresis is maintained. Hypotonic fluids, such as half-normal saline or D_5W, should not be given. Dialysis should be considered if renal function is severely impaired or if the saline load is poorly tolerated because of underlying cardiovascular or renal disease; it is not, however, the therapy of first choice. Both hemodialysis and peritoneal dialysis have been successful.

If efforts to promote calcium excretion fail and the clinical situation deteriorates as a result of sustained severe hypercalcemia, alternative modes of therapy must be considered. Intravenous phosphate, although effective, is not without hazard. It may lead to precipitation of calcium phosphate in tissues, including the heart and blood vessels, and therefore should not be used if the serum phosphorus level is greater than 4 mg/dl. The usual dosage is 0.5–1.0 mmol phosphorus/kg in 500 ml normal saline during a period of 6–8 hours. Oral phosphate is also effective at times but not as emergency treatment since response to it is much slower. Calcitonin is an acceptable and fast-acting second-line mode of therapy. The usual dosage is 8 MRC units/kg intramuscularly or intravenously every 6 hours.

Other forms of therapy, which are handicapped because they elicit slower responses, should not be used as initial therapy but are acceptable after the emergency has passed. Mithramycin, an antineoplastic agent, may be effective in lowering the level of serum calcium in any disorder involving increased bone turnover, especially malignancy. Its onset of action is 12–48 hours. An initial dose of 25 μg/kg as an intravenous bolus in a small volume of normal saline may be followed by a second dosage 48–72 hours later if necessary. Toxicity, which may result from thrombocytopenia and derangement of liver function, is not a problem if excessive and frequent dosages are avoided. *Corticosteroids* do not show any effect until days or weeks after they are administered and therefore should not be chosen as primary therapy for patients with severe hypercalcemia. They should be considered only as adjunctive therapy for patients with multiple myeloma and the vitamin D mediated syndromes of sarcoidosis and vitamin D intoxication; patients with some tumors, such as metastatic carcinoma and hematopoietic malignancies, may also respond. The usual regimen is 40–60 mg of prednisone (or its glucocorticoid equivalent) a day in divided dosages.

ADRENAL INSUFFICIENCY

The clinical presentation of adrenal insufficiency is quite variable, and the diagnosis is often not entertained. Physicians must, however, be alert to its possibility since rapid diagnosis and therapy for critically ill patients are crucial. Adrenal insufficiency arises from disease of the adrenal glands (primary insufficiency) or of the hypothalamic–pituitary axis (secondary insufficiency). Of the causes of adrenal insufficiency, listed in Table 27.3, the most common is the chronic use of exogenous glucocorticoids, which suppress the hypothalamic–pituitary axis; true Addison's disease and previous surgical ablation are the most common causes of primary insufficiency.

PATHOPHYSIOLOGY

Clinically, adrenal insufficiency is attributable to deficiencies of cortisol, aldosterone, and adrenal androgen. In primary disease of the adrenal gland, production of all three hormones has stopped or is severely diminished; in secondary insufficiency, aldosterone secretion is adequate even though adrenocorticotropic hormone (ACTH) secretion is decreased. Hypotension, hyponatremia, hyperkalemia, and hypoglycemia are only some of the possible consequences of these various deficiencies. Hypotension in patients with adrenal insufficiency is due to sodium diuresis (aldosterone) and loss of peripheral arteriolar tone associated with a lack of cortisol. Hyponatremia results from a loss of sodium in the absence of aldosterone and a reduced ability to generate a hypotonic urine because of lack of cortisol. Hyperkalemia, which occurs only during primary adrenal insufficiency that is secondary to loss of aldosterone, is accompanied by a severe reduction in glomerular filtration rate. Hypoglycemia is a consequence of the fasting state coupled with impaired gluconeogenesis in the liver when cortisol is not present.

It is important to remember that the unfolding of the syndrome is often related to a stressful illness, which must always be carefully sought when evaluating patients with adrenal insufficiency. The ability of the adrenal glands to withstand stress, normally mediated by increases in ACTH secretion, is lost during both primary and secondary insufficiency; patients with marginal hypothalamic, pituitary, and adrenal function may do quite well for long periods only to be tipped into a disastrous crisis by any of a variety of stressful illnesses, some seemingly trivial, such as a mild respiratory infection. Patients who are undergoing chronic steroid replacement must be carefully instructed on managing steroid dosages during intercurrent illnesses.

DIAGNOSIS

The symptoms of adrenal insufficiency may suggest a variety of illnesses and vary depending on the etiology of the insufficiency and the tempo of evolution of the crisis. The symptoms can be divided into two types: acute and chronic.

Increasing malaise and fatigue are common *acute complaints*. Gastrointestinal symptoms with nausea, vomiting, and anorexia often predominate. Muscular weakness and a change in mental status, from lassitude to frank coma, are frequent signs. Salt craving and change in the taste for salt are valuable clues and are symptoms exclusive to primary insufficiency. Fasting hypoglycemia with changes in mentation, nervousness, tremor, diaphoresis, palpitations, and hunger may be encountered. Abdominal pain is occasionally observed.

Weight loss is a frequent *chronic complaint*. The patient may have noticed increasing hyperpigmentation or easy sun tanning, which are clues to primary insufficiency. Hair loss, especially in women, in the axillary or pubic regions is common. During the initial evaluation, the physician should carefully determine whether the patient's history suggests another endocrine hypofunction, such as hypothyroidism or hypogonadism, that may be related to a disease of the hypothalamic–pituitary axis.

The physical examination may yield important clues for making the diagnosis. Hypotension (which may be only mild postural hypotension but may be severe enough to cause frank shock) accompanied by tachycardia is usual. Fever is very common, but it should strongly suggest the presence of infection. Changes in the integument may predominant. Dehydration with decreased skin turgor, dry mucous membranes, and no axillary sweat may be evident. The patient should be ex-

---

TABLE 27.3 Causes of Adrenal Insufficiency

Primary insufficiency
  Addison's disease (idiopathic atrophy)
  Surgical removal of the adrenal glands (palliation of breast
    carcinoma, therapy for Cushing's syndrome)
  Tuberculosis
  Hemorrhage into adrenal glands (disseminated intravascular
    coagulation, anticoagulants, postvenography)
  Congenital enzyme defects
  Metastatic carcinoma, a rare cause of adrenal insufficiency
  Drugs (metyrapone, aminoglutethimide)
Secondary insufficiency
  Exogenous glucocorticoid use
  Hypopituitarism [secondary to tumor, infiltrative disease, trauma,
    pituitary hemorrhage (apoplexy)]

amined for hyperpigmentation (particularly of flexion creases, elbows, buccal mucosa, and scars), which is a sign of primary insufficiency, because of an increase in the production of melanocyte stimulating hormone (MSH) that accompanies primary adrenal failure. Hair loss in the axillary or pubic regions should be noted as well, but it does not differentiate primary and secondary insufficiencies. Calcification of the pinnae may point to primary adrenal disease. The physician should also carefully look for evidence of glucocorticoid excess, which suggests the use of exogenous corticosteroids; these manifestations of Cushing's syndrome include centripetal obesity, increases in supraclavicular and nuchal adipose tissue, thin skin with purpura from insignificant trauma, pink or purple abdominal striae, muscle wasting, hirsutism, and facial plethora. A careful examination for evidence of other endocrine hypofunction, particularly hypothyroidism and hypogonadism, is necessary.

LABORATORY EVALUATION

Routine laboratory determinations may offer several valuable clues for diagnosing adrenal insufficiency, but none is absolutely diagnostic. Ultimately the diagnosis depends on the plasma cortisol level. Although decisions for therapy have to be made in the emergency setting without the benefit of the test results, blood for cortisol determination should always be drawn before therapy. A plasma cortisol level of less than 20 μg/dl in the severely ill and stressed patient is virtual proof of at least some degree of adrenal insufficiency.

The hematocrit may be spuriously elevated if dehydration is extreme. The white blood cell count is generally greater than 10,000/mm^3. Two features of the differential count may be valuable clues: relative lymphocytosis and eosinophilia (50–200/mmm^3).

Serum sodium may be low in patients with either primary or secondary insufficiency. In the former the low level is due to sodium diuresis with aldosterone lack and the inability to generate a water diuresis with cortisol lack; in the latter the effects of the lack of cortisol are predominant. Serum potassium is generally normal; if its level is extremely high, as it is at times, primary insufficiency with loss of aldosterone is almost always involved. A mild hyperchloremic acidosis may be observed, which is due to a proximal renal tubular acidosis that occurs when mineralocorticoid is absent and hydrogen shifts out of cells. An anion-gap metabolic acidosis may result if hypotension with secondary reduction of glomerular filtration rate is severe and accompanies tissue hypoxia with secondary lactic acidosis. Renal function generally diminishes when the BUN level rises disproportionately to the level of creatinine;

the imbalance reflects severe ECF volume reduction. Hypoglycemia as a result of cortisol lack may be present in patients with either primary or secondary insufficiency. Measurements of urine electrolytes may show an inappropriate increase in the urine sodium and a decrease in the urine potassium relative to serum values, but the urine values vary with the severity of the reduction in the glomerular filtration rate.

Roentgenographic studies may reveal a small cardiac silhouette or adrenal calcifications; the latter suggests tuberculous disease of the adrenals.

THERAPY

The cardinal rule in treating patients with adrenal insufficiency is that if the diagnosis is suspected, treatment should be initiated immediately and not deferred for laboratory test results. Blood for a plasma cortisol determination should always be drawn before therapy. A brief course of corticosteroids while diagnostic studies are underway does no harm and may be lifesaving.

The *glucocorticoid dose* and route of administration should be based on the principle of giving dosages of glucocorticoid that approximate the maximal stress responses of the normal adrenal cortex. The intravenous route should be used initially to avoid the potential problem of slow mobilization from an intramuscular depot in the hypotensive patient. Several preparations of glucocorticoid are equally effective if given in dosages of equal potency. These include 100–300 mg of hydrocortisone, 20–40 mg of methylprednisolone, and 4–8 mg of dexamethasone, all as an intravenous bolus. If necessary, repetitive intravenous bolus dosages must be given every 60–90 minutes to maintain a therapeutic effect. Therapy may also proceed as a continuous intravenous infusion; such a regimen is hydrocortisone diluted in normal saline and administered at a rate of 25–50 mg/hr. After initial therapy and normal blood pressure and tissue perfusion are restored, the route should be changed to an intramuscular one. Dosages in the "stress" range (such as 25–50 mg cortisone acetate every 6 hours, 5–10 mg methylprednisolone every 6 hours, or 1–2 mg dexamethasone every 6 hours) should be continued for 1–2 days after the crisis has passed. Depending on the clinical state of the patient, corticosteroids may then be rapidly tapered to the previous maintenance dosage or to the pharmacologic dosage. Overtreatment with high dosages does little harm in the short course; therefore, low or marginal dosages should be avoided.

Intravenous fluids are an extremely important part of therapy. Normal saline is the fluid of choice. Sodium diuresis with obligatory water excretion will have led to significant depletion of total body sodium and water during the evolution of the illness, especially in patients with primary insufficiency. One to two liters of normal saline should be administered rapidly to restore blood pressure; additional amounts and the rates of their administration are dictated by the clinical response of the patient.

Replacing *mineralocorticoid* is usually not necessary as a part of the emergency treatment. Patients with hyperkalemia usually respond to saline rehydration plus glucocorticoid, which restore urine output. If the hyperkalemia is severe and potentially life threatening, it should be treated like any other case of hyperkalemia (see Chapter 10). Mineralocorticoid can be replaced in this setting with 3–5 mg deoxycorticosterone (DOC) acetate intramuscularly, but the long-acting preparation of DOC available as trimethylacetate should be avoided. Fludrocortisone (Fluirinef), 50–200 µg, may be given orally, but because the onset of action is much slower, it is generally used only for treating patients with chronic primary adrenal insufficiency.

Glucose replacement may be necessary in boluses of 50% dextrose if severe hypoglycemia is present or of 5% dextrose-containing intravenous fluids during rehydration.

The final aspect of management involves a careful search for the precipitating cause of the adrenal crisis. Infection ranks high on the list of stressful illnesses to be excluded. In addition, the physician is obligated to secure a card, bracelet, or necklace for the patient that identifies the patient as having adrenal insufficiency or being on chronic glucocorticoid therapy so that future crises can be quickly recognized and the patient treated.

SUGGESTED READINGS

Diabetic Ketoacidosis—General

Alberti KGMM and Hockaday TDR: *Clin Endo Metab* 6, 421, 1977.
Alberti KGMM and Nattrass M: *Med Clin N Amer* 62, 799, 1978.
Hockaday TDR and Alberti KGMM: *Clin Endo Metab* 1, 751, 1972.
Kreisberg RA: *Ann Int Med* 88, 681, 1978.

Diabetic Ketoacidosis—Specific Issues

COMA

Fulop M et al: *Lancet* II, 635, 1973.
Fulop M, Rosenblatt A, Kreitzer SM, et al: *Diabetes* 24, 594, 1975.
Ohman JL: *New Engl J Med* 284, 283, 1971.

LOW DOSE vs HIGH DOSE INSULIN

Alberti KGMM, Hockaday TDR and Turner RC: *Lancet* II, 515, 1973.
Kitabchi AE, Ayyagari V, Guerra SMO et al: *Ann Int Med* 84, 633, 1976.
Padilla AJ and Loeb JN: *Am J Med* 63, 843, 1977.
Sacks HS, Shahshahani M, Kitabchi AE, et al: *Ann Int Med* 90, 36, 1979.

HYPOKALEMIA

Biegelman PM: *Am J Med* 54, 419, 1973.
Fulop M: *New Engl J Med* 300, 1087, 1979.

HYPOPHOSPHATEMIA

Keller U and Berger W: *Diabetes* 29, 87, 1980.

PARADOXICAL ACIDOSIS

Posner JB and Plum F: *New Engl J Med* 277, 605, 1967.

CEREBRAL EDEMA

Clements RS et al: *Lancet* II, 671, 1971.
Lufkin EG, Reagen TJ, Doan DH et al: *Metabolism* 26, 363, 1977.

Hyperosmolar Coma

Arieff A and Carroll HJ: *Medicine* 51, 73, 1972.
Foster DW: in *Adv Int Med* (Stollerman GH, ed), 19, 159, 1974.
Podolsky S: *Med Clin N Amer* 62, 815, 1978.

Alcoholic Ketoacidosis

Cooperman MT, Davidoff F, Spark R, Pallotta J: *Diabetes* 23, 433, 1974.
Levy LJ, Duga J, Girgis M and Gordon EE: *Ann Int Med* 78, 213, 1973.

Hypercalcemia

Binstock ML and Mundy GR: *Ann Int Med* 93, 269, 1980.
Deftos L and Neer R: *Ann Rev Med* 25, 323, 1974.
Goldsmith RS: *Med Clin N Amer* 56, 951, 1972.
Neer RM and Potts JT Jr: in *Endocrinology* (DeGroot L, ed), 1979, p 725ff.
Suki WW et al: *New Engl J Med* 283, 836, 1970.

Adrenal Insufficiency

Axelrod L in *Handbook of Drug Therapy* (Miller RR and Greenblatt DJ, ed), 1979, chapter 49.

Axelrod L: *Medicine* 55, 39, 1976.

Irvine TJ and Barnes EW: *Clin Endo Metab* 1, 549, 1972.

Irvine WJ, Toft AD and Feek CM: in *The Adrenal Gland* (James VHT, ed), 1979, pp 131ff.

Nelson DH: in *Major Problems in Internal Medicine*, 1980.

Other Endocrine Emergencies

THYROID STORM

Eriksson M et al: *New Engl J Med* 296, 263, 1977.

Ingbar S: *New Engl J Med* 274, 1252, 1966.

Lee TC et al: *Ann Surgery* 177, 643, 1973.

MYXEDEMA COMA

Blum M: *Am J Med Sci* 264, 432, 1972.

Dowling JT: *Arch Int Med* 113, 89, 1964.

DIABETES INSIPIDUS

Cobb WE, Spare S and Reichlin S: *Ann Int Med* 88, 183, 1978.

Hockaday TDR: *Brit Med J* 2, 210, 1972.

PHEOCHROMOCYTOMA CRISIS

Gitlow SE, Pertsemlidis D and Bertani LM: *Am Heart J* 82, 557, 1971.

Remine WH et al: *Ann Surgery* 179, 740, 1974.

28

INFECTIONS AND THE FEBRILE PATIENT

Donald H. Rubin
Gerald H. Friedland

The evaluation and treatment of patients with life-threatening infections is challenging and often gratifyingly successful. In few areas of medicine are the physician's diagnostic skills so tested, the detection of specific disease etiology so clearly possible, and the specific effective therapy so readily available. Successful diagnosis and therapy usually require only a careful and thorough history and physical examination combined with a few relevant laboratory examinations. However, familiarity with the presentation of infections in many organ systems, as well as knowledge of the relevant characteristics of possible infecting agents, is essential. Appropriate understanding and use of microbiologic diagnostic laboratory techniques are necessary and the indications, efficacy, pharmacology, and toxicology of antimicrobial agents must be known if therapy is to be successfully instituted. Additionally, in emergency situations the physician must be able to distinguish quickly between acute infections and noninfectious diseases presenting with similar clinical manifestations and must be able to differentiate expeditiously between severe life-threatening infections requiring immediate therapy and minor self-limited infectious diseases. This chapter provides a general outline for focused clinical and laboratory evaluations of patients with severe life-threatening infectious diseases and a guide to the choice and use of specific antimicrobial agents. Emphasis is placed on acute bacterial infections. Although these are less common than nonbacterial infections, they comprise the great majority of life-threatening, specifically treatable, infections.

In evaluating a patient with a life-threatening infection, the physician should keep the following five basic questions in mind and attempt to answer them in an orderly and logical fashion:

1. Is the patient septic or is there another explanation for the patient's presentation?
2. What is the involved organ system or portal of entry of the infection?
3. What are the likely pathogens in this portal of entry?
4. Are there clinical or epidemiologic circumstances that may modify these likely pathogens?
5. What is the optimal therapy?

To find the answers to these questions, a thorough but relevant and focused history and physical examination combined with a small number of selected and readily available laboratory examinations must be performed.

EVALUATION OF THE PATIENT

History

A careful and detailed chronological exploration of the patient's presenting complaint is essential. Specific attention should be paid to the areas discussed below.

DURATION AND TEMPO OF THE ILLNESS

When was the patient last completely well? Is the present illness acute and rapidly progressive over hours or is it chronic, indolent, and slowly progressive over months? The answers to these questions will tell the physician how rapidly to proceed with the diagnostic workup, and the tempo of the illness will suggest certain diagnostic possibilities. For example, acute pyogenic bacterial infections are explosive in onset, whereas granulomatous infections are insidious.

PATTERN AND HEIGHT OF THE FEVER

Fever represents the cardinal manifestation of infectious diseases. Certain types of fever patterns should be sought since these may suggest specific infections. *Intermittent or hectic fever* is characterized by widely varying temperature with high fever, interrupted by return of the temperature to normal, usually during each 24-hour period. Pyogenic abscesses are most often responsible for this type of fever pattern, but administration of salicylates to patients when their temperatures exceed a predetermined level, such as 40°C (104°F), also commonly causes this pattern. *Sustained or continuous fever* is characterized by the absence of swings and is seen in patients with heat stroke, typhoid, tuberculosis, pneumococcal pneumonia, and streptococcal infections. *Relapsing or recurrent fever* is characterized by several days of temperature elevation followed by several days of normal temperature. This pattern is frequently seen in patients with ascending cholangitis, malaria, chronic meningococcemia, and lymphoma.

Not all infections produce fever in proportion to their severity. The febrile response is blunted by uremia and by the administration of corticosteroids and other immunosuppressive agents. Neonates and the very elderly can have significant life-threatening infections without having a febrile response. Hypothermia may be seen in viral infections and during the course of gram-negative sepsis with shock.

RESPONSE TO FEVER

Many patients experience a sensation of cold or chilliness with fever. This should not be confused with rigors, which are characterized by gross shaking and chattering teeth. Although the presence of true rigors is sometimes a feature of noninfectious diseases or non-life-threatening viral infections, it should raise the spector of severe and serious infection. Among the diagnoses that should be considered in patients with true rigors are pneumococcal pneumonia, streptococcal or staphylococcal sepsis, pyogenic abscesses, pyelonephritis, osteomyelitis, endocarditis, and cholangitis. Specific inquiry should be made about the use of aspirin since it may produce rigors in febrile patients as well.

CHANGES IN MENTAL STATUS

Disorientation, confusion, and changing levels of consciousness are historical findings of grave importance in an infected patient. They may be present in any serious infection as a nonspecific manifestation, or they may connote the presence of intracranial or meningeal infection.

PRESENCE OF ORGAN SYSTEM SPECIFIC SYMPTOMS

The patient's presenting complaint as well as a review of systems should be evaluated with a view toward determining the predominant organ system involved in the infectious process. This will direct the physician's further efforts in the most economical and effective manner. Additionally, defining the portal of entry and involved organ system will allow the clinician to make a reasonable guess as to the likely infecting pathogens (Table 28.1).

UNDERLYING DISEASES THAT PREDISPOSE TO SPECIFIC INFECTIOUS DISEASES

Some obvious examples of patients with underlying diseases that predispose to infectious diseases include patients with granulocytopenia or hypogammaglobulinemia, who are at increased risk of pyogenic infections; patients with sickle cell disease, who are at increased risk of pneumococcal and *Sal-*monella infections; and patients with known valvular heart disease, in whom the presence of endocarditis must always be considered.

RECENT ADMINISTRATION OF THERAPEUTIC AGENTS

The clinical presentation of infection may be blunted or otherwise altered by antimicrobial therapy, and bacteriologic confirmation of the etiologic agent may be rendered difficult. Certain agents may be the cause of the presenting febrile illness. Those frequently associated with hypersensitivity reactions (barbituates, sulfonamides, penicillins, alpha methyldopa) may be responsible for a clinical illness that mimics an infectious disease.

EPIDEMIOLOGIC SETTING

The presence of similar disease or symptoms in household members or other close associates of the patient may be very helpful in suggesting the etiologic agent. Diseases that occur in epidemic clusters include viral respiratory and gastrointestinal (GI) infections, streptococcal skin and pharyngeal infections, *Salmonella* and *Shigella* infections, tuberculosis, Legionnaire's disease, and gonococcal and meningococcal infections.

Certain diseases are associated with occupational environment or animal exposure and may not be considered unless the patient is asked specific questions. Examples include brucellosis in abattoir workers and tularemia in hunters and farmers. The diagnosis of psittacosis, Rocky Mountain spotted fever, plague, and many other zoonoses requires suspicion and inquiry about animal contact.

Do not shy away from asking about sexual preference or the use of illicit drugs. Male homosexuals have a high incidence of sexually transmitted disease, gastroenteritis, hepatitis, and a newly described, lethal acquired immunodeficiency syndrome. Similarly, users of illicit drugs may have a predilection for endovascular infection, pneumonitis, or acquired immunodeficiency. (See acquired immunodeficiency.)

Physical Examination

As with the history, the physical examination should be directed toward assessing the seriousness of the illness and defining the focus or portal of entry of the infection. A series of maneuvers should be routine in examining every patient with a serious infection.

RAPID BEDSIDE APPRAISAL OF TOXICITY

Most patients with life-threatening infection appear profoundly toxic. This is evident from a combination of several general physical findings that experienced clinicians are usually able to recognize, including fever, flushing or pallor, profuse sweating, rapid breathing, disorientation, agitation or lethargy, and a look of apprehension. Patients with this constellation of findings require immediate evaluation and rapid institution of therapy. Although this clinical syndrome is most frequently a result of sepsis, it may be mimicked by cardiovascular collapse secondary to pulmonary embolus, myocardial infarction, or blood loss. Patients with fever as a result of noninfectious etiologies usually do not present with profound toxicity. Notable exceptions to this general rule are patients with heat stroke. Conversely, in patients at the extremes of age—the very old and very young—and in those receiving corticosteroids or those with uremia, the toxic manifestations of severe infection may be quite blunted. Although desperately ill, these patients may appear deceptively well.

VITAL SIGNS

The presence of hypotension is of obvious importance and may signal the presence of septic shock. Extreme hypertension is similarly important as a finding in patients with intracranial infection. Tachycardia is present in most patients with infection and is usually in proportion to the height of the fever. Relative bradycardia, if present, raises the possibility of the patient having typhoid fever, intracranial infection, or factitious fever. Increased respiration rate is an invariable finding in patients with respiratory infections, but it is also a common early sign of septic shock.

MENTAL STATUS EXAMINATION

Disorientation and altered state of consciousness are extremely important findings. They connote serious systemic infection or the presence of encephalitis or meningitis.

EXAMINATION OF THE SKIN

The skin is readily accessible to examination but is frequently bypassed as clinicians turn their attention to visceral structures. The skin may give clues to the presence of life-threatening infection (jaundice, pallor, vasoconstriction, cyanosis, infarction, bleeding) or it may be the site of a rash that may be characteristic or pathognomonic for certain diseases. The character of a rash, if not pathognomonic, may still suggest a general area of diagnosis. For example, vesicular, maculo papular, diffuse eruptions are common in patients who have viral infections and drug hypersensitivity reactions and generally do not suggest life-threatening infections, whereas hemorrhagic eruptions do (see Chapter 29). Rashes on the palms and soles are seen in patients with meningococcemia and Rocky Mountain spotted fever and should always be taken seriously.

EXAMINATION OF NONSTERILE ORIFICES

Unless there are historical findings pointing toward infections of the mouth, rectum, or vagina, physicians tend to overlook or to examine these areas only superficially. These areas are commonly infected with the normal contiguous microbial flora. Particularly in patients without an obvious source of sepsis and in leukopenic patients, careful examination, including systematic palpation of the teeth, the perirectal area, the uterine cervix, and the prostate gland is mandatory.

EXAMINATION OF INVADED OR MEDICALLY TRAUMATIZED AREAS

Careful inspection of intravenous or cutdown sites, surgical wounds, and the urinary tract in the catheterized patient is essential in patients who are hospitalized or have been recently discharged from the hospital.

The history and physical examination should be directed toward determining if the infection is life threatening and in uncovering a portal of entry or focus of infection. In most circumstances, both of these goals can be rapidly accomplished. Occasionally, the physician encounters a patient who is seriously ill but in whom a focus is not definable. Important diagnostic possibilities for patients in this group are recorded in Table 28.2. In the majority of patients in whom a portal of infection is defined, it is possible to make a reasonable judgment about the likely pathogens or infected organ system. This is the result of the well-known but poorly understood phenomenon of tissue tropism. Most mucosal surfaces are colonized with a predictable normal flora, and infections of those surfaces or contiguous sites often involve at least part of this flora. Additionally, sites that are normally sterile are in most circumstances infected with only a limited number of pathogens. The most likely organisms causing infection in each organ system are well known and therefore a reasonable bacteriologic prediction and therapeutic judgment can be based upon defining the primary site of infection. The normal and pathologic flora of each organ system is shown in Table 28.1. This

TABLE 28.1 Organ System Related Normal and Pathologic Flora

Organ System	Normal Flora	Infection	Usual Pathogens
Skin and subcutaneous tissues	Staphylococcus epidermidis Diphtheroids Staphylococcus aureus Propionibacterium acnes Anaerobic streptococci	Primary skin infections Erysipelas and lymphangitis Cellulitis Burns Decubiti Traumatic and surgical wounds Necrotizing fasciitis Synergystic gangrene Bacteremic skin infections	Streptococcus pyogenes (group A) Staphylococcus aureus Streptococcus pyogenes (group A) Staphylococcus aureus Aerobic and anaerobic streptococci Clostridium Enteric gram-negative bacilli Pseudomonas Staphylococcus aureus Neisseria meningitidis (meningococcus) Haemophilus influenzae Pseudomonas aeruginosa

Upper respiratory tract including mouth and pharynx	Streptococcus (nongroup A)
	Anaerobic streptococci and micrococci
	Neisseria (nonpathogenic species)
	Haemophilus parainfluenzae
	Bacteroides
	Fusobacterium
	N. meningitidis (meningococcus 5–20%)
	Streptococcus pyogenes (group A 5–10%)
	Streptococcus pneumoniae (pneumococcus 20–40%)
	Staphylococcus epidermis
	Staphylococcus aureus
		Otitis media
		
		Sinusitis
		
		Pharyngitis
		
		Epiglottitis
			Otitis media:
			<5 years old
			  H. influenzae
			>5 years old
			  Streptococcus pneumoniae (pneumococcus)
			Sinusitis:
			Streptococcus pyogenes (group A)
			Streptococcus pneumoniae (pneumococcus)
			H. influenzae
			Pharyngitis:
			Streptococcus pyogenes (group A)
			Neisseria gonorrhoeae (gonococcus)
			Corynebacterium diphtheriae
			H. influenzae
			Epiglottitis:
			H. influenzae

Lower respiratory tract	Sterile	Tracheobronchitis Pneumonia Aspiration pneumonia and aspiration lung abscess Empyema	Tracheobronchitis: Streptococcus pneumoniae (pneumococcus) H. influenzae Pneumonia: Streptococcus pneumoniae (pneumococcus) Staphylococcus aureus H. influenzae Enteric gram-negative bacilli P. aeruginosa Mixed mouth anaerobic flora Same as for pneumonia
Gastrointestinal tract	Upper GI tract Surviving ingested bacteria Lactobacillus Enterococcus Bacteroides Lower GI tract Bacteroides Anaerobic streptococci Escherichia coli Streptococcus faecalis (enterococcus) Klebsiella Other gram-negative bacilli including proteus, pseudomonas aeruginosa Staphylococcus epidermidis and aureus Candida albicans Other nongroup A streptococci	Intraabdominal abscess, peritonitis Biliary sepsis including ascending cholangitis and cholecystitis Bacillary dysentery	Enteric gram-negative bacilli Bacteroides fragilis Anaerobic streptococci Streptococcus faecalis (enterococcus) Enteric gram-negative bacilli Streptococcus faecalis (enterococcus) Clostridium Shigella Salmonella Camphyobacter

Body system	Normal flora	Condition	Organisms
Urinary tract	Sterile	Urinary tract infection Community acquired Hospital acquired	E. coli E. coli Klebsiella Serratia Enterobacter Proteus Streptococcus faecalis (enterococcus)
Female genital tract	Lactobacilli Nongroup A streptococci including enterococcus Staphylococcus epidermidis Diphtheroids Anaerobic streptococci Bacteroides E. coli Other gram-negative bacilli Hemophilus vaginalis C. albicans Neisseria (nongonococcal) Trichomonas vaginalis	Vaginitis	T. vaginalis C. albicans H. vaginalis
		Cervicitis Endometritis Pelvic abscess	N. gonorrhoeae (gonococcus) Anaerobic cocci Aerobic streptococci B. fragilis Enteric gram-negative bacilli Clostridia
		Salpingitis Tuboovarian abscess	N. gonorrhoeae (gonococcus) Anaerobic streptococci B. fragilis Enteric gram-negative bacilli
Male genital tract	Sterile	Urethritis Epididymitis	N. gonorrhoeae (gonococcus) Chlamydia
Musculoskeletal system	Sterile	Osteomyelitis	Staphylococcus aureus Salmonella (sickle cell disease)
		Septic arthritis	Staphylococcus aureus N. gonorrhoeae (gonococcus) N. meningitidis (meningococcus) H. influenzae (children) Enteric gram-negative bacilli (after surgery or trauma)
Central nervous system	Sterile	Meningitis	Streptococcus pneumoniae (pneumococcus) N. meningitidis (meningococcus) H. influenzae (children 6 mo–5 yr predominantly) Enteric gram-negative bacilli (neonates and after trauma or surgery) Streptococcus group B (neonates) Staphylococcus epidermiditis (with cerebrospinal fluid shunts) Listeria monocytogenes
		Brain abscess	Streptococcus pneumoniae (pneumococcus) Anaerobic streptococci Bacteroides Staphylococcus aureus Enteric gram-negative bacilli (posttrauma or surgery)
Endocardium	Sterile	Endocarditis	Streptococcus viridans Staphylococcus aureus Streptococcus faecalis (enterococcus) Gram-negative bacilli (prosthetic valves and heroin users)

TABLE 28.2 Life-Threatening Bacterial Infections with Occult Focus

Endocarditis
Typhoid fever and other *Salmonella* infections
Intraabdominal abscesses
Prostatic abscesses
Retroperitoneal abscesses
Biliary sepsis
Infections in leukopenic patients
Sepsis in newborns and the elderly
Nosocomial infections—intravenous sites, surgical wounds, catheterized urinary tract

principle must be tempered by a number of important variables that may modify the predictable flora. These variables, listed in Table 28.3, should be sought in the history taking, physical examination, and laboratory examination of the patients.

LABORATORY EVALUATION

General Procedures

A *complete blood cell count* is essential in the evaluation of febrile patients. Hematologic changes often suggest an infectious and more specifically, a bacterial, viral, or parasitic etiology. Changes in leukocytes are often helpful diagnostically. Both quantitative and qualitative changes in leukocytes are of importance. At the extreme, leukemoid reactions and leukopenia carry a grave prognosis in bacterial infections. Elevation in the white blood cell count of a moderate to marked degree (12,000–20,000) are found in most patients with bacterial infections. The qualitative changes in neutrophilic granulocytes, however, are more important. The presence of a "shift to the left," that is, more than 75% polymorphonuclear leukocytes

TABLE 28.3 Factors Altering Usual Infecting Organisms

Age
Hospital acquisition of infection
Previous administration of antibiotics
Travel history
Occupational history
Animal exposure
Local epidemiology
Underlying disease
Recent culture results

with many early forms, degranulation or vacuolization of leukocytes, or toxic granulations are all suggestive of acute bacterial infections. Recognizing changes in lymphocytes also helps in evaluating the febrile patient. Patients with viral infections often have a relative lymphocytosis, and the presence of more than 15% atypical lymphocytes suggests infectious mononucleosis or a mononucleosislike syndrome caused by cytomegalovirus or toxoplasmosis. Eosinophilia is usually found in tissue-invading helminthic infections and in hypersensitivity reactions. Conversely, it is of extreme importance to recognize that patients with granulocytopenia of less than 500/mm^3 are at great risk for bacterial infection. Fever in patients with granulocytopenia to this degree must always be assumed to be because of acute life-threatening bacterial infection until proven otherwise.

Changes in red blood cell count are common but usually nonspecific. Low grade anemias that are normochromic and normocytic are often found in patients with chronic infections. Hemolytic anemia is a feature of patients who have acute infections with bacteremia. A microangiopathic picture with partially destroyed red blood cells may be seen in the presence of disseminated intravascular coagulation.

Quantitative changes in platelets are of great importance in the evaluation of febrile patients. Thrombocytopenia in patients who have fever and hypotension suggests disseminated intravascular coagulation. In such circumstances the skin should be carefully examined for bleeding, and additional tests of clotting function, including the prothombin time, partial thromboplastin time, and fibrin split should be performed (Chapter 40).

Urinalysis must be performed carefully to detect protein, red blood cells, white blood cells, and white blood cell casts. Proteinuria may be a nonspecific finding in febrile patients. However, the presence of cells and casts suggests infection of the urinary tract. A semiquantitative appreciation of significant bacteriuria may be obtained by finding more than 100 bacteremia per high-power field on the spun sediment, or approximately 1 organism per high-power field on a Gram stain of the upspun urine.

Blood urea nitrogen (BUN), creatinine, electrolytes, and blood glucose should be measured in critically ill patients. Metabolic derangement, dehydration, and severe renal failure may all be present in patients with severe infections. Specific corrective therapy as well as modification of antibiotic choices and doses may be necessary if these abnormalities are present. Arterial blood gases will further define metabolic derangement and help guide therapy. The presence of diabetes mellitus may help suggest certain specific infections (fungal disease, tuberculosis, gangrenous gallbladder). The peripheral blood sugar level is important in evaluating the significance of glucose concentration in other body fluids.

At least two sets of blood cultures, obtained by separate venipunctures 10–20 minutes apart, should be obtained in patients suspected of having serious bacterial infections. The procedure should be done following a sterile technique of cleansing the skin first with povidone–iodine preparation and then with alcohol. Ten milliliters of blood should be obtained and 5 ml should be inoculated under sterile conditions into separate aerobic and anaerobic flasks. Therapeutic decisions cannot wait for the results of blood cultures in seriously ill patients, and the institution of antibiotic therapy must be based on clinical information that is at hand. However, the documentation of bacteremia and the isolation of a specific organism and knowledge of its antibiotic susceptibility will make subsequent therapeutic decisions more specific and rational. Wright's stain examination of the buffy coat occasionally reveals organisms with leukocytes in patients with high-grade bacteremia (i.e., staphylococcal sepsis, meningococcemia). The buffy coat may easily be obtained from the spun anticoagulated blood specimen used to perform hematologic studies.

Collection and Examination of Specimens

The proper collection and examination of samples of infected fluids or exudates are of major and obvious importance. Confirmation of the diagnosis of bacterial infection as well as determination of the specific agent(s) and subsequent institution of specific therapy requires appropriate and thoughtful handling and interpretation of specimens from these areas. Several general principles are set forth below:

1. Specimens should be obtained as an emergency procedure before initiating antimicrobial therapy.
2. Before obtaining a specimen, the physician should think of what tests will be performed. A sufficient sample to perform all required tests should be obtained, and appropriate containers, tubes, and slides should be available at the bedside.
3. The physician must be responsible for ensuring that the specimen is adequate. Delegation of specimen collection to inexperienced assistants without adequate supervision will often result in an inadequate specimen and possible incorrect diagnostic and therapeutic decisions.
4. In the common situation in which a specimen must be obtained through a normally unsterile area, such as the respiratory or urinary tract, there is always a danger of contaminating the specimen. To ensure an adequate and interpretable specimen, care must be taken to avoid or minimize contamination of the specimens during collection

or to bypass the contaminating area, for example, by performing a transtracheal aspiration or a single straight catheterization or a suprapubic aspiration of the bladder.

5. Specimens from infected areas should be examined grossly for the presence of blood, cloudiness, and purulence. The odor of the sample should be noted. (The presence of anaerobic organisms will impart an offensive, foul odor to collected specimens.)
6. Cell counts, differential white blood cell count, and determination of the concentration of glucose and protein should be performed on all fluids.
7. Specimens should be appropriately cultured on media designed to isolate and identify potential pathogens. The recommended media for various specimens are outlined in Table 28.4.

GRAM STAIN

Gram stain should always be performed on collected specimens from the infected area (Table 28.5). These include samples from the respiratory tract, skin, urinary tract, and all other sites that are usually sterile, that is, joints, peritoneum, pleural space, cerebrospinal fluid (CSF). It is not usually useful to Gram stain pharyngeal exudates or stool. A careful evaluation of the Gram stain allows the clinician to determine if the specimen obtained is adequate and truly representative of the infected area. The Gram stain features that suggest a true sampling of the infected area include the presence of many polymorphonuclear leukocytes, large numbers of organisms, the predominance of a single type of organism, and the absence of epithelia cells from the contiguous mucosal surface. If these findings are present, an acute bacterial infection is highly likely. In the absence of these features on Gram stain, the physician should strongly consider obtaining another specimen for Gram stain and culture and should hesitate to base therapy upon bacteriologic results from the original specimen.

The Gram stain is uniquely useful in guiding the selection of initial antibiotic therapy. It gives the clinician an appropriate etiologic answer at the time when he or she first sees the patient. Additionally, it gives an estimate of the relative numbers of organisms present in a specimen, and it may demonstrate organisms that by virtue of their fastidiousness, may not grow in the bacteriology lab, for example, gonococci, pneumococci, and anaerobes.

Interpretation of the Gram stain should include the following steps:

1. Evaluate adequacy of specimens from infected areas under low power magnification. Properly collected specimens

TABLE 28.4 Specimen Examination and Culture

Specimen	Examination[a]	Culture Media[a]
Blood	Buffy coat smear[b]	5 ml each into 100 ml dextrose phosphate broth and thioglycolate
Throat		
Streptococcus group A		BAP
Gonococcus		TM
diphtheroid		Loeffler's slant
		Tellurite plate
Middle ear and sinuses	Gram stain	BAP
		CAP
Sputum		
Expectorated	Gram stain	BAP, MAC, CAP
Nasotracheal suction		LJ
Bronchoscopy washings	AFB stain[b]	Sab[b]
Transtracheal aspirate	Gram stain	BAP, MAC, CAP
Lung aspirate	AFB stain[b]	Primary anaerobic plate
		LJ[b]
		Sab[b]
Urine	Urinalysis	BAP, MAC
	Gram stain	
Urethra, cervix	Gram stain	BAP, TM, MAC
Wound or abscess	Gram stain	BAP, MAC
		Primary anaerobic plate and thioglycolate
Fluid	Cell count and	BAP, MAC, CAS
CSF, joint, pleural,	differential	Nutrient broth
peritoneal	Protein and glucose	Primary anaerobic plate
	Gram stain	LJ[b]
	AFB stain[b]	Sab[b]
	Fungal stain[b]	
Stool	Wet preparations for cells and ova and parasites Methylene blue stain for leukocytes	BAP, MAC, CM, SS, or XLD

Adopted from Gardner P, Provine HT: *Manual of Acute Bacterial Infections.* Boston, Little Brown Company, 1975.

[a]Abbreviations: AFB, acid fast bacilli; BAP, blood agar plate; CAP, chocolate agar plate; CAS, chocolate agar slant; SS, Salmonella shigellae agar plate; TM, Thayer-Martin agar plate; MAC, MacConkey agar plate; LJ, Lowenstein-Jensen slant for tuberculosis; Sab, Sabouraud's slant for fungi; CM, Campylobacter agar plate; XLD, xylose, lysine, desoxycholate.

[b]If clinically indicated.

should contain large numbers of polymorphonuclear leukocytes and few epithelial cells.

2. Evaluate adequacy of stain under oil emersion. If the staining has been properly carried out, polymorphonuclear leukocytes should appear red. If they are blue, there has been inadequate decolorization.

3. Evaluate the presence of bacteria. Gram-positive organisms appear dark blue to purple, and gram-negative organisms appear pink to red. Most infections from normally sterile areas will show a single organism. The presence of several different types of organisms is common in aspiration pneumonia and lung abscesses, peritonitis, abdominal abscesses, gynecologic infections, and peripheral ulcers.

4. Examine several areas of the smear before drawing conclusions. Consider obtaining another specimen or repeating the procedures if the results are equivocal.

TABLE 28.5 Gram Stain Technique

Preparation
1. Using a sterile swab or loop, make a thin smear of material on a clean glass slide.
2. Air dry.
3. Heat fix by passing slide over flame two or three times.
4. Place a wax mark near the smear.

Staining
1. Flood slide with crystal violet for 10 seconds. Rinse with water.
2. Flood slide with Gram's iodine for 10 seconds. Rinse with water.
3. Decolorize with ethanol–acetone or ethanol (95%) until the thinnest parts of the smear are colorless. Rinse with water.
4. Flood with safranin for 10 seconds. Wash with water. Air or blot dry.

5. Consider performing an acid-fast stain and procedures for demonstrating fungi and parasites if the clinical presentation suggests the possibility of these agents.

CULTURE OF THE SPECIMEN

The details of the multiplicity of culturing techniques and material available are beyond the scope of this chapter. Table 28.4 outlines a reasonable selection of media for specimens from different sites. The clinician should be aware of a few general principles of microbiologic culturing as outlined below:

1. All specimens should be planted as soon as possible after being obtained. Delay may result in the loss of fastidious flora or an overgrowth of contaminants. Specimens should be refrigerated if delay is anticipated.
2. Media may be either nonselective (will support the growth of most common pathogens, i.e., blood agar) or selective (contain special nutrients that will promote the growth of certain organisms and inhibit that of others, e.g. *Salmonella–Shigella* and Thayer-Martin agars). Selective media are invaluable in identifying pathogens in areas of mixed flora, but they may occasionally suppress the growth of the desired pathogen as well. Therefore a combination of several types of media is usually inoculated to give the optimum yield.
3. Specimens should be streaked on agar plates in order to increase the likelihood of isolation of discrete colonies. This is best accomplished by four overlapping streakings.
4. Anaerobic cultures are necessary in specimens in which anaerobes are likely to be significant pathogens. These in-

clude infections in proximity to a mucosal surface (pharynx, colon, vagina), those associated with malignancies, necrotic tissues, and foreign bodies, and infections in which there is a fetid odor, gas in tissues, or septic phlebitis. In these circumstances, specimens should be processed immediately for anaerobes specifically. Many devices and media are available for removing oxygen and preserving anaerobic growth. An anaerobic culturing system should be available in most bacteriology laboratories.

5. Obtaining a quantitative estimate of the number of bacteria is helpful in evaluating patients with urinary tract infections. Techniques to evaluate whether a significant number of bacteria are present in urine samples include the use of calibrated loop and a dip stick method. More than 10^5 bacteria are visible after 18 hours with these techniques. Both of these methods allow for the determination of colonial morphology and Gram stain characteristics. More rapid means of determining whether significant bacteriuria exists are available in automated laboratories using machines that detect bacterial growth by optical density or detection of radiolabeled gas produced by bacterial metabolism of a radioactive substrate.

Routine cultures are generally examined after 18–24 hours of incubation. Anaerobic cultures are examined after 48 hours. Definitive identification of organisms and antimicrobial sensitivity patterns usually are available in each instance after an additional 24–48 hours.

6. Diagnostic and therapeutic errors often result from assuming that growth of organisms is equivalent to infection from these organisms. Table 28.1 lists the normal flora in various anatomical sites that may grow in clinical specimens. The presence of bacterial growth must be interpreted in the light of all available clinical information, and the possibility of contamination with normal flora must always be considered. This is especially true with the automated rapid diagnostic laboratory techniques mentioned above.

7. The clinical characteristics of the patient's infection may suggest the need for special cultures for mycobacteria, fungi, or fastidious organisms. The use of special cultures for viruses, mycoplasmas, rickettsiae, and chlamydiae is sometimes also useful, although they are usually only available in research or referral laboratories.

THERAPY

Use of Antibiotics—General Principles

The selection of the optimal therapy for the infected patient is based upon those diagnostic maneuvers elaborated upon in preceding sections of this chapter. If the portal of entry and likely pathogens are defined and demonstrated, specific and effective therapy can usually be selected. The following general therapeutic principles should be borne in mind before initiating therapy:

1. All possible attempts should be made within the confines of the tempo and seriousness of the situation to collect adequate diagnostic material before instituting therapy.

2. Antimicrobial therapy should only be administered if a significant infection is felt to be present or is highly likely.

3. Patients should be questioned about allergies to the specific agents to be administered before they are given and should be monitored for antimicrobial toxicity during therapy. This is particularly true of patients who exhibit hypersensitivity to penicillins, nephrotoxicity to aminoglycoside agents such as gentamicin, kanamycin, tobramycin, and amikacin, and hematologic effects to chloramphenicol, or moxolactam.

4. The pharmacology of the drug(s) to be used should be considered. Its route of administration and diffusion into the infected site should be taken into account. In seriously ill patients with life-threatening infections, antimicrobial agents should be given parenterally, preferable by intravenous route. We favor high-dose therapy administered by intermittent bolus, the interval determined by the pharmacology of the individual agent. The appropriate dose and dosage interval for commonly used agents are outlined in Table 28.6.

5. The toxicity of drug(s) to be used should be considered in the individual patient. Patients at risk for serious side effects of certain agents should be considered for therapy with alternative agents (Table 28.7).

6. The selection of antimicrobial agent(s) should be specific. A shotgun, unthinking approach with broad spectrum agents or fixed combinations of drugs should be avoided. The choice of agent(s) should be on the basis of all of the assembled data on the individual patient and not on a preset formula.

7. Drug incompatibilities or antagonisms should be avoided. More than one agent should not be mixed in the same administration apparatus.

8. Undue and exclusive reliance upon antimicrobial agents may be dangerous in patients with serious infections. Surgical intervention is often essential, for example, drainage of abscesses, removal of foreign bodies, relief of obstructed viscera, and debridement of necrotic tissue.

9. Specific and appropriate antimicrobial therapy must be combined with sound supportive care and physiologic management. For example, fluid and electrolyte balance must be maintained, acidosis and hypotension corrected, and pulmonary secretions drained.

10. Efficacy and toxicity are the major factors to consider in the selection of antimicrobial agents. If several agents are equivalent for the treatment of an infection in an individual patient, the comparative cost of the agents should be considered and the least expensive one chosen.

Table 28.6 provides the usual recommended doses of selected, commonly used antimicrobial agents and their spectrum of activity, common indications, and important adverse effects. For many organisms and infections there is controversy about antimicrobial agents of choice. Some selections represent our bias, although in most cases in which controversy exists, the most generally accepted agent has been recommended or several agents have been recorded. The choices are recorded for initial therapy before laboratory confirmation of susceptibility is available. For certain organisms in which susceptibility is so variable, initial choices must always be confirmed by laboratory testing. Refer to the standard reference texts noted in the selected reading for more detailed information on antimicrobial use.

Treatment of Fever

In most adult patients, fever does not require specific therapy. Most patients, particularly young adults, will tolerate fever quite well without adverse effect or morbidity. High or prolonged fever may cause increased tissue catabolism or dehydration, may increase or precipitate congestive heart failure, and may cause convulsions (in infants and children). Specific antipyretic therapy is therefore indicated in the following clinical circumstances: in children under the age of 3 to reduce the likelihood of febrile convulsions; in older adults if the fever and the ensuing hypermetabolic and high output state are judged to have dangerous cardiovascular consequences; in patients with heat stroke; and in uncomfortable patients with minor febrile illness, that is, viral respiratory infection in which the febrile pattern is not essential for diagnostic or therapeutic assessment. In most other circumstances in which the patient is seriously ill, the attempt to eliminate or suppress the febrile response is unnecessary and may lead to clinical confusion by obscuring the fever pattern or clouding the assessment of response to specific antimicrobial therapy. Antipyretics may occasionally be dangerous to the patient as well; hypotension and hypothermia may result from overzealous antipyretic use in febrile patients with gram-negative bacteremia, typhoid fever, and other bacterial infections. If the patient is uncomfortable from fever-related symptoms such as myalgias or head-

TABLE 28.6 Selected Antibiotic Dosages, Spectra, and Adverse Effects

Agent Generic Name (Brand Name)	Usual Adult Dosage	Usual Pediatric Dosage	Spectrum of Activity	Adverse Effects	Common Indications
Penicillins *Penicillinase susceptible* Penicillin G Aqueous crystalline	500,000–4 million units q4h IV	10–75,000 units/kg every 4 hrs IV 50–400,000 units/kg/ day)	Gram(+) cocci including Streptococci (enterococcus less susceptible) Pneumococci Not most staphylococci Gram(−) cocci including Meningococcus Gonococcus	Hypersensitivity reactions including rash fever Rarely Anaphylaxis (1/30,000 usages) Hemolytic anemia Interstitial nephritis	Upper and lower respiratory tract infections Impetigo Erysipelas Cellulitis Meningitis and endocarditis Gonorrhea Syphilis
Procaine	Higher doses for meningitis and endocarditis 600,000–1.2 million units q12h IM	10–25,000 units/kg q12h IM 20–50,000 units/kg/d)			
Benzathine	600,000–1.2 million units every week–month IM	10–25,000 units/kg IM	Gram(−) bacilli including *Shigella.* Most strains of indole (−) *Proteus* Some strains of *E. coli* and *H. influenzae* Not *Pseudomonas, Klebsiella, Enterobacter, Serratia* Gram(+) bacilli including *Clostridium Listeria T. pallidum* (syphilis)		
Phenoxymethyl penicillin (penicillin V)	0.25–1 g q6h PO (before meals)	10–15 mg/kg q6h PO (40–60 mg/kg/d)	Gram(+) cocci as above Gram(+) organisms less susceptible including Gonococcus Meningococcus *H. influenzae* Gram(−) bacilli	As above	Oral treatment of above skin and respiratory tract infections
Ampicillin	0.25–1.0 g q6h PO 0.5–2 g q4–6h IV (Higher doses for meningitis and endocarditis)	10–25 mg/kg q6h PO (40–100 mg/kg/d) 15–100 mg/kg c4h IV (50–400 mg/kg/d)	Gram(+) cocci as above Not most staphylococci Gram(−) organisms including *H. influenzae* (5–20% strains may be resistant) Meningococcus Gonococcus *Salmonella Shigella* (amp > amox) Many strains of indole(−) *Proteus E. Coli* Not *Pseudomonas Klebsiella Enterobacter Serratia*	As above Rash 3 times more frequent than with penicillin G Diarrhea ? amp > amox	Respiratory tract infections, particularly otitis in children Meningitis GI and GU infections Gonorrhea *Salmonella* and *Shigella* infections (amp > amox)
Amoxicillin (Amoxil, Larotid)	0.25–0.50 g every 8 hr PO	7.5–15 mg/kg every 8 hr PO (20–40 mg/kg/ day)			
Carbenicillin (Pyopen–Geopen)	5 g q4h IV	25–100 mg/kg/q4h IV (100–500 mg/kg/d)	Gram(+) cocci Not most staphylococci, not enterococci Gram(−) bacilli including	Hypersensitivity as with other penicillins Thrombocytopenia Hypokalemia	*Pseudomonas* infections (with aminoglycoside) Mixed anaerobic

TABLE 28.6 (Continued)

Agent Generic Name (Brand Name)	Usual Adult Dosage	Usual Pediatric Dosage	Spectrum of Activity	Adverse Effects	Common Indications
			Pseudomonas Proteus E. coli Enterobacter including many Bacteroides fragilis Not Klebsiella Gram(−) anaerobes	Hemolytic anemia Salt overload	infections Urinary tract infections, including prostatitis
Ticarcillin (Ticar)			Same as Carbenicillin	Less salt overload	Same as Carbenicillin
Penicillinase Resistant Penicillins (PRP)					
Oxacillin (Prostaphlin)	0.5–2.0 g q4–6h IV	25–100 mg/kg/q4–6h IV (100–200 mg/kg/d)	Staphylococcus aureus Other Gram(+) cocci including Pneumonococci Streptococci (Not enterococci)	Hypersensitivity as with other penicillins Rarely interstitial nephritis, granulocytopenia	
Nafcillin (Unipen)	Same	Same			
Methacillin (Staphcillin)	Same	Same			
Cloxacillin (Tegopen)	0.25–0.5 g q6h PO	10–25 mg/kg q6h PO (50–100 mg/kg/d)			
Dicloxacillin (Dynapen, Pathocil)	0.125–0.25 g q6h PO	5–25 mg/kg q6h PO (20–50 mg/kg/d)			
Cephalosporins					
Cephalothin (Keflin)	0.5–2 g q4–6h IV	15–40 mg/kg q4–6h IV (60–250 mg/kg/d)	Gram(+) cocci including Staphylococcus aureus Pneumococci Streptococci Not enterococci Gram(−) bacilli including many strains of E. coli Klebsiella Proteus Not H. influenzae Meningococci Gonococci Enterobacter Serratia Pseudomonas B. fragilis	Hypersensitivity reactions including Rash and fever Phlebitis Rarely Anaphylaxis Granulocytopenia Nephrotoxicity	Second choice agents after penicillins or in penicillin-allergic patients for respiratory, skin and soft tissue Gi, Gu tract infections, and endocarditis (Not to be used in CNS infections)
Cephazolin (Kefzol, Ancef)	0.5–2 g q6–8h IV or IM	8–25 mg/kg q6–8h IV or IM (25–100 mg/kg/d)			
Cephalexin (Keflex)	0.25–1 g q6h PO	8–15 mg/kg/q6h PO (25–60mg/kg/d)			
Cephapirin (Cephadyl)	0.5–2g q4–6h IV or IM	15–40 mg/kg/q4–6h IV (60–240 mg/kg/d)			
Cephradine (Velosef, Anspor)	0.25–1g q6h PO 0.5–2 g q4–6h	5–15 mg/kg q6h PO (20–50 mg/kg/d) 15–40 mg/kg q4–6h IV (60–250 mg/kg/d)			
Cefamandole (Mandol)	0.5–2 g q4–6h IV	15–40 mg/kg q4–6h IV 60–240 mg/kg/d	As above but more active against H. influenzae and other Gram(−) organisms		
Cefoxitin (Mefoxin)	0.5–2 g q4–6h IV	15–40 mg/kg q6h IV (60–240 mg/kg/d)	As above, but more active against B. fragilis and other Gram(−) organisms		
Cefotaxime (Claforan)	1–2 g q4–6h IV	Not established	As above, but more active against H. influenzae, B. fragilis, and most other Gram(−) organisms		As above, and CNS infections
Moxalactam (Moxam)	0.5–3 g q8h IV	15–60 mg/kg q8h IV	Not active against enterococci and Pseudomonas Streptococcus pneumoniae	Bleeding diathesis	As above, and CNS infections

Drug	Dose	Dose	Susceptible organisms	Side effects / Precautions	Clinical uses
Aminoglycosides Gentamicin (Garamycin)	1–2 mg/kg q8h IM or IV 5 mg intrathecal q12h	1–2.5 mg/kg q8h IM or IV (3–7.5 mg/kg/day) 1–2 mg intrathecal q12h	Gram(−) bacilli including most strains of E. coli Klebsiella Proteus Enterobacter Serratia Pseudomonas Acinetobacter Not B. fragilis Gonococci Meningococci H. influenzae Gram(+) cocci including Staphylococcus aureus Streptococci (with penicillin) Not pneumococci	Nephrotoxicity and ototoxicity dose and serum level related 1. Monitor renal function and serum levels; safe level = peak—7–10 µg/ml through < 2 µg/ml 2. Avoid simultaneous use of ethacrynic acid, furosemide, cephalosporins 3. Adjust dose in renal failure by Levels Nomogram Formula Dose Intervals = 1–2 mg/kg × creatine × 8 Rare: Neuromuscular blockade, rash	Life-threatening infections of GI and GU tract and sepsis of undetermined origin in immunocompromised or hospitalized patients
Kanamycin (Kantrex)	7.5 mg/kg q12h IM or IV	7.5 mg/kg q12h IM or IV	Gram(−) bacilli As above (fewer strains susceptible) Not Pseudomonas Gram(+) cocci As above	Same, adjust dose by Levels Nomogram Formula–dose interval 7.5 mg/kg × creatine × 9	Non-hospital-acquired gram-negative infections
Tobramycin (Nebcin) Amikacin (Amikin)	1–2 mg/kg q8h IV or IM 7.5 mg/kg q12h IV or IM	1–2 mg/kg q8h IV or IM 7.5 mg/kg q12h IV or IM	Most strains of Gram(−) organisms as above, including Pseudomonas Acinetobacter Not B. fragilis Gonococci Meningococci H. influenzae	Same	
Streptomycin	0.5–1 g q12h IM	10–15 mg/kg q12h IM	Few strains of Gram(−) bacilli Brucella Yersinia pestis Franciscella tularensis M. tuberculosis	Same	Brucellosis Plague Tularemia Tuberculosis
Tetracyclines Tetracycline	0.25–0.50 g q5h PO before meals (absorption interfered with by Fe^{2+}, Ca^{2+}, Al^{2+}, Mg^{2+})	Not recommended	Many strains of Gram(+) and (−) organisms including H. influenzae Gonococci B. fragilis	GI distress Negative nitrogen balance (↑ BUN) Teeth and bone staining (children < 8 years) Rare	Minor respiratory tract infections, including Mycoplasmal pneumonia Urinary tract infections
Doxycycline (Vibramycin)	0.1 g q12h PO or IV × 24 hr then 0.1–0.2 g/d (can use in renal failure)	Not recommended	E. coli T. pallidum Not Staphylococcus aureus Pseudomonas Many group A streptococci	Hepatotoxic	Gonorrhea Other GU infections Syphilis in penicillin-allergic patients

TABLE 28.6 (Continued)

Agent Generic Name (Brand Name)	Usual Adult Dosage	Usual Pediatric Dosage	Spectrum of Activity	Adverse Effects	Common Indications
Minocycline (Minocin)	100 mg PO	Not recommended	Mycoplasma Rickettsiae Chlamydiae	Same + vestibular toxicity	
Erythromycin	0.25–0.50 g q6h PO 0.25–1 g q6h IV	7.5–15 mg/kg q6h PO (30–50 mg/kg/d) 15 mg/kg q6h IV (50 mg/kg/d)	Gram(+) cocci including Staphylococcus aureus Pneumococci Streptococci Gram(+) bacilli including Diphtheria Clostridia Gram(−) cocci including Gonococci Meningococci Bacteroides H. influenzae Legionella T. pallidum (syphilis) Chlamydiae Mycoplasma	Gastrointestinal distress Rare Rash Cholestatic Jaundice with estolate preparation	Skin and respiratory and GU infections in penicillin-allergic patients Mycoplasmal pneumonia Legionnaire's disease
Clindamycin (Cleocin)	0.150–0.450 g q6h PO 0.150–0.900 g q6h IV or IM	2.5–6 mg/kg q6h PO (10–25 mg/kg/d) 2.4–10 mg/kg q6h IV or IM (10–40 mg/kg/d)	Gram(+) cocci including Staphylococcus aureus Pneumococci Streptococci (not Enterococci) Gram(−) anaerobes including B. fragilis Not Gonococci Meningococci H. influenzae Mycoplasma Chlamydiae Gram(−) aerobes	Diarrhea Rare Pseudomembranous colitis	Staphylococcus aureus Infections in penicillin-allergic patients, mixed anaerobic GI and GU infections including peritonitis and abscesses
Chloramphenicol (Chloromycetin)	0.25–0.75 g q6h PO 0.25–1 g q6h IV (do not give IM)	10 mg/kg q6h PO 10–25 mg/kg q6h IV (50–100 mg/kg/d)	Gram(+) organisms including Staphylococcus aureus (not agent of choice) Pneumococcus Streptococci (some enterococci) Clostridia Gram(−) organisms including Many E. coli Klebsiella Enterobacter Proteus Salmonella H. influenzae Meningococci Gonococci B. fragilis Not Pseudomonas Rickettsiae Chlamydiae	Bone marrow depression (dose related—reversible) Keep levels < 25 μg/ml Monitor serum Fe, retic count CBC[a] (q3d) Bone marrow aplasia (idiosyncratic—rare N 1/30,000 usages) Gray baby syndrome	CNS infections in penicillin-allergic patients Life-threatening H. influenzae infections Mixed anaerobic GI and GU infections including peritonitis and abscesses Typhoid fever

Drug	Dosage	Spectrum	Toxicity	Clinical use
Vancomycin (Vancocin)	0.5 g q6h IV 0.5 g q6h PO (topical—not absorbed)	Gram(+) organisms including *Staphylococcus aureus*, *Staphylococcus epidermidis*, Pneumococci, Streptococci including enterococci	Fever Rash Ototoxicity (unusual) Nephrotoxicity (rare)	Staphylococcal and enterococcal endocarditis in penicillin-allergic patients Pseudomembranous colitis
Trimethoprim Sulfamethoxazole (Bactrim, Septra)	2 tabs bid (400 mg SMZ[b]; 50 mg TMP[c]) 25–50 mg/kg/d SMZ 5–10 mg/kg/day TMP divided into q8–12h intervals	Gram(+) organisms including Pneumococci, Streptococci (not enterococci), Not *Staphylococcus aureus* Gram(−) organisms including *E. coli*, *Salmonella*, *Shigella*, Many *H. influenzae* Not *Pseudomonas*, *B. fragilis*, *Pneumocystis carinii*	Hypersensitivity reactions Rash Fever Rare Hemolytic anemia Bone marrow depression	Respiratory and urinary tract infections Pneumocystic pneumonia

[a]CBC, complete blood count

[b]SMZ, Sulfamethoxazole

[c]TMP, Trimethoprim

TABLE 28.7 Antimicrobial Choices for Selected Pathologic Organisms

Infecting Organism	Drug of Choice	Alternative
Gram-positive cocci		
Staphylococcus aureus		
Non-penicillinase producing	Penicillin G	Cephalosporin[b] Clindamycin Vancomycin
Penicillinase producing	PRP[a]	Cephalosporin[b] Clindamycin Vancomycin
Staphylococcus epidermidis	Vancomycin	PRP[a,c] Cephalosporin[b,c] Gentamicin
Streptococcus pyogenes (group A) and groups B, C, G	Penicillin G	Erythromycin Cephalosporin[b] Clindamycin
Streptococcus viridans	Penicillin G	Cephalosporin[b] Vancomycin Erythromycin
Streptococcus faecalis (enterococcus)		
Endocarditis	Ampicillin with gentamicin	Vancomycin with gentamicin
Urinary tract	Ampicillin	Chloramphenicol[c] Tetracycline[c] Erythromycin[c]
Streptococcus, anaerobic	Penicillin G	Clindamycin Erythromycin Tetracycline
Streptococcus pneumoniae (pneumococcus)	Penicillin G	Erythromycin Cephalosporin[b] Chloramphenicol
Gram-negative cocci		
Neisseria meningitidis (meningococcus)	Penicillin G	Chloramphenicol Sulfonamide
Neisseria gonorrhoea (gonococcus)	Penicillin G	Ampicillin Tetracycline Spectinomycin Erythromycin
Gram-positive bacilli		
Clostridium perfringens	Penicillin G	Tetracycline Erythromycin Chloramphenicol
Clostridium tetani	Penicillin G	Tetracycline
Corynebacterium diphtheriae	Erythromycin	Penicillin G
Listeria monocytogenes	Ampicillin with or without gentamicin	Penicillin G Tetracycline Erythromycin
Gram-negative bacilli		
Acinetobacter (Mima, Herellea)[c]	Gentamicin	Tobramycin Amikacin Kanamycin Chloramphenicol
Bacteroides		
Oropharyngeal strains	Penicillin G	Clindamycin Ampicillin Chloramphenicol Tetracycline
Gastrointestinal and genital strains	Clindamycin	Chloramphenicol Metronidazole Tetracycline

TABLE 28.7 (Continued)

Infecting Organism	Drug of Choice	Alternative
Bordetella pertussis (whooping cough)	Erythromycin	Ampicillin
Brucella (brucellosis)	Tetracycline with or without streptomycin	Chloramphenicol with or without streptomycin Trimethoprim–Sulfamethoxazole
Enterobacter[c]	Gentamicin	Tobramycin Amikacin Kanamycin Chloramphenicol Tetracycline Carbenicillin
Escherichia coli Community acquired[c]	Ampicillin or sulfasoxazole	Gentamicin Cephalosporin[b] Tetracycline Chloramphenicol
Hospital acquired[c]	Gentamicin	Ampicillin Cephalosporin[b] Tobramycin Kanamycin Tetracycline Chloramphenicol
Francisella tularensis (tularemia)	Streptomycin	Tetracycline Chloramphenicol
Haemophilus influenzae Meningitis, epiglottitis or other life-threatening infection[c]	Chloramphenicol	Ampicillin
Other infections	Ampicillin or amoxicillin	Trimethoprim Sulfamethoxazole Tetracycline Cephamandole Sulfonamide
Klebsiella pneumoniae[c]	Gentamicin	Tobramycin Kanamycin Cephalosporin[b] Chloramphenicol Amikacin
Pasteurella multocida	Penicillin G	Tetracycline Cephalosporin[b]
Proteus mirabilis[c] (indole negative)	Ampicillin	Kanamycin Cephalosporin[b] Gentamicin Tobramycin Chloramphenicol Amikacin
Other Proteus[c] (indole positive)	Gentamicin	Kanamycin Tobramycin Amikacin Chloramphenicol Tetracycline Carbenicillin
Pseudomonas aeruginosa Urinary tract infection[c]	Carbenicillin	Gentamicin Polymyxin Tobramycin Amikacin

TABLE 28.7 (Continued)

Infecting Organism	Drug of Choice	Alternative
Other infections[c]	Gentamicin or tobramycin with carbenicillin or ticarcillin	
Providencia[c]	Gentamicin	Cephalosporin[b] Kanamycin Amikacin Chloramphenicol Trimethoprim–Sulfamethoxazole
Salmonella typhi[c]	Chloramphenicol	Ampicillin Amoxicillin Trimethoprim Sulfamethoxazole
Other Salmonella	Ampicillin	Chloramphenicol Trimethoprim–Sulfamethoxazole
Serratia marcescens[c]	Gentamicin	Tobramycin Amikacin Chloramphenicol Cephalosporin Carbenicillin
Shigella[c]	Ampicillin	Trimethoprim–Sulfamethoxazole Chloramphenicol Tetracycline
Yersinia pestis (plague)	Streptomycin	Tetracycline Chloramphenicol
Other Organisms		
Legionella	Erythromycin	
Leptospira (leptospirosis)	Penicillin G	Tetracycline
Treponema pallidum (syphilis)	Penicillin G	Tetracycline Erythromycin
Campylobacter fetus	Erythromycin	Tetracycline
Pneumocystis carinii	Trimethoprim-Sulfamethoxazole	Pentamidine
Rickettsia (Rocky Mountain spotted fever, typhus, Q fever)	Tetracycline	Chloramphenicol
Chlamydia (psittacosis, trachoma, nonspecific urethritis)	Tetracycline	Erythromycin Chloramphenicol
Mycoplasma pneumoniae	Tetracycline	Erythromycin

[a]Pencillinase-resistant penicillin—oxacillin, nafcillin, methacillin; 85–95% of *Staphylococcus aureus* are resistant to penicillin G, which should therefore be used only if susceptibility has been demonstrated.

[b]Cephalosporins–cephalothin, cefazolin, cephapirin, cefamandole, cefoxitin, cefotaxime, moxalactam. Cephalosporins have similar spectra of activity. Cephalothin, ceazolin, and cephapirin are somewhat more active against gram-positive organisms. Cefamandole has increased activity against *H. influenzae* and other gram-negative organisms. Cefoxitin has increased activity against *Bacteroides fragilis* and other gram-negative organisms. Cefotaxime and moxalactam are both active against many strains of antibiotic-resistant enteric gram-negative organisms and *H. influenzae* and *B. fragilis*. About 5% of patients with hypersensitivity to penicillin will have hypersensitivity reactions to cephalosporins. These agents should be used with caution in patients with immediate-type penicillin allergy.

[c]Antibiotic susceptibility varies and must be determined in the laboratory.

[d]Surgical drainage is usually necessary in addition to antibiotic therapy.

[e]Enteric gram-negative include *E. coli, Klebsiella, Proteus, Enterobacter.*

ache, it is often wiser to administer agents such as codeine or sedatives, which will suppress these symptoms without altering the fever. Particularly to be frowned upon in seriously ill patients in the hospital is the all too common practice of administering antipyretics on an "as required" basis when fever exceeds a certain level. This results in swinging fever pattern that is of great discomfort to the patient, because it causes rigors and sweats, and that is most confusing to the physician.

If it is necessary to reduce or suppress a fever, it is wisest to give antipyretic agents in low doses, every 2–4 hours. This will often produce a sustained lower temperature without causing dangerous and uncomfortable peaks and valleys.

Two classes of antipyretic drugs are commonly used: salicylates and paraaminophenol derivatives (acetaminophen). Aspirin is the most commonly used antipyretic agent. It may be given orally, intravenously, or per rectum as the clinical need dictates. Important side effects are gastrointestinal irritation, decreased platelet function, and tinnitus. Aspirin should not be given to patients who have bleeding disorders, who are on anticoagulant drugs, or who have ulcer disease. The usual adult dosage is 0.3–1 g every 2–4 hours. The rectal dosage is one or two 0.3g suppositories every 2–4 hours. Intravenous aspirin may be given in a dosage of 0.5 g every 8 hours. Paraaminophenol derivatives (acetaminophen) are being used with increasing frequency as antipyretic agents because of their relative safety. Side effects include methemoglobinemia and hemolytic anemia, both of which are rare. Acetaminophen is not a gastric irritant and has no effect upon the coagulation system. Usual adult dosages are 0.3–0.6 g usually every 3–6 hours.

In addition to antipyretic agents, tepid sponge baths may be used. They are more commonly used and more effective for children than adults. Hypothermia blankets are commonly used for febrile patients in the hospital setting. They are quite effective but cause shivering and are extremely uncomfortable. Additionally, careful hourly monitoring of rectal temperature is required since precipitious drops in temperature may occur. Hypothermia blankets should be discontinued if the patient's temperature falls below 38°C (100.4°F). It is extremely difficult to lower temperature with ice baths, and their use is generally reserved for patients with heat stroke. Maintenance of adequate hydration by intravenous or oral route is an important adjunct measure that should be routinely carried out in all febrile patients.

SPECIFIC INFECTIOUS DISEASES

Infectious emergencies frequently require both medical and surgical expertise. Many acute febrile emergencies are dis-

cussed in other chapters. Emphasis in this chapter is given to the presentation, complications, and management of specific diseases and life-threatening noninfectious febrile illnesses not discussed elsewhere in this book. Infections are grouped by organ system. Those diseases that are not primarily organ-system related are discussed as a group at the end of the chapter. Emphasis is placed upon the life-threatening infections or the life-threatening, albeit unusual, complications of commonly benign infections. This orientation is, of necessity, highly selective; for further in-depth reading, see the selected readings at the end of this chapter.

INFECTIONS OF THE SKIN AND SUBCUTANEOUS TISSUE

Primary Skin Infections

Primary skin infections are invariably characterized by warmth, erythema, swelling, pain, and tenderness. Since very few organisms are capable of penetrating unbroken skin, a primary penetrating break in the skin surface is usually present, for example, insect bite, abrasion, or laceration. Most primary skin infections are caused by gram-positive cocci (*Staphylococcus aureus* and group A streptococci). These and other pathogens may be suspect in certain clinical and epidemiologic circumstances (Table 28.8). More precise diagnosis is often possible by staining aspirated or draining pus. Most primary skin infections are associated with proximal tender lymphadenopathy. In certain clinical situations these may be aspirated and also yield a specific infective agent.

Erysipelas, a superficial rapidly spreading erythematous infection with raised margins and lymphangitis, is a clinically distinct and recognizable entity. It is invariably a result of group A streptococci and can therefore be treated with penicillin G alone.

Furuncles, unless in the perineum, are usually staphylococcal in origin. Treatment with a semisynthetic penicillinase-resistant penicillin or alternative is indicated if systemic signs and symptoms are present, the lesions are multiple, or there is spreading cellulitis. Surgical incision and drainage are often indicated.

Most common primary *cellulitic skin infections* are caused by staphylococci or streptococci. It is often difficult to distinguish clinically between a streptococcal and staphylococcal etiology. Treatment for both is indicated with a semisynthetic penicillinase-resistant penicillin unless a specific diagnosis is possible by examination of aspirated or draining pus or the epidemiologic setting suggests another infecting agent.

Rarely, unusual pathogens may be introduced into the skin

TABLE 28.8 Diagnostic and Theraputic Features of Skin Infections

Clinical Lesion	Epidemiologic Setting	Organism	Other Features	Drug of Choice	Alternatives
Primary skin infection					
Erysipelas	Any age	Group A Streptococcus	Lymphangitis, Raised margins, Draining lymphadenopathy	Penicillin g	Cephalosporin, Erythromycin, Clindamycin
Carbuncle Furuncle	Any age	Staphylococcus aureus	Gram-positive cocci in clusters	Oxacillin or nafcillin	Cephalosporin, Clindamycin
Bullous impetigo (scalded skin syndrome)	Infants	Staphylococcus aureus	Gram-positive cocci in clusters	Oxacillin or nafcillin	Cephalosporin, Clindamycin
Cellulitis	Any age, Most settings	Group A Streptococcus or Staphylococcus aureus	Gram-positive cocci in clusters or in chains, Draining lymphadenopathy	Oxacillin or nafcillin	Cephalosporin, Clindamycin
	Children < 5	H. influenzae	Purple color, Gram-negative coccobacilli, Bacteremia likely	Chloramphenicol	Ampicillin
	Dog and cat bites	Pasteurella multocida	Small gram-negative coccobacilli	Penicillin G	Cephalosporin, Tetracycline
	Hunters and farmers	Francisella tularensis (tularemia)	May be bacteremic, Suppurating nodes, Gram-negative rods	Streptomycin	Tetracycline, Chloramphenicol
	Fish and meat handlers	Erysipelothrix	Small gram-positive rods	Penicillin	Cephalosporin, Erythromycin, Tetracycline, Chloraphenicol
	Southwest United States, Rodent contact	Yersinea pestis (plague)	May be bacteremic, Large suppurating nodes, organism seen in Giemsa stain	Streptomycin	Tetracycline, Chloramphenicol
Traumatic skin infection					
Synergistic gangrene	After surgery or trauma	Staphylococcus aureus Streptococcus	Marked systemic toxicity, immediate surgical therapy	Oxacillin or nafcillin	Cephalosporin
Necrotizing fasciitis	Posttrauma	Staphylococcus aureus Streptococcus Gram-negative bacilli	Minimal systemic toxicity, immediate surgical therapy	Oxacillin or nafcillin plus gentamicin	Clindamycin or cephalosporin plus gentamicin
Bronze edema with bullae with myonecrosis	After trauma or surgery	Clostridium perfringens	Marked systemic toxicity, gram-positive rods, Immediate surgical therapy	Penicillin g	Chloramphenicol
Bacteremic skin infection					
Icthyma gangrenosum	Immunocompromised host with granutopenia	Pseudomonas aeruginosa	Bacteremic infection with vasculitis	Carbenicillin or ticarcillin with gentamicin or tobramycin	
Palpable purpura or skin infarcts	Any age	Staphylococcus aureus	Consider endocarditis	Oxacillin or nafcillin	Cephalosporin, Vancomycin
	Child or young adult	N. meningitidis	Consider meningitis	Penicillin G	Tetracycline
	Sexually active adult	N. gonorrhoeae	Consider genital source	Penicillin G	Tetracycline
Hemorrhagic pustules	Sexually active adult	N. gonorrhoeae	Arthritis, tenosynovitis may be present	Penicillin G	Tetracycline
Diffuse petechiae	Child or young adult	N. meningitidis	Consider meningitis	Penicillin G	Chloramphenicol
	Dog contact in endemic area	Rickettsial infections (Rocky Mountain spotted fever)		Tetracycline	
Rose spots (macular lesions on abdomen)	Travel to endemic area	Salmonella typhi	Diagnosis Lesions, blood, stool cultures—positive	Chloramphenicol	Ampicillin, Trimetoprim-sulfamethoxazole

through animal vectors. These include *Francisella tularensis* (tularemia), *Yersinea pestis* (plague), *Pasteurella multocida,* and *Erysipelothrix* (erysipeloid). Each of these has a specific epidemiologic setting noted in Table 28.8. Each is associated with cellulitis at the inoculation site and with tender, often draining, nodes. A high index of suspicion and early recognition are imperative in diagnosing plague and tularemia since both are associated with significant mortality when untreated. Plague is treated with streptomycin and/or tetracycline. Chloramphenicol may be used as an alternative agent. Streptomycin is also the agent of choice for the treatment of tularemia. Erysipeloid and *Pasteurella* infections are less serious, rarely life threatening, and effectively treated with penicillin.

THERAPY

Most primary skin infections can be treated in the emergency room with local measures, incision and drainage as indicated, oral antibiotics, and careful follow-up. Warm soaks and elevation and rest of the affected limb are palliative and may speed resolution. Therapy of choice and alternative drugs may be selected from Tables 28.6 and 28.7. Occasionally, primary skin infections may require hospitalization, intravenous antibiotics, and/or other emergency measures for the conditions listed below:

1. Infections in which there are crepitus and/or obvious necrosis of skin and underlying structures. In this circumstance extensive and immediate surgical debridement is essential.
2. Infections in which there are marked systemic toxicity, suspected bacteremia, and metastatic spread of infection.
3. Infections in which there are serious suspicions of underlying infection of bone, tendon, or joint or of a retained foreign body.
4. Infections in patients whose host defenses are compromised (granulocytopenia, extremes of age, vascular insufficiency in the affected limb).
5. Infections in patients who are likely to be unreliable and/or unable to comply with a medical outpatient regimen (i.e., alcohol or drug abusers, debilitated patients).
6. Infections in which there are suspicions of unusual etiologic agents (i.e., tularemia, plague).

Infections in Traumatized Skin

Infections in traumatized skin are often more complex bacteriologically than are primary skin infections and are more difficult to treat. These include infections in burns, wounds, and decubitus ulcers. Mixed aerobic and anaerobic bacterial etiol-

ogies are common, and therefore it is of major therapeutic importance to attempt a specific bacteriologic diagnosis. Often anaerobic organisms (clostridia or anaerobic streptococci) are present that are of clinical significance but will not be appreciated unless Gram stains and anaerobic cultures are taken.

Clostridial skin infections can be divided into two groups: anaerobic cellulitis and anaerobic myositis. The former is less severe and is characterized by local pain and systemic fever. Crepitation in the subcutaneous tissues and a spreading bronze-colored cellulitis are often present. There may be a pink, foul-smelling discharge from the lesion that on Gram stain shows large gram-positive rods without polymorphonuclear leukocytes. The latter, true gas gangrene, is abrupt in onset and characterized by severe local pain and marked systemic signs and symptoms of toxicity. The wound rapidly becomes necrotic, and dusky grey nonviable muscle can be seen at its base (see Chapter 13).

Synergistic (Meleney's) gangrene may occasionally follow surgery or trauma. An enlarging painful central area of necrosis surrounded by bright red cellulitis develops gradually over days. The slow development of the lesion sets it apart from classic gas gangrene. *Staphylococcus aureus* and anaerobic streptococci are the usual etiologic agents.

Necrotizing fasciitis progresses rapidly and differs from the other two infections in that there is usually minimal or no pain in the infected area, although an area of central necrosis is apparent. Systemic symptoms are minimal but fever is usually present. This infection is caused by mixed aerobic and anaerobic streptococci and is often found in tissue in which there is a compromised vascular supply.

THERAPY

Patients who have infections in traumatized skin require immediate hospitalization. Immediate extensive surgical debridement is the cornerstone of therapy; this is combined with appropriate antibiotic selection and administration. Since many of these infections are mixed, it is common for therapy to require several antimicrobial agents. The usual pathogens and the recommended antibiotic therapy for each agent are outlined in Table 28.8. The management of noninfected skin wounds including antimicrobial, tetanus, and rabies prophylaxis are discussed in detail in Chapters 13 and 14.

Bacteremic Skin Infections

The presence of bacteremic skin infections should be considered in patients who are systemically ill and have petechial and/or palpable purpuric lesions. These may be single or multiple and are characterized by bleeding into the skin and the later development of skin necrosis. Macular, papular, and vesicular eruptions are far less likely to be life threatening. They are usually not the result of bacterial infection but are more commonly seen in patients with viral and allergic illnesses. Bacteremic infection of the skin almost invariably indicates a severe life-threatening infection. Signs and symptoms of the primary site of infection should be carefully sought. The bacteria that are most likely to cause bacteremic infection metastatic to skin include *Staphylococcus aureus*, particularly in infectious endocarditis; *Pseudomonas*, in the setting of granulocytopenia; *Neisseria meningitidus*, in association with meningitis; *Neisseria gonorrhoeae*, in association with septic arthritis; and *Haemophilus influenzae*, in children under the age of 3. An immediate etiologic diagnosis is often possible by aspiration and Gram stain of purpuric or necrotic lesions. Blood cultures are usually positive, but therapy must be instituted before the results are known.

THERAPY

The treatment of bacteremic skin infections is essentially that of the underlying systemic bacteremic illness. Immediate hospitalization and the administration of high-dose systemic antibiotics (selection being based upon the clinical situation) are always indicated (Tables 28.6, 28.7). Appropriate hematologic studies to determine if disseminated intravascular coagulation is present should always be performed. Careful attention to physiologic life support to combat shock, congestive heart failure, and renal failure is essential.

Toxic Shock Syndrome

Toxic shock syndrome is a clinical entity characterized by fever; hypotension; a prominent generalized erythroderma; involvement of mucous membranes with resultant conjunctivitis, stomatitis/pharyngitis; diarrhea; and vaginal erythema. The disease is clearly the result of a *Staphylococcus aureus* produced toxin and in recent years has been most frequently associated with the use of vaginal tampons in menstruating women with vaginal *Staphylococcus aureus* carriage. The disease characteristically appears during or a short time after menses, although cases may occur when the patient has any staphylococcal infection. The major complications of the disease, as well as the substantial mortality in unrecognized cases, is the result of hypotension.

THERAPY

Treatment is directed immediately at volume expansion. Several liters of normal saline should be rapidly infused during the first hour after recognition. Further fluid administration depends upon the clinical course, but usually 6–8 liters will be required during the first 24 hours. Antistaphylococcal antibiotics should be administered as well. Their effect on the clinical course during an acute case may be minimal, but the substantial recurrence rate will be reduced. Women who recover from the disease should be advised against the subsequent use of vaginal tampons.

INFECTIONS OF THE RESPIRATORY TRACT

Upper Respiratory Tract Infections

Upper respiratory tract infections are among the most common medical problems seen in ambulatory practice. Most are viral in etiology and are self-limited. Rarely, an upper respiratory tract infection will result in threat to life by virtue of airway obstruction, spread to contiguous vital structures, or bacteremia.

Ludwig's angina is a rapidly advancing cellulitis of the floor of the mouth, base of the tongue, and anterior compartment of the neck. It is usually found in patient's with poor dental hygiene and is discussed in detail in Chapter 32.

Streptococcal pharyngitis is most commonly encountered in children and adolescents. Most cases occur in winter months in temperate climates. Streptococcal pharyngitis and its suppurative complications (peritonsillar or lateral pharyngeal abscesses) are discussed in Chapter 32.

Bacterial infection of the epiglottis, *epiglottitis,* is a frequently fatal illness if not recognized early and treated aggressively. It is most frequently encountered in children under 5 years old; however, cases occuring in adults are being increasingly recognized. Almost all cases are due to *H. influenzae,* type B. The infection is usually explosive in onset, with fever, marked dysphagia, barking cough, inability to handle secretions, and, most prominently, stridor and air hunger. In young children, epiglottitis must be distinguished from viral croup. Croup is insidious in onset accompanied by upper respiratory tract infections (URI) symptoms. Croup is also associated with a distinctive barking cough, and inspiratory stridor may be present. Epiglottitis is acute in onset, and patients are frequently more acutely ill than are patients with croup. In suspected cases of epiglottitis, it is safest to avoid directly visualizing the epiglottitis, as this may result in airway occlusion in the presence of epiglottitis. Lateral films of the neck should be performed immediately. The diagnosis of epiglottitis is established if the epiglottis is demonstrated to be enlarged and impinging on the airway. Blood cultures should be obtained (90% of patients are bacteremic) and cultures of the pharynx avoided. High-dose intraveneous (IV) chloramphenicol should be started (25 mg/kg every 6 hours). Ampicillin (75–100 mg/kg IV every 4 hours) may be given simultaneously. If the isolated organism is demonstrated to be sensitive to ampicillin, this agent may be substituted, or it may be continued and the chloramphenicol may be stopped. Since death from suffocation is a frequent complication, early tracheostomy should strongly be considered if respiratory embarrassment is severe. (See Chapters 32 and 44 for details of treatment.)

Acute bacterial sinusitis and otitis media are common and usually minor infections. Both are the result of spread of organisms commonly found in the upper respiratory tract when drainage of secretions is obstructed. Hence most cases occur in the context of colds or allergic rhinitis. Pain is a common presenting complaint, and its locations usually suggests the affected site. In patients with frontal sinusitis, the pain is located in the forehead, above the eyebrow. In patients with maxillary sinusitis, the pain is over the cheek and upper teeth. In patients with sphenoidal sinusitis, the pain may be in the suboccipital region, whereas in patients with ethmoidal sinusitis the pain may be in the temporal area or over the distribution of the trigeminal nerve. In patients with otitis media, the pain is usually within the ear, at the angle of the jaw, or over the mastoid bone.

In adults, acute bacterial sinusitis and otitis media are usually due to *Streptococcus pneumoniae* or other streptococci. In children, particularly under the age of 5, *H. influenzae* is the most common pathogen. Most of these infections are uncomplicated and respond easily to antibiotics and drainage. Rare but life-threatening complications of these infections are caused by their spread to contiguous structures resulting in orbital cellulitis, periorbital abscesses, cavernous sinus thrombosis, osteomyelitis, lateral vein thrombosis, brain abscess, and meningitis. Choice of antibiotic therapy is age dependent. Penicillin G is usually sufficient in adults, but ampicillin or trimethoprim sulfamethoxazole should be used in children. The choice of antibiotics in children ultimately will depend upon the prevalence of strains of *H. influenzae* that are resistant to ampicillin and typically seen in a particular community. Drainage is essential for curing sinusitis and is best accomplished with local heat, inhalation of heated mist, and oral decongestants. The role of decongestants in otitis media remains controversial. Most studies have not demonstrated their efficacy.

DIPHTHERIA

Although rarely encountered, *diphtheria* is an important disease to consider in severe upper respiratory tract infections in which exudate or membrane is present in the pharynx. Diphtheria is seen in individuals who have not been vaccinated or in whom vaccination has lapsed. These people include immigrants from developing countries and the urban or rural poor.

In the typical case, there is a low grade fever rarely over 38.3°C (101°F), pharyngeal pain, cervical lymphadenopathy, and a grey to black adherent membrane in the pharynx. Patients seen late in the course of the illness may present with suffocation from membrane extension, myocarditis, and late-appearing neurologic complications. An important feature that distinguishes diphtheria from mononucleosis, an illness in which pharyngeal membrane may also be present, is that in the former bleeding results when the membrane is removed. Milder forms of the disease, with minimal or no membrane formation, are exceedingly difficult to diagnose.

In all suspected cases a Gram stain of the exudate should be performed. Palisading gram-positive coccobacillary forms having the appearance of Chinese characters are typically seen. Special media Löffler's tellurite is required for culture, and therefore the bacteriology laboratory should be informed of the possibility of diphtheria when the specimen is submitted.

Therapy

Therapy is aimed at the neutralization of the toxin and elimination of the toxin-producing organism. Equine antitoxin, with appropriate precautions, is given in a dose of 40,000–80,000 units, half intramuscularly (IM) and half by slow intravenous infusion. If the membrane is causing respiratory embarrassment it should be removed. Bronchoscopy is the preferred approach to removal of the membrane from the trachea. Erythromycin is the drug of choice and should be given by intravenous route and continued for 2 weeks. Antibiotics probably offer little benefit to the sequalae of diphtheria, but they eliminate the carrier state.

Prognosis

The prognosis for patients with diphtheria is dependent upon the severity of infection and the degree of toxin. Illness associated with pharyngeal and laryngeal involvement has a more severe course than illness associated with nasal involvement alone. Myocarditis with atrioventricular (AV) block and left bundle branch block is associated with 60–100% mortality rate. Bleeding from the upper airway is also ominous. All patients with a tentative diagnosis of diphtheria should be isolated, and unimmunized contacts should be sought. These people should have throat cultures performed and should receive oral erythromycin prophylaxis.

Lower Respiratory Tract Infections

Lower respiratory tract infections—pneumonia and tracheobronchitis—are the most common infections for which patients require hospitalization and are the major infectious causes of death in the United States. Most patients with lower respiratory tract infections (LRTI) present with fever, cough, and shortness of breath. Major life-threatening complications include respiratory failure, bacteremia, and extrapulmonary spread of infection. The etiologic agents that cause infection of the lower respiratory tract are multiple. For purposes of clinical diagnosis and therapy it is useful to categorize infections into bacterial and nonbacterial etiologies. The latter are further divided into viral and mycoplasma and the former into the large number of possible bacterial etiologies on the basis of epidemiologic

clinical and laboratory findings (Table 28.9). Bacterial pneumonia represents the most life-threatening and specifically treatable entity and, as such, will be emphasized in this section. The major bacterial species responsible for pneumonia are *Streptococcus pneumoniae, Staphylococcus aureus*, gram-negative enteric bacilli, and *H. influenzae*.

CLINICAL CONTEXT

The *route of infection* of lower respiratory tract infection is twofold: aspiration of gastric, oral, and pharyngeal contents, or spread of microorganisms to the lungs through the bloodstream. The former is the most common route of bacterial infection and occurs most often in neonates and the elderly, particularly in the context of poor dental hygiene and/or the presence of anatomical or physiologic interference with normal swallowing, the gag reflex, and local host defenses. This includes the use of alcohol and sedatives and cigarette smoking. Pneumonia may occur during the course of a bacteremia, but this is relatively uncommon. Conversely, lower respiratory tract infections due to viruses are commonly the result of both extension from an upper respiratory infection and systemic viremia and not from aspiration.

TABLE 28.9 Differential Features of Common Pneumonias

	Bacterial	Viral	Mycoplasma
Age	Older adults Infants	Children Young adults	Young adults Children
URI[a]	Recent past	Present	Variable
Epidemic illness	No	Yes	Variable
Rigors	Common	Rare	Rare
Cough	Productive Sputum purulent	Nonproductive	Productive Sputum purulent
Pleuritic chest pain	Yes	No	No
Consolidation on physical examination	Yes	No	Variable
WBC	Elevated (shift to left)	Normal or diminished	Normal
X-ray film Infiltrate	Lobar or segmental	Patchy	Patchy
Effusion	Common	No	Occasional (very small)
Respiratory failure	Occasional	Uncommon	Rare
Sputum Gram stain	Many polys Predominant organism seen	No sputum or if obtainable, few inflammatory cells, few organisms	Polys Few organisms

Sputum culture	Pathogen isolated as predominant organism	Negative	Negative
			  Special cultures
			  Serologic tests

Blood cultures	Positive 30%	Negative	Negative

[a]URI, upper respiratory tract infection

Age is an important determinant of both the frequency and etiology of pneumonia. Patients at the extremes of age—neonates and the elderly—are at greater risk. Age further allows for some separation of bacterial etiologies. *Staphylococcus aureus*, group B streptococci, and enteric gram-negative bacilli are important bacterial pathogens in neonates. In children under the age of 5, *H. influenzae* and *Staphylococcus aureus* are significant pathogens. The major bacterial pathogen in adults that causes community-acquired pneumonia is *Streptococcus pneumoniae* (pneumococcus). In debilitated patients who acquire their infections in the hospital or after antibiotic administration, *Staphylococcus aureus* and gram-negative bacilli again become important pathogens. Children most commonly have nonbacterial etiologies, predominantly viral, for lower respiratory tract infection, and the most common cause of pneumonia in young adults is Mycoplasma pneumoniae.

Seasonal variations in lower respiratory tract infections are the rule in viral infections, most notably influenza. Therefore, viral pneumonia often involves many people simultaneously. Bacterial pneumonia is usually sporadic in occurence, although the majority of cases occurs during the colder months, often closely following influenza and other respiratory viral infections. *Mycoplasma pneumoniae* is less seasonal in occurrence and spreads slowly through a susceptible population.

DIAGNOSIS OF BACTERIAL PNEUMONIA

The history may give useful clues to both the presence and the etiology of the pneumonia. The tempo of the illness is helpful. Bacterial pneumonias arise abruptly and often are associated with rigors. In streptococcus pneumoniae there is classically one rigor that heralds the onset of the disease. A history of multiple rigors increases the likelihood of other bacterial pathogens. Pleuritic chest pain occurs in more than 75% of patients with bacterial pneumonia, whereas it is distinctly uncommon in patients with viral pneumonia and is infrequent in patients with mycoplasma pneumonia. The pleuritic chest pain associated with bacterial pneumonia is often severe enough to result in marked splinting of the affected side.

Bacterial pneumonia, except in dehydrated, debilitated patients and infants, is invariably associated with a painful cough productive of purulent sputum. In pneumococcal pneumonia the sputum is characteristically rusty although this may occasionally be seen with other bacterial etiologies as well. Green colored sputum is common in *H. influenzae* and *Pseudomonas aeruginosa* infections. Viscid, mucoid, bloody sputum is common in *Klebsiella* and staphylococcal infection. The sputum in patients with aspiration pneumonia and putrid lung abscess is characteristically thick and foul smelling. In the latter case,

the sputum may layer into distinctive bands. Viral pneumonia is most commonly associated with a dry, hacking, nonproductive cough. If sputum is produced, it is invariably yellow-white in color.

Nonrespiratory symptoms, including nausea, vomiting, and ileus, are common with bacterial pneumonia. Patients who have bacterial pneumonia, particularly when their lower lobes are involved, may present with abdominal pain, tenderness, or ileus. Pneumonia should be considered in all febrile patients with the acute onset of atypical abdominal pain. Neurologic findings, including delirium, are not uncommon, particularly in older people. Pneumonia caused by *Legionella pneumophila* (Legionnaire's disease) is characteristically associated with multisystem involvement including the liver, kidneys, and central nervous system.

Patients in whom a bacterial pneumonia occurs as a superinfection of a viral lower respiratory tract infection will often have a biphasic illness. The symptoms of the bacterial process will become prominent several days after seeming recovery from the viral infection has occurred. An exception to this general rule is superinfecting *Staphylococcus aureus* pneumonia, which may rapidly progress without an intervening recovery period and must be suspected in severely ill patients with a clinical picture of viral pneumonia.

The *physical examination* offers additional clues to the etiology of pneumonia. Most patients with acute bacterial pneumonia have the toxic appearance described earlier in this chapter. Patients are febrile, tachypneic, and often either anxious and agitated or lethargic. They may be cyanotic and hypotensive. This condition is variable and much less common in patients with nonbacterial pneumonia. Evidence of upper respiratory tract infection is common in patients with viral pneumonia, and bullous myringitis has been described as a useful, although not pathognomonic, finding in patients with *Mycoplasma* infection.

Findings of lobar consolidations are frequently present in patients who have bacterial pneumonia (bronchial breath sounds, percussion dullness, and increased fremitus accompanied by moist rales). Splinting on the involved side is common, and elevation of the ipsilateral hemidiaphragm occurs. The patient often sits up, leans forward, and breathes rapidly but shallowly in order to avoid pain. Signs of pleural effusion may be present as well; occasionally a pleural friction rub will be heard. Cyanosis of the lips and nail beds may be present. Patients with nonbacterial pneumonia will often have diffuse rales involving more than one anatomical segment. Friction rubs are not heard and their presence should suggest bacterial superinfection or pulmonary embolus, not nonbacterial pneumonia. It is common to appreciate only minimal physical findings in the presence of extensive viral pneumonia. Again it is important to point out that in pneumonia caused by *Staphylococcus aureus* the physical examination of the lungs may be deceptively normal.

Laboratory evaluation may help differentiate between various etiologies of pneumonia and aid in the management of patients with pneumonia. The complete blood count should always be performed in patients with suspected pneumonia. Although the results are not specific, they are helpful in suggesting etiology and prognosis: Bacterial pneumonias tend to produce white blood cell counts greater than 12,000/mm³ with a predominance of polymorphonuclear leukocytes and many band forms. The presence of fewer than 5,000 white blood cells per cubic millimeter is a poor prognostic sign in bacterial pneumonia and is associated with a mortality rate approaching 70%. The neutrophil population in the presence of leukopenia is still mostly polymorphonuclear and band forms. In contrast,

nonbacterial pneumonias may not elevate the white blood cell count and may produce relative lymphocytosis. Indeed, mild neutropenia may commonly be seen in patients with viral pneumonia. In some patients who have an overwhelming bacterial infection, marked neutropenia may be present.

At least two sets of blood cultures should be obtained in patients suspected of having bacterial pneumonia before therapy is instituted since bacteremia is present in about one-third of patients with bacterial pneumonia. Subsequent antibiotic therapy will be more rational if blood cultures are taken initially.

Arterial blood gases are often of great value in management of all forms of pneumonia. In the presence of marked hypoxia (PO₂ 50 mm H₂O), intubation and assisted ventilation must be considered.

Bedside cold agglutinin determination (agglutination of 4–5 drops of heparin in 1 ml blood, held on ice) should be per-

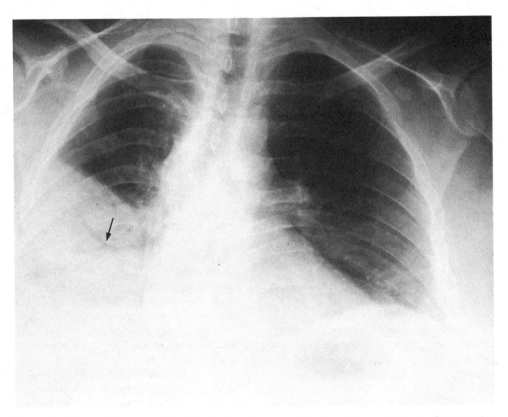

Figure 28.1 Bacterial pneumonitis with bulging fissure and air bronchiogram (arrow). The causative organism was *Streptococcus pneumoniae*.

formed in patients with nonbacterial pneumonia. Cold agglutinins are present in approximately 70% of patients with mycoplasmal pneumonia by the second week of illness. The test is useful but not pathognomonic since it may be positive in 15% of patients with viral pneumonia.

The chest film is indispensible in evaluating the patient with suspected pneumonia. Both posterior–anterior and lateral films should be obtained to allow for precise anatomical localization of any infiltrate and to best determine if fluid is present. Initially, in patients with pneumonia or who are markedly dehydrated, the chest film may be negative. In such cases, the history and physical examination must be relied upon more heavily. Repeat chest films after rehydration will usually show characteristic patterns. It is worth noting that patients with underlying chronic lung diseases may have atypical chest film appearance.

Bacterial pneumonias usually result in lobar and segmental consolidation that respects anatomical boundaries. An air bronchogram is usually observed, indicating fluid in the alveoli. The lobar pattern starts from the periphery and extends toward the hium. The predominant site of *Streptococcus pneumoniae* infection is in the lower lobes, but any lobe may be involved (Fig. 28.1). The same is true of most gram-negative pneumonias except for *Klebsiella pneumoniae,* which often involves the upper lobes, causing a downward bulging of the fissure. Aspiration pneumonia most commonly involves the apical segment of the right lower lobe or the posterior segment of the right or left upper lobe if the patient aspirates while on his or her back or side. The lower lobes are most frequently involved if aspiration occurs while the patient is in a sitting position. Multilobe involvement may be seen in all forms of bacterial pneumonia and carries a worse prognosis than involvement of a single lobe (Fig. 28.2). The x-ray appearance of *Staphylococcus aureus* pneumonia differs from other bacterial pneumonias in that infiltrates are often patchy and multiple and may cavitate.

Cavitary pneumonia may also result from gram-negative bacilli, aspiration pneumonia, and reactivation of *Mycobacterium tuberculosis* infection (Fig. 28.3). The cavities in gram-

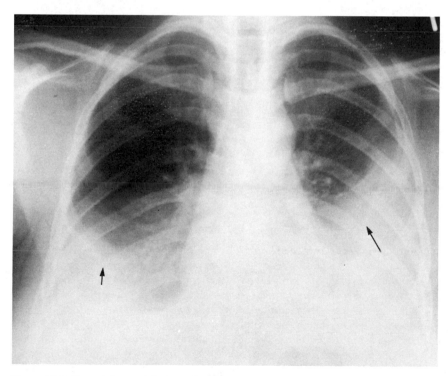

Figure 28.2 Bacterial superinfection of viral pneumonia with bilateral pleural effusions (arrows). The causative organism was *Hemophilus influenzae.*

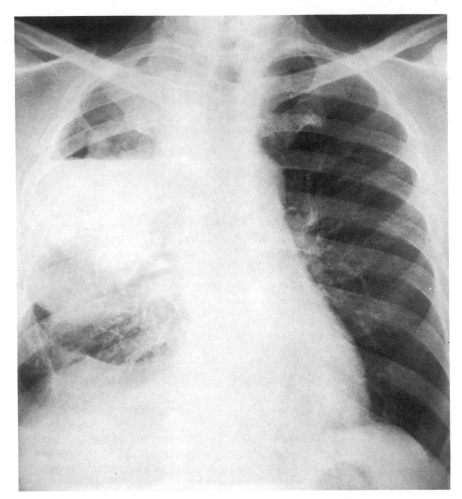

Figure 28.3 Lung abscess associated with aspiration pneumonia; an air fluid level is evident (arrow). The infection was a mixed one.

negative and *Staphylococcus aureus* pneumonia are often multiple. Whereas aspiration pneumonia usually results in a single large centrally cavitating lesion with an air fluid level in the locations noted above, the cavities in *Mycobacterium tuberculosis* disease are almost always in the upper lobes and are not associated with air fluid levels. Fungal pneumonias will demonstrate a radiologic appearance indistinguishable from tuberculosis. Many bacterial pneumonias are accompanied by pleural effusions. If fluid is evident, lateral decubitus films should be taken to assess whether the fluid is free or loculated. Loculated fluid should be further localized and drained under the guidance of ultrasound.

Nonbacterial pneumonias usually have a different radiologic appearance. Viral pneumonias are almost always interstitial in character. Pneumonia caused by *Mycoplasma pneumoniae* and *Legionella pneumophila* may show a mixed alveolar interstitial pattern. In pneumonia caused by these agents the infiltrates cross anatomical boundaries and are diffuse and patchy. They may be single or multiple, usually begin at the hilum and progress toward the periphery. The radiographic findings are frequently more prominent than are the physical findings. Viral and *Mycoplasma* pneumonias do not cavitate. Viral pneumonia is not associated with pleural effusions, and their presence should immediately raise the possibility of bacterial superinfection (Fig. 28.2). Mycoplasmal pneumonia may be associated with pleural effusions, but these are usually quite small. In addition, atypical pneumonias are virtually impossible to distinguish from each other by radiography pattern (Figs. 28.4, 28.5, and 28.6).

Sputum examination is the cornerstone of accurate diagnosis of pneumonia. Although all of the above noted epidemiologic, clinical, and radiographic findings are useful diagnostically, a properly obtained and correctly interpreted sputum specimen is crucial for the specific diagnosis of pneumonia. In most patients with bacterial pneumonia an adequately coughed specimen can be obtained with little difficulty. Measures that aid in the production of sputum are hydration, pulmonary therapy, and warm or ultrasonic nebulizer therapy. Unless the patient is desperately ill, it is usually possible to wait 1 or 2 hours until these measures are effective before proceeding to more invasive procedures or instituting empirical antibiotic therapy. If efforts to obtain an adequate expectorated specimen fail, and bacterial pneumonia is strongly suspected, nasotracheal or transtracheal aspiration should be performed. Patients with viral pneumonia usually will not produce sputum despite aggressive attempts to obtain a specimen.

The absence of sputum in an otherwise healthy patient who has pneumonia, is coughing, and is not markedly dehydrated is good evidence for an interstitial, not intraalveolar, process and strongly suggests a viral etiology. There are exceptions to this rule, but in general it is reliable. Conversely, it is worth repeating that patients with most bacterial pneumonias should be able to produce an adequate sputum specimen with proper encouragement and technique.

An adequate sputum specimen should contain fewer than 10 squamous epithelial cells and more than 25 leukocytes per

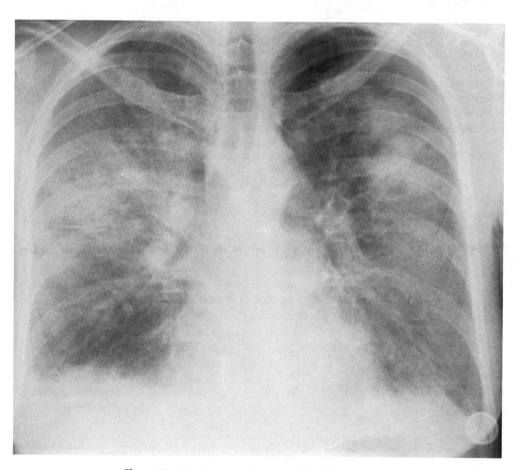

Figure 28.4 Viral pneumonitis caused by influenza virus.

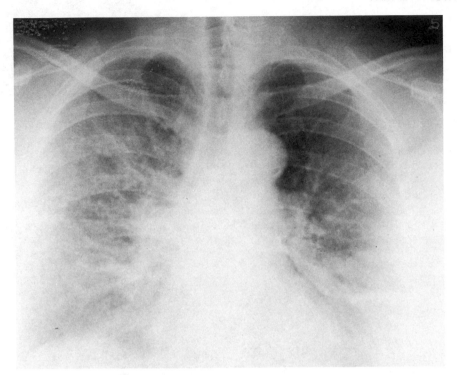

Figure 28.5 Radiographic pattern of *Legionella pneumoniae* infection (Legionnaire's disease).

low power field (× 100) on Gram stain in the presence of pneumonia. Bronchial mucosal cells and alveolar macrophages, if present, are additional supportive evidence of an adequate sample.

A Gram stain should be performed on all sputum specimens. *Streptococcus pneumoniae* appears as gram positive, lancet-shaped diplococcus; *Staphylococcus aureus* forms larger gram-positive grapelike clusters; *H. influenzae* is seen as small faintly staining gram-negative mixed coccal and bacillary organisms. Gram-negative plump rods are typically seen in *Klebsiella, Escherichia coli, Proteus,* and other enteric bacillary pneumonias. *Pseudomonas aerugionsa* are often similar in appearance. Aspiration pneumonia and lung abscesses will demonstrate a mixed predominantly gram-positive coccal flora.

In patients with pneumonia in whom inflammatory cells are seen on sputum Gram stain but organisms are absent, tuberculosis, fungal diseases, Legionnaire's disease, mycoplasmal pneumonia, *Chlamydia,* and rickettsial infection should be considered. Acid-fast stains of sputum should be performed to rule out tuberculosis in selected patients.

Transtracheal aspiration is the most reliable method of obtaining an excellent sputum specimen. Nasotracheal aspiration may produce sputum that is contaminated by mouth flora, whereas transtracheal aspiration will bypass the normal upper airway flora. This procedure is indicated particularly in a seriously ill patient with suspected bacterial pneumonia who may be infected with an usual pathogen and from whom sputum is unobtainable. This includes patients with hospital-acquired pneumonia, immunocompromised patients, patients who develop pneumonia while on antibiotics, and patients with cavitary pneumonias. Lack of experience with the transtracheal approach and concern about the small risk of complications has made it less commonly used than it should be as a routine diagnostic procedure.

Before performing a transtracheal aspiration, a history of bleeding disorder, and, if quickly available, a brief check of hemostasis should be made. (Prothrombin time should be within 3 seconds of control, and the platelet count should be greater than 50,000/mm^3.) The neck is hyperextended by placing a pillow under it and the cricothyroid cartilage is identified. The area is antiseptically prepared with iodophor and alcohol. The skin and subcutaneous tissue to the cricothyroid membrane is infiltrated with lidocaine (Xylocaine) and an Intracath needle (14 or 15 gauge) is introduced with bevel up, pointing toward the thorax. When the needle "pops" into the trachea, the catheter is quickly inserted and the needle is withdrawn. Introduction of air into the mediastinum and laceration of the trachea are thereby avoided. The catheter is attached to a sterile 10-ml syringe; 1 or 2 ml of nonbacteriostatic sterile saline is injected, inducing a vigorous cough. The syringe is aspirated, withdrawing a small amount of sputum into the catheter. The catheter is then removed; the tip and aspirated sputum are stained and cultured. Vigorous cough usually continues after the procedure, and additional expectorated specimens may be obtained. Complications of the procedure include introduction of air into the mediastinum and bleeding. The former is a common occurrence and is usually self-limited with eventual absorption. The latter complication is more serious but is much less frequent. Extratracheal bleeding can usually be controlled with minimal direct pressure. If bleeding into the trachea per-

sists for more than 30 minutes, it may require endotracheal intubation for control.

Other procedures may be appropriate in selected patients. In patients with progressive diffuse interstitial pneumonia or focal infiltrates without sputum production, more invasive diagnostic procedures may be indicated. This is particularly true in immunocompromised patients in whom the infective agents may be unusual and who may require unconventional therapy. These procedures include direct lung puncture, transbronchial brushing and biopsy, and open lung biopsy. Each procedure has its place and its own advantages and disadvantages. The choice and timing is best made with the help of pulmonary and infectious disease consultants and will often depend upon their expertise and familiarity with each of these procedures.

Sputum culture is outlined in Table 28.4. *Streptococcus pneumoniae* (Pneumococci) are fastidious organisms, often requiring increased carbon dioxide to grow, and therefore the sputum culture may be negative in the face of classic *Streptococcus pneumoniae* pneumonia. Blood cultures may be positive more readily in *Streptococcus pneumoniae* pneumonia.

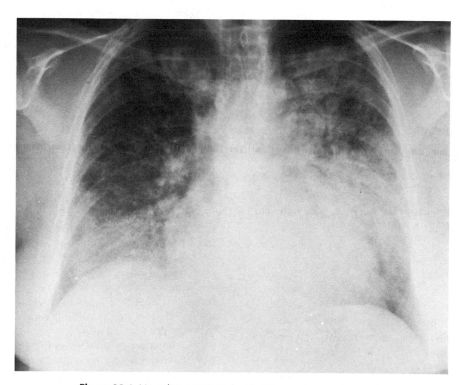

Figure 28.6 Vasculitis associated with Wegener's granulomatosis.

Most other bacterial pathogens, including *Staphylococcus aureus* and gram-negative bacilli, grow easily and should confirm the initial Gram stain diagnosis. In the case of true pathogens, abundant and predominant growth, not few or scant organisms, should be obtained on culture. The growth of normal upper respiratory tract flora is expected in patients with aspiration pneumonia and lung abscesses. Special cultures are required for mycoplasmal, chlamydial, and rickettsial infections. Serologic tests are available for *Mycoplasma* and *Legionella* infections.

COMPLICATIONS OF PNEUMONIA

Complications of pneumonia depend upon the infecting agent and the underlying health of the host. Those host factors that increase the likelihood of complications and mortality are listed in Table 28.10. Bacterial pneumonias caused by organisms other than *Streptococcus pneumoniae* (*Staphylococcus aureus*, gram-negative bacilli) are much more frequently associated with pulmonary and extrapulmonary complications.

General complications of pneumonia include the following:

1. Acute gastric dilation and paralytic ileus associated with nausea, vomiting, and aspiration
2. Congestive heart failure, usually as a result of hypoxia, toxic myocarditis, and/or increased cardiac work
3. Respiratory failure manifested by cyanosis, hypoxia, and/or carbon dioxide retention

Septic complications of pneumonia include the following:

1. Septic shock.
2. Empyema—Infected pleural fluid or pus in the pleural space is uncommon at present in infections with *Streptococcus pneumoniae* when treated early. Pleural effusions are very common in the course of *Streptococcus pneumoniae* pneu-

TABLE 28.10 Host Factors Associated with Complications in Pneumonia

Extremes of age
Chronic lung disease
Alcoholism
Congestive heart failure
Diabetes mellitus
Carcinoma or other malignancy
Multiple myeloma and/or hypogammaglobulinemia
Immunosuppression or chemotherapy
Hemoglobinopathy
Asplenia

monia and are usually sterile transudates. Empyema, however, is a frequent (20–30%) complication of pneumonia as a result of *Staphylococcus aureus* and gram-negative bacilli and in patients with aspiration pneumonia. The prognostic and therapeutic consequences of empyema mandate that all pleural effusions in the presence of pneumonia be sampled by thoracentesis. Therapy for empyema is discussed below.

3. Lung abscess is very unusual in *Streptococcus pneumoniae* pneumonia but is common in *Staphylococcus aureus* and gram-negative and aspiration pneumonia. In the latter a single large abscess is typical whereas in the former two, multiple abscesses are the rule.
4. Purulent pericarditis is an unusual but lethal complication of bacterial pneumonia if unrecognized. Enlarged heart shadow and signs of cardiac tamponade are clues to the diagnosis.
5. Meningitis is a dreaded complication of bacterial pneumonia and is often fatal despite appropriate therapy. Early diagnosis is essential for survival. Any patient with pneumonia and an altered mental status should have a lumbar puncture performed. This is true even if the examination does not reveal a stiff neck.
6. Endocarditis is an unusual but similarly dreaded complication of bacterial pneumonia. It should be suspected in patients who have pneumonia and prolonged or continual bacteremia and in all patients who have *Staphylococcus aureus* pneumonia.

GENERAL THERAPY

Hospitalization is generally required for patients with bacterial pneumonia. This is particularly true if the risk factors noted in Table 28.10 are present. All patients with bacterial pneumonia as a result of organisms other than *Streptococcus pneumoniae* or with any of the complications noted above should be hospitalized. Young, otherwise healthy, individuals with nonbacterial pneumonia or uncomplicated *Streptococcus pneumoniae* pneumonia may be treated as outpatients if adequate follow-up can be assured.

Correction of hypoxia is essential. Administration of oxygen by nasal catheter or face mask should be tried initially, and arterial blood gases should be carefully monitored. If severe hypoxia (PO_2 50mm H_2O) or carbon dioxide retention persists, considerations should be given to intubation and assisted ventilation. Hydration by the intravenous or oral route is important in maintaining adequate tissue perfusion and in aiding liquefaction and expectoration of sputum. *Chest physical therapy,* postural drainage, and other measures to promote sputum production and reduce atelectasis are important adjunctive measures.

SPECIFIC THERAPY

Antibiotic therapy for pneumonia is outlined in Table 28.11.

Uncomplicated *Streptococcus pneumoniae* pneumonia can be treated with low dose parenteral or oral penicillin. Therapy is usually continued for 10 days or for 4–5 days after the patient becomes febrile. *Streptococcus pneumoniae* pneumonia with septic complications should always be treated with intravenous penicillin in a dose of 10–20 million units per day and for a more prolonged course. Patients who are allergic to penicillin

may be treated with erythromycin, clindamycin, or a cephalosporin.

Staphylococcal pneumonia requires high dose intravenous therapy with semi-synthetic penicillinase-resistant penicillin usually for 2–3 weeks but longer if septic complications are present.

Gram-negative bacillary pneumonia is usually treated initially with an intravenous aminoglycoside. The choice of agent depends upon the local epidemiology of antibiotic resistance. In most areas, gentamicin is a safe initial choice. It may be combined with a cephalosporin. In immunocompromised hosts with gram-negative pnuemonia, carbenicillin or ticarcillin should be added to gentamicin initially to provide maximum coverage for *Pseudomonas aeruginosa*. The duration of therapy is usually

TABLE 28.11 Antibiotic Therapy of Pneumonia[a]

Bacteria	Drug of Choice	Alternative
Streptococcus pneumoniae	Penicillin G 500,000u IV q4–6h or procaine penicillin 1.2 million units IM q12h or pen VK 500 mg PO q8h	Cephalosporin Erythromycin Clindamycin
Staphylococcus aureus	Oxacillin or nafcillin 1 g IV q4h	Cephalosporin Clindamycin Vancomycin
Enteric gram-negative bacilli[b,c]	Gentamicin 1.5–2 mg/kg or 60 mg/m² IV q8h	Cephalosporin Tobramycin Amikacin Chloramphenicol
Pseudomonas aeruginosa[b]	Carbenicillin or ticarcillin with gentamicin or tobramycin	
Aspiration (mixed anaerobes)	Penicillin G 1–2 million units IV q4h	Clindamycin
Haemophilus influenzae[b]	Chloramphenicol 0.5–1 gm IV q6h	Ampicillin Cefamandole
Legionella pneumophilia (Legionnaire's disease)	Erythromycin 1 gm IV q6h	
Mycobacterium tuberculosis[b]	Isoniazid Rifampin	Isoniazid and ethambutol with or without streptomycin
Nonbacterial		
Mycoplasma pneumoniae	Tetracycline 500 mg PO q6h	Erythromycin
Chlamydia	Tetracycline 500 mg PO q6h	Erythromycin Chloramphenicol
Rickettsiae (Q fever)	Tetracycline 500 mg PO q6h	Chloramphenicol

[a]Adult doses. See Table 28.6 for pediatric doses.

[b]Antibiotic susceptibility varies and must be determined in the laboratory.

[c]*Eschericia coli, Klebsiella, Proteus,* and *Enterobacter.*

in the range of 2–3 weeks but may be longer if septic complications are present.

Aspiration pneumonia and aspiration lung abscesses can be successfully treated with penicillin alone in moderately high doses given intravenously (8–10 million units). Therapy is often maintained for 3–4 weeks. Once the patient improves, the dose of penicillin may be reduced and oral penicillin may be used to complete the course if the patient responds well to initial therapy. Treatment with corticosteroids has not been proven to be effective.

Mycoplasmal pneumonia, if uncomplicated by respiratory failure, can be treated with oral erythromycin or tetracycline for 7–10 days. Pneumonia caused by *Legionella pneumophila* requires high doses of intravenous erythromycin, 4 g per day. Specific antimicrobial therapy for viral pneumonia is not indicated.

Empyema generally requires aggressive surgical therapy to avoid continuing sepsis and/or fibrothorax. Initial drainage with a chest tube may be attempted (Procedure 19). However, if multiple loculations are present or tube drainage ceases in the face of residual pleural fluid, open drainage is required. Definitive drainage should be attempted with the initial procedure. Lung abscess will usually respond to medical therapy if adequate postural drainage through the bronchial tree can be established. Surgical drainage procedures are rarely necessary. Bronchoscopy should be considered in nonclearing or recurrent solitary lung abscesses to rule out bronchial obstruction with a foreign body or an endobronchial tumor.

INFECTIONS OF THE CENTRAL NERVOUS SYSTEM

Meningitis

Meningitis is a life-threatening medical emergency. Immediate recognition is critical. Fever, headache, stiff neck, altered level of consciousness, and seizures are the cardinal manifestations of meningitis. Early recognition before the disease fully develops is most important if a favorable outcome is to be achieved. Differentiation between bacterial and nonbacterial etiologies, determination of specific bacterial pathogens, and rapid institution of appropriate antibiotic and supportive therapy are essential once infection of the meninges has been recognized (Table 28.12, 28.13, and 28.14). The following organisms are recognized as causes of acute bacterial meningitis in decreasing order of frequency: *Streptococcus pneumoniae, H. influenzae, N. meningitidis, Listeria monocytogenes,* and gram-negative enteric bacilli. In patients with suspected acute bacterial meningitis, only a brief and focused history should be taken.

This may need to be obtained from friends or family members because of the patient's mental status. A brief physical examination, emphasizing the nervous system but including the head, neck, and skin, and an assessment of the patient's circulatory and ventilatory status should be quickly performed. The physician should then proceed directly to the performance of a lumbar puncture and an analysis of the CSF. Further historical details can be obtained and the physical examination completed once the diagnosis is excluded or established and appropriate therapy has been instituted. The details of these procedures and their interpretation are elaborated upon below and are outlined in Table 28.12.

CLINICAL CONTEXT

The patient's age is a useful, albeit nonspecific, determinant of the etiology of meningitis. Bacterial meningitis is more common in neonates and the elderly. Viral etiologies more frequently occur in children and young adults. More specifically, bacterial meningitis in neonates is likely to be caused by the group B streptococci or gram-negative bacilli. Bacterial meningitis in children under the age of 5 is most commonly a result of *H. influenzae*. In children beyond the age of 6, *H. influenzae* is a rare cause of meningitis, and *N. meningitidis* (meningococcus) is the predominant bacterial pathogen in people 7–40 years old. After age 40, *Streptococcus pneumoniae* accounts for most cases of bacterial meningitis. Together, meningococci and pneumococci account for 90% of bacterial meningitis in adults. In many patients at the extremes of age, bacterial meningitis may initially present with atypical or less-explosive features. In children under 2 years of age, restlessness, agitation, or minimal changes in behavior may be the only early presenting symptoms. In the elderly, fever and lethargy may be the sole initial complaints. Delirium may be the only early manifestation at any age. Partially treated bacterial meningitis may present with subtle and blunted manifestations as well.

The epidemiologic setting is of importance in meningitis and is sometimes helpful in diagnosis. *Neisseria meningitidis* may cause epidemic disease, particularly in closed populations of susceptible people (military bases, schools, colleges, etc.), and both *N. meningitidis* and *H. influenzae* have an increased secondary attack rate on people who have household contact with patients with meningitis due to these pathogens. These two bacterial etiologies should therefore be strongly suspected in the above mentioned epidemiologic settings. Both of these pathogens are more likely to cause disease during the winter and early spring months. *Streptococcus pneumoniae* meningitis is usually sporadic in occurence and without secondary cases. Viral meningitis, on the other hand, is much more likely

TABLE 28.12 Differential Features of Central Nervous System Infections

	Meningitis Viral	Meningitis Bacterial	Meningitis TB and Fungal	Brain abscess	Encephalitis
Age	Children Young adults	Any age Neonates—Staphylococcus aureus Enteric gram-negative bacilli Infants—H. influenzae Children—N. meningitidis Adults—Streptococcus pneumoniae	Any age	Children Young adults	Children Young adults
Season	Summer	Winter and spring N. meningitidis H. influenzae Any season Streptococcus pneumoniae	Any season	Any season	Summer
Epidemics	Yes—enterovirus	Yes—N. meningitidis	No	No	Yes
Onset	Rapid	Usually explosive	Insidious	Gradual	Rapid
Headache	Severe	Severe	Severe	Severe	Severe
Altered sensorium	Mild	Severe	Mild	Mild—progressive	Severe
Cranial nerve involvement	Rare	Occasional	Frequent	Frequent	Occasional Common in H. simplex
Seizures	Unusual	Frequent	Occasional	Frequent	Frequent
Underlying illness					
Contiguous focus	No	Yes	No	Yes	No
Surgery or trauma	No	Yes	No	Yes	No
Immunocompromise	No	No	Yes	No	No
Extremes of age	No	Yes	No	No	No
Right-to-left shunt	No	No	No	Yes	No
Splenectomy	No	Yes	No	No	No
Dermal defects (lower spine midline)	No	Yes	No	No	No
CSF					
Opening pressure	Usually normal	Elevated	Elevated	Elevated	Elevated
WBC[a]	Usually <500/mm³	1,000–20,000/mm³	<1000/mm³	Usually 500/mm³	<500/mm³, RBC in H. simplex
Differential[a]	Usually >80% mononuclear (polys may predominate during first 48 hours)	>95% polys	>80% mononuclear	Variable but usually >80% mononuclear	>80% mononuclear
Protein	Moderately elevated (50–100 mg%)	Elevated (75–500 mg%)	Elevated (75–500 mg%)	Elevated (100–500 mg%)	Moderately elevated (50–100 mg%)
Sugar[b]	Normal or slightly depressed (40–50 mg%)	Depressed (20–40 mg%)	Depressed (0–50 mg%)	Normal or slightly depressed (40–50 mg%)	Normal or slightly depressed (40–50 mg%)
Gram stain	Negative	Positive—80% of patients	Negative—do AFB smears and india ink preparations	Negative	Negative
Other examinations	Serological studies Viral isolation from stool	Countercurrent immunoelectrophoresis	Positive cryptococcal antigen	Mass lesion on CT scan	Temporal lobe focus in H. simplex on EEG and CT scan

[a]Values may be quite variable in patients with partially treated bacterial meningitis.
[b]Always do simultaneous blood sugar. Values may be deceptively normal or elevated in diabetics.

to occur during the summer months when enteroviral diseases (ECHO and coxsackie) are prevalent. Furthermore, patients with viral meningitis are more likely to be without predisposing factors and to present with meningitis in the context of an antecedent or coexisting viral syndrome (i.e., myalgia, arthralgia, malaise, URI, or gastroenteritis).

DIAGNOSIS

The clinical features of meningitis are sometimes associated with signs and symptoms referable to the route of infection of the meninges. The route of bacterial seeding of the meninges may be either by way of the bloodstream or by direct extension from a contiguous focus of infection. In approximately one-third of patients, bacterial meningitis follows sinusitus, otitis media, or other local infections; in one-third, a more distant focus of infection may be present (i.e., pneumonia, intraabdominal sepsis); in the final third a primary site of infection may not be apparent. Clinical features of use to the physician are associated with specific etiologic agents.

Meningococcal meningitis is suspected in a young adult with meningitis. It is marked by a rapidly evolving course accompanied by a petechial or purpuric cutaneous lesion, and it is likely to cause hypotension and circulatory collapse. Pneumococcal meningitis is frequently seen in the elderly, in alcoholics, in patients after splenectomy, in patients with multiple myeloma or sickle cell disease, and in patients who have pneumococcal infection elsewhere. Pneumococci often gain access to the meninges by extension from contiguous infected foci as in cases of otitis, sinusitis, or mastoiditis, or when skull fracture exposes the nasal cavity or paranasal sinuses to the meninges. Staphylococcal and gram-negative meningitis in adults are rare and occur in the context of bacteremia, after neurosurgical procedures, or by extension from a parameningeal focus. Gram-negative bacillary meningitis is the rule in infants under 6 months of age but is rare thereafter, except after trauma or neurosurgical procedures. *Listeria* meningitis most commonly occurs in patients with underlying lymphoproliferative disorders or immunosuppression.

Physical Examination

Physical examination reveals an altered sensorium and signs of meningeal irritation. The latter is most easily demonstrated by encountering resistance to passive neck flexion and is confirmed by Kernig's and Brudzinski's signs. Kernig's sign is the resistance to knee extension when the hip and knee are flexed to 90 deg. Brudzinski's sign is elicited by passively flexing the neck to 45 deg with resultant hip flexion. When these signs are present they are helpful, but they may be absent or equivocal in early meningitis or in very young and very old patients. Obtundation and cervical osteoarthritis may obscure these findings as well (see Chapter 10).

Other neurologic manifestations of importance are the presence of localizing or lateralizing signs, particularly those involving the cranial nerves, and the presence of papilledema. Both may be present in acute bacterial meningitis and would be highly unlikely in viral meningitis. Their presence raises the important possibility of a mass lesion such as a brain abscess. If a slow tempo and focal neurologic findings make brain abscess a likely possibility, an emergency brain scan or computed tomographic (CT) scan should be considered before a lumbar puncture is performed to avoid the risk of acute herniation. The brain scan may be positive before the CT scan. If a mass lesion is found, lumbar puncture should be withheld. An alternative approach is to administer mannitol and proceed with the lumbar puncture. If the findings do not suggest meningitis, a CT scan is then performed. Basilar meningitis is produced by *Mycobacterium tuberculosis* and fungal agents and will often involve the cranial nerves early in the disease process. These diseases are usually much more subacute in tempo than is pyogenic bacterial meningitis. Early cranial nerve involvement is a feature of meningovascular syphilis as well.

Notable nonneurologic findings are common in the presence of infection in contiguous foci or in disruption of the dura in bacterial meningitis. A diligent search should be made for infection of the ears, mastoid, sinuses, teeth, and face for previously unrecognized congenital malformation (e.g., meningomyelocele) and for trauma to the skull and face. Nasal discharge should be examined for glycorrhea since fracture of the cribriform plate may result in CSF leakage and secondary infection. Careful examination of the skin for rashes characteristic of meningococcemia (petechial or purpuric) or enteroviral infection (maculopapular or vesicular) may give a clue to the etiology of the meningitis.

The lumbar puncture is the crucial diagnostic test. It should be performed in all patients who are suspected of having meningitis, even if the likelihood of a positive result is small. All patients with fever and/or altered sensorium, seizures, and nuchal rigidity must have a lumbar puncture performed. It is safest to err on the side of excessive zeal in performing the examination on patients with less dramatic findings since unrecognized meningitis is often fatal.

The patient should be on the side with head and hips flexed in the fetal position. In difficult procedures the patient may alternatively be seated and the trunk flexed forward. The region around L-4 to L-5 is cleansed with povidone–iodine (Betadine) and alcohol and is infiltrated with 1% lidocaine down to the intervertebral disc. The performance of the puncture at a disc space higher than L-3 will increase the risk of traumatic injury to the spinal cord and should be undertaken only in extreme situations by experienced physicians when more distal punctures are unsuccessful. It is safest to use a small-gauge needle, that is, 21 gauge or 22 gauge. The bevel is pointed perpendicular to the long axis of the spine and the needle is inserted between the vertebral processes and is angled toward the umbilicus. Slow insertion with frequent removal of the stylet helps avoid a traumatic lumbar puncture. A "pop" can sometimes be felt upon entering the dura, but it is not always present. When fluid is obtained, the manometer is quickly attached. If the pressure is greater than 400 mm Hg, only 1 or 2 ml of fluid is withdrawn, which is divided for cell count and differential, Gram stain, and culture (see Chapter 10). If the pressure is lower, 2 ml are collected in each of four tubes. The first and third tubes are used for cell counts, Gram stains, and chemistries. The second tube is sent for bacteriologic culture. The last tube is held or sent for special tests if they are indicated.

The spinal fluid cell count is done on the unspun sample in a counting chamber in the standard manner. An accurate and reliable differential count requires the performance of a Wright stain on the spun sediment. Chamber differential counts are notoriously misleading. The spinal fluid cell count is normally 0–5 lymphocytes per cubic millimeter. The presence of more than this number, particularly if the cells are polymorphonuclear leukocytes, should raise the possibility of central nervous system bacterial infection. When a traumatic lumbar puncture occurs, the cell count should fall between the first and third tubes. Seven hundred red blood cells to one white blood cell is the appropriate anticipated ratio, and the white blood cell differential count is reflective of the peripheral count. If the white blood cell count to red blood cell count ratio is increased or the differential count is altered, then true infection rather than a traumatic tap should be suspected. In bacterial meningitis a white blood cell count of 1,000–20,000/mm³ is expected. Polymorphonuclear cells are usually present in excess of 85%. Viral meningitis is usually associated with a white blood cell count of 100–1,000/mm³, the majority of which are lymphocytes. Early in the course of viral meningitis up to 75% of the white blood cells may be polymorphonuclear leukocytes; however, in most cases the ratio will shift within 6 hours to a majority of lymphocytes. In equivocal cases it is often useful to observe the patient without giving him or her antibiotics and perform a second lumbar puncture after 6 hours. If a shift to mononuclear cells has occurred, viral meningitis

is most likely. In fungal and tuberculous meningitis, the cell count and differential is similar to that seen with viral meningitis. Eosinophilia in the cerebrospinal fluid, although rare, is found in patients with helminthic or fungal infection of the central nervous system. Patients with partially treated bacterial meningitis will exhibit variable findings, with blood cell counts usually above 1,000/mm³ and differential counts that are predominantly polymorphonuclear. Table 28.13 lists the most important causes of CSF pleocytosis aside from bacterial meningitis.

The spinal fluid chemistries are useful in the evaluation of patients but are not in themselves specific. Spinal fluid glucose is normally greater than 45 mg% or two-thirds that of a simultaneously obtained serum glucose. The glucose will be reduced in 50% of patients with acute bacterial meningitis and less frequently in patients with viral meningitis. A mildly reduced CSF glucose does not therefore distinguish between bacterial and viral meningitis. Extremely low values (5–20 mg%) are seen in listerial meningitis, tuberculous meningitis, and carcinomatous meningitis. The glucose may be normal or low in partially treated bacterial meningitis.

A CSF protein is normally less than 45 mg%. In bacterial meningitis, values of 100–1,500 mg% are usually seen. Extremely high CSF protein levels are seen in CSF block and central nervous system malignancies. The protein may be normal but is usually moderately elevated in partially treated bacterial meningitis. It is useful to know that the CSF protein will be raised 1 mg% for every 1,000 red blood cells and therefore may be significantly elevated in traumatic taps.

A Gram stain should be made of spun sediment (10–15 minutes at 1,500 rpm) and looked at immediately. In approximately 80% of patients with bacterial meningitis, the causative organism will be seen and antimicrobial therapy can be im-

TABLE 28.13 Differential Diagnosis of Asceptic Meningitis

Viral meningitis
Parameningeal infection
Tuberculous meningitis
Fungal meningitis
Partially treated bacterial meningitis
Leptospirosis
Bacterial endocarditis
Syphilitic meningitis
Carcinomatous meningitis
Cerebral vasculitis
Subarachnoid hemorrhage

mediately instituted. *Streptococcus pneumoniae* appear as gram-positive lancet-shaped diplococci, occasionally in chains. *Listeria monocytogenes* are also gram positive. Although they are usually more bacillary in appearance, they may be confused with pneumococci, as may over decolorized *H. influenzae*. *Hemophilus influenzae* appear as faint-staining gram-negative pleomorphic coccobacillary organisms. Meningococci are intensely gram-negative bean-shaped diplococci that are aligned with their long axes abutting one another. The quelling reaction, if antiserum is available, will clearly and specifically distinguish between *Streptococcus pneumoniae* and other organisms.

If the Gram stain is negative, the cells are predominantly lymphocytic, and there are suggestive clinical and epidemiologic features for tuberculous or fungal meningitis. Then stains for acid-fast bacillus (AFB) and an india ink preparation should be made. Both use the spun sediment. For tuberculosis a thick smear is made by placing 20 successive drops of the spun sediment on a slide and allowing it to dry between each drop. A Ziehl-Neelsen stain is then performed. To test for cryptococci, a drop of spun sediment is placed on a slide next to a drop of india ink. A cover slip is then placed over the two drops and the preparation is examined for cryptococci.

Cultures of the spinal fluid should be performed as outlined in Table 28.4. When clinically indicated and available, viral isolation may be attempted from the CSF. A small amount of the specimen (tube 4 may be used) may be innoculated into a 50% mixture of a balanced salt solution of bacteriostatic normal saline and frozen at 70°C until isolation can be performed.

Other CSF tests are of use in special circumstances. Countercurrent immune electrophoresis (CIE), if available, may rapidly diagnose *H. influenzae* or *N. meningitidis* infection. Antigen can be detected in blood and urine as well as CSF using this test. It is particularly useful in partially treated meningitis in which the cultures may be negative but bacterial antigen is still present. Cryptococcal antigen determination may be similarly useful in appropriately selected patients.

Other laboratory tests are indicated. At least two sets of blood cultures should be obtained in all patients suspected of having bacterial meningitis. Cultures of all other infected sites should be carried out as well. Serum electrolytes should be obtained since the syndrome of inappropriate antidiuretic hormone (SIADH) secretion is quite common in meningitis. A clotting profile should be obtained to determine if disseminated intravascular coagulation is present. To determine if associated sites of infection exist, chest, sinus, and skull films should be obtained as early in the course of the disease as the patient's condition allows. Serology for syphilis, leptospirosis, entero-

viral, and other viral agents may be helpful in selected cases in which an etiology is unclear. Finally, a PPD should be placed in all individuals in whom tuberculous meningitis is considered.

THERAPY

Bacterial meningitis requires immediate antimicrobial therapy. (Specific recommendations are outlined in Table 28.14.) An agent or agents should be chosen that will reach concentration in the CSF sufficient to kill or inhibit the causative organisms. This requires very high doses, intravenously administered agents, given by intermittent but frequent bolus. The penicillins and chloramphenicol are the most frequently used agents in the treatment of *Streptococcus pneumoniae*, *Neisseria meningitidis*, and *H. influenzae* meningitis. First- and second-generation cephalosporins do not achieve adequate levels in the CSF and should not be used to treat central nervous system infection. However, some of the new cephalosporins (third generation) achieve good CSF levels. Preliminary data in adults are encouraging for the treatment of gram-negative meningitis with cefotaxime and moxalactam. A note of caution has been raised because of a failure to cure meningeal infection with these agents when used alone in the pediatric age group. Until further data are obtained for gram-negative infection, intrathecal administration of an aminoglycoside must be strongly considered either by the lumbar or ventricular route in addition to parenteral administration of the aminoglycoside. A third-generation cephalosporin should be given in addition.

The dose of antibiotic should *not* be reduced as the patient improves but should be kept at a high level for the duration of the usual 10- to 14-day course of therapy. Repeat lumbar puncture is often performed within the first 48 hours of therapy to ensure that the organisms are cleared and that the cell count and chemistries are returning to normal. The timing of subsequent lumbar punctures is dependent upon the patient's clinical course. In most uncomplicated cases a repeat lumbar puncture is performed before hospital discharge at the completion of a 10- to 14-day course of antibiotic therapy. Corticosteroids are indicated early in the course of meningitis in those patients who have signs of increasing intracranial pressure. Dexamethasone sodium phosphate (Decadron) 4mg/kg IV every 6 hours is given for several days. In individuals with suspected acute bacterial meningitis in whom an etiologic agent cannot be readily determined, initial antimicrobial coverage is based upon the statistically likely organisms in the individual patient. This, in turn, is largely dependent upon the patient's age and the presence of special clinical circumstances (Table 28.12).

TABLE 28.14 Antimicrobial Therapy for Bacterial Meningitis

	Drug of Choice	Alternative
Known Organisms		
N. meningitidis *Streptococcus pneumoniae* (pneumococcus)	Penicillin G Adults: 4 million units IV q4h Children: 75,000 units/kg IV q4h	Chloramphenicol Adults: 1 g IV q6h Children: 25 mg/kg IV q6h
H. influenzae	Chloramphenicol Adults: 1 g IV q6h Children: 25 mg/kg IV q6h	Ampicillin Adults: 2 g IV q4h Children: 100 mg/kg IV q4h Selected only when organism known to be sensitive
Staphylococcus aureus	Oxacillin or nafcillin Adults: 2 g IV q4h Children: 100 mg/kg IV q4h	Vancomycin Adults: 0.5 g IV q6h Children: 10 mg/kg IV q6h
E. coli and other enteric gram-negative organisms	Gentamicin Adults: 2 mg/kg or 60 mg/m^2 IV $\quad$ q8h $\quad$ 5 mg intrathecal q12h Children: 2 mg/kg or 60 mg/m^2 $\quad$ IV q8h $\quad$ 1–2 mg intrathecal $\quad$ q12h and Moxalactam Adults: 4 g IV q8h Children: 100 mg/kg IV q8h or Cefotaxime Adults: 2 g IV q4h Children: 50 mg/kg IV q4h	Ampicillin or chloramphenicol (doses as above—select only when organism known to be sensitive)
Pseudomonas aeruginosa	Gentamicin (as above) and carbenicillin Adults: 5 g IV q4h Children: 100 mg/kg IV q4h	Tobramycin and ticarcillin
Unknown Organisms (see doses above)		
Premature and neonate	Ampicillin and gentamicin	Chloramphenicol (monitor blood levels—keep below 25 µg/ml)
2 months to 6 years	Chloramphenicol	
6 years and over	Ampicillin	Penicillin G or chloramphenicol
Skull fracture or postsurgery or prosthesis	Oxacillin or nafcillin and gentamicin	Vancomycin and chloramphenicol or moxalactam or cefotaxime

In patients in whom a clear distinction between bacterial and viral meningitis cannot initially be made, it is best to begin antibiotics for bacterial meningitis and await the results of cultures of the CSF and blood before discontinuing therapy.

The therapy for tuberculous and fungal meningitis is outlined in the texts listed in the selected readings.

Viral Encephalitis

Viral infections of the brain are most commonly a result of arthropod borne agents (arboviruses) and herpes simplex virus. The former is often an epidemic zoonosis, whereas the latter is sporadic in occurrence, affecting individuals with either primary or recurrent herpes simplex disease. It is now of great importance to attempt to specifically identify patients with herpes simplex encephalitis since therapy is available for this agent.

Many patients will manifest only mild and self-limiting illness. Full-blown encephalitis of any viral etiology presents with the rapid onset of severe headaches, fever, and vomiting and progresses to change in mental status, including stupor and acute organic psychosis. Signs of meningeal irritation may be present as may seizures and increased intracranial pressure. Of great importance is the common finding in herpes simplex encephalitis of signs localized to the temporal lobes.

The CSF shows a moderate pleocytosis that is predominantly mononuclear, a normal sugar, and elevated protein. The Gram stain and cultures are negative. In herpes simplex encephalitis, there are often large numbers of red blood cells in the CSF. If local findings suggesting temporal lobe involvement are present and red blood cells are found in the CSF, immediate electroencephalogram (EEG) and CT scans should be performed. Confirmation of predominant temporal lobe involvement increases the likelihood of herpes simplex. No specific therapy is available for encephalitis other than that caused by herpes simplex (with a definitive diagnosis). Current recommendations for encephalitis are that a brain biopsy of the temporal lobe be performed and the patient be placed on intravenous adenine arabinoside in a dosage of 15 mg/kg/day. The biopsy is cultured and stained for herpes simplex virus and, if positive, the drug is continued for a full 10-day course. If viral cultures are negative, the drug is stopped. If brain biopsy is not obtainable, therapy is given presumptively with intravenous adenine arabinoside for a full 10-day course.

Brain Abscess

Localized bacterial infection of the brain is far less common than is meningitis. It occurs predominantly in children and young adults and has a more gradual onset than bacterial meningitis. Seizures and focal neurologic findings are common. The infection is usually the result of spread of infection to the brain from contiguous foci or by way of the bloodstream. The CSF findings are similar to those of viral meningitis. The bacteriology within the abscess is most often that of a mixture of anaerobic organisms (Table 28.12). The CSF is almost invariably sterile. The diagnosis requires a brain scan or CT scan demonstrating a mass lesion. High dose intravenous antibiotics directed at the likely flora are given. Penicillin G and chloramphenicol are usually used in combination unless the brain abscess develops in the course of a documented bacteremia with a known organism. Antibiotics in this situation are directed at the isolated organism. Surgical drainage is strongly recommended in addition to antibiotic therapy, but excision of the abscess is usually unnecessary.

INFECTIONS OF THE HEART

Acute Bacterial Endocarditis

Acute bacterial endocarditis is a life-threatening infection clinically characterized by multiple organ system signs and symptoms. Although it is more likely to occur in individuals with valvular heart disease, many patients with acute endocarditis may have no underlying valvular pathology.

DIAGNOSIS

The cardinal clinical manifestations of acute bacterial endocarditis are fever, tachycardia, murmurs signifying valvular insufficiency, septic emboli resulting in classic skin infarcts or vasculitis (Osler's nodes, splinter hemorrhages, petechiae), neurologic abnormalities (aseptic meningitis, cerebral vasculitis with encephalitis, major vessel cerebrovascular accidents), and congestive heart failure (valve perforation and/or myocarditis).

In comparison to subacute bacterial endocarditis, which is often present for weeks to months before recognition, the tempo of acute bacterial endocarditis is rapid. Valve destruction and/or septic emboli with metastatic infection may result in fatality within days to a week of onset of symptoms.

The diagnosis is definitely confirmed only at surgery or autopsy, but the clinical syndrome described above accompanied by repeatedly positive blood cultures is highly suggestive of the diagnosis. Acute endocarditis is usually caused by virulent bacteria that are known to cause rapid tissue destruction: *Staphylococcus aureus, Streptococcus faecalis* (enterococci), *Streptococcus pneumoniae,* and gram-negative bacilli. Occasionally, less virulent organisms such as *Streptococcus viridans* may cause typical acute destructive disease. Prosthetic valve infections usually are caused by staphylococci or gram-negative bacilli when infection occurs within 1 month of surgery and are caused by relatively nonvirulent organisms when infection occurs more than 1 month after surgery. Intravenous drug users are prone to acute endocarditis with *Staphylococcus aureus, Pseudomonas,* and other gram-negative bacilli.

At least three separate sets of blood cultures should be obtained over a 1-hour period. With proper technique, positive venous blood cultures can be expected in essentially all patients with acute bacterial endocarditis. Fungal endocarditis, in contrast, will often be culture negative. Additionally, in patients with acute bacterial endocarditis, virtually all obtained blood cultures will be positive. This demonstration of a continual bacteremia is a strong indication of endothelial infection. Continual or persistent bacteremia is so characteristic of endocarditis that this finding in the absence of a defined primary focus mandates treatment for endocarditis even in the absence of other typical clinical findings. Occasionally, the diagnosis may be made by aspiration, Gram stain, and culture of peripheral infarcts of the skin.

TREATMENT

Intravenous high dose bactericidal antibiotics should be given for at least 4 and usually 6 weeks.

Staphylococcus aureus endocarditis is treated with a penicillinase-resistant penicillin such as oxacillin or nafcillin in a dosage of 2 g intravenously every 4 hours.

Gram-negative endocarditis is treated with an aminoglycoside with the addition of a cephalosporin if synergistic by laboratory determination.

Enterococcal endocarditis is currently best treated with a combination of ampicillin (2 g IV every 4 hours) and gentamicin.

Acute bacterial endocarditis of undetermined etiology should be treated first with nafcillin, penicillin, and gentamicin and appropriate changes made when final identification of the organism is accomplished.

Special bacteriologic procedures are important in guiding therapy for this disease. Minimal inhibitory and bactericidal concentrations of the infecting organism to the administered drug(s) should be determined in the laboratory. The patient's serum is used to determine if an effective level of antibiotics has been obtained. Synergistic combinations of antibiotics should be sought for patients with infections with usual organisms. Cardiac function must be carefully assessed and atrioventricular conduction abnormalities monitored particularly if aortic insufficiency is present. Surgery to remove the infected valve should be strongly considered in the following circumstances:

1. Inability to control infection by antibiotics (i.e., blood cultures remain positive after 48 hours of appropriate bactericidal antibiotic therapy)
2. The development of congestive heart failure that is unresponsive to medical management in the presence of valvular insufficiency
3. The development of heart block
4. The occurence of major life-threatening large vessel emboli (i.e., cerebrovascular accident, large vessel emboli to the extremities)
5. Fungal or gram-negative bacillary endocarditis

Pericarditis

Infection of the pericardium is most commonly a benign disease that presents with characteristic anterior chest pain (see Chapter 4). Physical findings include a pericardial friction rub and diminished heart sounds. Chest film may show evidence of an enlarged cardiac silhouette. The echo cardiogram will demonstrate pericardial fluid. The electrocardiogram (ECG) findings of diffuse ST segment elevations are typical but infrequent.

Purulent pericarditis, though rare, may result from bacterial seeding of the pericardium or spread from contiguous pneumonic or mediastinal infection. This is a medical emergency. Patients invariably are desperately ill and require immediate surgical drainage of the pericardium as well as high dose, parenteral antimicrobial agents. The most common bacterial etiologies are *Staphylococcus aureus, Streptococcus pneumoniae, N. meningitidis,* and *H. influenzae.*

Tuberculous pericarditis should always be considered in the differential diagnosis of pericarditis. The diagnosis can usually be excluded if there are no typical systemic signs and symptoms of tuberculosis (fever, sweats, weight loss) and no active pulmonary disease exists. Tuberculous pericarditis almost always occurs in the context of active pulmonary tuberculosis. A purified protein derivative (PPD) tuberculin skin test should be planted in all patients with pericarditis and the diagnosis strongly considered if it is positive.

Benign viral pericarditis is usually enteroviral in etiology and rarely serious in nature.

Noninfectious etiologies that enter into the differential diagnosis of pericarditis include collagen vascular disease (usually accompanied by inflammation of other serious surfaces), metastatic disease (usually in patients with known intrathoracic malignancy or lymphoproliferative disorders), uremic pericarditis, Dressler's syndrome (postmyocardial infection), and acute rheumatic fever.

Occasional benign viral pericarditis will result in sufficient pericardial effusion to cause cardiac tamponade. This is signaled by tachycardia, hypotension, low cardiac output, and pulsus paradoxus. Pericardiocentesis may be lifesaving in this situation. An open pericardial drainage procedure and pericardial window may be necessary if pericardial fluid accumulation continues. Pericardial fluid obtained by these maneuvers should be Gram stained and cultured. Attempts to culture the fluid for enteroviral agents are also worthwhile. A pericardial biopsy should always be performed if surgical intervention is necessary. Atrial and ventricular arrhythmias may complicate viral pericarditis. Extensive myocardial inflammation, if present, may result in congestive heart failure.

TREATMENT

Treatment of bacterial pericarditis is directed toward the most likely organisms based upon Gram stain of pericardial fluid. Adequate surgical drainage is required in all instances of bacterial pericarditis (see Chapter 4).

There is no specific therapy for benign or complicated viral pericarditis. The disease is almost always self-limiting with complete recovery, although recurrences may occur. Some authorities recommend corticosteroid therapy in complicated cases, although there are no controlled trials that demonstrate their efficacy, and experimental evidence suggests that they may, in fact, be deleterious. Similarly, nonsteroidal antiinflammatory agents have been anecdotally successful and are probably safer. Therapy for complications include usual measures to treat arrhythmias and bed rest, digitalization, and administration of oxygen for congestive heart failure. Occasionally, more unusual measures may be necessary if extensive myocarditis results in severe, nonresponsive heart failure. The intraaortic balloon pump and left ventricular assist devices have been successfully used in extreme cases. Young patients need not be hospitalized if the diagnosis is clearly established, if there are no signs and symptoms of heart failure and/or arrhythmias, and if there is no apparent evidence of large pericardial effusion and tamponade. Careful follow-up of patients with complications over several weeks is, however, mandatory.

INFECTIONS OF BONES AND JOINTS

Bone and joint infections require rapid diagnosis, institution of specific antibiotic therapy, and often surgical drainage procedures. Diagnostic and therapeutic measures are aimed at location of the source of infection since these infections often arise as a consequence of bacteremic spread from distant foci. Therapy must be aimed at the eradication of the acute bacterial skeletal infection and primary site of infection, if found, and also at the preservation of bone and joint function and the avoidance of chronic skeletal infection.

Osteomyelitis

Acute bacterial infections of bone are most common in childhood. Individuals at high risk for acquisition of osteomyelitis include intravenous drug users and patients with sickle cell disease. Acute osteomyelitis is usually a result of *Staphylococcus aureus* when caused by hematogenous spread. When caused by spread from contiguous infected foci, the bacteriology may be more complex. This is particularly true if spread is from an adjacent mucosal surface with a mixed normal and pathologic flora or if infection is acquired from a traumatic wound. Patients with sickle cell disease have a predilection for development of *Salmonella* osteomyelitis, and heroin users are prone to develop *Pseudomonas* osteomyelitis.

CLINICAL EVALUATION

The onset of osteomyelitis is usually explosive. Local pain, tenderness, and limitation of movement are characteristic, and often swelling, redness, and warmth point directly to the site of infection. This is particularly true of the long bones and legs but less so of the vertebral column, infections of which may be relatively occult. Systemic signs of infection are usually marked. The initial presentation of bone and joint infections much less frequently may be indolent; pain is the predominant symptom and there is a remarkable absence of systemic illness. The differential diagnosis includes trauma, gout, viral arthritis, collagen vascular disease, and hypersensitivity reactions. Leukocytosis with marked shift to the left is invariably present, and blood cultures are usually positive. Patients suspected of pyogenic skeletal infections should have at least two sets of blood cultures drawn before any therapeutic measures are undertaken.

Bone films will rarely show significant lesions earlier than 2 weeks after onset of the illness, but experienced radiologists will suspect the infection on the basis of soft tissue swelling and alteration of normal fat lines. *Bone scans* should be positive at the time the patient is first seen, but are not specific for osteomyelitis.

Whether infection is by hematogenous or local spread, a direct attempt should be made in most cases to achieve a specific bacterial diagnosis. This is accomplished by needle biopsy or, preferably, if there is evidence of periosteal elevation, by open surgical biopsy. In the latter instance, surgical drainage of pus under pressure will dramatically relieve symptoms and may result in diminished likelihood of chronic osteomyelitis. Material obtained by either aspiration or open biopsy and drainage should be examined by Gram stain and should be cultured. Blood cultures will usually be positive in infections resulting from hematogenous spread.

THERAPY

Antibiotic therapy should be directed at the organisms seen on Gram stain and may be modified by subsequent blood and tissue culture results. Initially, high dose parenteral antibiotics are indicated. Patients with acute osteomyelitis are usually treated for 4–6 weeks. Completion of the therapeutic course with oral agents is reasonable if a good response has been achieved and compliance with the regimen can be assured.

Septic Arthritis

Septic arthritis is most commonly the result of hematogenous seeding of the joint space. The larger joints (hips, knees, ankles, shoulders, elbows, wrists) are most frequently involved, and in most instances the process is monoarticular. In contrast to acute osteomyelitis, the bacteriologic agents are quite varied. *Neisseria meningitidis, Streptococcus pneumoniae, Staphylococcus aureus,* and, in small children, *H. influenzae,* are all important pathogens. At present, in young adults, *N. gonorrhoeae* arthritis is by far the most common. Gonococcal arthritis is typically preceded by a short period of arthralgias involving multiple joints and low grade fever. Tenosynovitis, pustules, and hemorrhagic bullae are often present.

CLINICAL EVALUATION

The clinical presentation of septic arthritis is one of warmth, swelling, and limitation of motion of the affected joint. The diagnosis of septic arthritis is confirmed by the examination of aspirated joint fluid. This procedure should be performed as soon as possible since in all cases of suspected septic arthritis a delay in diagnosis and therapy may result in rapid joint destruction. Examination of the joint fluid should include Gram stain and white blood cell count. A differential should be performed on a Wright's-stained smear. Septic arthritis is almost always associated with joint fluid white blood cell counts of greater than 30,000/mm^3. Usually more than 80% of cells are polymorphonuclear leukocytes. The glucose level in the joint fluid is usually less than 50% of the peripheral venous blood sugar, and the mucin clot is poor. The fluid should be cultured as outlined in Table 28.4. The major differential diagnostic possibilities—gout, rheumatoid arthritis, viral arthritis, and trauma—are usually excluded by careful joint fluid examination.

In any patient suspected of having septic arthritis, at least two sets of blood cultures should be drawn. In addition, a careful search for possible extraskeletal primary foci should be performed.

THERAPY

Therapy for septic arthritis involves administration of appropriate antibiotics in high doses intravenously, drainage of purulent joint effusions, and joint immobilization. Antibiotics initially may be selected on the basis of the Gram stain. Gram-positive coccal joint infections are usually easily seen on Gram stain, and oxacillin or nafcillin should be given. The Gram stain is less likely to be positive in neisserial infections. In such cases, the local and systemic clinical features of the infection dictate antibiotic choice. High doses of penicillin G are appropriate for both gonococcal and meningococcal arthritis. *Haemophilus influenzae* arthritis initially should be treated with chloramphenicol until the antibiotic susceptibility of the organism is known. The intraarticular administration of antibiotics is unnecessary and should be avoided. Infected joints must be adequately drained. In most instances this may be accomplished by repeated aspirations. The hip joint may require open drainage because of the difficulty of aspiration and possibility of compromise of blood supply.

SEPTIC SHOCK

Septic shock is a clinical syndrome most commonly associated with gram-negative bacteremia and thought to be a result of the effect of endotoxin on the microcirculation. It represents a true medical emergency.

Septic shock usually occurs in the context of bacterial infection in a specific organ system. These infections are often apparent and should be quickly sought with a focused history and physical examination. Infections of the urinary tract, intraabdominal sepsis, intravenous line sepsis, and pneumonia are the most common sources of bacteremia. Patients on immunosuppressive therapy are at particular risk.

DIAGNOSIS

The diagnosis of septic shock is apparent in a typical well-developed case. The patient is febrile, hypotensive, and agitated, and a focus of infection is apparent. The clinical characteristics of septic shock may be varied, however, largely depending upon the time sequence of vascular events. Additionally, septic shock may be indistinguishable from shock because of myocardial infarction, pulmonary embolus, or acute hemorrhage. Initially there is peripheral vasodilation and increased cardiac output, which results in fever, warm skin, and warm extremities. Tachycardia is present, and the blood pressure will initially remain normal if cardiac output is sufficient. However, if vasodilation persists, and there is vascular pooling and diminished blood return to the heart, the cardiac output will fall and hypotension invariably will develop. The patient's temperature may then fall to hypothermic levels. Peripheral vasoconstriction will develop; the skin and extremities will become cold and clammy. Hyperventilation is a frequent initial and persistent finding in patients with septic shock. Altered mental status, including lethargy, agitation, and delirium, are common.

Laboratory evaluation includes a complete hemogram and blood cultures (at least two sets if time allows). Clotting factors and degree of hypoxia and acidosis should be determined. Laboratory findings early in the syndrome include leukocytosis with a shift to the left, clotting abnormalities, hypoxia, mixed respiratory alkalosis, and lactic acidosis. Renal, cardiac, and respiratory failure may be apparent within hours to days of the onset of the syndrome.

TREATMENT

The major features of therapy that are essential are discussed below.

Measures to combat circulatory failure (Chapter 3, treatment of shock) are undertaken immediately. Rapid expansion of intravascular volume is the mainstay of therapy. A central venous line or pulmonary artery (Swan-Ganz) catheter should be placed. Fluid for volume expansion should be initially infused at a rate sufficient to bring the central venous pressure above 15 cm H_2O or pulmonary–capillary pressure above 20 mm Hg. Bicarbonate should be administered to correct acidosis, and vasopressors should be administered if shock persists despite rapid volume infusion. Several agents are used: First, dopamine should be given at a rate sufficient to maintain tissue perfusion (2–20 mg/kg/min initially). Perfusion is monitored by the patient's sensorium and urine output. If left ventricular pressure appears to be adequate, isoproterenol may be given (5–10 mg/min) with care to maintain normal blood volume with intravenous fluids. Levarterenol and metaraminol should be avoided since these agents may decrease tissue perfusion and deepen acidosis by virtue of their vasoconstrictive action.

Diagnosis is followed by treatment of the underlying infection with high doses of intravenously administered antibiotics appropriate to eradicate infection in the suspected organ system. A broad spectrum bactericidal agent (gentamicin, tobramycin) active against most gram-negative organisms is usually given in initially high dose (i.e., 2 mg/kg IV or 60 mg/m^2) and is combined with a semisynthetic penicillinase-resistant penicillin or cephalosporin at a dosage of 1–2 g IV every 4 hours. In immunocompromised patients and/or patients with hospital-acquired septic shock, carbenicillin or ticarcillin (4–5 g every 4 hours) are added as well to cover possible *Pseudomonas* bacteremia. Antibiotic therapy should be combined with emergency surgery to drain abscesses, remove necrotic tissue, or free obstructed viscera.

Corticosteroid administration remains a controversial issue in the treatment of septic shock. Corticosteroids clearly increase cardiac output and improve tissue perfusion experimentally, and they have been shown to be effective in one controlled clinical trial. They have numerous side effects that may complicate the clinical course of the disease, including gastrointestinal hemorrhage and acute psychosis. They are given in pharmacologic rather than physiologic doses. Dexamethasone 3 mg/kg IV initially, followed by 10–20 mg IV every 4–6 hours or methylprednisolone 30 mg/kg IV followed by 100–200 mg every 4 hours may only be effective if started early in the course, if at all.

Disseminated intravascular coagulation, which often accompanies septic shock, is usually not specifically treated. All of the above measures are usually sufficient to restore normal coagulation without specific therapy. Heparin or fresh frozen plasma may be considered if significant life-threatening hemorrhage continues (see Chapter 40).

PROGNOSIS

Mortality is clearly related to underlying host factors. For example, gram-negative septic shock, when occuring in individuals who have a rapidly fatal underlying disease (i.e., leukemia, widely metastatic carcinoma), carries with it a mortality rate of 40–70%; in patients with an underlying disease that will ultimately be fatal (i.e., congestive heart failure, renal failure), the mortality rate is 20–40%; and in patients with nonfatal underlying disease, the mortality rate is less than 20%. In each category, early recognition of septic shock is crucial since delay of appropriate antimicrobial and supportive therapy decreases chances for survival.

ACQUIRED IMMUNODEFICIENCY SYNDROME

The acquired immunodeficiency syndrome (AIDS) is a newly described life threatening illness. A patient is considered to have AIDS if the presenting illness suggests a defect in cell-mediated immunity without predisposing reason for diminished immunity. The types of presenting diseases are listed in Table 28.15. A patient is considered to have the syndrome if he or she has the appropriate infection at any age less than 80, or Kaposi's sarcoma at an age less than 60.

Epidemiologic investigation has revealed that there are several groups at risk (Table 28.16). Homosexual males living in major metropolitan centers on the east and west coasts account

TABLE 28.15. Acquired Immunodeficiency: Associated Diseases

Infections
  Pneumonia, meningitis, encephalitis
    Pneumocystis carinii pneumonia
    Aspergillosis
    Candidiasis
    Cryptococcosis
    Cytomegalovirus
    Nocardiosis
    Strongyloidiosis
    Toxoplasmosis
    Zygomycosis
    Atypical mycobacteriosis *(Avirium intracellulare)*
    Progressive multifocal leukoencephalopathy

  Diarrheal disease
    Cryptosporidiosis
    Isospora belli

  Esophagitis
    Candidiasis
    Cytomegalovirus
    Herpes simplex

  Mucocutaneous disease
    Herpes simplex of more than 5 weeks duration

Tumors
  Kaposi's
  Burkitt's

for approximately 75% of all cases. Midwestern cities have had fewer cases. A homosexual patient with a high number of sexual partners has an increased risk of developing AIDS. However, no particular type of sexual activity has been correlated with the disease. The immune defect appears to be infectious and transmitted by blood products or intimate personal contact. Patients have been identified who have had contact with

TABLE 28.16 High-Risk Groups

Male homosexuals
Intravenous drug users
Haitians
Blood transfusion recipients[a]
Cryoglobulin recipients
Children born to AIDS patients
Household contacts of patients with AIDS

[a]Possible risk greater than risk to general population.

other known patients. Such contacts suggest that the incubation time from initial exposure to clinical illness is approximately 8 months to $1\frac{1}{2}$ years. Some infants born to AIDS patients have had a slightly shorter incubation period, suggesting that transplacental infection may occur. Approximately 5% of all cases do not fit any known high-risk group. Since no agent has been identified, there is no definitive diagnostic test to determine whether a subclinical illness exists.

Diagnosis

Clinical Features

Patients may have prodromal symptoms marked by malaise, oral condidiasis, lymphadenopathy, weight loss greater than 10 kg, and diarrhea. To be a prodromal case, the lymph nodes when biopsied should have no evidence of an infectious agent. Patients with AIDS frequently will not have granulomas, and biopsied lymph nodes should routinely be cultured and stained for acid fast organisms. For cases of AIDS, the presenting complaints will vary depending on the site of infection and the infectious agent. An aggressive diagnostic approach is required for AIDS patients to determine if infection is present. *Pneumocystis carinii* pneumonia should be suspected in patients with atypical pneumonitis who are at high risk for AIDS. To determine if *Pneumocystis carinii* is present, bronchoscopy and transbronchial lung biopsy is the preferred diagnostic procedure. Chronic diarrhea for more than 4 months may be due to unusual organisms, such as the parasite *Cryptosporidium*. Patients who have cutaneous or systemic lesions of Kaposi's sarcoma or non-Hodgkin's lymphoma most likely will develop infections during the course of their illness.

Laboratory Evaluation

There is no laboratory test definitive for the diagnosis. A total lymphocyte count less than 1500 cm^3 is frequently encountered. Extensive lymphocyte studies have revealed an inversion of the normal concentrations of helper thymus-derived (T) lymphocytes to suppressor/cytotoxic T lymphocytes in peripheral blood. The normal helper T lymphocyte ratio is 1.8 (range 1.1–2.8), whereas AIDS patients have levels less than 1.1. Normal patients with viral or bacterial illness that is not life threatening may have similar inverse ratios of helper to suppressor/cytotoxic T lymphocytes, and it is not suggested that studies of lymphocytes be performed as a routine screening test. Normal individuals with an inverse ratio of helper to suppressor/cytotoxic T lymphocytes during an acute illness have a return to a normal ratio after recovery. Patients with AIDS have a persistent abnormality of helper to suppressor/cytotoxic T lymphocytes. Cutaneous anergy is usually seen and is a reasonable screening test.

Risk to Medical Personnel

To date there have been no cases of AIDS in medical personnel caring for AIDS patients. However, prudent care should be taken with all body secretions and blood. Blood and other body fluids are probably infectious, based upon epidemiologic data. It is incumbent on the initial examining physician to alert the laboratory workers that AIDS is a potential diagnosis. The epidemiologic data strongly suggest blood borne transmission, and laboratory workers are conceivably at high risk. Additional risk groups include surgeons and dentists. Dentists and oral hygienists in particular should take precautions to wear gloves during oral procedures. Stool and needle precautions are needed for hospitalized patients.

Clinical Course, Therapy, and Prognosis

There is no effective therapy for the underlying immunodeficiency in AIDS patients. Treatment is aimed at the infecting agent or concurrent tumor (i.e., Kaposi's sarcoma). In view of the high incidence of *Pneumocystitis carinii* pneumonia in this group, *Pneumocystitis carinii* pneumonia should be considered in every AIDS patient with atypical pneumonia. For these patients, sulfamethoxazole-trimethoprim is the initial treatment of choice. The dose is calculated on the basis of body weight and the trimethoprim moiety of the fixed drug combination (20 mg trimethoprim/kg). If at 5 days of therapy the blood gases show continued deterioration and bronchoscopy specimens are still positive for *Pneumocystis,* then treatment should be changed to pentamidine (4 mg/kd/d) intramuscularly. Patients with one course of *Pneumocystitis carinii* pneumonia may relapse after apparent effective therapy. The role of prophylaxis with sulfa-trimethoprim either for protection from *Pneumocystitis* or after an episode of the disease has not been adequately studied. Treatment of mucocutaneous herpes simplex with acyclovir may be life saving. Adenine arabinoside is not effective for mucocutaneous herpes simplex in this patient population. The AIDS patients do not respond to therapy as rapidly as normal hosts, and therapy for any infection may need to be extended for prolonged periods to obtain a cure. The prognosis is grim for patients with AIDS; the mortality rate from infection and tumors approches 100%. The survival from the time of diagnosis is usually less than 2 years.

HEAT-INTOLERANCE SYNDROMES

Three heat-intolerance syndromes are recognized clinically. They differ substantially in presentation, severity, and therapy (Table 28.17).

Heat Stroke

Heat stroke is an acute medical emergency. Mortality rates of 17–70% have been reported. Early recognition and immediate corrective measures are imperative. Heat stroke is caused by excessive and unrelieved body heat storage. This is the result

TABLE 28.17 Heat-Intolerance Syndromes

	Heat Stroke	Heat Exhaustion	Heat Cramps
Age	Usually elderly	Young adults	Young adults
Rectal temperature	40°C (104°F)	40°C (104°F)	40°C (104°F)
Skin	Hot and dry	Sweating present	Sweating present
CNS abnormalities	Confusion Disorientation Seizures Coma	Headache Dizziness Nausea Mild confusion	Absent
Muscle cramps	Absent	Infrequent	Present
Associated findings	High output CHF renal, hepatic, and coagulation abnormalities	Dehydration Salt depletion	Minimal
Treatment	Emergency cooling	Salt and water replacement	Salt replacement

of a paralysis of normal body thermoregulatory mechanisms. Heat dissipation and cooling by radiation or convection fails and cooling by sweat evaporation ceases.

Clinically, heat stroke is manifested by three cardinal signs (1) extreme hyperpyrexia, (2) hot, dry skin, (3) central nervous system disturbance. The rectal temperature is usually in excess of 41°C (106°F) and is never below 40°C (104°F). There is no sweating. The skin is characteristically hot and bone dry to the touch. The skin may be pink or ashen, depending upon the patient's circulatory state. Disturbance in central nervous system function initially may be mild, consisting of headache, dizziness, and confusion. Rapid progression to delirium, euphoria, stupor, and finally coma occurs in untreated patients. Generalized convulsions, muscle flaccidity, focal neurologic abnormalities, including cranial nerve palsies and hemiplegia, and extensor plantar responses have all been observed and may be present singly or in combination. Many associated abnormalities may develop in patients with advanced heat stroke. These include high output cardiac failure, disseminated intravascular coagulation, and renal and hepatic failure.

Heat stroke usually occurs on hot, humid, windless days. It may occur in young healthy individuals, such as military personnel, athletes, or laborers, who are exposed to extensive and prolonged physical stress during such climatic conditions. It is far more common, however, in elderly persons with underlying cardiovascular disease, in alcoholics, in patients with Parkinson's disease, and in those who are taking anticholinergic drugs. Patients in each of these circumstances seem to predispose to the failure of their heat dissipation mechanisms, which characterizes the disease.

DIAGNOSIS

The diagnosis of heat stroke is usually easily made when susceptible individuals present with the triad of extreme pyrexia, absence of sweating, and mental status changes during hot weather. Central nervous system infection is the major differential diagnosis. Consequently, blood cultures and a lumbar puncture and examination of the spinal fluid should be performed. Assessment of cardiac and renal function, electrolyte status, and clotting parameters are all important. It is important to emphasize, however, that none of these diagnostic studies should delay the immediate application of emergency cooling measures by any means available.

TREATMENT

The elimination of hyperpyrexia in heat stroke is imperative and should be begun once the diagnosis is clinically suspected. The most effective measure is total immersion of the patient in an ice water bath. Ice cubes should be added. If a total immersion bath is not available, ice water should be splashed and sponged on the patient and fans directed toward the patient to aid evaporation. Vigorous massage of skin and muscles should be carried out to promote surface circulation and further dissipation of heat. The patient should be removed from the bath when rectal temperature is reduced to 38.8°C (102°F) and should be kept in a cool, shaded area with careful monitoring of rectal temperature. Because of the possibility of multiple organ system damage, observation in an intensive care setting is essential once the patient improves. A secure intravenous line should be placed while the temperature is being lowered, and studies to assess the state of oxygenation and of renal, hepatic, and clotting function should be performed.

Ancillary therapeutic measures include maintenance of the high output state until the hyperpyrexia is corrected. Dehydration, hypovolemia, and electrolyte derangement are not usually prominent. The cautious administration of 1–1.5 liters of half-normal saline or lactated Ringer's solution is required during the first 4 hours. Of course, more rapid volume expansion is necessary if hypotension is present. Digitalization is indicated if congestive heart failure is present, and antiarrhythmic drugs should be given if necessary. Oxygen should be administered by mask or nasal catheter if hypoxemia exists. If present, electrolyte abnormalities should be corrected and seizures treated with intravenous diphenylhydantoin or diazepam. It is essential to *avoid* all anticholenergic agents since they inhibit sweating. Vasopressors that may produce peripheral vasoconstriction and therefore further decrease heat dissipation are also contraindicated. Some authorities recommend that patients with marked shivering and agitation receive intravenous phenothiazines. Mannitol is recommended if there are signs of increased intracranial pressure. Convalescent care should include restriction of activity and avoidance of exposure to sunlight or excessive heat for several weeks. Individuals who have recovered from heat stroke are at continued risk for subsequent episodes and demonstrate long-term abnormalities of thermoregulatory mechanisms

Heat Exhaustion

Heat exhaustion, or heat prostration, occurs as the result of excessive salt and water depletion. As opposed to heat stroke, this entity is not the result of a paralysis of heat dissipation mechanisms, but rather is the result of excessive sweating in which there is replacement of lost electrolytes and fluid with only hypotonic solutions. It occurs in young, physically active individuals in hot, humid weather and is usually insidious in onset—over hours to days. The symptoms are those of progressive lassitude and inability to perform work. In severe cases, this may be followed by headache, dizziness, vomiting, and occasionally syncope. In rare cases, hypovolemia may be profound and result in oligemic shock. The patient's temperature is at most slightly elevated, and sweating is usually present. These two findings easily distinguish this entity from heat stroke. Laboratory examinations are usually not necessary. Hemoconcentration, hypernatremia, hyperchloremia, and a highly concentrated urine are found.

Treatment consists of rest, rehydration with administration of salt-rich solutions such as Gatorade or bouillon or the addition of 1 teaspoon of salt in 0.5 liter of water or juice. Patients rarely need to be hospitalized and should be told to liberalize their salt intake during hot and humid periods.

Heat Cramps

Heat cramps are painful muscle cramps experienced by individuals engaged in strenuous activity in which profuse sweating occurs over a short period of time. Marathon runners, for example, are at particular risk. Cramps usually involve the leg and abdominal muscles. Sweating is preserved, and there is usually little fever and no central nervous system abnormalities. Treatment is directed at salt replacement with electrolyte-rich fluids, as for heat exhaustion. Hospitalization is not indicated. Patients at risk should be advised to increase salt intake during periods of excessive sweating.

SUGGESTED READINGS

Beeson PB, McDermott W (eds): *Textbook of Medicine*, ed 14. *Microbial Diseases*. Philadelphia, WB Saunders Co, 1979, part 8.

Beneson AS (ed): *Control of Communicable Diseases in Man*, ed 12. Washington, D.C., American Public Health Association, 1975.

Braude A (ed): *Medical Microbiology and Infectious Diseases*. Philadelphia, WB Saunders Co, 1981.

Clowes GHA Jr, O'Donnell TF Jr: Heat stroke. *N Engl J Med* 1974; 291:564–567.

Gantz HM, Gleckman RA: *Manual of Clinical Problems in Infectious Diseases*. Boston, Little Brown & Co, 1979.

Gardner P, Provine HT: *Manual of Acute Bacterial Infections: Early Diagnosis and Treatment*. Boston, Little Brown & Co, 1975.

Garrod LP, Lambert HP, O'Grady F: *Antibiotic and Chemotherapy*, ed 5. New York, Churchill Livingstone Inc, 1981.

Hoeprich PD (ed): *Infectious Diseases: A Modern Treatise of Infectious Processes*. Hagerstown, MD, Harper & Row Publishers Inc, 1977.

Krugman S, Ward R, Katz, SL: *Infectious Diseases of Children*, ed 6. St. Louis, The CV Mosby Co, 1977.

Kucers A, Bennet NM: *The Use of Antibiotics: A Comprehensive Review with Clinical Emphasis*, ed 3. Philadelphia, JB Lippincott Co, 1979.

Mackowiak PA: The normal microbial flora. *N Engl J Med* 1982; 307:83–93.

Mandell GL, Douglas JV, Bennett JE (eds): *Principles and Practice of Infectious Diseases*. New York, John Wiley & Sons Inc, 1979.

Medical Letter Drugs and Therapeutics. *Handbook of Antimicrobial Therapy*. New Rochelle, NY, The Medical Letter, 1980.

O'Donnell TF Jr: Acute heat stroke. Epidemiologic, biochemical, renal and coagulation studies. *J Am Med Assoc* 1975; 234:824–828.

Proulx RP: Heat stress disease, in Schwartz GR, Safar P, Stone JH, et al (eds): *Principles and Practice of Emergency Medicine*. Saunders, Philadelphia, 1978, p. 815.

Schuman W: Steroids in the treatment of clinical septic shock. *Ann Surg* 1976; 184:333.

Shubin H, Weil MH, Carlson RW: Bacterial shock. *Am Heart J* 1977; 94:112.

Top FH Sr, Wehrle PF (eds): *Communicable and Infectious Diseases*, ed 8. St. Louis, The CV Mosby Co, 1976.

Weinstein L: Chemotherapy of microbial diseases section XIV, in Goodman LS, Gilman AG (eds): *The Pharmacological Basis of Therapeutics*, ed 5. New York, Macmillan Inc, 1975.

Wheeler M: Heat stroke in the elderly. *Med Clin North Am* 1976; 60:1289.

29
SKIN MANIFESTATIONS OF ACUTE DISORDERS

Robert S. Stern
Kenneth A. Arndt

As many as 15% of all patients who are evaluated in emergency rooms have cutaneous changes. The skin condition may be the sole reason for seeking care, or it may be one of several presenting complaints. Many dermatologic conditions are acute, and although they require immediate attention, the patients are otherwise well. A few disorders, however, are signs of underlying systemic illnesses, some of which may be life threatening. Every skin abnormality must therefore be thoroughly evaluated.

Because an emergency room serves not only as an entry point for critically ill patients but also as a source of care for many patients with acute but not serious conditions, physicians should be familiar with a variety of dermatologic disorders (Table 29.1). In addition to diagnosing and treating underlying problems, they must also be prepared to begin treating acute symptoms regardless of etiology.

The ability to differentiate various kinds of lesions, as well as knowing which type of lesion is characteristic of a particular condition, is extremely important. Promptness in establishing a diagnosis and in initiating therapy is sometimes crucial. For example, some patients presenting primarily with cutaneous complaints have a vesiculobullous disorder (toxic epidermal necrolysis, erythema multiforme, or disseminated herpes infection) and are seriously ill. Unless the disease is diagnosed early in its course and appropriate therapy initiated, the patient may remain at substantial risk. Rocky Mountain spotted fever and gonococcemia can be treated effectively once diagnosed. On the other hand, an eruption caused by a drug and accompanied by a fever often resolves if the medication is simply withdrawn or another agent substituted; thus, unnecessary therapy can be avoided. At the same time, the physician must be able to distinguish among conditions, such as contact der-

matitis and impetigo, that are clinically similar but for which treatment and prognosis are quite different.

The approach to a patient with cutaneous changes is no different from the approach to other patients. Data from history, physical examination, and laboratory studies must be synthesized in order for a sound clinical diagnosis to be established.

There are many kinds of cutaneous lesions, each associated with a characteristic etiology and manner of presentation. Papulosquamous and vesiculobullous diseases primarily involve the epidermis or the immediate subepidermal region of the skin. Exanthems, erythemas, and purpuras, on the other hand, are due to changes in the vasculature; for example, purpura results if red blood cells leak from the capillary endothelium. Erosions cause only superficial skin damage and affect the epidermis; ulcers, however, involve all layers of the skin, may extend to underlying bone, and always leave scars. Nodules result from the accumulation of material in dermis or subcutaneous tissue (e.g., metastatic cancer) or from localized inflammation (e.g., erythema nodosum). Urticaria is produced by dermal edema that accompanies histamine and other mediators of inflammation release. It can be localized to the skin or can be a manifestation of life-threatening systemic anaphylaxis (Chapter 7). Table 29.1 presents a classification of cutaneous diseases commonly seen in the emergency room, by severity and anatomical structure principally affected.

The most severe systemic problems often present with no specific physical features. The pruritus caused by some malignancies or by hepatic or renal disease, for example, is not accompanied by specific physical findings; it can, nevertheless, be agonizing.

EVALUATION OF THE PATIENT

History

The nature of the onset of illness, the associated systemic symptoms (fever, malaise, pruritus), and whether a systemic or topical medication is being used are essential parts of the history. In addition, it should include specific information about a personal or family history of cutaneous disease and about exposure to infectious agents; for example, if a child is living in an institution, he or she is at higher risk for impetigo, or if a patient has scabies, other household members may also be infested.

Drugs must be considered as possible etiologic agents in almost every cutaneous eruption. Any one of a number of prescription and over-the-counter drugs, systemic as well as topical, may cause an eruption. Because a physical examination usually cannot distinguish a viral eruption from a drug-induced rash, a carefully taken history often provides the most useful diagnostic information.

TABLE 29.1 Cutaneous Diseases Seen in the Emergency Room

Life Threatening	Commonly Seen in Emergency Room
Vesiculobullous Eruptions	
Erythema multiforme	Herpes simplex
Toxic epidermal necrolysis	Herpes zoster
Disseminated viral infections	Impetigo
of the skin	Contact dermatitis
	Pressure bullae
	Miliaria
	Sunburn
Urticaria	
Urticaria with anaphylaxis	Chronic urticaria
	Serum sickness
Exanthems and Erythemas	
	Drug eruptions
	Butterfly rashes
	Viral exanthems
Purpuric Eruptions	
Septic vasculitis	Trauma
Systemic vasculitis	
Ulcers	
	Primary syphilis
	Traumatic
	Stasis
	Aphthous stomatitis
Papulosquamous Eruptions	
	Secondary syphilis
	Pityriasis rosea
Nodules	
	Erythema nodosum
Infestations and Bites	
	Scabies
	Pediculosis
	Tick bites

Physical and chemical agents such as sunlight and household and industrial chemicals commonly affect the skin directly and trigger acute changes. Many are potentially toxic. The sun itself may damage the skin, or its effects may be augmented by a systemic or topical medication. For example, phototoxic reactions, indistinguishable from sunburn, can result without excessive exposure to the sun in an individual using a photosensitizing medication (Table 29.2). Many rashes result from chemicals contacting the skin. Poison ivy is the most common cause of contact dermatitis, but a number of irritant dermatoses are due to chronic contact with a mildly irritating compound.

Physical Examination

All skin surfaces, including mucous membranes, nails, scalp, hair, and genitalia, must be viewed. The patient should disrobe completely, and adequate illumination is essential. The distribution, character, and extent of the dermatosis are important. Using the terminology in Table 29.3, observers can communicate with others about what they have seen and thus may provide additional insight into the pathophysiology of the rash.

Laboratory Evaluation

In the emergency room, infectious processes can be differentiated from noninfectious ones, and skin eruptions resulting from systemic illness can be identified if the proper laboratory studies are performed.

GRAM STAIN

A Gram stain of tissues and exudates is useful for diagnosing bacterial and some fungal disorders quickly. Thus therapy can be instituted promptly, that is, days before culture results would be available.

TZANCK TEST

A *Tzanck test* can identify the multinucleated giant cells of varicella, herpes zoster, and herpes simplex (Table 29.4). Simple to perform, this technique in conjunction with a Gram stain can provide a definitive diagnosis of many vesiculobullous eruptions.

OTHER TESTS

Occasionally, a specialized laboratory procedure such as a *skin biopsy* may be required for an acutely ill patient. Disseminated intravascular coagulopathy, septic and allergic vasculitis, and some infectious processes can be diagnosed from a biopsy specimen. Frozen sections may be useful in differentiating drug-induced from staphylococcus-induced toxic epidermal necrolysis. To minimize scarring, a skin biopsy should be performed along the skin's natural tension lines. (See Chapter 14, Fig. 14.14.)

At times, a culture of the blood and tissue from a wound should be taken to check for bacteria and viruses. Microscopic examination for yeasts and fungi can rapidly establish the cause of many otherwise puzzling eruptions. The white blood cell

TABLE 29.2 Common Photosensitizing Agents

Type of Agent	Found in
Sulfonamides (Gantrisin)	
Sulfonylureas (Orinase)	
Chlorothiazides (Diuril)	
Phenothiazines (Thorazine)	
Demethylchlortetracycline (Declomycin)	
Furocoumarins (Oxsoralen, Tripsoralen)	Treatment of psoriasis, vitiligo Naturally occurring in parsnip, lime, dill, bergamot, perfumes
Halogenated salicylanilides	Deodorant and antibacterial soaps

count is frequently increased in infection. Eosinophilia often accompanies drug eruptions and parasitic infestations that cause chronic urticaria. The platelet count may be altered by vasculitis or there may be purpuric eruptions. Determining the sedimentation rate and testing for leukopenia and anemia help differentiate systemic lupus erythematosus (SLE) from other butterfly eruptions (Table 29.5). Reliable tests for syphilis, both primary and secondary, are available and are described later in this chapter. Tests of liver function, which is altered in patients with hepatitis, have also been developed and can confirm the diagnosis in a patient presenting with urticaria and generalized malaise.

TABLE 29.3 Lexicon of Commonly Encountered Dermatologic Terminology

Macule	A flat, circumscribed lesion in the plane of normal skin.
Papule	A raised, discrete lesion smaller than 1 cm in diameter.
Plaque	A raised, discrete lesion larger than 1 cm in diameter.
Pustule	An elevated lesion filled with purulent material.
Nodule	A discrete, palpable, solid lesion elevated or flat.
Wheal (hive)	A transitory (less than 24 hours), usually white or pink, elevated lesion resulting from edema in the dermis
Vesicle	A circumscribed, fluid-filled, raised lesion 0.5 cm in diameter.
Erosion	A moist lesion that results when the roof of a vesicle or bulla is lost; does not extend through the epidermis; heals without scarring.
Ulcer	A lesion resulting from the loss of all layers of the epidermis; heals with scarring.
Crust	A collection of dried exudate that often includes serum and inflammatory cells.
Atrophy	A loss of substance in any or all components of the skin. Epidermal atrophy is a loss of epidermal thickness that results in increased skin transparency. Dermal atrophy is a loss of dermis that results in decreased skin thickness.
Fissure	A small break in the normal continuity of skin often because of cracking in dry or inelastic epidermis.
Excoriation	A superficial loss of tissue owing to trauma, usually scratching.
Scale	Adherent stratum corneum cells often seen in diseases of increased epidermal turnover such as most papulosquamous disorders (e.g., psoriasis).
Bulla	A circumscribed, fluid-filled, raised lesion 5.0 cm in diameter (see vesicle).
Purpura	A purple discoloration resulting from the extravasation of blood into the skin.
Morbilliform	An eruption resembling that in rubella, characterized by a symmetrically distributed, erythematous, maculopapular rash.

TABLE 29.4 Tzanck Test

1. A specimen, preferably a scraping of a blister roof and base, is smeared on a slide.
2. The smear is fixed with gentle flaming.
3. The slide is covered with Wright's stain (90 sec).
4. An equal amount of buffer is added (150 sec).
5. The slide is washed with water and dried.
6. Under a high, dry lens the smear is examined for multinucleated giant cells of herpes simplex, herpes zoster, and varicella infections.

VESICULOBULLOUS ERUPTIONS

Vesicle and bulla formation within the skin can be the result of injury, infection, or immunologic events. Such disorders can be serious and of acute onset. Disorders of this type include erythema multiforme, disseminated viral infections of the skin, bacterial infections of the skin, and toxic epidermal necrolysis.

Vesiculobullous eruptions are important not only because of their reflection of an underlying process, but also because with the formation of vesicles and bullae the epidermal barrier of the skin is breached and the patient is at higher risk for secondary infection or, in cases of extensive or deeper vesicles or bullae, is at risk for fluid and electrolyte loss.

Erythema Multiforme

In its most severe form erythema multiforme is known as Stevens-Johnson syndrome. Erythema multiforme is thought to be a hypersensitivity syndrome. Several types of lesions including the characteristic iris, or target, lesion may develop; a lymphohistiocytic infiltrate and subepidermal or intraepidermal vesiculation are common histologic findings. Although the exact immunologic mechanism is not known, several precipitating factors have been identified: infections, drugs (penicillin, barbiturates, sulfonimides), endocrine changes, and underlying malignancies. Herpes simplex infections are an antecedant infectious cause of erythema multiforme, but many other viral, bacterial, and microbacterial agents have also been implicated.

DIAGNOSIS

General malaise and sore throat are often associated with erythema multiforme in its earliest stage before lesions appear, and drugs prescribed to relieve the discomfort are sometimes erroneously blamed for the subsequent eruption. Individual lesions may sting or burn, and large bullae may be painful. Fever is common, and lesions on mucous membranes are frequently quite prominent. Typically, lesions are distributed symmetrically on extensor surfaces, distal limbs, palms and soles, face, and oral mucous membranes. Bright reddish purple annular, macular, and papular areas and some lesions similar to those of urticaria may appear. Most often on the hands, the iris lesion consists of a central vesicle or a livid erythema surrounded by alternating concentric pale and red rings (Plate 1).

The history should include information about prior infections (especially herpes simplex), drug administration, and other illness. Among the infectious diseases that must be considered

TABLE 29.5 Butterfly Rashes of the Face

Diagnosis	Incidence	Clinical Features
Seborrheic dermatitis	Very common	Yellowish-red scaly papules and plaques; other areas (scalp, eyebrows, behind ears, groin) often involved.
Rosacea	Very common	Erythema, telangiectasia with papules and pustules; nose may be involved.
Bacterial infection (erysipelas, cellulitis)	Common	Acute onset, local warmth and tenderness, often fever. May follow trauma. Often recurrent.
Photosensitivity dermatitis	Infrequent	
Systemic lupus erythematosus	Very infrequent	Predominantly seen in females; erythematous, edematous blush of cheek and nose, often provoked by sun. Fever, lymphadenopathy, nephritis, CNS symptoms, and arthritis may accompany.

are streptococcal, mycoplasmal, or deep fungal conditions (histoplasmosis, coccidioidomycosis), hepatitis, infectious mononucleosis, and tuberculosis. In the emergency room, an x-ray film of the chest should be made to determine whether the patient has mycoplasmal or fungal pneumonia or a tuberculous infection. Cultures for streptococci and fungi should be made if the clinical history indicates the need.

Conditions that have clinical features in common with erythema multiforme include vascular reactions such as urticaria and vasculitis and blistering eruptions such as pemphigus and bullous pemphigoid. The skin and mucous membrane changes accompanying toxic epidermal necrolysis, acute herpetic gingivostomatitis, hand-foot-and-mouth disease, and Behçet's syndrome can sometimes be mistaken for signs of erythema multiforme.

TREATMENT AND PROGNOSIS

A mild case of erythema multiforme can be treated with oral antihistamines and open wet compresses applied to bullous or erosive lesions. Any underlying infections should also be treated. If mucous membranes are affected, the patient should rinse his or her mouth with hydrogen peroxide. A topical anesthetic (dyclonine hydrochloride or lidocaine) or an analgesic is useful for treating discomfort.

A severe case of erythema multiforme mandates immediate hospitalization and administration of fluid intravenously. Some clinicians advise prednisone, 80–120 mg/day (or an equilavent dose of another corticosteroid), be given until the patient responds. Then the dosage should be gradually decreased over 2–3 weeks.

Although a mild case of erythema multiforme resolves without treatment in 2–3 weeks, a severe case may last as long as 2 months and can be fatal unless adequately treated. Reexposure to the precipitating agent can result in a new episode of erythema multiforme.

Toxic Epidermal Necrolysis

Toxic epidermal necrolysis (TEN) is characterized by the sudden loss of large areas of epidermis; in children the staphylococcal infection is also known as scalded skin syndrome. This disorder does indeed resemble a burn. The cause in infants is a prior staphylococcal infection with an organism of phage group 2; in adults, the syndrome is usually the result of an allergic reaction to medication. Although both types of TEN are clinically similar, each has its own histopathology and prognosis. In staphylococcal TEN, the bacteria elaborate an exfoliative toxin that causes epidermal cells to separate high

in the epidermis. As a result, healing is rapid. Drug-related TEN, on the other hand, causes the epidermis to split at a lower point or the split may even occur below the epidermis; healing is slow, scarring may result, and the mortality rate is higher.

DIAGNOSIS

In staphylococcal TEN, the antecedent infection is often not clinically apparent. Profuse erythema appears rapidly, and the skin becomes very tender in the areas of erythema. The perioral, perinasal, and periorbital skin is usually affected early. Bullae may be present in any erythematous region, the Nikolsky sign (stripping of skin with light lateral pressure) is common (Plate 2) and a purulent conjunctivitis is noticeable in most patients; fever and general malaise usually accompany this eruption.

Drug-related TEN is more common in patients over 10 years old. It presents with painful skin and sudden extensive loss of epidermis. Except that the patient has a history of taking drugs, its clinical picture is similar to staphylococcal TEN.

TREATMENT AND PROGNOSIS

In infants and children, TEN should be treated with an antibiotic effective against staphylococci, phage group 2. Compresses should be applied and the skin protected. It is crucial to compensate for fluid loss and prevent superinfection of damaged skin. In adult TEN, all drugs should be discontinued, if possible, and skin care such as that for second-degree thermal burns can be lifesaving. Because much of the epidermal barrier is lost in both types of TEN, patients have problems in common with patients who have severe burns. Any pressure or trauma to the skin must be prevented because skin can be lost quite easily. Although most children recover, the mortality rate for drug-related TEN is approximately 15%.

Disseminated Viral Infections of the Skin

Disseminated, or widespread, viral infections of the skin include herpes simplex (eczema herpeticum) (Plate 3), herpes zoster (disseminated zoster) (Plate 4), and vaccinia (eczema vaccinatum). Patients who have atopic dermatitis or who have a skin disease such as pemphigus or keratosis follicularis (Darier's disease) and those with compromised immune status because of disease (for example, patients with Hodgkin's disease or those being treated with immunosuppressive drugs) have a much higher risk for such an infection.

DIAGNOSIS

A localized eruption from herpes simplex, herpes zoster, or vaccination usually precedes dissemination by 2–10 days. Cutaneous viral infections may spread to other organs or to the central nervous system. Lesions may have spread gradually or disseminated explosively. The characteristic lesions are umbilicated vesicles or pustules, fever is usually present, and the disseminated eruption typically lasts 3–4 weeks. Bacterial superinfection must be guarded against and treated if it does occur. A Tzanck test and a viral culture aid in differentiating vaccinia from herpes simplex; giant cells are present in herpes simplex and zoster–varicella but not in vaccinia. Because eczema herpeticum may affect the eyes, an ophthalmologic examination should be an integral part of the evaluation. The differential diagnosis includes erythema multiforme, other vesiculobullous disease (dermatitis herpetiformis, pemphigoid), and, rarely, smallpox.

TREATMENT AND PROGNOSIS

Treatment of a water or an electrolyte abnormality must be initiated immediately. Additional therapy should consist of isolation, wet compresses applied to vesicular lesions, and treatment of bacterial superinfection. Isolation from the surrounding environment is necessary to protect the patient from secondary infection and also to protect others, especially immunologically suppressed individuals, from viral infection. The role of immunoglobulins and drugs is still not well established. But if herpes simplex has affected the face, the eyes should be treated with topical adenosine arabinoside (ara-A).

Although most patients recover, death can result from bacterial infection, fluid loss, electrolyte imbalance, viral encephalitis, or cardiovascular collapse. The presence or severity of an underlying skin disease is not directly correlated with the susceptibility to disseminated viral infection. Once an individual with atopic dermatitis has an episode of disseminated herpes simplex, the condition is likely to recur whether or not the eczema is under control at the time of the recurrence.

Herpes Simplex

Zoster–varicella, and herpes simplex, cytomegalic, and Epstein-Barr viruses, are all members of the herpes virus family. Herpes zoster and herpes simplex infections differ in their epidemiology and clinic presentation. Herpes zoster occurs in older patients, usually involves a greater skin area, is more often confined to a single dermatome, and is far less likely to recur than is herpes simplex.

Herpes simplex is a DNA virus that infects only humans. Two types of the virus exist: Type 1 usually causes nongenital herpetic infections, and type 2 commonly results in genital infections. With either type, the infection may be primary or recurrent. The primary form is a severely painful and often disabling eruption that appears only in previously uninfected individuals; the recurrent form, on the other hand, occurs only in previously infected patients who present with cold sores or fever blisters on the face or with a vesicular eruption on the genitalia.

Most individuals have a subclinical primary herpetic infection. After primary infection, the virus enters into a latent phase during which it resides in sensory nerve ganglia, but it can be reactivated at any time if it is triggered by factors such as emotional stress, physical trauma, sunlight, fever, sexual activity, or systemic infection.

The earliest symptom of a primary herpetic infection, oral or genital, is tenderness of mucocutaneous surfaces that lasts 1–2 days. Lesions form and become extremely painful (Plate 5); discomfort may, in fact, be so severe that the patient limits normal activities. If the primary infection is oral, gingivostomatitis develops, and vesicles, erosions, and macerations appear on the entire buccal mucosa; fever and cervical adenopathy are common. In men, a primary genital infection usually results in a painful cutaneous penile lesion but it can also cause urethritis or discharge. In women, a primary genital infection may present with vulvovaginitis, consisting of widespread vesicles and erosion and edema of the labia, vulva, and surrounding skin. Vaginal discharge is profuse, and spasm of the sphincter or urinary retention may result from the pain associated with urination. Bilateral adenopathy and fever are usually present.

A recurrent episode of herpes simplex is often preceded by several hours of a burning or tingling sensation. Although lesions are uncomfortable when they form, they are much less painful than those of a primary infection. Recurrent infection presents with many small vesicles clustered on an erythematous, edematous base. The clear vesicles rapidly become cloudy and purulent, and dried crusts form within 7–10 days. Regional adenopathy is common. A yellow or gold crust on older herpetic lesions usually suggests bacterial superinfection.

DIAGNOSIS

A Tzanck test made with a smear from the base of a vesicle is a helpful diagnostic tool; multinucleated giant cells are observed if the virus is present. Viral cultures, which require 24–48 hours, can also confirm infection. Herpes simplex lesions sometimes resemble those of aphthous stomatitis, herpes zoster, or impetigo.

TREATMENT AND PROGNOSIS

There is no known prophylaxis for primary or recurrent infection with herpes simplex virus. Primary infection is treated symptomatically with analgesics, cleansing mouth washes for gingivostomatisis, and sitz baths for vulvovaginitis. Women with painful vulvar lesions are often able to urinate more easily while sitting in a bathtub, but catheterization is occasionally necessary. Hospitalization and intravenous fluid administration are sometimes necessary. Therapy for a recurrent infection is aimed at drying the lesions and preventing secondary bacterial infection. Agents containing alcohol (for example, Blistex) may be useful, and wet compresses and topical antibiotics help prevent bacterial superinfection.

Three groups of patients who have a herpes simplex infection require special attention: individuals with eye symptoms should be examined with a slit lamp and treated with ara-A or idoxuridine if any evidence of herpetic keratitis is found; they should also receive ophthalmologic consultation (see Chapter 31). Pregnant women with active vulvar lesions may require delivery by cesarean section; a neonatal herpes infection, acquired by direct innoculation in the birth canal, can be life threatening. As discussed above, patients with atopic dermatitis or immunodeficiency may develop disseminated viral infection.

Herpes Zoster

Herpes zoster (shingles) is a painful vesicular eruption that appears in a dermatomal distribution (Plate 4). After a varicella (chicken pox) infection has resolved, the zoster–varicella virus enters a latent period during which it resides in the dorsal root or cervical nerve ganglia. Herpes zoster results when the reactivated virus migrates down the nerve and infects the skin overlying the nerve ending.

DIAGNOSIS

The rash is frequently preceded by mild or severe pruritus, and all or part of the affected dermatome may be tender or painful. Lesions usually first appear posteriorly and then on the anterior and peripheral distributions of the nerve; erythematous macular and papular plaques are seen initially, and grouped vesicles appear almost invariably within 24 hours, although occasionally blisters never develop. Mucous membranes within the dermatome are also affected. The vesicles become puru-

lent, crust, and fall off within 1–2 weeks. Vesicles often form outside the affected dermatome, but such an occurrence is not indicative of dissemination unless the lesions are quite numerous.

The Tzanck test with a smear from a vesicle base aids in establishing the diagnosis. The differential diagnosis of herpes zoster includes herpes simplex, impetigo, and pressure bullae.

TREATMENT AND PROGNOSIS

Debilitated or immunosuppressed patients in whom the herpes zoster infection is widespread should be hospitalized and strictly isolated. Most individuals, however, require only symptomatic treatment with analgesics and compresses. A topical antibiotic reduces the possibility of secondary infection, and ocular involvement should be evaluated as in herpes simplex. Postherpetic neuralgia, persistent pain after the eruption has subsided, is much more common in patients over the age of 60 years than in young patients. Some clinicians advise a 3-week regimen of a systemic steroid early in the clinical course, which may inhibit perineural fibrosis and subsequent pain. The neuralgia usually lasts for 2–3 weeks but may persist for months or years.

Impetigo

Impetigo is a vesicular and crusted eruption that develops most frequently in children. The condition, which is a superficial bacterial infection of the skin, is usually caused by staphylococci or streptococci.

DIAGNOSIS

Streptococcal impetigo presents initially with small erythematous macules that develop rapidly into fragile vesicles; later these vesicles ooze and form a yellowish crust. Satellite pustules are common. In bullous staphylococcal impetigo the lesions are flaccid blisters, which are clear at first and then are cloudy. The eruption is usually pruritic, and scratching can spread the infection. Although they present most often as crusted plaques, the primary lesions of nonbullous impetigo are subcorneal pustules that initially contain only group A β-hemolytic streptococci. Later in the disease staphylococci frequently colonize the lesions. Because most cases of impetigo can be diagnosed clinically, cultures are usually not necessary. If the diagnosis is uncertain, however, a Gram stain should be made to determine whether the organism is present.

Impetigo is most common in warm climates or during the

summer in temperate climates. Any skin injury or eruption that compromises the integrity of the epidermis is a possible predisposing event. Nummular eczema, herpes simplex, and herpes zoster should be considered in the differential diagnosis of impetigo.

TREATMENT AND PROGNOSIS

Impetigo should be treated systemically with antibiotics. Such treatment decreases the healing time, the likelihood of recurrence, and the number of streptococcal carriers in the community. For nonbullous impetigo, a 10-day course of penicillin or erythromycin is appropriate. One injection of benzathine penicillin G intramuscularly (adults and children weighing more than 45 kg—1.2 million units; children weighing 27–45 kg—0.6 million units) is excellent treatment and avoids the uncertainty of patient compliance. Bullous eruptions should be treated with semisynthetic penicillin, such as dicloxacillin, or with erythromycin.

Contact Dermatitis

Contact dermatitis is an inflammatory response of the skin to a substance; it may be irritating because of its physical properties, or it may elicit an allergic, cell-mediated, delayed hypersensitivity reaction. Any unprotected person may develop an irritant reaction to certain chemicals if contact is of sufficient duration. On the other hand, the rash of allergic contact dermatitis occurs only in people sensitized to specific antigens, although a history of previous exposure is not always forthcoming.

DIAGNOSIS

Allergic contact eruptions are often weeping, vesicular, and extremely pruritic. The patient's history and the distribution of the dermatitis are essential for making a direct diagnosis. For example, poison ivy and poison oak reactions, the most frequent causes of contact sensitization encountered in emergency room practice, are usually seen on exposed parts of the body (extremities and face) as linear lesions. The presence of such lesions is an excellent clue to the diagnosis of contact dermatitis. Other common contact sensitizers include industrial chemicals and drugs such as topical antipruritics containing antihistamines (for example, Caladryl, which contains diphenhydramine hydrochloride).

Proper treatment depends on determining whether the condition is a true allergic contact dermatitis, an irritant contact dermatitis, or atopic dermatitis. Extensive contact dermatitis with an accompanying autosensitivity reaction can also be mistaken for a drug reaction or a viral exanthem.

TREATMENT AND PROGNOSIS

Treatment of contact dermatitis is much the same for all patients. Identifying the offending agent and preventing contact with it are, of course, essential whether the reaction is an irritant or an allergic contact dermatitis. Acute dermatitis with edema, erythema, and oozing responds if compresses moistened with saline or Burow's solution diluted 1:20 with tap water are applied four times a day. Antihistamines usually relieve itching. After the acute weeping eruption has subsided, a potent topical corticosteroid may speed resolution of the dermatitis (Table 29.6). Severe cases of contact dermatitis with extreme pruritis and edema of face or genitalia or with widespread lesions should be treated with prednisone for 10–14 days. In an adult, 60–80 mg/day is the usual initial dosage. If the offending agent cannot be identified, patch testing should be considered after the acute eruption has resolved.

Pressure Bullae

If a patient has been immobile for a prolonged period, erythematous urticarial plaques and erosions, a result of ischemic necrosis, may appear at pressure sites (Plate 6). Although the lesions are most common in patients comatose from drug overdose, they can form when any condition produces prolonged stupor or insensitivity to pain or pressure. The underlying cause of coma should, of course, be treated, and the comatose patient should be rotated frequently. In addition, sterile aspiration of large bullae facilitates healing and helps prevent secondary bacterial infection.

Miliaria

Miliaria is a skin eruption resulting from the blockage of eccrine sweat ducts. The clinical form depends to a great extent on the level at which the ducts are blocked. Miliaria rubra (prickly heat), the type seen most frequently in the emergency room, is a pruritic eruption; its small erythematous macules, usually on the trunk and neck, may be topped with central vesicles. Most individuals, both infants and adults, are susceptible to miliaria rubra if exposed to heat and humidity extreme enough to result in duct blockage. A cooler, drier environment is generally the only treatment that is required. Occlusion from nonabsorbent clothes and bed linen and from topical medications must be avoided.

TABLE 29.6 Common Topical Medications in Dermatology

Indication	Agent	Supplied as	Dosage
Antibacterial	Bacitracin	Ointment	After cleaning wound, 4–6 times a day
Antiyeast	Nystatin	Cream (100,000 units / g), vaginal suppositories	2 or 3 times a day
	Clotrimazole (Lotrimin)	Cream (1%), lotion (1%)	3 times a day
	Miconazole (Micatin) (Monistat)	Cream (2%)	3 times a day
Antifungal	Clotrimazole	Cream (1%), lotion (1%)	3 times a day
	Miconazole (Micatin)	Cream (2%)	3 times a day
	Tolnaftate (Tinactin)		
Scabicides	Gamma-benzene hexachloride (Gamene, Kwell)	Cream (1%), lotion (1%), shampoo (1%)	
Pediculicides	Gamma-benzene hexachloride (Gamene, Kwell)	Cream (1%), lotion (1%), shampoo (1%)	
Antiinflammatory nonsteroids	Burow's solution (aluminum acetate)	Solution	Open wet dressings for 8–10 min 4–6 times a day
	Iodochlorhydroxyquin	Cream (3%)	3 times a day
Antiinflammatory steroids	Fluocinonide	Cream (.05%), ointment (0.05%)	3 times a day
	Betamethasone dipropinate (Diprosone)	Cream (.05%), ointment (0.5%)	3 times a day
	Valerate (Valisone)	Cream (1%), ointment (1%), solution (1%)	3 times a day
	Fluocinolone acetonide (Fluonid, Synalar)	Cream (0.01%, 0.025%), ointment (0.002%), solution (0.25%, 0.01%)	3 times a day
	Triamcinolone (Aristocort, Kenalog)	Cream (11.5%), ointment (0.1%, 0.5%), solution (0.1%)	3 times a day
	Hydrocortisone	Cream (0.5%, 1.0%, 2.5%), solution (1%), ointment (1%)	3 times a day
Emollient	Eucerin	Cream	As necessary
	Keri	Cream, lotion	As necessary
	Cetaphil	Lotion (lipid free)	As necessary
Antipruritic	0.25% menthol and 1% phenol in Eucerin	Cream Phenolated (1%) calamine lotion	As necessary
Anesthetic	Dyclonine hydrochloride (Dyclone)	Solution	As necessary up to 4 times a day
	Lidocaine (Xylocaine)	Ointment, solution	As necessary up to 4 times a day
	Dimethisoquin hydrochloride (Quotane)	Ointment, lotion	As necessary up to 4 times a day

Sunburn

Sunburn is the reaction caused by extensive exposure to ultraviolet light, most often midwave length ultraviolet radiation (UVB) . The initial erythema that is produced fades somewhat but recurs later. This erythema is most intense 14–20 hours after exposure and lasts 1–3 days. Exposure for only 1 hour at midday in a temperate climate can moderately or severely burn a fair-skinned person. The patient's pigmentation, the intensity of the sunlight, and the duration of the exposure determine the severity of the reaction.

DIAGNOSIS

The earliest sign of sunburn is a pink or scarlet hue with mild edema, which may progress to vivid erythema, intense edema, or blistering. During the repair phase, the skin peels and the newly exposed layers have increased pigmentation. Mildly sunburned skin is tender, warm, and taut; a severe burn, however, may be extremely painful and accompanied by nausea, tachycardia, chills, and fever. If the history of sun exposure does not account for the severity of the burn, the physician must determine whether an underlying illness or a drug has increased the patient's sensitivity to sunlight. The most common photosensitizers in the United States are drugs in the sulfonamide family, including thiazide diuretics (Table 29.2). The differential diagnosis of sunburn includes contact dermatitis caused by airborne substances, photosensitivity eruption such as phototoxic and photoallergic drug reactions, and viral exanthems, which are sometimes exacerbated by exposure to sun.

TREATMENT AND PROGNOSIS

Preventive measures for sunburn include shielding and sun-protective medications that contain chemical substances that absorb ultraviolet light. In addition to opaque sun screens such as reflecta or zinc oxide paste, there are a variety of agents that absorb ultraviolet light. The most effective are p-aminobenzoic acid (PABA) preparations that absorb midwave length radiation often in combination with the broader-spectrum benzaphenone sun-screen agents (PreSun 15, Total Eclipse, Super Shade 15) that absorb a broader range of ultraviolet radiation.

A mild sunburn should be treated with compresses moistened with cool tap water or with dilute Burow's solution and applied 3 or 4 times a day. A topical steroid, such as a lotion or a cream, sometimes reduces inflammation and pain, and an emollient may sooth and relieve dryness. Because the risk of contact sensitization is so great, over-the-counter preparations containing local anesthetics such as benzocaine or diphenhydramine hydrochloride should not be used.

If a severe sunburn is treated early with oral prednisone, 40–60 mg/day or its equivalent, its effects may be significantly diminished. Severe sunburn may also be treated topically with continuous cool compresses or baths, local corticosteroids, and emollients. Analgesics may be required, and hospitalizations for patients with severe cases of sunburn is sometimes necessary. Because the normal protective barrier furnished by the skin is compromised, secondary bacterial infection is a risk if sunburn is severe. Occasionally a severe sunburn heals with scarring.

URTICARIA

Urticaria (hives) consists of pruritic areas of localized skin edema. Urticaria can be confined to the skin or can occur as part of a systemic reaction; anaphylaxis, which results from vasodilatation and local edema, can involve the cardiovascular system, the respiratory tract, and the gastrointestinal tract. As part of this reaction, hypotension, bronchospasm, cardiac failure, laryngeal edema, nausea, and vomiting can occur. Anaphylaxis can be life threatening and demands immediate attention. The treatment is outlined in Chapter 7.

The systemic reactions are the result of so-called immediate hypersensitivity reactions with IgE and histamine playing essential roles. Antigenic stimuli responsible for such reactions include drugs, food, insect bites, and infections. The mast cell has an important role in anaphylaxis. Most frequently, we see urticaria confined to the skin or with minor associated noncutaneous symptoms, such as mild bronchospasm or nausea. Hives may also accompany collagen vascular disease and malignant tumors. When urticaria occurs in submucous or deep dermous, the lesions are termed angioedema. Urticaria and arthritis may be seen as a prodromal symptom in patients with hepatitis or vasculitis.

Urticaria can also be induced by a variety of physical events including cold and ultraviolet light. If urticaria lasts longer than 6 weeks, it is considered chronic. The etiology of chronic urticaria is difficult to pinpoint; in fact, the causative agent can be identified in less than 10% of the cases.

DIAGNOSIS

Intense pruritus is the typical symptom of urticaria, but at times tingling and stinging sensations are also described. Urticarial wheals are raised erythematous, edematous plaques with sharp borders that may be millimeters or many centimeters in diameter. Individual lesions may last for 8–12 hours. If they persist for longer than 24 hours they are not true urticaria. A detailed history often uncovers the cause of an acute urticarial reaction. If the condition is persistent and its etiology cannot be determined, the patient should be referred for a laboratory workup and a possible biopsy to determine whether the condition is a urticarial vasculitis or is associated with systemic disease.

TREATMENT AND PROGNOSIS

Acute or severe urticaria with limited associated systemic symptoms can be treated with 0.3–0.5 ml epinephrine 1:1,000 intramuscularly or subcutaneously every 1–2 hours (if there are no cardiac contraindications) or with an antihistamine given orally or intramuscularly. Sublingual isoproterenol also may be useful. An antipruritic agent, such as phenolated calamine lotion or 0.25% menthol and 1% phenol in Eucerin may relieve the itching. Systemic corticosteroid is only rarely necessary.

Identifying and removing the trigger factor is the only effective long-term therapy for patients with chronic urticaria. For patients with short-term intermittent urticaria, an antihistamine, such as hydroxyzine or chlorpheniramine maleate, can inhibit the formation and itching of lesions. The regimen should begin with 10–25 mg hydroxyzine (Atarax) or 4 mg chlorpheniramine maleate (Chlor-Trimeton), and the dosage should be increased slowly until the drug becomes effective or side effects such as drowsiness develop.

EXANTHEMS AND ERYTHEMAS

Erythema of the skin reflects increased blood flow through the skin. Persistent erythema usually reflects dilitation of the dermal blood vessels that frequently accompanies inflammation in the skin. Although erythema is seen as one component of many types of skin lesions, including urticaria and the vesiculobullous disorders, when it occurs over wide areas of the body without other specific cutaneous changes in a symmetrical distribution, it is usually called an exanthem or erythema. In the emergency room, exanthems and erythemas of the skin are most often associated with drug eruptions or infectious illness. Distinguishing between these two etiologies is often extremely difficult.

Drug Reactions

The most common form of drug reactions seen in patients in the emergency room is an exanthematous, morbilliform eruption, usually the result of a hypersensitivity response to a foreign antigen. The predominant symptom of this type of drug reaction is pruritis, either mild or severe.

DIAGNOSIS

The eruption begins as macules, which gradually become brighter red, more extensive, and edematous. Usually in a symmetrical pattern, the lesions appear first on the head and proximal extremities and then on distal areas; palms, soles, and mucous membranes may be involved. Severe eruptions may produce purpuric lesions on the lower extremities without thrombocytopenia or vasculitis, or occasionally bullae may develop.

First episodes of hypersensitivity drug reactions of the exanthematous type occur most often within 1 week after the patient has started taking the drug; occasionally, however, the rash appears as long as 14 days after the drug has been discontinued. It is possible that the patient has been treated with the drug many times before without developing reactions. Typically the eruption is severe for 3–7 days but rarely lasts longer than 2–3 weeks. The morphology of the eruption gives no clue to the specific causative agent. Thus, a carefully taken history of all medications, both prescription and over the counter, and all other substances having entered any body orifice is essential in making the proper diagnosis. Exanthematous drug eruptions are often difficult to distinguish from viral exanthems.

Drugs can also cause urticaria or trigger anaphylactic reactions. Other types of drug eruptions include fixed drug eruptions, photosensitivity and photoallergic drug eruptions, urticaria, pustular eruptions, and vasculitis and are discussed separately. In addition, a specific eruption can develop when a specific drug is administered to a patient with a specific disease. This most commonly occurs when ampicillin is administered to patients with infectious mononucleosis who then develop a morbilliform eruption. Table 29.7 lists skin reaction rates to commonly used drugs with reaction rates of greater than 1 per 1,000 in hospitalized recipients. Table 29.8 lists specific drugs associated with characteristic eruptions.

TREATMENT AND PROGNOSIS

The sensitizing agent should, of course, be discontinued. Milder cases usually require only antihistamines, compresses moistened with cool tap water or Burow's solution, oatmeal baths, or lubricating antipruritic emollients (0.25% menthol and 1% phenol in Eucerin, Keri lotion) to alleviate pruritus. If the drug eruption is severe, 60 mg prednisone a day or an equivalent dose of another systemic steroid usually relieves symptoms;

TABLE 29.7 Allergic Skin Reactions to Drugs

Drug	Reaction Rate (Reactions/1,000 recipients)[a]
Ampicillin	52
Semisynthetic penicillins[b]	36
Blood, whole human	35
Penicillin G	16
Gentamicin sulfate	16
Cephalosporins[c]	13
Quinidine	12
Dipyrine	11
Mercurial diuretics[d]	9.5
Packed red blood cells	8.1
Heparin	7.7
Trimethobenzamide hydrochloride	6.6
Nitrazepam	6.3
Barbiturates[e]	4.7
Chlordiazepoxide	4.2
Diazepam	3.8
Propoxyphene	3.4
Isoniazid	3.0
Guaifenesin[f]	2.9
Chlorothiazide	2.8
Furosemide	2.6
Isophane insulin suspension	1.3
Phenytoin	1.1

Adapted from Arndt KA and Jick H: *J Am Med Assoc* 1976; 235:918–922.

[a]Only drugs with allergic reaction rates exceeding 1 reaction per 1,000 recipients are included.

[b]Carbenicillin, cloxacillin sodium monohydrate, dicloxacillin, methicillin, nafcillin.

[c]Cephalexin monohydrate, cephaloglycin dihydrate, cephaloridine, cephalothin sodium

[d]Meralluride, mercaptomerin sodium

[e]Amobarbital, barbital, butabarbital, butethal, mephobarbital, phenobarbital, secobarbital

[g]Guaifenesin and theophylline

the dosage should be decreased gradually over a 2-week period.

Infectious Diseases

Infection as a result of a variety of viral, rickettsial, and bacterial agents can lead to the development of exanthems or enanthems

TABLE 29.8 Common Drugs Associated with Characteristic Eruptions

Type of Eruption	Drugs
Erythema multiforme	Penicillin, phenothiazides, sulfonamides, thiazides, chlorpropamide
Erythema nodosum	Sulfonamides, oral contraceptives
Fixed	Barbiturates, phenolphthalein, quinidine, sulfonamides, gold, tetracycline, phenacetin
Lichen planus like	Chloroquine, gold, thiazides, quinidine
Purpuric	Barbiturates, chlorothiazide, gold, sulfonamides, quinidine, griseofulvin
Bullous	Bromides, phenolphthalein, salicylates

that may be indistinguishable in appearance from drug eruptions. The cutaneous manifestations of some infectious processes that are of critical clinical importance begin as erythemas or exanthems and progress to purpuric lesions. These include pseudomonal sepsis, meningococcemia, gonococcemia (Plate 7) and Rocky Mountain spotted fever (Plate 8). The clinical presentation of these disorders are discussed in greater detail in the section on purpura. Table 29.9 presents clinical characteristics of other common enanthems and exanthems with infectious etiologies.

PURPURA

Purpura is a discoloration of the skin as a result of extravasation of red blood cells from the vascular space and can result from several alterations in the vasculature or circulating elements (Table 29.10). Of special concern in the emergency room is purpura related to thrombocytopenia, intravascular coagulopathy, infection, or hypersensitivity. Thrombocytopenia and hypersensitivity reactions to drugs may be clinically indistinguishable.

Purpura fulminans, which is rare, results from intravascular thrombosis and necrosis of superficial blood vessels (disseminated intravascular longulopathy). Large areas become necrotic; anemia, fever, and malaise are common. Purpura fulminans usually presents 2–10 weeks after an infection of the upper respiratory tract.

Three purpuric eruptions that present with hemorrhagic infarcts sometimes preceeded by erythematous macules or papules are related to systemic bacterial infection: disseminated gonococcemia, meningococcemia, and bacterial endocarditis. Urethritis, arthritis, and fever are common in patients with

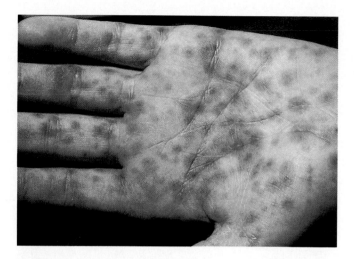

Plate 1   *Erythema multiforme.*

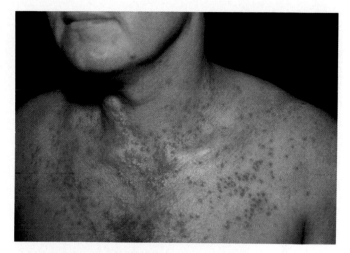

Plate 3   *Eczema herpeticum.*

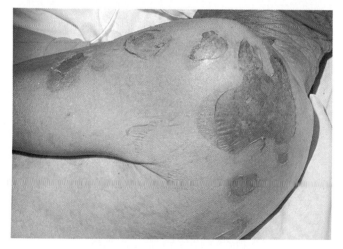

Plate 2   *Toxic epidermal necrolysis (staphylococcal).*

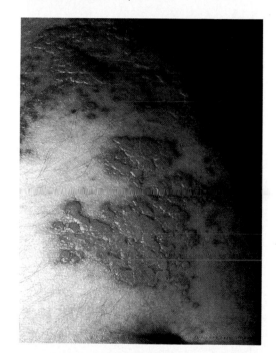

Plate 4   *Herpes zoster.*

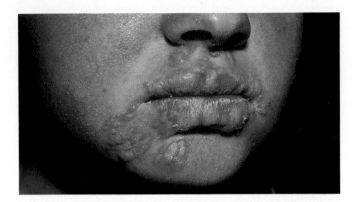

Plate 5 *Herpes simplex.*

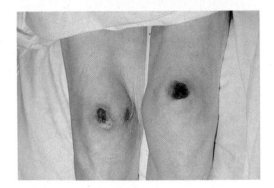

Plate 6 *Pressure bullae.*

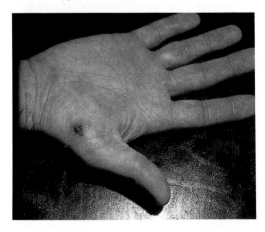

Plate 7 *Gonococcemia.*

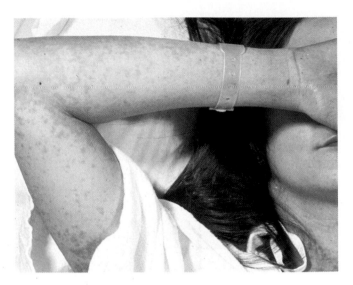

Plate 8 *Rocky Mountain spotted fever.*

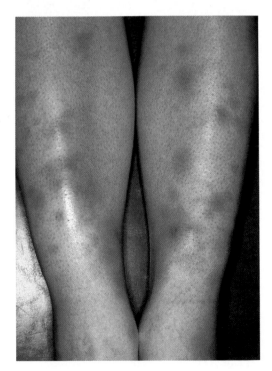

Plate 9 *Erythema nodosum.*

gonococcemia. Meningococcemia often is accompanied by fever, headache, and meningeal symptoms, and purpuric lesions are larger and more numerous. Cardiac signs and symptoms in patients with bacterial endocarditis are essential in establishing the proper diagnosis and instituting prompt treatment. Appropriate smears and cultures are crucial for documenting each of these infections. Rocky Mountain spotted fever, a rickettsial disease transmitted by a tick, begins with erythematous macules that begin centripetally and spread centrally.

Purpuric lesions that seem to be a hypersensitivity reaction may in fact be a result of a drug or an infection; at times, however, no precipitating factor can be identified. Because Henoch-Schönlein purpura, a classic hypersensitivity vasculitis that occurs most often in children, often involves other organs, such as the gastrointestinal tract, the joints, or the kidneys, any patient who presents with purpuric eruptions should be examined thoroughly to rule out infection and to determine whether other organs are involved.

DIAGNOSIS

Table 29.10 presents the differential diagnosis of purpuric lesions.

TREATMENT AND PROGNOSIS

The key to treating this heterogeneous group of diseases is determining the etiology. Prognosis varies greatly both among and within diagnostic categories. Hospitalization of the patient in order to establish the diagnosis and to initiate therapy is often desirable.

TABLE 29.9 Common Exanthems and Enanthems of Infectious Etiology

Disease	Agent	Clinical Characteristics
Measles (Rubeola)	Myxovirus	Incub. 10–11 days; mild URI followed by more toxic 4-day prodrome with headache, conjunctivitis, photophobia. Rash begins in scalp as red macules, extends, becomes papular, desquamates, Koplick spots of buccal mucosa (white spots) characteristic.
German measles (Rubella)	RNA Myxoviey	Incub. 12–24 days, 1–5 day mild prodrome, rash begins at hairline, spreads downward, lasts 2–3 days, resolves with desquamation.
Roseola infantum	?	Incub. 5–15 days, 3–5 days of high fever, which decreases with onset of rash, mainly of trunk, red papules with surrounding blanch.
Chicken pox (Varicella)	Zoster–varicella virus	Incub. 10–20 days, 0–2 day prodrome fever, begins on thorax as red macules that become umbilicated vesicles, very pruritic, mainly face and trunk, vesicles crust in 24–48 hours.
Erythema infectiosum (Fifth disease)	?	Incub. 6–10 days, prodrome uncommon, low fever, cough, coryza accompanying rash on face that spreads over cheeks with circumoral pallor (slapped cheeks), mottled erythema or extensor surfaces of body.
Scarlet fever	Streptococci (group A)	Sudden onset fever, sore throat, headache 2–4 days duration, 2 days of rash begins on base of neck and spreads over body, fine red papules that are blanchable except in body creases (Pastia's lines), palatal petechiae are characteristic, desquamation follows acute eruption.
Hand-foot-and mouth-disease	Coxsackievirus A16, A5	Incub. 3–5 day, prodrome 12–24 hours, low fever, abd. pain, malaise; macules and papules with central vesicles—hands, feet, buttocks, mouth most frequent locations.
Herpangina	Coxsackievirus group A	Childhood summertime illness, fever, myalgias, anorexia with blister of posterior pharynx.
Secondary syphilis	*T. pallidum*	Incub. 6–12 weeks.
Mucocutaneous lymph node syndrome (Kawasaki's disease)	?	High fever 1–4 days, followed by onset of rash with erythema and edema of acral areas, desquamation of hands and feet, exfoliation of lips, red lips and strawberry-like tongue, scarlatiniform eruption may occur, lymphadenopathy prominent. Assoc. findings: carditis, arthritis, aseptic meningitis, diarrhea, jaundice.

TABLE 29.10 Conditions Producing Purpura

Metabolic
  Cushing's syndrome
  Steroid therapy
  Scurvy
  Diabetes mellitus
Mechanical
  Trauma
  Increased intraluminal pressure (stasis)
Infectious
  Gonococcemia
  Meningococcemia
  Purpura fulminans
  Endocarditis
  Other miscellaneous infections
Immunologic
  Drug reactions
  Henoch-Schönlein purpura
  Collagen vascular disease
  Allergic cutaneous venulitis
Thrombocytopenic
  Decreased production
  Increased destruction
  Dysfunction
Coagulopathic
  Hemophilia and other congenital disorders
  Vitamin K deficiency
  Anticoagulants
  Cryoglobulinemia
  Macroglobulinemia
  Disseminated intravascular coagulopathy (purpura fulminans)

ULCERS

Of all skin ulcers seen in patients in the emergency room, pressure and traumatic ulcers are by far the most frequent and should be readily identifiable by their location and appearance and the patient's clinical history. Traumatic and pressure ulcers are often secondarily infected or may be a portal of entry for systemic bacterial infection. In addition, physicians should be cognizant of a common painless ulcer—the chancre of primary syphilis.

Primary Syphilis

The lesion of primary syphilis is the chancre, a painless ulcer that develops 10–20 days after sexual contact with an infected partner. It lasts 1–5 weeks and disappears without treatment. Although the chancre is most common on the genitalia, it may occur on any mucous membrane or on skin of any area that has been exposed to the spirochete. Usually only a single lesion

forms; it is covered with a crust, is quite firm, and is surprisingly nontender. Except for regional nontender adenopathy, the patient seems to be well.

DIAGNOSIS

Direct examination with a dark-field microscopy for spirochetes is essential for establishing the diagnosis since serological tests are often not positive in primary syphilis. If the dark-field examination is negative, serologic tests should be made weekly for 3 weeks and then at 6-week intervals. Primary syphilis can be confused with traumatic ulcers, chancroid, furuncles, and herpes simplex. The lesions of these conditions are usually painful, whereas a chancre is not.

TREATMENT AND PROGNOSIS

An adult patient who is not allergic to penicillin should be started with a single 2.4 million unit dose of benzathene penicillin intramuscularly or with 600,000 units of procaine penicillin G per day for 10 days. An alternative regimen is 500 mg tetracycline four times a day for 15 days or 500 mg erythromycin 4 times a day for 15 days. Follow-up serologic tests for syphilis should be performed 3, 6, and 12 months later; if the test at 12 months is positive, repeating the treatment regimen should be considered. Any person with whom the patient has had sexual contact should also be treated with benzathene penicillin G (1.2 million units intramuscularly). Treatment protocols are published regularly by the Center for Disease Control.

PAPULOSQUAMOUS ERUPTIONS

Common papulosquamous disorders of the skin include psoriasis, seborrheic dermatitis, tinea corporis, chronic eczema, and tinea versicolor. These chronic papulosquamous disorders usually increase slowly in extent and are far more likely to be seen in patients in dermatologists' offices than in patients in emergency rooms. Two common papulosquamous disorders, secondary syphilis and pityriasis rosea, have more rapid onset and are more likely to be seen in patients in emergency rooms.

Secondary Syphilis

Secondary syphilis is the second clinically evident stage of the infection by the spirochete *Treponema pallidum*. Many patients present with influenzalike symptoms: headache, malaise, sore throat, lymphadenopathy, fever. The rash of secondary syphilis consists of disseminated plaques or faint, reddish-brown macules and papules. The lesions may be scaling papules on the palms or soles, white mucosal plaques on the oral mucosa (mucous patches), or moist, vegetative anogenital growths (condyloma lata). The rash, which almost never itches and never forms blisters, develops on the average about 9 weeks after initial infection or about 6 weeks after the appearance of the chancre of primary syphilis.

DIAGNOSIS

Although the organism can sometimes be demonstrated by dark-field examination, serologic evidence and physical findings are most often the key to diagnosis. Infected individuals produce two major types of antibodies that are the basis for the serologic tests for syphilis. One type includes nonspecific antibodies that are directed against a lipoidal antigen; they result when the host and parasite interact. The Venereal Disease Research Laboratory (VDRL) test and the rapid plasma reagin (RPR) tests, which are flocculation tests that are very sensitive, easily performed, and inexpensive, are based on this type of antibody and should always be used for initial screening. The spirochete also causes infected patients to produce specific treponemal antibodies whose presence can be detected by the flourescent treponemal antibody (FTA) and *T. pallidum* immobilization (TPI) tests.

Secondary syphilis must be differentiated from pityriasis rosea, superficial fungal infections, drug eruptions, viral exanthems, and nummular eczema.

TREATMENT AND PROGNOSIS

Secondary syphilis should be treated with benzathene penicillin G (a single dose of 2.4 million units) or with procaine penicillin G (600,000 units a day for 10 days). A patient who is allergic to penicillin can often be treated effectively with tetracycline (500 mg four times a day for 15 days) or erythromycin (500 mg four times a day for 15 days). Some patients, however, are allergic to all of these drugs. Periodically the Center for Disease Control publishes up-to-date accepted treatment regimens. Serologic tests should be performed every 3 months for any patient who has been treated for syphilis to determine whether the treatment has been adequate or whether the infection has been reacquired.

If the disease is not treated, evidence of syphilis, both clinical and serologic, disappears in approximately one-third of patients. Serologic tests continue to be positive for another one-third, yet they enjoy good health. The final one-third later develop signs of late syphilis; of this group, approximately 25%

die as a result of the disease, and 80% of such deaths are due to cardiovascular disease caused by syphilis.

Pityriasis Rosea

Pityriasis rosea is a self-limiting, mild, scaling eruption that appears most frequently in young adults during spring or fall. The condition is thought to be viral in origin, but this hypothesis has yet to be substantiated.

DIAGNOSIS

Although pityriasis rosea sometimes presents initially with mild malaise and symptoms similar to those of a viral infection of the upper respiratory tract, most patients have no systemic complaints. The initial lesion is a 2–6-cm erythematous scaling plaque known as a herald patch. Other lesions appear 2–10 days later on the trunk and proximal extremities, but the face, hands, and feet are usually spared. These lesions are 1–2 cm in diameter, pale red, oval or round, macular or papular, and are characterized by a wrinkled surface such as that of a fine cigarette paper and a rim of fine scale. The condition is most often asymptomatic, but at times the rash may be very pruritic.

Pityriasis rosea must be distinguished from disorders such as secondary syphilis, tinea corporis, seborrheic dermatitis, acute psoriasis, and tinea versicolor. All patients should receive a serologic test for syphilis.

TREATMENT AND PROGNOSIS

Most patients with pityriasis rosea require no treatment. Exposure to sun or ultraviolet radiation (UVB) frequently relieves severe itching, and emollients or antihistamines are sometimes beneficial for symptomatic relief. Ordinarily, topical steroids do not help. Lesions usually heal in 8–12 weeks, and the resulting slight changes in pigmentation are only temporary.

Aphthous Stomatitis

Recurrent, painful, mucosal erosions of the oropharynx characterize aphthous stomatitis, also known as canker sores. Although trauma, food and drug allergies, and physical and emotional stress have been implicated in the pathogenesis, cause has not been definitely established. Herpes simplex virus is not found in the aphthae; α-hemolytic streptococci, however, are common and may, through immunologic mechanisms, have an etiologic role. One or more aphthae may be seen. They appear as small, shallow, sharply defined erosions covered with a gray membrane and surrounded by an erythematous halo. Extremely large lesions are rare, and only occasionally are aphthae extremely numerous. Tingling or burning may precede the lesion by 24 hours, and during the first 2–3 days they are so painful that they may interfere with eating and speaking.

DIAGNOSIS

The differential diagnosis of aphthous stomatitis includes acute (primary) herpes simplex gingivostomatitis, Vincent's angina, traumatic ulcers, and herpangina. The erosions of Behçet's syndrome and of aphthous stomatitis may be identical; indeed, the two conditions may represent the same entity.

TREATMENT AND PROGNOSIS

Treatment of aphthous stomatitis should be aimed at controlling the pain and minimizing the duration of the lesions. A topical anesthetic such as dyclonine hydrochloride (Dyclone) or a solution of 2% lidocaine (Xylocaine Viscous) usually numbs the ulcers. Streptococci in the mouth can at times be suppressed with an antibiotic. For example, compresses moistened with a tetracycline solution (250 mg tetracycline dissolved in 30 ml water) are often effective if applied to the affected area for 10 minutes four times a day. A topical steroid such as triamcinolone acetonide (Kenalog in Orabase) or fluocinonide (Lidex ointment) is sometimes useful. It is used when the lesions first appear. Topical therapy should always be tried before systemic steroids are given, although systemic treatment is occasionally justified for a brief period when ulcers are debilitating. Left untreated, lesions usually heal in approximately 10 days.

NODULES

Erythema Nodosum

Erythema nodosum is a hypersensitivity reaction characterized by tender, red nodules usually seen on the legs (Plate 9). Since it is an immune complex disease, pathologically, a lobular panniculitis occurs. Although it generally affects young women, the disorder may occur in males and females of any age. It is associated with several conditions, but in the United States the most common cause is a prior streptococcal infection. Drugs, particularly sulfonamides and birth control pills, and sarcoidosis are also associated with this reaction pattern.

A single or many lesions may form, but ulcerations are never seen. Bright red, oval or round, slightly raised nodules are several centimeters in diameter and have indistinct borders.

As the redness fades, the lesions become blue and then yellowish-green. They may be distributed unilaterally or bilaterally. Although they are most common on the pretibial surfaces, other sites such as sides, arms, face, or neck may be involved. The lesions are extremely tender and are often accompanied by ankle edema.

DIAGNOSIS

The diagnostic workup must be directed toward identifying the etiology and therefore requires a detailed history of the present illness. In cases with no known predisposing factor, fever, malaise, and arthralgia that last 7–15 days may preceed the development of the nodose lesions. Diagnostic studies should include a complete blood count, a determination of sedementation rate, urinalysis, chest film, antistreptolysin O titer, and throat culture. Deep fungal and tuberculosis skin tests should also be considered. Trauma and other types of panniculitis may result in pretibial nodose lesions similar to those of erythema nodosum.

TREATMENT AND PROGNOSIS

Essential to the treatment of patients with erythema nodosum is the removal or treatment of the causative factor, be it drug, infection, or an underlying disease. Rest with elevation alleviates pain and edema, and aspirin often is useful to alleviate both pain and inflammation. In most cases, pain and swelling decrease as lesions resolve within 2 weeks once the underlying cause has been treated. In refractory cases, however, potassium iodide or prednisone may be prescribed. The appropriate dosage is 4 drops of saturated solution of potassium iodide (SSKI) four times a day until the lesions have cleared. Then the dosage should be decreased gradually over 3 weeks. If other therapies fail and infectious etiologies are excluded, a short course of prednisone orally can be considered as therapy for patients with severe cases.

INFESTATIONS AND BITES

Scabies and Pediculosis

The most common cutaneous infestations are scabies and pediculosis. *Scabies* is an infestation by the mite *Sarcoptes scabiei* and is usually acquired through close personal contact. Scabies may be transmitted by clothing, linen, or towels. Severe pruritus, most pronounced in the evening, is its hallmark. The diagnosis is suggested by the location and character of the lesions: papules, papulovessicles, and burrows form in the interdigital webs of the hand or on the wrists, axillae, nipples, umbilicus, lower abdomen, genitalia, or gluteal cleft. Impetigo as a secondary bacterial infection is common.

Pediculosis is an infestation by either of two species of blood-sucking lice. These obligate parasites, similar in appearance but with different feeding habits, inhabit the patient's scalp or another hairy area of the body. The head louse is transmitted by shared clothing and brushes, the body louse by bedding or clothing, and the pubic louse by direct contact with an infested person or by shared clothing, bedding, or towels.

DIAGNOSIS

Extreme pruritis is the primary presenting feature of pediculosis. In the scalp, nits are seen most easily on hairs of the occiput and above the ears; adult lice, however, are often difficult to find. Lymphadenitis and secondary impetigo, as well as excoriations, are common complications.

Pediculosis corporis is characterized by linear scratch marks, eczematous changes, and persistent erythematous papules. These body lice are found in the seams of clothing and are only rarely seen on the skin. With pediculosis pubis, on the other hand, nits are present in the hair of the pubic and thigh areas, and adult organisms are less difficult to find. Body, axillary, eyelash, or beard hair may be infected with pubic lice.

A diagnosis of scalp lice should be considered if pruritis of the scalp cannot be explained; similarly, unexplained pubic itching may be a result of pubic lice. In either case, a careful examination for nits should be made. Body lice bites are difficult to distinguish from bites of other insects, including bed bugs. Pediculosis is most common in communal environments when housekeeping standards are less than scrupulous.

TREATMENT AND PROGNOSIS

For both pediculosis and scabies, the treatment of choice is topical gamma-benzine hexachloride (GBH, Gamene or Kwell) which is a 1% concentration of the pesticide, lindane. A shampoo is available for treating pediculosis capitis and a cream or lotion for scabies or any other form of pediculosis. Topical GBH also repels tics and other arthropods and kills chiggers. Because as much as 10% of the drug may be absorbed through the skin if administered topically, an alternative or a limited treatment regimen should be considered for infants, young children, and pregnant women. An oral antihistamine is often useful for relieving pruritus. Clearing of scabitic and pediculosis infections ultimately depends on eliminating the parasite from all family members, close friends, and sexual contacts, as well as from clothing, sheets, and towels that may serve as reservoirs for reinfestation.

Pediculosis capitis or pubis should be treated with 30 ml of shampoo lathered and left on for 5 minutes; dead nits should be removed with a fine-toothed comb. This procedure can be repeated if necessary 4 days later. Lice on clothing should be killed by boiling and ironing, by dry cleaning, or by applying dry heat. Pediculosis pubis responds to GBH cream or lotion that is left on for 12–24 hours. Scabies also can be treated with GBH cream or lotion applied to the entire body from the neck down with particular attention to the interdigital webs and to the axillary and inguinal areas. Again, the medication should remain on for 12–24 hours, and the treatment should be repeated 4–7 days later. Postscabies pruritus, an allergic sensitization to the organism, often continues for weeks. It is treated most effectively with a topical or, occasionally if the case is very severe, a systemic corticosteroid.

Tick Bites

Ticks are large mites that live by sucking blood from mammals, birds, and reptiles. They are found in trees, grass, and bushes and on animals. After attaching itself to human skin, a female tick feeds for 7–14 days and then drops off. Some ticks are capable of transmitting rickettsial diseases such as Rocky Mountain spotted fever or viral encephalitis.

DIAGNOSIS

The bites are painless and often are discovered only when itching develops or when an engorged tick, which may be as large as a pea, is found on the body. A local urticaria or necrosis may occur at the site of a bite.

TREATMENT AND PROGNOSIS

A tick should be removed without being crushed. The easiest method is to grasp it near its mouth with forceps and lift it gently upward and forward. A needle or other sharp pointed object can be inserted between the tick and the skin to help pry it out. Touching a tick with a hot object (a match head that has just been extinguished or a hot nail) or applying a few drops of a solvent (chloroform, gasoline) induces it to loosen its grip. A patient should be followed for the development of any systemic illness and should be instructed to inform the physician of the history of recent tick bites if an illness develops within 3 weeks.

SUGGESTED READINGS

Braverman I: *Skin Signs of Systemic Disease*. Philadelphia, WB Saunders Co, 1981, p 965.

Chanda JJ, Callen JP: Erythema multiforme and the Stevens-Johnson syndrome. *South Med J* 1978; 71:566–570.

Fitzpatrick TB, Eisen AZ, Wolff K, Freedberg IM, Austen KF (eds): *Dermatology in General Medicine,* ed 2. New York, McGraw-Hill Book Co, 1979, p 1884.

Hirsch MS, Swartz MN: Drug therapy: Antiviral agents (first of two parts). *N Engl J Med* 1980; 302:903–907.

Mathews KP: Management of urticaria and angioedema. *J Allergy Clin Immunol* 1980; 66:347–357.

Musher DM, McKenzie SO: Infections due to staphylococcus aureus. *Medicine (Baltimore)* 1977; 56:383–409.

Neefe LI, Tuazon CU, Cardella TA, et al: Case report. Staphylococcal scalded skin syndrome in adults: case report and review of the literature. *Am J Med Sci* 1979; 277:99–110.

Peter G, Smith AL: Group A streptococcal infections of the skin and pharynx (first of two parts). *N Engl J Med* 1977; 297:311–317.

Rogers RS: Recurrent aphthous stomatitis: clinical characteristics and evidence for an immunopathogenesis. *J Invest Dermatol* 1977; 69:499–509.

VanArsdel PP Jr: Drug allergy, an update. *Med Clin North Am* 1981; 65:1089–1103.

30
ACUTE NEUROLOGIC DISORDERS

Dennis M.D. Landis

A bewildering variety of pathologic processes can cause a catastrophic change in the capacity of the nervous system to perform its usual functions. In this chapter we will discuss disorders that affect the nervous system directly. Our emphasis is on the recognition and initial management of the problem in the emergency room. A thorough assessment of many neurologic disorders often requires careful physical examination. A detailed discussion of the maneuvers of a neurologic examination together with a brief description of the significance of some of the physical findings has been presented in Chapter 10.

SEIZURES

About 0.5–2% of the population of the United States experiences repeated seizures, and a greater percentage of people have a seizure at least once in their lives. A seizure may be such an obvious and sometimes frightening departure from good health that patients are often taken to the emergency room in the throes of a seizure or shortly thereafter. The seizure itself is rarely damaging, but it can be a manifestation of a threatening underlying disorder such as metabolic derangement, intracranial infection, drug withdrawal, drug intoxication, or hypertensive encephalopathy.

Diagnosis

There are several different types of seizures that vary in their manifestations and in the disorders associated with them. In general, a *seizure* represents the repetitive firing of neurons, spreading contiguously and by fiber pathways. The clinial manifestations of the seizure reflect the type of neurons involved: repetitive firing of neurons in the motor cortex gives rise to uncontrollable movement in the contralateral limbs, whereas abnormal activity restricted to a small neuronal population in the medial temporal lobe may simply result in an "absence" spell. Clinically, we usually distinguish generalized and focal seizures. In a *generalized seizure*, abnormal electrical activity spreads over both cerebral hemispheres and is attended by loss of consciousness. A generalized *grand mal* seizure usually begins with abrupt loss of consciousness and stiffening of the body and is followed by tonic–clonic movements of body and limbs. Commonly there is loss of sphincteric control and occasionally biting of the tongue. About one-half of patients with recurrent epilepsy experience generalized seizures with major motor manifestations. By contrast, a generalized *petit mal* seizure usually causes an abrupt loss (or suspension) of consciousness and minimal motor movement. These spells are most common in children and adolescents and have a characteristic electroencephalogram (EEG) pattern. They are usually not associated with underlying metabolic or structural disease.

Focal seizures are varied in their manifestations and appear to reflect abnormal electrical activity that begins in one region and may then spread. A focal motor seizure, for example, may cause rhythmic, clonic movement of one group of muscles in the body. Focal motor seizure activity can spread to nearby muscle groups and can involve all of the muscles on one side of the body. This spread is often described as a "Jacksonian march." If the region of abnormal electrical activity is restricted to the parietal cortex, the patient may experience odd sensations in a portion of the body. These, too, can seem to spread if the neuronal activity spreads. A focal seizure in the occipital cortex may be manifest as a sensation of light, darkness, or other visual disturbance. In focal psychomotor seizures, the abnormal neuronal firing is confined to the temporal lobe, but the manifestations are highly variable. Commonly there is an aura preceding the seizure that consists of an olfactory or visceral hallucination. During the seizure the patient may appear to be awake, though he or she is out of touch, and can walk or perform complicated movements. The seizure may last from seconds to hours.

Management

It is presently uncertain whether the abnormal neuronal activity that causes a single generalized seizure can directly cause brain damage. There is therefore little reason to attempt to interrupt the course of a single generalized seizure. Initial management should instead be focused on supportive measures and diagnostic evaluation. On the other hand, generalized seizures that recur before the patient recovers consciousness—status epilepticus—require immediate therapeutic maneuvers.

GENERAL SUPPORTIVE MEASURES AND DIAGNOSTIC TESTS

It may be startling and even frightening to see a patient writhing unconsciously in the throes of a grand mal generalized motor seizure, but the seizure itself is rarely threatening. The seizure almost always will stop within 1–3 minutes of its onset, and then the patient may manifest postictal stupor or agitation. The initial responses to patients who are having seizures are to protect them from slamming into objects and to have them maintain lateral decubitus or prone position to prevent aspiration. In the postictal interval, position a bite block (never attempt to force a bite block into position during a seizure—you are more likely to knock out teeth than to prevent tongue biting).

The patient should remain in lateral decubitus or prone position in a bed with padded and raised bedrails and body restraints to prevent a fall from the bed. Blood should be drawn for determinations of glucose, sodium, potassium, calcium, and blood urea nitrogen (BUN). Twenty-five grams glucose must be given intravenously immediately (add 50 mg thiamine intravenously as soon as possible). If the cause of the seizure is not immediately obvious, obtain an electrocardiogram (ECG) and arterial blood gases, x-ray the neck and skull, and establish intravenous access that will persist despite further seizure activity.

It is not necessary to institute intravenous anticonvulsant therapy empirically after a single convulsion unless the patient is at special risk because of a recent myocardial infarction or respiratory failure (generalized motor seizures often result in hypoxemia and sometimes in a combination of metabolic and respiratory acidosis) or an unhealed wound. If seizure activity occurs again before the patient recovers consciousness, however, proceed with therapy for status epilepticus.

THERAPY FOR STATUS EPILEPTICUS

A patient who remains unconscious and who suffers repeated generalized motor seizures is at risk for aspiration, trauma, hypoxemia, hyperpyrexia, and sometimes hyperkalemia. The emergency room physician should first protect the patient against the hazards posed by unconsciousness and motor activity, as described above, and then proceed to establish rapidly effective levels of anticonvulsants. Intravenous access should be established so that it will not be shaken loose by seizure activity. A 12-inch large-bore plastic catheter placed in the antecubital fossa is fairly reliable and avoids the hazards of longer central venous pressure (CVP) lines. An alternative site is the cephalic vein higher on the upper part of the arm. Normal saline is the initial infusion, but the rate must be less than 100 ml/hr until the possibility of concomitant cerebral edema has been eliminated.

If it is absolutely necessary to stop a seizure, intravenous diazepam is the most rapidly effective anticonvulsant. This is a hazardous approach and should be reserved for patients who require intubation or who are already manifesting hyperthermia, acidosis, or hyperkalemia from seizure activity. The principal hazard of intravenous diazepam is respiratory arrest, especially in elderly patients or in people using barbiturates. Respiratory arrest can occur within seconds of drug administration or up to 30 minutes thereafter; the patient must be watched continuously and preparation for intubation should be made. Diazepam should be infused at a rate of 2 mg/min until the seizure stops, or up to a maximum dose of 20 mg.

The present drug of choice for patients with status epilepticus is phenytoin given intravenously. Even if one elects to use diazepam to abort a seizure, intravenous phenytoin should be started concomitantly. There are two approaches to administration. Preferably, undiluted phenytoin should be injected into a fairly rapid (10–25 ml/min) normal saline infusion as close as possible to the vein. The rate of infusion is no faster than 50 mg/min, and the dose is 10–15 mg/kg, not to exceed 1,000 mg in the first hour. A less satisfactory technique is to dilute the total dose in 100 ml of normal saline and to infuse by a volume-control set. This frequently causes problems, though, since the propylene glycol buffer in the phenytoin may be diluted beyond effectiveness, and the drug may precipitate in the line. Phenytoin directly suppresses cardiac automaticity and may increase atrioventricular (AV) block; in patients with cardiac conduction system disease or in the elderly it can cause bradycardia and asystole. Continuous cardiac monitoring is thus indicated during rapid, large intravenous infusions. Cardiac toxicity is usually apparent within 5 minutes but is rapidly reversible, and an infusion may be resumed at a slower rate after bradycardia clears. The onset of anticonvulsant activity may require 15–30 minutes. If seizures continue 30 minutes after the total phenytoin dose has been given, an additional anticonvulsant is probably required.

If the patient is allergic to phenytoin or if seizures continue 30 minutes after the completion of the phenytoin infusion, one can turn to an infusion of phenobarbital or diazepam. Phenobarbital is safer but slower in its onset of efficacy. If the patient has already received diazepam, that drug should be used at this point since phenobarbital and diazepam should not be given to the same patient because they mutually potentiate respiratory depression. A reasonable dosage schedule for a patient having recurrent seizure activity, but is not yet acidotic or hyperthermic, is to infuse intravenously 150 mg phenobarbital at 50 mg/min and to repeat the dose at 20-minute intervals. Do not exceed 450 mg in 2 hours, 600 mg in 4 hours, or a total dose of 20 mg/kg. When phenobarbital is being used as the primary drug or when the patient is becoming systemically ill from the uncontrolled seizure activity, the rate of infusion can be increased to 50 mg/min and maintained until the seizure stops or a maximum dose of 20 mg/kg is reached. If diazepam is used instead of phenobarbital, the dosage of diazepam is 5–8 mg/hr by continuous infusion. Phenytoin, phenobarbital, and diazepam all may cause systemic hypotension, so blood pressure must be checked frequently.

Continuous infusion of a combination of phenytoin and phenobarbital or phenytoin and diazepam is nearly always effective in arresting status epilepticus. Persistence of focal seizure activity is not an indication for further therapy if the patient recovers consciousness. On the other hand, diminution of the motor manifestations of the seizure in the context of vigorous intravenous anticonvulsant therapy does not mean that the abnormal electrical activity in the brain has ceased. One should look for recovery of consciousness as the best clinical indication that drug therapy has been effective. Cessation of motor activity is a less reliable indicator of success. For example, if the seizures had been caused by hypoglycemia or hypoxia, these insults would eventually damage the brain sufficiently so that the various fiber paths would be unable to conduct the abnormal neuronal firing. The abnormal electrical activity might therefore continue but as the spinal cord became progressively unable to direct muscular movement, tonic–clonic convulsions might give way to barely evident eye twitching. There is evidence that persistent abnormal neuronal firing, preventing recovery of awareness but not necessarily causing motor manifestations, is itself dangerous for the brain, even in the absence of systemic metabolic derangement. If possible, obtain an EEG if a patient remains obtunded despite cessation of motor activity to determine whether cortical seizure activity persists. If it does, continue to add anticonvulsant drugs. On the other hand, it is not yet clear that continued cortical seizure activity in the absence of motor activity is sufficient indication for general anesthesia.

If seizure activity is judged to persist despite therapy with phenytoin and phenobarbital or phenytoin and diazepam, paraldehyde is the next drug to be added. The dosage must be arrived at empirically, using respiratory depression as the toxic endpoint, particularly because paraldehyde is usually employed as a final resort in addition to several other drugs. If available, a 1% solution in D_5W can be infused at about 500 ml/hr (or 5 ml paraldehyde per hour). Such a large volume of hypotonic fluid, however, could exacerbate preexisting cerebral edema, and so one must be sure that cerebral edema is not a complicating factor in the patient's presentation. An infusion may be continued to a total dose of 100 ml of paraldehyde, though that would almost never be required. Paraldehyde may also be administered by nasogastric tube (flush the tubing immediately or the paraldehyde may dissolve it) or by rectum, although that route runs the risk of unreliable absorption.

If generalized motor seizures persist despite the therapy outlined above, general anesthesia is the last resort. In general, it takes about 2 hours from the onset of therapy to the institution of paraldehyde. If seizures have become intermittent, one can wait another 2 hours to assess whether abnormal electrical activity has been blocked. If the patient develops metabolic acidosis, hyperthermia, or hyperkalemia to a threatening degree, general anesthesia should be instituted. If the combination of anticonvulsant medications has caused respiratory insufficiency, consider general anesthesia to simplify management as effective levels of anticonvulsants are established.

ETIOLOGIC CONSIDERATIONS IN THE EMERGENCY ROOM

The major task in the emergency room is to determine the probable etiology of the seizure. This is especially true when the seizure is the first one experienced by the patient. Particular attention should be paid to the following etiologies:

- Hypoglycemia
- Hyponatremia
- Hypocalcemia
- Hypoxia
- Hypertensive encephalopathy
- Hyperthermia
- Drug intoxication or withdrawal, especially alcohol
- Meningitis or other intracranial infections
- Intracranial neoplasm
- Encephalitis, especially herpes simplex
- Cortical vein or sinus thrombosis

If the patient is known to have a seizure disorder, anticonvulsant levels should be checked.

It should be noted that generalized petit mal seizures in children or adolescents are rarely associated with significant underlying disease. The diagnosis of seizure in the context of fever is one of exclusion, even in typical clinical settings. It is important to consider the etiologies listed above and to proceed with a lumbar puncture.

Unfortunately, it is rarely possible to determine the nature of the underlying lesion from the clinical manifestations of the seizure. A focal seizure and the characteristics of an aura often are useful indications for deciding where the trouble began, but they are less useful in assessing the cause. Seizures in the context of severe hypoglycemia or hyponatremia tend to be generalized. The possibility of meningitis must be considered in every case of new onset of seizures. This, of course, requires lumbar puncture, which in turn requires that efforts be made to exclude the presence of an intracranial mass. Many seizures in alcoholic patients will be withdrawal seizures (see below), but alcoholics are also especially vulnerable to infection, hyponatremia, and hypoglycemia, and therefore the diagnosis of "rum fits" should be one of exclusion.

EXCEPTIONAL TYPES OF SEIZURES

Rum fits are seizures that affect alcoholics within the first 48 hours of abstinence from alcohol. They are virtually always self-limited. The motor manifestations of the seizure usually can be interrupted by an infusion of diazepam, but this intervention should be reserved for the exceptional instances in which one wishes to proceed with intubation or to protect the patient's heart or a wound. Phenytoin is ineffective in preventing alcohol withdrawal seizures, and probably even therapeutic levels of phenytoin will not prevent the second or third of a flurry of seizures. Alcohol withdrawal seizures occurring 2–4 days after the cessation of alcohol intake, often in the context of full-blown delirium tremens, tend to be brief and of little danger in themselves. Therapy should be directed toward the withdrawal syndrome, as described in Chapter 43, though one should also consider the possibility of intracranial infection.

Never dismiss seizures in an alcoholic as the sequelae of alcohol abstinence, especially when the exact history of recent alcohol intake is uncertain. Many alcoholics have chronic seizure disorders, and others are vulnerable to head trauma, meningitis, subdural empyemas, and so forth. If the patient's history is uncertain and one anticipates delirium tremens, a prudent approach is to use paraldehyde early in the management of the alcohol withdrawal syndrome.

Patients with *barbiturate withdrawal* seizures respond well to phenobarbital. The dose is tailored to the requirements of the withdrawal syndrome.

Epilepsia partialis continua is a syndrome of incessant focal motor seizures, usually caused by major cerebral cortical trauma, infection, or infarction. The seizure activity is by definition resistant to anticonvulsant therapy and can continue for weeks. The physician should be careful not to confuse this focal motor seizure with status epilepticus—the latter is associated with loss of consciousness and is usually generalized. Drug therapy using intravenous phenytoin and intravenous phenobarbital should be prompt. These drugs may be followed with oral valproic acid or carbamazepine. Failure of complete control is the rule, even with time.

Psychomotor and petit mal seizure activities may become essentially continuous. These may present a perplexing problem for diagnosis, but they rarely constitute an emergency. Recurrent temporal lobe (psychomotor) seizures can cause an altered state of awareness or automatic, repetitive oral movements. The patient may be able to walk or even carry on a conversation, but memory is usually compromised for the interval of the seizure and the patient appears to be out of touch even to the casual observer. The condition is easily mistaken for a psychiatric disorder, and the diagnosis may require a careful history or a very high index of suspicion. The new onset of psychomotor seizures requires consideration of the several metabolic and structural etiologies listed above. Petit mal status similarly can cause an isolated clouding of the sensorium with little or no motor behavior, and repetitive absence spells may persist for weeks. These spells usually do not require emergency therapy, and the diagnosis is readily made with an EEG.

CEREBROVASCULAR DISEASE

The abrupt onset of aphasia, hemiplegia, or other neurologic deficit caused by a vascular event may be the most tragic event of a lifetime, but it represents an emergency only when obtundation can be expected or when a specific therapeutic modality is available. At the present time, cerebellar hemorrhage, some instances of carotid artery occlusion, and certain types of dissecting aortic aneurysms can be treated surgically and therefore must be recognized in the emergency room. Certain forms of occlusive disease in the basilar and carotid arteries and some forms of embolic disease may benefit from immediate anticoagulation, and therefore these also must be differentiated from other causes of stroke. Hemispheric infarction, basilar artery occlusion, some instances of subarachnoid hemorrhage, and all hypertensive parenchymal hemorrhages can lead to coma and must be treated expectantly.

The arterial lesions causing central nervous system damage fall into four major patterns: (1) occlusion by embolic material; (2) in situ thrombosis of a large vessel, usually at the site of atherosclerotic stenosis; (3) rupture and leakage, causing parenchymal hemorrhage or, in the case of ruptured aneurysms, subarachnoid hemorrhage often accompanied by a parenchymal hematoma; and (4) occlusion of an extracranial vessel by a dissecting aortic aneurysm. It can be very difficult to distinguish between the several etiologic possibilities, but the effort is justified by the importance of recognizing treatable neurologic catastrophe and also because we sometimes stumble across evidence of treatable disease elsewhere such as subacute or acute bacterial endocarditis. The different vascular pathologies tend to occur in recognizable clinical constellations, and sometimes the diagnosis can be made by attending to the mode of onset, evolution of the deficit, general clinical context, and specific class of deficit.

Although patterns exist there are no hard and fast rules, and it is important to remember that in the following discussion we suggest only the outlines of diagnostic considerations. When specific clinical features are present, they are most useful in arriving at a diagnosis.

Diagnosis

In the emergency room the differential diagnosis of stroke is facilitated by considering four issues: (1) the mode of onset, (2) the progression of the deficit, (3) the clinical context, and (4) the character of the deficit.

The *mode of onset* is an important clue in differential diagnosis. The abrupt, painless onset of a deficit that evolves to a stable loss of function in less than 15 minutes suggests embolic disease. If the deficit has been heralded by one or more transient spells of similar dysfunction, we should first consider the possibility of large vessel atherosclerotic disease, either causing repeated embolization or occlusion at the site of atherosclerotic stenosis. Rapidly worsening, unfamiliar, severe headache associated with clouding of the sensorium and frequently a focal neurologic deficit is the typical clinical presentation of subarachnoid hemorrhage from a ruptured berry aneurysm. Severe headache associated with a more obvious focal deficit in an hypertensive person should suggest hypertensive parenchymal hemorrhage.

The *manner in which the neurologic deficit progresses* over time offers additional information. If the deficit seems not to be changing after an hour, the etiology is probably embolism or completed large vessel occlusion. Remember that all clinically significant ischemic lesions will worsen to a variable degree over the ensuing 72 hours as focal cerebral edema develops. A focal neurologic deficit that waxes and wanes in its severity over the first few hours suggests incomplete or progressing occlusion of a large vessel. It is extremely important that one be alert for this clinical presentation because emergency anticoagulation may prevent a major occlusion in the carotid or basilar artery. If a patient presents with a fairly stable neurologic deficit and then develops a new, distinct deficit,

one should consider two etiologic mechanisms: the first is repeated embolism from an extracranial source, in which case the new deficit is not necessarily in the same arterial territory as the original deficit. The second is progressing occlusion in a carotid or basilar artery, in which case the thrombus is occluding more and more branches or giving rise to repeated emboli in the same arterial territory. In both cases, anticoagulation is a potential therapeutic intervention. A severe neurologic deficit, usually developing in association with headache, that steadily worsens over hours is the hallmark of hypertensive parenchymal hemorrhage. The probable cause of the worsening is severe, local cerebral edema and continuing spread of the extravasated blood. The actual leak of blood from the vessel is thought to stop quite early unless the patient is wildly hypertensive or has been given an anticoagulant.

Most vascular disorders have a characteristic *clinical context*. Embolic disease is often associated with intermittent or constant atrial tachyarrhythmia, especially in the presence of mitral stenosis. Other disorders associated with embolic disease include subacute bacterial endocarditis, recent (less than 6 months) myocardial infarction, left atrial myxoma, marantic endocarditis, and paradoxical embolism through a patent foramen ovale in the presence of pulmonary emboli. Usually subarachnoid hemorrhage results from the rupture of a berry aneurysm in the circle of Willis; these aneurysms are more common in patients who have polycystic renal or polycystic hepatic disease.

Subarachnoid hemorrhage infrequently is caused by the rupture of a mycotic aneurysm (in the setting of subacute bacterial endocarditis or other intermittent systemic bacteremia) or by rupture of an arteriovenous malformation.

Intraparenchymal hemorrhage is virtually always associated with clinically significant arterial hypertension and is rare in people younger than 55 years. Unfortunately, there are few clinical settings that reliably point toward carotid occlusive disease except that the patients are usually over 60 years old and have evidence of atherosclerotic disease elsewhere.

The *character of the neurologic deficit* sometimes is a key to the pathogenesis. The dysfunction caused by occlusive (embolic or thrombotic) vascular disease reflects the brain territory supplied by the vessel, the presence or absence of other lesions, the availability of collateral blood supply, the presence or absence of associated cerebral edema, and so on. The list of neurologic syndromes caused by occlusive vascular disease is too long to be reviewed here, but a few generalizations may be useful. Infarction in the territory of the anterior, middle, or posterior cerebral artery is nearly always caused by emboli to the vessel or its branches. However, carotid occlusion can mimic anterior or middle cerebral artery disease, producing a spectrum of deficits ranging from minimal paresis to virtually complete hemispheric destruction. A history of transient neurologic deficits before the onset of the stroke should always be sought in patients in whom dysfunction is referable to the anterior or middle cerebral arterial territories since such transient ischemic events may indicate underlying carotid disease. The deficits caused by hypertensive parenchymal hemorrhage are distinctive and are discussed below.

Initial Management and Evaluation

CEREBRAL EMBOLISM

Emboli in cerebral vessels commonly lodge in the major branches of the middle, anterior, and posterior cerebral arteries. They abruptly cause the onset of a neurologic deficit that reflects the loss of function in the portion of the brain deprived of its blood supply. There is probably nothing available in the therapeutic armamentarium that directly alters the extent of injury that the embolus causes. The emergency room physician has to initiate the search for the source of the emboli and should correct any general medical disorder (hypotension, dehydration, etc.), but there is little to be done about the stroke itself. The essential reason for haste in determining the source of the embolus is to avoid a second or third insult to brain vasculature. Appropriate tests should be obtained to assess the likelihood of the following conditions:

1. Recent myocardial infarction
2. Acute or subacute bacterial endocarditis
3. Hypercoagulation (thrombocytosis, leukemoid reaction, etc.)
4. Intermittent or persistent supraventricular tachyarrhythmia (especially atrial fibrillation)
5. Valvular heart disease or cardiac prosthetic valve

CEREBRAL THROMBOSIS

Thrombotic occlusion of the carotid or basilar arteries is a common complication of atherosclerotic disease. Over many years, the lumen of the vessel becomes increasingly narrowed as atherosclerotic material accumulates in the vessel walls. Stroke syndromes, however, usually develop because of thrombosis at the site of the vessel stenosis. The clinical manifestations of thrombotic occlusion of the carotid artery are extremely varied: Many are entirely asymptomatic (presumably collateral circulation supports the deprived brain region), whereas carotid occlusion in some people may result in ischemic infarction of the ipsilateral hemisphere. The principal task in the emergency room is to decide whether or not to anticoagulate

the patient acutely. The rationale for such therapy is that we may avoid progressive accumulation of thrombus and total block of the vessel.

There are really only two sets of clues to the presence of thrombotic disease available in the emergency room. One should seek a history of waxing and waning, or stepwise progression, in the evolution of the neurologic deficit. Such a stuttering onset presumably reflects repeated embolization from a forming thrombus or intermittent obstruction of the vessel by thrombus at a stenotic region. In such cases, all of the neurologic deficits should be referable to one or another carotid artery territory or to the region irrigated by the basilar artery. The second major clue is a history of one or more transient ischemic attacks in the same brain region before the presenting episode. Such transient neurologic deficits may result from emboli arising at the thrombus in the stenotic or ulcerated major vessel.

If carotid thrombotic disease is suspected, listen for a bruit in the vessel. Interpretation of this particular aspect of the physical examination is uncertain, however. The absence of a bruit could simply indicate that the vessel is now occluded, or that stenosis is not sufficiently bad to cause a bruit. The apparent presence of a bruit may in fact reflect a bruit in a stenotic external carotid vessel or radiation from a cardiac murmur. Finally, a vessel may have a bruit yet not be involved in the pathogenesis of the stroke syndrome in that patient.

If the onset and progression of the neurologic disorder suggest thrombotic occlusive vascular disease, consider immediate anticoagulation with intravenous heparin while the patient is still in the emergency ward. If the diagnosis is correct, such therapy may or may not be helpful. However, if the diagnosis is wrong, anticoagulation could result in disaster. Before anticoagulation is initiated, it is necessary to exclude the possibility that one of the following conditions exists:

1. Hypertensive intraparenchymal hemorrhage
2. Subarachnoid hemorrhage from an aneurysm
3. Acute or chronic subdural hematoma
4. Acute epidural hematoma
5. Dissecting aortic aneurysm

All of these disorders are easily detected by cranial computed tomography (CT) scanning, and if available, that test should be obtained within 4 hours of the patient's arrival in the emergency room. Also obtain the several laboratory determinations discussed under the heading Cerebral Embolism.

In some major medical centers, vascular surgeons or neurosurgeons may be available to undertake emergency carotid endarterectomy in the setting of progressing stroke. The efficacy of this approach is still uncertain, but diagnosis in the emergency room is the key to the prompt initiation of such therapy.

TRANSIENT ISCHEMIC ATTACKS

We often encounter patients who have suffered the sudden onset of a definite neurologic deficit but who have regained normal neurologic function by the time they have arrived in the emergency room. Often these transient deficits mimic in detail a stroke syndrome such as aphasia, hemiplegia, or hemiparesthesias. The formal definition of a *transient ischemic attack* is a neurologic deficit referable to ischemia that disappears without residue in less than 24 hours. In practice, however, most episodes last less than 15 minutes. The importance of recognizing transient ischemic attacks in the emergency room derives from two possible etiologies: First, repeated embolism from a thrombus in an atherosclerotic carotid or basilar artery can give rise to several minor, transient spells of dysfunction before the major episode caused by occlusion of the atherosclerotic vessel. Second, an extracranial source of emboli may give rise to several minor emboli, reflected in transient cerebral dysfunction, before a major embolus breaks loose. Doubtless, these clinical situations account for the common observation that major strokes may be preceded by one or many transient ischemic attacks. It is also true, however, that many patients experience transient ischemic attacks, but even exhaustive inquiry fails to define the presence of atherosclerotic occlusive disease or a source of emboli. Perhaps such patients suffer from intermittent, incomplete "spasm" in cerebral vasculature. The issue is not yet settled.

The evaluation in the emergency room of a patient presenting with one or more transient ischemic attacks is straightforward. Obtain the tests listed above to evaluate the possibility of cerebral embolism and cerebral thrombosis. Be aware that several other disease categories such as those listed below can cause syndromes similar to transient ischemic attacks:

1. Focal seizures
2. Chronic subdural hematoma
3. Cardiac arrhythmia
4. Severe hypoxemia or hypoglycemia
5. Arterial hypotension

INTRACEREBRAL HEMORRHAGE

Intracerebral hemorrhage is virtually always associated with long-standing arterial hypertension. The hemorrhage tends to occur in one of four brain regions, giving rise to a fairly characteristic deficit. Putamenal hemorrhage is the most common.

The patient is usually hemiparetic, and gaze is deviated conjugately toward the side of the hemorrhage (away from the paresis). Thalamic hemorrhage also causes hemiparesis, but the patient's eyes tend to be deviated downward and the pupils are small and unreactive. Presumably the deviation downward is caused by pressure of the midbrain tectum; in its mildest form it may be evident only as paresis of voluntary upward gaze or paresis of upward gaze induced by oculocephalic (doll's head) testing. The absence of the pupillary reflex to light in patients with thalamic hemorrhage is caused by interruption of visual pathway fibers converging on the tectum. Both putamenal and thalamic hemorrhages act like supratentorial masses and often progress to more extensive paralysis and brainstem dysfunction by causing transtentorial herniation. The clinical picture is thus a hypertensive patient who suffers the abrupt onset of headache and paralysis, becomes progressively obtunded, and then may die of brainstem compression.

Pontine hemorrhage, by contrast, creates its havoc without transtentorial herniation. Hemorrhage into the pons often compresses the motor nucleus of the sixth cranial nerve (abducens) and the medial longitudinal fasciculus, causing paralysis of lateral gaze. The eyes become fixed in central position and occasionally exhibit a peculiar bobbing movement. Compression of the sympathetic pathways by the hematoma causes the pupils to be tiny, but parasympathetic tracts are intact and pupillary response to light persists. Continuing expansion of the hematoma and associated edema eventually can cause bilateral decerebrate posturing, coma, and respiratory arrest. Only about 10% of intracerebral hemorrhages occur in the cerebellum, but these are potentially curable by surgery, and one must therefore be able to recognize them in patients in the emergency room. The patient usually complains of the abrupt onset of dizziness (vertigo), nausea, and occipital headache. The patient is usually unable to walk because of severe truncal ataxia. Blood dissecting into the brainstem along the middle cerebellar peduncle can cause conjugate lateral gaze deviation to the opposite side by pressing on the pontine gaze center. Less often there may be an isolated sixth cranial nerve weakness. Otherwise, extraocular movements and pupillary reaction to light are preserved. The expanding hematoma in the posterior fossa can sometimes result in catastrophic herniation of the cerebellar tonsils toward the foramen magnum, which compresses the medulla and results in respiratory arrest.

A cranial CT scan demonstrates putamenal, thalamic, pontine, and cerebellar hemorrhage with incredible precision. The test should be obtained as soon as possible. If cerebellar hemorrhage is suspected but CT scanning is not available, resort to angiography as soon as possible. The posterior fossa hematomas pose great hazard if lumbar puncture is undertaken.

Patients with intracerebral hemorrhage almost invariably have a long history of hypertension, and their systolic blood pressures are characteristically very elevated in the setting of acute hemorrhage. Steps to control this should be instituted in the emergency room since uncontrolled intracranial hypertension in the ischemic–necrotic brain will worsen cerebral edema. Patients with arterial hypertension should be treated with propranolol, alpha methyldopa, or nitroprusside if necessary. Avoid agents such as hydralazine or diazoxide, which are effective in controlling pressure but also tend to cause elevated left ventricular stroke work (dp/dt). Systemic pressure tends to decline within 4–6 hours of the onset of the hemorrhage, and we have to be wary of overtreatment.

Usually the hemorrhage itself has stopped by the time the patient arrives in the emergency room. Continued progression reflects accumulating cerebral edema and further spread of extravasated blood. Emergency therapeutic maneuvers should include intravenous dexamethasone in anticipation of cerebral edema. A sodium and fluid restriction should be initiated, again to control intracerebral pressure. If the hemorrhage has been sufficiently severe to cause coma, hyperosmotic therapy with mannitol should be instituted and hyperventilation should be considered as well, as discussed in Chapter 10. Intracerebral hemorrhage can cause hydrocephalus by compression at several points. Usually the patient has arrived in the emergency room before hydrocephalus has contributed to the clinical picture. The diagnosis is made by CT scanning or angiography; therapy for acute hydrocephalus is usually a ventricular shunt that is placed by a neurosurgeon.

SUBARACHNOID HEMORRHAGE

The rupture of an aneurysm on an intracranial vessel floods the subarachnoid space with blood under arterial pressure. If the leak is minor, the blood dilutes into the cerebrospinal fluid (CSF) and may cause nothing more troubling than a moderate headache. In worse situations, the jet of blood dissects into the brain, forming a clot and compressing local structures. Blood spurting from the ruptured aneurysm in the circle of Willis can erode upward and burst into the ventricular system, causing loss of consciousness and leading to later obstructive hydrocephalus. Even when the stream of blood is directed away from the brain, there may be a dramatic rise in intracranial pressure that leads to obtundation.

The diagnosis of subarachnoid hemorrhage is most easily made by cranial CT scanning. The next best test is lumbar puncture to look for blood in the CSF. Unfortunately, if there is a hematoma associated with the ruptured aneurysm or acute obstructive hydrocephalus, lumbar puncture may lead to tran-

stentorial herniation. If the patient is awake and does not have a focal deficit, lumbar puncture is probably safe. If the clinical situation is less clear, proceed with lumbar puncture in the setting of possible increased intracranial pressure as discussed in Chapter 10.

The initial management of subarachnoid hemorrhage is focused on control of systemic blood pressure since we want to avoid hypertension and additional rupture of the aneurysm. The pharmacologic agents of choice are propranolol, alpha methyldopa, or nitroprusside. Intravenous dexamethasone and hyperosmotic therapy can be instituted in patients who manifest severe local cerebral edema around a clot. We have to remember that subarachnoid hemorrhage also may be caused by arteriovenous malformations; inspection of skull films for calcifications and auscultation for an intracranial bruit should be routinely performed.

DISSECTING AORTIC ANEURYSMS

Dissection of the thoracic aorta can cut off carotid or vertebral circulation causing focal cerebral ischemia. This is a very uncommon cause of cerebrovascular disease. It is worth mentioning in the present context only because dissection can be recognized by its clinical presentation (sharp chest pain radiating into the back) and occasionally by observing a widened aorta on a chest x-ray film. Therapy is often unsatisfactory. If instituting anticoagulation is considered, however, be sure that dissection is not a potential etiology of the disorder.

SPINAL CORD SYNDROMES

Compression, ischemia, or an infectious process involving the spinal cord usually causes loss of sensory function and motor power below the level of the lesion and some derangement of bladder and bowel function. The duration of spinal cord compression may be an extremely important factor in determining whether irreversible cord injury will result. The abrupt onset of spinal cord compression is an emergency and we will have to make a decision about immediate myelography and laminectomy. Acute spinal cord ischemia can be caused by a dissecting aortic aneurysm, and occasionally it is the only clinical clue to that process.

Diagnosis

The following are the six major causes of acute spinal cord compression:

1. Traumatic dislocation of a vertebra
2. Vertebral body collapse
3. Hematoma—traumatic or spontaneous
4. Epidural abscess
5. Tumor
6. Ruptured intervertebral disc

In each case there may be pain radiating in a dermatomal fashion or radicular paresthesias at the level of the lesion caused by distortion of the spinal roots. All of these may cause back pain discretely localized to the involved vertebra; often percussion of the spinous process of the vertebra will cause severe local pain. Compression of the spinal cord from one side initially causes ipsilateral paresis and contralateral sensory loss below the lesion (the Brown-Séquard syndrome). Cord compression by a posteriorly located mass sufficiently severe to cause weakness will also be accompanied by evidence of posterior column sensory dysfunction.

The location of the lesion is established by examining motor power and by particular attention to mapping pain sensation by pinprick. Initially, the patient should be immobilized, and spine films should be obtained immediately. Vertebral body collapse should be readily apparent, although both abscess and tumor may cause erosion of bone and the presence of a paraspinous soft tissue density. If the nature of the lesion is not apparent from plain spine films, we have to consider myelography as the next step in the diagnosis. In general, two major hazards attend lumbar myelography in an emergency setting. First, we may inadvertently penetrate the lesion itself in the process of the lumbar puncture. Second, an abrupt decrease in CSF pressure at the site of the lumbar puncture may precipitate herniation of the cord past a block higher up in the spinal cord canal. If the lesion is likely to be in the lumbar cord, therefore, introduction of the myelography dye should be done by cisternal or C-1–C-2 puncture.

As noted earlier, obstruction of the arteries arising in the low thoracic aorta can cause focal spinal cord ischemia. Clinically, this may be manifest only as painless, symmetric or asymmetric paraplegia. In every case of low thoracic or lumbar spinal cord dysfunction, therefore, we should palpate for an abdominal aortic aneurysm and examine the peripheral pulses.

Management

The initial steps in the management of spinal cord syndromes are immobilization and obtaining spine films; myelography has to follow unless the diagnosis is firmly made by plain films. Evidence of acute cord compression in the setting of trauma is indication for emergency laminectomy; in extraordinary cases the surgeon may wish to operate even without the information provided by a myelogram. Cord compression by vertebral body collapse or by traumatic dislocation of a vertebra also requires immediate surgical care. On the other hand, cord compression by an extradural neoplasm may not require emergency surgery. Once the patient has been immobilized and preparations have been made for spine films and subsequent myelography, the help of a neurosurgeon will be required for diagnostic and therapeutic planning.

MUSCULAR WEAKNESS

Patients who do not complain of weakness in the emergency room are the exception rather than the rule, and the physician is often tempted to seek another, more useful complaint in an effort to define the presenting illness. Weakness, however, is the real complaint in two illnesses—myasthenia gravis and the Guillain-Barré syndrome—that cause a fulminating loss of motor power and that may threaten respiratory insufficiency. These often go unrecognized in early states, and the patient is returned home to face inexorably worsening weakness, possibly at a fatal pace. Several other illnesses, fortunately rare, also cause weakness and will be briefly considered. These include poliomyelitis, polymyositis, transverse myelitis, botulism, amyotrophic lateral sclerosis, and tick bite paralysis.

Diagnosis

Disorders causing diffuse, severe, rapidly worsening weakness fall into three major categories: (1) loss of spinal cord function, (2) peripheral neuropathy, (3) neuromuscular junction blockade.

Loss of spinal cord function will result in loss of voluntary movement below the lesion, usually with simultaneous loss of sensation and derangement of bladder and bowel function. The several causes of acute spinal cord dysfunction have been discussed earlier in this chapter. The possibility of spinal cord damage should be the first consideration in the initial evaluation of patients presenting with weakness.

A rapidly worsening demyelinating *peripheral neuropathy* can interrupt the conduction of action potentials from the spinal cord to skeletal muscles and thus results in weakness of voluntary movement. Practically speaking, the *Guillain-Barré syndrome* of inflammatory polyradiculitis is the only major cause of fulminant neuropathy, though in past years diphtheria would have had that dubious distinction. The Guillain-Barré syndrome probably results from an autoimmune attack on the myelin-forming cells of the spinal roots and peripheral nerves. The patient manifests a striking contrast between obvious muscular weakness and relative preservation of sensory function. The weakness is usually symmetrical and involves proximal and distal musculature. It tends to ascend from the legs and can evolve in hours or days. Sensory complaints are minimal, but we can usually elicit a history of paresthesias in the involved regions, and the weakened muscles are tender when squeezed. Autonomic dysfunction, including cardiac arrhythmias, occurs in more severe cases. Cerebrospinal fluid pressure is usually normal; the CSF protein is always elevated 48 hours after the onset of weakness (but may be normal before then), and lymphocytic pleocytosis occurs in less than 10% of patients. Often a history can be obtained of a viruslike infection 1–3 weeks before the onset of weakness, and specific inquiry and tests for hepatitis and mononucleosis should be undertaken.

The third major category of disorders causing weakness is *neuromuscular junction blockade*. The major diseases in this category are myasthenia gravis and botulism.

Myasthenia gravis is probably caused by antibodies that bind to acetylcholine receptor sites at neuromuscular junctions in skeletal muscle. As a result, the muscle is not depolarized by normal nerve stimulation and does not contract. The resulting weakness affects cranial and pharyngeal musculature before other groups, causing a bewildering array of ophthalmoplegia, ptosis, and facial, jaw, and pharyngeal paralysis. Women are affected about twice as frequently as men. Oropharyngeal weakness leading to difficulty with speech and threatening aspiration can be a presenting problem, but it is unusual for respiratory insufficiency because of compromised thoracic musculature to be an initial difficulty. Sensation is unaffected.

Myasthenia gravis causes abnormally rapid fatigue in affected muscles performing repetitive work, a phenomenon easily tested by instructing the patient to squeeze a ball repeatedly, maintain gaze upward, and the like. A more definitive test is to examine the response to an injection of a short-acting anticholinesterase. The anticholinesterase blocks enzymatic degradation of acetylcholine at the neuromuscular junction, thus permitting the acetylcholine released by the nerve terminal to depolarize the muscle over a longer interval. The drug usually employed is edrophonium chloride (Tensilon); 1 mg is injected intravenously as a test dose and 60 seconds later—in the absence of anaphylactic reaction—the remaining 9 mg are given intravenously over a 15-second period. In a positive response, which is diagnostic of myasthenia gravis, increased motor power is evident within 30 seconds and begins to dissipate 2 minutes after the injection. The assessment of improvement in ptosis,

ophthalmoplegia, or facial weakness is often highly subjective, and even experienced observers prefer to perform this test in a double-blind fashion using normal saline as a control.

Botulism results from ingestion of a toxin produced by *Clostridium botulinum* growing in improperly canned, often home-preserved, foods. The toxin blocks release of acetylcholine at the neuromuscular junction. Blurred vision because of mydriasis, diplopia, dysphagia, and weakness usually precede respiratory paralysis, but the whole gamut can be covered in less than 24 hours. Neither myasthenia gravis nor Guillain-Barré syndrome causes mydriasis. Edrophonium chloride does not improve the weakness. The diagnosis is usually confirmed by history or analysis of the ingested food, but no laboratory tests are useful after the intoxication has occurred. Polyvalent antitoxin is available and should be given promptly.

In general, the only form of weakness that requires prompt recognition and response is that which will proceed to respiratory insufficiency within hours. Several *unusual causes of fulminant weakness* are briefly described below in an effort to provide some clues to their diagnoses.

Infectious *poliomyelitis* is a viral disease that attacks motor neurons in the spinal cord, causing profound weakness and fasciculations with no sensory loss. The weakness is usually accompanied by fever, meningeal irritation, and cramping pain in the affected muscles. Characteristically, the weakness is asymmetrical. The Babinski sign is absent. Involvement of the brainstem can cause life-threatening respiratory irregularity and associated paralysis of the oropharyngeal musculature.

Transverse myelitis is caused by a poorly understood necrotizing or demyelinating process that can effectively transect the spinal cord in less than 48 hours, resulting in paralysis and sensory loss below the level of the major lesion. If the lesion occurs in cervical segments C-3–C-5 or above, fatal respiratory insufficiency can ensue. The diagnosis should be entertained in patients who have recently received radiotherapy that may have included the spinal cord in a field or in patients who are known to have multiple sclerosis. Acute spinal cord compression by trauma, disc disease, epidural abscess, or spontaneous epidural hematoma can produce a similar picture. Thallium intoxication also causes radicular back pain and myelitis and sometimes can proceed to coma. Presently the only therapeutic response to transverse myelitis is supportive care, but we must be careful that the possible cord compression etiologies have been throughly considered.

Amyotrophic lateral sclerosis is a disease of unknown etiology characterized by progressive destruction of motor neurons in the spinal cord, brainstem, and cerebral cortex. It results in weakness, increased deep tendon reflexes, fasciculations, and eventually muscle atrophy. Respiratory insufficiency may be a terminal event but occurs only after long-standing involvement elsewhere. There is no known effective treatment.

Tick bite paralysis is a result of a toxin injected by any one of several species of tick while they feed. The tick, found mainly in the Southwest, must feed for several days before symptoms develop, but then flaccid paralysis of the extremities, brainstem motor dysfunction, and direct effects on brainstem regulation of respiration can evolve over 24–48 hours. Children are the usual victims. The diagnosis and definitive therapy are accomplished by finding and removing the tick, including the mouth parts that tend to stick in the flesh.

The differential diagnosis to be considered in the case of the weakened but not dying patient can include several other diseases. Most of these will not cause rapid respiratory insufficiency, and a more leisurely pace is permissible in their recognition. They include diphtheritic polyneuropathy, acute intermittent hepatic porphyria, polymyositis, the Eaton-Lambert syndrome, periodic paralysis, and hyperthyroidism or hypothyroidism.

Management

GULLAIN-BARRÉ SYNDROME

There is presently no direct therapy for Gullain-Barré syndrome. Steroids are not of proven benefit. Plasmaphoresis is under investigation, but no clear conclusions have been reached yet. The patients must be closely watched, and frequent measurements of their vital capacities must be taken until the progression of weakness has clearly halted. Cardiac monitoring is indicated to detect supraventricular bradyarrhythmias and tachyarrhythmias. There may be an increased vulnerability to pressure or entrapment neuropathies, and so footboards must be provided along with scrupulous efforts to avoid anterior tibial nerve compression or passive extreme wrist extension.

MYASTHENIA GRAVIS

It is rarely necessary to initiate therapy of patients newly diagnosed as having myasthenia gravis in the emergency room, but in the unusual situation in which the patient is threatened by aspiration or respiratory insufficiency, 0.5–2 mg of neostigmine may be given intravenously or intramuscularly. The effect is evident within 15 minutes, and the dose may be repeated after 60 minutes but should not exceed 2 mg/hr. Oral neostigmine can be used on an initial schedule of 15 mg/3 hr. In general, the use of drugs is of secondary importance and attention should first be directed toward respiratory support, including endotracheal intubation if necessary. Remember that anticholinesterase medications will have the muscarinic side effects of excessive salivation and increased bronchial secretions that may further embarrass respiratory function; these side effects may be ameliorated by the use of atropine (0.4–1 mg IV, repeated as necessary).

Corticosteroids can cause an improvement in patients with myasthenia gravis in a few days, but the initial effect is often paradoxical worsening and steroids should be avoided until respiratory support is assured. Certain antibiotics may cause a partial neuromuscular blockade and are relatively contraindicated in myasthenic crises. These are neomycin, polymyxin B, colistin, kanamycin, gentamicin, streptomycin, and dihydrostreptomycin. Any agent causing respiratory depression is obviously to be avoided. Quinine is another drug contraindicated in severe myasthenia.

The evaluation of increasing weakness is doubly difficult in people known to have myasthenia gravis and to be receiving anticholinesterase medication because of the entity called *cholinergic crisis*. When too much anticholinesterase is given, acetylcholine accumulates at the neuromuscular junction and causes a depolarization blockade—the resulting weakness is indistinguishable from that caused by insufficient anticholinesterase medication, that is, myasthenia. Cholinergic crisis is usually (but not always) accompanied by muscarinic side effects of excess acetylcholine, including nausea, abdominal cramps, diarrhea, sweating, lacrimation, pallor, and miosis (the presence or absence of fasciculations is not a reliable differentiating feature). Severe acetylcholine excess in the context of anticholinesterase overmedication can lead to hypotension, confusion, and coma. Bradycardia is unusual, but intravenous anticholinesterase mistakenly administered during cholinergic crisis can cause cardiac arrest.

Edrophonium chloride sometimes is useful in distinguishing myasthenia from cholinergic crisis in patients with moderate weakness—myasthenic weakness improves transiently and cholinergic crisis worsens only slightly. The results are often equivocal, however, and an occasional patient will present with some muscle groups weakened by myasthenia whereas others will simultaneously be poisoned by depolarization blockade. In all patients with severe weakness and in patients with confusing pictures, the most prudent emergency responses are endotracheal intubation, vigorous pulmonary therapy, and withdrawal of medications. We can sort out the etiology later in comparative safety.

In patients with myasthenia gravis, fluctuating strength can reflect the effects of hypothyroidism or hyperthyroidism, and thyroid parameters should be routinely assessed. Worsening myasthenia often develops in the context of infection, pregnancy, injury, and ill-advised use of muscle relaxants. A common history is that a patient perceives increasing weakness and takes additional anticholinesterase medication—the cycle repeats and develops into cholinergic crisis.

OTHER CAUSES OF MUSCULAR WEAKNESS

The only direct therapy for *botulism* is polyvalent antitoxin, and this should be given as soon as the diagnosis is made. *Tick bite paralysis* is still rare. Removal of the tick will start the recovery process, although supportive care may be necessary for hours to days.

HEADACHE

Headaches are common and in the vast majority of cases, they are neither damaging nor do they reflect an underlying threatening process. When headache is the chief complaint of a patient in the emergency room, it can pose a diagnostic problem of bewildering complexity. Among the many patients who complain of head pain, there are a few who have significant disease, and among them there are a handful who require immediate help. The quality or severity of the discomfort is entirely subjective, and only rarely does a description of the pain lend any help in the diagnostic evaluation. In the following section, first we will describe some of the features of disease processes that commonly present as headache. Then, we will suggest a group of clinical characteristics that can aid the physician in diagnosing significant disease.

Clinical Features and Contexts of Disorders Causing Headache

SUBARACHNOID HEMORRHAGE

Subarachnoid hemorrhage results from rupture of an aneurysm in one of the large intracranial arteries, usually in the circle of Willis. A jet of blood spews from the site of rupture under arterial pressure and rapidly floods the subarachnoid space. Intracranial pressure abruptly rises. Depending on the site of rupture and the direction of the jet of blood, the stream can dissect into the parenchyma of the brain causing a hematoma, or it may actually penetrate the brain substance and burst into the ventricular system. The blood in the CSF commonly clogs the arachnoid villi, the site of CSF resorption, and many patients will develop a rapidly evolving communicating hydro-

cephalus. Blood in the ventricular system itself may cause an obstructive hydrocephalus. Four to seven days after the hemorrhage, arterial vessels bathed in the extravasated blood may develop spasm, causing an additional ischemic insult.

Most patients have no warning before the hemorrhage. In a few patients, the aneurysm itself may have pressed on the opthalmic nerve or on the third, fourth, or sixth cranial nerves, causing symptoms days or weeks before the rupture. The hemorrhage typically occurs while the patient is active, and it is common to obtain a history of unusual emotional stress, physical exertion, or sexual activity immediately before the hemorrhage. When the aneurysm ruptures, the headache is very abrupt in onset and reaches a maximum intensity in seconds to minutes. When the headache is severe, the pain is generalized and excruciating, and the patient may abruptly lose consciousness. Presumably this correlates with the abrupt increase in intracranial pressure. A few patients lose consciousness at the onset, but preceding headache is the rule. Unconscious patients develop frightening attacks of extensor rigidity, much like decerebrate posturing, during which there may be respiratory arrest and vagal bradycardia. Less severely affected people may awake in a few moments and are usually confused or amnestic about the onset. In patients who do not lose consciousness or who awake a short time after the onset, the headache remains severe and becomes associated with a stiff neck.

Most patients, particularly those who remain conscious or who have regained consciousness before arrival in the emergency room, have no major focal neurologic deficits. Isolated cranial nerve palsies can result from the aneurysm itself. In more severe cases, however, hematomas can cause hemiplegia, aphasia, and so forth. The diagnosis in most cases can be promptly established by a cranial CT scan. If that is not available, lumbar puncture to demonstrate blood in the CSF is the next best test. Lumbar puncture can be hazardous if a clot has formed in the cranial vault or if there is acute obstructive hydrocephalus, and so one should make every effort to identify these potential relative contraindications. Initial management of subarachnoid hemorrhage includes measures to protect the unconscious patient—prone or decubitus position, ECG monitoring, and so forth. High blood pressure should be brought to normotensive levels rapidly with nitroprusside, propranolol, or alpha methyldopa. Nausea and vomiting should be controlled with intramuscular phenothiazines. A neurosurgeon should be alerted as soon as possible since it may prove necessary to deal with rapidly evolving hydrocephalus. In most instances, it is possible to make the diagnosis with CT scanning or lumbar puncture; emergency angiography is rarely necessary.

CEREBRAL HEMORRHAGE

Intraparenchymal hemorrhage almost invariably occurs in people with long-standing severe or poorly controlled hypertension. The hemorrhage is caused by the rupture of a medium-caliber penetrating artery; such vessels occur in the basal ganglia, in the pons, and in the white matter of the cerebellum. The hemorrhage causes a local blood clot, which compresses and distorts neighboring brain, resulting in a focal neurologic deficit. In addition, the sudden addition of the volume of the clot to the closed intracranial space causes an abrupt increase in intracranial pressure. Usually the blood leak from the ruptured artery has stopped by the time the patient arrives in the emergency room. The subsequent clinical course reflects accumulating cerebral edema, obstructive or communicating hydrocephalus, and the mass effect of the clot.

At least half of the patients with hypertensive intraparenchymal hemorrhage complain of rapidly worsening severe headache at the outset. The characteristics of the pain are varied. If there has been leakage of blood into the ventricular system, the discomfort is often generalized. More commonly, the clot somehow causes ipsilateral dull severe discomfort. Diagnosis is rarely a major difficulty. The neurologic deficit is severe and more troubling to the patient than the head pain, and the sensorium is invariably clouded. The exact nature of the neurologic deficit reflects the location and size of the clot, as described above in the discussion of cerebrovascular disease. Cranial CT scanning is the diagnostic procedure of choice. If CT scanning is not available, cerebral angiography would be the only other procedure of diagnostic value. Usually the clinical constellation is typical, and angiography should be employed on an emergency basis only if we are concerned about the possibility of subdural or epidural hematoma. Lumbar puncture is hazardous in the setting of intraparenchymal hemorrhage because it entails the risk of transtentorial or cerebellar herniation. Since not every hemorrhage gains access to the CSF, lumbar puncture may not necessarily contribute to the diagnostic process.

INTRACRANIAL MASS LESION

Patients who experience an unfamiliar headache, and are sufficiently troubled by it to come to the emergency room, often harbor the awful fear that they are suffering from a brain tumor. Because headache can be an accompaniment of intracerebral neoplasm, the physician in the emergency room has to share their concern. Unfortunately, the quality and severity of headache associated with an infectious or neoplastic mass lesion is highly varied. The mechanism of the pain is presumed to be distortion of the meninges or of innervated blood vessels or, less commonly, to be some manifestation of generally increased intracranial pressure. The severity of the pain is not a very useful indicator; the pain of migraine, subarachnoid hemorrhage, sinusitis, and concussion all may be more severe. Features that are more suggestive of a mass include chronicity, presence of the discomfort upon awakening, and worsening of the pain with coughing, straining at stool, and so forth.

The diagnostic evaluation of a patient with a possible intracranial mass should begin with skull films and CT scanning, as discussed in Chapter 10. In most instances, careful examination will disclose focal neurologic deficits, and the patient may manifest some depression of his or her usual level of awareness. Unless the patient is obtunded, however, the evaluation of a possible intracranial mass lesion in the emergency room does not require emergency angiography. On the other hand, patients with intracranial neoplasms often manifest many of the same problems as patients with subdural hematomas or brain abscesses. Until that differential diagnosis is settled, the patient has to be watched carefully.

SUBDURAL HEMATOMA

A subdural hematoma occurs when bleeding forms a clot between the membranes of the outer portion of the dura mater. The bleeding is usually initiated by trauma, but the trauma itself can be so trivial as to be promptly forgotten, especially in elderly patients. Subdural hematomas vary greatly in size from a few drops of blood to a clot occupying the volume of half a hemisphere. The pressure of the hematoma on the adjacent brain causes focal neurologic dysfunction. Increased intracranial pressure is commonly associated with stupor or confusion. There are two general, long-term hazards with subdural hematoma: transtentorial herniation and destruction of the chronically compressed brain tissue.

In patients under age 35, the trauma sufficient to cause a subdural hematoma will be memorable (unless, of course, the patient is amnestic of the episode because of a concomitant concussion). The great problem in diagnosis arises when elderly patients complain of headache. In elderly patients, trauma sufficient to initiate the formation of a hematoma may be trivial and forgotten. Chronic subdural hematomas sometimes cause a peculiar waxing and waning neurologic deficit. The patient may complain of head pain that comes and goes and may exhibit a fluctuating level of awareness. Often such patients will be taking pain relievers of moderate potency and so their fluctuating neurologic status is incorrectly ascribed to inadvertent overdosage. In the most troubling cases, the principal manifestation of the hematoma may be a compromise of the intellect not unlike mild or moderate dementia.

The diagnostic evaluation of possible subdural hematoma begins with a careful neurologic examination, paying special attention to alertness and level of intellectual function. Skull x-ray films may reveal an associated fracture, but they are more useful in that lateral displacement of the pineal gland may be visualized. As is usually the case in neurologic diagnosis, CT scanning is the procedure of choice. Angiography is the next best test. If CT scanning is not available, angiography need not be done in the emergency room unless one fears that the subdural is of recent origin and may still be enlarging.

GIANT CELL ARTERITIS

Giant cell arteritis is a peculiar inflammation of certain arteries that has a characteristic pathology, including invasion of the arterial media by giant cells. The temporal arteries and the occipital arteries are the usual sites of clinically evident inflammation. The inflamed arteries are tender and seem thickened when palpated, and the patient may also have the clinical syndrome of polymyalgia rheumatica. The importance of recognizing giant cell arteritis is that the inflammation may proceed to involve the ophthalmic artery or its branches in the orbit, leading to precipitous and permanent blindness in that eye.

Giant cell arteritis occurs in people over 55 years old. The pain is worse at the site of the involved artery—temporal or occipital—and the patient is often aware of local tenderness to the touch. In most instances, the headache is well in advance of any local neurologic dysfunction. The diagnosis is accomplished when a heightened index of suspicion leads the physician to obtain an erythrocyte sedimentation rate (ESR). The ESR is invariably elevated in patients with active arteritis, and there may also be a mild anemia.

ANGLE CLOSURE GLAUCOMA

Acute angle closure glaucoma can cause severe ipsilateral ocular and facial pain, as well as nausea and vomiting at times. The diagnosis is made by measurement of the intraocular pressure. Though vision in the involved eye may be affected, there is no other related neurologic deficit. The importance of recognizing the syndrome in the emergency room is that one may be able to avoid permanent visual impairment.

MIGRAINE

Migraine headache may present as severe debilitating pain, but there is no threat to life and no hazard to neurologic func-

tion. The essential problem posed by patients with migraine in the emergency room is that it enormously complicates the process of differential diagnosis.

Classic migraine is the most stereotypic of the migraine syndromes and occurs in about 10% of all people thought to have migraine headaches. The headache is preceded by a prodrome of neurologic dysfunction. Typical neurologic manifestations are often visual—patients often describe "positive" visual phenomena such as jagged white lines, bars of light, lines like the battlements of a castle, or variously sized bursts of white or colored light. In addition, there are "negative" visual events such as scotoma in which vision is absent or blurred. The key aspect of the description of these visual phenomena is that they move over the visual field—the lines march, the balls of light expand and shift position, and the scotoma drift. This is to be differentiated from ischemia in the retina or occipital cortex, which may also cause negative or positive experiences but which have a steady position in the visual field. Nonvisual neurologic prodromes include hemiparesis and hemiparethesias. These are experienced as migrating over the body—numbness may be felt first in the fingers, then in the hands, then after minutes creep up the arm, then be accompanied by the same sensation in the foot and leg. The prodrome requires 3–10 minutes to occupy the entire side of the body; essentially no other neurologic event has the same time course. The whole prodrome lasts no more than 30 minutes and is then followed by headache, usually hemicranial, on the side opposite the prodrome experience. The pain is severe, pounding, and associated with photophobia, nausea, and vomiting. Patients typically seek dark, quiet places and lie quite still until the pain passes. A family history of migraine can be obtained in over one-half of the patients. In women, headaches may be associated with onset of menses or with pregnancy.

The clinical constellation of classic migraine is uncommon in its complete form. The prodrome may occur but the headache never develops, or typical hemicranial pain may occur without a prodrome. These incomplete syndromes are described as *common migraine*. Family history is less often obtained, and the discomfort is less stereotypic.

Patients may be able to identify precipitating events leading to the headache. Many note that headache predictably follows ingestion of red wine, chocolate, or tyramine-containing cheese. Even though the mechanism is not known, it has been found that the pain will respond to administration of ergot alkaloids if they are administered before the peak of the discomfort. In practice, patients who know they have migraine headaches tend to take the medication immediately upon experiencing the prodrome. In the emergency room when the diagnosis of migraine is clear, there should be no hesitation to use opiate analgesia, perhaps in association with an antinausea preparation.

One uncommon type of migraine is described as a *cluster headache*. This occurs almost exclusively in young men. The pain is extremely severe and is always localized over one eye. Attack follows attack in clusters of episodes. More than one attack can occur in a day. The pain is often accompanied by tearing of the ipsilateral eye or ipsilateral rhinorrhea. Sufferers can be made so desperate by the pain that suicide is not unknown.

Diagnosis

The basic problem in the emergency room is to recognize the patients who may have significant diseases in association with their headaches. The screening processes are history and physical examination. The following clinical constellations should alert us to the necessity for special attention:

1. Headache in association with specific neurologic abnormalities such as behavior change, neurologic deficit, seizure, or altered vision
2. Abrupt onset of severe, unfamiliar headache
3. Worsening in the severity of the pain with straining at stool, coughing, stooping, or other maneuvers that may be expected to increase intracranial pressure
4. Headache in association with fever or stiff neck
5. Recurrent focal pain
6. Change in the quality or distribution of chronic headache

We should also be aware of the special problems of headache following trauma and headache in the elderly. Headache after significant head trauma is common at any age, but it should alert us to the possibility of fracture and subdural or epidural bleeding. Headache in the elderly should always be taken seriously. Usually it will be found to reflect depression or other emotional events, but subdural hematomas and intracranial mass lesions are more common in the elderly.

The laboratory determinations available for help in the evaluation of headache include the following:

1. Complete blood cell count for evidence of infection
2. ESR for giant cell arteritis
3. Skull films

    Fractures
    Sinus infection
    Focal bone erosion
    Displacement of the pineal
    Abnormal intracranial calcifications
4. Cranial CT scanning
5. Lumbar puncture
    Cell count
    Culture
    Pressure
6. Cerebral angiography

The relevance of each test to the various pathologic entities presenting as headache has been presented in the previous section. There is no laboratory determination that is diagnostic for migraine.

SELECTED READINGS

Adams RD, Victor M: *Principles of Neurology,* ed 2. New York, McGraw-Hill Book Co, 1981.

Cranford RE, Leppik IE, Patrick B, Anderson CB, Koolick B: Intravenous phenytoin in acute treatment of seizures. *Neurology* 1979; 29:1474–1479.

Dalessio DV: *Wolff's Headache and Other Head Pain,* ed 3. New York, Oxford University Press, 1972.

Delgado-Escueta AV, Wasterlain C, Freeman DM, Porter JR: Management of status epilepticus. *N Engl J Med* 1982; 306:1337–1340.

Donadio JA, Gangarosa EJ, Faich GA: Diagnosis and treatment of botulism. *J Infect Dis* 1971; 124:108.

Drachman DB: Myasthenia gravis, *N Engl J Med* 1978; 298:136–142, 186–193.

Fauchald P, Rygvold O, Oystese B: Temporal arteritis and polymyalgia rheumatica, clinical and biopsy findings. *Ann Intern Med* 1972; 77:845.

McLeod JG, Walsh JC, Prineas JW, Pollard JD: Acute idiopathic polyneuritis. *J Neurol Sci* 1976; 27:145.

Millikan CH: Reassessment of anticoagulant therapy in various types of occlusive cerebrovascular disease. *Stroke* 1971; 2:201.

Plum F, Posner JB: *The Diagnosis of Stupor and Coma,* ed 3. Philadelphia, FA Davis Co, 1980.

Samuels MA (ed): *Manual of Neurologic Therapeutics.* Boston, Little Brown & Co, 1978.

31
ACUTE NONTRAUMATIC EYE DISORDERS

Alfredo A. Sadun
Don C. Bienfang

Ophthalmologists treat an organ that can be almost totally inspected. However, some of the examination is partly dependent upon sophisticated equipment that may be unfamiliar to many physicians and unavailable in an emergency. This chapter is written in the hope of presenting an approach to ocular emergencies that uses equipment that is available in any general emergency ward. Emphasis will be on recognition of the nature of the problem. In many instances, the emergency ward physician will be comfortable in managing such eye problems as allergic and viral conjunctivitis or a lid stye, whereas at other times elective referral to an ophthalmologist is appropriate (Table 31.1 column B). In a third group of patients (Table 31.1, column A) therapy should be instituted immediately even though future referral is expected. The emergency ward physician should be able to recognize such emergencies quickly and initiate therapy.

Specific areas of history need to be addressed with each set of presenting complaints. Similarly, certain physical examinations and tests are required for specific presentations. These are discussed, together with special tests, in connection with different presentations. However, there are a few basic aspects to ophthalmic history taking and to the physical examination of the eye, that apply to almost every patient with an ocular complaint.

EVALUATION

History

Serious eye diseases usually decrease vision. The patient should be asked about the vision in the affected eye as compared to the vision before the injury. The time course and tempo from first symptoms to emergency room visit will be useful information for the differential diagnosis. The extent and nature of the pain needs to be explored. When severe pain is the over-

whelming symptom, it is usually generated in the anterior segment of the eye, often in the iris or cornea. A history of any significant medical problem (i.e., diabetes or systemic lupus erythematosus) and a list of current and past medications should be obtained.

Examination of the Eye

It should be remembered that eyes retain a remarkable beauty and clarity even when patients are elderly. In the evaluation of the cornea, anterior chamber, and iris, obscuring of crisp details usually means something is wrong. An attempt should be made to document at least the following five findings.

CENTRAL VISION

Since serious eye disease usually decreases vision and since vision is the primary function of the eye, it would logically follow that the measurement of this ocular function is the most important part of the eye examination. Unfortunately, it is a piece of information that is often missing from an emergency room evaluation. The measurement of central visual acuity is important data for diagnosis, for later evaluation of the course of the eye problem, and for medicolegal purposes. The visual acuity can be measured on a Snellen chart at any distance over 6 ft, as a numerator (distance in feet from chart) and denominator (value of the smallest line read). Any common item and distance can be substituted such as counting fingers at 8 ft or reading 2-in. high print at 10 ft. Thus, an ophthalmologist may document the steady deterioration of a patient's vision as follows: 20/20 to 20/50 to 20/200 to counting fingers at 6 ft to counting fingers at 1 ft to light perception only. Each eye needs to be recorded separately and with usual glasses worn. The measurement of close reading vision is less useful because it requires accommodation, but this, too, is of value if the patient's reading glasses are available. Visual fields provide useful neuroophthalmologic data but rarely contribute to emergency room management.

PUPILS

Are the pupils equal and round? Is there brisk constriction to light directed to each eye? Compare the constriction to direct illumination to the consensual response brought on by illuminating the other eye. This is the swinging flashlight or Marcus Gunn test. If when swinging a light from eye to eye, one pupil consistently dilates while the fellow pupil constricts, the first pupil is said to have a relative afferent defect. This is almost always a sign of optic nerve disease and suggests serious trouble. Advanced cataracts and retinal diseases may markedly

TABLE 31.1 Priorities in Eye Emergencies

A. Immediate Treatment	B. Quick Referral
The emergency room physician must recognize condition and be able to begin treatment without ophthalmic consultation	If necessary, there is time to discuss the case with an ophthalmologist
1. Chemical injuries	1. Retinal detachment
2. Penetrating injuries	2. Blunt injury
3. Central retinal artery occlusion	3. Corneal abrasion
4. Angle-closure glaucoma	4. Corneal foreign body
	5. Corneal ulcer (infected)
	6. Spontaneous intraocular hemorrhage
	7. Optic neuritis
	8. Uveitis

decrease visual acuity but usually fail to give a positive Marcus Gunn test, yet subtle neurologic lesions provoke a positive test.

CONJUNCTIVA

During inspection of the bulbar conjunctiva (that portion applied to the globe), one should assess the color and apparent depth of any inflammation present. When the superficial vessels are dilated, as in infections of the conjunctiva, the visible vessels are bright red. Conjunctival edema (chemosis) can be dramatic with folds of conjunctiva literally spilling out between the eye lids.

CORNEA

The cornea is the source of most severe eye pain. One should attempt to examine the normally smooth surface with a flashlight. Look carefully for embedded foreign bodies or roughened areas of epithelium. Abrasions or epithelial defects often appear as shadows moving across the iris when the flashlight beam is scanned across the cornea.

FUNDUS AND OPTIC DISCS

Mastery of direct ophthalmoscopy is not difficult. After assessing the pupil, the eyes should usually be dilated with tropicamide 0.5% (Mydriacil). The risk of provoking an angle closure attack is small, and because it is diagnostic of narrow angles, this serves the patient. Tropicamide only lasts 2–3 hours and is easily reversed with pilocarpine (see angle closure glaucoma section).

Most fundi are best seen with the ophthalmoscope set on the minus (red) numbers 2–4. If the eye is aphakic (after cat-

aract extraction), plus (black) 6–8 lenses are usually best. Examine the patient's right eye with your right eye and the left with your left. Keep close to the patient's eye. The optic disc should be examined for pallor, margin clarity (the nasal margin may normally be a little blurred), cupping (the central white area should occupy less than one-half of the disc), and spontaneous venous pulsations (seen best where the vein bends into the cup), which help rule out increased cerebrospinal fluid (CSF) pressure.

CLINICAL SETTINGS

Painless Loss of Vision

Significant visual loss is the most ominous sign for the ophthalmologist. The most important element to extract from the history is whether the loss was acute or gradual; specifically, what was the nature and time course of the visual loss?

Often a patient becomes suddenly aware of an eye that has not seen well for a long time (sometimes years or a lifetime). The patient may have casually covered the good eye while rubbing it and noted that he or she could not see well. In taking a history the physician must bring this out and must avoid discarding any suspicion of a chronic or slowly progressive disorder such as cataracts, amblyopia, open angle glaucoma, or refractive error.

The most common error in the evaluation of painless loss of vision is failure to document an accurate measure of visual acuity. One of the first things to do is to test the true visual acuity (Fig. 31.1). While the visual acuity is being assessed, a simple test determines if much of the visual loss is a result of refractive error. This is done by placing a small hole in a

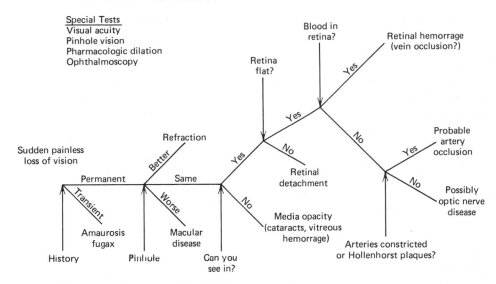

Figure 31.1 Flow chart of differential diagnosis for causes of painless loss of sight.

darkened piece of paper or cardboard (can be made with a 20-gauge needle) and asking the patient to look through the small hole at the eye chart a second time. If the visual acuity is strikingly improved by this maneuver, the visual loss is, at least in large part, because of a *refractive error,* which is probably correctable with glasses. Further tests that help in making the differential diagnosis in painless visual loss are reviewed in Figure 31.1.

CENTRAL RETINAL ARTERY OCCLUSION

If the visual loss is not refractive and the change was sudden and a dramatic uniocular event, then the emergency room physician must immediately suspect a central retinal artery (CRA) occlusion. This is more likely to occur in older people, particularly in those with hypertension or vascular disease.

Diagnosis

There is a history of sudden, complete, and painless loss of vision in one eye. The visual acuity is counting fingers or worse. The pupil does not react briskly to light. There is a positive Marcus Gunn pupil. Ophthalmoscopic examination reveals a clear vitreous. The fundus may appear normal or pale, often yielding the appearance of a cherry-red macula (Plate 10). One might note bloodless arterioles that may be difficult to see.

There may be "box car" segmentation of the stagnant blood in the veins. A Hollenhorst plaque (embolus from a sclerotic plaque) may be seen by ophthalmoscopy as a glistening yellow spot lodged in the central retinal artery or in bifurcations of branch arterioles (Plate 11).

Therapy

The physician should not delay while awaiting any special test results. The goals of management are to try to lower the intraocular pressure rapidly and to dilate the retinal arteries in the hope that an obstruction will move distally to allow return of blood flow to part of the retina. Lowering of the intraocular pressure can be accomplished by several maneuvers as follows:

1. The globe is pressed through the closed lids for a count of 5 and released for a count of 3. This should be done for 5 minutes. It is best done by the patient, who will be less reluctant to press firmly.

2. Acetazolamide (Diamox), 250–500 mg, should be given piggy back intravenously in 100 ml D_5W or saline, over 5–10 minutes.

3. Osmoglyn (lime-flavored glycerol), 75–150 ml on crushed ice should be given orally. This osmotic agent is better tolerated than intravenous mannitol or urea. This agent may

cause nausea, which can be treated with prochlorperazine (Compazine) 5 mg intramuscularly.

4. The retinal arteries may dilate if the patient breathes a mixture of 90% oxygen and 10% carbon dioxide for 20–45 minutes to raise blood Pco_2. The high blood Po_2 may also help protect ischemic retinal ganglion cells.

5. Finally, the *ophthalmologist* may elect to lower the pressure rapidly by withdrawing 0.2 ml of aqueous humor through a peripherally located corneal puncture (paracentesis).

6. Referral to evaluate sources of emboli can be carried out later.

7. Several hours after onset there is little that can be offered for the patient (experiments with monkeys suggest 90 minutes of ischemia is all the retina can tolerate).

8. Visual acuity may return promptly if a clot becomes dislodged. Further improvement may develop over a course of days as retinal edema subsides. However, if the CRA remains occluded, the visual potential of the eye is largely lost.

TEMPORAL ARTERITIS

Temporal arteritis (TA) can produce a picture of CRA or present less dramatically and less completely. The patient is usually over 65 years old. The history may reveal scalp tenderness or jaw pain for days to weeks. There may have been weight loss and malaise. Temporal arteritis is but one manifestation of polymyalgia rheumatica. The consideration and early diagnosis of TA remains extremely important for the following three reasons:

1. The disease process is very treatable.
2. Visual loss can be precipitous.
3. The second eye is at immediate risk.

Diagnosis

The patient is almost invariably elderly and often gives a variety of complaints of recent poor general health. The patient may complain of headache or scalp or brow tenderness exacerbated while masticating. On examination, the temporal arteries should be palpated for tenderness. They may feel cordlike, firm, or lumpy. If there is any doubt of TA, a sedimentation rate should be sent for immediately. Values greater than 40 mm should be regarded as suspicious and values over 70 as highly suggestive.

Therapy and Prognosis

If a diagnosis of probable TA is made, the patient should be started on prednisone, about 80 mg orally every day immediately. The vision in both eyes is at immediate risk, and there is no justification for delay. Further workup by the ophthalmologist may include a temporal artery biopsy, which will remain positive for a few weeks after steroid treatment. The ophthalmologist will probably continue high doses of steroids until the sedimentation rate falls to lower levels. Fortunately, most patients respond quickly to steroids and will do well clinically once their sedimentation rates come down. The patients may be kept on lower doses of steroids for 6 months to several years.

RETINAL DETACHMENTS

Retinal detachments are especially frequent following injuries to the eye or cataract surgery. They may also be spontaneous, particularly in patients with high myopia. History often reveals, for example, episodes of flashing lights or of showers of sparks. The patient may describe a shade climbing up over his or her view.

Diagnosis

Central visual acuity may be normal or very poor if the macula is detached. Ophthalmoscopy may reveal billowing grey sails (Plate 12). Peripheral retinal detachments are difficult to see without an indirect ophthalmoscope. A cataract or other media opacity may also make the diagnosis difficult.

Therapy and Prognosis

The patient should be instructed to remain inactive and should be sent to an ophthalmologist immediately. If surgery is performed before the macula becomes detached, the prognosis remains good.

CENTRAL RETINAL VEIN OCCLUSION

Central retinal vein occlusion is usually caused by compression of the veins against a rigid arterial wall. Thus many of the same predisposing factors of CRA occlusion (by arteriosclerosis, diabetes) apply. In addition, high intraocular pressure (glaucoma) often is a factor. Less frequently, conditions of hyperviscosity of the blood, such as polycythemia, cryoglobulinemia, or leukemia, play a role.

Diagnosis

The history of visual loss is often less dramatic than with CRA. The patient usually has counting fingers vision. Ophthalmoscopy reveals a "blood and thunder" fundus from widespread hemorrhage often radiating from the optic disc (Plate 13).

Therapy and Prognosis

Treatment consists of lowering the intraocular pressure if it is elevated. Timoptic 0.5% twice a day is a good starting medication if the patient does not have chronic obstructive pulmonary disease or congestive heart failure. Pilocarpine 1% four times a day is a good alternative. Referral within 24 hours is indicated. If the intraocular pressure is lowered, an impending (not complete) central vein occlusion may resolve with excellent recovery of vision. If the central vein occlusion is complete, vision generally remains poor. New vessel growth in the iris (rubeosis) and retina (Plate 14) may develop 3–4 months later, leading to glaucoma and detached retinas, respectively, both of which tend to be refractory to treatment.

VITREOUS HEMORRHAGE

Vitreous hemorrhage may be secondary to retinal arteriole or venous disease. Vasculitis, diabetes, and phlebitis of the local vasculature may produce a hemorrhage that progresses into the vitreous. Patients with new vessel growth in the retina from diabetes, retinal degenerations, and vessel occlusions are particularly prone to vitreous hemorrhage. The posterior vitreous detachment seen in those patients over 55 years old may also produce a vitreous hemorrhage.

Diagnosis

The patient usually describes a dark red cloud developing over a course of hours and obscuring vision. Vision may be as bad as bare light perception if the hemorrhage is extensive. Ophthalmoscopy reveals a dark red obscuration of the media behind the lens. Ultrasound can be used to assess the extent of the hemorrhage.

Therapy and Prognosis

There is little that can be offered in the emergency room, and there is no urgency unless an etiologic factor can be identified and treated. Generally there is little the ophthalmologist can do while he or she waits for the hemorrhage to settle inferiorly and clear. Small hemorrhages may clear in a few weeks. Extensive and repeat hemorrhages may never clear and may lead to vitreous condensations and traction on the retina. A vitrectomy may then be attempted to salvage some vision.

Painful Loss of Vision

The combination of a reasonably acute loss of vision and a painful eye that is not red suggests a rather limited set of alternatives. We are presently excluding those injuries of the eye caused by trauma, which are discussed in Chapter 18. Whereas painless loss of vision is often seen in the elderly, painful acute visual loss is found in all age groups, often in young adults. Once again, an accurate description of the temporal course of both the visual loss and the pain is indispensable. It is useful to get a sense of whether the pain is in front of the eye, in the eye, or behind the eye. If the pain is of very sudden onset to the front of the eye and the eye is red, visual loss is probably minimal (i.e., from 20/20 to 20/30); these conditions will be described in the discussion about the red eye.

IRITIS

The pain of iritis is sharp or aching and is often localized to the front of the eye. The inflammation is usually limited to the anterior part of the eye or, less frequently, to part of a generalized uveitis. There exists a myriad of etiologies for iritis, though most often, despite extensive testing, no underlying abnormality is found. There seems to be a slight preponderance of teenagers and young adults presenting with iritis. Iritis often is seen in connection with mild trauma or corneal irritation.

Diagnosis

There is an acute onset of sharp or aching continuous pain almost always uniocularly. The patient usually complains of photophobia. Visual acuity at a distance may be near normal or moderately affected (20/80). The eye may be red, especially that part of the sclera abuting the limbus, forming a delicate pink halo around the cornea termed *ciliary flush*. The pupil may be miotic and sluggish to light. There is no Marcus Gunn sign. If a slit lamp is available, examination will reveal the pathognomonic presence of cells and flare (aqueous light scattering because of a high protein content) in the anterior chamber.

A large number of tests such as complete blood cell count (CBC), erythrocyte sedimentation rate (ESR), calcium levels, and chest x-ray films may be ordered later if episodes of iritis have been recurrent. These tests have a very low yield of positive results. Since the test results will not change the treatment, they can be ordered later.

Therapy and Prognosis

Fortunately, iritis responds well to current therapy regardless of the etiology. Cycloplegia and steroids in combination work very effectively. However, unless the diagnosis can be made with assurity, it is better to treat with cycloplegia alone since steroids may aggravate conditions with similar pictures such as herpes simplex keratitis. Cyclopentolate hydrochloride (Cyclogyl) 1% twice a day is an excellent choice of cycloplegic. When steroids are given (such as prednisolone 1%) initially they are administered frequently (four times daily or every 4 hours) and then are tapered over the next several days. Most cases of mild iritis resolve well with cycloplegia alone but an ophthalmology consult in a day or two is appropriate.

ACUTE ANGLE-CLOSURE GLAUCOMA

Acute angle-closure glaucoma is a serious condition brought on by a change in the fluid dynamics in the anterior chamber of the eye (Figs. 31.2 and 31.3). Contrary to common belief, it does not start with obstruction of the aqueous outflow at the angle by iris folds. Instead, it usually begins when aqueous is trapped posterior to the iris. Its normal route of flow is from

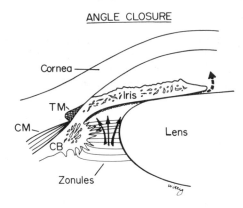

ANGLE CLOSURE

Figure 31.3 Angle closure. Cross section of a shallow anterior chamber and a closed angle. The iris is appositioned over the trabecular meshwork (filtration area), obstructing outflow. Aqueous is trapped in the posterior chamber bowing the peripheral iris forward and causing the intraocular pressure to rise. TM, trabecular meshwork; CM, ciliary muscle; CB, ciliary body.

the posterior to the anterior chamber through the pupil. However, in patients with shallow anterior chambers (often seen in hyperopes—those with smaller eyes who are farsighted) the iris gets "stuck" in a middilated position and there is no room for the aqueous to get between the iris–pupillary margin and the lens. The pressure behind the iris builds up, bowing the iris forward (Fig. 31.3). Occlusion of the anterior chamber angle may then occur secondarily.

Diagnosis

The patient may be of any age. Patients with shallow anterior chambers (Plate 15) are especially prone to such attacks. The patient frequently describes the attack as beginning in a dark room while he or she was awake (e.g., in a movie theater). The pain is very severe, boring, and often associated with headache, nausea, and vomitting. The patient may describe halos around lights. There is marked loss of vision (sometimes to counting fingers level) with the patient complaining of "smoky" vision. The eye may be quite red (scleral and conjunctival injection). The cornea may appear hazy or steamy. The pupil is fixed in a middilated position and is often oval instead of round. If the patient has had previous episodes of high intraocular pressure, there may be less pain and little inflammation.

Schiötz tonometry should be employed to verify the high (35–65 mm Hg) intraocular pressure (Procedure 32).

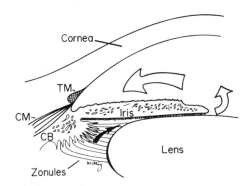

Figure 31.2 Open angle. Cross section of a deep anterior chamber and a wide open angle to the trabecular meshwork (filtration area). Aqueous passes from the posterior chamber, between the iris and the lens, to the anterior chamber, through the pupil, and out through the angle filtration area. TM, trabecular meshwork; CM, ciliary muscle; CB, ciliary body.

Therapy and Prognosis

The goal of therapy is reduction of intraocular pressure, thus releasing the iris and permitting normal fluid dynamics to be restored. This is done with osmotic agents, drugs that decrease aqueous production and agents that enhance outflow facility. All of the below can be initiated in quick sequence:

1. Acetazolamide (Diamox) 250 mg (500 mg for a heavy person) should be given IV piggy back (in D_5W or saline) over 10 minutes.
2. Acetazolamide (Diamox) 500 mg should also be given orally to become effective as the IV dose dissipates.
3. Prochlorperazine (Compazine) 5 mg IM can be given to alleviate the nausea that may preclude oral administration of medications.
4. Lime-flavored glycerol (Osmoglyn) 75–150 ml can be given on crushed ice to be sipped slowly.
5. Pilocarpine 2% or 4% eye drops move the pupil (miosis) and enhance outflow facility. They should be given at a rate of 1 drop every 15 minutes up to a maximum of six administrations.
6. Timolol maleate (Timoptic) 0.5% may also be useful given once and repeated in 30 minutes (after checking for a history of COPD or CHF).
7. The ophthalmologist should be contacted as soon as possible.

Since an angle closure attack is more easily broken sooner than later, it is advantageous to initiate therapy while locating an ophthalmologist. The attack can usually be broken (the pressure will drop to 10–20 mm Hg) medically, as described above, within an hour or two. After the inflammation has subsided, the ophthalmologist will usually perform a peripheral iridectomy (or laser iridotomy) to preclude future attacks. An iridotomy is often performed on the other eye as well since it probably shares the anatomical predisposition to angle closure. Certain other pathologies may produce angle closure and need to be addressed separately by the ophthalmologist.

OPTIC NEURITIS

Optic neuritis (ON) may occur in all age groups; however, young adults seem to predominate. Approximately one-fourth of males and almost one-half of females presenting with ON go on to develop multiple sclerosis (although these figures vary with age). There is a wide spectrum of descriptions of pain and diminished visual acuity in patients with ON. Generally, young patients complain more of both symptoms.

Diagnosis

The patient may describe pain behind the eye exacerbated on lateral eye movements. The condition may worsen during periods of high temperature (e.g., baths or menses). The visual acuity may be almost normal or as bad as counting fingers. The key finding is a Marcus Gunn pupil. This may be obvious even with little or no discernable visual loss. The external eye examination will be normal. The fundus examination may be normal (retrobulbar ON) or there may be engorgement of the optic disc with hyperemia noted (papillitis) (Plate 16).

The patient can often describe a small paracentral scotoma while looking, with the normal eye occluded, at a fixation spot in the center of a piece of graph paper. Often an area 1 or 2 inches from fixation will be seen by the patient as fuzzy. The patient may describe colors (particularly red) as less bright or saturated when viewed through the affected eye. A bright red pen or bottle cap can be shown to each eye separately for comparison. Extensive testing to rule out cranial mass lesions can be initiated at a later date by an ophthalmologist or neurologist.

Therapy and Prognosis

The neuroophthalmologist occasionally may choose to put the patient on systemic steroids which may hasten recovery. Most patients show almost complete resolution of symptoms within several weeks.

Red Eye

Inflammation of the conjunctiva in a mildly or moderately painful eye is a common reason for a visit to the emergency room. Most causes of red eye are not serious and are self-limiting, but since corneal infections can lead to loss of the eye, the diagnosis remains important. Frequently, the cause of a red eye is obvious from the history (e.g., corneal abrasion) and a description of the pain (e.g., sharp, burning, or itching). Refer to the flowchart on red eye (Fig. 31.4).

CORNEAL INJURY

The sudden onset of sharp severe pain in the front of the eye is almost invariably a sign of epithelial loss of the cornea. There usually is only minimal loss of visual acuity. The most common causes of corneal injury are discussed below.

A foreign body may be under the lid (the upper lid should be everted, Fig. 31.5) or embedded in the cornea (Plate 17). Topical anesthetic (proparacaine) should be instilled. The for-

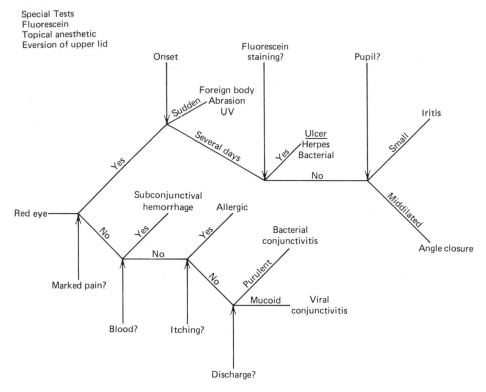

Figure 31.4 Flow chart of differential diagnosis for causes of red eye.

eign body may be removed with a cotton-tipped applicator or a small sterile spatula tip. If the foreign body cannot be removed easily, the patient should be referred to an ophthalmologist. If a foreign body is removed from the cornea, there remains a corneal abrasion.

Sun lamps or welder's arcs may be the source of ultraviolet (UV) radiation producing an *ultraviolet keratitis*. The severe pain usually begins 8–12 hours after exposure to the UV light. The deepithelialization of the cornea can be seen by fluorescein staining (see below) as a diffuse punctate injury. It is treated as a corneal abrasion.

A corneal abrasion can be very painful and often provokes a sensation of a foreign body though none is there. Most larger abrasions (Plate 18) are easily detected by fluorescein staining (placing the end of a fluorescein paper strip under the lower lid for 2 seconds). Blue light causes the fluorescein-stained deepithelialized corneal cells to fluoresce bright green. Most ophthalmoscopes have a blue light filter that can be used in combination with the magnification afforded by peering through

the ophthalmoscope at a setting of plus 10 (black) at a distance of 3 inches from the eye.

Therapy

Corneal abrasions are treated with a mydriatic agent such as cyclopentolate hydrochloride (Cyclogel) 1%, an antibiotic such as erythromycin ophthalmic ointment, and tight patching. Two eye pads on top of one another are held in place by tape running from the center of the forehead diagonally onto the cheek. Such a patch should remain in place for 24–36 hours. Most abrasions will be largely healed by then, and the patch may be removed. If the patient feels only moderate irritation after 24 hours and if he or she continues to feel improvement, follow-up is not necessary. The patient should return if there is any lack of improvement or any regression. Many patients will need a pain or sleeping medication for the first night. Be sure to warn the patient that the topical anesthetic used will wear off soon. Never give topical anesthetic for repeated use!

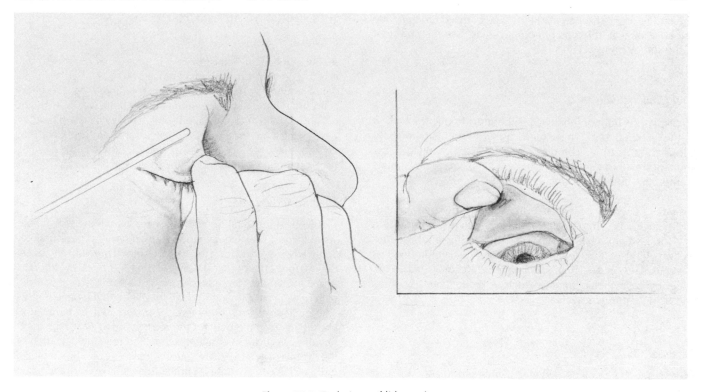

Figure 31.5 Technique of lid eversion.

If the patient has persistent pain, an ophthalmology referral is advised.

CORNEAL ULCERS

Occasionally an infectious process can cause symptoms similar to those from a foreign body. The difference is that the onset of the symptoms is rather insidious compared to mechanical trauma so that a patient with an infectious process causing the symptom is likely to seek help a day or two after symptoms begin, whereas a patient with a foreign body almost always appears shortly after the insult.

Bacterial Ulcers

DIAGNOSIS. Bacterial ulcers usually have a regular oval or irregular geographic epithelial defect that stains with fluorescein (Plate 19). The margins of the ulcer are frequently surrounded by an intracorneal white area representing subepithelial leucocytic infiltrates.

THERAPY. Corneal ulcers, particularly those caused by *Pseudomonas,* can very quickly devastate the eye. Immediate referral to an ophthalmologist is recommended. The ophthalmologist will take corneal scrapings for staining and culturing and give appropriate antibiotics. Hospitalization may be required in serious cases.

Herpes Simplex

DIAGNOSIS. Herpes simplex infections of the cornea have a characteristic pattern when stained with fluorescein. The delicate, branching pattern is termed a *herpes dendrite* (Plate 20).

THERAPY. Corneal herpes is a serious infection requiring an ophthalmologist's attention. Antiviral agents such as vidarabine (Vira-A) have proven efficacious. Steroids may aggravate the infection.

CONJUNCTIVITIS

Infection or irritation of the conjunctiva is manifested by injection of the superficial blood vessels and some discharge.

The nature of the discharge and the type of discomfort provide valuable clues to the type of conjunctivitis. See the flowchart of the red eye (Fig. 31.4).

Viral Conjunctivitis

DIAGNOSIS.   Viral conjunctivitis is the most frequent infection of the external eye. The patient usually complains of mild burning and tearing. The discharge is watery or mucoid. Examination without slit lamp usually fails to reveal any abnormality other than hyperemic conjunctiva.

THERAPY.   There is no effective treatment. However, an antibiotic such as erythromycin ointment is often given (twice a day for 1 week) as prophylaxis to avoid a bacterial superinfection. Viral conjunctivitis is self-limited (usually lasting less than 10 days) but is highly contagious. Recommend to the patient good hygienic practices such as frequent hand washing and using separate towels.

Bacterial Conjunctivitis

DIAGNOSIS.   Bacterial conjunctivitis often produces a purulent discharge. A conjunctival culture should be obtained with a sterile cotton swab placed into a beef broth tube or culturette.

THERAPY.   Erythromycin or bacitracin ophthalmic ointments or chloramphenicol (Chloroptic) drops can be given four times a day until the culture reports return. Ophthalmic referral is advised if the conjunctivitis proves to be bacterial or does not respond promptly to therapy.

Allergic Conjunctivitis

DIAGNOSIS.   Allergic conjunctivitis produces itching and minimal or watery discharge. There may be a dramatic reaction to an allergin in one eye, which produces marked chemosis. Seasonal allergies (e.g., hayfever) may produce seasonal bilateral inflammation called vernal conjunctivitis.

THERAPY.   Allergic conjunctivitis is managed best with cold compresses and topical decongestants/antihistamines (Vasocon-A three times a day is recommended). Topical steroid therapy is rarely necessary and is best left to an ophthalmologist.

SUBCONJUNCTIVAL HEMORRHAGE

Diagnosis

A subconjunctival hemorrhage will present as a red eye, but it has such a distinctive appearance (Plate 21) that it should not be confused with true inflammatory conditions. The characteristic finding of a subconjunctival hemorrhage is its bright red appearance as though a red splotch with very sharp borders were painted on the eye. On close inspection, it is clear that the eye is not red because of dilated blood vessels but rather because there is blood in the subconjunctival space.

Therapy and Prognosis

Most subconjunctival hemorrhages are seen in the elderly, are spontaneous, and require no therapy other than reassurance. Some advocate checking the patient's blood pressure and questioning for hematuria and easy bruising.

The most common serious error in the management of a red painful eye is to provide topical anesthetic to the patient. This anesthetic gives such relief that the patient may be tempted to pocket an available bottle. One must guard against such theft. Regular use of such an agent retards the reepithelialization of the cornea. Moreover, an anesthetized eye is vulnerable to further injury. Devastating corneal ulcers have been the result of patients taking topical anesthetics home with them.

Another serious error is the treatment of an inflamed eye with steroids before the diagnosis is established. Though the eye may look and feel better with steroids, an infection that is not properly covered may become much worse with steroid use. This is especially true of herpes and fungal keratitis.

Swollen Lids

The skin of the eyelids is remarkably thin and elastic. There is also very little subcutaneous fat to conceal pathology. Thus relatively minor processes can produce noticeable and even dramatic effects. For example, the slight generalized edema seen in patients preceding menses or in patients who are fatigued can be discerned in the periocular lid swelling (this and vasocongestion produce the transient look of dark, tired eyes). Fortunately, most lid swellings are of a very benign nature. The most common exception to this, especially in children, is cellulitis of the lids.

CELLULITIS

Cellulitis can be localized superficially in the lids and is then termed preorbital cellulitis, or it can occur behind the septum

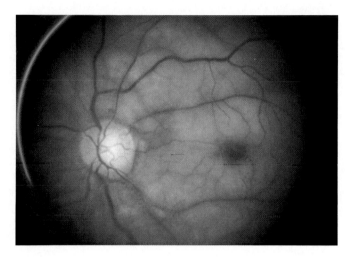

Plate 10 *Central retinal artery occlusion.*
The arterioles are attenuated; the retina is pale and edematous making the macula appear darker by comparison (cherry red spot).

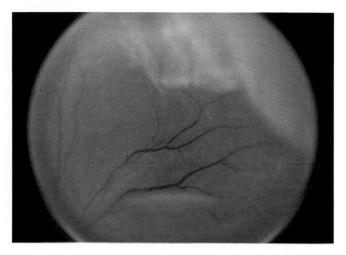

Plate 12 *Retinal detachment.*
Pale billowing folds of detached retina are seen superiorly.

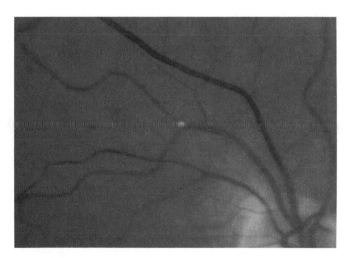

Plate 11 *Hollenhorst plaque.*
A highly reflective plaque is seen at an arteriole bifurcation blocking arterial blood flow distally.

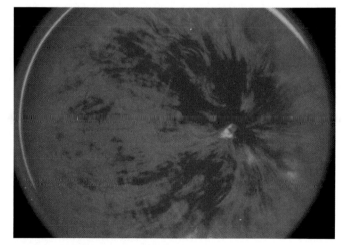

Plate 13 *Central retinal vein occlusion.*
Blockage of venous return produces this characteristic blood and thunder fundus appearance.

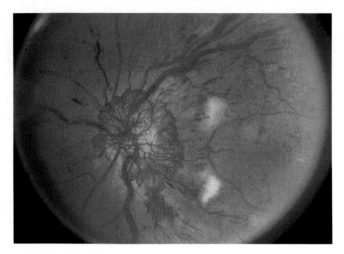

Plate 14 *Neovascular net.*
Diabetic retinopathy (proliferative) is a common cause of new vessel growth seen here about the nerve head.

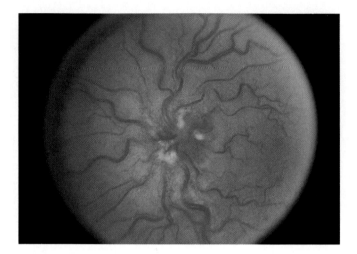

Plate 16 *Papillitis.*
Engorgement of the optic nerve head can occur unilaterally secondary to inflammation of the nerve (as in optic neuritis) or a partial central retinal vein occlusion.

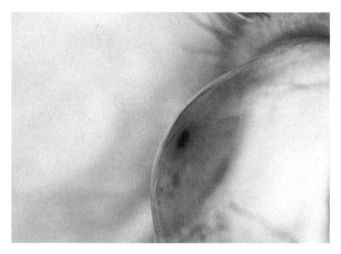

Plate 15 *Narrow angle.*
The anterior chamber is extremely shallow (there is very little distance between the iris and cornea). Such a patient is prone to acute angle-closure glaucoma.

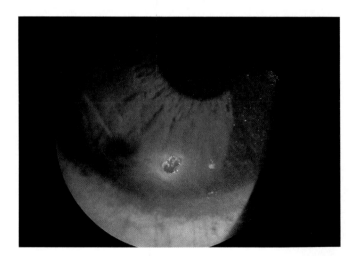

Plate 17 *Corneal foreign body.*
A rusting metallic foreign body is embedded in the anterior cornea provoking a leukocytic infiltration in the surrounding subepithelium. Note the shadow of the foreign body on the iris.

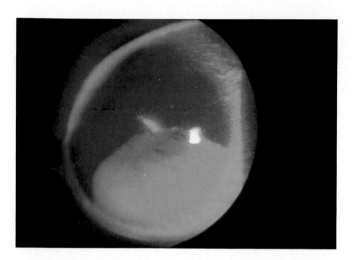

Plate 18 *Corneal abrasion.*
A large abrasion of the cornea picks up fluorescein stain and is seen easily in blue light.

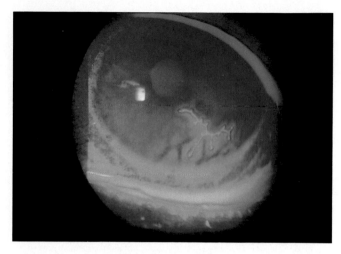

Plate 20 *Herpes simplex keratitis dendrite.*
A herpes infection of the cornea produces a delicate branching dendrite when stained with fluorescein.

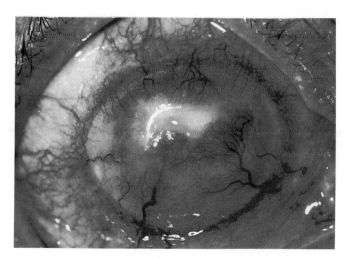

Plate 19 *Corneal ulcer.*
The central cornea is opaque, necrotic, and excavated. There is profuse vascular ingrowth toward the central ulcer.

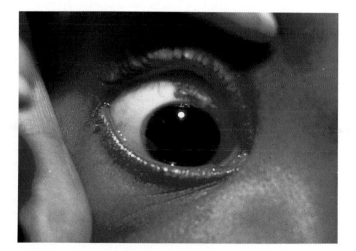

Plate 21 *Subconjunctival hemorrhage.*
The blood is trapped under the conjunctiva giving a bright red painted appearance. Note the absence of injected vessels.

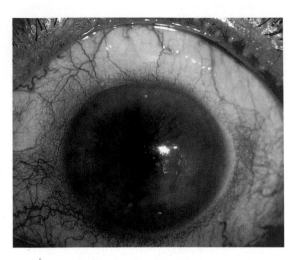

Plate 22 *Bullous keratopathy with corneal edema.*
Corneal endothelial dysfunction results in edema of the cornea that produces marked reduction of visual acuity and conjunctival injection.

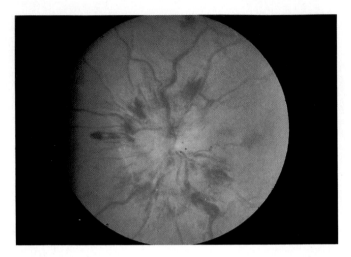

Plate 24 *Papilledema.*
High CSF pressure has led to swelling of the optic disc with peripapillary hemorrhages.

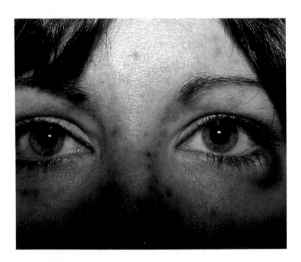

Plate 23 *Hordeolum (stye).*
There is a tender firm lump in the left lower lid caused by blockage of a meibomian gland duct.

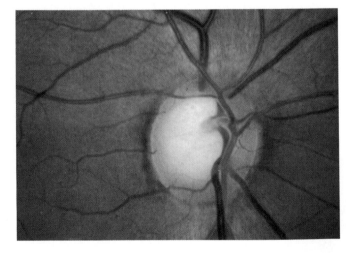

Plate 25 *Glaucomatous cupping.*
The optic disc has a large pale cup resulting in only a thin rim of neural tissue temporally.

and then becomes a very dangerous orbital cellulitis. Orbital cellulitis is one of the most frequent causes of proptosis (exophthalmos) in children and requires urgent attention.

Diagnosis

The patient or the parent of the patient often complains of progressive lid swelling over several days. There may be a source of the infection revealed by history (scratch, insect bite, or history of staphylococcus boils). Visual acuity is usually not affected until very late. The lids are firm, hot, and erythematous.

Temperature and white blood cell count often are raised with orbital cellulitis. Sinus films can help rule out adjacent sinus involvement.

Therapy and Prognosis

Common bacterial pathogens are staphylococci and streptococci. Dicloxacillin or cephalexin (Keflex) given by mouth four times a day are suitable initial antibiotics. If there is a question of the cellulitis being orbital, the patient should be referred to an ophthalmologist immediately. Orbital cellulitis usually requires hospitalization for intravenous antibiotic treatment.

Warm compresses over the lids four times a day may help localize and drain an abscess. Antibiotics (i.e., Bacitracin) are given in the eye to prevent draining puss from establishing a bacterial conjunctivitis. Patients who are sent home on such therapy and with a diagnosis of preorbital cellulitis should be told to take their temperature twice a day. Close follow-up is mandated. Most cases of orbital and preorbital cellulitis resolve nicely with conservative medical management.

CONJUNCTIVITIS

Swollen lids are often seen with conjunctivitis (see section on red eye), especially allergic conjunctivitis and epidemic keratoconjunctivitis (EKC). The conjunctiva will, of course, show marked injection (Plate 22).

LOCALIZED LID INFECTION (STYE)

Lid infections often begin as a diffuse swelling with pain or tactile hypersensitivity. The diffuse swelling then condenses to a hard, less painful abscess. These almost always drain spontaneously, especially if the inflammatory process is intense. An early "hot" infection of a skin, lid, or conjunctival gland is termed a *hordeolum* (stye) (Plate 23) and may "point" inwardly or to the skin side of the lid. Long-term blockage and infection of the meibomian glands of the lids may lead to a granulomatous reaction, termed a *chalazion*.

Diagnosis

The initial inflammatory phase (hordeolum) lasts a few days and the patient complains of pain and tenderness. The granulomatous phase (chalazion) begins after a history of a lump in the lids for a few weeks. The hordeolum appears as a localized lump on the lid and is soft and tender. A chalazion will be harder and less tender. There is no need for a special diagnostic test.

Therapy

1. A hot compress consisting of a moist hot cloth (e.g., a washcloth) should be used with a dry towel on top to keep the heat in. This not only cleans the lid and eye, but also makes it more comfortable and seems to speed the resolution of the abscess. The more frequently hot compresses are used, the better, but three times a day for 5 minutes at a time is a reasonable regimen. This treatment usually produces a complete resolution of the hordeolum in 2 weeks.

2. Topical antibiotics (erythromycin three times a day) are of limited value but are advocated by some to prevent a bacterial conjunctivitis from the purulent discharge.

3. If the hordeolum does not respond to the above management in 2 or 3 weeks, it will have become a chalazion and may require excision by an ophthalmologist. A patient with a cold, nontender lump without an antecedent inflamed lid may have a lid tumor and should also be referred.

Diplopia and Pupil Abnormalities

The evaluation of neuroophthalmologic problems can be subtle and complex. Fortunately, true neuroophthalmic emergencies are rare and the emergency room physician can simply concentrate on ruling these out. The most common neuroophthalmic presentations to the emergency room are diplopia and anisocoria (pupils of unequal size). The latter often are urgently brought to the neurosurgeon's attention unnecessarily, causing undue fright to the patient. Only in combination with other neurologic signs does a large pupil usually indicate serious pathology.

MONOCULAR DIPLOPIA

The patient with monocular diplopia complains of double vision in one eye. Alternately covering each eye often eliminates the diplopia and reveals it as, in fact, binocular.

If the diplopia proves to be monocular, a pin-hole test should be employed. If the diplopia is eliminated, this implicates the cornea as part of a refractive problem producing the two images. If the diplopia persists (or sometimes gets worse) with the pin-hole test, there may be a refractive problem with the lens (secondary to a cataract or subluxation) or, rarely, with the macula. By far, the most common cause of monocular diplopia is a cataract. The patient may wish to have tape covering the spectacle lens in front of the offending eye. Even transparent tape blurs the image sufficiently to alleviate symptoms. Referral to an ophthalmologist may lead to a more permanent resolution of the problem (e.g., cataract extraction).

BINOCULAR DIPLOPIA

In patients with binocular diplopia, the diplopia disappears when the patient covers either eye. Ask the patient whether the two images lie horizontally, vertically, or diagonally separated. In both children and adults, the most common ocular nerve palsy is derived from the sixth cranial nerve leading to a simply horizontal diplopia, which is made worse upon looking in the direction of the offending eye.

Diagnosis

Establish the tempo of onset, associated pain, and position of diplopia. Does the diplopia come on only with fatigue? Is the pupil examination normal? Are the eye movements full? Does each eye fully abduct, adduct, move vertically, and converge? Are the eye movements conjugate?

Conjugate eye movements seen in patients without pain or pupil abnormalities whose diplopia gets worse with fatigue, indicate an old, decompensated phoria (latent strabismus).

Disconjugate eye movements of sudden onset in association with pain or abnormal pupils suggest an ocular cranial nerve palsy. Though the most common nerve palsy is derived from the sixth cranial nerve, pupil involvement or vertical diplopia speaks for a third cranial nerve palsy. With trauma and diagonal diplopia, fourth cranial nerve palsy may be implicated. Viral infections (in young children), diabetes, vascular accidents, aneurysm, tumor, myasthenia gravis, and Graves' disease are common causes of binocular diplopia.

Therapy and Prognosis

The patient should be referred to an ophthalmologist. More extensive testing to establish the diagnosis will usually begin when the initial blood tests return. The emergency room physician may wish to get blood electrolytes and a complete blood count. Old decompensated phorias are usually quite benign. Most reversible lesions of the ocular nerves (e.g., diabetes or childhood viral) lead to recovery of nerve function within 6–10 weeks.

ANISOCORIA

Often patients presenting with asymmetric pupil sizes generate high levels of anxiety in the emergency room. The association of a "blown pupil" with a large intracranial mass lesion and uncal herniation has been grossly overplayed. In the absence of other neurologic signs, a large pupil rarely portends such a serious problem. Between 5% and 10% of the population has a "normal" anisocoria.

A history of pain and possibly diplopia with a dilated pupil raises the suspicion of an aneurysm as the cause of third cranial nerve palsy. This is fortunately rare.

A frequent cause of a dilated pupil, especially in young adults, is purposeful or accidental use of a mydriatic agent such as atropine. The nurse who rubs her eyes after administering such a drug or someone who uses a roommate's eye drops may present with a widely dilated pupil and have trouble focusing for near vision. A second common cause of pupil asymmetry is Adie's tonic pupil. This is a benign denervation of the parasympathetic innervation of the iris sphincter, occasionally associated with trauma. Sometimes the smaller pupil is the pathologic one, as with Horner's syndrome. Old photographs often help in establishing the real time of onset. See the flowchart for a differential diagnosis of pupil asymmetry (Fig. 31.6).

Diagnosis

Elicit a history of the onset of pupil changes and associated pain or trouble reading. Visual acuity for near objects should be measured, as well as visual acuity for distant objects. Asymmetries of the pupil size should be assessed in bright light, room light, and dim light. The illumination under which the pupillary asymmetry is most marked indicates which eye is abnormal and whether the pathology is in the sphincter control system (parasympathetic) of one eye or the dilator control system (sympathetic) of the other eye.

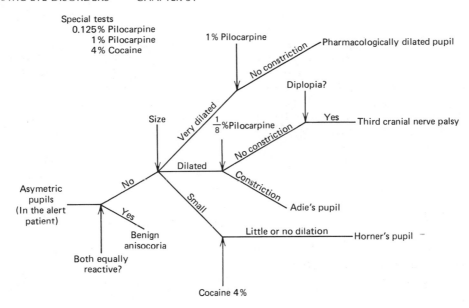

Figure 31.6 Flow chart of differential diagnosis for causes of asymmetric pupils in alert patients.

During an evaluation for an abnormal pupil, the following considerations must be borne in mind:

1. Pilocarpine 0.125% will not constrict a normal eye but will constrict an Adie's pupil.
2. Pilocarpine 1% will constrict a normal eye but will not constrict an atropinized eye.
3. Cocaine 4% will not easily dilate a Horner's pupil.

Therapy

In the absence of accompanying neurologic signs, none of the above diagnoses requires therapy or urgent referral unless there is suspicion of a third cranial nerve palsy with a dilated pupil. In such a case, even if the patient is a known diabetic, she or he should be immediately referred to a neurosurgeon because of the possibility of a posterior communicating artery aneurysm. Such an aneurysm can often be successfully clipped.

Optic Disc Abnormalities

There exists a myriad of optic disc abnormalities, some congenital, such as tilted disc or staphyloma, others that develop with the onset of adulthood, such as optic drusen or myopic degeneration and still others that manifest a new onset of pathology. It is only this latter group that needs to be addressed by the emergency room physician. There remains a dictum that the visual field always matches the disc findings. Unfortunately, this can only hold true for carefully done fields on a tangent screen or Goldman perimeter by an experienced perimetrist. This is usually not possible in the emergency room. Nonetheless, fairly reliable, if not detailed, fields can be obtained by confrontation techniques. In this method, the examiner faces the patient, who has one eye occluded. The examiner closes his or her own opposite eye and looks directly at the patient's open eye to confirm fixation. The patient is asked to fix on the tip of the examiner's nose. The patient is then asked if he or she can see all parts of the examiner's face *equally well*. The patient may note that one ear is darker than the other, which would suggest a paracentral scotoma. The examiner then holds his or her fingers in each quadrant of the periphery and asks the patient to count the total number of fingers presented. Take into account the patient's refractive error and correction (e.g., cataract glasses produce a ring scotoma).

PAPILLEDEMA

In papilledema, the disc appears swollen and congested (Plate 24). There are no spontaneous venous pulsations. The disc margins and marginal vessels are blurred. There are usually hemorrhages about the disc. The condition is almost always bilateral, though one can be fooled especially if the "normal" flat disc is in an eye with very poor vision. Papilledema entails high CSF pressure and represents a neurologic as well as ophthalmic emergency (it may lead to loss of vision).

PAPILLITIS

In papillitis, the optic disc may appear hyperemic (Plate 16). There may be an unusually large number of fine blood vessels spreading from the disc onto the retina. Central visual loss may be profound. The process is usually uniocular. Occasionally we can see cells in the vitreous over the disc. Papillitis may be just an anterior form of optic neuritis.

ISCHEMIC OPTIC NEURITIS

Ischemic optic neuritis is a vascular problem usually affecting only a segment of the optic disc. Thus there often is an altitudinal visual field loss. The disc characteristically is pale, slightly swollen, and seen in conjunction with peripapillary splinter hemorrhages. Often, subsequent vascular accidents will compromise the fellow disc.

OPTIC DRUSEN

Optic drusen are hyalinelike bodies embedded in the disc substance. They may give the appearance of a "lumpy" swollen disc and can produce visual field defects often seen as a Bjerrum scotoma or an enlarged blind spot.

CENTRAL RETINAL VEIN AND ARTERY OCCLUSION

These have been previously discussed.

DISC CUPPING

Disc cupping may be "physiologic," in which case it is usually mild, bilateral, and not associated with visual field defects. Marked disc cupping (Plate 25) is pathologic and is usually seen in open-angle glaucoma, a progressive insidious disease not usually seen in the emergency room. In such an eye, it is particularly important that the intraocular pressure be measured (see procedures section) and that the patient be referred to an ophthalmologist.

Fluoroscein angiography performed by the ophthalmologist often contributes to the differential diagnosis of the swollen disc.

SELECTED READINGS

Chandler PA, Grant WM: *Lectures on Glaucoma*. Philadelphia, Lea & Febiger, 1965.

Cogan DG: *Neurology of the Visual System*. Springfield, Ill, Charles C Thomas Publisher, 1966

Duane TD (ed): *Clinical Ophthalmology*. Hagerstown, Md, Harper & Row Publishers Inc, 1980, Vol 1–5.

Gass JDM: *Stereoscopic Atlas of Macular Diseases: A Fundoscopic and Angiographic Presentation*. St. Louis, The CV Mosby Co, 1977.

Goldberg MF (ed): *Genetic and Metabolic Eye Disease*. Boston, Little Brown & Co, 1974, chaps 5 and 6.

Havener WH: *Ocular Pharmocology*, ed 3. St. Louis, The CV Mosby Co, 1974

Hogan JM, Alvarado JA, Weddell JE: *Histology of the Human Eye*. Philadelphia, WB Saunders Co, 1971.

Rubin ML: *Optics for Clinicians*, ed 2. Gainesville, Fla, Scientific Publishers, 1974.

Schlaegal TF Jr: *Essentials of Uveitis*. Boston, Little Brown & Co, 1969.

Walsh FB, Hoyt WF: *Clinical Neuro-Ophthalmology*, ed 3. Baltimore, The Williams & Wilkins Co, 1969, vols 1–3.

Yanoff M, Fine BS: *Ocular Pathology*. Hagerstown, Md, Harper & Row Publishers Inc, 1975.

Zinn KM: *The Pupil*. Springfield, Ill, Charles C Thomas Publisher, 1972.

32

ACUTE NONTRAUMATIC DISORDERS OF THE EAR, FACIAL STRUCTURES, AND UPPER AIRWAY

Edward E. Jacobs, Jr.
Leonard B. Kaban

Approximately 20% of primary care problems are related to the head and neck. Fortunately, this region is easily examined with instruments commonly found in emergency rooms and primary care facilities. In most cases, plain films of the head and neck are sufficient to aid in the confirmation of a diagnosis. With few exceptions, most diagnoses can be made with the help of routine laboratory tests. Therefore most problems in the head and neck area can be managed initially by the primary care physician. Follow-up of routine problems and more complete evaluations can be performed by the otolaryngologist or dentist whenever a difficult problem arises.

EXAMINATION OF FACIAL STRUCTURES

Facial structures are evaluated by inspection, palpation, and transillumination. In general, the facial region is inspected for symmetry, erythema, or obvious swelling that is related to soft tissue or underlying structures such as sinuses. Palpation of the face is done to elicit tenderness overlying specific sinuses, the temporomandibular joints, and orbital structures (Fig. 32.1). Frontal sinus tenderness may be elicited by applying gentle pressure along the medial floor of the frontal sinus and pressing superiorly with the index finger; ethmoid sinus tenderness may be appreciated by palpating over the superior and lateral aspects of the nose on the affected side; and maxillary sinus tenderness may be observed by palpating over the anterior and

lateral aspects of the maxillary sinus. Percussion of the involved sinuses, performed with index or middle finger with minimal force, may also elicit tenderness. If sinusitis is suspected, transillumination is performed in a darkened room; it may be accomplished with the otoscope if a transilluminating light is not available. To examine the frontal sinuses, the light source is placed on the skin in the supraorbital region, and the left and right frontal sinus area illumination is compared (Fig. 32.2). The maxillary sinuses are transilluminated by placing the light source on the skin over the maxillary sinus in its anterior aspect and viewing the inferior aspect of the sinus through the patient's open mouth. The left and right maxillary sinus transillumination is compared. Decreased transillumination in an involved sinus is considered to be a positive sign for sinus opacification and sinusitis. Radiographic confirmation of this finding is indicated since transillumination is not as reliable as the plain sinus films.

Physical Examination

SALIVARY GLANDS

The parotid gland is examined by palpating anterior to and below the auricle. It normally lies anterior to the sternomastoid muscle and posterior to the anterior border of the masseter muscle (Chapter 17, Fig. 17.2). Normally the tip of the index finger can be placed medial to the angle of the mandible in palpating the parotid gland. If the finger does not pass easily into this region, an abnormal parotid gland should be suspected.

The submandibular gland should be palpated directly beneath the ramus of the mandible, midway between the chin and the angle of the mandible. The size and consistency of the submaxillary gland can be determined by bimanual palpation, using the gloved index finger to palpate the floor of the mouth while the opposite hand palpates externally. Tenderness of the gland, a mass within it, or calcification of the duct can usually be detected in this way. The parotid and submaxillary glands can be "milked" by massaging externally, thereby expressing saliva from their respective duct orifices intraorally. The character of the saliva expressed from the duct should be noted and any purulent discharge should be cultured.

ORAL CAVITY AND PHARYNX

Examination of the oral cavity and pharynx is best performed with the patient in an upright position. A wooden tongue depressor and a light source are used to inspect the tongue, oral mucosa, Stensen's and Wharton's duct orifices, teeth, floor of the mouth, palatine tonsils, palate, and pharynx. Care should

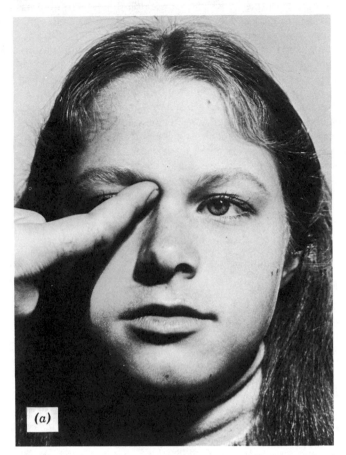 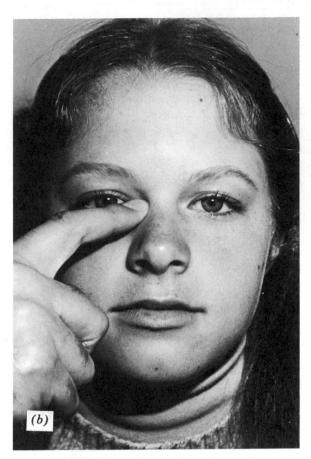

Figure 32.1 Palpation of (a) frontal sinus, (b) ethmoid sinus, and (c) maxillary sinus. Unilateral sinusitis usually produces marked differences in tenderness when comparing left and right sides. Percussion of sinuses may also elicit marked tenderness when compared to the normal side.

be taken to avoid touching the posterior third of the tongue with the depressor since this will elicit the gag reflex. When the patient elevates the anterior portion of the tongue, the floor of the mouth and the frenulum can be seen. The submaxillary (Wharton's) duct from each side has its orifice near the base of the frenulum in the sublingual papilla (Fig. 32.3). The parotid (Stensen's) duct orifice may be seen on the buccal mucosa opposite the upper second molar on each side. As described above, saliva can be expressed from the Wharton's or Stensen's duct orifice by massaging the submaxillary or parotid gland, respectively.

The teeth may be inspected for obvious carries and can be easily percussed with a wooden tongue depressor in order to test for tenderness associated with periapical or other dental infection. The palatine tonsils and pharyngeal mucosa can be easily inspected and any sign of inflammation, exudate, or ulceration noted. The apparent size of the tonsils is usually unimportant unless there is marked asymmetry or massive enlargement producing airway obstruction.

NOSE

Examination of the nose is best accomplished when the patient is in a sitting position and by using a headlight and nasal speculum. Children under the age of 10 frequently object to being examined with a nasal speculum; an alternative method of examining the anterior 2 cm of the nasal septum in a child is to place the four fingers of one hand on the frontal region and gently lift the tip of the nose with the thumb, thereby exposing the interior of the nose. If a nasal speculum is used,

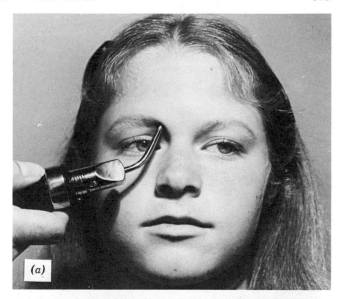

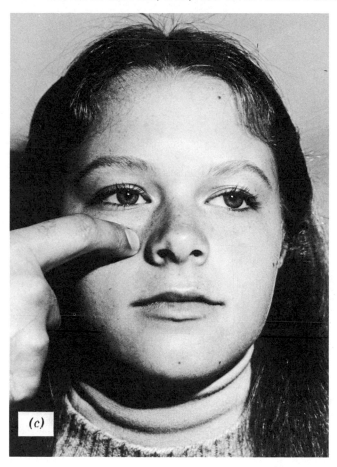

Figure 32.1 (*continued*)

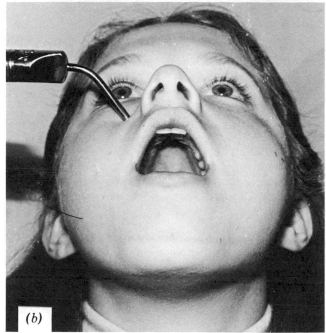

care should be taken to avoid touching the nasal septum with the tips of the speculum blades and to avoid opening the speculum blades too widely since both of these maneuvers may cause unnecessary pain (Fig. 32.4). If nasal discharge or epistaxis is the problem, the Frazier suction may be used to aspirate secretions or blood gently in order to obtain a better view of the nasal cavity. If inspection of the deeper portions of the nasal cavity is desired, spray the nose with 0.25 or 0.5% phenylephrine (Neo-Synephrine) solution and wait 10 minutes for vasoconstriction and decongestion of the nasal mucosa. If the nasal septum is not markedly deviated, the observer may see the entire length of the cavity and can easily see the nasal portion of the soft palate move into view when the patient repeats the letter "K" several times.

A headlight or head mirror greatly aids in the examination

Figure 32.2 Transillumination of (*a*) frontal sinus and (*b*) maxillary sinus. Unilateral sinusitis of the maxillary antrum frequently produces decreased transillumination of the affected side when viewing the intensity of the light that appears intraorally in the region of the palate. In contrast, asymmetric frontal sinus transilluminations may also be due to variations in the size and shape of the left and right frontal sinuses. Transillumination should be accomplished in a darkened room with a small, intense light source. The standard otoscope may be used.

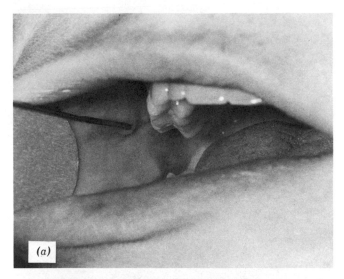

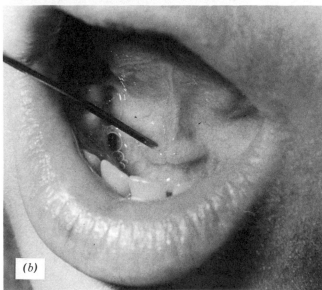

Figure 32.3 Parotid duct (Stenson's) and submaxillary gland duct (Wharton's) orifices. (a) Probe in Stenson's duct; (b) Probe in Wharton's duct.

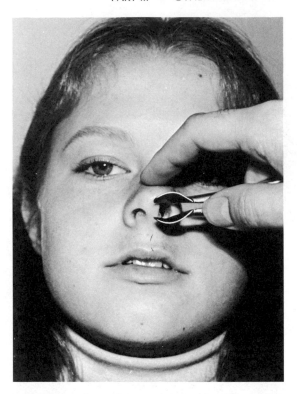

Figure 32.4 A nasal speculum gently inserted into the nostril is stabilized with the index finger on the nasal tip. Inspection reveals anterior nasal septum medially and anterior aspect of inferior turbinate laterally. Normally the septum is in the midline, the left and right turbinates are about equal in size, there is no intranasal discharge, the space between the inferior turbinate and the nasal septum is 1–2 mm, and the lining has a moist, pale red appearance similar to normal oral mucosa.

of the headlight allows the examiner to have both hands free for instrumentation. This is especially valuable in the treatment of epistaxis. If a headlight is unavailable, then a handheld flashlight or a head mirror may be used to aid in the nasal examination.

EAR

The ear examination is best accomplished when the patient is in a sitting position. An infant may be stabilized in the supine position after wrapping the child in a blanket to control movement of the extremities. A small child may be examined by having the child sit on the parent's lap with the child's legs trapped between the parent's legs and the child's arms and hands restrained by the parent's hands. An assistant is usually

of the nasal cavity (Fig. 32.5a–c). The best view is obtained when the headlight is positioned low on the forehead near the examiner's glabella and the light beam is directed straight ahead between the forward-looking visual axis of the examiner. In this way, coaxial vision is possible along the light beam. Use required to stabilize the child's head during an otoscopic examination of the ear. The otoscope is used for examining the ear canal and tympanic membrane (Fig. 32.5 *d, e*). Care should be taken to insert the ear speculum gently into the canal after gently straightening the ear canal by pulling upward and posteriorly on the auricle. Observers should note the caliber of the external ear canal, the nature of the skin of the ear canal, and whether any foreign bodies are present. The landmarks of the tympanic membrane, including the long process of the malleus and the color and consistency of the tympanic membrane, should be noted (Fig. 32.6).

The whisper test is a rapid and useful screening assessment

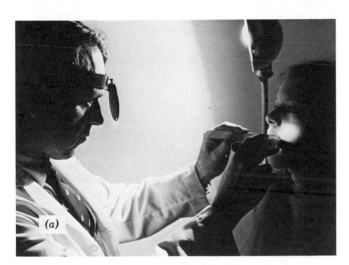
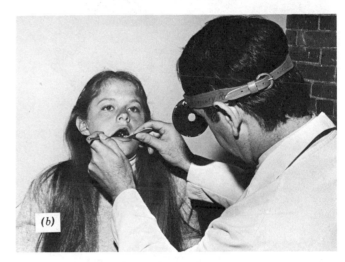

Figure 32.5 (*a*) Examination of the nasopharynx, hypopharynx, larynx, ear canal, and tympanic membrane. If a head mirror is used, a fixed light source located near the patient's head is necessary to provide adequate illumination. The head mirror is positioned in front of the observer's stronger eye and is adjusted so that the reflected light is cast forward directly to the place where the stronger eye is gazing through the central head mirror hole. Ideally, the head mirror shadows both eyes from the direct rays of light from the source, and the examiner's head is held upright with the field of gaze directly forward and both eyes open. A head-mounted light source also enables the examiner to use both hands to hold instruments and to cast the light beam deeply into the nose or pharynx directly in the line of vision. With the head erect and gaze forward, the light and the eyes should be parallel to the floor so that the observer has coaxial vision using one or both eyes to look along the light beam. (*b*) Examination of the nasopharynx is accomplished by depressing the tongue with a tongue blade and gently inserting a small mirror behind the free border of the soft palate without touching the tongue or the posterior pharyngeal wall. The mirror may be rotated to provide a view of the nasopharynx in this way. (*c*) Indirect mirror examination of the hypopharynx and larynx may be achieved by holding the patient's tongue forward with a dry sponge using gentle traction. The patient is instructed to pant through the mouth and to project the chin slightly forward during this maneuver. The laryngeal mirror should be warmed to body temperature with hot water or by brief contact with a light bulb to prevent fogging of the mirror. The mirror is held against the uvula and angled at approximately 45 deg to view the epiglottis, true vocal cords, and hypopharynx. (*d*) Otoscopic examination of the ear is accomplished by gently inserting the otoscope tip into the ear canal while gently retracting the auricle superiorly and posteriorly. The observer should view the ear canal through the otoscope while inserting this instrument to ensure that no pain is caused by intrusion too far into the ear canal. When the otoscope is in place it is not necessary to retract the auricle. (*e*) Pneumatic otoscopy of the ear is accomplished with a closed-head otoscope and a small pneumatic bulb attachment that allows the examiner to massage the tympanic membrane pneumatically. Repetitive insufflation of small bursts of air allows the examiner to view the to-and-fro excursions of the tympanic membrane, thereby determining whether normal mobility is present.

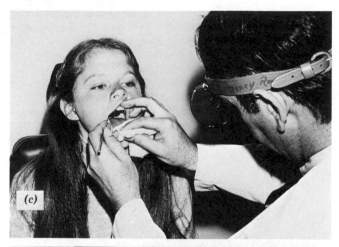

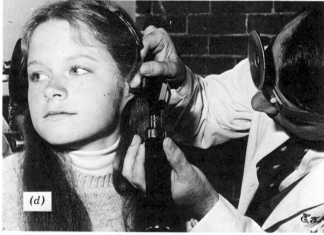

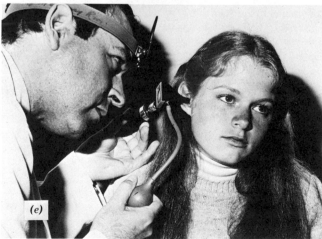

Figure 32.5 (continued)

of hearing acuity in the speech range and may be performed without special equipment and in ambient noise conditions. The test consists of covering one ear, having the examiner whisper a test word into the patient's other ear, and asking the patient to repeat the test word to the observer. Common phonetically balanced test words such as "hot dog," "cowboy," "ice cream," and "baseball" are whispered at first inaudibly and then with gradually increasing intensity until the observer hears the test word with his or her own ear. Assuming that the observer has normal hearing, the patient should hear the test word before the intensity is increased to the point where the observer hears the test word. If the observer hears the test word before the patient, the patient's hearing is abnormally decreased. The advantage of this test is that background noise will have the same masking effect on both the subject and the observer. This test does not detect high-frequency hearing loss (i.e., above 4,000 cps) or decreases in single-frequency thresholds since the test word is a multifrequency stimulus with an average intensity for all of the frequencies covered.

Otoscopic examination of the ear may be difficult or impossible if there is a large amount of wax in the ear. If examination of the eardrum is not necessary at the time of the emergency visit, the patient should be started on glycerin and peroxide drops (Debrox) twice a day and should be seen again in approximately 10 days for removal of wax. If it is necessary to clean out the earwax, the best method is to syringe the ear gently with body-temperature water using an ear syringe or a bulb syringe, taking care to keep the nozzle point from entering the ear canal at any time. Unless the physician has experience in mechanical removal of wax from the ear using a wax curet, curettage is not recommended because of the possibility of damage to the ear canal or the tympanic membrane.

Radiographic Examinations

Radiographic examinations may be performed in the emergency room or primary care setting to further evaluate a patient's head and neck problems. In general, plain films of the sinuses, neck, and nasal bones are the most commonly ordered films that are used to assist primary care personnel in evaluations. Less commonly, plain films of the mandible, dental structures, temporomandibular joints, and mastoid bones are used to supplement the findings on physical examination in order to arrive at a diagnosis.

Sinus films generally consist of four projections—Caldwell, Waters, base, and lateral—that provide a composite visualization of the soft tissue and bony structures of the face (Fig. 32.7). Sinus films are helpful in cases of suspected sinusitis, sinus neoplasms, and facial bone fractures. The Caldwell view is helpful in identifying frontal and ethmoid sinusitis and pos-

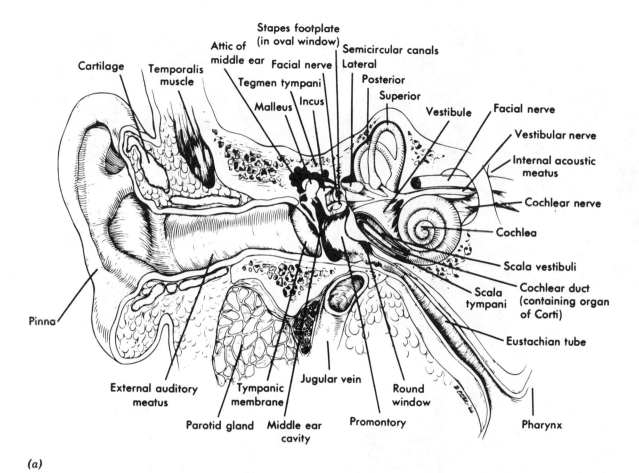

Figure 32.6 (a) Coronal section of the ear with normal anatomy. (b) Otoscopic view of left tympanic membrane with normal anatomy. (Used with permission from Saunders WH, Paparella MM and Miglets AW: *Atlas of Ear Surgery*, ed. 3. St. Louis, C.V. Mosby Co., 1980.)

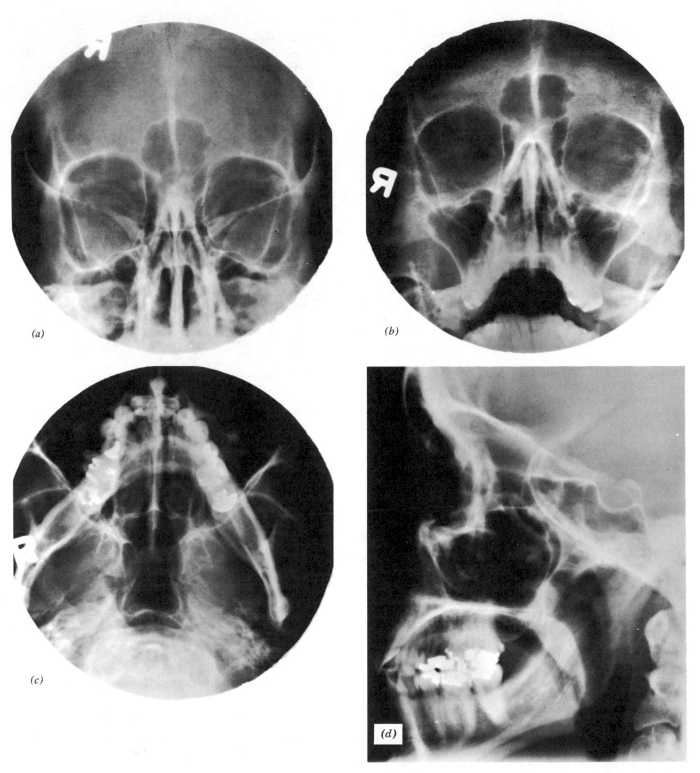

terior orbital floor fractures. The Waters view is valuable in documenting maxillary sinusitis and fractures involving the zygoma, orbital rim anteriorly, and maxilla. The base view helps to visualize the maxillary sinuses and the zygomatic arches along with the nasopharynx and sphenoid sinus. The lateral view is used to provide visualization of the nasopharynx, ethmoid sinuses, and sphenoid sinuses. In general, sinus films should be viewed with respect to symmetry of the bony structures and whether there is opacification that lateralizes to one side or the other. Not infrequently, there are anatomical variations that produce normal differences in the density of the two frontal sinuses and the two sphenoid sinuses.

The lateral and anteroposterior neck films are indicated in cases of airway obstruction, suspected foreign body, dysphagia, and neck trauma. When ordering these films, it is important to specify that soft tissue detail is desired since too much penetration in the radiographic technique will prevent adequate visualization of the soft tissues. The anteroposterior view is helpful in visualizing the cervical trachea, subglottic area, and vocal cords and may be used to document subcutaneous emphysema in cases of suspected trauma (Fig. 32.8). The lateral view is used to visualize the base of the tongue, epiglottis, glottis, infraglottis, trachea, and cervical esophagus.

Nasal bone plain films are ordered in cases of nasal trauma or suspected nasal fracture. In these cases, nasal bone films should be ordered routinely to document nasal bone or maxillary fractures with or without displacement. Not all nasal fractures can be demonstrated on radiographic examinations, and clinical judgment is required to make the diagnosis of nasal fracture in addition to the radiographic findings. The nasal bone films are important documentations of the existence of a nasal fracture and should be ordered whenever this diagnosis is entertained.

Less frequently ordered plain films include mandibular, floor of mouth, orthopantomograph, (mandibular and dental), in-

dividual dental (bitewing), temporomandibular joint views and mastoid series. Mandibular films are ordered in cases of suspected fracture, neoplasm, or infectious invasion of the mandible. Dental films are helpful in identifying periapical abscesses and traumatic dental injuries. Temporomandibular joint films are usually interpreted as being within normal limits unless there is severe derangement of the temporomandibular

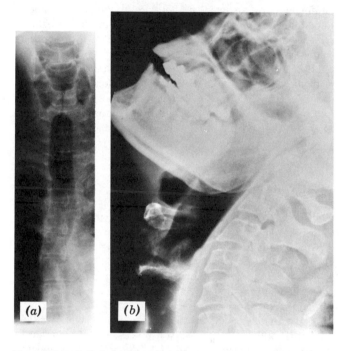

Figure 32.8. Soft tissue films of the upper airway. (a) The anteroposterior soft tissue view of the neck shows the tracheal air column and the vocal cords. Just inferior to the vocal cords are the symmetrical shoulders of the subglottic region, which angle sharply laterally to merge with the tracheal walls in the healthy patient. In cases of laryngotracheitis (croup) the normal sharp angulation is lost and there is a much more gradual funneling of the shoulders into the tracheal region. Tracheal obstruction and intratracheal foreign bodies may be seen on this view. (b) Soft tissue lateral view of the neck. The parallel tracheal walls, dark ventricular shadow immediately above the true vocal cords, and epiglottis superiorly are best seen on this view. The epiglottis is usually thin and may be slightly curved. The inlet to the larynx at the base of the epiglottis is usually about one-half the diameter of the tracheal lumen diameter. The thyroid cartilage and hyoid bones may have varying degrees of calcification in the healthy patient and may lead to a source of confusion in trying to determine the presence of a foreign body in this region. Normally, there is no air in the cervical esophagus, and the presence of an air shadow in this area indicates the likelihood of a retained foreign body.

Figure 32.7. Normal films of the paranasal sinuses. (a) The Caldwell projection. The frontal and ethmoid sinus and posterior orbital floors are seen to best advantage on this view. Differences in apparent opacification of the left and right frontal sinuses may be a result of fluid collection or to anatomical differences in sinus cavity depth or thickness of the frontal or posterior bony walls of the sinuses. (b) The Waters projection. The maxillary sinuses, anterior infraorbital rims, zygomas, bony nasal arch, and nasal septum are usually seen best on this view. (c) The base view helps to localize pathology in the nasopharynx, maxillary, and sphenoid sinuses. (d) The lateral projection is the best view to examine the nasopharynx, sphenoid sinus, and anterior and posterior walls of the frontal sinuses.

joints, which is clinically identifiable. Plain films of the mastoid are used less frequently to confirm the presence of mastoiditis, having been replaced by polytomographic films of the temporal bones. However, mastoid films may be ordered if polytomographic films are unavailable.

Special radiographic studies, including salivary gland sialography to document salivary duct stricture or calculus and specific salivary gland lesions, are usually ordered as specific examinations by a specialist after careful clinical evaluation. Sialography is contraindicated for patients with acute infections of the salivary glands and should be postponed for approximately 4 weeks after the acute inflammatory episode. Laryngeal fluoroscopy, barium swallow, and polytomographic studies of the ear, sinuses, and trachea are usually not ordered when the patient is in the emergency setting. Other special studies (e.g., computed tomography and ultrasonography) are generally reserved for more sophisticated diagnostic evaluations in the nonemergency setting.

FACIAL PAIN AND SWELLING

Acute facial pain associated with swelling most commonly occurs with facial trauma with or without facial fractures and with advanced infection of the paranasal sinuses, nose, orbits, salivary glands, and oral cavity structures, including teeth, tongue, and floor of the mouth. Chronic pain and swelling are more frequently associated with neoplasia and occasionally with an inflammatory process.

Facial pain may occur alone or in combination with swelling of intraoral and external facial soft tissues. Facial pain that is not associated with swelling is usually due to localized inflammation of the deeper facial structures, such as the paranasal sinuses, nasal cavity, and teeth, and frequently will be accompanied by other symptoms, such as localized tenderness, nasal obstruction, rhinorrhea, and intraoral bleeding, which help to define the etiology. Occasionally, facial pain is caused by dysfunction of cranial nerves after trauma or infection or may occur idiopathically; trigeminal, sphenopalatine, auriculotemporal, glossopharyngeal, and other neuralgias may occur in the absence of physical abnormalities. Less frequently, facial pain may be referred from an adjacent or distant site (e.g., eye, temporomandibular joint, or larynx).

Facial swelling without pain is usually localized to the soft tissues of one region. Acute or recurrent swelling confined to the parotid or submaxillary (submandibular) gland area suggests salivary duct obstruction. In contrast, acute swelling not localized to salivary glands is usually due to allergic reactions, minor trauma, or insect bites. Chronic painless swelling commonly is due to benign and malignant neoplasms, enlarged lymph nodes, and more rarely, to indolent infections (e.g., actinomycosis and tuberculosis).

Because facial pain and/or swelling may be related to significant pathology, a careful history and physical examination of the facial structures and oral cavity, together with appropriate radiographic and laboratory studies, are indicated to evaluate and manage patients with these symptoms (Fig. 32.9).

Sinusitis

Sinusitis of the maxillary, ethmoid, frontal, or sphenoid sinus may occur singly or in combination. It may be caused by obstructing nasal pathology alone, allergic inflammation of the sinus mucosa, or frank infection. It is usually associated with inflammation of the nose (rhinitis) but may occur in the absence of nasal congestion and pain. Acute sinusitis usually produces a feeling of pressure and tenderness localized to the involved sinus. It may be associated with referred pain to the retroorbital area, vertex, ear, occiput, or teeth. These symptoms may be a result of obstruction of the paranasal sinus osteum, acute inflammation of the sinus mucosa alone, or suppuration within the sinus.

Acute rhinosinusitis occurs more frequently in people who smoke cigarettes and people exposed to high-density air pollution (e.g., firefighters or chemical workers) during the winter months. Patients with known allergic symptoms (e.g., sneezing and watery rhinorrhea) are more likely to suffer from nasal obstruction because of hyperplastic nasal mucosa and polyps together with allergic and obstructive sinusitis, which may be complicated by acute episodes of infectious sinusitis. Sinusitis occurs less frequently in children under the age of 15 and may be associated with nasal obstruction (nasal polyposis, cystic fibrosis, hyperplastic adenoids) or as part of an allergic constellation of symptoms.

DIAGNOSIS

Typically, the patient complains of increasing pain, beginning in the morning after arising, which lasts most of the day. The pain is increased by placing the head in the dependent position and by straining. The pain commonly is of a steady dull nature but may be throbbing in quality and quite severe. Malaise, lethargy, and dizziness may be associated symptoms. There may be soft tissue swelling over the involved sinus, and decreased transillumination may suggest the presence of pus. Body temperature usually is minimally elevated to 37.5°C or 38.5°C (100°F or 101°F); the white blood cell count commonly is not increased although a moderate leukocytosis is the rule.

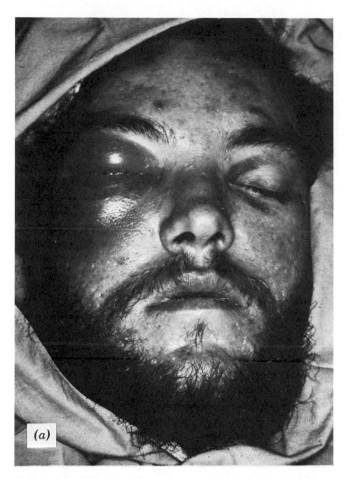

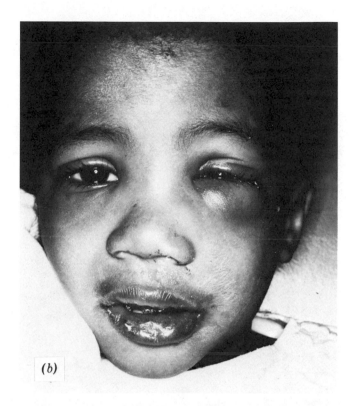

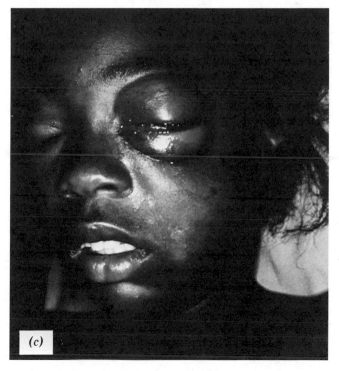

Figure 32.9 Differential diagnosis of facial swelling. (a) Periorbital infection secondary to trauma. (b) Periorbital cellulitis secondary to skin infection. (c) Periorbital cellulitis secondary to an infected maillary tooth. (d) Periorbital and cheek swelling and infection secondary to infected maxillary molar tooth and sinusitis. (e) Ludwig's angina secondary to an infected mandibular molar.

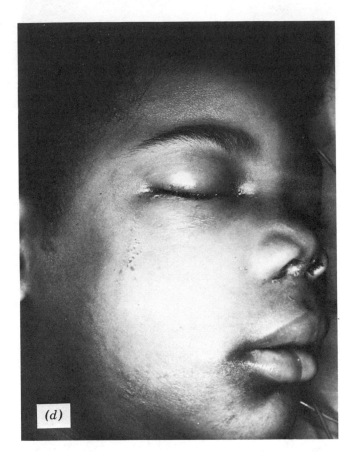

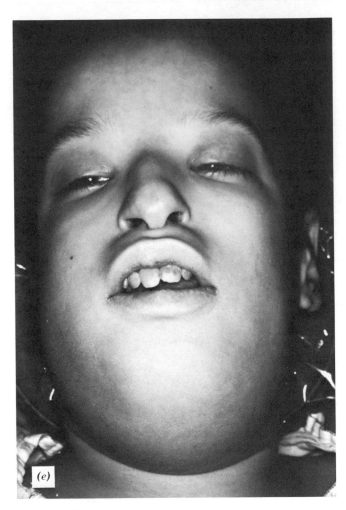

Figure 32.9 (continued)

Sinusitis may be complicated by intracranial or intraorbital extension with or without osteomyletitis. Proptosis, decreased occular mobility, or visual defects are signs of orbital cellulitis or abscess.

Frontal sinusitis may be associated with exquisite tenderness on palpation of the supraorbital region medially (floor of the frontal sinus) or on gentle percussion directly over the frontal sinus. Ethmoid sinusitis is commonly associated with edema of the adjacent upper eyelid. Particularly in children, isolated acute upper eyelid swelling, without ocular findings, may be the earliest sign of ethmoiditis. Sphenoid sinusitis usually oc-

curs with inflammation of the other sinuses or nasopharynx. Pain from the sphenoid sinus often is referred to the vertex or occiput.

Maxillary sinusitis, in addition to localized pain, may refer pain to the upper teeth. Conversely, upper dental problems (e.g., periapical abscesses) may be the source of isolated sinusitis in the adjacent maxillary antrum. Since the maxillary teeth from the premolars to the third molar all communicate with the maxillary sinus, acute maxillary sinusitis may present in a similar fashion to acute odontogenic infection in the maxilla. There are several differences, however: (1) pain and tenderness to percussion in all the teeth in the maxillary quadrant is usually evidence of involvement of the sinus; (2) purulent drainage around all the teeth is also evidence of sinus involvement; (3) an air–fluid level on a Water's film also indicates maxillary sinus involvement, which may be primary or secondary to odontogenic infection.

TREATMENT

Humidification

General treatment measures for sinusitis are directed toward relieving obstruction of the sinus ostea and nasal cavities in order to promote intranasal drainage, since inspired air with low relative humidity increases nasal mucosal congestion. A program for humidification should be recommended to the patient. This may be accomplished by using a cool-mist humidifier or a vaporizer in the bedroom at night and, if possible, in the work area during waking hours. This measure is particularly recommended during cold weather since heated indoor air retains a very low relative humidity. Ideally, the inspired air should have a relative humidity of at least 65%. More intensive humidification can be accomplished by frequent hot showers or by inspiring the water vapor from a pan of boiled water. The latter is accomplished by taking a pan of boiled water to the stove and placing a large bath towel over the head to provide a hooded enclosure over the hot water, which enables a higher concentration of water vapor to be inspired. Each treatment should last for 10–15 minutes and may be repeated at least four times a day.

Decongestants

Oral antihistamines, such as Chlorpheniramine (Chlor-Trimeton) may be prescribed if allergy is suspected as the primary etiology. Sympathomimetic nasal decongestants, such as pseudoephedrine (Sudafed) 30–60 mg, orally, three times a day, may be prescribed if nasal mucosal congestion is a dominant finding. Combination antihistamine–sympathomimetic decongestant medication (e.g., Dimetapp, Actifed, Fedahist) may also be used to promote sinus drainage if an allergic component is suspected.

Topical nasal sprays are useful primarily to diminish nasal mucosal inflammation and to shrink enlarged turbinates, thereby promoting decongestion of the nose. Sympathomimetic sprays (e.g., Neosynephrine 0.25 or 0.5% two sprays in each nostril every 6 hours as needed, or Afrin, two sprays in each nostril every 12 hours as needed provide more immediate relief, but

their use should be limited to 5 days since prolonged use is often associated with a rebound phenomenon, which is a manifestation of loss of nasal vasomotor control. The rebound phenomenon is characterized by reactive nasal mucosal inflammation and turbinate swelling following the initial decongestion caused by the topical sympathomimetic spray. Topical steroids and nasal sprays (e.g., dexamethasone—Turbinaire Decadron—one spray in each nostril four times a day) should be used for more prolonged periods of time and are useful in treating patients with allergic rhinitis as well as nonspecific inflammations of the nose. Aerosol steroid sprays used in recommended dosages are not associated with significant systemic absorption and may be used for several weeks without harmful side effects. The disadvantage of the steroid sprays is that the onset of action may be delayed and therefore relief from nasal obstruction may not occur until 24–48 hours after initiating treatment.

Antibiotics

Specific medical treatment of infectious sinusitis requires the use of antibiotics. Infectious sinusitis is frequently a result of gram-positive (streptococcal, pneumococcal) organisms; however, penicillin-resistant and mixed infections are becoming more prevalent. Initial treatment consists of doxycycline (Vibramycin) 100 mg twice a day for the first day followed by 100 mg every day for 9 days or cephalexin 500 mg orally, three times a day for 10 days. If the patient fails to improve within 24–48 hours, admission to the hospital for intensive intravenous antibiotic therapy is indicated.

Other Considerations

Surgical management of patients with acute and chronic sinusitis and its complications are normally handled by an otolaryngologist and/or an oral surgeon if a dental etiology is evident.

If the maxillary sinus is involved secondary to dental infection, the patient is treated in a manner similar to that for acute alveolar abscess, and the sinusitis will resolve as the dental infection subsides. If the patient has primary sinusitis and pain in the teeth secondary to this, the sinusitis should be treated and the dental pain will subside as the sinusitis resolves.

PROGNOSIS

The prognosis for patients with sinusitis depends on the specific etiology. If sinusitis is due to a chronic condition such as allergy, then complete control of symptoms may or may not occur within several days after institution of treatment. Usually patients with infectious sinusitis will respond to treatment within 48 hours, and complete control of the infection may be expected within 10 days. Occasionally, patients do not respond to oral medication and have to be hospitalized for intravenous therapy and, occasionally, surgical management of the infectious sinusitis. Patients should be instructed to contact an otolaryngologist within 24 hours if their symptoms are progressive despite oral medication and the general treatment measures outlined above.

Salivary Gland Obstruction and Infection

ACUTE OBSTRUCTIVE SIALADENITIS

Acute enlargement of the major salivary glands, parotid and submandibular (submaxillary), most frequently occurs in healthy adults without antecedent symptoms or associated disease. Quite often this problem is caused by acute obstruction of the salivary duct by one or more calculi and to a lesser extent by other pathologic problems such as strictures and neoplasms. Submandibular glands are more frequently involved than are the parotid.

Diagnosis

Typically patients give a history of sudden enlargement beginning at mealtime and localized to the involved gland associated with a feeling of pressure. Usually, there is minimal or no pain associated with these symptoms. These symptoms may subside in several hours, only to recur at mealtimes; occasionally the swelling may persist more chronically. In the case of acute submaxillary sialadenitis, physical examination will reveal erythema and edema in the area of the salivary gland duct and diminished or no salivary flow upon massaging the gland. In some cases, purulent material can be expressed from the duct, and in other cases a stone will be palpable intraorally.

It is recognized that chronic and recurrent salivary obstruction with stasis, because of calculi, strictures, and so on, is associated with an increased incidence of inflammation and infection of the salivary gland parenchyma. Therefore, in an otherwise healthy adult, an acutely inflamed salivary gland must be suspected of having an antecedent ductal abnormality. In contrast, as discussed below, acute salivary inflammation and infection may occur spontaneously in patients with de-creased salivary flow as a result of systemic problems (e.g., dehydration and debilitation).

Films will often reveal a radiopaque stone along the course of the submaxillary duct. A lateral oblique film of the mandible, panoramic view of the mandible, or dental film will show the stone. In the parotid area, a dental film placed on the cheek can often show the stone. Radiographically, it is much more difficult to show a stone in the parotid duct than in the submaxillary duct because of the smaller size of the parotid duct and the interference of other superimposed skeletal structures.

Sialograms should not be done during an acute episode because of the possibility of driving stones more proximally into the duct and the possibility of rupturing small ductules and acini and spreading the infection when the dye is injected under pressure. Three or four weeks after the acute episode is resolved, a sialogram should be done to detect the presence of other stones or strictures in the duct.

Treatment

ANTIBIOTICS.   Since most organisms in obstructive sialadenitis are penicillin sensitive, the drug of choice is penicillin, VK 250–500 mg by mouth every 6 hours. External heat and intraoral warm saline rinses promote resolution of the infection.

REMOVAL OF STONES.   Obstruction of major salivary glands usually does not require emergency treatment in the absence of infection. However, the patient should be referred to a specialist within 24 hours so that the obstruction may be relieved since an obstructed salivary gland frequently becomes infected and may be complicated by abscess formation. The patient should be reassured and referred to an otolaryngologist or oral surgeon for appropriate diagnosis and treatment. No specific emergency treatment is indicated for this condition, but if pain is present, it may be relieved by appropriate analgesics.

ACUTE SUPPURATIVE PAROTITIS

Acute suppurative (sometimes known as *acute postoperative*) parotitis is a distinct clinical entity. It usually occurs in elderly, debilitated, dehydrated patients who may have had a recent surgical procedure. The patient presents with marked preauricular swelling, erythema, and tenderness. Intraorally there is swelling and erythema around the parotid orifice as well as purulent drainage. The patient will have a fever and is often markedly dehydrated. *Staphylococcus aureus* is almost universally responsible for this infection.

Acute suppurative parotitis is a very virulent infection, and before the antibiotic era, carried a very high mortality rate. Patients with this infection must be treated early and aggressively with high dosages of intravenous oxacillin (10–12 g per day in divided doses) or another penicillinase-resistant drug. The purulent drainage from the parotid duct should, of course, be cultured before antibiotics are started, and the patient usually needs to remain on intravenous antibiotics for 10 days. During the course of intravenous therapy it is helpful to dilate the parotid duct and massage the gland in order to promote drainage. The role of the emergency room physician in treating patients with acute suppurative parotitis is to make the diagnosis early, to culture the purulent drainage from the parotid duct, and to see that the patient is admitted to the hospital under the care of a specialist, such as an oral surgeon or otolaryngologist, who will manage the intravenous antibiotics and local care of the gland.

RECURRENT ACUTE PAROTITIS

Recurrent acute parotitis is a salivary gland infection that usually occurs in children from 9 years of age through adolescence. The patient characteristically develops multiple episodes of unilateral or bilateral parotid swelling. They present to the emergency room with pain, erythema, and swelling in the preauricular regions. They may have fever and an elevated white blood cell count. Intraorally, there is usually no purulent drainage from the parotid duct. The organism responsible for recurrent acute parotitis is usually a penicillin-sensitive α-streptococcus. There is no detectable underlying etiology such as a stone or other duct obstruction. The patient usually has multiple episodes of infection during childhood, but usually responds to oral penicillin (1–2 g per day), heat, and sialogogues such as lemon drops to promote salivary flow. Erythromycin, in the same dosage schedule, can be used for patients who are allergic to penicillin. Multiple episodes of acute infection usually subside when the patient is in the late teens, and the only sequelae is the presence of sialangectasis visible on parotid sialograms.

Acute Odontogenic Infection

The most common dental emergency consists of pain related to odontogenic infection, that is, dental caries or periodontal disease. The patients are often treated in the dental office and do not appear in emergency room statistics. Nevertheless, as patients begin to use emergency facilities for many of their primary complaints, an understanding of acute odontogenic

infections is important for the emergency room physician. Since advanced odontogenic infections may spread to adjacent structures, such as the soft tissues of the neck, base of the tongue, larynx, paranasal sinuses, orbits, and salivary glands, the evaluation of a patient with intraoral or facial pain and swelling should include a careful history and intraoral examination.

ACUTE ALVEOLAR ABSCESS

Acute alveolar abscess is the end result of advanced dental caries. The most common organism is *Streptococcus viridans*. When the acute alveolar abscess is accompanied by facial cellulitis, the patient will present with extraoral swelling as well as pain. In the early stages of dental caries, pain is precipitated by thermal or chemical stimuli; in more advanced cases, there may be spontaneous severe pain (acute pulpitis).

In addition to dental caries and loss of tooth structure, intraoral swelling in the gingiva or alveolar mucosa adjacent to the tooth is also present. If a posterior mandibular tooth is involved, the swelling may spread to the lingual side of the alveolar ridge causing elevation of the tongue and floor of the mouth. If this progresses untreated, the lingual swelling will cross the midline and produce the classic signs of Ludwig's angina: severe swelling of the entire floor of the mouth and elevation of the tongue with respiratory obstruction (Fig. 32.9). There may be extraoral swelling overlying the jaw bone. In the maxilla, swelling may spread to the cheek and the periorbital area. Infection may also dissect posteriorly to the area of the pterygomaxillary fissure and the inferior orbital fissure, resulting in orbital cellulitis. Tenderness will be elicited on percussion of the offending tooth, and dental films will reveal a periapical radiolucency at the root of the tooth.

Treatment of acute alveolar abscess consists of (1) surgical drainage if the swelling is fluctuant; (2) removal of the tooth if it is nonrestorable; and (3) antibiotic therapy with penicillin or erythromycin. If the swelling is not fluctuant, the emergency room physician should start the patient on penicillin VK 250–500 mg by mouth every 6 hours and refer the patient to his or her local dentist as soon as possible. If the patient is febrile, dehydrated, and has an elevated white blood cell count, the patient should be admitted for intravenous antibiotic therapy and fluids. Treatment with warm saline intraoral rinses and external heat will help the infection localize or resolve.

PERICORONITIS

Pericoronitis, an extremely common periodontal infection in teenage patients, is an infection in the gingiva around a partially erupted third molar tooth. It occurs because food and bacteria stagnate in the cul-de-sac produced by a flap of gingiva over the partially erupted tooth. The patients commonly present with pain and swelling without any prior history of toothache. The symptoms are usually localized to the mandible in the retromolar area. There will be no evidence of dental caries, but there will be a partially erupted third molar tooth with soft tissue swelling around it. These patients should be treated with penicillin VK 250 mg by mouth every 6 hours and warm saline rinses. They should be seen by an oral surgeon as soon as possible, and once the infection is under control (usually within 48–72 hours), the third molar tooth can be removed. In the penicillin-allergic patient, erythromycin in the same dosage can be used.

ACUTE PERIODONTAL ABSCESS

Acute periodontal abscess is also characterized by pain, swelling, and toothache, particularly when the patient bites down on the tooth. Examination will usually reveal the absence of dental caries, but will show a very mobile tooth with extremely inflammed gingiva and purulent drainage around the tooth. Patients with a periodontal abscess should also be started on penicillin VK 250 mg by mouth every 6 hours and warm saline rinses. The patient should be referred to his or her local dentist for gingival curettage to eliminate the calculus that is usually the underlying cause or for extraction if the tooth is not salvageable.

ACUTE GINGIVAL MUCOUS MEMBRANE CONDITIONS

Vincent's infection (trench mouth, acute ulcerative gingivitis) is characterized by the acute onset of severe pain in gingiva along the teeth, accompanied by swelling and bleeding. Examination will reveal severe edema, erythema, and bleeding in the gingiva around the necks of the teeth, in particular in the areas of the gingival papillae. Some of these gingival papillae may be frankly necrotic, and there will be a white necrotic slough overlying the gingiva.

Vincent's infection often occurs when there is a major anxiety-producing event in the life of the patient such as examinations, engagement, or divorce. The disease most commonly occurs in teenagers and young adults, and the common bacterial organisms are intraoral fusospirochetal bacteria. These patients should be started on penicillin VK 250 mg by mouth every 6 hours and warm saline intraoral rinses. They should be referred to their dentists to have their teeth cleaned within

48 hours to 1 week. There is a complex interrelationship between soft debris around the teeth and the other psychosomatic factors mentioned above in the production of acute Vincent's infection, and, therefore, antibiotics, dental prophylaxis, and some counseling are all required for successful treatment of this infection.

Acute primary herpetic gingival stomatitis is an intraoral mucous membrane disease that usually occurs in young children but may occur in teenagers and young adults. It is caused by the herpes simplex virus. The patients present with severe intraoral pain and necrotic ulcerative lesions that encompass not only the gingivae but the palate, buccal mucosa, tongue, and floor of the mouth. The generalized nature of the inflammatory process and ulcerative lesions distinguish it from Vincent's infection. The patients very often have fever and lymphadenopathy and are dehydrated. The patients are usually treated with a bland diet, intraoral saline rinses for hygiene, and penicillin VK 250 mg by mouth every 6 hours if it looks as though the ulcerative lesions are becoming secondarily infected. For symptomatic treatment for the pain, a mixture of diphenhydramine (Benadryl) (25 mg per 5 ml) and Kaopectate mixed in a ratio of 1:1, with 5 ml of each, may be used as a rinse. This disease, like most viral illnesses, is self-limited, and patients begin to feel better in 7–10 days. In some patients, the disease is so severe that it requires admission to the hospital for intravenous fluid therapy.

Other Causes of Facial Pain or Swelling

TUMORS

We should always keep in mind the fact that intraoral tumors exposed to the contaminated oral environment may often become infected and result in acute facial pain and swelling. If on examination all of the teeth and salivary gland structures look normal, we should suspect any ulcerated or fungating lesion in the area of the intraoral swelling. If the ulcer remains after the inflammatory component has been treated, a biopsy should be done.

ALLERGIES

Allergic swelling of the face may be a result of local reactions (e.g., insect bites or contact dermatitis) or part of a systemic response (e.g., drug reaction). For localized swelling, ice packs may be applied for 24 hours and oral antihistamines (e.g., diphenhydramine 50 mg orally every 8 hours) administered;

in addition, the patient should avoid the suspected offending allergen. If facial swelling is part of a systemic allergic reaction, there may be edema of the tongue, floor of the mouth, pharynx, and larynx, as well as varying degress of airway obstruction. In these cases, maintenance of airway obviously becomes the most important consideration, and endotracheal intubation or cricothyrotomy may be necessary if the process cannot be controlled with subcutaneous administration of 0.3 ml epinephrine 1:1,000 dilution for adults. Intravenous corticosteroids and vigorous cardiopulmonary support may also be required. Parotid and submaxillary glands may swell painlessly and periodically if their ducts are obstructed by calculi or strictures. Characteristically an obstructed gland will swell at mealtimes and may remain distended for several hours or days. The patient with this problem should be referred to a specialist for evaluation and management of the underlying problem.

SOFT TISSUE INFECTIONS

Infections of the soft tissues of the face are usually evident because of localized tenderness, swelling, and erythema. Infected sebaceous or dermal cysts, furuncles, or suppurative lymph nodes are the most common causes of soft tissue infections. The usual pathogen is *Staphylococcus aureus*. A localized infection is fluctuant, and incision and drainage are indicated. Cultures should be taken whenever possible, and the patient should be started on antibiotics for this organism. Dicloxacillin sodium 250 mg orally, four times a day, erythromycin 250 mg orally, four times a day, or cephalexin 250 mg orally, four times a day for 10 days are the drugs of choice. The patient should be advised to apply a heating pad or hot-water bottle to the infected area for 15 minutes four times a day. Appropriate analgesics are also prescribed.

AURICULOTEMPORAL NEURALGIA

Auriculotemporal neuralgia is commonly associated with temporomandibular joint dysfunction (Costen's syndrome). Frequently, patients with this problem will present with an earache; however, not infrequently, referred pain from the temporomandibular joint to the side of the head, jaw, neck, and mastoid region is the presenting complaint. Palpation of the temporomandibular joint when the patient's jaw is open and closed usually demonstrates point tenderness of the joint. Treatment consists of a program of mechanical soft diet, aspirin every 4 hours, and local heat applications four times a day for 5 days. If the pain persists, referral to an oral surgeon is indicated.

TRIGEMINAL NEURALGIA

Trigeminal neuralgia (tic douloureux) is characterized by a history of episodic and sudden lancinating pain in the distribution of the trigeminal nerve. Typically, the pain is elicited by stimulating a trigger point in the mouth or on the face. Patients with this problem should be given analgesics and referred for complete neurologic evaluation and management.

HERPES ZOSTER DERMATITIS

Herpes zoster dermatitis (shingles) may occur along the distribution of any or all of the divisions of the trigeminal nerve. The pain is usually intense, steady, and frequently has a burning quality. Pain may precede appearance of the vesicular rash, which is diagnostic. Patients with suspected herpes zoster along the ophthalmic division of the trigeminal nerve are at risk for corneal herpetic infections and should be referred for evaluation by an ophthalmologist.

ACUTE NASAL PROBLEMS

Patients with acute nasal problems commonly present with symptoms of obstruction, rhinorrhea (discharge), pain, and epistaxis. These symptoms may be associated and may overlap with complaints referable to the adjacent structures (e.g., sinuses and maxillary teeth). Therefore the nose is frequently examined in conjunction with evaluation of these structures.

Epistaxis

Nose bleed is a common problem that usually requires immediate treatment since active bleeding may vary in degree from slight to exsanguinating hemorrhage. Often the patient will arrive in an alarmed state, actively bleeding, with blood clots in both nasal cavities, nauseated at having swallowed an unknown quantity of blood and, less frequently, anemic from blood loss.

Fortunately, 90% of epistaxis cases occur from localized, single arterial bleeding from one side of the anterior nasal septum within 2 cm of the nasal tip; therefore, bleeding can be controlled with relatively simple measures such as cautery or anterior nasal packing. In 10% of the cases in which bleeding is more posterior or the specific origin cannot be located, more active bleeding may require anteroposterior packing and/or surgical ligation of the arterial supply.

Although epistaxis is frequently associated with underlying nasal or systemic disorders, spontaneous nasal hemorrhage commonly occurs without apparent etiology and as an isolated event. This problem is particularly prevalent during the winter months and during periods of excessively dry air. Idiopathic epistaxis occurs in all age groups: children between 5 and 12 years old are the most frequent pediatric patients, but adults over 50 years old are more commonly affected. Almost all pediatric patients have anterior septal epistaxis (frequently associated with rhinitis). Posterior epistaxis, although rare in children, is invariably associated with specific conditions (e.g., postadenoidectomy, nasal trauma, nasopharyngeal angiofibroma, blood dyscrasias). Adults are more likely to have epistaxis associated with other disorders; therefore, when indicated, an appropriate investigation should be undertaken and proper management should be instituted after bleeding is controlled.

Traumatic injuries of the nose and sinuses, including intranasal lacerations, foreign bodies, and fractures frequently cause epistaxis. Facial injuries with paranasal sinus fractures may cause epistaxis as intrasinus hemorrhage escapes into the nasal cavity.

Inflammatory conditions of the nose and sinuses, including all forms of rhinitis and sinusitis, may be associated with epistaxis secondary to the associated hypervascularity that accompanies these conditions.

Abnormalities of the cardiovascular system, particularly in the elderly population, are associated with increased incidence of epistaxis. Commonly, arterial hypertension and atherosclerosis are underlying factors that require concomitant treatment in control of epistaxis. Decreased arteriole elasticity and elevated systolic and diastolic blood pressure predispose patients to spontaneous epistaxis. As expected, patients with these problems typically are elderly and have multisystem abnormalities. Although initial blood pressures for most patients are elevated because of the excitement surrounding acute hemorrhage, in the majority of cases, after control of epistaxis the patient will become normotensive again. If hypertension persists, concurrent control of the hypertension may be necessary to control epistaxis.

Iatrogenic causes such as intranasal trauma (e.g., passage of nasogastric tubes, nasal surgery) or use of drugs with primary or secondary anticoagulent effects (e.g., warfarin, aspirin, phenothiazines) may be associated with epistaxis.

Coagulopathies related to blood dyscrasias (e.g., thrombocytopenia, leukemia, drug ingestion, hepatic and renal disease) may be encountered and may be associated with hemorrhage elsewhere in the body.

Other less common conditions that may present as epistaxis are nasal polyps, benign and malignant tumors of the nose, nasopharynx, and paranasal sinuses, intranasal foreign bodies, hereditary telangiectasias (Rendu-Osler-Weber syndrome), granulomatous disease, and syphilis.

MANAGEMENT

Successful management of epistaxis is achieved by following a simple stepwise procedure using (1) optimal patient position, (2) proper equipment, (3) fundamental knowledge of nasal anatomy, and (4) a treatment method ranging from no treatment to arterial surgery scaled to the severity and location of the epistaxis.

Patient Position

During treatment the patient should be sitting upright in a chair or on a stretcher; the examiner's head should be slightly below the patient's and the patient's head should be tilted forward so that the floor of the nose is inclined anteriorly. This position allows the examiner to see the rate of blood loss and the site of the bleeding and also prevents blood from passing posteriorly into the pharynx. Blood pressure is taken, and if anemia or coagulopathy is suspected, appropriate blood studies are taken (CBC, prothrombin time, partial thromboplastin time, platelet count, bleeding time). The patient should be reassured that in most cases bleeding can be controlled within a few minutes. The patient should be covered with a gown, bib, or towel, and the examiner should also put on a gown to prevent blood staining of clothing. The patient is given several 4-by-4 inch gauze sponges folded once to clinch gently in his or her teeth while breathing through the mouth with open lips. If there are clots in the nose, the patient is asked to blow his or her nose to clear the clots before holding the gauze sponge in the teeth with head inclined forward.

Equipment

A light source (head-mounted light), vacuum suction with narrow tip (e.g., Frazier type), nasal speculum, bayonet forceps, and cotton pledgets dampened with 4% cocaine solution, or a mixture of one part tetracaine 2% (Pontocaine) and one part phenylephrine 0.5% should be available (Fig. 32.10). Cauterization can be best accomplished using silver nitrate sticks. Anterior packing requires approximately 3–12 ft of 0.5- or 1-in. gauze ribbon impregnated with petrolatum or petrolatum-

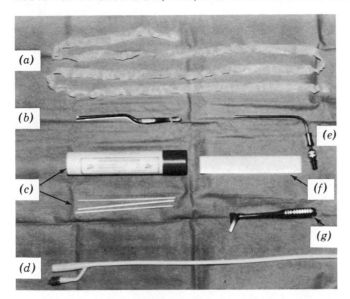

Figure 32.10 (a) 1-inch petrolatum gauze packing; (b) bayonet forceps; (c) silver nitrate sticks; (d) Foley catheter with 30 ml balloon; (e) Frazier's suction tip; (f) cotton strip pledget; (g) nasal speculum.

antibiotic ointment (e.g., bacitracin ointment). Anteroposterior packing, in addition to the anterior packing, requires a No. 16 or No. 18 Foley-type catheter with a 30-ml balloon.

The basic anatomy of the nasal cavity and blood supply is shown in Figure 32.11. The arterial anastomosis (Kisselbach's plexus) supplying the anterior septum (Little's area) is the location of 90% of epistaxis and commonly produces mild-to-moderate hemorrhage. Epistaxis occurring from rupture of the ethmoid or the larger sphenopalatine arteries posteriorly may be more severe and may be exceedingly difficult to identify since the adult nasal cavity is about 9 cm deep. Epistaxis with a source more than 5 cm posterior to the nasal tip should be considered to be posterior for treatment purposes.

Treatment

Treatment of patients with epistaxis may be divided into four steps: (1) localization of bleeding site; (2) initial control of active bleeding; (3) definitive control of bleeding; and (4) follow-up care.

LOCALIZATION OF BLEEDING SITE. The bleeding site may be located by inspecting the nasal cavity with the headlight and nasal speculum after clots are cleared from the nose. In the majority of cases, the bleeding site will be an active arterial bleeder found within 2 cm of the nasal tip on the anterior nasal septum. If no active bleeding is seen on inspection, then a small cotton-tipped applicator may be used to gently rub Kisselbach's area to promote active epistaxis. If no epistaxis can be elicited using this maneuver, the patient may be asked to blow his or her nose forcefully or perform a Valsalva maneuver to raise the blood pressure temporarily. It is important to localize the bleeding site before any measures of control are instituted. If there is no active bleeding, no cauterization should be attempted. In these cases, the patient is usually discharged and instructed to return at the first sign of recurrent epistaxis. In unusual cases in which severe hemorrhage or prolonged or recurrent hemorrhage suggests that the patient's cardiovascular stability is threatened, the patient may be admitted for observation.

If there is active epistaxis and the bleeding site is not in Kisselbach's plexus, the Frazier suction tip is passed from the nasal tip along the floor of the nose posteriorly while inspecting the nasal cavity (Fig. 32.12). The suction tip will remove all of the active blood as it is passed in a posterior direction along the floor of the nose, which is tilted forward. Once the suction tip is more posterior than the origin of the bleeding site, blood will begin to appear at the anterior tip of the nose. At this point if the suction tip is retracted more anteriorly, the blood will again be suctioned into the aspirating tip. In this manner, a rough estimate of the depth of the bleeding site can be made by measuring the length of the suction tip that is in the nasal cavity. If the bleeding site is more than 5 cm from the nasal tip, an anteroposterior pack will be required to control the hemorrhage. If it is less than 5 cm from the nasal tip, an anterior nasal pack will usually control the bleeding.

INITIAL CONTROL OF ACTIVE BLEEDING. Initial control of active bleeding may be accomplished by packing the nasal cavity with cotton pledgets dampened with 4% cocaine or a tetracaine–phenylephrine mixture. The nasal cavity should be packed tightly with the cotton packs so that the nasal mucosa will become anesthetized and adequate vasoconstriction will control the bleeding vessel. The cotton packs are left in place for approximately 10 minutes. If bleeding recurs, the nasal cavity is packed again for another 10 minutes. It is possible to control epistaxis initially by placing cotton pledgets deeply into the nasal cavity to reach areas that cannot be adequately seen but are suspected sites of epistaxis. When using cocaine care should be taken that the total amount does not exceed 200 mg (5 ml 4% cocaine solution) and that cardiopulmonary resuscitation equipment is readily available to treat the patient if any adverse

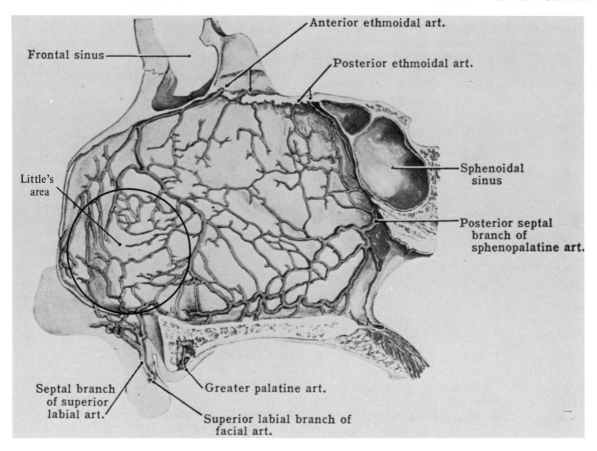

Figure 32.11 Anatomy of the nasal cavity. The location of the arterial blood supply to the nasal septum is shown. The main arterial supply is (a) anterior ethmoidal artery and (b) branches of the sphenopalatine artery. Ninety percent of nose bleeds occur in Little's area within 2 cm of the anterior septal margin. (Used with permission from Grant JCB: *Grant's Atlas of Anatomy, Sixth Edition*. Baltimore, Williams and Wilkins Co, 1972, Figure 607.)

cardiopulmonary or central nervous system reactions to cocaine or tetracaine and sympathomimetics occur. After initial control of active bleeding is accomplished, a more definitive method of control should be instituted. If initial control cannot be accomplished using cotton pledgets, definitive control should be instituted.

DEFINITIVE CONTROL OF BLEEDING.   Cauterization with silver nitrate is usually the first method of choice for definitive control of small bleeding vessels in the anterior nasal septum (Fig. 32.13). Cauterization should be done only after sufficient top-

ical anesthesia has been achieved and should be directed specifically to the bleeding site. Silver nitrate cauterization is less successful when applied to vessels that are actively bleeding and optimally should be applied to bleeding sites that have been controlled with the initial control methods. Cauterization is contraindicated if no specific bleeding site can be found or if there is diffuse mucosal hemorrhage (e.g., blood dyscrasias) since cauterization may produce epistaxis in patients with poor coagulation.

Anterior nasal packing should be attempted if cauterization is unsuccessful in controlling epistaxis or if there is a more

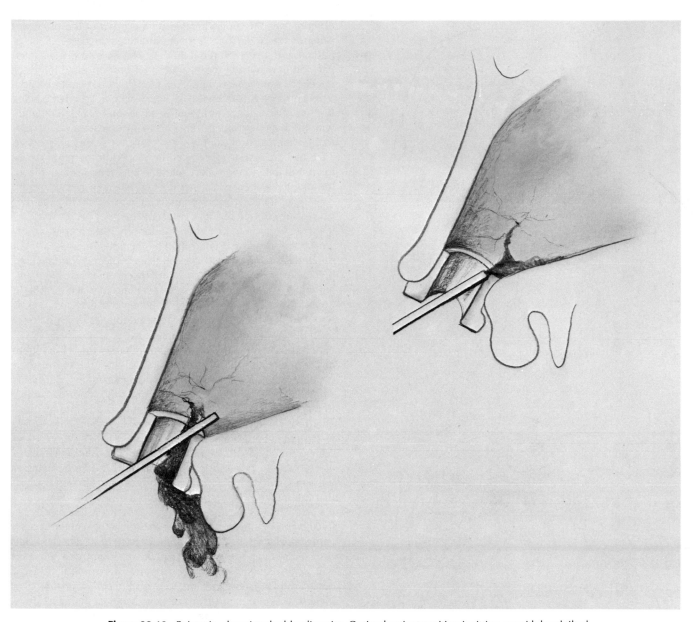

Figure 32.12 Epistaxis—locating the bleeding site. Optimal patient position is sitting up with head tilted forward so that blood runs out the front of the nose and is not swallowed. (a) Using a headlight or headmirror and Frazier suction, the bleeding site is located 90% of the time in Little's area (anterior nasal septum). If the bleeding site is more posterior, the suction tip is advanced posteriorly along the nasal floor until the site is passed and anterior nasal bleeding resumes. When this occurs the depth of the suction tip is noted. If the bleeding site is greater than 5 cm from the nasal tip an anterior–posterior pack will be required; if it is less than 5 cm, an anterior pack will usually control the epistaxis.

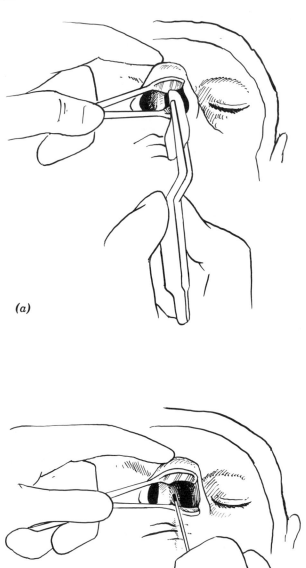

(a)

(b)

Figure 32.13. Control of epistaxis with silver nitrate cautery. After initial control of known epistaxis site with cocaine and cotton packs (a) the packs are removed and (b) the bleeding site is cauterized with silver nitrate sticks. Only known sites are cauterized. Cautery is contraindicated if no bleeding origin can be located.

obscure bleeding point located within 5 cm of the nasal tip. Anterior nasal packing is contraindicated in cases of nasal trauma or if a cerebrospinal fluid (CSF) leak is suspected since packing may increse the chance of cribriform plate injury or infection. Anterior nasal packing alone will not control a posterior epistaxis. Anterior nasal packing is accomplished by placing layered ribbon gauze in the nasal cavity and packing it tightly with the bayonet forceps (Fig. 32.14). In most anterior packs that are properly placed, a minimum of 3 ft and often up to 12 ft of 1-in. ribbon gauze can be placed in the nasal cavity to control anterior epistaxis. After the anterior pack is in place, the mouth is checked to see if there is active hemorrhaging into the nasopharynx and pharynx, which would indicate unsuccessful control of the epistaxis. This may be because of inadequate packing or a more posteriorly placed epistaxis origin. If the bleeding is controlled by the anterior pack, a small dry sterile dressing is placed over the tip of the nose and secured by tape, and the patient may be followed-up as an outpatient. Normally, an anterior pack should remain in place for 48–72 hours. Since epistaxis may recur when the anterior pack is removed, the patient is usually referred to an otolaryngologist for removal of the nasal pack.

Anteroposterior (AP) packing is used when there is a failure of the anterior packing alone to control nasal hemorrhage or when a posterior epistaxis has been diagnosed (Fig. 32.15). A simplified method for achieving an anteroposterior packing is to place a Foley catheter with the 30-ml balloon into the nose after lubricating it with a petrolatum or lubricant jelly. Before inserting the Foley catheter, its tip, distal to the balloon, is cut off and the balloon is tested with water. After sliding the catheter tip to the posterior pharyngeal wall, the Foley catheter balloon is inflated to 20 ml and the catheter is pulled back so that the inflated balloon is lodged in the posterior choana of the nose. While an assistant keeps steady tension on the retracted Foley catheter, the nose is packed with an anterior pack in the usual fashion. After the anterior pack is placed, the Foley catheter is clamped with a urinary catheter clamp or a hemostat that is cushioned from the soft tissues of the nasal tip by a dental roll, a gauze packing, or a short section of tubing to prevent pressure necrosis of the soft tissues of the nasal tip.

Anteroposterior packing may produce significant hypoxia in patients because of edema and depression of the soft palate. Therefore patients are admitted to the hospital and placed under close observation; their heads should be elevated and they should be in a humidified atmosphere. The pharynx is frequently inspected to determine whether active hemorrhaging is occurring in the pharynx posteriorly. Anteroposterior packs are usually kept in place 4 or 5 days before removal by an otolaryngologist. Hemorrhaging on removal of an anteropos-

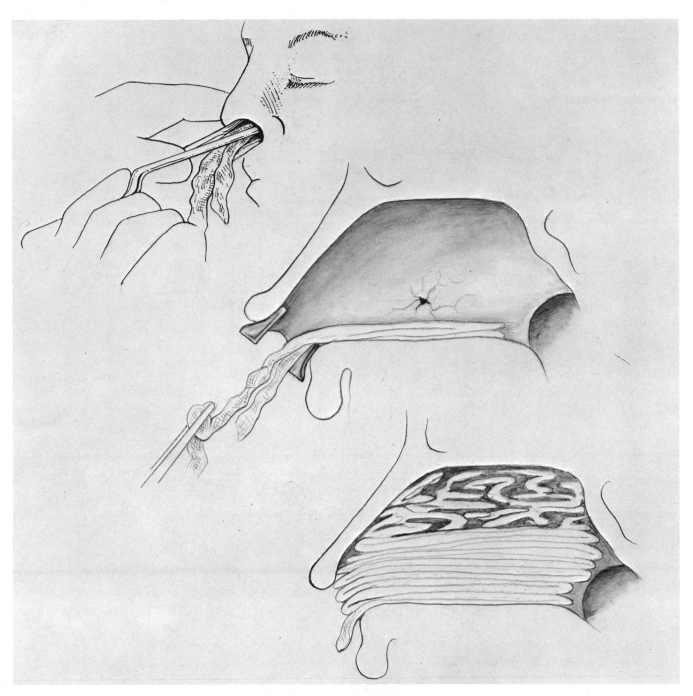

Figure 32.14 Anterior nasal packing is used when cautery is unsuccessful or bleeding is believed to be coming from a location in the anterior 5 cm of the nasal cavity. After topical anesthesia with cocaine, the packs are removed and a ribbon gauze lubricated with petrolatum or antibiotic ointment is inserted in accordion fashion into the nasal cavity with bayonet forceps. Beginning at the nasal floor the gauze is tamped down tightly, taking care to fill the more posterior part of the nasal cavity first. From 3 to 12 ft of ribbon gauze are used for one side of the nose. Bilateral nasal packing is rarely required.

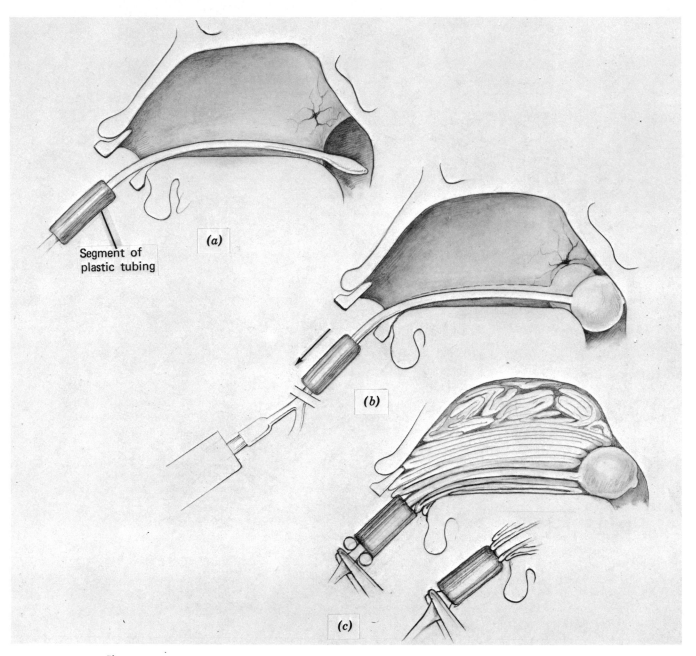

Segment of plastic tubing *(a)*

(b)

(c)

Figure 32.15 AP packing may be required if bleeding is clearly from a posterior site or whenever anterior packing fails to control the hemorrhage. (a) A No. 16 or No. 18 Foley-type catheter with 30-ml balloon and distal tip cut off is inserted along the floor of the nose until it reaches the nasopharynx (about 9 cm). (A 1-inch segment of suction line plastic tubing should be passed over the catheter before nasal insertion.) (b) The balloon is inflated with about 20 ml water, and the catheter is pulled anteriorly until the balloon wedges firmly in the posterior choana of the nose. (c) While an assistant maintains steady forward traction on the catheter, an anterior pack is placed. After placement of the anterior pack, traction on the posterior pack (balloon) is maintained by sliding the suction tubing segment up against the anterior packing and securing the catheter with a clamp. Care should be taken to avoid any direct pressure from the plastic tube or clamp on the nasal tissues since necrosis of the nasal tip may be a complication of an improperly placed AP pack.

terior pack usually is an indication for arterial ligation of the internal maxillary artery and/or the ethmoid artery.

FOLLOW-UP CARE.   Follow-up care of epistaxis patients requires an appropriate investigation of any underlying disorders that may be associated with epistaxis, as detailed above. Patients with epistaxis who are discharged to be followed-up as outpatients should be given instructions to avoid excessive activity, nose blowing, alcoholic beverages, smoking, and excessively hot or spicy foods for 48 hours. Patients should be instructed to breathe humidified air and should be given antibiotics if an anterior pack or an anteroposterior pack has been placed. Penicillin or erythromycin, 250 mg orally four times a day, is usually sufficient for 5 days.

In most cases, epistaxis occurs as an isolated event that can be managed successfully without referral by using the techniques described here. In patients in whom anterior epistaxis occurs repeatedly, routine referral is indicated. If the epistaxis has required placement of an anterior pack, the patient should be referred for pack removal in 48–72 hours. If epistaxis control requires an anteroposterior pack, the patient should be admitted to the hospital for care.

No definitive treatment for epistaxis is required for most nasal fractures since in these cases epistaxis usually stops spontaneously within 1 hour of the injury. In unusual nasal fractures, bleeding may continue, and control of epistaxis then requires reduction of the nasal fracture. These types of nasal fractures are usually more extensive and require the management of an otolaryngologist. Also, if there is no active bleeding and if no specific bleeding site can be identified, no specific treatment should be instituted since cauterization and packing produce a certain amount of intranasal mucosal trauma that can make subsequent management more difficult.

Nasal Obstruction

The most common causes of acute nasal obstruction are due to acute inflammation (e.g., upper respiratory infections, allergies) and trauma. Acute obstruction may occur in the context of more chronic nasal obstruction, which is commonly due to a deviated nasal septum, nasal polyps, vasomotor and allergic rhinitis, enlarged adenoids, and, more rarely, intranasal tumors and granulomatous infections or atresia of the choana.

ACUTE INFECTIOUS RHINITIS

Obstruction of the nasal passageway as a result of acute inflammation is most commonly seen in the setting of upper respiratory tract infection. This syndrome is caused by a variety of viruses that cause an inflammatory reaction in the upper respiratory tract. Typically, after a short prodromal period of malaise, headache, and a nonspecific irritating sensation in the nose, the nose becomes obstructed in association with watery rhinorrhea with or without sneezing. There may be a low-grade fever and an associated sore throat that lasts for several days. If secondary bacterial superinfection occurs, the nasal discharge may become mucopurulent and change in color from clear to yellow or greenish. At this point, the patient may complain of increasing nasal and facial pain because of an associated suppurative sinusitis. An uncomplicated upper respiratory tract infection usually lasts 3–5 days but may persist for a much longer period of time if bacterial superinfection occurs or if infection is complicated by sinusitis or otitis media.

General treatment measures for the common cold consist of symptomatic treatment including salicylates or acetaminophen (Tylenol), humidification of inspired air, sympathomimetic drugs (e.g., pseudoephedrine 30–60 mg orally, four times a day), and topical nasal sprays (described in the section on sinusitis). If bacterial superinfection is suspected, appropriate cultures of the mucopurulent nasal discharge should be taken and the patient should be started on penicillin VK or erythromycin 250 mg orally, four times a day for a 7-day course.

ALLERGIC RHINITIS

Allergic rhinitis is usually chronic and is associated with an itchy sensation in the nose, nasal obstruction, paroxysmal sneezing, and copious, watery nasal discharge. Episodes of acute obstruction may occur seasonally or at times of exposure to specific allergens (e.g., cats, feathers). Allergic rhinitis may also be a result of food allergens (e.g., milk, chocolate, eggs, citrus fruits) or ingestion of certain drugs (e.g., salicylates, iodides).

The clinical signs of allergic rhinitis include pale and swollen turbinates associated with varying amounts of clear and watery nasal discharge. Nasal obstruction is usually bilateral and may be associated with intranasal polyps.

Treatment of allergic rhinitis in the emergency situation is limited to the prescription of an antihistamine (e.g., chlorpheniramine 4 mg orally, three times a day) and a topical steroid nasal spray (e.g., dexamethasone, one spray in each nostril four times a day). The patient should be referred to an allergist or an otolaryngologist for routine evaluation.

VASOMOTOR RHINITIS

Vasomotor rhinitis is usually chronic, and commonly there is no known etiology for this condition. It is believed to be a result of neurovascular dysfunction of the nasal parasympathetic and sympathetic nervous systems that control the size of the turbinates. Various etiologies have been identified that contribute to vasomotor rhinitis; these include (1) hormonal alterations (e.g., pregnancy and use of oral contraceptives); (2) psychological factors (e.g., depression); and (3) secondary effects of drugs (e.g., reserpine and other antihypertensive medications) and (4) environmental factors (e.g., extremes of temperature change, low relative humidity, and cigarette smoke).

In patients with vasomotor rhinitis, the nasal mucosa is inflammed and the turbinates are swollen. The nasal mucosa is more characteristically erythematous and dry, sometimes associated with crusting of the mucosa.

Treatment of vasomotor rhinitis consists of the prescription of a sympathomimetic (e.g., pseudoephedrine 30–60 mg orally, three times a day), unless this is contraindicated, and the use of humidified, inspired air. The patient should be referred for evaluation to determine the etiology of the condition.

RHINITIS MEDICAMENTOSA

Rhinitis medicamentosa is iatrogenic and is basically a chemical rhinitis caused by the excessive sympathomimetic nasal sprays (e.g., Afrin, Neo-Synephrine, Dristan). The use and abuse of these sprays has been discussed in the section dealing with the general treatment of sinus conditions. These sprays are notorious for depleting adrenalin stores in the local nasal tissues, and their continued use very commonly leads to a rebound phenomenon that is manifested by severe nasal congestion after the initial vasoconstrictive effect of the spray. The rebound phenomenon characteristically occurs after these sprays are used more than 5–7 days.

Treatment of this form of rhinitis consists of humidification, oral antihistamine–decongestants (e.g., Dimetapp, Drixoral, Actifed), and a topical steroid spray such as Decadron Turbinaire, one spray in each nostril six times a day. The patient should be warned that it may take several weeks to reverse the chemical rhinitis and that sympathomimetic sprays should be avoided. Cauterization of the inferior turbinates and other minor surgical procedures may be required to control this condition; such treatment is usually handled by the otolaryngologist in a follow-up situation.

NASAL TRAUMA

Acute obstruction of the nose may occur after trauma to the nose with or without a clinical fracture. The cause of the nasal obstruction may be a result of any or all of the following, singly or in combination: (1) reactive mucosal edema; (2) acutely displaced nasal septum; (3) septal hematoma or abscess; (4) blood clot in the nasal cavity; (5) fracture displacement of the nasal pyramid. Traumatic injuries of the nose may be associated with considerable damage to the cartilaginous and soft tissues of the nose without a fracture of the bony structure of the nose. If nasal obstruction is not clearly a result of retained blood clots or mucosal swelling, a displaced nasal septum and/or an intraseptal hematoma should be suspected.

A septal hematoma may be diagnosed by inspecting the nose and comparing the position of the septal mucosa in its superior aspect while looking into the left and the right nostrils. If the left and right sides of the nasal septal mucosa appear to be more than 3 mm apart, a nasal septal hematoma should be suspected and a consultation with an otolaryngologist should be requested (see Chapter 17).

NASAL FOREIGN BODIES

The most common objects found in the nasal cavities are beads, small parts of toys, stones, peanuts, and vegetable matter. An intranasal object usually does not cause obstruction or pain and typically presents as unilateral nasal discharge beginning 24–48 hours after insertion. Intranasal foreign bodies are usually self-induced by children under the age of 10 or by psychiatric patients.

Treatment of this condition should only be attempted with a cooperative patient and if the foreign body lies within 1 cm of the anterior nasal opening. If the patient cannot discharge the object by simply blowing his or her nose, removal may be attempted, first, by aspirating the nasal secretion with a Frazier suction and, then, by removing the foreign body with a bayonet forceps under direct vision. This maneuver may be facilitated by first instilling 2 or 3 drops of 4% cocaine solution to produce topical anesthesia, vasoconstriction, and shrinkage of the nasal mucosa. Removal of foreign bodies may be quite difficult; the object may accidentally be pushed back into the nasopharynx, thereby increasing the danger of aspiration, may be impacted in the nasal cavity by reactive swelling, or may be associated with epistaxis during removal. Therefore if the foreign body cannot be removed on the first or second attempt, the primary care examiner should refer the patient to an otolaryngologist. Frequently, general anesthesia and specialized instruments are required to remove objects safely from the nose; therefore, early consultation is advised in difficult cases.

CHRONIC NASAL OBSTRUCTION

Chronic nasal obstruction is commonly due to rhinitis, deviated nasal septum, intranasal adhesions, nasal polyps, enlarged adenoids, or, more rarely, tumors, granulomatous infections, or congenital problems. The evaluation of a patient with chronic nasal obstruction is beyond the scope of the emergency room physician and the patient should routinely be referred to an otolaryngologist.

Nasal Discharge (Rhinorrhea)

The respiratory epithelium of the nose and paranasal sinuses normally produces mucus that humidifies inspired air and helps trap inhaled contaminants. In a healthy adult during a 24-hour period, about 1 liter of mucus is generated and transported by ciliary action posteriorly to the nasopharynx, where it is swallowed unnoticed. However, if the nasal passage is *obstructed* (e.g., enlarged adenoids) and/or if nasal mucus production is increased (e.g., inflammation due to allergy or infection), anterior nasal discharge may become a dominant symptom. Therefore, the examiner should look for associated symptoms of obstruction and pain in the nose and sinuses since these symptoms may not be associated with the underlying pathology.

MUCOPURULENT DISCHARGE

Mucopurulent discharge is most frequently associated with infectious rhinitis and rhinosinusitis and occasionally with isolated sinusitis (e.g., maxillary sinusitis due to dental problem). Bilateral discharge frequently accompanies the common cold and occurs episodically in patients with chronically obstructed noses, which are more prone to repeated suppurative infections. The most common pathogens are streptococci, pneumococci, and staphylococci; a thick yellow or greenish character to the mucus usually signifies bacterial infection.

Unilateral Mucopurulent Discharge

In a child, unilateral mucopurulent discharge is a classic presenting symptom of intranasal foreign body; therefore, this diagnosis must be held with a high index of suspicion until a complete evaluation can be undertaken. This diagnosis is discussed above.

CLEAR NASAL DISCHARGE

Clear nasal discharge is usually due to inflammation or to nasal obstruction without infection. In children under 12 years old, the most common cause of chronic discharge is hypertrophied adenoids. In adults, the most common cause of clear nasal discharge is acute and chronic rhinitis.

Cerebrospinal fluid rhinorrhea is an unusual cause of clear nasal rhinorrhea that may occur as a complication of traumatic injuries of the nose and sinuses, after nasal operations, and rarely spontaneously. Clear and copious nasal discharge after a facial injury or nasal surgery should alert the examiner to the possibility of CSF rhinorrhea, and the patient should be referred for a comprehensive evaluation, which is beyond the scope of the primary care setting.

Pain

Acute pain that localizes in the region of the nose is usually due to infections of the nasal soft tissues on the external surface (e.g., cellulitis or furuncle) or localized infection within the nasal cavity (nasal vestibule). Nasal pain may be associated with inflammation of the superior portion of the nasal cavity and is frequently described by patients as having an associated sensation of pressure localized in this region. Not uncommonly this type of pain–pressure symptom may not be associated with restricted airflow if the inferior portion of the nasal cavity is not obstructed. Treatment of this problem is the same as for rhinitis.

NASAL SOFT TISSUE INFECTIONS

If the patient presents with a soft tissue infection on the external nose, nasal septum, or nasal vestibule, a careful neurologic examination (including an examination of the eye fields) should be conducted. Because the venous drainage from the nasal area is to the cavernous sinus on each side, cavernous sinus thrombosis is a serious and very often fatal complication of nasal cellulitis or abscess. The potential for this complication dictates that the patient be started on high dosages of antistaphylococcal antibiotics and be placed under close observation of a specialist within 24 hours. Frequently patients with this type of problem are admitted for intensive intravenous antibiosis.

Anosmia

Anosmia, or loss of smell, may occur acutely and may be a result of primary neurologic dysfunction of the olfactory nerve or superior nasal cavity obstruction. When this symptom occurs as a result of intracranial or other pathology, it is usually overshadowed by other signs and symptoms. The evaluation of this problem may require an extensive investigation and is beyond the scope of the emergency room physician.

ACUTE EAR PROBLEMS

Common symptoms encountered in the emergency room are earache, ear discharge and bleeding, hearing loss, and vertigo. Acute earache is usually associated with obvious ear pathology such as external otitis, serous otitis media, acute suppurative otitis media, or acute eardrum perforation; occasionally, an earache may be the result of a referred pain from an abnormality of an adjacent or distant structure (e.g., temporomandibular joint, larynx). Otorrhea may consist of purulent discharge from acute or chronic infections of the middle ear or external ear structure. Acute bleeding from the ear canal is usually the result of traumatic injury of the ear canal or tympanic membrane or more severe head injuries that produce basilar skull fractures. Frequently the bleeding is associated with CSF otorrhea as well. Acute hearing loss usually is unilateral and may be a result of decreased sound conduction from obstruction of the external ear canal with cerumen or decreased middle ear sound transmission because of middle ear serous effusion or suppuration. Occasionally acute hearing loss is due to acute tympanic membrane rupture or acute hemorrhage in the middle ear space (barotrauma). In addition, sudden hearing loss may be due to dysfunction of the inner ear or acoustic nerve structures. Vertigo may be the dominant symptom associated with inner ear disease, central nervous system disorders, or systemic problems; frequently vertigo will be associated with characteristic symptoms and signs that help to identify the origin of the symptom.

Earache with Abnormal Ear Findings

EXTERNAL OTITIS, CELLULITIS, AND FURUNCLE

Diffuse and localized soft tissue infections of the ear canal are common, particularly in the summer months. External otitis, commonly called swimmer's ear, usually progresses gradually over several hours and may produce severe pain. Typically there is a history of prolonged water immersion associated with recent cleaning of the ears with cotton-tipped applicators. The auricle is quite tender and manipulation of the auricle or tragus produces exquisite pain. The ear canal is usually quite swollen compared to the opposite side, and the lumen may be completely occluded by the local inflammatory edema. The tympanic membrane may not be visible because of canal swelling. Occasionally tenderness and pain may be localized to a small furuncle in the ear canal or an infected sebaceous cyst in the periauricular area.

Treatment

Treatment of external otitis consists of water precautions, otic combination antibiotic–steroid drops, analgesics, and, in more severe cases, the insertion of an ear canal cotton wick and the administration of systemic antibiotics. The patient should be advised to avoid water contamination of the involved ear (i.e., swimming and bathing) for approximately 4 weeks. A simple way to keep water from entering the ear canal is to have the patient place cotton mixed with a small amount of petrolatum (Vaseline) into the ear as an oily plug that will prevent water from entering the ear during showers or shampooing. The oily cotton plug should be discarded after bathing. Ear drops are used to retard surface bacterial growth and to decrease a local soft tissue swelling. Cortisporin otic suspension, VoSoL HC, and Pyocidin are popular eardrops that are usually prescribed to be given 3 drops in the ear three times a day for about 10 days. In severe cases of external otitis, the canal lumen may be narrowed more than 50% as compared to the normal size; in these cases it is advisable to insert gently a small rolled cylinder of cotton to a depth of about 1 cm in the ear canal. The purpose of this ear wick is to aid in the penetration of the eardrops for the first 48 hours. The patient should be instructed to remove the wick after 48 hours but to continue the drops for the full 10 days. If a wick is inserted and/or there is regional cervical adenopathy, the patient should be started on a 10-day course of systemic antibiotics with penicillin or erythromycin as the drug of choice. It is important to warn the patient that the pain associated with external otitis may continue to increase 12–24 hours after treatment is started before it begins to subside in response to treatment. Because of this, analgesics equivalent to or more potent than codeine are frequently prescribed during the first 24–48 hours after a treatment is begun. If a localized, fluctuant infection is identified (e.g., furuncle, infected sebaceous cyst), a routine incision and drainage with a culture of the contents is indicated. In these cases, there is a high incidence of staphylococcal or penicillinase-resistant organisms and the patient should be treated with an appropriate antibiotic (e.g., erythromycin, dicloxacillin).

MALIGNANT EXTERNAL OTITIS

Malignant external otitis is a severe form of external otitis that occurs in diabetics and is frequently associated with an osteitis of the temporal bone. This infection frequently has an extremely rapid course and may progress to a fatal outcome. Malignant external otitis generally is due to a *Pseudomonas* cellulitis of the ear canal and requires that the patient be admitted to the hospital for intensive intravenous antibiosis and special otologic care.

SEROUS (SECRETORY) OTITIS MEDIA

Serous otitis media may occur in adults but is usually seen in children 3–7 years old and is usually bilateral. The middle ear space is filled with a serous effusion of variable viscosity; this condition is associated with poor ventilation of the middle ear space because of eustachian tube dysfunction. The most common reasons for eustachian tube dysfunction are allergy, inflammatory and developmental factors, and nasopharyngeal obstruction (e.g., hypertrophied adenoids). The effusion produces variable degrees of conductive hearing loss that may have an insidious onset and fluctuating intensity. Commonly, children complain of intermittent earaches lasting from a few seconds to a few minutes, which usually are not associated with fever. Otoscopically the eardrum appears to be retracted and may be slightly amber to pink in color. The tympanic membrane blood vessels are usually slightly injected, and pneumatic massage usually reveals decreased mobility of the tympanic membrane. A slight to moderate hearing loss can be detected by means of the whisper test discussed earlier.

Treatment

Treatment of patients with serous otitis media is directed at improving eustachian tube function with systemic antihistamine–decongestant therapy, humidification, and control of regional inflammatory conditions (bacterial tonsillitis). Antihistamine–decongestant medications such as Dimetapp, Actifed, Fedahist, and Triaminic, administered in the liquid form three times a day, have been found to be quite helpful in resolving this problem in children. Extended time-release forms of these and similar medications may be given to adults every 12 hours. Since low or relative humidity is frequently associated with reactive inflammation of the nasal and eustachian tube mucosa, humidification with a cool-mist humidifier is recommended if there is significant exposure to air that is artificially heated or air conditioned. From a practical point of view, humidification of the patient's bedroom at night is a reasonably acceptable way to achieve this goal. Since serous otitis media may either resolve within a few days or become chronic and require more specialized otologic care, the initial treatment should include decongestant therapy and humidification for 2 weeks and a follow-up examination scheduled at the end of this period.

ACUTE SUPPURATIVE OTITIS MEDIA

Acute suppurative otitis media usually presents as progressive pain in one ear that lasts for more than a few minutes and is associated with fever and signs of systemic toxicity. It often follows the onset of an upper respiratory tract infection. Otoscopic examination reveals a bulging and reddened tympanic membrane with hypervascularity. The mastoid may be slightly tender. If the eardrum is ruptured, there will be pus in the ear canal.

Treatment

The management of acute suppurative otitis media requires systemic antibiotics for 10 days. Penicillin or erythromycin is the drug of choice in children 6 years or older, and broad-spectrum antibiotics, such as ampicillin, amoxicillin, or Bactrim, are usually prescribed for children under 6 years old. Antibiotics are prescribed for a 10-day course and an antihistamine–decongestant combination for a 3-week period. Appropriate analgesics should be given and the patient should be cautioned about water contamination in the ear. In patients in whom acute perforation has occurred, an addition of an antibiotic eardrop to the treatment program is indicated. Routine follow-up for this problem is usually scheduled after 10 days.

The prognosis for patients with acute suppurative otitis media is usually complete resolution after 10 days; however, some ears will fail to resolve completely and will show signs of chronic serous otitis media that persists beyond this time.

AEROTITIS MEDIA

Aerotitis media is caused by sudden pressure changes (e.g., scuba diving or airplane descent), which suddenly stretch the eardrum causing capillary rupture within the middle ear space and resulting in painful hemotympanum and hearing loss. The eardrum may appear to be hemorrhagic, dark blue, purple, or almost black. Treatment and prognosis are similar to that for serous otitis media.

BULLOUS MYRINGITIS

Bullous myringitis is an inflammation of the tympanic membrane that produces small amber bullae on the tympanic membrane that are quite painful. This condition is thought to be a result of a localized viral infection, but it may be secondarily infected by bacterial contamination. Analgesics and penicillin or erythromycin are given for a 10-day period. Bullous myringitis often produces a mild hearing loss because of poor movement of the tympanic membrane.

MASTOIDITIS

Mastoiditis usually occurs 10–14 days after acute suppurative otitis media or at any time during chronic suppurative otitis media. It is usually painless, but mastoiditis with mastoid pain may signify abscess formation. In the vast majority of cases, the tympanic membrane is thickened, inflamed, and may be perforated. If mastoiditis is suspected, an otolaryngologist should be consulted immediately since early surgical exploration may be indicated. Infection from an infected mastoid occasionally may extend intracranially to cause meningitis, epidural abscesses, or middle or posterior fossa abscesses. Rarely, extension from the mastoid tip into the neck causes a deep-neck abscess (Bezold's abscess), or extension anteriorly into the zygomatic bone root produces a preauricular abscess.

Red Eardrum

A diagnostic problem that commonly presents itself to the clinician is the red eardrum. The eardrum may appear pink or red in cases of early acute suppurative otitis media or possibly serous otitis media. Similar appearance of the eardrum may be seen if the ear has been recently syringed and the blood vessels of the tympanic membranes are dilated. A young child who is crying forcefully may also have bright red tympanic membranes that can further confuse the diagnostic investigation. If the clinician is confronted with the red eardrum and an infectious process cannot be definitely excluded on the basis of history and physical examination, the best course of action is to start the patient on antibiotic and decongestant therapy as if he or she were suffering from an early acute suppurative otitis media.

Tumors of the Ears

Tumors of the ears are uncommon and rarely cause pain unless they are malignant. The mass is usually seen otoscopically, and early referral is indicated. Frequently facial paralysis, hearing loss, tinnitus, and vertigo are associated with the symptoms.

Herpes Zoster Oticus

Herpes zoster oticus is an infection of the external ear that may cause severe pain in the ear and that is usually associated with a vesicular eruption of the external ear and ear canal.

Earache without Ear Signs (Referred Pain)

If the patient complains of earache and there are no findings on otoscopic examination, other sources of ear pain should be considered. The ear is innervated by cranial nerves V, VII, IX, and X and by cervical nerves II and III; therefore disorders of any regions supplied by these nerves can produce referred pain to the ear. Thus a careful search of the entire ear, nose, and throat area needs to be made in patients who complain of earache but in whom no ear abnormality can be found. The most common etiologies of pain that are referred to the ear are temporomandibular joint arthralgia (Costen's syndrome), dental problems (caries, periapical abscesses, impacted wisdom teeth), sinusitis, and laryngeal and pharyngeal inflammation and tumors.

TEMPOROMANDIBULAR JOINT INFLAMMATION

Temporomandibular joint (TMJ) inflammation may be diagnosed by palpating both temporomandibular joints while the patient opens and closes his or her mouth. Tenderness of the joints on one side is often elicited in this manner. Radiographs of the joints often do not show an abnormality. The pain and tenderness may be referred from the TMJ to the vertex, the lower jaw, the neck, and posteriorly into the mastoid region. The TMJ arthralgia is usually due to myofascial dysfunction of the masticatory muscles.

The treatment of patients with TMJ arthralgia can be initiated by telling patients to have a soft diet for 5 days. Patients should also take a mild analgesic such as aspirin every 4 hours for 5 days and should apply a heating pad or hot-water bottle to the affected joint three or four times a day. Most patients with TMJ disorders will respond to this treatment within the 5-day period. Occasionally TMJ pain will be a result of malocclusion or badly fitting dentures. A referral to an oral surgeon is indicated if the patient does not respond to the measures described here.

Acute Hearing Loss

Most patients who complain of hearing loss in an emergency room setting will give a history of sudden partial or complete hearing loss in one or both ears. Sudden bilateral profound hearing loss without obvious cause (e.g., skull fracture, wax impaction) is extremely rare but occasionally is associated with psychotic and drug-related mental abberations. Chronic hearing loss may be a result of a variety of conditions that often require sophisticated audiometry and evaluation that are beyond the skills of the emergency room physician. Acute hearing loss may be associated with disorders of the external, middle, or inner ear mechanisms.

EARWAX, EAR CANAL DEBRIS, AND FOREIGN BODIES

Obstruction of the external ear canal may cause a conductive hearing loss because sound is prevented from reaching the middle ear. Earwax and natural squamous epithelial debris may produce hearing loss by completely occluding the canal or by touching the eardrum; gentle syringe lavage is the method of choice for removal. Foreign bodies should not be removed from the ear canal unless they are easily extracted under direct vision on the first try. Repeated attempts to remove a foreign body may result in trauma to the ear canal or damage to the tympanic membrane or other middle ear structures. Removal of foreign bodies from the ear canal frequently requires general anesthesia and specialized instrumentation.

EAR TRAUMA

Transcanal injuries (e.g., with cotton-tipped applicators), compression injuries to the ear, explosion rupture of the eardrum, ossicular discontinuity, and sensorineural hearing loss may be the result of direct trauma to the middle ear and inner ear structures. Basilar skull fractures with temporal bone fractures frequently are associated with hearing loss. Immediate treatment for these types of injuries requires water precautions and notification of an otolaryngologist since the management frequently requires emergency surgery.

INFECTION AND INFLAMMATION OF THE EXTERNAL AND MIDDLE EAR

External otitis, acute suppurative otitis, and serous otitis media may be associated with acute hearing loss. Chronic suppurative otitis media is chronic infection in the middle ear space and mastoid cavity, which is invariably associated with a chronic perforation of the tympanic membrane. This disorder usually produces a gradual hearing loss but may also be associated with a sudden hearing loss if the infection causes erosion of the middle ear ossicles or inflammatory debris obstructs sound transmission. Chronic suppurative otitis media is usually painless and may be associated with recurrent drainage from the ear.

ROUND WINDOW RUPTURE

Acute rupture of the round window membrane produces a sudden hearing loss that may be associated with vertigo. There is usually a history of exertion and straining with a sudden loss of hearing and, frequently, a popping sensation in the ear. Patients with profound, unilateral, and sudden hearing loss with a history of exertion or straining before the loss should be evaluated by an otolaryngologist immediately to determine whether immediate surgical exploration is indicated.

ACOUSTIC TRAUMA

Exposure to impulse noise (e.g., explosion or air blast) produces a temporary threshold shift that may produce varying degrees of hearing loss, often associated with tinnitus, because of changes in the sensorineural function of the cochlea. Usually complete recovery occurs within 8–12 hours, but there may be some permanent sensorineural hearing loss. No specific treatment is required, but a complete otologic evaluation is indicated if hearing fails to return to normal or if tinnitus persists.

OTOTOXIC DRUGS

Drugs such as aspirin, gentamicin, kanamycin, nitrogen mustard, and ethacrynic acid may produce a sudden hearing loss. Patients should be questioned closely about their use of medications before the hearing loss. Reversal of the hearing loss frequently occurs when the medication is stopped.

SYPHILIS

Congenital or acquired syphilis may cause sudden hearing loss, vertigo, tinnitus, singly or in combination. Since the diagnosis and treatment of this disorder fall outside of the emergency setting, an early otologic referral is needed if syphilis is suspected.

IDIOPATHIC SUDDEN HEARING LOSS

Some cases of sudden hearing loss are without identifiable cause. Viral, allergic, microvascular, and other mechanisms have been postulated to explain these cases, but no definite explanation has been established.

Discharging Ear (Otorrhea)

The most common causes of drainage from the ear are chronic external otitis and chronic suppurative otitis media. Chronic external otitis is usually associated with recurrent and chronic itching in the ear canals. Inspection reveals thickened ear canal skin and crusting and debris. The hearing may be diminished because of severe thickening of the ear canal skin and partial or complete occlusion of the ear canal. Chronic suppurative otitis media produces discharge from chronic, purulent, or mucopurulent infection in the middle ear space that discharges through a chronic perforation into the ear canal. After trauma to the ear or temporal bone, there may be bloody discharge and/or CSF otorrhea.

Treatment of patients with mucopurulent or purulent discharge from the ear usually consists of otic drops and water precautions. Referral for an otologic evaluation is indicated since the long-term management of patients with these disorders goes beyond the emergency room setting.

Bleeding from the Ear

The most common causes of bleeding from the ear are middle ear infection; traumatic injuries of the ear canal, temporal bone, or tympanic membrane; foreign bodies in the ear canal; pressure equalization ventilating tubes; and, rarely, neoplasms of the ear.

Acute and chronic infections of the middle ear may produce episodic and recurrent bleeding because of the hypervascularity associated with the inflammatory condition. Bleeding usually occurs in conjunction with purulent discharge in these conditions and patients are treated with otic drops and systemic antibiotics as indicated by the primary infection site.

TRAUMATIC INJURIES OF THE EAR ASSOCIATED WITH BLEEDING

Traumatic injuries of the ear are usually severe and are associated with some hearing loss because of disruption of middle ear structures. Simple lacerations of the ear canal require no treatment except for dry sterile cotton to be placed in the external ear to absorb the blood. Eardrops are contraindicated for bleeding from the ear associated with trauma. Battle's sign is ecchymosis over the mastoid after skull fracture or temporal bone fracture and indicates bleeding within the temporal bone and over the mastoid cortex. This may be the earliest sign of a basal skull fracture, and appropriate neurosurgical consultation is indicated if this disorder is seen in a patient with a head injury.

FOREIGN BODIES IN THE EAR

Foreign bodies may produce ear canal laceration and bleeding. Removal of foreign bodies should not be attempted unless they can be removed on the first try without causing further trauma to the ear canal. Pressure equalization ventilating tubes that have been inserted into the tympanic membranes will some-

times cause local bleeding if the tympanic membranes become infected. Treatment of patients with this condition consists of otic drops for 10 days and referral to an otolaryngologist for evaluation.

NEOPLASMS

Rarely, tumors of the ear may present as bleeding. Usually there is hearing loss and an obvious mass in the ear canal that may appear friable. Referral of the patient for biopsy and management is indicated.

Vertigo

Vertigo is a sensation of turning or spinning in space and should be distinguished from other forms of dizziness that may be described as lightheadedness or disequilibrium or unsteadiness. True vertigo may be divided into two types based on the origin of the vertigo: peripheral and central. *Peripheral vertigo* originates in structures within the temporal bone and may be considered labyrinthine in type. *Central vertigo* originates from a disorder in the central nervous system. About 90% of vertigo is peripheral and may be associated with specific ear problems such as acute suppurative otitis media, chronic suppurative otitis media, Ménière's disease, labyrinthitis, and vestibular neuronitis.

Peripheral vertigo is often associated with nausea, vomiting, tinnitus, hearing loss, and nystagmus that is horizontal or rotary in nature. Central vertigo occurs in about 10% of vertigo cases and is often due to central nervous system neoplasms, demyelinating or degenerative diseases, and metabolic cardiovascular disorders.

Peripheral vertigo is often associated with pain and tinnitus in the affected area and may also give a feeling of fullness and blocking. It is usually associated with nausea and vomiting, and physical examination may reveal middle ear pathology or horizontal and rotary nystagmus. Aside from blurriness of vision, no particular visual problems are associated with peripheral vertigo.

Central vertigo is frequently associated with neurologic symptoms such as dimming of vision, diplopia, paresthesias, paralysis, and cardiac arrhythmias. In contrast, lightheadedness and other forms of dizziness may be a result of numerous causes that involve endocrine deficiencies, metabolic problems (e.g., hypoglycemia), drug ingestion, or emotional tension and stress.

Central vertigo may or may not be associated with tinnitus. The nystagmus seen in this type of vertigo may be vertical, direction changing, or disconjugate. Frequently there are other cranial nerve dysfunctions, and visual disturbances are common. There may also be cerebellar signs.

Acute demyelinating and degenerative disease may also be heralded by vertigo. Metabolic and cardiovascular disorders may also produce vertigo and varying degrees of dizziness.

PERIPHERAL VERTIGO

There are several common causes of peripheral vertigo. These are frequently associated with other symptoms referable to the ear. Viral labyrinthitis and vestibular neuronitis are disorders of the labyrinth and vestibular nerve that are thought to be a result of viral infection. There may or may not be associated tinnitus, and usually there is normal hearing. The otoscopic examination is normal. Frequently there is horizontal nystagmus with the fast component directed away from the affected ear. Placing the affected ear in the dependent position will increase the feeling of vertigo and the amplitude of the nystagmus. Viral labyrinthitis and vestibular neuronitis are often associated with nausea and vomiting; these symptoms begin suddenly and may last for several days before tapering off to a gradual feeling of unsteadiness that may persist for several weeks.

Ménière's syndrome is a clinical syndrome characterized by recurrent bouts of vertigo, frequently associated with tinnitus and hearing loss, and may also be associated with nausea and vomiting. The attacks begin suddenly and are sometimes associated with a prodromal feeling.

Vertigo may be associated with middle ear infection that may be either acute or chronic. Acute suppurative otitis media is sometimes associated with vertigo as a result of a sympathetic labyrinthitis in the infected ear. Treatment directed at the acute suppurative otitis media is usually sufficient to control the vertigo. In patients with chronic suppurative otitis media, active infection may produce vertigo through a suppurative labyrinthitis. There also may be erosion of the lateral semicircular canal by cholesteatoma with the occurrence of a labyrinthine fistula. Rarely cerebellar abscess may be the result of a progressive cholesteatoma and chronic suppuration in the middle ear space, but vertigo in this situation is also associated with classical cerebellar dysfunction signs.

BENIGN POSITIONAL VERTIGO

Benign positional vertigo occurs when the patient's head is tilted backward or far forward, characteristically when the patient is in the supine position; it is most prominent when the affected ear is in the dependent position. Placing the patient in a supine position with the left or the right ear in the dependent position will produce rotary or horizontal nystagmus that has its onset several seconds after assuming the position and that lasts for 15–60 seconds. The nystagmus and vertigo will fatigue with each successive assumption of the supine position so that after the third or fourth try, the nystagmus and vertigo are minimal or absent. No specific treatment is needed for this entity since it will clear spontaneously in 4–8 weeks; the patient should avoid assuming the aggravating position in the meantime.

Other causes of vertigo are related to more unusual causes such as syphilis and postconcussion syndrome.

CENTRAL VERTIGO

Central vertigo is often associated with dysfunction of other cranial nerves, and patients frequently have symptoms of dysarthria, diplopia, sensory loss, and, occasionally, paralysis.

Cerebrovascular accidents, vertebrobasilar insufficiency, and subclavian steal are causes of central vertigo. These diagnoses are suggested by appropriate history and physical examination. Treatment is directed toward the underlying cause.

Cerebellopontine angle tumors and cerebellar neoplasms may produce vertigo. Depending upon the severity of the problem, hearing may be affected and other cranial neuropathies may be evident.

ACUTE ORAL AND PHARYNGEAL PROBLEMS

Life-Threatening Emergencies

AIRWAY OBSTRUCTION

A complete discussion of airway obstruction is found in Chapters 1 and 2. Sudden airway obstructions without prodrome is usually due to a foreign body or trauma, whereas progressive obstruction is usually associated with inflammation such as epiglottitis or tumor. The management of inflammatory obstruction is discussed in Chapters 2 and 44.

PHARYNGEAL HEMORRHAGE

The most important consideration in patients with pharyngeal hemorrhage is preventing aspiration of blood. Even in the most massive hemorrhages, proper patient position, adequate suctioning of the pharynx, and adequate intravenous replacement will stabilize the patient until he or she can be moved to the operating room for primary control of the hemorrhage. Deaths that occur during pharyngeal hemorrhage are usually due to airway obstruction from aspiration of blood, not from blood loss itself.

Common causes of this disorder are penetrating injury to the pharynx and intraoral or intrapharyngeal tumor with hemorrhage. Patients will usually have a history of intermittent hemorrhage from the mouth (which may be slight or massive). Patients sometimes experience pharyngeal bleeding 7–10 days after a tonsillectomy because the catgut suture ligatures used to control hemorrhage at the time of the operation generally dissolve in about 1 week. Hemorrhage resulting from penetrating injuries of the pharynx (e.g., knife wounds) can be located by placing a probe or gloved finger into the wound. Injuries of the posterior pharyngeal wall, usually seen in children, may result from direct penetration by objects held in the mouth during a fall, such as popsicle or lollipop sticks.

Management of pharyngeal hemorrhage is best accomplished when the patient is lying down with the head in a dependent position. If the site of the bleeding can be determined, place the hemorrhaging side in the dependent position as well. An intravenous line should be established immediately and blood replacement begun if necessary. The first step in the control of bleeding is to determine the location of the hemorrhage. A light source attached to the head allows the clinician to use both hands in the examination. A tongue blade is inserted with one hand and the tongue is depressed while the other hand is used to introduce a tonsil suction tip (Yankauer) (Fig. 32.16). The suction tip should be placed well into the back of the pharynx and clots and blood should be suctioned out (Fig. 32.17). If the bleeding site can be seen, the suction tip is placed directly over it and is kept there until definitive tamponade can be performed.

In a post tonsillectomy patient, if the bleeding site cannot be determined, it is probably the inferior pole of one of the tonsillar fossae. The inferior pole is located near the base of the tongue on either the left or the right side of the tongue. The suction tip is placed blindly on one side of the pharynx to see if the suction tip is effectively directing the blood out of the pharynx. If the bleeding does not appear to be lessening with this maneuver, the site is probably on the opposite tonsillar fossa and the suction tip should be directed to this area.

Tamponade of pharyngeal bleeding can be accomplished with a curved hemostatic clamp (Kelly) and a 2-by-2 inch gauze sponge folded into a small ball. The sponge ball can be held tightly against the hemorrhaging vessel by a Kelly clamp. This maneuver can be made more effective by applying counterpressure against the tonsillar fossa externally if the opposite fingertips are directed medially just posterior to the ramus of the mandible. This method of bimanual tamponade is effective

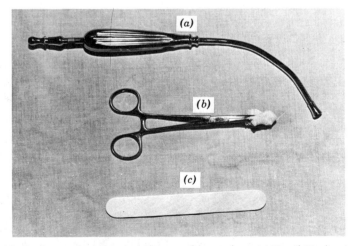

Figure 32.16 Equipment for control of pharyngeal hemorrhage (a) Tonsil (Yankaur) suction tip, (b) long hemostatic clamp (Kelly) with 2-by-2-in. folded sponge tampon and tongue blade. A head mirror or headlight is also necessary.

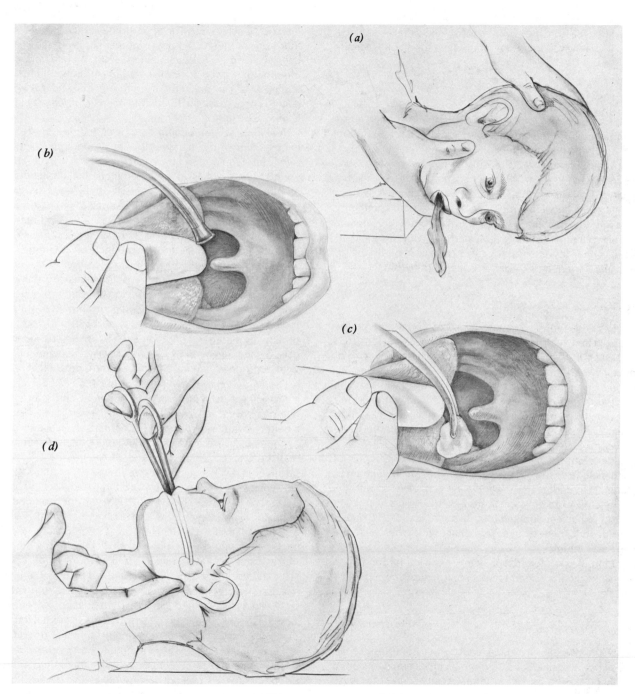

Figure 32.17 Method for emergency control of pharyngeal hemorrhage. (a) Position patient to prevent aspiration—either sitting up and leaning forward or lying down with head lower than chest. (b) Depress tongue with blade and place suction tip in posterior pharynx (tonsillar fossa) near base of tongue to remove blood continuously from airway. (c) Tamponade bleeding site by direct pressure with sponge held in hemostatic clamp. (d) Additional tamponade is provided by the external index finger posterior to the ramus of the mandible.

in controlling massive posttonsillectomy hemorrhages until the patient can be moved to an operating room for definitive treatment.

Throat Pain

Acute throat pain may originate from a localized pharyngeal problem (e.g., bacterial tonsillitis) or it may be referred from distant structures that are innervated by cranial nerves IX or X (e.g., myocardial angina). The most common causes of sore throat are bacterial and viral infections that primarily involve the pharynx and are often associated with tenderness and enlargement of the cervical lymph nodes. Throat pain commonly radiates into the ears along the distribution of the glossopharyngeal nerve and is usually aggravated by swallowing (odynophagia). Other less common causes of pain include foreign bodies, tumors, cricoarytenoid arthritis, and thyroiditis.

INFECTIOUS THROAT PAIN

Pharyngitis is the most common cause of throat pain and is often associated with fever, malaise and anorexia, localized physical signs of pharyngeal inflammation, and tender cervical adenopathy. Although identifying the type of infection on clinical evidence alone is impossible, a general rule is that the more rapid the onset and the more severe the symptoms and findings, the more likely it is that the infection is due to group A β-hemolytic streptococci. Throat cultures should be made whenever possible.

General treatment measures of patients with pharyngitis of any kind include the use of analgesics (aspirin, acetaminophen, or codeine), humidification, and saline gargles (½ tsp salt dissolved in a tall glass of warm water) every 4 hours. The adult patient should be encouraged to drink more than 2,000 ml per 24-hour period. In cases of severe pharyngitis when pain and swelling may inhibit swallowing, there is danger of progressive dehydration. If complete dysphagia has existed for more than 24 hours, hospitalization of the patient for intravenous therapy is indicated.

Bacterial Infections

Bacterial pharyngitis is usually caused by gram-positive organisms (e.g., staphylococci, streptococci, pneumococci) but occasionally may be caused by gram-negative organisms (e.g., gonococci, *Haemophilus influenzae*, coliform bacteria).

Bacterial infections of the throat should be treated with antibiotics. Penicillin or erythromycin is the drug of choice for patients older than 5 years unless a gram-negative bacterial infection is suspected. The appropriate adult dosage is 500 mg, four times a day for 10 days; the pediatric dosage should be chosen according to the patient's weight. A child under 5 years old should be given a broad-spectrum antibiotic, such as amoxicillin, or a combination of erythromycin and sulfisoxazole (Gantrisin) because the likelihood of an *H. influenzae* infection is increased in this age group.

Tonsillitis, which is manifested by erythema and, frequently, enlargement of the palatine tonsils, in addition to the other signs and symptoms of pharyngitis, is common in children and young adults and has an increased incidence during the winter months. Typically, tonsillitis is associated with pharyngitis and tender cervical adenopathy. The onset may be insidious or rather sudden over a course of 2 or 3 hours and may be associated with temperature as high as 40°C (104° F). Acute follicular tonsillitis has the appearance of inflamed tonsils with small, punctate yellowish discoloration of the crypts of the tonsillar surfaces. This form of tonsillitis is usually due to streptococcal infection. Necrotizing tonsillitis produces tonsillar ulcerations and exudate. Since this form of tonsillitis may indicate a severe infection and may be associated with an underlying systemic condition such as infectious mononucleosis, a careful general history and physical examination along with appropriate laboratory studies are indicated.

Diphtheria pharyngitis is seen rarely and is characterized by a pharyngeal exudate, which is adherent and gray in color. The pharyngeal mucosa bleeds easily when it is rubbed with a culture swab. Typically the patient has cervical adenopathy, a moderate fever, tachycardia, and moderately severe malaise with headache. Gram-stain and throat culture tests will be positive for *Corynebacterium diphtheriae*. Hospitalization and intravenous penicillin therapy are indicated.

Peritonsillar abscess develops between the pseudocapsule of the tonsil and the muscles of the pharyngeal wall. Typically a peritonsillar abscess develops as a complication of simple bacterial tonsillitis, which frequently occurs during the course of treatment with antibiotics. The development of a peritonsillar abscess is associated with localized pain on the involved side that usually becomes progressively severe and is associated with dysphagia and trismus. The patient usually develops a peculiar "hot potato" voice secondary to poor palatal movement. Inspection of the pharynx reveals medial displacement of the affected tonsil toward the midline, an edematous uvula, trismus, and a flucuant tender mass palpable in the soft palate near the superior pole of the involved tonsil. Treatment of patients with a peritonsillar abscess usually requires surgical drainage by a specialist and intravenous antibiotics.

Viral infections, including coxsackievirus A, adenoviruses, and influenza viruses, are common pathogens that infect the pharynx. In most cases, the nose, nasopharynx, larynx, and trachea are also involved. The symptoms are those of the familiar viral syndrome, and usually the pharyngeal findings do not dominate the clinical picture. The general treatment regimen of analgesics, humidification, saline gargles, and adequate oral fluid intake is usually all that is required.

Herpetic infections of the oral and pharyngeal mucosa typically produce severe pain and well-defined, pale grey, shallow ulcerations with erythematous margins. There may be single or multiple ulcerations that tend to resolve spontaneously in 10–14 days. Usually no special treatment is needed for patients with herpetic ulcerations. If ulcers are numerous and pain is severe, the patient may be treated with systemic analgesics. Topical analgesics (viscous lidocaine—Xylocaine—solution, 5 ml, mouthwash rinse, ½ hour before meals) may provide some relief for local pain.

Aphthous stomatitis, a poorly understood condition of the oral and pharyngeal mucosa, is typified by a single ulcer or by several shallow and painful ulcers. They may be indistinguishable from herpetic lesions and usually resolve spontaneously in 10–14 days.

Infectious mononucleosis may be manifested initially by a nonspecific throat inflammation or by a rapidly progressing necrotizing tonsillitis with foul breath, cervical adenopathy, and systemic symptoms of fever, malaise, and anorexia. Tonsillitis that is resistant to routine medical treatment strongly suggests infectious mononucleosis, which can be confirmed by appropriate blood tests (e.g., heterophil and CBC). Although mononucleosis tonsillitis usually occurs in young adults, it is not uncommon in young children. Frequently, infectious mononucleosis is associated with secondary gram-positive bacterial tonsillitis, which requires treatment with penicillin or erythromycin.

The pharynx is rarely infected by a *fungus,* but when it is, the most common pathogen is *Candida albicans.* In this form of pharyngitis the mucosa is coated with a whitish exudate that looks like cottage cheese. Diabetics and patients whose resistance has been lowered by immunosuppressive drugs, antibiotic or steroid therapy, or debilitating diseases (e.g., leukemia) are susceptible to monilia infections. The appropriate treatment consists of nystatin (Mycostatin) oral suspension (100,000 units/ml) 5 ml mouthwash. The patient should be instructed to rinse the mouth and swallow the suspension four times a day for 10 days.

NONINFECTIOUS THROAT PAIN

Foreign bodies lodged in the hypopharynx and cervical esophagus may cause pain in varying degrees. This diagnosis is suggested by history and is often confirmed by plain roentgenographs of the neck. The lateral neck plain film may show a radiopaque foreign body (e.g., chicken bone) in the hypopharynx or cervical esophagus, but it may fail to show a foreign body if the object is not radiopaque (e.g., meat or vegetable matter). Careful evaluation of the cervical esophageal region of the film may reveal air in the cervical esophagus. This finding is abnormal and is invariably associated with a foreign body in the postcricoid region of the esophagus. If a foreign body is suspected, appropriate consultation with a specialist is advised.

Cricoarytenoid arthritis is a rare cause of throat pain and is often associated with systemic forms of rheumatoid arthritis. This type of throat pain is aggravated by swallowing and may be associated with hoarseness. The diagnosis can be made by indirect (mirror) laryngoscopy.

Thyroiditis may produce pain referred to the throat. Thyroiditis is usually associated with tenderness of the thyroid gland.

Tumors of the hypopharynx and larynx may produce pain that may not be detectable by ordinary examination techniques. Carcinomas of the tonsil, base of the tongue, hypopharynx, and larynx may have throat pain as the first symptom. Typically these tumors are associated with a history of cigarette smoking and alcohol usage. Indirect laryngoscopy, direct laryngoscopy, and fluoroscopy may be required to evaluate the patient with a suspected tumor in this region; therefore appropriate referral is indicated.

Intraoral Bleeding

The most common causes of intraoral bleeding are trauma to the teeth and intraoral soft tissue structures, which has been dealt with previously, and postextraction hemorrhage owing to lack of adequate compression of the socket and lack of a suture across the interdental papillae on either end of the extraction site. The large jelly clot protruding from the socket should be removed and the area should be rinsed with cold saline. A moist gauze sponge should be placed over the socket, and the patient should compress this by biting down for approximately a half hour. If the bleeding continues, a 3-0 plain gut suture should be placed across the interdental papillae on either end of the socket. The gauze pressure dressing should then be replaced and the patient should bite down again for a half hour. If the bleeding persists, it may be evidence of a small bone bleeder at the base of the socket. The socket should again be irrigated and then gelfoam should be placed and packed into the socket and a pressure dressing with gauze reapplied.

If sutures have to be placed or the socket has to be packed with gelfoam, a local anesthetic should be infiltrated in the maxilla on the buccal and palatal side of the extraction socket. The agent of choice is lidocaine 2% with epinephrine 1:1,000,000. The same procedure could be carried out on the mandible, but anesthesia is better achieved by an inferior alveolar nerve block. It is usually necessary to obtain the help of an oral surgeon in treating postextraction bleeding. If bleeding persists after this local treatment, the possiblity of some primary abnormality in the coagulation system should be considered and the patient should be worked-up for this.

Chronic gingival bleeding is most commonly caused by chronic inflammatory periodontal disease. However, patients with acute leukemia may present with gingival enlargement and bleeding, and this diagnosis should be entertained for any patient who exhibits malaise, weight loss, and ecchymosis on the skin.

Other Problems

NONTRAUMATIC NECK PROBLEMS

The management of neck trauma is discussed in Chapter 19. Chronic neck masses may be a result of soft tissue infection, inflammation, obstruction, or hypertrophy of endocrine, salivary, or lymphoid glands, metastatic or primary neoplasms, or cysts of the neck. The differential diagnosis of chronic neck masses requires a complete examination of the nose, paranasal sinuses, nasopharynx, hypopharynx, and larynx, since about 80% of solitary adult neck masses are found to be metastatic lymph nodes from primary tumors located in the head and neck region. Therefore, referral for evaluation, including nasopharyngoscopy and indirect laryngoscopy, is indicated.

Acute neck masses are usually due to salivary gland obstruction or extension of bacterial infections from the oral cavity, pharynx, or salivary glands into the cervical lymph nodes or soft tissues of the neck. Although streptococci are common pathogens, mixed infections and penicillinase-resistant staphylococcal infections are becoming more prevalent. Lymph node suppuration frequently leads to deep cellulitis and even abscess formation in the neck. Salivary gland obstruction and infection have been discussed elsewhere in this chapter.

Deep neck infections are usually due to extension from pyogenic infections of the teeth, pharynx, or salivary glands. Typically the patient presents with a tender mass in the upper neck often associated with high fever, trismus, painful tongue motion, and sometimes stridor. Commonly the patient has been taking oral antibiotics for tonsillitis or a dental infection. Consequently neck infections may develop as a rapidly expanding area of cellulitis or abscess resistant to penicillin. The causative

bacteria are usually staphlococci or mixed infections. Cephalosporin (e.g., Keflin 2 g intravenously every 4 hours) or comparable antibiotic coverage is indicated, and surgical drainage is usually necessary under general anesthesia.

HOARSENESS (DYSPHONIA)

Dysphonia is usually caused from chronic or acute inflammation of the vocal cords, but it may also result from a variety of other conditions (e.g., tumor, vocal paralysis). The proper evaluation of this disorder requires indirect laryngoscopy. If the hoarseness has persisted for more than 2 weeks, appropriate referral for a complete ear, nose, and throat examination is indicated.

DYSPHAGIA

Acute dysphagia is usually the result of a foreign body in the hypopharynx or esophagus. The most common item causing acute dysphagia is a fish or chicken bone. Progressive dysphagia may be a result of a tumor, diverticulum, web inflammation, or neuromuscular disorder of the esophagus. If the dysphagia is progressive, a barium swallow is indicated to determine the cause of the problem; if the dysphagia is acute, lateral and AP views of the neck are indicated to detect a foreign body. If the dysphagia is so complete that the patient is unable to swallow saliva, endoscopy will usually be necessary to determine the cause of the problem and to effect removal of the foreign body.

FACIAL NERVE PARALYSIS

Facial nerve paralysis may be classified as either central or peripheral, according to the location of the lesion in relation to the facial nucleus in the brainstem. Central facial nerve paralysis results from a lesion proximal to the facial nucleus in the brainstem and produces ipsilateral paralysis to the lower two-thirds of the face. The ipsilateral forehead functions normally because of bilateral crossed enervation. Disorders of the central nervous system, such as multiple sclerosis, cerebrovascular accidents, and neoplasms, may present as facial paralysis. Usually there are other associated neurologic signs; these cases will be discovered by careful neurologic evaluation.

BELL'S PALSY

Diagnosis of idiopathic facial paralysis (Bell's palsy) should be made only when there are no specific causes of facial nerve paralysis. This disorder is more common in adults, especially women. It is thought to be a result of ischemia and edema of the facial nerve within the fallopian canal at the temporal bone. Viral infection, vascular disorders, allergy, and autoimmune mechanisms have been postulated as possible causes for Bell's palsy. The onset of facial paralysis may take several hours or several days and may be partial or complete. Most cases are unilateral, seldom recur, and recover spontaneously within 2–8 weeks regardless of treatment.

In the primary setting treatment of patients with Bell's palsy is directed toward protection of the involved eye with its diminished blink reflex. The eye is closed and a dry sterile patch is placed over it to prevent corneal drying. Referral to an otolaryngologist or a neurologist is indicated; hence, a careful search should be made to exclude more occult causes of the paralysis. Although early surgical decompression of the facial nerve has been advocated in cases of Bell's palsy, a more conservative and expectant course is generally accepted. Use of systemic corticosteroids is controversial and of questionable effectiveness. A 5-day course of tapered oral corticosteroids (e.g., prednisone 60 mg, 50 mg, 40 mg, 30 mg, 10 mg, on successive days) may be tried.

If the onset of facial paralysis is associated with an identifiable etiology (e.g., blunt or penetrating trauma, temporal bone fracture, acute suppurative otitis media, chronic suppurative otitis media), then immediate consultation with an otolaryngologist is advised since emergency surgical treatment may be indicated. Trauma associated with facial nerve paralysis may be a result of temporal bone fracture compression of the facial nerve within the fallopian canal and/or a laceration of the nerve within the soft tissues of the face. As discussed in Chapter 17, penetrating injuries may cause divisions of the branches of the facial nerve and the parotid duct.

SELECTED READINGS

Ballenger JJ: *Diseases of the Nose, Throat and Ear,* ed 12. Philadelphia, Lea & Febiger, 1977.

Converse JM: *Surgical Treatment of Facial Injuries,* ed 3. Baltimore, The William and Wilkins Co, 1974.

Dayal VS: *Clinical Otolaryngology.* Philadelphia, JB Lippincott Co, 1981.

DeWeese DD, Saunders WH: *Textbook of Otolaryngology,* ed 6. St. Louis, The CV Mosby Co, 1982.

English G: *Otolaryngology: A Textbook.* New York: Harper & Row Publishers Inc, 1976.

Frost EAM: Respiratory problems associated with head trauma. *Neurosurgery* 1977; 1:300–305.

Jennett B, Teasdale G: *Management of Head Injuries.* Philadelphia, FA Davis Co, 1981.

May M: Penetrating neck wounds. *Laryngoscope* 1975; 85:57.

Montgomery WW, Fabian RL, Lavelle WG: Fundamental otolaryngologic procedures, *Principles and Practice of Emergency Medicine.* Philadelphia, WB Saunders Co, 1978, chap 16.

Montgomery WW, Fabian RL, Lavelle WG, Witte JM: Nontraumatic otolaryngologic emergencies, in *Principles and Practice of Emergency Medicine.* Philadelphia, WB Saunders Co, 1978, chap 45.

Newman M, Haskell et al: *Handbook of Ear, Nose and Throat Emergencies.* Flushing, New York, New York Medical Examination Publishing Co, 1973.

Newman MH, Travis LW: Frontal sinus fractures. *Laryngoscope* 1975; 85:1.

Paparella, Shumrick (eds): *Otolaryngology.* Philadelphia, WB Saunders Co, 1980.

Torg J (ed): *Athletic Injuries to the Head, Neck and Face.* Philadelphia, Lea & Febiger, 1982.

33

THE ACUTE ABDOMEN

Lynn M. Peterson

Evaluation of the patient with acute, recent onset of abdominal pain is one of the most challenging responsibilities of the emergency physician. The physician's initial approach and early management can play a critical role in the final outcome because of the potentially catastrophic yet completely recoverable conditions that can produce acute abdominal pain.

Although attempts at establishing an accurate and early diagnosis in patients with an acute abdomen are laudable, the most important consideration is to achieve a suitable working diagnosis leading to appropriate diagnostic measures, treatment, and ultimately a successful outcome. Overemphasis on diagnostic accuracy can actually be harmful when time-consuming procedures are carried out that interfere with prompt attention to life-threatening concerns. Diagnostic technology has expanded dramatically in the past two decades, whereas therapeutic modalities and the need for urgent laparotomy for diagnosis and treatment of certain acute abdominal conditions has remained the same. Special procedures (e.g., laparoscopy, peritoneal lavage, ultrasound, computerized body scan) may be useful in certain difficult cases, but it is extremely unlikely that they will improve outcome on a routine basis.

An important aspect of the initial approach to a patient with an acute abdomen is a careful and thorough evaluation of the clinical data—history and examination—with a determination to seek a prompt resolution of the problem. Although urgent or rapid action is occasionally demanded, the majority of acute abdominal conditions require meticulous attention to the details of history and examination and repeated observation, first, to establish a working diagnosis and, then, in a deliberate and methodical fashion, to institute appropriate therapy. Although consultation from peers and other physicians may be helpful, it is essential that one physician remain in charge.

A major issue that must be confronted immediately in every patient with an acute abdomen is the possible need for an operation. The timing of such an operation could be critical and must influence the diagnostic measures and therapeutic modalities considered. For example, a patient with generalized peritonitis should receive fluid and blood volume repletion as well as appropriate broad-spectrum antibiotics immediately while anesthesia and operating personnel are in preparation. However, a patient with possible appendicitis will need a more detailed history, repeated examinations, and repeated determinations of temperature and blood count to help confirm or repudiate the physician's initial impression.

This chapter first covers general aspects of abdominal pain and then discusses important considerations in patient evaluation regarding history, examination, and laboratory data. Next, a framework is provided for the emergency room physician to help categorize acute abdominal conditions according to the urgency of and need for an operation. Finally, pitfalls are listed that emphasize practical matters with which the emergency room physician must be particularly concerned.

PATHOPHYSIOLOGIC CONSIDERATIONS

Awareness of abdominal pain arises from both visceral and somatic sensory nerve endings. Visceral afferent receptors are located on the peritoneal surface (both visceral and parietal peritoneum) as well as within the muscular coat of the bowel, gallbladder, bile duct, ureter, and bladder. These receptors respond to changes in tension within the muscular coat of the viscera, traction on the root of the mesentery, and any irritation provoked by tissue injury. They are not capable of recognizing touch or sharp pain (e.g., cutting) and are also unable to localize various stimuli discretely. Characteristically, in the cerebral cortex they produce a vague awareness of discomfort or, in the case of colic, a more acute and sharper feeling of abdominal pressure. Visceral afferent fibers travel with sympathetic and parasympathetic fibers, and some visceral stimuli reach the level of cortical awareness. However, many visceral afferents are involved in poorly understood viscero-visceral reflexes rather than signaling derangements to the level of consciousness. Hence abnormalities in motility, secretion, and blood flow and their clinical consequences (e.g., ileus, nausea, vomiting, tachycardia, bradycardia) are often prominent early evidence of noxious stimuli to the visceral nerve endings. Compared to the visceral efferents there is less known about the precise function and neuroanatomical pathways of visceral afferents even though they comprise 30–90% of the autonomic nerve trunks.

Somatic receptors and their axons innervate the parietal peritoneum as well as the outer levels of the abdominal wall. They are capable of discrete localization of noxious stimuli and are likely responsible for involuntary and voluntary muscle spasm, rigidity, and guarding. Therefore, appendicitis is initially recognized through visceral afferents when the patient has a vague awareness of discomfort or even pressure in the midabdomen, but later, when parietal peritoneum and somatic afferents are involved, the pain can be localized in the right lower quadrant and produces characteristic local muscle spasm.

When a noxious stimulus in the abdomen produces awareness of pain in an extraabdominal location it is called *referred pain*. The precise neurophysiologic explanation of this phenomenon is lacking, but the dermatome where pain is felt has a common embryologic origin with the affected part of the abdomen. Common pairs of pain sites and referred locations are as follows: (1) subdiaphragmatic—ipsilateral shoulder; (2) ureter—ipsilateral flank, groin, medial thigh, and scrotum or labia; and (3) gallbladder—right subscapular region. Pancreatic pain is often felt in the back, but this could be a result of direct involvement of contiguous posterior parietal peritoneum and surrounding structures rather than distant referral.

The degree and type of pain are also related to the noxious stimulus. Receptors located in the muscular coat of viscera respond to tension in the wall; the degree of tension is determined by the intraluminal volume as well as factors (e.g., hormonal and neural) controlling the state of muscular contraction or tone. Thus intestinal distention caused by muscular paralysis (ileus) produces little pain compared to that associated with intestinal obstruction when muscular contraction is greatly increased. Pain from fluid escaping into the free peritoneal cavity is proportional to the amount of tissue damage or irritation the particular fluid produces. Gastric juice, with its low pH, causes more irritation and pain than blood, which produces little irritation. Pancreatic juice contains various hydrolytic enzymes, but those capable of tissue damage (the proteolytic and phospholipolytic enzymes) are synthesized and secreted into pancreatic juice in an inactive form (zymogens or proenzymes) and hence must be activated before causing tissue damage. Activation occurs upon contact with the duodenal lumen or with inflammation—pancreatitis. Therefore, leakage of pure pancreatic juice can produce relatively little pain (e.g., pancreatic ascites) or can produce severe destruction and pain when associated with a duodenal leak or inflammation. Urine, bile, intestinal fluid, feces, and pus produce varying degrees of tissue damage and pain, depending on their volume and composition at the time of leakage. Oftentimes a viscus or abscess can become very tense just before rupture. Rupture then relieves the tension or pressure and thus can be associated with a sudden diminution in pain, especially if the leaking fluid is not irritating to the peritoneal surface, followed by a more disastrous condition resulting from generalized peritoneal sepsis.

EVALUATION OF THE PATIENT

It is important that the patient evaluation be carried out with thought and attention paid to the patient's comfort and anxiety. A quiet examining area, comfortable room temperature, and a bed that allows a relaxed, comfortable position are important considerations. Gentleness will also allow a more accurate evaluation.

History

The type of pain, its duration, constancy or intermittency, and its relationship to meals, activity, or sleep are important and obvious initial considerations. Pain that has lasted more than 6 hours and has interfered with sleep is more likely to be serious. Intermittent pain, if cramplike, is more likely to be associated with obstruction of a hollow viscus, whereas pain from peritoneal irritation is more likely to be continuous. Previous similar attacks are more likely associated with an underlying chronic disorder, for example, cholelithiasis, peptic ulcer, pelvic inflammatory disease, and less likely to be acute appendicitis. The onset of pain before vomiting is more likely related to a "surgical" condition (e.g., intestinal obstruction or appendicitis), whereas vomiting before the onset of pain often indicates gastroenteritis. In patients with proximal intestinal obstruction vomiting usually occurs within 1 or 2 hours after the onset of pain, however, in patients with distal obstruction vomiting may be delayed for many hours.

Severity of pain does not necessarily correlate with the gravity or seriousness of the underlying disorder. Intestinal and ureteral colic (associated with obstipation and renal calculi) can produce excruciating pain that is capable of spontaneous, nonoperative resolution. On the other hand, mesenteric vascular occlusion may produce little pain yet be of life-threatening severity.

Underlying medical conditions can play a significant role. Patients with diabetes or renal failure and patients who are receiving chronic steroid therapy can have advanced intraabdominal pathology with relatively mild clinical manifestations; the inflammatory response in these patients is blunted, and even mild symptoms can be significant. Drugs with anticholinergic and antispasmotic effects (e.g., amitriptyline—Elavil) can produce ileus and abdominal distention making intestinal obstruction difficult to evaluate. Diuretics producing potassium depletion have a similar effect. Serious abdominal conditions in the elderly also tend to be more subtle.

Physical Examination

The patient's general appearance can be very important. Patients with obstruction and colic tend to be restless and move during episodes of pain, whereas those with inflammatory conditions lie still. Evidence of poor cerebral or cutaneous perfusion—confusion, listlessness, cyanosis, pallor—are important indications of shock that may not be obvious in the initial blood pressure and pulse determinations. Vital signs, including rectal temperature, are important and should be carefully recorded in all patients with acute abdominal pain.

Examination of the abdomen itself should be carried out in a methodical, gentle manner. Careful observations can disclose subtle but important evidence of distention or discoloration around the umbilicus (Cullen's sign) or in the flanks (Grey Turner's sign). A bluish discoloration seen in these areas is a result of retroperitoneal hemorrhage from conditions such as pancreatitis; extravasated blood spreads to dependent regions (flank) or it is easily visible because skin and peritoneum are least separated by musculofascial layers (umbilicus). Auscultation, often best performed early in the examination, is important but should not be overemphasized; bowel sounds may be present and normal in patients with major intestinal infarction or perforation, whereas a quiet abdomen may reflect ileus secondary to an extraabdominal process.

The findings of peritoneal irritation are important since they generally indicate the presence of a surgical acute abdomen. Oftentimes during auscultation the physician is able to identify areas of discrete abdominal tenderness that can be further delineated by subsequent palpation. Observation of the patient's facial expression during palpation can help localize the area of maximal tenderness. Asking the patient to cough and gently shaking the abdomen are useful ways of demonstrating areas of peritoneal irritation as well. Tenderness elicited by gentle palpation does not require more forceful pressure for confirmation.

Rebound tenderness—pain elicited by sudden release of abdominal pressure—can be a sign of peritoneal irritation but also may be found with intestinal distention from a variety of causes. *Referred tenderness*—pain felt in one area as a result of pressure in another—is a more helpful indication of localized peritoneal irritation than is rebound tenderness. Rebound and referred tenderness can be disclosed by gentle maneuvers and do not require forceful pressure.

Involuntary muscle spasm is a very helpful indication of localized peritoneal irritation and is detected by gentle palpation and careful comparison of the tension or resistance in various regions of the abdominal wall. Distracting the patient's attention can help prevent voluntary and generalized muscle contraction or guarding that can mask areas of discrete localized spasm. Boardlike rigidity of the abdomen is a result of involuntary spasm of all of the abdominal wall muscles and occurs when there is severe irritation of the entire parietal peritoneal surface. Perforation of a peptic ulcer with release of gastric acid into the peritoneal cavity produces such an irritation with a boardlike abdomen; blood is much less noxious and the abdominal muscle tone is more relaxed. Generally the abdominal findings of peritoneal irritation tend to be constant and reproducible, whereas those due to gastroenteritis are variable.

Searching for an occult incarcerated hernia is important since occasionally the hernia itself may be asymptomatic and unnoticed yet still produce proximal intestinal obstruction and volvulus. The umbilical and femoral areas are the most notorious in this regard, but inguinal, incisional, and spigelian (at the lateral border of the rectus abdominus and the semilunar line which is approximately one-third the distance below the umbilicus to the pubis) regions must also be carefully examined.

Rectal and pelvic examinations must be performed in every patient with acute abdominal pain. This allows palpation of the lower pelvic peritoneum and, importantly, the prostate in males. Cervical smear and culture should be carried out whenever there is any possibility of pelvic inflammatory disease. Pain elicited by motion of the cervix must be sought since this suggests parametrial inflammation. Testing stool on the examining finger for occult blood should also be done.

Laboratory Evaluation

All patients should have a blood cell count with differential and urine analysis. An elevated hematocrit can be an important indication of hemoconcentration because of plasma loss in patients with pancreatitis and generalized peritonitis, whereas a low hematocrit suggests bleeding that has occurred several hours ago. Leukocytosis can be an important clue to abdominal inflammation and/or tissue damage; in patients with intestinal obstruction, leukocytosis suggests compromise of bowel viability and possible impending perforation. Serial white blood cell counts can be very helpful when the diagnosis is uncertain; initial leukocytosis can be a result of dehydration or acute stress, whereas normal counts can be present in the early stages of appendicitis, cholecystitis, or diverticulitis. The peripheral smear can show an important shift to the left in patients with acute appendicitis and normal total leukocyte count and can indicate the possibility of a blood dyscrasia in patients with leukopenia or marked leukocytosis. A normal blood count and peripheral smear do not exclude the possibility of a serious abdominal condition urgently requiring an operation. Urine analysis provides important information about a possible urinary tract infection if leukocytes and renal calculi are present when erythrocytes are found. These microscopic findings can rarely be seen secondary to retroperitoneal inflammatory conditions (e.g., psoas abscess, retrocecal appendicitis). Glucosuria suggests diabetes and ketonuria dehydration; glucosuria and ketonuria together indicate diabetic ketoacidosis requiring urgent metabolic therapy. Serum amylase is the most important chemistry test and should be done routinely. In patients with abdominal pain and elevation of serum amylase, the clearance ratio of amylase:creatinine (urine amylase × serum creatinine ÷ urine creatinine × serum amylase × 100), obtained by determining both amylase and creatinine on serum and urine samples obtained simultaneously, can provide helpful confirmatory evidence of pancreatitis when elevated (greater than 6%). Patients with right upper quadrant pain should have liver function tests ordered in the emergency room to look for evidence of hepatocellular disease or biliary obstruction. Blood urea nitrogen (BUN) and/or serum creatinine are useful to assess renal function, and blood sugar to look for diabetes. It is important to remember to determine the serum calcium in patients who are thought to have pancreatitis because of its therapeutic and prognostic implications.

Extensive laboratory testing is generally unnecessary, and all laboratory data must be interpreted in terms of their relevance to the clinical situation. A patient with an acute perforated duodenal ulcer may have completely normal laboratory tests yet require emergency surgery, whereas a patient with alcoholic hepatitis can have dramatic leukocytosis and not require surgery.

Radiologic Evaluation

Plain adbominal x-ray films are frequently helpful along with an upright chest film. The presence of free air (Fig. 33.1), abnormal intestinal gas shadows (Fig. 33.2–33.5), calcified stones in ureter or biliary tree, suggestion of an abdominal mass, thumbprinting in the bowel wall (Fig. 33.6), free intraabdominal fluid, obliteration of the psoas shadow and peritoneal fat line, and appendicolithiasis are the common things for which we should look. Abdominal films are most helpful for patients suspected of perforation or intestinal obstruction and for patients in whom the diagnosis is uncertain. The presence of free intraperitoneal air is best seen subdiaphragmatically in an upright chest film centered low enough to include both diaphragms. The patient must be upright for at least 10 minutes

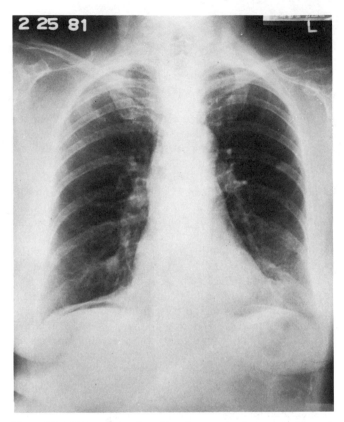

Figure 33.1 This upright chest film shows a small amount of free air beneath both hemidiaphragms. Gastric and colonic gas can produce an air shadow under the left diaphragm but not on the right. Therefore free intraperitoneal air will generally be most reliably seen under the right diaphragm.

to allow the air to rise to the subdiaphragmatic location. Lateral decubitus films, taken with the patient lying on the side, can be used to demonstrate free air in patients unable to sit up, but adequate time must still be allowed for the air to rise to the lateral abdominal wall. A chest x-ray film is essential in almost every patient being prepared for laparotomy.

Contrast studies of the intestinal tract are generally not necessary in patients suspected of having intestinal obstruction but can be helpful in some specific instances and should be ordered by the surgeon. Barium enema is useful in patients with distal small bowel or colonic obstruction since colonic cancer is a relatively common underlying cause. Such a study helps in planning the operative approach and in preparing the patient for the possibility of a colostomy. Upper intestinal studies are

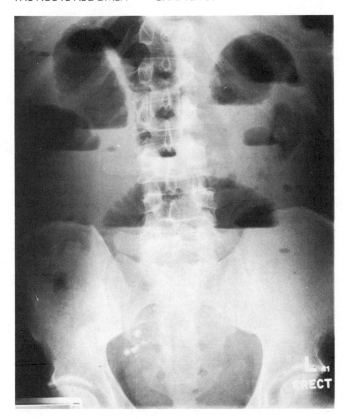

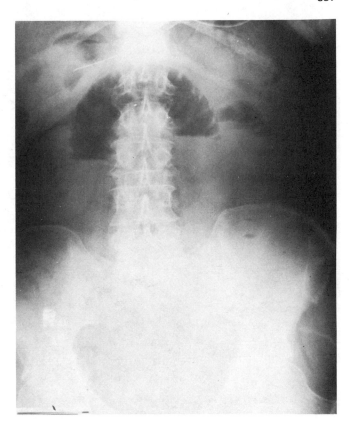

Figure 33.2 Paralytic ileus is illustrated in this upright film showing multiple loops of dilated small intestine with air–fluid levels. There is some gas in the right and left colon. Obstruction cannot be excluded on the basis of this x-ray. This patient had a distended, painless abdomen with absent bowel sounds. The condition resolved after 2 days of gastric suction and parenteral fluids.

Figure 33.3 Mechanical small bowel obstruction with a single dilated loop of small intestine in the midabdomen with air–fluid levels. This patient had obstruction secondary to a jejunal twist (volvulus) around an adhesive band.

less likely to be helpful as "emergency" examinations except in unusually difficult cases; demonstration of complete obstruction indicates the need for immediate operation because of the possibility of a volvulus and compromised intestinal viability. The presence of barium proximal to an obstructive lesion can cause problems because of the difficulty in evacuation and tendency to become inspissated. Even with operative relief of the obstruction, delayed transit because of postoperative ileus can cause the barium to be "sticky," difficult to evacuate and impacted. In cases of suspected intestinal perforation, barium should be avoided and gastrograffin or a water-soluble contrast agent used instead.

Ultrasound examination is helpful in patients suspected of acute biliary disease since it can be done on an emergency basis and can often demonstrate the presence of gallstones or ductal obstruction. Ultrasound is also helpful in evaluating pelvic masses and in searching for intraabdominal abscesses. Clinical judgment is extremely important in deciding on the meaning or relevance of a particular ultrasonographic finding.

Special diagnostic studies are worth considering in certain individual cases. Sigmoidoscopy can be helpful in patients with intestinal obstruction, diarrhea, or hematochezia, (see Chapter 34). Peritoneal tap or paracentesis can be helpful in patients with free peritoneal fluid and acute abdominal pain but should probably be performed by the surgeon. Fluid obtained should be examined for the presence of blood, bile and feces and microscopically examined for white blood cells and microorganisms. A pH determination is helpful; if found to be low,

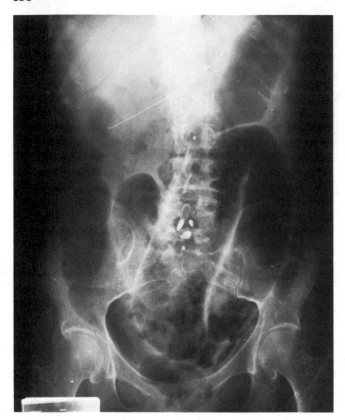

Figure 33.4 Sigmoid volvulus: a large loop of dilated bowel extends from the pelvis upward to the left midabdomen representing the twisted sigmoid colon. There is air in the ascending, transverse, and descending colon surrounding the volvulus.

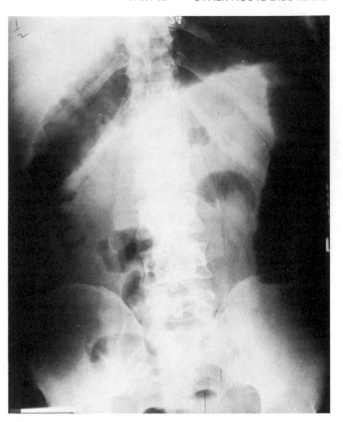

Figure 33.5 Toxic megacolon in which virtually the entire colon is abnormal, with greatest distention of the transverse and descending colon. The normal haustral pattern is lost, the bowel wall is thickened, and there are multiple lobulated filling defects representing pseudopolyps or sloughing colonic mucosa.

it indicates gastric or duodenal perforation. The fluid should be cultured. Peritoneal tap or lavage in patients without free fluid is more hazardous; it should not be routinely used in these patients.

CLINICAL SETTINGS

It is probably most helpful for the emergency room physician to categorize diseases producing abdominal pain according to the urgency of the need for operative intervention. In some patients a few hours delay can significantly impair the likelihood of successful treatment, whereas for other patients a few hours delay can be very helpful in making appropriate decisions. The following organization attempts to help physicians categorize diseases in this way.

Conditions That Require Urgent or Immediate Operation

The major nontraumatic abdominal conditions that require immediate or urgent operation are hemorrhage and ischemia.

HEMORRHAGE

The nontraumatic conditions producing intraperitoneal hemorrhage include ruptured aortic aneurysm, ruptured ectopic pregnancy, ruptured visceral artery aneurysms (splenic, hepatic, etc.), hemorrhagic pancreatitis, ruptured hepatic tumors (hepatoma or adenoma), delayed hemorrhage from a traumatized spleen especially in the context of diseases involving the spleen (e.g., mononucleosis and leukemia), and, rarely, massive hemorrhage from an ovarian cyst. Aortic and visceral

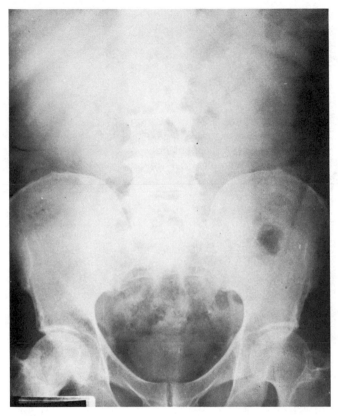

Figure 33.6 Ischemic colitis with multiple smooth defects impinging on the narrowed air column of the splenic flexure and descending colon. These smooth, submucosal defects produce a thumbprint appearance.

aneurysms are more common in men over the age of 50, whereas ectopic pregnancy and ruptured ovarian cysts occur in women in the child-bearing age group. Hepatic adenomas are more common in young women, especially those taking birth control pills. Patients taking anticoagulants are more susceptible to spontaneous intraperitoneal or retroperitoneal hemorrhage without any pathoanatomical deformity.

Diagnosis

Free intraperitoneal hemorrhage is often associated with syncope and abdominal distention in addition to abdominal pain, although the pain itself may not be severe. Because intraperitoneal blood is relatively nonirritating, at least initially, the abdomen may be surprisingly soft in spite of the presence of a large volume of blood. Vital signs may demonstrate hypo-

tension or tachycardia, but when they are normal, comparison of blood pressure and pulse in supine and sitting positions (postural changes) is a more sensitive index of hypovolemia. An increase in pulse of more than 20 beats/min and a decrease in systolic blood pressure of more than 10 mm Hg upon sitting indicates a significant volume loss (greater than 1,000 ml). Hematocrit changes may not be apparent with brisk bleeding because approximately 4 hours are required for significant hemodilution. Peritoneal tap or culdocentesis can help secure the diagnosis and avoid needless delay in getting the patient to the operating room. When there is evidence of brisk intraperitoneal bleeding, the time spent getting "routine" tests (e.g., electrocardiograms and films) is generally not worthwhile and may cause hazardous delay in stopping the bleeding.

Management

Initial management of hemorrhage must include establishment of secure and adequate venous infusion lines, matching blood for transfusion, and preparation of the operating room. The surgeon should be notified as soon as the diagnosis of intraperitoneal hemorrhage is strongly suspected.

ISCHEMIA

Patients likely to have intestinal arterial ischemia would be those who are elderly and those with other evidence of cardiovascular disease, for example, atherosclerotic changes causing loss of pedal pulses, atrial fibrillation, or a past history of arterial emboli. Mesenteric venous occlusion occurs rarely and is generally found in patients with cirrhosis or pancreatitis and characteristically produces bloody peritoneal fluid.

Diagnosis

Intestinal ischemia is one of the most difficult diagnostic categories because the symptoms and findings can be vague and nonspecific. Pain may be severe, but severe pain is not always present. Systemic changes may precede definitive abdominal evidence of bowel ischemia and the patient may look very ill with tachycardia and hypotension yet have few abdominal findings. There are few, if any, specific abdominal findings with early ischemia so the diagnosis frequently depends on a strong suspicion and ruling out other acute abdominal conditions. Later, as the bowel wall undergoes more complete necrosis, peritoneal signs associated with inflammation are found, for example, rebound tenderness, muscle spasm, and guarding. Bloody diarrhea or the presence of occult blood in the stool obtained on rectal examination is a helpful finding when present. Plain abdominal films can be very helpful when they show an abnormal gas pattern with thumbprinting of the bowel wall as a result submucosal edema and/or hemorrhage (Fig. 33.6). If arteriography is done, it can demonstrate arterial occlusion by a thrombus or embolus and, in patients with nonocclusive ischemia, evidence of vasoconstriction and reduced splanchnic flow.

Management

In the emergency room all patients suspected of having intestinal ischemia should be treated by prompt correction of any underlying circulatory compromise (shock) with adequate parenteral fluid administration, and patients with cardiac failure should be treated with inotropic support with agents such as dopamine or isoproterenol. Digitalis preparations should probably be avoided because of their possible adverse effects on splanchnic vascular resistance and blood flow. A Foley catheter and central venous line should generally be inserted to help monitor hydration and cardiac output. A nasogastric tube will usually need to be inserted in the emergency room in order to relieve the fluid accumulation in the upper gastrointestinal tract produced by the concomitant paralytic ileus. The surgeon should be involved early in the management since in patients with vascular occlusion immediate operation is the only hope for survival. In patients with nonocclusive ischemia demonstrated arteriographically, local arterial infusion of a vasodilator (papaverine) may offer the best chance for recovery.

Conditions That Require Early Operation

The most common conditions that require early operation are perforation, intestinal obstruction, appendicitis, abdominal abscess, and incarcerated hernia. The diagnosis is more likely to be obvious for patients in this group since they are likely to have fully established findings of peritoneal irritation (peritonitis). The major threat to these patients is impending or already present abdominal sepsis. The emergency room physician must remember to correct deficits in circulating blood volume as a result of plasma loss as well as the vasodilatation and pooling that occurs in the septic state. These deficits must be corrected promptly in order to support visceral function as well as to prepare for an operation that will require general anesthesia with its impairment of supportive sympathoadrenal reflexes. Although surgery is the most important element in controlling the septic process, broad spectrum antibiotics—an aminoglycoside (e.g., tobramycin or gentamicin) to cover the aerobic and clindamycin to cover the anaerobic bowel organisms likely to be present—should be administered in adequate doses before surgery to individuals thought to have an established bac-

terial infection. Prophylactic antibiotics (a cephalosporin given parenterally for 24–48 hours) should be started preoperatively in other patients in this group who have a high risk of intraoperative bacterial contamination of the surgical wound.

PERFORATION

Patients who require an early operation may have a past history of disease involving the perforated organ, for example, gallstones in patients with gallbladder perforation, peptic ulcer disease in those with ulcer perforation.

Diagnosis

Gastric or duodenal perforation generally produces dramatic pain and generalized abdominal rigidity. Intestinal, colonic, or appendiceal perforation may not produce the same sudden and severe degree of pain and rigidity, but subsequent bacterial peritonitis will produce a septic and critically ill patient. The site of perforation may not be easy to specify preoperatively in patients with perforation of a pancreatic pseudocyst or pelvic or diverticular abscess. Occasionally patients will not seek medical attention for several hours or even days after the perforation has occurred. At this time the pain may be less intense and more localized and an abscess may have formed (see below). When a localized abscess does not form, patients with an old perforation may have abdominal findings that are diffuse and less striking; these patients are often lethargic and moribund.

Management

Nasogastric suction, in addition to parenteral fluids and broad spectrum antibiotics (see above), will usually be necessary in the emergency room. A Foley catheter and central venous pressure line may also be needed in patients requiring vigorous fluid resuscitation. Since an operation will be required soon, the surgeon should be notified promptly.

INTESTINAL OBSTRUCTION WITH EVIDENCE OF ISCHEMIA

Individuals who have had previous abdominal operations (adhesions) or abdominal wall hernias are generally susceptible to develop intestinal obstruction. As a result of the obstruction, volvulus, or intestinal vascular compromise can develop, creating an urgent need for an operation.

Diagnosis

Patients with intestinal ischemia usually start with crampy abdominal pain and vomiting. Later as the intestinal ischemia develops, the pain becomes more constant or continuous rather than crampy or intermittent. The presence of signs of peritoneal irritation and fever along with leukocytosis strongly suggests this diagnosis. Plain abdominal films will help to establish the diagnosis and suggest the site or level of obstruction, but detailed gastrointestinal studies and prolonged attempts at preoperative decompression are not indicated.

Management

Parenteral fluid administration to replace external (vomiting) and internal (peritoneal as well as intraluminal fluid) losses is the most important initial consideration. Nasogastric suction to decompress the upper gastrointestinal tract and Foley catheter to monitor fluid replacement will often be useful in the emergency room. Since bacterial contamination by way of the compromised bowel is likely to occur pre- or intraoperatively, administration of an antibiotic with broad gram-negative coverage (e.g., a cephalosporin) would be useful in the emergency room in preparation for operation.

DEFINITE APPENDICITIS

The relatively common condition of appendicitis can occur in patients of any age, but it is more common in people between the ages of 7 and 17. Although a past history of right lower quadrant pain is occasionally present, most patients with acute appendicitis have not had chronic or recurrent attacks of pain.

Diagnosis

Periumbilical pain moving to the right lower quadrant along with anorexia, nausea, and vomiting are the usual historical features of appendicitis. Examination will often disclose localized tenderness and muscle spasm in the right lower quadrant, and the patient will have a temperature of 38°C (100–101°F). The major laboratory finding is a mild leukocytosis ranging from 11,000–15,000. Rectal and pelvic examinations may occasionally reveal localized tenderness when the abdominal examination is not striking. Difficulty in diagnosis depends on the stage of the disease, location of the appendix, and various individual factors such as age. Abdominal films are of little value when the diagnosis seems certain since they are generally normal, but when there is uncertainty, abdominal film can be helpful in suggesting another possible diagnosis.

Management

Prompt appendectomy is the treatment of choice for patients with acute appendicitis, but intravenous fluids for rehydration and a preoperative antibiotic (cephalosporin) should be administered in the emergency room. If the appendix has become gangrenous or perforated there is usually a walled off abscess in the right lower quadrant and a longer history of illness (more than 48 hours), higher fever (greater than 39°C or 102°F), and marked leukocytosis (greater than 15,000). Occasionally a mass or abscess can be palpated in the right lower quadrant. In this condition an aminoglycoside (gentamicin or tobramycin) and an antibiotic effective against anaerobic organisms should be given in preparation for operation.

ABDOMINAL ABSCESS WITH SEPTICEMIA

An abdominal abscess can arise from a variety of organs, such as colon, fallopian tube, appendix, pancreas, or duodenum. Regardless of its origin, prompt operation to establish drainage must be considered since the septic process may not be controlled by antibiotics and there is a threat of abscess rupture with intraperitoneal spread of the infection.

Diagnosis

Patients with abdominal abscess generally have abdominal pain, fever, and leukocytosis, characteristically associated with shaking chills or rigor. If the septic process is advanced or occurs in a compromised host, hypothermia, thrombocytopenia, and even leukopenia can ensue. Occasionally a tender mass may be palpable. Emergency ultrasound can be helpful in locating the abscess, but it is not completely accurate and false-negative and false-positive results are possible. Gallium or computerized tomographic scanning is not suitable on an emergency basis.

Management

Preoperative hydration, antibiotics, and early drainage are critical since rupture with peritoneal soilage could be disastrous.

INCARCERATED HERNIA

Patients with incarcerated hernias have generally had a previously reducible hernia. They come to the emergency room when the hernia becomes painful or tender and is no longer reducible. The emergency room physician should not attempt reduction by applying forceful pressure but should help the patient lie comfortably and should notify the surgeon. Urgent operative intervention may be necessary because of the threat of injury to the bowel or its blood supply.

Obstructive Conditions for Which Operation Is Delayed

In obstructive conditions in which operation should be delayed, observation (usually in the hospital) for a period of time helps clarify the diagnosis and allows the best decision for operative or nonoperative therapy. If an operation is needed, the patient is often better prepared.

GASTRIC OUTLET OBSTRUCTION

A past history of peptic ulcer disease is common in patients with a gastric outlet obstruction. Gastric and pancreatic neoplasms can also produce this condition, in which case there may be no history of antecedent difficulty.

Diagnosis

Vomiting, upper abdominal pain, and tenderness are characteristic features of gastric outlet obstruction. The vomitus contains undigested food and clear yellow gastric secretions but nothing green or bile stained. There may be a succussion splash in the left upper quadrant produced by the air-and-fluid-filled stomach. Upper gastrointestinal series and/or endoscopy are needed to confirm the diagnosis. Electrolyte abdnormalities with hypochloremic, hypokalemic alkalosis can be profound.

Management

Gastric suction, parenteral fluids, and efforts to correct acid–base and electrolyte deficits should be initiated in the emergency room. If there is a history of peptic ulcer disease, cimetidine, could also be started in the emergency room.

Often the edema of an acute ulcer will diminish and the obstruction will be relieved in 48–72 hours. The need for an operation will depend on consideration of multiple factors including the possibility of treating underlying peptic ulcer disease with healing of the ulcer and resolution of the obstruction.

SMALL BOWEL OBSTRUCTION

The most common causes of small bowel obstruction are adhesions from a previous operation, an incarcerated hernia, and a colonic neoplasm. Previous attacks are not uncommon.

Diagnosis

Patients with small bowel obstruction have crampy abdominal pain and vomiting but without evidence of peritoneal irritation, fever, or leukocytosis. If the latter findings become manifest, then the possibility of ischemia exists (see above section Intestinal Obstruction with Evidence of Ischemia). Pain abdominal films, ordered by the emergency room physician, should be done with the patient in the supine and upright positions. When there is small bowel obstruction there will be gas-filled small bowel loops with air–fluid levels and a stepladder pattern (Fig. 33.3); the absence or paucity of colonic gas helps localize the obstructive site to the small intestinal level.

Management

Initially, patients with small bowel obstruction can usually be treated with nasogastric suction and parenteral fluids. Careful observation in the hospital, including serial abdominal films, repeat abdominal examinations, temperatures monitoring, and white blood cell counts, can be carried out over the next 12–24 hours. If there is no evidence of relief of the obstruction, an operation will probably be necessary.

COLONIC OBSTRUCTION

Carcinoma of the colon, diverticulitis, and volvulus are the major causes of colonic obstruction.

Diagnosis

Crampy abdominal pain and abdominal distention are common, but nausea and vomiting are less common with colonic than with small bowel obstruction. Obstipation is usually present, but diarrhea is not an uncommon feature of partial colonic obstruction. Plain films will show varying amounts of colonic gas and distention. Sigmoid volvulus often has a characteristic appearance on plain roentgenograms of the abdomen (Fig. 33.4). If the ileocecal valve becomes incompetent, distention of the small bowel will be seen; decompression of colonic pressure into the small bowel reduces the intracolonic pressure and the risk of colonic perforation. However, if cecal dilatation reaches a critical level (diameter of 10 cm on film), there is a serious risk of colonic perforation.

Management

Patients with colonic obstruction should receive parenteral fluid and nasogastric suction in the emergency room. The nasogastric suction relieves vomiting if present, and, more importantly, prevents further air and fluid from reaching the obstructed colon. Gastric suction will not decompress the dilated colon. Sigmoid volvulus can be relieved by sigmoidoscopic or colonoscopic intubation but probably should be done by the surgeon in the emergency room. Antibiotics (a cephalosporin) should be administered prophylactically to patients undergoing emergency colonic surgery because of the high risk of bacterial contamination.

Inflammatory Conditions for Which Operation Is Delayed

POSSIBLE APPENDICITIS

Patients in whom the diagnosis of appendicitis is not clear can usually be safely observed for 8–12 hours. This allows repeat examination as well as repeat determinations of temperature and white blood cell count. This would be especially applicable for patients in whom the initial temperature and white blood cell count were normal.

DIVERTICULITIS

Patients with diverticulitis are usually over 50 and frequently have a past history of constipation.

Diagnosis

Acute diverticulitis presents with left lower quadrant pain, tenderness, low-grade fever, and leukocytosis. Obstipation or diarrhea may be present. Usually there is no vomiting.

Management

Uncomplicated diverticulitis can be successfully treated with liquid diet or parenteral fluids and antibiotics. Most patients with acute diverticulitis can be successfully treated with a single antibiotic effective against gram-negative bacteria (e.g., ampicillin or cephalosporin). However, life-threatening septic conditions (e.g., an abscess or perforation) should be treated with optimal doses of an aminoglycoside (gentamicin or tobramycin) as well as an agent to control anaerobic bacteria (lincomycin or chloramphenicol). There should be progressive improvement over 2–4 days, after which the diet can be advanced. Stool softeners can be added at this time to prevent any increase in intraluminal colonic pressure. Lack of improvement would suggest development of more complicated disease, for example, local perforation and abscess formation,

and would indicate potential need for operative intervention. Barium enema is best done after the acute inflammatory process has subsided.

ACUTE CHOLECYSTITIS

Patients with acute cholecystitis will sometimes have a history of fatty food intolerance and past episodes of upper abdominal pain or discomfort.

Diagnosis

Right upper-quadrant pain, tenderness, fever, and leukocytosis are usually present when the gallbladder is acutely inflamed. Pain from cholecystitis is usually slowly progressive and constant in intensity, whereas biliary colic (without inflammation) has a sharp, sudden onset often related to eating and tends to fluctuate in intensity. The results of liver function tests, including bilirubin and amylase, can be mildly elevated without implicating hepatic or pancreatic disease. Ultrasound and radionuclide scanning are the two most useful diagnostic tests in an emergency setting because they do not rely on gastrointestinal absorption of a contrast agent as does oral cholecystography nor do they depend on normal liver function as does intravenous cholangiography. Ultrasound can demonstrate the gallstones while radionuclide scanning confirms the diagnosis by failing to visualize the gallbladder because of obstruction of the cystic duct. Both tests occasionally can be helpful for patients seen in the emergency room but, generally, treatment is initiated on the basis of a clinical diagnosis and these tests are done later to confirm the clinical impression.

Management

Parenteral fluids and an antibiotic (ampicillin or cephalosporin) will usually allow the acute process to subside. Nasogastric suction is useful in patients who are vomiting. If improvement occurs, waiting for 2 or 3 days will often allow more stable circumstances for a semielective cholecystectomy. If improvement is not obvious in 12–36 hours, empyema, gangrene, or perforation of the gallbladder must be suspected and operation undertaken.

CHOLANGITIS

Infection in the biliary tree and liver generally occurs in patients with obstructive jaundice produced by gallstones rather than malignancy.

Diagnosis

Fever, leukocytosis, right upper-quadrant pain, and tenderness in a jaundiced patient are the usual clinical features. Shaking chills are often present. Liver function tests may indicate hepatocellular dysfunction along with an elevated bilirubin. Demonstration of gallstones and biliary tract dilatation by ultrasound can be very helpful.

Management

Initially, antibiotics, parenteral fluids, and nasogastric suction, if there is any vomiting, are given. Elevation of serum amylase would suggest obstruction at the level of Vater's ampulla and the possibility of coexistent pancreatitis. Often there is dramatic improvement in 24–48 hours with the above measures, and operation can be performed in a more deliberate and definitive manner after the acute infection has come under control. If improvement does not occur, urgent decompression of the biliary tree is needed.

INFLAMMATORY BOWEL DISEASE

Patients with inflammatory bowel disease often have a past history of diarrhea, especially with blood, but absence of such a history does not exclude this diagnosis. Without past documentation of Crohn's disease or ulcerative colitis, these disorders can be difficult to diagnose in the emergency room in patients with acute abdominal pain.

Diagnosis

Abdominal pain, tenderness, fever, nausea, vomiting, diarrhea, and leukocytosis are the usual clinical features in patients with inflammatory bowel disease. Terminal ileitis can be impossible to distinguish from acute appendicitis and can be associated with an intraabdominal abscess requiring operative drainage. Careful examination of the perianal region for fistula tracts and sigmoidoscopy can be very helpful in establishing a correct working diagnosis. Plain abdominal films should be ordered in the emergency room to look for evidence of intestinal obstruction, an abdominal mass, perforation, and so forth. Excessive dilatation of the colon (transverse colon greater than 10 cm) can also be seen and suggests megacolon, which can be present in patients with either ulcerative or Crohn's colitis (Fig. 33.5).

Management

If Crohn's disease seems likely based on past documentation and there is no evidence of an abscess, parenteral steroids would be indicated. If an abscess is likely to be present, antibiotics would also be used initially but operative drainage and/or resection would be likely to be necessary later. Initial treatment of toxic megacolon is with steroids and antibiotics. If improvement in colonic distention and toxicity of the patient is not seen in 24–48 hours, an emergency colectomy will be needed.

PANCREATITIS

Patients with pancreatitis often have a history of excessive alcohol intake or cholelithiasis.

Diagnosis

Upper abdominal pain, tenderness, and vomiting are the usual clinical features. The pain from pancreatitis is often severe and sharp and frequently radiates to the midback region. Patients sometimes find that sitting with hips and knees flexed and bending forward relieves their pain. Marked elevation of serum amylase (at least twice normal) and an increased amylase clearance helps confirm the diagnosis, but a normal amylase does not rule it out. Hyperglycemia and hypocalcemia are confirmatory if present. Abdominal films and upright chest film help rule out perforation.

Management

The most important initial management is adequate parenteral fluid administration including both colloid and crystalloid. Nasogastric suction should also generally be used. Close observation, intensive care, and special attention to renal and pulmonary function are essential. Marked temperature rise (greater than 39°C or 102°F) and leukocytosis (greater than 15,000) suggest the possibility of a pancreatic abscess, and antibiotics should be used after blood cultures are obtained. Evidence of underlying biliary disease (gallstones) is also an indication for the use of antibiotics after blood cultures are obtained. Operation is generally not indicated unless there is evidence of an abscess, pseudocyst, massive hemorrhage, bowel infarction, or perforation.

Conditions for Which Operation Should Be Avoided

GASTROENTERITIS

In patients with gastroenteritis, vomiting and diarrhea are often present from the onset. Pain is diffuse and variable, the abdomen is soft, and there is little if any tenderness. Fever is often present, but the white blood cell count and differential are generally normal.

URINARY TRACT INFECTION

Pyelonephritis can produce abdominal pain and tenderness, and there is usually associated flank tenderness. Fever and leukocytosis are present. Urine analysis shows pyuria and frequently white blood cell casts. Cystitis, urethritis, and prostatitis may produce abdominal pain secondary to bladder distention from urinary retention. Urine analysis shows pyuria. Prostatitis is demonstrated by prostatic tenderness on rectal examination or epididymal and testicular tenderness on examination of the groin and scrotum.

RENAL CALCULI

Severe intermittent attacks of abdominal pain, often most marked in the flank and referred to the testicle or labia, are the hallmark of renal calculi. Hematuria is generally present.

MESENTERIC ADENITIS

Mesenteric adenitis can mimic appendicitis completely, but the white blood cell count can be very high (greater than 20,000) and the differential show lymphocytosis. This condition occurs oftentimes immediately after a viral upper respiratory tract infection.

MITTELSCHMERZ

Ovarian bleeding at the time of ovulation can cause abdominal pain and tenderness. This usually occurs at midcycle. Temperature and white blood cell count are generally normal. If the right ovary is involved, differentiation from appendicitis can be difficult. It can also be confused with ectopic pregnancy.

HEPATITIS

Right upper quadrant pain and tenderness occurs as a result of tension and irritation of Glisson's capsule. The patient is often jaundiced, but jaundice is not necessarily present. Anorexia can be profound, and nausea and vomiting are not uncommon. Degree of fever and leukocytosis are variable. Elevated serum transaminases (especially if greater than 1,000) confirm the diagnosis.

CONGESTIVE HEART FAILURE

Abdominal pain and tenderness can occur because of hepatic congestion with pressure on the peritoneal covering of the liver, similar to hepatitis. Fever and leukocytosis are absent. Other signs of congestive heart failure—especially pulmonary edema—are present.

ACUTE MYOCARDIAL INFARCTION

Upper abdominal pain is occasionally present but there is no tenderness or fever. Usually there are cardiac findings (rub, gallop, tachycardia, electrocardiographic changes, etc.).

PNEUMONIA

Lower lobe pneumonia or pleurodynia can produce upper abdominal pain. Abdominal examination is negative. There is often a pleuritic component to the pain. Chest examination and film are critical in making this diagnosis.

PARALYTIC ILEUS

Abdominal pain is generalized, vague, and associated with distention. There is no tenderness, fever, or leukocytosis. Bowel sounds are diminished or absent. Plain films (Fig. 33.2) show general gaseous distention of the small and large bowel.

PRIMARY PERITONITIS

Usually free peritoneal fluid is present, and this condition often occurs in the context of other disease such as cirrhosis, nephrotic syndrome, collagen disease, and pneumococcal pneumonia. Fever, tenderness, and leukocytosis are often present. Paracentesis demonstrates polymorphonuclear leukocytes and/or bacteria. Gram-positive bacteria in conjunction with a disease known to predispose to primary peritonitis and without evidence of visceral perforation or abscess can be treated with antibiotics alone. Gram-negative bacteria, mixed bacterial flora, or evidence of abscess or perforation generally require laparotomy.

UNEXPLAINED (PSYCHOGENIC) ABDOMINAL PAIN

Patients with unexplained abdominal pain have usually had multiple previous hospitalizations or operations for abdominal pain without a specific disease being found. Hysterectomy, appendectomy, and cholecystectomy may have been done previously without relief. It is important to avoid both under—and over—treatment of these patients. Prescription of narcotic analgesics can be detrimental. Further surgery should be avoided without a specific diagnosis or disease requiring an operation.

FAMILIAL MEDITERRANEAN FEVER

Patients with familial Mediterranean fever have abdominal pain, fever, tenderness, and leukocytosis. They are usually young, have a family history of abdominal pain, and are of Mediterranean extraction. There is often a past history of appendectomy. Diagnosis is difficult without this background and often requires laparotomy and appendectomy to rule out the possibility of appendicitis. Colchicine is the specific treatment of choice to prevent further attacks, but it does not relieve current pain.

PORPHYRIA

Abdominal examination and temperature are normal. The pain is severe. There is a history of previous attacks of pain, and a diagnosis can be made with a positive Watson-Schwartz test or urinary porphobilinogen.

SICKLE CELL DISEASE

Young black patients with anemia are the most likely to have sickle cell disease. The pain is often in the left upper quadrant because of splenic infarction and can be associated with tenderness and slight fever.

DIABETIC KETOACIDOSIS

Abdominal examination of patients with diabetic ketoacidosis is negative. Diabetes is out of control, and the pain disappears after medical control of the diabetes.

LEAD INTOXICATION

Patients with lead intoxication have crampy abdominal pain, nausea, and vomiting. There is no fever or localized abdominal tenderness. The pain usually subsides spontaneously and is thought to be because of either spasm of intestinal or abdominal wall muscles.

INTESTINAL PSEUDOOBSTRUCTION

The history and examination of patients with intestinal pseudoobstruction are typical of intestinal obstruction. There tend to be recurring attacks that subside spontaneously. Barium films of the upper intestine or colon fail to show evidence of obstruction, although plain films may suggest its presence. This condition occurs spontaneously as well as in some patients on vincristine chemotherapy for malignancy, myxedema, collagen diseases, and diabetes.

PITFALLS

The following are pitfalls emphasizing practical matters with which the emergency room physican must be particularly concerned:

1. Failure to analyze carefully the type of pain and to note the hour-by-hour history of the pain
2. Reliance on a history taken by someone else
3. Use of oral rather than rectal temperatures
4. Failure to recognize the significance of early abdominal distention
5. Hurried and rough rather than gentle palpation of the abdomen
6. Failure to detect an incarcerated hernia in a patient with small bowel obstruction
7. Failure to consider appendicitis in all patients and ectopic pregnancy in all female patients with lower abdominal pain
8. Reliance on laboratory tests to make a specific diagnosis and to determine whether operation is necessary
9. Failure to examine the chest and get a chest film to rule out pneumonia
10. Failure to get an upright abdominal film for fluid levels when the supine film is negative, and failure to get an upright chest film when looking for free air under the diaphragm

SUGGESTED READINGS

Angell JC: *The Acute Abdomen for the Man on the Spot.* Kent, England, Pitman Medical Publishing Co Ltd, 1978.

Beal JM, Raffensperger JG: *Diagnosis of Acute Abdominal Disease.* Philadelphia, Lea & Febiger, 1979.

Botsford TW, Wilson RE: *The Acute Abdomen.* Philadelphia, WB Saunders Co, 1969.

Cope Z: *A History of the Acute Abdomen.* London, Oxford University Press, 1965.

Jones PF: *Emergency Abdominal Surgery.* Oxford, Blackwell Scientific Publications, 1974.

Raymond HW: *Fundamentals of Abdominal Sonography.* New York, Grune & Stratton, 1979.

Silen W: *Cope's Early Diagnosis of the Acute Abdomen.* New York, Oxford University Press, 1979.

34
GASTROINTESTINAL BLEEDING

Stephen E. Hedberg

Despite the recent sophisticated advances in endoscopy, radiology, and pharmacology, gastrointestinal (GI) bleeding remains a challenge for primary physicians and specialists alike. Many etiologies are responsible for GI bleeding (Table 34.1).

At times it is impossible to distinguish immediately between life-threatening hemorrhage and trivial bleeding. A bleeding patient must, therefore, be considered in mortal danger until proven otherwise. Homeostatic mechanisms may compensate for extensive blood loss, but *only to a point,* beyond which even slight depletion may cause circulation to deteriorate rapidly. Patients who are elderly or who have arteriosclerosis or heart disease are hemodynamically less resilient than others in hypovolemia; therefore, the hypovolemia must be corrected rapidly to prevent heart or kidney damage, but with particular care not to overload.

For management purposes, it is usually less crucial to know the pathology of a bleeding lesion than it is to know its location. Because all decisions after the initial evaluation depend on an opinion about the general location and the rate of bleeding, primary care physicians should be familiar not only with the means of gathering the essential data but also with their relevance to further management. Diagnostic maneuvers thus assume great importance in overall management. Ultimately, the exact site of the bleeding lesion must be established; otherwise, medical or surgical treatment may fail. Bleeding, whatever its extent or rate, can usually be managed successfully once its source is known. Major exceptions to this rule are patients with hepatic cirrhosis or malignant blood dyscrasias, for whom survival depends as much on effective treatment of the underlying disease as it does on control of bleeding.

It is the responsibility of the primary care physician to resuscitate the patient, perform the initial therapeutic and diagnostic maneuvers, assess the status of the stabilized or unstabilized patient, and make the decision regarding further therapy, diagnosis, or consultation. In many cases, the primary physician must decide whether to call first for a surgeon, an angiographer, an endoscopist, a psychiatrist, or a Sengstaken-Blakemore tube. How unhappy is the primary physician who must explain to the angiographer, the surgeon, or the endoscopist why the GI tract is full of barium suspension that failed to demonstrate a bleeding point on an emergency GI series. A barium study can never prove bleeding from a visualized lesion and does, in fact, frequently interfere with more effective diagnostic or therapeutic measures.

PATHOPHYSIOLOGY

Bleeding that arises above the ligament of Treitz or, occasionally, from a lower point if the intestine is obstructed, may result in hematemesis. When bleeding in the gastroesophagus is relatively slow, gastric acid converts red hemoglobin to brown hematin, which is responsible for vomitus that resembles coffee grounds. Bleeding that originates high in the gut frequently is accompanied by melena (the passing of dark tarry stools), although a slowly bleeding lesion in the colon also may cause stools to be dark and tarry. Melena almost always follows hematemesis but can occur alone; in fact, whenever as little as 60 ml of blood has been lost from any point along the GI tract, melena may result. Slow bleeding of the intestine or rapid bleeding in the duodenum is typically signaled by hematochezia (passing of bloody stools). Slow bleeding in the upper GI tract also may result in hematochezia when intestinal activity increases.

EVALUATION OF THE PATIENT

The presentation of GI bleeding depends on the source of bleeding, the amount and rate of loss, and the coexistence of other diseases. Pallor, headache, insomnia, and "nervous legs," for example, may result from iron-deficiency anemia as a result of chronic bleeding, whereas shock or renal failure is common with massive hemorrhage. Before definitive management can be instituted, the general location of the bleeding point and the rate and volume of loss must be determined. A complete history and physical examination, blood studies for coagulation abnormalities or liver malfunction, and repeated measurements of the hematocrit are essential.

History

The patient's history should focus on the occurrence and nature of hematemesis. For example, effortless welling of blood clots is typical of esophageal bleeding, whereas vomiting of "quarts of coffee grounds" is usually associated with gastritis or pyloric obstruction. Painful vomiting of nonbloody material followed by hematemesis is characteristic of Mallory-Weiss syndrome. A personal history suggesting peptic ulcer or liver disease is

TABLE 34.1 Causes of Gastrointestinal Bleeding

Common
  Peptic ulcers
  Diffuse gastric mucosal bleeding (gastritis)
  Gastroesophageal varices in portal hypertension
  Colonic carcinomas
  Hemorrhoids
  Diverticulitis coli
  Gastric carcinomas
  Meckel's diverticulum
  Colonic polyps
  Ulcerative colitis
  Gastroesophageal lacerations of Mallory-Weiss syndrome
Less Common[a]
  Blood swallowed from an oronasopharyngeal, respiratory, or
    external source (e.g., during birth)
  Tumors in any part of the gut
  Tuberculosis at any level
  Hematobilia (usually posttraumatic)
  Complications of surgery
  Foreign bodies
  Drugs
  Dysentery
  Intussusception
  Volvulus
  Vascular occlusion
  Angiodysplasia
  Blood dyscrasias
  Coagulopathy
  Vasculoenteric fistulas
  Miscellaneous lesions

[a]Together responsible for about 2% of cases.

valuable information, and a family history of similar trouble may furnish a shortcut to a diagnosis. GI bleeding of an emergency nature is, in general, manifested by hematemesis, melena, or hematochezia. Iron deficiency anemia or minimally guaiac-positive stools, on the other hand, usually accompany less rapid hemorrhage.

Physical Examination

The physical examination should assess the patient's general condition. Especially important are signs reflecting the extent of blood loss: color, pulse, blood pressure. Existing volume depletion can usually be estimated from clinical manifestations. Pallor, sweating, or postural dizziness indicates a volume loss of at least 15%. A volume loss of 25% is suggested if two or more large tarry stools have been passed in 24 hours, if postural hypotension is found in the range of 20–30 mm Hg, or if central venous pressure is abnormally low. The volume loss is probably 50% or more if hematemesis has been massive, if palmar creases are pale, or if signs of shock are present when the patient is recumbent; a systolic blood pressure below 100 mm Hg in a previously normotensive patient or a decrease greater than 30 mm Hg in a previously hypertensive patient also means that at least 50% of the normal volume has been lost.

Cutaneous signs of systemic disease often signal an underlying condition that will suggest a particular site of bleeding. Jaundice, spider angiomata, or caput medusae may accompany varices. Buccal spots characteristic of Peutz-Jeghers syndrome imply intestinal polyps as the source. Unusual ecchymoses are often associated with coagulation disorders. Café-au-lait spots may indicate von Recklinghausen's disease, telangiectases are associated with Rendu-Osler-Weber disease, and loss of axillary hair may be a result of cirrhosis. In addition to cutaneous signs, point tenderness in the epigastrium suggests peptic ulcer disease, and hepatomegaly indicates portal hypertension. A rectal examination should not be deferred.

Laboratory Evaluation

The hematocrit level of blood drawn after a massive hemorrhage does not fall until the intravascular volume becomes diluted by influx of extracellular fluid. Equilibration to a lower level that accurately reflects the true extent of the loss takes 12–30 hours, more or less depending on the amount of additional fluid that may be furnished orally or parenterally.

The stool guaiac test may remain positive for 3 or 4 days after bleeding has stopped, depending on the rate of intestinal activity. Nonhemorrhagic melena as a result of ingestion of iron, bismuth, berries, greens, or beets can be distinguished from true bleeding by testing for occult blood.

Diagnostic Procedures

GASTRIC ASPIRATION AND IRRIGATION

The systematic use of other diagnostic maneuvers for upper GI bleeding is based on the nature of the returns on aspiration and irrigation, which are, in fact, the sine qua non of diagnosis and management. The cessation or the persistence and the rate of hemorrhage can be ascertained from the nature of irrigant returns once all clots have been cleared. For example, if the returns are clear or if only a few "coffee grounds" are seen in a stable patient who has reported hematemesis, bleeding has ceased; observation and waiting are more appropriate than a vigorous diagnostic approach. On the other hand, clear returns and only a few "coffee grounds" in a patient with continuing melena and ongoing need for volume replacement strongly suggest a persistent hemorrhage below the pylorus but above the ligament of Treitz; immediate duodenoscopy is justified.

RADIOACTIVELY TAGGED RED BLOOD CELL SCAN

The radioactively tagged red blood cell scan is a simple, quick, relatively noninvasive study that can pinpoint the source of bleeding and that is especially helpful in identifying the general location of sources below the ligament of Treitz. Because of peristaltic activity pushing shed blood rapidly around the intestine, there can be misinterpretation as to its exact point of origin. However, it is so valuable to be able to distinguish small bowel from right colon and left colon as sources and it is so important to know whether bleeding has stopped or continues, that tagged erythrocytic scans are being done with increasing frequency very early in the management of bleeding.

ANGIOGRAPHY

If blood is being lost at a rate of 0.5 ml/min or faster from any point in the GI tract, angiography can locate the lesion. In combination with vasopressin infusion, this procedure may also stop bleeding and obviate emergency surgery. Angiography is the only practical way to locate a bleeding point between the lower reach of the gastroduodenoscope and the upper reach of the colonoscope; the procedure can also reveal vascular malformations, such as aneurysms and hemangiomas, even if they are not bleeding. A patient with blood in the stomach should undergo endoscopy before angiography so that the angiographer will know which artery to catheterize. Caution must be exercised, however, if a patient has iliofemoral atherosclerosis.

FIBEROPTIC ENDOSCOPY

Lesions bleeding too slowly to be seen angiographically can be detected by fiberoptic endoscopy. This procedure, which reveals not only the location of the bleeding point but also the nature of the lesion, is also useful for determining whether associated nonbleeding lesions are present and whether more than one lesion is bleeding. It should be performed in patients with blood in the stomach, but it may be unsuccessful if bleeding is torrential. On the other hand, since massive bleeding from esophageal varices can now virtually always be controlled by injection sclerosis through the fiberscope this diagnostic–therapeutic maneuver is being given early priority in patients suspected of varices. Extreme caution must be exercised if endoscopy is performed within 7–10 days after gastroduodenal surgery.

BARIUM STUDIES

Although barium studies are often able to demonstrate lesions that cannot be diagnosed by endoscopy or angiography, they should *never* be performed as an emergency diagnostic procedure on a bleeding patient; any barium remaining in the intestine will interfere with the interpretation of angiography or endoscopy, should either become necessary. Another disadvantage is that in patients with gastritis or esophagitis barium studies fail to show a potentially bleeding lesion, and they cannot prove that a visualized lesion is the source of bleeding. Barium studies are most appropriately used after the danger of recurrent bleeding has passed, that is, several days after the last hemorrhage, and they should always be performed before elective GI surgery, even if angiography or endoscopy has located the bleeding point.

BALLOON TAMPONADE

As a diagnostic technique, balloon tamponade with a Linton or Sengstaken-Blakemore tube (Procedure 23) is of limited value; it is difficult to estimate the true rate of bleeding just before and after the tube has been inserted. Another disadvantage is that an incorrect diagnosis of variceal bleeding can be made; for example, spontaneous cessation of bleeding from a source other than a varix may coincide with tamponade or the balloon may tamponade a source other than varices, such as a high gastric ulcer or a Mallory-Weiss mucosal tear, that is the actual bleeding point. Balloon tamponade is a high-risk procedure for all patients. Its chief value nowadays is in patients whose endoscopically proved bleeding varices have been incompletely controlled by injection sclerosis or in patients for whom sclerosis cannot be performed immediately.

RIGID ESOPHAGOSCOPY

A bleeding lesion in the esophagus can be demonstrated by rigid esophagoscopy. It should therefore be performed under general anesthesia and at the time of surgery if a diagnosis has not previously been established for a patient with torrential bleeding. In a massively bleeding patient, suction with an esophagoscope permits direct visualization of a variceal or Mallory-Weiss bleeding point and control of bleeding by tamponade with an epinephrine-soaked swab or by injection sclerosis of the varices. Topical anesthesia may be sufficient in this situation; it should also be used when variceal bleeding is suspected and surgery would be performed only if injection sclerosis or balloon tamponade failed to control bleeding.

SIGMOIDOSCOPY

Sigmoidoscopy should be performed in the emergency room on any patient with hematochezia even though a higher source may appear obvious. No patient should be operated upon without having had a recent sigmoidoscopy even though the bleeding may have been manifest rectally only by melena or guaiac-positive stool.

COLONOSCOPY

Colonoscopy is being done with increasing frequency as an emergency diagnostic test in patients who can be estimated to have bled more than 1,000–1,500 ml. It should be done by a specialist in the field. If the source is estimated by gastric aspiration, upper GI endoscopy, or erythrocyte scan to be below the ligament of Treitz, then emergency colonoscopy can be diagnostic. Preparation under these conditions is by means of a saline flush given through a nasogastric tube over the course of 2 or 3 hours. An additional advantage of colonoscopy is that many of the angiodysplastic lesions of the right colon can be controlled by cauterization through the scope.

STRING TEST

Although the string test is useful when bleeding is intermittent or too slow to be revealed by gastric aspiration, it should not be used if aspiration has demonstrated active bleeding. The procedure may be diagnostic for a slowly bleeding duodenal ulcer, for duodenitis not seen on barium studies, or for a small lesion in the bowel that is bleeding too slowly to be seen angiographically.

MANAGEMENT

Initial Management

If a patient presents with massive bleeding or if at any time it becomes evident that bleeding is or has been more than trivial, resuscitative measures are mandatory.

INTRAVENOUS THERAPY

When resuscitative measures are necessary, a large-bore intravenous cannula should be inserted immediately. A flexible plastic tube should be used because a rigid needle can become dislodged quite easily. Although the effects of volume repletion can be monitored with a central venous line, its length creates such resistance to flow that rapid infusion may be impossible. Therefore infusion should begin through a short plastic cannula after blood has been drawn for laboratory tests and cross-matching. A solution of serum albumin, or crystalloid if serum albumin is unavailable, may be infused initially to raise blood pressure, but fresh, frozen plasma should be substituted as soon as it can be thawed if a large volume may be required or if coagulopathy may be present. Replacement of red blood cells should begin immediately once cross-matched blood is available.

The appropriate transfusion rate is 500 ml every 15–30 minutes, with a pump if necessary, until signs of shock have been corrected. The hematocrit need not be restored to normal but should be maintained at 32–35% so that oxygenation is optimal, and in case surgery becomes necessary.

MONITORING

Because of oliguria, or even anuria, resulting from hypotension, a catheter should be inserted into the bladder of a briskly bleeding patient. The volume drained initially should be recorded, and additional measurements should be made at frequent intervals. Satisfactory output must be established and maintained.

A rapid change in volume may cause the serum concentration of potassium and calcium to vary so greatly from normal that cardiac function is threatened, especially in patients taking digitalis. Continuous monitoring of the electrocardiogram (ECG) is required for a patient in shock, especially if the patient is elderly, has a history of cardiovascular symptoms, or is being treated with drugs for a heart condition.

GASTRIC ASPIRATION AND IRRIGATION

A nasogastric tube no smaller than a No. 18 or No. 20 French gauge should be used to aspirate the stomach. If clots are found, lavage with iced saline is required until the stomach has been cleared. If the stomach cannot be completely emptied in 10–15 minutes with a Levin tube, a No. 30 French Ewald tube should be substituted to remove massive clots, which aggravate bleeding from gastritis by stretching the friable mucosa. After clots are removed, rapid irrigation with iced saline is considerably more effective in chilling the stomach, which reduces blood flow and can slow or stop bleeding. Furthermore, only after all clots are evacuated can the true rate of continuing blood loss be estimated accurately.

Management Decisions

Once the patient's general condition has been assessed, the general site of bleeding determined, and the rate and amount of blood loss estimated, the physician has all of the necessary data to choose the appropriate course of management. However, even when the history or physical findings suggest a bleeding lesion, definitive therapy is hazardous if based on evidence less secure than actual visualization of the bleeding point. Therefore, the system of diagnosis and management that we propose is purposely not dependent on history or physical examination. Some of the diagnostic maneuvers have a measurable risk that must be factored into the management decision process. The mortality rate of severe bleeding is so high compared with the risk of any diagnostic procedure, however, that the maneuver selected as appropriate on the basis of the basic data is rarely contraindicated. Exceptions are patients who have recently undergone gastric surgery, in whom endoscopy may be traumatic, and atherosclerotic patients, whose vessels may be unsuitable for angiography.

Although the parameters of the patient status may be considered infinitely variable, site and rate of bleeding and tactical considerations combine, for practical purposes, in only a few ways. Thus, a system based on the advantages, capabilities, disadvantages, and dangers of each diagnostic test can be devised for selecting the appropriate diagnostic sequence for any possible combination of hematemesis, melena, findings on gastric aspiration, results of ice-water irrigation, and transfusion requirement.

This decision process, whose purpose is to guide diagnosis and therapy, is summarized in Figure 34.1. "Clear," "pink," "red," and "bloody" denote the possible nature of returns on irrigation. Under Action, letters in each column indicate the order in which the tests should be considered for each combination of conditions.

Some assumptions underlie the construction of the table. Bleeding at a rate faster than 5 ml/min is assumed to require control, by angiographic infusion of vasopressin, balloon tamponade, injection sclerosis of varices, or, if the patient is a good candidate or if other methods have failed, by surgery. Other assumptions are that diagnosis by fiberoscopy may be difficult or impossible when grossly bloody returns are seen

on irrigation and may be missed by angiography when bleeding is slower than 5 ml/min. Balloon tamponade, injection sclerosis, or angiography may be considered as a first method for a poor-risk candidate for surgery who is bleeding massively and shows signs of portal hypertension; a good-risk patient, on the other hand, may usually be safely and more definitively managed by emergency surgery (see discussion of balloon tamponade).

If bleeding is originating in the upper GI tract, emergency surgery should always be preceded by conventional esophagoscopy unless the esophagus has been exonerated by fiberoscopy. Sigmoidoscopy should be considered first in patients with hematochezia but may be rejected if upper GI bleeding is obviously active. Although all patients should undergo sigmoidoscopy at some time, if only as a matter of routine, a letter appears under Action only if sigmoidoscopy is considered a logical procedure for determining the site of bleeding (e.g., in all patients with hematochezia). Not listed in the table is endotracheal intubation, which should be considered a protective measure in obtunded patients who are in danger of aspirating vomitus.

The timing and coordination of these examinations obviously cannot follow such a rigid protocol as implied in a decision table. The judgmental function and flexibility of the emergency room physician are of utmost importance. The facilities and specialists actually available will often determine the order of procedure with a validity equal to that of the decision table.

All but a very few patients with significant GI bleeding require hospitalization. Management by the primary physician should therefore be oriented in that direction from the beginning. When hospitalization is not possible, hypotension and vasoconstriction often seem to cause bleeding to stop. However, to attempt hemostasis by calculated exsanguination when blood is available cannot be justified today. Replacement should be started as soon as the need is apparent and blood is available. At all times the amount of blood in the bank is a vital consideration in the overall plan. If iced-saline irrigation, vasopressin infusion, and antacid therapy are ineffective, surgery may be necessary; thus, enough blood must be available to support the patient during surgery as well as during diagnostic procedures. If blood supply is low, endoscopy should be done sooner. Only rarely is it necessary to operate without a sufficient blood supply or a diagnosis. Fortunately, GI bleeders rarely confront such grim circumstances today; the problem is more often one of too much blood and too many tests. But a prepared primary physician is well able to escort patients accurately through the maze of options presently available.

Condition																
Guaiac + aspirate or hematemesis	N			Y												
Continuing Blood Loss (5 ml/min)	N	Y		N					Y							
Result of Gastric Irrigation																
Clear	—	—				Y				Y						
Pink								Y				Y				
Red														Y		
Bloody																Y
Hematochezia	N	Y	*N	Y	N	Y	N	Y	N	Y	N	Y	N	Y	N	Y
Action																
Sigmoidoscopy	A	A		A	D	A	C	A		A		A		a		a
Fiberoptic endoscopy	C			C	D	A	B	A	B	A	B	A	A	A	A	A
Angiography	F	D		D					(B)	(C)	(B)	(C)	(B)	(B)	+	+
Balloon Tamponade													?	?	?	?
Esophagoscopy (Rigid)															B	B
Operation	H			F					C	D	C	D	C	C	C	C
Observation	G				A E	B E	D	E								
Barium Studies	B	C		E	B	C	B	C								
Colonoscopy	D	B		C												
String Test	E															
Red Cell Scan				B												

Figure 34.1 Algorithm for diagnosing the source of gastrointestinal bleeding. Each combination of *conditions* presents four leads to a particular combination and sequence of diagnostic/therapeutic *actions*. The usual sequence is indicated alphabetically. Actions in parentheses may be omitted in good risk patients when the diagnosis is established endoscopically. *indicates a combination of conditions that could not occur. "a" acknowledges the fact that sigmoidoscopy may be logical in hematochezia but is not practical or necessary when irrigation of the stomach gives red or bloody returns. "+" denotes that angiography for vasopressin therapy may be preferable to esophagoscopy and surgery in a poor risk patient. "?" indicates that balloon tamponade may be the first choice in massive bleeding when varices are suspected.

HEMATEMESIS

Diagnosis and Initial Management

A reliable history of hematemesis is accepted as solid evidence that bleeding is originating above the ligament of Treitz. The stomach should be immediately aspirated with a large-bore Levin tube; further diagnostic or therapeutic maneuvers depend on the findings on aspiration (Figs. 34.2 and 34.3).

Blood in the Levin-tube Aspirate

If aspiration demonstrates blood in any form—brown guaiac-positive gastric juice, "coffee grounds," clots, or bright red blood—the stomach should be completely emptied as rapidly as possible by irrigation with iced saline. If massive clots prevent evacuation in a reasonable time through the Levin tube, an Ewald tube should be substituted and irrigation continued vigorously by two people until all of the clots have been cleared. The rate of bleeding into the stomach can then be assessed from the color of the irrigation returns.

TORRENTIAL HEMORRHAGE

Balloon tamponade of the esophagogastric junction is a reasonable diagnostic or therapeutic choice for a patient known to have esophageal varices or advanced liver disease provided

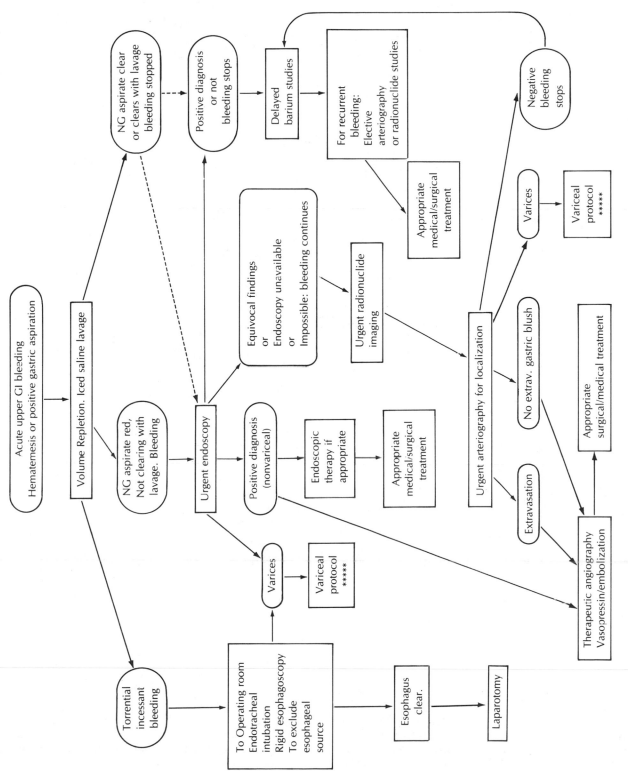

Figure 34.2 Acute upper GI bleeding with hematemesis or positive gastric aspiration.

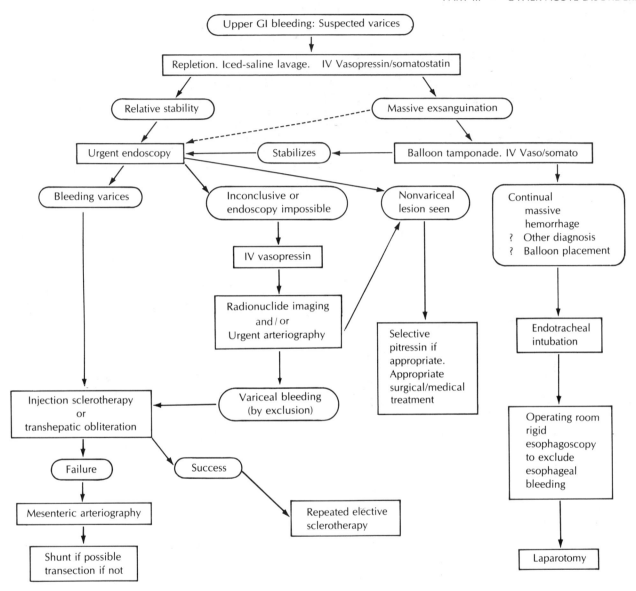

Figure 34.3 Upper GI bleeding: suspected varices.

that the stomach has been cleared of clots by irrigation. However, if a skilled endoscopist is available, injection sclerosis of the varices through the fiberscope carries a lower risk and a greater chance of successful control of bleeding. An endotracheal tube should be inserted immediately in a weakened and possibly comatose patient to prevent aspiration of blood. An alternative approach, before a balloon tube is inserted, is rigid esophagoscopy. This procedure is quite useful, however rapid the bleeding, to determine whether bleeding is originating in the esophagus before an incision is made. In either case, the surgeon can at least be confident that the incision will be made into the correct body cavity, even if problems occur after the incision is made. For patients with truly massive bleeding, conventional esophagoscopy should be done under the general anesthesia to be used for surgery. (Surgery would already have been elected on the basis of the rate of hemorrhage determined from Ewald returns.)

Angiography or barium studies should not be used when massive exsanguinating hemorrhage is diagnosed in patients for whom surgery is appropriate.

BRISK LOSS

Many patients with continuing, rapid blood loss despite cold irrigation should be considered for early surgery. Fiberoptic endoscopy should be performed to determine whether blood is entering the stomach from above, refluxing from below, or arising from within; the procedure may furnish valuable information for the angiographer as well as for the surgeon. However, if a lesion that is difficult to manage surgically (e.g., gastritis) is found, the physician may elect to continue medical treatment longer than if another type of lesion were seen (e.g., a gastric ulcer). For patients who are poor-risk candidates for surgery, angiography may be selected for diagnosis and vasopressin for therapy. The situation becomes dangerous, however, if bleeding becomes uncontrollable in the radiology suite during the procedure, and the surgeon and the operating room should be alerted to this potential emergency.

PERSISTENT PINK OR RED RETURNS

If there are pink or red returns, the patient is a good candidate for endoscopy or angiography. Endoscopy is preferable because it is the simpler and more direct way to locate the bleeding point exactly; in addition, information about important associated lesions may be provided. Angiography, on the other hand, may be desirable in an elderly or poor-risk patient. Although intraarterial vasopressin may be selected as initial treatment for a patient with any bleeding lesion, preliminary endoscopy should be considered to locate the site for the angiographer; thus only one vessel, rather than three has to be demonstrated. Endoscopy should definitely be elected when bleeding is relatively slow because the amount of contrast material extravasated may be too small to be seen by angiography.

CLEAR RETURNS WITH CONTINUED REQUIREMENT FOR TRANSFUSION

Bleeding from a duodenal ulcer is virtually certain when a patient with clear returns continues to require transfusion. Irrigation with iced saline, although often effective for stopping bleeding from a duodenal ulcer, may cause spasm of the pylorus while the ulcer continues to bleed. The choice between angiography and surgery should be based on the patient's history and condition. Immediate surgery may be indicated for a patient with a documented intractable ulcer, previous hemorrhage, or other prior indication for surgery. On the other hand, angiographic demonstration of bleeding from an uncommon location in the duodenum may indicate that the surgeon faces a difficult technical problem.

In evaluating GI bleeding, surgery is always a possibility. Some generalizations can be considered during the decision process. When perforation and hemorrhage coexist, surgery is mandatory. A patient whose bleeding stops and then recurs during treatment should also be operated on. Surgical therapy also must be seriously considered for chronic alcoholics and for patients who have persistent pain during hemorrhage. Older patients have less tolerance for hypovolemia, and repeated transfusions are less likely to stop bleeding from an ulcer in these patients than in younger ones. Operation for gastric ulcer is safe and effective compared with surgical treatment of gastritis, which may require total gastrectomy. Bleeding gastritis tends to be self-limiting, like bleeding from an ulcer, which often stops permanently without surgery. Ulcers seen endoscopically to have a visible vessel in the base have a higher risk of rebleeding than ulcers without a visible vessel. Failure to stabilize hemodynamically after 2,500 ml of blood is given or a continuing requirement for blood after that much initial replacement usually indicates the need for surgical intervention. A younger patient who has had no previous symptoms and who is bleeding from a potentially treatable lesion may be allowed up to 7,500 ml of blood over a 24-hour period in an effort to obviate surgery, whereas a patient over 50 years old who has major hemorrhage from, for example, a chronic ulcer, is considered a candidate for surgery as soon as his condition permits.

BLEEDING STOPPED

No immediate diagnostic procedure is indicated after bleeding has stopped. Barium studies, in fact, are contraindicated because they may interfere not only with medical treatment, but also with angiography or endoscopy should bleeding recur and necessitate either procedure. Tube drainage should be continued, usually for 24 hours, for monitoring purposes.

No Blood in the Aspirate

FURTHER BLEEDING AND HISTORY OF HEMATEMESIS

The source of bleeding in hematemesis is definitely between the pylorus and the ligament of Treitz; that is, a duodenal ulcer is bleeding. Gastroscopy will not demonstrate the bleeding point if the gastric returns are clear, but duodenoscopy may show the lesion; barium studies offer, at most, further presumptive evidence. If persistent bleeding that is well localized by circumstances is vigorous enough to require blood transfusion, a definite advantage may be gained by using angiography. Not only can it precisely locate the lesion, but it may also provide vasoconstrictive treatment. The angiographer can then catheterize the hepatic artery; in a good-risk patient, however, endoscopy should usually precede angiography.

NO FURTHER BLEEDING

In a patient who has bled from above the ligament of Treitz and in whom the bleeding has stopped, a reasonable course is the same as the regimen for a patient with a bleeding peptic ulcer: cimetidine, sucralfate, and antacids (not, however, ones containing carbonate or aluminum hydroxide, which may combine with blood to form concretions in the intestine), and either milk or egg products. Anticholinergic drugs should not be used until the presence of a duodenal ulcer has been proven; the delayed GI motility they cause may have adverse effects on an esophagogastric lesion, such as gastritis or gastric ulcer, and they slow the clearing of shed blood by the intestine. After the patient has been treated medically, he or she should undergo barium studies of the upper GI tract. If delayed barium studies do not establish a diagnosis, esophagogastroduodenoscopy should be considered even if bleeding has stopped. No advantage is gained by doing these studies urgently; in fact patients who undergo immediate barium studies have recurrence of bleeding more often than patients who receive vigorous medical treatment first.

BLEEDING DETECTED ONLY RECTALLY (Fig. 34.4)

Melena or Hematochezia with Brisk Bleeding

BLOOD IN THE STOMACH

The patient who has blood in the stomach should be managed exactly as a patient without melena or hematochezia.

NO BLOOD IN THE STOMACH

If bleeding is rapid, angiography is likely to demonstrate the bleeding point and, if sigmoidoscopy is normal, is probably the only method that can be diagnostic. However, tagged red blood cell scan before angiography can be very informative.

If the source is identified angiographically, bleeding may be controlled by infusing vasopressin through the angiographic catheter, but only after medical measures have been initiated or perhaps after the bowel has been evacuated and prepared for surgery. Barium studies may be done after mesenteric arteriography, but they can demonstrate, at most, only possible sources of bleeding not an actual bleeding point. Again, such studies done initially greatly hinder angiographic interpretation.

Continuing Rectal Loss

Determining by immediate or possibly by repeated gastric aspiration whether any trace of blood is in the stomach is most important in diagnosing the source of continuing rectal loss.

BLOOD IN THE STOMACH

A patient with blood in the stomach would be managed exactly as would a patient in whom guaiac-positive stools, melena, or hematochezia was not found, as described above under HEMATEMESIS.

NO BLOOD IN THE STOMACH

If bleeding continues from below the stomach, if hematemesis is not present, and if repeated aspiration reveals that the stomach is free of blood, bleeding may be originating at any point below the pylorus. Reflux of yellow bile into the stomach, however, indicates that the source must be below the ligament of Treitz if hemorrhage is still occurring when the bile is noted. Sigmoidoscopy should be done first, followed immediately by either angiography or colonoscopy. The appropriate choice depends on the rapidity of the bleeding, but one or the other should be done promptly when the volume lost exceeds 1,500 ml. Angiography should be selected if the rate is estimated to be greater than 30 ml/hr. A patient bleeding more slowly is better managed with colonoscopy at once or with barium studies after a few days of no tests. The disadvantage of barium in the gut if angiography becomes necessary is much greater than the hazard of a slow loss of blood.

Guaiac-Positive Stools and Slow Chronic Bleeding

If the rate of bleeding is less than 30 ml/hr, even gastric aspiration may not reveal blood. Neither angiography nor endoscopy of the upper GI tract is likely to demonstrate the

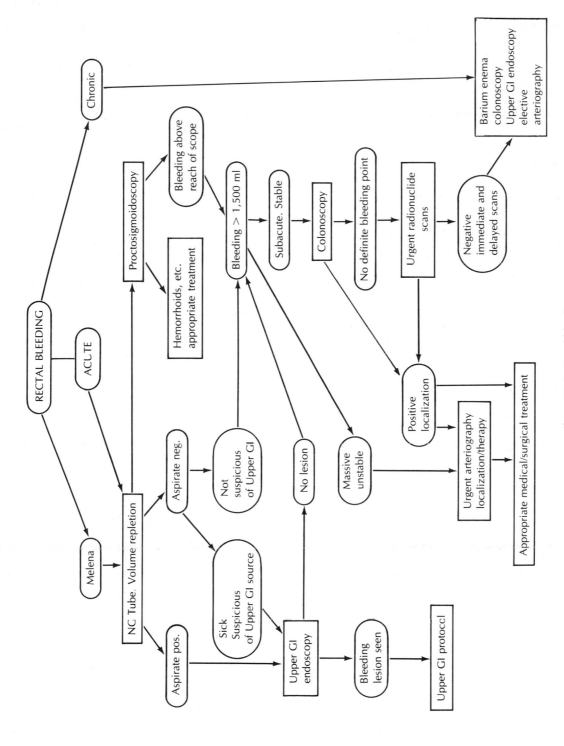

Figure 34.4 Rectal bleeding.

bleeding point. Red blood cell scans, especially with delayed follow-up scans, may show the point in the abdomen at which bleeding arises. Sigmoidoscopy, barium enema, or upper GI series may demonstrate an abnormality. If no evidence of disease is found, other tests should be performed in order of increasing risk and expense: string test, esophagogastroduodenoscopy, colonoscopy, and angiography.

SELECTED REFERENCES

Babb RR: The value of upper gastrointestinal endoscopy. *J Am Med Assoc* 1973; 223:189.

Baird RA: Diagnosis of upper gastrointestinal hemorrhage. *J Am Med Assoc* 1970; 214:598.

Baum S: Angiography: Super sleuth. (editorial) *N Engl J Med* 1972; 286:484.

Bray RS: An improved G.I. cord for the detection of upper gastrointestinal bleeding. *Am J Proctol* 1967; 18:277.

Conn HO, Smith HW, Brodoff M: Observer variation in the endoscopic diagnosis of esophageal varices: A prospective investigation of the diagnostic validity of esophagoscopy. *N Engl J Med* 1965; 272:830.

Crampton RS, Cali JR, Shutello DJ, Glaubitz JP: Observations on the duration and results of local gastric hypothermia in the management of active hemorrhage. *Surgery* 1966; 59:673.

Dagradi AE: Endoscopic examination of the gastroesophageal area. *Gastrointest Endosc* 1969; 15:175.

Dagradi AE: Gastrointestinal hemorrhage. (Editorial) *J Clin Gastroenterol* 1981; 3:215.

Dagradi AE, Stempien SJ, Juler G: The Mallory-Weiss lesion: An endoscopic study of thirty cases. *Gastrointest Endosc* 1967; 13:18.

Frey CF, Reuter ST, Bookstein JJ: Localization of gastrointestinal hemorrhage by selective angiography. *Surgery* 1970; 67:548.

Griffiths WJ, Neimann DA, Welsh, JD: The visible vessel as an indicator of uncontrolled or recurrent gastrointestinal hemorrhage. *N Engl J Med* 1979; 300:1411.

Heckman BA, Colker JL: The endoscopic diagnosis of isolated gastric varices. *Gastrointest Endosc* 1968; 15:24.

Hedberg SE: Early endoscopic diagnosis in upper gastrointestinal hemorrhage: An analysis of 323 cases. *Surg Clin North Am* 1966; 46:499.

Hedberg SE: Endoscopy in gastrointestinal bleeding: A systematic approach to diagnosis. *Surg Clin North Am* 1974; 54:549.

Hedberg SE, Fowler DL, Ryan RLR: Injection sclerotherapy of esophageal varices using ethanolamine oleate. A pilot study. *Am J Surg* 1982; 143:426.

Holland RR: Decision tables: Their use for the presentation of clinical algorithms. *J Am Med Assoc* 1975; 233:455.

Katz D, Douvres P, Weisberg H, McKinnon W, Glass GB: Early endoscopic diagnosis of acute upper gastrointestinal hemorrhage: Demonstration of relatively high incidence of erosions as a source of bleeding. *J Am Med Assoc* 1964; 188:405.

Kinard HB, Powell DW, Sandler RS, Callahan WT, Lapis JL, Levinson SL, Jones JD, Drossman DA, Jackson AL: A current approach to acute upper gastrointestinal bleeding. *J Clin Gastroenterol* 1981; 3:231.

Levinson SL, Powell DW, Callahan WT, Jones JD, Kinard HB, Jackson AL, Lapis JL, Drossman DA: A current approach to rectal bleeding. *J Clin Gastroenterol* 1981; 3(suppl 1):9.

McKhann CF, Wilson ID: A rational approach to GI bleeding emergencies. *Hosp Prac* 1971; 6:125.

Mitty WF Jr, Befeler D, Grossi C, Bonanno CA, Rusicki FF, Rossi P: Combined approach to upper gastrointestinal bleeding. *Am J Gastroenterol* 1969; 51:377.

Moore FD: Transcapillary refill, the unremaired anemia, and clinical hemodilution (Editorial). *Surg Gynecol Obstet* 1974; 139:245.

Morello DC, Klein NE, Wolferth CC Jr., Matsumoto T: Management of diffuse hemorrhage from gastric mucosa. II. Effects of selective intra-arterial infusion of vasopressin and/or epinephrine. *Am J Surg* 1972; 123:160.

Moss G: Technic of iced saline gastric lavage in upper gastrointestinal hemorrhage. *Am J Surg* 1971; 122:656.

Palmer ED: *Diagnosis of Upper Gastrointestinal Hemorrhage*. Springfield, Illinois, Charles C Thomas Publisher, 1961.

Palmer ED: The vigorous diagnostic approach to upper-gastrointestinal tract hemorrhage: A 23-year prospective study of 1,400 patients. *J Am Med Assoc* 1969; 207:1477.

Peterson WL: Evaluation and initial management of patients with upper gastrointestinal bleeding. *J Clin Gastroenterol* 1981; 3(suppl 2):79.

Tedesco FJ: Endoscopy in the evaluation of patients with upper gastrointestinal symptoms: Indications, expectations, and interpretation. *J Clin Gastroenterol* 1981; 3(Suppl 2):67.

Welch CE, Hedberg SE: *Polypoid Lesions of the Gastrointestinal Tract*, ed 2. Philadelphia, WB Saunders Co, 1975.

35

NONSURGICAL ACUTE GASTROINTESTINAL DISORDERS

Americo A. Abbruzzese

DIARRHEA

Diarrhea, an excessive fecal loss of water, may occur from an increase in bowel movements, or from increased fluidity or weight of stool. By definition, *acute diarrhea* occurs in previously healthy individuals, lasts for a few days to several weeks, is generally benign and self-limiting, and resolves without sequelae.

Acute diarrhea has plagued us since the dawn of history and continues to do so. The World War II battle of El Alamein was lost because the Germans were incapacitated by dysentery. In 1966–1967, acute diarrhea accounted for more than 4 million lost working days.

Pathophysiology of Acute Diarrhea

Under normal day-to-day living, approximately 10 liters of fluid enters the gut. The volume is derived from diet (2–3 liters) and from the enterosystemic circulation (7 liters). As this volume moves down the gastrointestinal (GI) tract, 98% is absorbed, chiefly in the small bowel, and the remaining 200 ml is eliminated in fecal waste. Water passively moves from the bowel lumen across the intestinal mucosa in response to osmotic gradients created by electrolytes and other osmotically active solutes. However, there is a less rapid but simultaneous secretion of water and electrolytes in the opposite direction. A wide variety of acute mucosal injuries can interfere with the gut's ability to preserve this finely integrated bidirectional flux and thus precipitate diarrhea.

The majority of acute diarrheas are caused by infectious agents that vary from a few viruses, to many bacteria or their toxins, to protozoa. Unfortunately, 80% of acute cases cannot be ascribed to a specific pathogen despite advances in laboratory technology. The most common agents are viruses that are not detectable by our present routine laboratory methods.

The schema below lists some of the most frequent causes of acute diarrhea. The following may cause diarrhea commonly associated with blood in stool:

- Infections
  - *Salmonella*
  - *Shigella*
  - Invasive *Escherichia coli*
  - *Yersinia enterocolitica*
  - *Campylobacter*
  - *Vibrio parahaemolyticus*
  - *Chlamydia trachomatis*
  - *Entamoeba histolytica*
- Noninfections
  - Inflammatory bowel disease
  - Ischemic colitis
  - Antibiotic associated colitis

The following are associated with diarrhea without blood in stool:

- Viral gastroenteritis
- Enterotoxin
  - Toxigenic *E. coli*
  - Cholera
  - *Clostridium perfringens*
  - *Staphylococcus aureus*
- Parasitic
  - *Giardia*
- Hormonal
  - Zollinger-Ellison syndrome
  - Pancreatic cholera
  - Carcinoid syndrome

Evaluation of the Patient

HISTORY

Because a wide variety of insults affect the gut and provoke diarrhea, a comprehensive history is central for the diagnosis, treatment, and cure of all patients presenting with diarrhea. Enquiry into the following areas will help clarify the etiology of the diarrhea.

Onset

Acute diarrhea, beginning 1–6 hours after a meal, is the gut's reaction to preformed toxins produced during bacterial growth in contaminated food. A more gradual onset of diarrhea, 12–24 hours after infection, indicates that the offending organism must first colonize the gut and then either produce a toxin or become invasive.

Associated Symptoms

Nausea, vomiting, abdominal pain, and cramps are common to many offending viral, bacterial, and protozoal agents. Fever and leukocytosis are signs of an invasive organism. However, a noninvasive organism, food-borne *Staphylococcus,* can cause high fever and leukocytosis in a severely dehydrated patient.

Pattern and Character

In shigellosis, the patient first has abdominal pains and then diarrhea. Watery diarrhea suggests a toxin-producing or non-invasive agent. Mucus, pus, and blood are indications of mucosal irritation and injury. Osmotic diarrhea will stop dramatically within 24 hours if the patient takes nothing by mouth.

Volume

Large-volume diarrhea, 2 liters or more daily, reflects either small bowel disease or humorally mediated diarrheas. Low-volume diarrhea, 500 ml or less daily, indicates colonic disease.

Food, Animal, Medication, Sexual, and Travel Exposure

Exposures to poorly prepared poultry products and to uncooked or undercooked meats and seafood are common causes of diarrhea. Domestic and household pets are an important reservoir of diarrheal agents. Recent exposure to antibiotics should suggest either antibiotic-associated diarrhea or antibiotic-associated colitis. The sexual transmission of *Salmonella, Shigella, Giardia,* and *Chlamydia* among homosexual males makes it imperative that sexual preferences be considered. A history of foreign travel can be an important clue in exploring the spectrum of traveler's diarrhea.

PHYSICAL EXAMINATION

The physical examination of patients with acute diarrhea will rarely be of help in identifying the responsible agent. Occa-

sionally, acute diarrhea may herald the presence of a hitherto silent systemic infection or a chronic inflammatory bowel problem. Therefore a careful search for hepatosplenomegaly, rose spots, a mass in the right lower quadrant, or erythema nodosum may lead to important findings. In addition to specific findings, a general examination provides valuable information regarding the patient's state of hydration. Decreased skin turgor, resting tachycardia, dizziness, lightheadedness, postural hypotension, elevated hematocrit, and plasma–protein concentration are all reliable indicators of fluid and electrolyte losses. A rule of thumb is that when the gross clinical signs of dehydration are detectable, the patient has lost about 15% of his or her extracellular fluid or, for an adult, 2–3 liters of fluid. In the very young and the very old with other debilitating problems, this loss may represent a life-threatening situation.

In general, the abdomen is "sore" all over without guarding. "Whooshing" peristaltic sounds are audible, and the explosive passage of gas accompanies each watery movement.

Visual examination of the perirectal area may reveal hemorrhoids, fissures, fistulas, or abscesses, which are sometimes clues of inflammatory bowel disease. Digital examination for strictures and masses and to note the texture of the rectal mucosa will determine the need for proctosigmoidoscopy. However, all patients with rectal bleeding should have a proctosigmoidoscopy.

LABORATORY EVALUATION

Complete blood cell count (CBC), serum electrolytes, blood urea nitrogen (BUN), and urinalysis will provide quick information concerning the severity of the patient's illness and state of hydration. Blood cultures are low-priority examinations unless the patient is clinically septic. A plain film of the abdomen can be very helpful and at times diagnostic (perforation, toxic megacolon, thumbprinting) (see Chapter 33, Figs. 33.5 and 33.6). Stool cultures for enteric pathogens and a search for ova and parasites should be done in all patients with a positive travel history.

Stool Examination

While the studies just mentioned are being completed, examination of the diarrheal stool is very important and does not require a great expenditure of time. The clinical expression of the host–parasite relationship depends on whether the offending agent is invasive or noninvasive. This important question can be quickly resolved by a simple *Wright's stain.* A drop or two of fresh liquid stool or mucus is placed on a microscope slide and is thoroughly mixed with several drops of Wright's stain. A coverslip is added, and after several minutes the specimen is examined under the high dry objective of a microscope. An invasive organism will provoke the lumenal outpouring of inflammatory cells and macrophages. Thus a positive Wright's stain, the presence of clumps of fecal leukocytes, is the hallmark of an inflammatory process and excludes all other agents that cause diarrhea without mucosal injury. The sighting of only rare fecal leukocytes indicates a negative examination. A fecal *Gram stain* adds the dimension of characterizing bacteria and suggests a specific diagnosis in staphylococcal enterocolitis, clostridial food poisoning, cholera, and gonococcal proctitis.

A provisional diagnosis of the cause of the diarrhea may be made on the basis of the following discriminants:

- Infectious
  · Invasive: mucosal injury; Wright's positive
  · Noninvasive: no mucosal injury; Wright's negative

- Noninfectious
  · Mucosal injury; Wright's positive
  · No mucosal injury; Wright's negative

Infectious—Wright's Positive

Salmonella
Shigella
Escherichia coli (enteroinvasive)
Y. enterocolitica
Campylobacter fetus
V. parahaemolyticus
Chlamydia trachomatis
Entamoeba histolytica
Inflammatory bowel disease
Ischemic colitis
Antibiotic-associated colitis

Infectious—Wright's Negative

Viral gastroenteritis
Staphylococcus aureus (food poisoning)
Clostridium perfringens (food poisoning)
Traveler's diarrhea (toxigenic *Escherichia coli*)
Vibrio cholerae
Giardia lamblia
Zollinger-Ellison syndrome
Pancreatic cholera
Carcinoid syndrome

Treatment and General Measures

Clearly, the treatment of any diarrheal syndrome is ultimately directed at the underlying cause. However, until the various diagnostic tests have been reported, the patients will need supportive care. Whether or not that care is provided on an inpatient or outpatient basis depends on how "sick" the patient is when examined in the emergency room. In general, patients with systemic toxicity, vomiting, dehydration, high fever, steady abdominal pains, and persistent diarrhea should be admitted for observation, fluid–electrolyte replacement, and other diagnostic tests that changing clinical conditions may dictate.

Fortunately, most patients who are examined by emergency room physicians can be sent home to complete bed rest, which frequently is enough to provide symptomatic relief. Solidifying excessively watery stools and reducing stool frequency can be accomplished with psyllium seed preparations (Metamucil). Two teaspoons in a single glass of water, three times daily, will firm up the stool and decrease the number of movements. Kaolin and pectin (Kaopectate) has a similar effect. Although both compounds may provide a welcomed reduction in bowel action, total fluid loss is unchanged, and the risk of dehydration and metabolic acidosis remains high unless the diarrhea is resolved. Paregoric, diphenoxylate, and loperamide are commonly used to decrease bowel motility and abdominal cramps and to relieve tenesmus. However, these drugs delay the fecal excretion of *Shigella* and *Salmonella* and may provoke toxic megacolon in antibiotic-associated diarrhea or inflammatory bowel disease. Bismuth subsalicylate (Pepto-Bismol) is effective for patients with traveler's diarrhea or mild toxigenic gastroenteritis. A recommended schedule is 30–60 ml every half-hour for 8 doses. It is not effective against diarrhea due to *Salmonella* or *Shigella*.

Home care replacement of fluids and electrolytes can be accomplished with various fruit juices to which a pinch or two of table salt and baking soda has been added. Gatorade is a commercial preparation containing 23 mEq/liter sodium, 17 mEq/liter chloride, and 3 mEq/liter potassium. Glucose, which facilitates the absorption of water and electrolytes, may be obtained by adding 2 teaspoons of honey or corn syrup to 1 liter of water. Broths and decarbonated beverages are also desirable hydrating fluids. Drinking alternatively from these solutions 2–5 liters/day, depending on fluid losses, will hasten recovery. Good urine output is a sign that hydration is progressing satisfactorily. As the diarrhea lessens, small, frequent feedings of easily digested foods (bananas, rice, baked potato, or applesauce) should be encouraged. If the patient does not improve within 24–48 hours of the initial examination, he or she should be told to return to the emergency room or seek additional medical assistance at home.

CLINICAL SETTINGS OF DIARRHEA

Infectious Invasive Diarrhea

SALMONELLA

Salmonellae are gram-negative, motile, and aerobic micro-organisms that are widely distributed in nature and are a serious cause of human disease. Although there are 1,700 serotypes and variants of *Salmonella* genus, one in four cases of sal-monellal gastroenteritis are caused by the species *S. typhi-murium*. Other common isolates are *S. enteritidis*, *S. newport*, and *S. heidelberg*. Salmonellae vary in their invasive potential and capacity to produce disease. *Salmonella typhi* and *S. chol-eraesuis* are the most invasive serotypes causing bacteremia and metastatic complications. Although infection by *S. typhi* is a classic example of enteric fever and the most severe type of *Salmonella* infection, the other nontyphoidal forms can be severe and clinically indistinguishable from typhoid fever.

Pets (dogs, cats, turtles, chicks) and domestic animals (chickens, turkeys, pigs, goats) are important reservoirs of infection. Contaminated drink or food (raw or undercooked meat, meat and fish by-products, egg and egg products, dried or frozen foods) and person-to-person contact are common vehicles of contagion. About 3% of people in the United States are chronic carriers of *Salmonella* organisms.

Diagnosis

After an incubation period that may be as brief as 10 hours, fever, chills, nausea, vomiting, headaches, colicky abdominal pain, and watery diarrhea with mucus/blood may abruptly begin. The frequency and severity of these symptoms depends on the virulence and dose of the *Salmonella* organism and the patient's resistance. If the patient is toxic, hepatosplenomegaly is common, but otherwise the liver and spleen are rarely palpable. Rose spots, characteristic of enteric fever, appear on the chest and upper abdomen about 2 weeks after the patient becomes infected. These eruptions are ephemeral, erythematous maculae, 2–4 mm in diameter, which rarely last more than 3 days and may be easily missed.

The only characteristic laboratory finding associated with *S. typhi* infection is leukopenia. Blood cultures are rarely positive but should be drawn on toxic patients. Fecal leukocytes are present. Stool cultures, plated on sterile solution (SS) agar, will identify the infecting organism.

Treatment and Prognosis

In the majority of cases, salmonellosis is a benign self-limiting infection, and an uneventful recovery can be expected in 7–10 days. Fluids and electrolyte problems can be managed with oral feedings. Antibiotics and antidiarrheals are not indicated and may, if given, delay recovery. Whether or not hospitalization is necessary depends on the clinical assessment of the patient when first seen. As a rule, all patients showing systemic toxicity, dehydration, and fever should be admitted. In the presence of bacteremia, ampicillin, 4–6 g orally or chloramphenicol, 2–5 g daily in divided doses should be started.

Salmonellal gastroenteritis has a death rate of less than 1% except in infants and elderly debilitated patients. Patients with hemolytic states, such as sickle hemoglobinopathy, are at risk of developing septic arthritis or osteomyelitis.

TYPHOID FEVER

Typhoid fever is the most severe form of salmonellal infection. *Salmonella typhi* is a highly invasive organism that provokes an acute systemic reaction leading to metastatic foci of infection, intestinal bleeding, and perforation.

Diagnosis

The *S. typhi* are ingested in contaminated food or liquids. After an incubation period of 1–2 weeks, longer than for most salmonellal infections, an insidious flu viruslike syndrome unfolds. Slight fever, malaise, headache, and chilly sensations are common. After 1 week the fever rises and becomes continuous or remittent, headaches worsen, abdominal pains become a problem, and bronchitic symptoms are common. Constipation, common in the early phase, gives way to diarrhea. The liver and spleen become palpable and abdominal tenderness is prominent. The patient's temperature is at 39°–40°C(103°–105°F), and a paradoxical bradycardia is noted in 40% of patients. Unrecognized, the febrile toxic course may continue for up to 8 weeks.

Leukopenia is typical of the febrile phase, and sudden increases in leukocytes suggest intestinal perforation. The yield of positive blood cultures is greatest during the first week of infection. Although fecal shedding is continuous, positive stool cultures peak in the third week and urine cultures are positive at about the same time.

Treatment

Chloramphenicol is the treatment of choice. In divided oral doses of 50 mg/kg/day, the infection can be brought under control in 2–5 days. Ampicillin, 6 g/day in divided doses, is an alternative treatment. However, the response is not as predictable as with chloramphenicol. With adequate antibiosis, the mortality rate has been reduced to under 2% from a high of 20%.

SHIGELLA

Shigellosis is a common infection of the colon caused by a slender, gram-negative, nonmotile rod. The organism is found worldwide, and the disease is common in areas in which sanitation and personal hygiene are poor. In the United States, the infection is spread by careless handling of food. Once ingested, shigellae colonize the colon, invade the epithelium, and cause a range of symptoms varying from mild diarrhea to bloody mucous colitis. Of the four species of *Shigella*, *S. sonnei* is the most common causative agent. In general, shigellosis is a benign disease and healing is complete in 7–10 days. However, in children and elderly patients the disease must be viewed with more caution. Patients suspected of *S. dysenteriae* type I should be hospitalized because of the virulent potential of this organism.

Diagnosis

The high-risk patients include children, foreign travelers, homosexuals, and those whose environments include poor sanitation and poor personal hygiene. After an incubation period of 1–4 days, fever, colicky abdominal pain, and headaches are common. Diarrhea is usually mild and watery. Later fecal urgency, tenesmus, and blood loss may appear. In children, seizures and meningismus are seen. Dehydration is common when the diarrhea is severe. Liver and spleen enlargement are rare unless the patient is toxic.

Leukocytosis and anemia are not the usual findings. A stained wet mount stool preparation reveals numerous leukocytes with a normal but scant flora. Sigmoidoscopy shows mucosal ulcerations not unlike that noted in infectious and noninfectious inflammatory bowel diseases. The immediate plating (SS agar) of swabbed rectal mucosa provides the highest diagnostic yield. Blood cultures are very low-yield procedures.

Treatment and Prognosis

Treatment of shigellosis is directed toward the correction of fluid and electrolyte losses. In general, this can be accomplished at home with the oral intake of juices, decarbonated beverages, liquid gelatin, or Gatorade. Patients with fever and voluminous watery stools will require hospitalization to guard against dehydration. Antidiarrheals are not indicated and may delay the excretion of the *Shigella* organism. Antibiotics should be reserved for those patients with systemic toxicity or positive

S. dysenteriae cultures. Ampicillin, 2 g in divided doses per day, may be given for 5–7 days. Tetracycline, 2.5 g as a single oral dose, is also effective. In areas in which resistant shigellae have been documented, trimethoprim (Bactrim) and sulfamethoxazole (Septra) are indicated: for adults, 160 and 800 mg, respectively, orally, every 12 hours for 5 days; for children, 8 and 40 mg/kg/day, respectively, every 12 hours for 5 days.

Fatalities are rare and are limited to children and to elderly debilitated patients infected with *S. dysenteriae* type I.

ESCHERICHIA COLI

Escherichia coli is a gram-negative nonsporing rod and a normal commensal in the gastrointestinal tract. These bacteria are the most numerous aerobic members of the normal intestinal flora. In the 1950s, strains of enteropathogenic *E. coli* were recognized and delineated into enteroinvasive and enterotoxigenic *E. coli*, both sharing a major role in the pathogenesis of traveler's diarrhea. The enteroinvasive strain causes a shigellosislike diarrhea. Although enteroinvasive *E. coli* is not as common a cause of traveler's diarrhea as is the noninvasive *E. coli*, it should be suspected in any recent traveler complaining of diarrhea, tenesmus, and rectal blood loss. The infection is spread through contaminated food, water, and fecal–oral route. After a short incubation period of 1–3 days, there is an abrupt onset of watery, blood-stained diarrhea. In general, it is unusual to pass more than 5–6 stools per day. Fever, nausea, abdominal cramps, and rectal urgency are common, but vomiting is not.

Diagnosis

At the present time, stool cultures are of no value because invasive *E. coli* cannot be distinguished from commensal *E. coli*. Fecal leukocytes and red cells are detectable with Wright's and Gram-stains.

Treatment and Prognosis

Treatment is supportive, and bed rest is required in about 20% of patients. Hospitalization is rare. The infection is benign, self-limited, and complete in about 7 days. Oral fluids are generally sufficient to overcome any dehydration problems. In the majority of cases, antibiotics and antidiarrheals have little positive influence. Recently bismuth subsalicylate (Pepto-Bismol) 30 ml every 30–60 minutes for 8 doses, has been reported to be helpful. If the disease persists beyond 1 week without signs of improvement, a careful search for other gut pathogens must be undertaken.

YERSINIA ENTEROCOLITICA

Yersinia enterocolitica is an invasive, pleomorphic, gram-negative rod that causes seasonal outbreaks of diarrhea similar to salmonellal and shigellal syndromes. Contaminated food and drink (usually dairy products) are the chief vehicle of transmission in schools, hospitals, and homes.

Diagnosis

Temperature of 39°C (102°F), abdominal pain, and watery diarrhea that is occasionally bloody are the rule. Erythema nodosum and polyarthritis have been recorded. Invasion of the mesenteric lymph nodes causes right lower-quadrant pain indistinguishable from acute appendicitis or Crohn's disease. Organomegaly is rare. Except for Wright's and Gram-stains of the feces to identify leukocytes and red cells, other laboratory studies are not helpful. The organism may be isolated from stool by plating on pectin agar at room temperature. A diagnosis can be made by documenting high antibody titers, greater than 1:160, during the acute phase of the illness. In the event of laparotomy, nodes should be cultured.

Treatment

Treatment is generally supportive, except in severe cases. Ampicillin, 2–4 g/day or chloramphenicol, 2–5 g/day in divided doses, may be given in life-threatening situations.

CAMPYLOBACTER FETUS SS JEJUNI

Campylobacter fetus ss *jejuni* is a gram-negative vibrio that has only recently been recognized as an important human enteric pathogen and a major cause of an acute severe dysenteric syndrome. Recent studies have shown that the organism was isolated from diarrheal stool cultures more often than either *Salmonella* or *Shigella*. *Campylobacter* is not part of the normal bowel flora of healthy adults living in developed countries. Natural reservoirs include domestic and wild animals. Transmission is through food (poorly cooked chicken), polluted streams, and untreated municipal water supplies. Person-to-person transmission is rare but does occur wherever sick children are incontinent of stools. The differential diagnosis of acute diarrheal illness or suspected ulcerative colitis should include *Campylobacter*.

Diagnosis

Fever, chills, malaise, cramping abdominal pain, and watery diarrhea characterize the illness. Generally 2–4 days after the onset of the illness either frank or occult blood appears in the stool. The majority of patients are 15 years old or younger.

A positive Wright's stain indicates the cytotoxic or invasive nature of the organism. The diagnosis is made by identifying motile, comma-shaped rods with phase microscopy of wet mounts of stool. The organism has a characteristic corkscrew-like motion.

Campylobacter may be isolated from stool cultures. It is important to request *Campylobacter* analysis specifically since this organism is not routinely cultured as are salmonellae and shigellae. Fecal material should be sent to the laboratory in a clean container and plated on selected antibiotic-containing media that inhibits normal flora. *Campylobacter* is a micro-aerophilic organism and must be incubated in 5% oxygen. Blood cultures are occasionally positive. A fourfold rise in serum IgG titer to this organism is diagnostic.

Treatment

As a rule, proven *Campylobacter* diarrhea is a mild infection requiring only supportive treatment, and runs its course in about 1 week. On the other hand, the disease may be a life-threatening illness. Bacteremic patients will respond to erythromycin, 500 mg every 6 hours for 7 days, and may require hospitalization.

VIBRIO PARAHAEMOLYTICUS

Vibrio parahaemolyticus is a marine organism that colonizes fish and shellfish. When contaminated raw or improperly cooked seafood is eaten, diarrhea begins within 24 hours. The disease usually occurs during the summer months and clinically resembles shigellosis. Fever, nausea, vomiting, and abdominal pain are common.

Diagnosis

The invasive nature of *V. parahaemolyticus* is proven by positive Wright's and Gram-stains. The diagnosis is made by plating either vomitus or a fresh rectal swab on a thiosulphate citrate bile salt (TCBS) agar, a selective agar; SS agar is of no value.

Treatment

As with nearly all patients who have acute diarrheas, only supportive care is necessary. Symptoms invariably resolve within 1 week. If otherwise, tetracycline, 2 g/day in divided doses may be used.

CHLAMYDIA TRACHOMATIS

Chlamydiae are obligatory intracellular microorganisms that cause a variety of infections in humans and animals. Two chlamydial species are pathogenic for humans: C. *psittaci* (psittacosis) and C. *trachomatis* (trachoma). *Chlamydia trachomatis*, in addition to causing blindness and a spectrum of urogenital tract diseases, has recently been proven to be a cause of hemorrhagic proctitis in homosexual males. The infection can mimic Crohn's disease, idiopathic ulcerative colitis, *Shigella, Salmonella, Yersinia, Campylobacter, V. parahaemolyticus,* and gonococcal proctitis.

Diagnosis

The typical patient presents with fever, anorectal pain, rectal bleeding, rectal discharge, diarrhea, and abdominal pain. The white blood cell count and sedimentation rate are elevated, but liver enzymes are normal. Sigmoidoscopy reveals a spectrum of mucosal changes that varies from diffuse friability with ulcerations to edematous and focal friability of the mucosa. A Gram stain of the rectal discharge shows many fecal leukocytes with no intracellular gram-negative diplococci. Ova and parasite studies are negative as are cultures for enteric pathogens.

Treatment and Prognosis

Tetracycline, 500 mg orally four times daily for 3 weeks is effective treatment. However, reinfection from an untreated sexual partner is a serious problem.

AMEBIASIS

The protozoan, *Entamoeba histolytica,* has a worldwide distribution. The infection is acquired through the ingestion of cyst-contaminated food and water. Excystation occurs in the area of the ileocecal valve in which the trophozoites establish either a commensal or parasitic relationship with the host. For this reason, the incubation period is variable, but 1–5 weeks is average. The infection begins insidiously with low-grade fever, flatulence, intermittent loose bowel movements, abdominal tenderness, and cramps. Vomiting is minimal. Bloody diarrhea indicates a more serious infection.

Diagnosis

Bowel sounds are frequent, and tenderness over the ileocecal valve and liver area is common. Stools are either positive for occult blood or grossly bloody. In the absence of frank rectal bleeding, sigmoidoscopy is positive in fewer than 20% of the cases. When gross bleeding is present, acute proctitis is seen in virtually all cases.

A moderate leukocytosis is present but eosinophilia is not characteristic. Hemagglutination and complement fixation tests may be helpful. Wright's and Gram stains show erythrocytes but only rare leukocytes. The immediate wet mount microscopic examination of stool, mucus, or mucosal scrapings obtained at sigmoidoscopy for motile trophozoites–cysts is a valuable study. Identical samples placed in polyvinyl alcohol and sent for laboratory examination will provide confirmatory results. Specimens must be obtained before any drug treatment is initiated or barium studies are done.

Treatment and Prognosis

Metronidazole (Flagyl), 750 mg orally three times a day for 10 days with diiodohydroxyquin, 650 mg orally three times a day for 20 days is effective against luminal and invasive disease. Metastatic dissemination to liver, lungs, and brain occur rarely.

Infectious Noninvasive Diarrhea

VIRAL DIARRHEA

Rotaviruses are a major cause of diarrhea in children whereas paraviruses (Norwalk and Hawaii) cause symptoms in both children and adults. These are highly infectious agents that have a seasonal pattern (summer and winter). After an incubation period of 1–3 days, symptoms begin abruptly with diarrhea, nausea, vomiting, headaches, abdominal pain, and low-grade fever.

Routine hematologic studies and blood cultures are rarely of any diagnostic value. Fecal leukocytes and red blood cells are absent reflecting the nonexudative character of the diarrhea.

Viral diarrheas are typically benign, self-limiting infections that last 3–4 days. Treatment is supportive and attention to personal hygiene is required. Antibiotics are not indicated.

STAPHYLOCOCCUS AUREUS: FOOD POISONING

Staphylococcus aureus is a common cause of food-borne diarrhea. Salads, (chicken, potato), cold cuts, and meat stews can become contaminated by a food handler who has staphylococcal infection. The organism produces a heat-stable neurotoxin while it is growing in undercooked or spoiled foods.

Diagnosis

Because the toxin is preformed, symptoms begin to show about 1 hour after ingestion of the contaminated food. Symptoms begin with vomiting followed by watery diarrhea. There is no fever. Wright's stain is negative but the Gram stain is positive, showing a predominance of staphylococci. A stool culture is also positive for the same organism.

Treatment and Prognosis

Treatment is symptomatic with attention to hydration. In otherwise healthy individuals, the illness is self-limiting and resolves within 24 hours.

CLOSTRIDIUM PERFRINGENS

Clostridium perfringens is another common cause of food-borne diarrhea. Transmission is through contaminated meat products. The ingested heat-resistant spore produces an enterotoxin in the gut.

Diagnosis

Symptoms begin later than in the case of *Staphylococcus aureus* food poisoning; they begin on the average 12 hours after ingestion of the spore. Nausea is common but vomiting is rare. A watery diarrhea can be severe but is free of inflammatory elements. The clostridial organism may be identified by Gram stain.

Treatment and Prognosis

Treatment is supportive and recovery is uneventful in 12–24 hours. The disease is benign and self-limiting but hydration, at times, may be a problem.

VIBRIO CHOLERAE

Cholera is a water-borne or contaminated food infection with an incubation period of 1–5 days or, in some cases, only a few hours. The gram-negative organism, *V. cholerae*, produces a powerful enterotoxin that stimulates a massive secretion of fluids and electrolytes from the entire small bowel through increased intracellular cyclic adenosine monophosphate (AMP) production.

In fulminant cases, the volume of fluid secreted—1 liter/hr is not uncommon—simply overwhelms the colon's absorptive capacity. In milder cases, the diarrhea may be clinically in-distinguishable from the diarrhea caused by toxigenic *Escherichia coli*, *Salmonella*, or the Norwalk virus.

Although cholera has long been considered an insignificant problem in the United States, a recent outbreak in Louisiana and the easy availability of travel to endemic areas has renewed our interest in this disease.

Diagnosis

In patients with cholera, a short interval of annoying borborygmy is replaced by diarrhea. Nausea, vomiting, and fever are uncommon. As in all secretory diarrheas, the passage of stools is painless. The characteristic stool is clear and has floating flecks of mucus suggesting rice in water—the "rice water" stool.

Fecal Gram stain will show abundant, small, occasionally curved, gram-negative rods. Fecal leukocytes are absent. A positive diagnosis may be made by the direct plating of fresh stool on an alkaline peptone media or by simply dipping a piece of filter paper into the "rice water," sealing it in a sterile container, and alerting the laboratory of the diagnosis.

Treatment

The key to treating patients with cholera is aggressive rehydration. A patient purging 1 liter every 1–2 hours cannot be stablized on 4–5 liters a day of Ringer's lactate or normal saline. In less critically ill patients, oral fluids containing 3.5 g sodium chloride, 2.5 g sodium bicarbonate, 1.5 g potassium chloride, and 20 g glucose per liter of water may be used. Blood electrolytes should be checked two to three times a day. Serum specific gravity (nl 1.025–1.027) will remain high in underhydrated patients, who may develop acute tubular necrosis if the situation is not corrected. Oral tetracycline, 500 mg every 6 hours, will attenuate the illness and halt the excretion of the vibrio.

GIARDIA LAMBLIA

Giardia lamblia, a flagellated protozoan of low pathogenicity, is the most frequently unidentifiable cause of food- and water-borne diarrhea in the United States. Although the disease is common in travelers to certain geographical areas (Leningrad, Rocky Mountains), it occurs in patients with no travel history and is especially common in patients with immunoglobulin deficiencies. Transmission of this disease among homosexuals has recently been documented.

Swallowed cysts parasitize the duodenum and upper jejunum where the alkaline pH favors excystation. Mobile flagellated trophozoites attach themselves to the epithelial surface with sucker discs and then feed and multiply. Over a period of 2–6 weeks, a wide variety of symptoms, depending on the magnitude of the infestation, occur. The exact pathogenic mechanism of giardial infection is unclear.

Diagnosis

There is little found from a physical examination to suggest giardiasis. Abdominal distention, tenderness, tympany, and hyperactive bowel sounds are present but nonspecific. Fever is uncommon but anorexia, nausea, and abdominal gurgling are common. Sulfuric belching, upper- to midepigastric bloating, pain, and cramps may be present. The diarrhea may be mild, watery, and transient or severe and prolonged. With prolonged infection, the stool tends to be of the malabsorptive type—bulky and foul smelling.

A history of foreign travel or backpacking and camping in the Rocky Mountains area provide important clues to the diagnosis.

Hematologic studies are of little value inasmuch as the organism does not provoke an inflammatory response. For the same reason, a Wright's fecal stain and sigmoidoscopy are also negative. Barium studies are nonspecific, but an edematous duodenal mucosa or spasm and irritability of the jejunum should suggest the possibility of giardiasis. A Sudan IV stain of the stool will document fat malabsorption. An experienced technician may find trophozoites–cysts in a fresh warm stool sample. However, parasite shedding may be intermittent, and one negative stool should never be considered adequate to rule out giardiasis. If several stools are negative and giardiasis is still a prime consideration, duodenal aspiration and/or a biopsy should be planned. The immediate microscopic search for fresh, warm duodenal fluid for trophozoites is a high-yield procedure. The histologic examination of duodenal biopsy material is also rewarding.

Treatment and Prognosis

Quinacrine hydrochloride, 100 mg three times daily for 10 days, is the treatment of choice. Metronidazole, 250 mg three times daily for 10 days, is an alternative and effective program. A complete resolution of symptoms may require up to 2 weeks.

The above program will cure 80–90% of cases. The stool should be reexamined in 2 weeks to ensure effective therapy.

TRAVELER'S DIARRHEA

Nearly one-half of North Americans traveling to tropical countries experience diarrhea. Traveler's diarrhea is a syndrome caused by a variety of infectious agents, the most common of which is the enterotoxigenic *Escherichia coli*. The organism produces a heat-liable and/or heat-stable enterotoxin that stimulates an outpouring of water and electrolytes beyond the colon's absorptive capacity. Other organisms implicated in this syndrome are *Salmonella*, *Shigella*, invasive *Escherichia coli*, *V. parahaemolyticus*, *Amoeba* and *Giardia*.

The constant feature of this syndrome is the sudden onset of watery diarrhea. Blood may also be recorded if the causative organisms are enteroinvasive. Malaise, anorexia, abdominal cramping, tenesmus, fever, nausea, and vomiting have been noted in varying degrees.

Diagnosis

Wright's and Gram stains will establish whether the traveler's diarrhea is secondary to an enterotoxigenic or enteroinvasive agent. Hemoglobin, hematocrit, and BUN are important in those patients whose diarrhea has been severe or prolonged.

Treatment and Prognosis

The oral replacement of fluids and electrolytes is the mainstay of treatment of traveler's diarrhea. All but the most severe cases can be managed on this regimen. Electrolytes may be replaced with Gatorade; broths; orange, apple, and pineapple juices; and carbonated drinks. Hospitalization and intravenous treatment is reserved only for seriously ill patients. Antibiotics are not indicated since, in general, the illness is of brief duration. In severe cases in which there is evidence that the causative organism is invasive, ampicillin, 2 g/day for 5 days, should be started. Drugs that reduce motility delay clearance of the infecting organism and prolong the illness. Kaolin and pectin (Kaopectate) does not reduce fluid loss but is innocuous and will make the stool more solid. Bismuth subsalicylate (Pepto-Bismol), with its antibacterial and antitoxin effect, is probably the best medication currently available. Thirty milliliters every half-hour for 8 doses is usually effective.

Most patients recover quickly, but 20% may have symptoms for as long as 2 weeks.

Noninfectious Diarrhea with Mucosal Injury

INFLAMMATORY BOWEL DISEASE

Ulcerative colitis (UC) and Crohn's disease (CD) are chronic recurring diseases of unknown etiology. Ulcerative colitis is limited to the colon where it may involve all of that organ—universal colitis—or part of it—right- or left-sided colitis. Ulcerative proctitis (UP) is a mild form of UC that is limited to the distal 15 cm of the rectum. Crohn's disease may be found anywhere in the gastrointestinal tract but is commonly identified at the terminal ileum and/or colon, where it is also known as granulomatous colitis. Both diseases have a predilection for the young, 10–30 years, for whites over blacks, and for Jews over non-Jews.

Although both diseases share many clinical, pathologic and epidemiologic features, the pathology in each case is distinctive. In UC, the inflammatory insult is transmucosal. However, when confronted with the active disease, the clinical separation of the two entities is difficult. Ten to fifteen percent of patients cannot be classified despite endoscopic, histologic, and radiographic analysis.

Diagnosis

Abdominal cramps, fever, bloody diarrhea, and weight loss are common to both entities. However, the clinical manifestations of these symptoms are directly related to the severity of the ulcerative process and the extent of bowel involvement. Since rectal involvement is more frequent in UC than CD, tenesmus is more commonly associated with UC. Conversely, right lower-quadrant pain is more common to CD than UC. Arthralgia, uveitis, and iridocyclitis occur in both diseases.

The physical findings are dictated by the degree and extent of bowel injury. A toxic patient with abdominal and rebound tenderness has severe colonic injury and requires plain films of the abdomen to exclude perforation or toxic megacolon. A transverse colon greater than 6 cm in diameter is cause for concern. Erythema nodosum on the legs, but occasionally on the arms, suggests inflammatory bowel disease (IBD). A right lower-quadrant mass is common in CD and indicates an abscess or matted bowel and omentum. Finger clubbing, although not a common finding, is five times more frequent in patients with CD than with UC. Extensive perianal disease, abscess, fistula, sinus tract, rectal stricture, cobblestoning, and thickening are indicative of CD.

Blood studies, hemoglobin, white blood cell count, sedimentation rate, proteins, electrolytes, and prothrombin time are not diagnostic, but they do define the severity of the disease.

Proctosigmoidoscopy is a valuable procedure to help separate these two entities. Ninety-five percent of patients with UC have diffuse rectal involvement either as edema–friability or frank ulcerations. Only about 50% of patients present with rectal involvement, and the mucosa tends to be cobblestoned and ulcerations more discrete. A rectal biopsy is one important adjunct, and if granulomata are histologically demonstrated, CD becomes the prime consideration.

Contrast studies to document the extent of disease and complications are important. However, they should be held in abeyance until the patient has been stabilized. Colonoscopy is another important but invasive tool that should not be attempted on acutely sick patients for fear of perforation. When available, gallium isotope scan of the colon is a simple, noninvasive procedure and will identify the extent of the inflammatory insult.

Treatment and Prognosis

The causes of both UC and CD are unknown, and therefore treatment remains empirical and directed toward adequate nutrition control of inflammation and replacement of fluid and blood losses. However, acutely sick patients must be identified as soon as possible and hospitalized. Severe colitis is characterized by fever, tachycardia, abdominal pain and tenderness, more than 10 bloody movements, electrolyte imbalance, decreased serum albumin, and hematocrit. Correction of fluid and blood losses should begin immediately. Antidiarrheals, especially those containing atropine and codeine may be harmful and should be avoided. Intravenous corticosteroids should be used when the diagnosis of IBD is fairly clear. Hydrocortisone, 100 mg every 8 hours, is an acceptable starting program. There is no place for sulfasalazine in the initial management of severe acute colitis.

Less critically ill patients can be cared for on an ambulatory basis. Oral steroids—prednisone, 20–60 mg/day, or sulfasalazine, beginning with 2 gm/day—can be very effective. Ulcerative proctitis and left-sided colitis respond well to both oral sulfasalazine and steroid enemas. Antibiotics are not indicated unless there is clear evidence of metastatic infection.

Ninety percent of patients presenting with their first attack of UC will respond to this regimen. Approximately 5% are not as fortunate and will die. Toxic megacolon is a serious complication of IBD with a mortality rate of about 30%. However, both entities are chronic recurrent diseases and require continued close supervision long after remission has been achieved.

The risk of colon cancer in patients with UC is 10 times that of a matched control population, and the risk parallels the duration of the disease. Therefore aggressive surveillance in patients with long-standing chronic UC is mandatory. Although the incidence of malignancy is also increased in CD, the risk is so low that cancer surveillance is not indicated in the same aggressive fashion as in UC. Ulcerative proctitis is a relatively benign disease with a low incidence of local and systemic complications. However, 10% of patients with UP will progress to UC.

ISCHEMIC COLITIS

Ischemic colitis is, in general, a reversible inflammatory lesion of the colon caused by inadequate tissue perfusion with secondary hypoxia. The lesion is most often encountered in patients over 50 years old because of the greater frequency of vascular disease in people in this age group. Although any area of the colon can be involved, the left transverse colon and splenic flexure are especially vulnerable as a result of limitations in blood supply. Predisposing factors include diabetes mellitus, connective tissue disorders, and arteriosclerosis. Young women on contraceptive steroids are also at risk.

Diagnosis

Patients in the acute fulminant stage of the disease present with severe abdominal pain, massive rectal bleeding, and cardiovascular collapse, findings not unlike those in patients with acute mesenteric infarction. Colonic perforation is common in this stage, and barium studies are contraindicated. Plain films of the abdomen can be diagnostic if thumbprinting is identified. In the subacute state, which is the most common type of ischemic colitis, patients present with a lesser degree of pain and rectal bleeding. Plain films of the abdomen may be all that is required for diagnosis. Although sigmoidoscopy is a primary diagnostic consideration in any patients with rectal bleeding, in this condition the rectum is rarely involved; a helpful clue in the differential diagnosis with ulcerative colitis, which shows rectal ulcerations in 95% of cases.

Treatment and Prognosis

Fluids and blood are administered according to the severity of the presenting symptoms and physical findings. Inasmuch as the majority of the patients suspected of ischemic colitis are elderly, hospitalization is essential. Perforation is always a possibility as is the further progression of the ischemic process. If perforation is not suspected, barium studies are useful and should be done early in the course of the disease because of the rapidity with which the pathologic process changes. It is not unusual to document the radiographic normalization of the previously affected colon in 5–10 days. Angiography, on occasion, may demonstrate an occlusive vascular lesion that can be surgically bypassed. Recently, in experienced hands, colonoscopy has been proven to be a safe, rapid, accurate, and simple means of diagnosing this condition.

Although subacute disease in the majority of patients runs a benign course over a period of 2–6 weeks, about 10% of the patients will require surgery either because of progression of the ischemic process, postischemic strictures, or chronic ulcer formations.

ANTIBIOTIC-ASSOCIATED COLITIS

Antimicrobial therapy has been a well-recognized cause of diarrhea for the past 30 years. An antibiotic-resistant strain of *Staphylococcous aureus* was regularly isolated from patients who developed diarrhea during neomycin bowel preparation. This problem was partially resolved by the addition of antibiotics that prevented the overgrowth of gram-positive organisms. Thus antibiotic diarrhea has been a minor and rather common side effect of antibiotic therapy.

However, the recent proliferation of newer broad-spectrum antibiotics has brought forth a flurry of reports describing a pseudomembraonous colitis or antibiotic-associated colitis (AAC). The diarrhea may vary from a mild, self-limiting afebrile illness to a persistent febrile dysentery. Almost all broad-spectrum antibiotics have induced AAC, especially those with anaerobic activity. A brief list includes amoxcillin, ampicillin, cephalothin, cephadex, cephalosporin, chloramphenicol, clindamycin, cortimoxazole, lincomycin, metronidazole, and tetracycline.

The development of AAC has been linked to the suppression of the normal bowel flora and the overgrowth of an antibiotic resistant, toxin-producing anaerobic bacterium, *Clostridium difficile*. The toxin-injured bowel responds with an outpouring of fluid, mucus, inflammatory cells, and occasionally blood. Patients can be of any age, but the very young, the elderly, and the postoperative patients are particularly susceptible.

Antibiotic-associated colitis may develop during antibiotic treatment or 3–4 weeks after therapy has ended. On the average, AAC begins 1 week after starting antibiotics administration.

Diagnosis

Patients with AAC present with diarrhea of varying severity that is characterized by watery, mucoid, and possibly bloody stools. Patients may be afebrile or have a temperature up to 40°C (104°F), with a leukocytosis. Cramps and abdominal tenderness depend on the degree of colon injury and the underlying disease that necessitated the antibiotic therapy.

Suspected AAC patients should have a CBC, electrolytes, BUN, and plain film of the abdomen. The diarrheal loss of potassium and bicarbonate predisposes to metabolic acidosis. Stool cultures for the common enteric pathogens, *Salmonella* and *Shigella*, must be obtained. Fecal leukocytes are usually present. Proctosigmoidoscopy is tbe simplest and most rapid means of diagnosis. Pseudomembranes—scattered, raised or flat, yellowish to white plaques—are virtually pathognomonic of AAC and can be seen in 90% of patients with the disease. If the diarrhea persists 4–5 days after cessation of all antibiotics and sigmoidoscopy is negative, a search for pseudomembranes beyond the rectosigmoid area (colonoscopy) or fresh stool specimens assayed for clostridial toxin are indicated. Twenty percent of patients with antibiotic diarrhea and some patients with severe relapsing ulcerative colitis also have positive toxin assays. Barium films are rarely helpful and may be harmful.

Treatment and Prognosis

The clinical course of untreated AAC is variable. With the onset of diarrhea, all antibiotics must be stopped. In many cases, this simple action alone will result in the patient's progressive improvement. Other patients develop a protracted course of remission and exacerbation, whereas others progress to fulminant dysentery. In these patients, oral vancomycin clearly reduces morbidity and mortality. Although the Food and Drug Administration (FDA) does not recognize vancomycin treatment of AAC, vancomycin effectively reduces *Clostridium difficile* in the gut and dramatically affects symptoms within 2–3 days.

Patients with persistent but clinically mild-to-moderate diarrhea may respond to low dosages of vancomycin—150 mg every 6 hours. Seriously ill patients will require full dosage—500 mg every 6 hours. Intravenous vancomycin treatment delivers low concentrations to the gut and is not indicated unless the oral route is impractical. The empiric use of vancomycin in critically ill patients with severe diarrhea may be justified if proctosigmoidoscopy is negative and enterotoxin assays are unavailable. However, a positive response should occur rapidly and dramatically with 24–48 hours. Preliminary studies indicate that another oral and poorly absorbed antibiotic, bacitracin, may also induce a clinical remission. Cholestyramine, 4 g/day orally for 5 days may bind *Clostridium difficile* toxin and control symptoms. The use of corticosteroids or adrenocorticotropic hormones (ACTH) is not indicated. Antidiarrheals, especially those containing atropine or codeine, may improve symptoms but will also delay the fecal elimination of clostridial toxins and may precipitate toxic dilatation of the colon.

Approximately 10% of treated patients will have a relapse and should be treated with longer courses of vancomycin. Approximately 33% of patients who suffer a relapse will have a second relapse. Relapse may be because of environmental exposure or remaining *Clostridium difficile* spores. The average mortality for patients older than 60 years is 40%.

Noninfectious Diarrhea without Mucosal Injury (Humorally Mediated Diarrheas)

Several endocrine tumors share diarrhea as a common symptom. In some cases the diarrhea is clearly related to a humoral agent, in others the diarrhea is associated less clearly with humoral abnormalities. The diarrheas are, in general, large-volume diarrheas, that is, volumes of 1 liter or more per day for several days.

ZOLLINGER-ELLISON SYNDROME

The diarrhea in patients with Zollinger-Ellison syndrome is a secretory diarrhea, meaning that it persists during fasting and remits only with severe dehydration. Pancreatic gastrin-producing tumors stimulate gastric hypersecretion of hydrogen ions. The large hydrogen ion volume in turn causes hypersecretion of pancreatic juices, bile, and Brunner's gland fluid, all of which contribute to the diarrheal syndrome. Large-volume diarrhea occurs in patients with peptic ulcer disease.

Diagnosis

Stool cultures and analysis are of no value. A carefully placed nasogastric tube aspirating all of the gastric output will stop the diarrhea and should prompt more definitive tests such as fasting serum gastrins and measurements of basal gastric acid.

Treatment and Prognosis

Cimetidine, 300 mg four times daily, will relieve the diarrhea. Surgery should be considered. Unfortunately, at the time of surgery, 50% of patients will already have metastases in regional lymph nodes and liver.

PANCREATIC CHOLERA

A nonbeta islet cell tumor causes watery diarrhea, hypokalemia, and achlorhydria. The WDHA syndrome is another example of large-volume secretory diarrhea; in proven cases, 3 liters/day is common. The majority of patients with WDHA are middle-aged women. All patients should be carefully screened for laxative, diuretic, and antacid abuse.

Symptoms are large-volume painless diarrhea with evidence of dehydration and hypokalemia. Fever is absent.

Diagnosis

The documentation of hypokalemia and achlorhydria–hypochlorhydia in the presence of a secretory diarrhea should suggest the diagnosis pancreatic cholera. A search for humoral substances is indicated. Hormones commonly associated with WDHA are the vasoactive intestinal polypeptide (VIP) and pancreatic polypeptide (PP). A tumor search may be undertaken with angiography, ultrasonography, and computer tomography (CT). Stool culture and analysis are negative.

Treatment and Prognosis

Surgical removal of localized tumors is the treatment of pancreatic cholera. Many tumors are large by the time the diarrhea is severe. The distinction between a benign or malignant tumor can only be made by the presence or absence of metastases. Histology of the primary tumor alone is not a reliable indication.

CARCINOID

Carcinoid is a clinical syndrome caused by midgut tumor, which includes explosive diarrhea, flushing, colic, telangiectasia, bronchospasm and valvular heart disease. Several substances are responsible for this constellation of findings; 5-hydroxytryptamine (5HT) (serotonin), kinin peptides, and prostaglandins are a few. Serotonin is responsible for gut hypermotility. A massively enlarged liver, cutaneous flushing, and diarrhea are the most common complaints.

Diagnosis

Urinary excretion of 5-hydroxyindoleacetic acid greater than five times normal is diagnostic.

Treatment and Prognosis

Methysergide maleate, a serotonin antagonist, 2 mg three times daily, has a beneficial affect on patients with diarrhea. Codeine and paregoric may also be tried. Surgical cures are rare and limited to tumors arising in testicular or ovarian teratomas. The large hepatic deposits of tumor indicate a poor prognosis.

ACUTE HEPATIC DISORDERS

Hepatitis—viral, toxic, or drug-induced—is a common problem for which patients seek medical attention. The liver is the chief organ for the metabolism and excretion of most drugs. By a process of oxidation, reduction, or hydrolysis and then conjugation, hundreds of endogenous and exogenous compounds are made soluble for excretion into bile or urine. Although nearly all drugs adversely affect the liver, the injury is of little clinical significance in the majority of cases. Unfortunately, with an ever-increasing number of drugs available for disease control, toxic and drug-induced hepatitis will continue to be a serious problem.

Toxic hepatitis refers to a predictable, acute liver injury caused by a true hepatotoxin such as carbon tetrachloride, phosphorus, or mushroom poisoning *(Amanita phalloides)*. *Drug-induced or alcoholic hepatitis* is an adverse, idiosyncratic hepatic reaction to a wide variety of medications. *Viral hepatitis* is an acute infection of the liver caused by one of at least three different viruses. In the United States the viruses type A (HAV), type B (HBV), and type non-A/non-B (HCV) are responsible for 500,000 cases of hepatitis annually.

Viral Hepatitis

HEPATITIS A

Hepatitis A (HAV) is an RNA-containing enterovirus, 27 nm in diameter with a short incubation period of 20–40 days. It is a highly contagious disease spread by fecal contamination of water and food and by person-to-person contact. The homosexual dissemination of the disease in men has added to the problem. Although this portion of the epidemiology is clear, the source of infection is obscure in 60% of cases.

Infected patients shed vast numbers of the virus in their stool, creating epidemic conditions wherever hygiene and sanitation are suboptimal. Viremia and fecal shedding of the virus peak several days before hepatitis is suspected and overt signs appear. It is during this period that patients are most contagious and close contacts are at great risk of infection. With the onset of symptoms, fecal shedding begins a rapid decline and ends within 2 weeks.

The serum markers of HAV infection are the hepatitis A antigen (HAAg) and the antibody against the type A virus (anti-HAV), which persists for life. Unfortunately, the serum concentration of the hepatitis A antigen is, for practical purposes, not measurable, and the diagnosis of acute hepatitis is based on the detection of serum antibodies (anti-HAV). However, because the hepatitis A virus is panendemic, the prevalance of anti-HAV is 40–80% depending on the age and socioeconomic background of the groups tested. Therefore the presence alone of anti-HAV is not diagnostic of acute infection. The recent laboratory ability to detect acute phase (IgM) and convalescent (IgG) antibodies radioimmunologically, has resolved this problem. The presence of IgM anti-HAV is diagnostic of acute infection, whereas the detection of IgG anti-HAV indicates past infection unrelated to a current bout of acute liver disease. Anti-HAV (IgM) peaks during the first week of infection and seldom persists beyond 6 months.

Hepatitis A infection is a benign disease with constitutional symptoms lasting 2–7 days and recovery, as a rule, within 4 weeks. Hospitalization should be reserved for those patients with fecal incontinence and severe nausea and vomiting. A carrier state and adverse sequelae have not been reported. Approximately 50% of sporadic hepatitis is caused by the type A virus.

Diagnosis

The prodromal phase of acute hepatitis is manifested by a wide variety of nonspecific constitutional symptoms affecting chiefly the gastrointestinal and respiratory systems. Anorexia, nausea, vomiting, fatigue, malaise, cough, and low-grade fever are common presenting symptoms.

A clinically icteric phase is not always detectable, although a brief period of dark urine is frequently mentioned by the patient. If there is an icteric phase, it is usually mild and of short duration.

Hepatic tenderness and mild enlargement are common findings in the early stages of the infection. The most useful test to confirm the diagnosis of acute hepatitis is the measurement of serum transaminases. Abnormal values should prompt a search for acute phase (IgM) antibodies. Their documentation confirms the diagnosis of acute hepatitis A.

Treatment and Prognosis

In general, treatment is symptomatic. Inasmuch as fecal shedding of the virus peaks *before* the onset of symptoms and rapidly declines thereafter, isolation of the patient after the diagnosis is established serves little purpose unless fecal incontinence or vomiting are problems. Wearing gloves and frequent hand washing are mandatory for all those who handle excreta and care for these patients. Small, frequent, well-balanced meals are indicated. Strict bed rest is not necessary unless the patient is clearly toxic.

Immune serum globulin (ISG) is effective against hepatitis A and should be administered to household members and close personal contacts. A single intramuscular injection of 0.02 ml/kg given within 2 weeks of exposure provides a high degree of protection. As a *general rule*, routine school and office contacts do not need ISG.

The prognosis is excellent in previously healthy patients. Patients with advanced age or serious underlying medical problems do less well.

HEPATITIS B

Hepatitis B (HBV) is a DNA-containing virus with a longer incubation period of 40–160 days and a lower contagion rate than HAV and is transmitted mainly by parenteral infusion of infected blood or blood products. The presence of the hepatitis B surface antigen (HB$_s$Ag) in nearly all human excreta (tears, sweat, saliva, bile, urine, stool, semen, and menstrual fluids) suggests that these fluids represent another vehicle of transmission. However, the infectious agent, the DNA virus, has not been identified in any fluid except blood.

The serologic indicators of HBV infection are hepatitis B surface antigen (HB$_s$Ag), the outer lipoprotein coat of the infectious virion (Dane particle); the hepatitis B core antigen (HB$_c$Ag), the dense inner core of the virion, and the hepatitis B e antigen (HB$_e$Ag) located within the inner core of the virion. Antibodies to these antigens are also identifiable. During the early incubation period of HBV, HB$_s$Ag is detectable in 80–90% of cases and persists from 1 week to as long as 5 months. Generally, the HB$_s$Ag rises parallel with the rising transaminases and the onset of symptoms.

The HB$_e$Ag appears soon after HB$_s$Ag and can be detected in nearly all acute cases along with the HB$_c$Ag core antigen. As hepatic healing begins, the reverse process occurs: HB$_s$Ag begins to fall, transaminases decrease, and symptoms improve. Convalescence is marked by the serologic clearance of HB$_s$Ag.

In general, patients with HBV have a favorable prognosis with complete recovery in 4–10 weeks. Depending on age and other concurrent medical problems, 1–2% of those afflicted with HBV will die. In transfusion-associated disease, however, the death rate is nearly five times greater. Although complete healing occurs in 90% of patients with acute HBV, 10% will remain HB$_s$Ag positive and may either remain asymptomatic carriers or progress to chronic active hepatitis. Chronic active hepatitis is probably the most widespread systemic viral disease in the world, affecting about 300 million people. Inherent in the disease are the serious sequelae of cirrhosis and hepatocellular carcinoma.

A third variant of this disease (less than 1%) takes the form of fulminant hepatitis, a rapid and severe form of liver failure with a high mortality (70–100%).

The routine serologic screening of all blood donors has all but eliminated posttransfusion hepatitis B. However, HBV remains a serious problem among the 15–30-year-old age group, presumably because of drug abuse, and among male homosexuals.

HEPATITIS C

Hepatitis C (HCV), type non-A/non-B, is a disease without antigenic markers. Therefore a diagnosis of hepatitis C can only be made by the exclusion of the other two forms of viral hepatitis. The serologic absence of surface antigen, anti-HAV, and anti-A IgM during the early phase of acute hepatitis rules out hepatitis A and B. Further confirmation may be obtained in serum collected during convalescence, which should contain *no* antibodies to the hepatitis B surface or core antigens. The average incubation period for HCV is 7–8 weeks, which is longer than that of HAV and somewhat shorter than that of HBV, otherwise the clinical and epidermiologic patterns of hepatitis C are similar to hepatitis B. Transmission is chiefly parenteral, and thus the high-risk groups are drug addicts, multiple-transfused patients, and dialysis patients. Nearly one-half of all the patients with HCV fail to recover completely and progress to chronic hepatitis, suggesting that hepatitis C is a leading cause of cirrhosis and possibly hepatic carcinoma. Clinically, this subgroup is identified by protracted fluctuations in transaminase levels. In the United States, HCV accounts for about 90–95% of all posttransfusion hepatitis cases and about 25% of sporatic hepatitis cases.

DIAGNOSIS OF VIRAL HEPATITIS

A diagnosis of hepatitis begins with an accurate and comprehensive history that explores diet, occupation, medication, drug abuse, and parenteral and physical exposure. There are few symptoms and clinical findings that are specific indicators of liver injury. Although anorexia, nausea, chills, fever, rashes, leukocytosis, and arthralgias are common extrahepatic manifestations of liver injury, they are equally common to a number of nonhepatic diseases. Jaundice indicates liver injury, and when it is associated with pruritus, severe cholestasis has developed. Jaundice and pruritis are common effects of drug injury, although viral injury may produce similar consequences. The symptoms of drug-induced hepatitis occur about 2–5 weeks after drug administration, whereas true liver toxins cause nausea and vomiting within hours of exposure.

It is estimated that 10 times as many patients have hepatitis as are seen by doctors. This suggests that in most cases, the clinical manifestation of liver injury are so mild as to go un-

detected. Those that do seek medical help present with some or all of the following: anorexia, nausea, fever, jaundice, tender hepatomegaly, and frequently splenomegaly. Spiders, ascites, and gastrointestinal bleeding are uncommon in patients with acute hepatitis and, if present, indicate a severe hepatic insult.

The many clinical features shared by all of the acute viral hepatitides prevents a reliable differentiation among them based solely on incubation time, type of prodrome, or levels of transaminases or bilirubin. If it were not for the serologic changes that follow HAV, HBV, and HCV infections, separation of the various hepatitides would be impossible.

The overall mortality rate for all reported cases is 2% for HBV, 3% for HCV, and 0.2% for drug-induced hepatitis. These figures are very likely too high considering the number of cases that are never reported.

Laboratory Tests for Viral Hepatitis

The most rapid and valuable tests for hepatic dysfunction are the serum transaminases—the serum glutamic-oxalocetic (SGOT) the serum glutamic-pyruvic transaminases (SGPT) tests. In cases of acute injury, these enzymes are already elevated before the bilirubin begins to rise. The half-life of these enzymes is about 21 days, making them useful indicators of day-to-day liver cell damage and healing. The prothrombin time (PT) is indispensable for accurately assessing the degree of liver injury and possible impending hepatic coma. An elevated white blood cell count is also an ominous sign; counts over 15,000 are associated with high mortality rates. The alkaline phosphatase and lactic dehydrogenase generally correlate poorly with acute injury.

The radioimmunoassay of the presently known serologic markers is the only means available for identifying the viruses responsible for the liver injury.

In a clinical setting of acute hepatitis, the serum identification of the HB_sAg is proof of type B hepatitis, and further tests are not necessary. Occasionally, the HB_sAg is rapidly cleared from the serum before hepatitis B is suspected. Thus, a gap or window exists between the disappearance of HB_sAg and the appearance of anti-HB_s. During this interval, which may last from 1 week to several months, anti-HB_c is detectable and may be the only serologic marker of HBV infection.

Without known specific serological markers, the diagnosis of hepatitis C is made only after the exclusion of hepatitis A and B.

TREATMENT OF VIRAL HEPATITIS

In nearly all cases of acute viral hepatitis, no specific treatment is required and the patient can be safely managed at home.

The illness produces lassitude, fatigue, and anorexia that limit the patient's activity and appetite. In general, these symptoms are of short duration, and strength and appetite return quickly. Therapy is supportive and all unnecessary medication discontinued. Bed rest and diet are tailored to the patient's response to the infection. Patients who are not seriously ill may be up and about but not to the point of excessive fatigue. Small, frequent feedings of a well-balanced bland diet are generally well tolerated. There is no evidence that rigid fat restriction has any predictable value.

However, excessive anorexia or vomiting require hospitalization for observation and intravenous therapy. Patients with prolonged PTs belong in the hospital and should receive a single injection of vitamin K. Repeated injections of this vitamin are rarely of any value, and if the PT remains uncorrected, consideration should be given to the use of fresh frozen plasma.

Patients suspected of having drug-induced hepatitis should have all drugs immediately discontinued. Treatment is supportive and recovery is the rule. In severe cases, steroids may be helpful but are not of consistently proven benefit.

The resumption of normal activity must be guided by lack of symptoms and of laboratory abnormalities.

PREVENTION OF VIRAL HEPATITIS

Recent clinical trials with highly purified formalin-inactivated vaccine against type B hepatitis have proven the vaccine to be safe and highly effective against acute hepatitis B, asymptomatic infection, and chronic antigenemia. Currently, however, the United States Public Health Service officially recommends hepatitis B immune globulin (HBIG) for postexposure prophylaxis in the following categories: (1) accidental needle sticks or lacerations, open abrasions, or mucosal membrane contact with fluids or secretions from known HG$_s$Ag patients. The recommended dosage is 0.05–0.07 ml/kg administered within 7 days of exposure and repeated in 1 month. No one need receive prophylaxis who is already antigen or antibody positive for HBV. (2) Neonates, born to mothers who had acute HBV during the third trimester of pregnancy or who are HB$_s$Ag positive at the time of delivery, should be given HBIG, 0.13 ml/kg, as a single dose immediately after delivery and again at 3- and 6-month intervals.

The recent identification of the type C virus is an important first step toward the future preparations of an anti-C vaccine. Presently there are no recommendations for immunoprophylaxis of HCV hepatitis, although there is anectodal evidence that standard ISG (5 ml) may attentuate the disease.

Alcoholic Hepatitis

There are approximately 10 million alcoholics in the United States, 1 million of whom will develop alcoholic hepatitis, a potentially lethal form of liver failure. In urban centers, alcoholic liver disease is the fourth most common cause of death.

Daily consumption of 160 g of alcohol for several years predisposes to severe hepatic dysfunction. This amount of alcohol is available in 1 pint of 86-proof whiskey, or 2 liters of wine, or 2 six packs of beer, quantities well within the capacity of a "social" drinker. However, only 35% of heavy abusers will develop acute hepatitis.

Diagnosis

Anorexia, weight loss, nausea, vomiting, fever, abdominal pain, and dark urine are common complaints of patients with alcoholic hepatitis. Hepatomegaly is invariably present and is accompanied by spider angiomata and splenomegaly in one-third of those examined. The triad of fever, jaundice, and ascites has been reported in one-half of these patients.

Laboratory

Leukocytosis (15,000–20,000) occurs in 50% of patients; a few patients show counts of 100,000 and above. The SGOT rarely exceeds the 300–500 unit range and may even be normal. When the SGOT is elevated, 90% of the time, it is higher than the SGPT. This has been such a consistent finding that the SGOT:SGPT ratio has been used not only to diagnose alcoholic hepatitis, but also to screen patients who deny their alcoholism. Elevation of the enzyme, γ-glutamyltranspeptidase (GGTP), originally proposed as a marker of alcoholic liver disease, is also helpful. Prothrombin time and albumin ratios should be recorded. The alkaline phosphatase may be markedly elevated, falsely suggesting extrabiliary tract surgical disease. Ultrasonography is extremely useful in resolving this dilemma. When possible, a liver biopsy should be done to confirm the diagnosis.

Treatment and Prognosis

Treatment is entirely supportive and designed to spare the liver further insult. Complete abstinence from alcohol coupled with a simple well-balanced diet is adequate in the majority of cases. Hospitalization may be necessary if complications arise (dehydration, severe nausea and vomiting, or gastrointestinal bleeding). The need for specific nutrients such as folic acid, thiamine, pyridoxine, magnesium, phosphate, zinc, potassium, and vitamin K depends on clinical and laboratory findings.

The parenteral use of glucose requires the concomitant administration of B vitamins. Nearly all chronic abusers have low reserves of B vitamins because of their predominately high carbohydrate diet. The use of intravenous glucose may further depress thiamine levels and precipitate mental and ocular disturbances (Wernicke's disease).

For the disruptive patient, diazepam (Valium) is useful and should be administered in small amounts with careful monitoring of the patient's clinical condition. Patients with ascites are always at risk of infection, and a diagnostic tap to exclude spontaneous bacterial peritonitis is indicated. The use of corticosteroids remains controversial since most of the studies indicate little or no benefit from their use.

About 15% of patients with proven alcoholic hepatitis die during the acute phase from variceal bleeding, azotemia, or infection. Ten percent will heal completely and 40% will continue to have recurrent bouts of acute alcoholic hepatitis without evidence of cirrhosis. The remaining survivors will progress to cirrhosis. Patients with serum bilirubins greater than 2 mg/dl, a serum albumin of less than 2 g/dl, and a PT prolonged by 5 seconds have a mortality rate of 75%.

Hepatic Coma

Although the liver may fail abruptly in acute viral or drug-related hepatitis, there are clinical neuropsychiatric warning signs that this event may occur. The syndrome may present as minor self-limiting disturbances in consciousness (stage I) or may progress to deep coma (stage III). Common precipitants of hepatic coma are hemorrhage, injudicious use of sedatives or diuretics, excessive protein intake, and infection.

Diagnosis

Asterixis (flapping tremor) is the most characteristic neurologic abnormality of hepatic coma. Although common in liver failure, asterixis is also found in uremia and advanced pulmonary and cardiac diseases. Changes in sleep pattern—sleeping longer than usual, reversal of the sleep pattern, sleeping during the day, remaining awake at night—are clues to early encephalopathy. Deterioration of mood, intellect, and personal care are also noted. Hyperactivity and noisy and violent delirium are seen in patients during acute encephalopathy. These changes are fluctuant and may appear only intermittently.

Prothrombin time is the most valuable test for impending coma. An elevated white blood cell count above 15,000 indicates a poor prognosis and presages gastrointestinal bleeding.

The electroencephalogram (EEG) is useful in doubtful situations because a pattern of encephalopathy may be discerned long before the onset of asterixis. Although EEG changes are nonspecific, the slowing of wave frequency in a patient with existing liver disease is virtually diagnostic. Blood ammonia levels correlate poorly with the patient's clinical status.

Treatment and Prognosis

The prognosis of hepatic coma depends largely on the virulence of the offending agents and liver reserve. Age is also a critical factor; anyone over 40, regardless of treatment modality, has virtually no chance of survival. Hepatic coma patients must be protected from all unnecessary medications, electrolyte imbalance, hypoglycemia, and infections. Any attempt to correct hyponatremia with sodium chloride should be shunned unless there is absolute evidence of excessive sodium loss. Lacking this information, hyponatremia should be corrected by sodium (10 mEq) and fluid (1000 ml/day) restrictions. Fluid overload must be rigorously avoided. The manically delerious patient will require sedation, and diazepam, 5 or 10 mg intravenously may be given slowly. This should not be a standing order. Additional sedation must be preceded by a careful examination of the patient. Oxazepam or lorazepam are not directly metabolized by the liver and deserve consideration as sedatives. Morphine and paraldehyde are contraindicated. Patients who show evidence of bleeding diathesis should be treated with fresh, frozen plasma. The use of antibiotics, nasogastric suction, protein restriction, lactulose–neomycin, or central venous monitoring is determined by the clinical assessment of the patient on a day-to-day basis. Exchange transfusions and steroids are of little if any therapeutic value.

Survival from coma (stage III) is inversely related to age. In the age group of 20 and under, 30% survive; between ages 20 and 40, 10% survive; and over age 40, recovery is rare. Fortunately there is some evidence that the spectrum of acute liver failure is decreasing.

SELECTED READINGS

Bryan, JA: Viral hepatitis. *Postgrad Med* 1980; 68:67.

Chang TW: Antimicrobial-associated diarrhea and enterocolitis. *Drug Therapy* 1981; 11:117.

Conn HO: Current diagnosis and treatment of hepatic coma. *Hosp Pract* 1973; 6:65.

DuPont HL: Enteropathogenic organisms. New etiologic agents and concepts of disease. *Med Clin North Am* 1978; 62:945.

Farmer RG: Clinical features and natural history of inflammatory bowel disease. *Med Clin North Am* 1980; 64:1103.

Krejs GJ, Fordtran JS: Diarrhea In Gastrointestinal Disease, ed 2. Sleisenger MH, Fordtran JS (eds) Philadelphia, WB Saunders Co, 1978, p 313.

Monroe PS, Baker AL: Alcoholic hepatitis. *Postgrad Med* 1981; 69:32.

Parks TG: Ischaemic disease of the colon. *Coloproctology*. International edition 1980; 2:213.

Phillips SF: Diarrhea: A current view of the pathophysiology. *Gastroenterology* 1972; 63:495.

Zimmerman HJ: Drug-induced liver disease: An overview. Seminars in liver. *Disease* 1981; 1:93.

36

ACUTE ANORECTAL DISORDERS

Edmund B. Cabot
David J. Sugarbaker

Complaints concerning the anorectal region are not uncommon from patients in emergency rooms. The physician must be prepared to deal with these in a compassionate and understanding manner, realizing that the patient may harbor considerable misgivings or even embarrassment about an area of the body often associated with social taboos, uncleanliness, anatomical ignorance, and great sensitivity.

The disorders of the anorectal region described in this chapter are those most commonly recognized. There are many variations of each of these, as well as many less-common conditions, that are not included here. This chapter is not intended to provide comprehensive descriptions of every known affliction of the anus and rectum. Rather, it is our intent to provide a rudimentary working knowledge of and approach to common problems in this area. Relatively few patients presenting with primary anorectal complaints will require immediate admission to the hospital. Broadly speaking, patients will fall into one of three categories: those with obviously acute problems, those with acute manifestations of chronic problems, and those with obviously long-standing and seemingly unchanged conditions who, for some inexplicable reason, have chosen this moment to present themselves for medical intervention.

Some patients will have significant pathology demanding hospital admission and urgent surgical intervention. But many can be managed on an outpatient basis. For the latter group, the physician's role is to make a tentative diagnosis, to provide some degree of symptomatic relief, to arrange the appropriate follow-up, and—perhaps most important—to reassure the patient.

A working knowledge of the anatomy of this region is extremely useful in understanding the nature of patient complaints and in determining the physician's approach to these problems. It is worth remembering that this region is where the gastrointestinal tract—with its autonomic innervation, portal venous drainage, involuntary musculature, and mucous-secreting epithelium—meets the body wall (perineum)—with its somatic innervation, systemic circulation, skeletal muscle, and keratinizing squamous epithelium. Figure 36.1 depicts the anatomy of this region.

The clinical disorders described in this chapter have been divided into three general categories: rectum, anus, and perianal region. The *rectum* is that portion of the colon below the pelvic floor (and therefore lacking a peritoneal covering) and above the pectinate line where, at the epithelial level, the mucocutaneous junction occurs. The latter is an important landmark since it is here that the transition from autonomic to somatic and from portal to systemic occurs. It is also where the anal crypts, separated by anal papillae, are located.

The *anus* itself extends from the pectinate line to the anal verge, where the skin of the anal canal, which is quite thin and lacks hair follicles, meets the normal skin of the perineum. This is a short region of only 1–3 cm in length. In terms of pathologic entities, there is obviously a good deal of overlap with both the rectum and the *perianal region*. The latter includes the skin and cutaneous appendages external to the anal verge, as well as the underlying space known as the ischioanal fossa. Some knowledge of these spacial relationships is an important step toward understanding anorectal diseases.

EVALUATION OF THE PATIENT

History

Patients with anorectal disorders may present with a variety of complaints. These symptoms may be of very recent onset, or they may be long standing and previously ignored. Broadly speaking, anorectal symptoms can be divided into four categories: those that are primarily sensory in nature; those that represent alterations of function; those that involve some kind of abnormal discharge, either from the anus itself or from the perianal region; and those that involve an abnormal protrusion.

Certainly one of the most common symptoms that brings patients to the emergency room is pain. This may vary from a mild discomfort or itching sensation to rather severe burning or aching pain that is often aggravated by walking, sitting, or defecation. The duration and nature of a patient's discomfort is often an important clue to the diagnostic evaluation, as well as an index of the patient's tolerance for whatever the problem turns out to be. The degree of discomfort may have important implications for the initial treatment and the need for reassurance.

Inquiry should always be made concerning the patient's bowel habits. It is useful to know the character and frequency of bowel movements. The patient's chief complaint may be constipation or diarrhea, but what is normal for one person may seem very abnormal to another. A history of the recent or regular use of

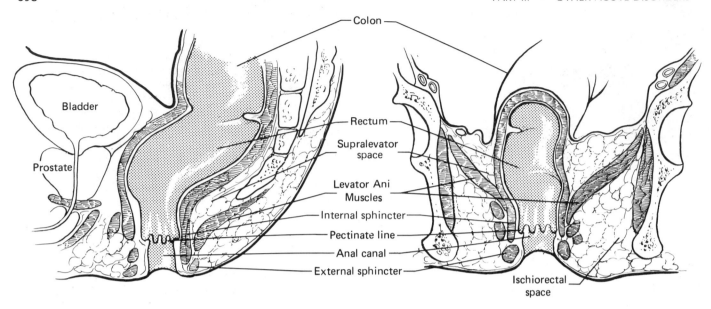

Figure 36.1 Anatomy of the rectum and perianal region.

stool softeners, cathartics, or enemas should be determined. It is most important to assess whether or not there has been any change in a given patient's bowel habits, as well as to determine the relationship of other associated symptoms with the act of defecation.

One of the most common and often significant presenting symptoms is that of bleeding. A tiny amount of blood on the toilet paper may be very alarming to many patients, whereas grossly melanotic stools may go unnoticed by others for many months and may not even be the presenting symptom. All patients should be questioned about rectal bleeding. If present, the color, duration, and amount of bleeding should be assessed. It is important to know if the bleeding is associated only with bowel movements and whether or not it is mixed with stool, streaked on the outside of stools, occurs after bowel movements, turns the toilet bowl red, or comes out as clots.

Other forms of anal or perianal discharge are also common presenting or associated symptoms. These may be purulent, fecal, or mucoid in nature. They may require constant wearing of a pad, and they may or may not be associated with pain. Under the appropriate circumstances, a history of trauma to the anorectal region or of regular anal intercourse must be elicited.

Finally, patients may complain of something protruding from the anus. It should be determined whether or not this is associated with pain or bleeding, what its relationship is to defecation, and whether or not the patient has been able to reduce the mass back up through the anus.

Physical Examination

Although the history relating to anorectal disorders may often suggest the diagnosis, a careful physical examination is invariably necessary. For this, it is imperative that the physician have adequate knowledge of the anatomy in this region, as well as an awareness of the patient's probable apprehension regarding the examination of this part of the body.

Some consideration should be given to the position of the patient and the examiner. Attention to the patient's sense of modesty can greatly enhance the physician's ability to diagnose and treat the problem. It is important to assure privacy, comfort, and adequate lighting whenever possible. The single best position for the anorectal examination is probably the knee–chest position with the patient kneeling on the examining table, head down, and the examiner standing at the foot of the table with an unobstructed source of light from behind. This can sometimes be modified by having the patient standing, legs apart, and leaning over with the head and chest on the table, while the examiner sits behind the patient between his or her legs.

The elderly, debilitated, or extremely ill patient may have to be examined in the lateral decubitus (Sims') position with the knees drawn up near the chest and the buttocks extending beyond the edge of the table.

Much can be learned and a diagnosis can often be made by simple external inspection of the perineum and perianal regions. This can be facilitated by gently drawing the buttocks apart for better exposure of the entire intergluteal region. In this way, the examiner can be alerted to the presence of external masses, protrusions, asymmetry, swelling, erythema, excoriations, sinus tracts, fistulous openings, and the like. This inspection, combined with the patient's presenting complaint, is often sufficient to make the diagnosis in several of the common conditions discussed below.

Palpation in the perianal region can sometimes provide further clues. When appropriate, the examiner should gently seek out any areas of tenderness, induration, or fluctuance by careful palpation in the perianal region.

Digital examination of the anal canal and rectal ampulla should be a part of every complete physical examination; but in the patient with anorectal complaints, it is not only critical but may also be somewhat more difficult because of tenderness or patient apprehension. Reassurance, ample lubrication, and the very slow introduction of the gloved index finger are the keys to success. Initially, the patient is asked to bear down as though to have a bowel movement, and the anus is inspected for any protuberance from above. Next, the finger is slowly introduced up the anal canal. This may be facilitated in some instances by asking the patient to intermittently bear down and relax in a fashion analogous to defecation. Care should be taken to avoid areas of the anal passage that are particularly sensitive by exerting greater pressure against the opposite side.

While introducing the examining finger, the examiner may be able to detect areas of irregularity or ulceration of the anal canal. At the pectinate line, an area of induration or tenderness may be detected. The presence of engorged or thrombosed hemorrhoidal tissue may also be discovered during this maneuver.

The examining finger is further introduced into the rectal ampulla, and palpation is directed circumferentially. Anteriorly, the size and consistency of the prostate is estimated in the male patient. Rectovaginal two-finger examination may be revealing in the female patient. It is important to direct the examining finger as far posteriorly as possible toward the coccyx since low rectal lesions in this area may otherwise be missed. If stool is present in the rectal ampulla, its consistency is noted and a specimen should be obtained on the examining glove for subsequent testing for occult blood.

Before removing the examining finger, the physician should estimate the degree of resting anal sphincter tone. The patient is also asked to tighten the anus voluntarily as a test of external sphincter competence.

In many instances, the proper diagnosis of anorectal disease requires visualization of the anal canal and rectal mucosa. Anoscopic examination is a very simple procedure, requiring minimal equipment and no special preparation, and may be of great benefit in defining the anatomical lesion. There are several different types of anoscopes. The most useful of these is the slotted variety. The instrument is copiously lubricated and gently inserted well into the anus with the fitted introducer in place. It is then rotated into position until the slot is over the area of suspected pathology in the anal canal. The introducer is then removed, allowing the overlying tissue to bulge slightly into the slot. By this means it is possible to visualize individual crypts, internal hemorrhoids, fissures, and so on. Before rotating the anoscope to another position, the introducer should be carefully replaced to prevent laceration of the epithelium.

Finally, sigmoidoscopy is a simple and relatively safe procedure that should be readily available to the emergency room physician for the diagnosis and possible treatment of disorders above the reach of the anoscope. It should not be considered as an alternative to anoscopy since the sigmoidoscope is not well suited for visualizing lesions of the anal canal itself. However, for higher lesions of the rectal mucosa, such as proctitis, rectal bleeding, rectal trauma, foreign bodies, and even fecal impaction, the sigmoidoscope may be invaluable. (For a description of the technique of sigmoidoscopy, see Procedure 28.)

Obviously, anorectal disease must be considered in the context of the patient as a whole. Disorders of the anorectum may be a window through which to detect disease elsewhere, particularly other disorders of the gastrointestinal tract such as inflammatory bowel disease. Other diagnostic studies, such as barium contrast radiographs, colonoscopy, or angiography, may be indicated in conditions that present initially as primary rectal disease. Such simple tests as a large vessel hematocrit or white blood cell count should not be overlooked in patients presenting with possibly significant rectal bleeding or infectious processes such as perirectal abscess.

After making a working diagnosis and initiating appropriate treatment, the emergency room physician is next responsible, in most cases, for providing some form of follow-up care. This may range from arranging for a return visit to the emergency room if the symptoms recur, to referral to a surgeon or internist for further evaluation and long-term care.

CLINICAL SETTINGS

Rectal

RECTAL TRAUMA

Injuries to the rectum and perineum carry a significant morbidity and mortality. Patients suffer both isolated rectal and perineal trauma, as well as rectal injuries associated with major pelvic trauma. The major effort of the emergency room physician is aimed at accurately diagnosing the type and extent of rectal injury. Rectal stab wounds (e.g., occuring through the rectum) can be devastating if they are not noted on physical examination and adequately treated. Gunshot wounds, impalement injuries, and knife wounds, along with crush injuries to the pelvis, are among the most common rectal and perineal injuries.

The accurate assessment of rectal trauma depends upon an accurate history and careful rectal examination, coupled with indicated radiologic procedures. The all-important digital examination is performed first, followed by a careful sigmoidoscopic examination. The appearance of blood in the rectum or a submucosal hematoma leads us to suspect mucosal perforation. The presence of free air under the diaphragm on KUB suggests perforation of the colon above the pelvic floor. Gas dissecting up the retroperitoneal space suggests perforation of the rectum. An enema using meglumine diatrizoate (Gastrografin enema) may be used to identify the site of perforation if sigmoidoscopy fails. Caution against the use of a barium enema is noted since barium has proven to aggravate the peritonitis that follows perforation.

All patients except those with the most superficial mucosal injuries require hospital admission for observation. The management of rectal trauma has been carefully studied in both military and civilian life. The treatment required for rectal perforation occuring at both the infra- and intraperitoneal areas is diverting colostomy, presacral drainage, closure of the perforated bowel, and washout of stool from the distal segment.

Lacerations and stab wounds to the perineum also mandate close examination to determine the extent and nature of the injury. Perineal stab wounds should be probed with a sterile gloved finger to assess the extent of injury. If communication with the peritoneal cavity is found, immediate admission of the patient for exploratory laparotomy is advocated. If rectal or sigmoidal injury is suspected from the perineal stab wound, sigmoidoscopy should be performed. Traumatic rectocutaneous fistulas are treated with diverting colostomy, presacral drainage, and closure of the perforated segment as stated earlier. If, however, the wound is confined to the subcutaneous tissue, it should be copiously irrigated and closed about a small Penrose drain. If further evaluation reveals this to be an isolated injury, the patient can be discharged with instructions to use a sitz bath three times a day. The drain is removed in 24–48 hours. The use of antibiotics in this setting is controversial and probably not warranted.

Lacerations of the external and internal anal sphincter are associated with several types of rectal trauma. These injuries can only be treated adequately with the aid of general anesthesia and the lighting of an operative suite. The treatment in the emergency room consists of gaining primary control of bleeding. This may be accomplished by packing the rectum with sterile gauze or clamping and ligating a bleeder if time and the patient's condition permits. Reconstruction of the internal and/or external anal sphincter should not be attempted in the emergency room.

FOREIGN BODIES IN THE RECTUM

Foreign bodies in the rectum have become a more common clinical problem for emergency room physicians. Foreign bodies are primarily of two types: Ingested foreign bodies such as chicken or fish bones, teeth, pins, coins, or toothpicks may impale themselves in the anorectal junction at the time of defecation. Patients who have ingested such items will present with acute rectal pain and may or may not have chronic abscess formation, depending upon the length of time the foreign body has been in situ. Foreign bodies that are introduced from below have been reported in all shapes and sizes, ranging from rectal thermometers to pieces of fruit. Patients may present with acute abdominal pain secondary to perforation or may simply complain of an inability to remove the object.

Digital examination will reveal the nature and position of low-lying foreign bodies. Small foreign bodies such as fish bones, toothpicks, and rectal thermometers that have been in situ for a period of time may look like a perirectal abscess or fistula in ano. Larger foreign bodies that are radiopaque can be seen on x-ray where their position can be better ascertained. Sigmoidoscopy should be used for all high-lying foreign bodies and all radiolucent foreign bodies. A careful abdominal examination should be performed in all patients to exclude the presence of perforation.

Treatment consists of the removal of smaller foreign bodies and drainage of any abscess formation. General or regional anesthesia is often required for adequate examination and drainage. Therefore, admission is mandated in these cases. Free-floating foreign bodies may be extracted in the emergency room by sedating the patient and placing him or her in the lithotomy position. The sigmoidoscope is used to visualize the foreign body; care must be taken not to move the foreign body cephalad inadvertently. Biopsy forceps, obstetric forceps, and a gloved hand may be used to deliver the object. Many ingenious methods have been devised to remove various objects. Filling hollow glass objects with plaster of paris or packing objects with cotton are methods that have been described. If the object is too high and cannot be reached, Barone found that if the patient was admitted, sedated, and placed on bed rest, within 12 hours the object descended to within reach. General or spinal anesthesia may be required to obtain adequate sphincteric relaxation. Sigmoidoscopy should be performed on all patients after removal of any foreign body to assess mucosal integrity and extent of any injury. Patients in whom mucosal injury is suspected or seen should be admitted for observation and further evaluation.

IMPACTION

Fecal impaction is found in all emergency room patient populations. It is most common in elderly, debilitated, and institutionalized patients, in patients whose diets are chronically low in bulk foods, or in patients who chronically abuse narcotics. Patients may present with diffuse crampy abdominal pain and/or diarrhea and incontinence. The ampulla is chronically distended with hard stool which relaxes the external sphincter allowing liquid stool to escape.

The diagnosis is made by rectal examination and is aided by a KUB showing a stool-filled colon. The absence of leukocytosis or fever helps differentiate simple impaction from diverticulitis causing spasm or other inflammatory conditions. The pain caused by an anal fissure or abscess can cause patients to avoid defecation thus causing impaction, and the presence of fissures and abscesses should be ruled out.

Manual disimpaction before the administration of enemas is mandatory since insertion of the anal canula into a distended thin-walled ampulla can lead to perforation. It is recommended that these initial evacuations be carried out in the emergency room, followed by a brief period of observation in debilitated patients for whom other causes of abdominal pain are being ruled out. Patients should be started on a regimen of stool softeners, bulk foods, and laxatives and enemas to prevent recurrence. Avoidance of narcotics, specifically codeine-containing medications, is also advised. Enemas that are commonly given in the management of fecal impaction or constipation are listed in Table 36.1.

PROCTITIS

Proctitis is an inflammation of the mucosa covering the anus and rectal ampulla. It may be a result of a variety of causes.

Patients present with pain on defecation and rectal bleeding, usually minor, occuring at the time of defecation. Stool is characteristically covered with mucus and blood. The diagnosis is established by sigmoidoscopic examination in the emergency room after a careful rectal examination has been performed. The inflammation may be chronic, as with chronic ulcerative colitis, or acute, appearing de novo.

Types of proctitis include radiation proctitis, infectious proctitis, nonspecific proctitis, and proctitis as a result of repeated mucosal trauma.

Radiation proctitis is an inflammation of the rectal mucosa secondary to radiation given in the treatment of pelvic malignancies. The rectal mucosa is more sensitive to radiation than is the vaginal mucosa, and it more easily develops chronic inflammation. Cancer of the endometrium, uterus, cervix, bladder, and prostate are commonly treated with radiation. The patient may have no external (cutaneous) effects from the radiation. The history of radiation therapy, along with a digital examination revealing a tender, indurated spastic anal canal, suggests the diagnosis of radiation proctitis. Craters or ulcers may form in the mucosa. Sigmoidoscopic examination reveals a friable, red, edematous mucosa that bleeds on palpation. Radiation proctitis may lead to chronic fistulous tract formation and strictures, and their presence should be looked for at the time of examination. Sigmoidoscopic biopsy of the mucosa confirms the diagnosis.

Patients are treated with a low-residue diet, antispasmotics, and sedation, as well as topical steroids. The patient's hematocrit must be checked before discharge from the emergency room to assess the need for iron-supplement therapy or possible transfusion. A follow-up barium enema will reveal the extent of disease. Further therapy depends upon the persistence and severity of the symptoms. Colostomy and/or resection of the affected bowel is performed for severe, well-localized lesions. If the malignancy treated with radiation therapy is irradicated, patients usually do well in the long term with resolution of the major symptomatology. However, late strictures of severely involved bowel are not uncommon.

Infectious proctitis is most commonly a result of bacillary infections, amebiasis, gonorrhea, or lymphogranuloma venereum. The clinical pictures seen with bacillary and gonorrheal infections are similar. Shigellosis, salmonellosis, and gonorrhea can all produce the classic changes of proctitis. Sigmoidoscopy, coupled with microscopic examination and culture of fecal discharge, will aid in the diagnosis. Treatment consists of the administration of proper antimicrobial agents.

In the acute phase of infectious proctitis, amebiasis is seen infecting the whole colon. Localization to the rectum occurs later. Acute amebic proctitis commonly presents with ulcerated

TABLE 36.1 Common Enemas

Type	Clinical Setting	Precautions and Contraindications	Administration	Action
Tap water	Fecal impaction Bowel preparation	Hyponatremia Hypokalemia Megacolon	500–1,000 ml at room temp; repeated PRN	Mechanical
Saline	Fecal impaction Bowel preparation	Fluid overload Congestive heart failure Megacolon	500–1,000 ml N.S. at room temp; repeated PRN.	Mechanical and mild cathartic
Phosphate (Fleet)	Mild constipation Routine pre-operation Preparation for film IVP, or anorectal procedures	Nausea/vomiting Abdominal pain Megacolon	4 oz commercial preparation at room temp	Cathartic
Soapsuds	High impaction	Colonic spasm Megacolon	Liquid soap in 500–1,000 ml luke-warm water	Mechanical and emollient
Oil retention	Low-impaction Dessicated stool Mucosal irritation	Nausea/vomiting Abdominal pain	4 oz mineral oil at room temp	Lubricant and emollient
Bisacodyl	Constipation 2° to colonic atony	Colonic spasm Abdominal pain	10 mg bisacodyl in 30 ml water	Stimulates peristalsis by direct irritant affect on colonic mucosa
Combination	Refractory constipation	Colonic spasm Abdominal pain	60 ml magnesium sulfate 60 ml glycerine 60 ml water	Cathartic, emollient, and mechanical

lesions resembling ulcerative colitis. The more chronic phase lacks these ulcers. The diagnosis may be made in the emergency room by microscopic examination of rectal scrapings. Treatment with proper antimicrobial agents is essential. Amebic proctitis is seen in the homosexual population with increasing frequency and therefore all sexual contacts should also be treated.

Proctitis secondary to lymphogranuloma venereum presents with all the features of infectious proctitis. The onset is usually acute. Sexual transmission is the rule. Strictures commonly develop in the later stages. Diagnosis can be made by serologic testing since physical findings are not helpful in differentiating it from the other forms of proctitis. Treatment is the same as in the other forms of noninfectious proctitis. Operative treatment of strictures as they form may be necessary in the late course of the disease.

Nonspecific proctitis may be the manifestation of rectal involvement in the spectrum of inflammatory bowel disease. *Ulcerative colitis* presents most commonly as localized proctitis since the rectum is the most common site of involvement in this disease. Women are more frequently affected than men. Patients present with rectal bleeding and increasing amounts of mucus in the rectum. Diarrhea may also be present if the disease involves the more proximal colon. Sigmoidoscopy re-

veals a friable mucosa that readily bleeds. A mucosal biopsy performed under controlled conditions will confirm the diagnosis. Microscopic examination in the emergency room is mandatory to rule out an infectious etiology. The emergency room physician should check the patient's hematocrit to assess the degree of chronic blood loss. No specific treatment may be warranted acutely, but close follow-up should be arranged to allow a formal treatment plan to be formulated. A preparation of sulfasalazine (Azulfidine) is used in symptomatic cases once the diagnosis has been firmly established. Ninety percent of cases may be treated conservatively with eventual regression of the disease.

Crohn's proctitis is seen in patients with or without coexistent inflammatory disease elsewhere in the bowel. Patients presenting with both terminal ileal disease and rectal disease are not uncommon. Sigmoidoscopic examination may resemble ulcerative proctitis, although the ulcerations are not as common nor as severe as in proctitis resulting from ulcerative colitis. Digital examination may suggest nodules of granulomatous infiltrates in the submucosa. Fistula in ano is associated with 80% of cases of Crohn's proctitis. The diagnosis of a coexistent fistula in ano is therefore helpful in making the diagnosis of Crohn's proctitis. The diagnosis is confirmed by a biopsy specimen. Treatment in the emergency room is again conservative. Patients are referred for close follow-up and continuing care. This disease often has a more fulminate course than ulcerative colitis. The development of severe strictures may require surgical intervention. Corticosteroid therapy also plays a role in the long-term management of this disease.

Traumatic proctitis is a frequent complication of repeated rectal prolapse. It may also be seen in cases of repeated digital disimpaction and in patients participating in anal intercourse. The presence of a single ulcer on the anterior rectal wall is sometimes seen on proctoscopic examination. This results from repeated trauma to the anterior rectal wall by offending objects. Treatment is usually conservative and consists primarily of reducing contact with the irritating factors. A biopsy specimen should be obtained for all patients with ulcerated lesions in the rectum. All such lesions should be considered malignant until proven histologically benign.

RECTAL PROLAPSE

Rectal prolapse (true procidentia) is a complete eversion of the entire rectal wall through the anus. False procidentia occurs when only the rectal mucosa is present outside the anus. The condition, although rare, is most often seen in elderly, institutionalized, nulliparous women. Weakness of pelvic musculature and suspensory ligaments of the rectum as a result of congenital anterior displacement of the rectum along with repeated straining at stool is thought to lead to prolapse.

The patient complains of incontinence and constant soiling of clothing from a bloody mucus discharge. The history of a mass protruding from the anus during defecation or strenuous activity leads us to suspect rectal prolapse. Early in the patient's course, the mass retracts spontaneously following defecation. Later, however, the mass persists and requires manual replacement.

Diagnosis is confirmed by demonstrating prolapse by having the patient strain or squat. We see mucosal folds in a telescoping circular fashion with the lumen directed posteriorly. Palpation will differentiate simple mucosal prolapse from a true procidentia containing an inner and outer rectal wall. Differentiation of prolapse from prolapsing hemorrhoids and rectal polyps can be made at this time.

The treatment of rectal prolapse is primarily surgical and several procedures are advocated. Immediate treatment primarily consists of efforts to relieve straining at stool by use of stool softeners and laxatives. The patient is then referred for surgical evaluation. A barium enema and sigmoidoscopy are performed before definitive operative therapy to rule out other intrinsic diseases.

Anal

HEMORRHOIDS

Hemorrhoids are dilations of the veins arising from the superior hemorrhoidal venus plexus and the inferior hemorrhoidal venus plexus (Fig. 36.2b). The anatomy of the area reveals that the superior plexus drains into the superior hemorrhoidal veins (portal circulation) and that the inferior plexus drains into the somatic (systemic) circulation. The dentate line distinctly separates the two plexuses. The differentiation between external hemorrhoids arising from the inferior plexus and internal hemorrhoids arising from the superior plexus has therapeutic importance (Fig. 36.2a). The etiology of these varicosities with ensuing mucosal irritation is debated. Straining at stool, which causes increased venous pressure and dilitation, which in turn causes thinning of the overlying mucosa, along with passage of hard stools that irritate the already thinned mucosa, is probably the oldest theory. Dietary factors have also been implicated. The so-called "Western diet," with its low residue leading to constipation and passage of hard stools, has been implicated. Some authors believe infection is the precursor to hemorrhoidal formation.

Internal Hemorrhoids

Patients may present at any age with symptomatic hemorrhoids. Most commonly, they are obese patients or postpartum women whose residual hemorrhoids are caused by increased pelvic venous pressure during pregnancy. Patients present with first-, second-, third-, or fourth-degree hemorrhoids. First-degree hemorrhoids present as painless bleeding on defecation and internal hemorrhoids protruding into the lumen of the anus on anoscopy. Second-degree hemorrhoids will protrude through the anus with straining and will spontaneously reduce when straining is stopped. When hemorrhoids no longer spontaneously reduce with cessation of straining, they are called third-degree hemorrhoids. These are replaced manually by the patient. If the patient can no longer manually replace the hemorrhoids and they are continuously prolapsed, they are said to be fourth degree.

The most common complaint of patients presenting with hemorrhoids is pain, primarily with defecation or straining. Patients may also complain of seeing bright red blood in the toilet bowl or on tissue paper after a bowel movement. Profound anemia in these patients is rare but has certainly been described.

The diagnosis of internal hemorrhoids is made by a gentle rectal examination followed by a slow and gentle proctoscopic examination. The patient is asked to strain after introduction

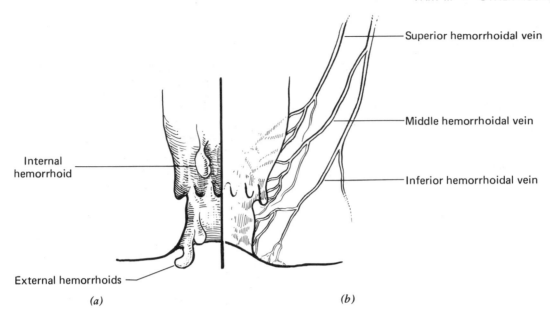

Internal
hemorrhoid

Superior hemorrhoidal vein

Middle hemorrhoidal vein

Inferior hemorrhoidal vein

External hemorrhoids

(a)   *(b)*

Figure 36.2 *(a)* Internal and external hemorrhoids. *(b)* Venous drainage of the anorectum.

of the anoscope, making the hemorrhoids more visible. The appearance of engorged, dilated, blue submucosal varicosities along with overlying irritated chronically inflamed mucosa confirms the diagnosis. Internal hemorrhoids characteristically appear at three cardinal positions: right anterior, right posterior, and left lateral positions. Small hemorrhoids may appear between these, but they seldom achieve the size of the ones at the cardinal positions. Patients may present with prolapsed internal hemorrhoids. These may be quite painful and must be differentiated from thrombosed external hemorrhoids.

Once the diagnosis of internal hemorrhoids is made, conservative treatment is the rule for emergency room care. If bleeding has been a problem, the hematocrit is checked while the patient is in the emergency room. This precaution is especially important in older patients, although young patients have presented with profound anemia secondary to hemorrhoidal bleeding. Therapy begins with alteration in the patient's diet to include increased amounts of bulk. Stool softeners and hydrophilic agents are also prescribed. A wide range of preparations for topical use are available. Anusol suppositories applied in the rectum after each bowel movement have been found to be very helpful. If a good deal of inflammation is present with edema, the patient is instructed to take a sitz bath

three times a day and to use Anusol-HC suppositories after each bowel movement. This steroid-containing suppository will help to quiet inflammation and edema. Its use is limited to about 1 week of therapy to avoid mucosal injury that follows the overuse of topical steroids. Proctofoam is also helpful when suppositories are difficult for the patient to use. A steroid-containing Proctofoam is also available. Along with this, patients are given adequate oral analgesics.

Patients are referred to a surgeon for follow-up. Patients who present with rectal bleeding require full proctosigmoidoscopy and barium enema to rule out concomitant colorectal neoplasias. Patients in whom pain persists may ultimately need hemorrhoidectomy. Conservative therapy is the correct initial treatment. Other modes of therapy include rubber band ligation, sclerotherapy, and, more recently, cryotherapy. The particular form of therapy should be performed by those adept at its use, and the patient must be followed-up on an on-going basis. Attempt at excision or incision of internal hemorrhoids should only be approached surgically in the operating room where proper lighting and anesthesia are provided. Usually, admission is required for those patients who present with profound anemia or who have strangulating, prolapsing internal hemorrhoids.

External Hemorrhoids

Dilation of veins in the inferior hemorrhoidal plexus below the dentate line are called external hemorrhoids. Thrombosis of these external hemorrhoids is a common presenting symptom. This is a result of rupture of one of these veins causing a hematoma that can be quite painful. This rupture is usually caused by straining secondary to coughing, lifting, sneezing, or strenuous exercise. This condition is more common in young patients and is not necessarily associated with internal hemorrhoids.

Pain is acute at the outset but gradually subsides. On examination, a dark blue perianal hematoma is present that is exquisitely sensitive to palpation. This lesion must be differentiated from prolapsing internal hemorrhoids since their treatment is entirely different. Early treatment consists of excision under local anesthesia in the emergency room. The patient is placed in the lithotomy position and the area about the hemorrhoid injected with 1% lidocaine (Xylocaine) with epinephrine. An elliptical incision is made around the base of the hemorrhoid, and it is entirely excised. Incision with clot extraction is more difficult, especially after 48 hours. During this period, the clot becomes organized and its removal is made more difficult. Patients presenting to the emergency room after 48 hours should be treated conservatively. Initial treatment consists of warm sitz baths followed by a cleansing of the area with witch hazel impregnanted pads after which 1% hydrocortisone cream is applied. Response to treatment is gradual and may take several days. Patients may be referred to a surgeon for general wound care and follow-up.

ANAL STENOSIS

Anal stenosis, or stricture, presents at any age with obstipation and/or pencil stools. Pain and discharge may be present secondary to chronic inflammation. The stenosis is caused by circumanal subepithelial scarring as a result of a variety of causes.

Anal stricture may be from a postoperative complication (primarily from hemorrhoidectomy) or from chronic inflammation caused by fissure in ano, ulcerative colitis, or proctitis. Anal stricture has been associated with the chronic use of laxatives as well as lymphogranuloma venereum. Gonorrhea and syphilis are rarely the cause of stricture. Carcinoma of the rectal region, as well as of the prostate, must always be ruled out as a primary cause of stricture.

Treatment in the emergency room consists of manual disimpaction and the administration of stool softeners and topical anesthetics if chronic inflammation is present. The definitive treatment is operative. Further workup should include sigmoidoscopy, barium enema, and a Frei test before definitive surgery.

FISSURE IN ANO

A primary fissure in ano is a linear ulceration of the epithelial lining of the anal canal. The cause is direct trauma, most commonly as a result of the passage of hard feces. It occurs in both sexes over a wide age range. The most common site is in the midline posteriorly. Women have a somewhat higher incidence of anterior fissures than males. Fissures usually occur singly but may occasionally be multiple. Secondary anal fissures associated with Crohn's disease are often multiple and are less often in the posterior midline.

Anal fissures may be either acute or chronic. The acute variety is very superficial with little ulceration and no "sentinel pile." They often heal spontaneously and usually respond to simple conservative management. They may, however, recur or develop into a chronic fissure. Chronic fissure in ano is a deeper ulceration with induration and heaped-up edges. This variety is often associated with an hypertrophied anal papilla and an edematous skin tag known as the *sentinel pile* because of its vague resemblance to an external hemorrhoid (Fig. 36.3).

The presenting symptom is almost always pain on defecation. The pain is sharp and may be quite severe. After defecation, the pain often changes to a dull ache that may last for several hours and is related to spasm of the underlying anal sphincter muscles. Patients occasionally report episodes of rectal bleeding consisting of a few traces of bright red blood on the toilet paper or underwear. There is sometimes an associated pruritis ani as a result of a chronic discharge from the ulcerated anus. Patients may occasionally complain of dyspareunia.

Diagnosis is usually easy to confirm by physical examination. However, the examiner must proceed very slowly and gently. Anal fissures are extremely painful, and once the pain has been induced the anal sphincters go into spasm and further examination becomes difficult, if not impossible. The fissure can usually be visualized by simple, gentle traction on the buttocks to draw them apart. The presence of a sentinel tag may be an important clue but may also serve to obscure the actual fissure from view.

Digital examination is sometimes impossible at this stage because of extreme tenderness. However, if the finger is well lubricated with an anesthetic jelly and is pressed against the opposite wall of the anal canal (usually anterior) as it is intro-

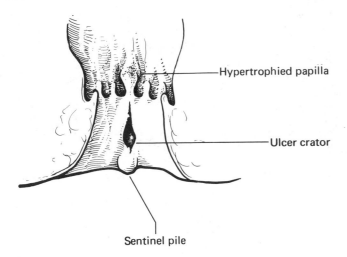

Hypertrophied papilla

Ulcer crator

Sentinel pile

Figure 36.3 Fissure in ano.

duced, it may then be possible to rotate the finger into position for palpating the fissure.

Occasionally, anoscopic examination to visualize the fissure should be considered. Usually, this must be postponed until healing has occured and should be performed in later follow-up to rule out other underlying anorectal diseases.

Initial treatment of the fissure in ano is conservative. The most important element is the avoidance of further trauma to the anal canal. This usually includes the rather aggressive use of stool softeners (such as Colace and Metamucil), as well as limited initial use of a bowel lubricant such as mineral oil. Topical anesthetic creams and jellies (e.g., dibucaine—Nupercaine) are sometimes of transient benefit, but suppositories are usually too painful to insert and rarely do any good. Warm sitz baths following defecation may be helpful in relieving the ache of sphincter spasm. Stool softeners and bulking agents should be continued for several weeks after healing of an acute fissure to prevent prompt recurrence. Associated pruritis may be treated with steroid creams.

Failure of the above methods to heal an anal fissure warrants referral for possible surgical intervention. Many surgical procedures have been advocated for chronic fissure in ano; their descriptions are beyond the scope of this chapter. Failure to heal may suggest the need for a biopsy specimen of the margin of the ulcer to rule out a malignancy or underlying Crohn's disease. In any event, the patient should be given a means for adequate follow-up and reassurance that proper treatment provides an excellent chance for permanent cure.

ANORECTAL ABSCESS

Acute anorectal pyogenic abscess is a relatively serious and not uncommon condition confronted by the emergency room physician. It occurs most commonly in otherwise healthy young adults. The peak age for its occurrence is 20–40 years, and it is somewhat more common in men than in women. Associated systemic and gastrointestinal diseases are the exception rather than the rule, the most common one being diabetes. Less common are Crohn's disease and intestinal tuberculosis.

There is an occasional association with chronic fissure in ano. Abscess in this region occurs rarely as a postoperative complication of anorectal surgery but may result from trauma or occasionally from a thrombosed hemorrhoid. As many as one-third of the patients will have a previous history of anorectal abscesses. Perianal hidradenitis suppurativa may be an obvious predisposing cause for abscess formation, but in the vast majority of patients the abscess appears to arise spontaneously.

The pathophysiology of most anorectal abscesses continues to be controversial. A commonly accepted hypothesis is that the abscess arises as an intermuscular infection of one of the tiny anal glands that discharge into the anal crypts at the pectinate line. Impaction of fectal matter in one of these crypts gives rise to a small crypt abscess as the primary focus. The resultant induration prevents drainage of pus back into the anal canal. As a result, the pus seeks an alternative route, giving rise to secondary abscess formation in one of several different tissue planes (Fig. 36.4).

Considerable confusion exists over the description of these secondary abscesses because of basically semantic arguments over the exact anatomy of the region. This controversy is more germane to the surgeon providing definitive treatment than to the emergency room physician. The latter must have a high index suspicion and low threshold for making the diagnosis, but the treatment is invariably surgical. For the purposes of this discussion, we will limit ourselves to two basic categories: the *perianal abscess,* presenting as a subcutaneous process near the anal verge, and the *perirectal abscess,* presenting as a deeper fluctuance palpable on digital rectal examination (see Fig. 36.4).

The most common presenting symptom is a persistent, throbbing pain, usually of recent onset and often exacerbated by defecation and sitting down. The pain is most noticeable when the abscess is low lying in the perianal subcutaneous region. Higher perirectal or supralevator abscesses may present with relatively little pain, but rather with signs of systemic toxicity. Fever is present in less than one-third of all patients with documented anorectal abscesses, but about two-thirds of patients

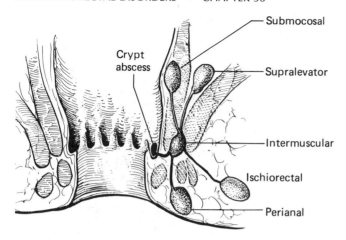

Figure 36.4 Anorectal abscesses.

will have a leukocytosis of more than 10,000 WBC/mm³. The diagnosis may easily be overlooked in the immunosuppressed or paraplegic patient.

Definitive diagnosis depends on a high index of suspicion and on the physical examination. Perianal abscess presents as an exquisitely tender, somewhat fluctuant, erythematous induration near the anal verge subcutaneously. It is usually to one side or the other of the midline and is said to occur slightly more often posteriorly than anteriorly. On digital rectal examination, the abscess can frequently be palpated between the finger and thumb.

The diagnosis of higher perirectal abscess may be more difficult, requiring deeper digital examination. The presence of a tender, fluctuant mass on either side of the rectum alerts the examiner to the presence of an abscess in the proper clinical setting. Although less common than perianal abscess, the higher perirectal abscess is more likely to be associated with systemic signs of fever and leukocytosis.

The treatment of anorectal abscess is surgical. Most patients require admission to the hospital for prompt incisional drainage under regional or general anesthesia. There is no role for conservative therapy with antibiotics alone since they serve only to mask the infection temporarily and promote resistent organisms. On the other hand, drainage should not be attempted by one who is unfamiliar with the details of anorectal anatomy and the sphincteric mechanisms.

FISTULA IN ANO

Anal fistula is a common sequela of anorectal abscess (see above). After external drainage of the abscess, either sponta-

neously or surgically, the potential exists for the formation of a chronic fistulous tract between the anal crypt, which was the primary source of abscess formation, and the perianal skin at the site of drainage of the secondary abscess. Such fistulae are usually single, well-defined, hollow, fibrous tracts communicating between the anal canal at the level of the pectinate line and the skin adjacent to the anal verge (Fig. 36.5).

Less commonly, anal fistulae may form multiple tracts in a more complex or horseshoe configuration with more than one external opening. These latter are associated with inadequately drained or multiply recurrent anorectal abscesses and should alert the physician to possible underlying disorders, notably Crohn's disease.

Patients most commonly present complaining of a malodorous drainage that soils their clothing. The problem may be intermittent over a period of months or years as a result of healing over of the external opening of the fistula, followed by formation of a small abscess in the infected tract with soreness and eventual rupture, recreating the cutaneous opening of the fistula and resulting in chronic drainage once again.

There is often a history of previous acute anorectal abscess, but in many patients the history will be one of low-grade, perianal infections, suggesting less-virulent organisms. In female patients, the same process may result in a rectovaginal fistula with the presenting complaint of passing flatus or feculent material through the vagina.

Physical examination characteristically reveals the chronically draining external fistulous opening in the skin of the perianal region. On digital rectal examination, the firm, fibrous, fistula tract is often palpable in the perianal tissue. Anoscopic examination may reveal an obviously involved anal

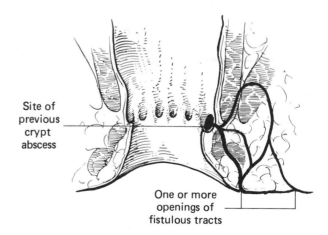

Figure 36.5 Fistula in ano.

crypt at the internal end of the fistula, and it is sometimes possible to detect the associated crypt by discharging purulent material from the fistula itself. In long-standing, chronic fistula in ano, however, it is often difficult to incriminate a particular crypt as the internal opening without passing a probe along the tract. This, in turn, may be difficult because of tortuosity of the tract; in the emergency room setting this maneuver is of limited value and may cause considerable patient discomfort.

The treatment of chronic fistula in ano is surgical. Rarely do these infected tracts heal completely on their own without recurrence. Initial treatment in the emergency room consists largely of reassurance, provided that anorectal abscess has been ruled out. Mild inflammatory soreness is usually relieved by sitz baths. Antibiotics are of no benefit, assuming that there is no underlying primary disease process. Patients with a long history of multiple recurrent fistulae should be evaluated for possible underlying Crohn's disease. The vast majority of patients will require referral to a surgeon for definitive fistulotomy.

Perianal

PILONIDAL SINUS

Pilonidal sinus is a complex of sinus tracts in the sacrococcygeal area. The origins of these epithelial-lined tracts are thought to be congenital or traumatized infected hair follicles. The follicle induces a foreign body reaction causing cyst and sinus tract formation. The condition is most common in young, white, hirsute males.

Pilonidal sinus becomes symptomatic after secondary infection sets in, inducing chronic, occasionally bloody discharge. In some cases, abscess formation occurs, and it is this presentation that is most likely to be seen in the emergency room. The abscess is usually surrounded by a varying degree of cellulitis.

On examination of the sacrococcygeal area, one or several small pores are noted in the area of fluctuance. The history of prior drainage and the presence of pores rule out simple furuncle.

Incision and drainage of the abscess under local anesthesia is the only treatment indicated in the emergency room. The use of antibiotics should be based on the physician's assessment of the adequacy of drainage and degree of cellulitis present. The patient is instructed to take sitz baths three times per day in warm soapy water. A follow-up appointment or referral is necessary in order that the chronic sinus tract may be dealt with in a definitive way after the acute inflammation has subsided since recurrence is almost inevitable. The definitive treatment of pilonidal sinuses is debated. Whereas excision with primary closure or marsupialization is advocated by some, simple fistulotomy with close outpatient follow-up is preferred by others.

CONDYLOMA ACUMINATUM

Perianal warts, or condylomas, are seen in male and female patients. They may be present on the genitalia as well. They generally occur in the anal canal and on the surrounding skin. The warts are viral in origin and are caused by the papovavirus. The virus is transmitted by sexual contact and is therefore considered to be a sexually transmitted disease (STD). In men this condition is associated with anal intercourse.

Examination may reveal a great number of lesions: some have large cauliflowerlike projections and some are less than 1 mm in diameter. Treatment of minor cases consists of reassurance and direct application of podophyllin to the specific lesions. Extensive involvement, however, can only be treated adequately by surgical removal under general or regional anesthesia. The warts tend to recur with continued exposure and are occasionally associated with squamous carcinoma of the anus.

PRURITIS ANI

Perianal itching of a chronic nature can be a perplexing problem because of a number of etiologies. Itching can be related to defecation, anxiety, food allergies, diabetes mellitus, dermatologic conditions, as well as chronic bacterial, fungal, and parasitic infections. Pruritis ani may also be caused by the irritation of scratching existing proctologic lesions such as anal skin tags, fissures, or intradermal carcinoma (Bowen's disease). The diagnosis of pruritis ani is made by a careful history and physical examination along with appropriate laboratory data. The perianal skin may show a great deal of thickening and excoriation, or changes may be minor. Evidence of anal fissures, skin tags, and possible malignant lesions should be looked for. Microscopic examination of the skin scrapings will help in the diagnosis of bacterial or fungal superinfection. The cellophane tape test is used in making the diagnosis of pinworm infection.

Emergency room treatment of pruritis ani is conservative. The patient will need long-term follow-up for this often unremitting condition. The patient is instructed to sitz bathe briefly four times a day in warm water without soap. The patient should clean the perianal region after each bowel movement with cloth impregnated with glycerine and witch hazel (Tucks) and should apply hydrocortisone cream 1% four times a day to the area. If a fungal etiology is suspected, a suitable antifungal cream may be added to the treatment regimen. Parasitic infections require specific oral drug therapy. The patients are then referred for follow-up and, if dermatologic conditions predominate, to a dermatologist. If symptoms are unremitting, a biopsy specimen should be obtained to rule out intradermal carcinoma. Often, the cause of pruritis ani is never found; its course is often long and the results of therapy can be frustrating to both the physician and patient involved.

SELECTED READING

Abcarian H: Surgical correction of chronic anal fissure. *Dis Colon Rectum* 1980; 23:31.

Abcarian H, Lowe R: Colon and rectal trauma. *Surg Clin No Am* 1978; 58:519.

Alexander-Williams J, Crapp AR: Conservative management of haemhorrhoids. Part I: Injection, freezing and ligation. *Clin Gastroenterol* 1975; 4:595.

Andrews NL: Impaction of rectum and colon. *Am Surg* 1955; 21:693.

Barone JE, Sohn N, Nealon TF: Perforations and foreign bodies of the rectum. *Ann Surg* 1974; 17:313.

Barron J: Office ligation treatment of hemorrhoids. *Dis Colon Rectum* 1963; 6:109.

Bartizal JF, Boyd DR et al: A critical review of management of 392 colonic and rectal injuries. *Dis Colon Rectum* 1974; 17:363.

Bascom J: Pilonidal disease: Origin from follicles of hair and results of follicle removal as treatment. *Surgery* 1980; 87:567.

Buls JG, Goldberg SM: Modern management of hemorrhoids. *Surg Clin North Am* 1978; 58:469.

Christian RL: Anorectal disorders, in *Office Practice of Medicine*. Philadelphia, WB Saunders Co, 1982, pp. 664–678.

Crapp AR, Alexander-Williams J: Fissure-in-ano and anal stenosis. *Clin Gastroenterol* 1975; 4:619.

Farmer RG: Clinical features of Crohn's disease and ulcerative colitis *Practical Gastroenterol* 1977; 1:17.

Farmer RG, Brown CH: Ulcerative proctitis course and prognosis. *Gastroenterology* 1966; 51:219.

Folley JH: Ulcerative proctitis. *N Engl J Med* 1970; 282:1362.

Goldberg SM, Gordon PH: Treatment of rectal prolapse. *Clin Gastroenterol* 1976; 62:119.

Goldberg SM, Leacock AG, Brossy JJ: The surgical anatomy of the anal canal. *Br J Surg* 1955; 43:51.

Goligher JC: Stricture of the rectum. *Dis Colon Rectum* 1976; 19:913.

Goligher JC: *Surgery of the Anus, Rectum and Colon*, ed 4. London, Bailliere Tindall, 1980.

Grunberg A: Acute urinary retention due to fecal impaction. *Am Surg* 1960; 83:801.

Haas PA, Fox RA: Civilian injuries of the rectum and anus. *Dis Colon Rectum* 1979; 22:17.

Hanley PH: Anorectal abscess fistula. *Surg Clin North Am* 1978; 58:487.

Howell HS, Bartizal JF, Freeark RJ: Blunt trauma involving the colon and rectum. *J Trauma* 1976; 16:624.

Keighley MRB, Buchmann P, Minervini S et al: Prospective trials of minor surgical procedures and high-fibre diet for haemorrhoids. *Br Med J* 1979; 2:967.

Kovalcik PJ, Peniston RL, Cross GH: Anorectal abscess. *Surg Gynecol Obstet* 1979; 149:884.

Lennond-Jones JE, Cooper GW, Newell A et al: Observations on idiopathic proctitis. *Gut* 1962; 3:201.

Moore GE, Norton LW, Meiselbaugh DM: Condyloma. *Arch Surg* 1978; 113:6360.

Nesselrod JP: Anatomy, pathogenesis and treatment of hemorrhoids and related anorectal conditions. *Rev Surg* 1966; 229:253.

Parks AG: Anatomical causes of rectal prolapse. *Proc R Soc Med* 1975; 66:26.

Parks AG, Gordon PH, Hardcastle JD: A classification of fistula in-ano. *Br J Surg* 1976; 63:1.

Parks AG, Thompson JPS: The rectum and anal canal, in Sabiston DC Jr (ed): Davis-Christopher, *Textbook of Surgery*, ed 11. Philadelphia, WB Saunders Co, 1977, pp 1134–1148.

Read DR, Abcarian H: A prospective survey of 474 patients with anorectal abscess. *Dis Colon Rectum* 1979; 22:566.

Shackelford RT, Zuidema GD: The anorectal tract, in *Surgery of the Alimentary Tract*. Philadelphia, WB Saunders Co, 1982, vol 3, p 327–689.

Shaver WA, Groh JR: Perianal region, anus, and anal canal.

Stone HH, Barian TC: Management of perforating colon trauma. *Ann Surg* 1979; 190:430.

Storer EG, Lockwood RA: Rectum and anus, in Schwartz SI (ed): *Principles of Surgery*. New York, McGraw-Hill Co, 1969, p 992–1015.

Suckling DV: The vall valve rectum due to impacted feces. *Lancet* 1962; 2:1147.

Sullivan ES, Garnjobst WM: Pruritis ani: A practical approach. *Surg Clin North Am* 1978; 58:505.

Theuerkaut FJ, Beahrs OH, Hill JR: Rectal prolapse: Causation and surgical treatment. *Ann Surg* 1970; 171:819.

Trunkey D, Hays RJ, Shires GT: Management of rectal trauma. *J Trauma* 1973; 13:411.

37
ACUTE GENITOURINARY DISORDERS

Peter T. Nieh
Stephen P. Dretler

The primary care physician is frequently called upon to evaluate and treat patients with acute nontraumatic urologic problems. In a study of over 5 million people who were hospitalized during a 2-year period, over 10% primarily had urologic diseases. The incidence of acute urologic disorders based on experience in our emergency rooms and screening clinics is similar. The leading problems are urinary tract infections, flank pain, and urinary retention; hematuria and scrotal masses trail well behind.

In this chapter, we will outline the basic pathophysiology, concentrate on the more common etiologies, describe helpful clues in the diagnostic evaluation, and provide guidelines in management to aid the emergency room physician in initiating proper medical therapy or in obtaining immediate urologic consultation.

Traumatic urologic emergencies are discussed in Chapter 21.

FLANK PAIN

Pain originating from the upper urinary tract is caused by acute distention of the renal capsule, renal pelvis, or ureter; the renal parenchyma itself is insensitive. Because the sensory innervation of the kidney arises from the tenth through twelfth thoracic nerve roots (T_{10}–T_{12}), the pain is typically experienced in the costovertebral angle and the flank. Calculi of the kidney and ureter are the most likely causes of flank pain, accounting for approximately one-third of acute urologic problems.

In the general evaluation of patients with flank pain, particular attention to the character of the pain is important: How severe or disabling is the pain? What about the rapidity of onset? Is the pain steady or spasmodic? Does it radiate away from the flank? Is the patient able to find any comfortable position? For diagnostic purposes, it is useful to distinguish between colicky pain and noncolicky pain. *Colic,* always acute in onset, is severe and unrelenting pain with spasmodic crescendo–decrescendo variations in pain; it may last from several minutes to hours at a time. Acute colic is usually associated with obstructed urinary drainage. *Noncolicky pain* is more steady in character but varies from patient to patient in its rapidity of onset and intensity. Acute noncolicky pain is often related to sudden alterations in renal blood flow, whereas *nonacute noncolicky pain* occurs with intrarenal swelling or perinephric infection. The common causes of flank pain may be classified under colicky pain, acute noncolicky pain, and nonacute noncolicky pain (Table 37.1). There are numerous exceptions and variations in the presenting pain patterns of these disorders. Thus such arbitrary grouping does not diminish the necessity for complete history, physical examination, urine analysis, intravenous pyelogram (IVP), or other appropriate diagnostic maneuvers.

The history should include inquiries regarding previous stones, dietary excesses, cardiac problems, hematuria, diabetes, and recent urinary tract infections or trauma. The physical examination should exclude an intraabdominal process by demonstrating fairly localized costovertebral angle and flank tenderness without signs of peritoneal irritation. The urine analysis may reveal hematuria with a stone, pyuria and bacteriuria with infection, or proteinuria suggesting renal disease. An IVP is the most informative study and is advisable in any patient with flank pain with few exceptions (e.g., those with dye allergy, renal insufficiency). Specific considerations will be detailed below.

Common nonurologic disorders must be differentiated from flank pain of renal origin; these include musculoskeletal disorders, cholecystitis, pancreatitis, pneumonia, pulmonary emboli, and duodenal ulcers.

Colicky Pain

Colic is a manifestation of urinary tract obstruction. As urine flow is blocked, intermittent distention of the renal pelvis and proximal ureter produces pain. Kidney stones are the most common cause of colic, but we must also consider blood clots or tissue from a tumor in the kidney or renal pelvis and sloughed renal papillae in patients with diabetes, urinary tract infection, sickle cell trait, or phenacetin analgesic abuse. Also, congenital ureteropelvic junction obstruction may present in adulthood with flank pain, which may be colicky following the diuresis induced by alcohol ingestion or diuretic antihypertensive medications.

Obstruction from calculus may occur at the ureteropelvic junction, at the midureter where it crosses the iliac vessels at the brim of the bony pelvis, or at the ureterovesical junction.

TABLE 37.1 Common Causes of Flank Pain

Colic
  Calculus
  Tumor
  Sloughed renal papilla
  Blood clot
  Ureteropelvic junction obstruction
Acute noncolicky
  Embolus to the renal artery
  Thrombosis of the renal vein
  Dissection of a renal artery aneurysm
Nonacute noncolicky
  Acute pyelonephritis
  Renal abscess
  Perinephric abscess
  Hemorrhage into a renal tumor

In addition to pain in the costovertebral angle and flank, obstruction in these locations produces a characteristic pattern of referred pain. Pain originating in the upper ureter or in the renal pelvis may be referred by way of the eleventh and twelfth thoracic nerve roots (T_{11}–T_{12}) to the groin or testicle in males or the labium majorum or round ligament in females. From the midureter, pain may be referred through the twelfth thoracic and first lumbar roots (T_{12}–L_1) to the right or left lower quadrant of the abdomen. The lower ureter is innervated by the third and fourth sacral nerves (S_3–S_4), which refer pain to the scrotal skin or perineum and may also cause symptoms of bladder irritability.

DIAGNOSIS

Colic in a younger patient is almost always because of stones. The patient may give a history of previous episodes of colic, gravel or sandlike particles in the urine, bouts of gouty arthritis, or excessive intake of dairy products. Acute colic in an older patient without history of calculi may be caused by a tumor. A history of diabetes, chronic pyelonephritis, sickle cell disease, or analgesic abuse raises the possibility that a sloughed papilla is causing the obstruction.

Obvious distress, agitation, diaphoresis, and writhing in an attempt to find a comfortable position all signal a patient with severe colic. In contrast, patients with peritoneal irritation from appendicitis or diverticulitis, for example, lie quietly, often with the ipsilateral lower extremity drawn up.

The patient with colic is tender in the costovertebral angle and along the flank but exhibits only mild abdominal guarding and no rebound tenderness or rigidity. Reflex ileus results in hypoactive bowel sounds. Fever, and even septicemia, may occur with concomitant infection above the obstruction; diabetics are particularly vulnerable to such infections.

Laboratory Examination

If obstruction is total, the urine may not contain any cellular elements. The norm, however, is microhematuria without gross clots in the urine. In the presence of pyuria and urine pH greater than 8, urea-splitting organisms (*Proteus* species) with magnesium ammonium phosphate calculi should be suspected. Crystals of uric acid (particularly with urine pH of 5), calcium oxalate, and cystine may be found. The white blood cell count is often slightly elevated if obstruction is uncomplicated, but a leukocytosis in excess of 15,000 cells/mm³ suggests active infection.

X-Ray Examination

A plain abdominal film is likely to demonstrate the calculus, since 90% of all stones contain calcium and are thus opaque (Fig. 37.1). Cystine and magnesium ammonium are somewhat less opaque but identifiable nonetheless. Calcified mesenteric lymph nodes, gallstones, or phleboliths may be confused with renal or ureteral calculi, so it is important to obtain oblique views. Uric acid calculi, sloughed papillae, blood clots, and tumors of the renal pelvis, on the other hand, are all radiolucent and cannot be detected on plain film. Thus, IVP is important.

All patients with colic, with rare exception, should undergo emergency IVP to identify the level and extent of obstruction unless pain abates or the stone is recovered. This study is imperative in patients with urinary tract infection or fever. Excretion of the dye may be delayed for only several minutes in acute or partial obstruction because of increased back pressure and diminished glomerular filtration. The usual radiographic findings in a patient who has just passed a stone are delayed and intensified nephrogram or cortical blush, followed by columning of dye above the edematous portion of the distal ureter (Fig. 37.2). In ureteropelvic junction obstruction, ballooning of the renal pelvis and calices without visualization of the ureter is characteristic (Fig. 37.3). During pyelography of acute occlusions, the caliceal fornices may be ruptured by the combined affects of back pressure and the sudden osmotic load of the contrast material. In this event, small amounts of urine may extravasate and be detectable near the renal pelvis.

In chronic or total obstruction, however, several hours may elapse before the dye appears; tomography and/or delayed films may therefore be required to visualize and delineate the dilated ureter and pyelocaliceal system.

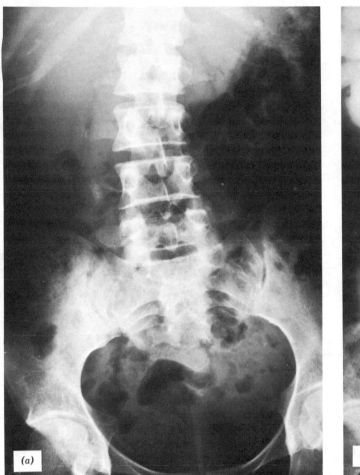
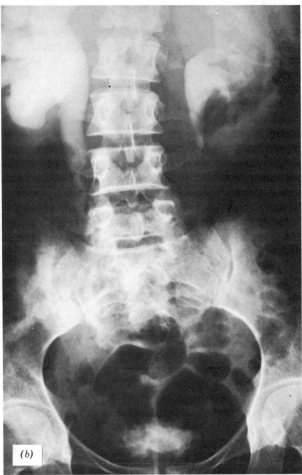

Figure 37.1 Obstructing ureteral calculus. (a) Plain abdominal film of a 29-year-old woman presenting with right flank pain and urinary tract infection. A large stippled calculus is visible just below the tip of the transverse process of the fourth lumbar vertebra (L-4). (b) Intravenous pyelogram demonstrating marked obstruction of the ureter and renal collecting system above the calculus.

MANAGEMENT

Most stones are passed either spontaneously or during urography. In the uncomplicated situation, patients require only oral analgesics and generous intake of fluids. If the stone is recovered, it should be sent for chemical analysis. If it is not recovered, the patient should strain all urines for a few days in the hope of accumulating fragments for analysis. When the patient is stable and has resumed a regular diet, the urologist will initiate the workup for the cause of stone formation.

Hospitalization and immediate urologic consultation are required in the following situations:

1. If pain is intractable and is accompanied by nausea and vomiting that prevent adequate hydration
2. If fever, leukocytosis, or pyuria is present since the risk of sepsis is high
3. If obstruction is complete or near completion, such that only a nephrogram appears on delayed films

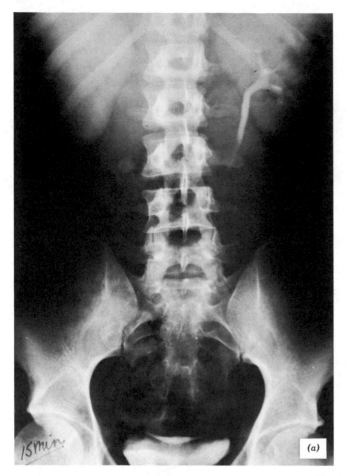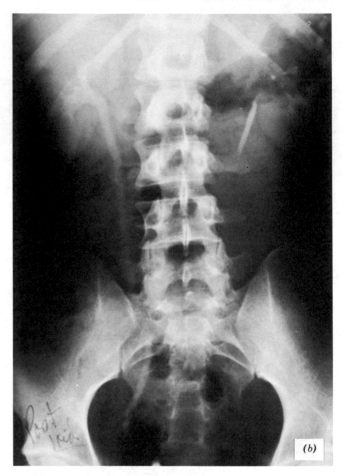

Figure 37.2 Passed ureteral calculus. (*a*) Early film during IVP showing delayed visualization of the right kidney with an intense nephrogram. (*b*) Later film, now demonstrating ureter with columning of contrast material down to the level of edema from the passed calculus.

4. If a calculus larger than 8 mm in diameter is producing symptoms or obstruction since spontaneous passage is then unlikely

Generous analgesia (meperidine 1–2 mg/kg or morphine sulfate 0.1–0.2 mg/kg intramuscularly every 3–4 hours), antiemetics, and intravenous hydration are necessary. Parenteral antibiotics (aminoglycosides, ampicillin, or cephalosporin), using adequate loading doses, should be started when the patient is in the emergency room if serious infection is present. Attempted extraction with a stone basket, bypass of the obstruction with a ureteral catheter, percutaneous nephrostomy, or surgical intervention may be required if symptoms persist or sepsis occurs. Extravasation observed in the urogram, but in the absence of infection, is not an indication for surgery. When calculi are asymptomatic and nonobstructing, they may be followed conservatively. Some uric acid calculi may be dissolved with alkalinization of the urine and allopurinol, whereas selected patients with magnesium ammonium phosphate stones have responded to acidifying irrigations or bacterial urease-inhibiting drugs in conjunction with antibiotic therapy. Treatment of colic due to sloughed papillae, blood clot, or tumor must also be aimed at controlling the primary disease process.

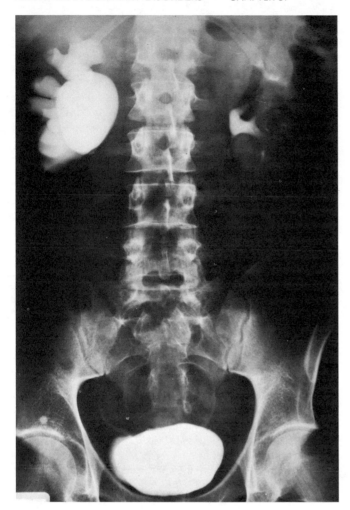

Figure 37.3 Ureteropelvic junction obstruction. An IVP in a 26-year-old man who complained of severe, right-sided colicky pain following alcohol consumption. The obstruction and symptoms responded to revision of the ureteropelvic junction.

Acute Noncolicky Pain

Acute flank pain that is not colicky, but severe and nonradiating, is usually associated with renal vascular disease. Most common in this category is pain caused by a renal artery embolus. This may be secondary to cardiovascular disease, especially rheumatic heart disease with atrial fibrillation, mural thrombus after a myocardial infarction, bacterial endocarditis, or replacement of an artificial heart valve. Dissection of an aortic aneurysm may extend into the renal artery, presenting with low back pain as well as flank pain.

Renal vein thrombosis is rare, but it can occur in patients with disseminated malignancy, deep venous thrombosis, or severe renal or perinephric infections. When renal vein thrombosis does occur, the kidney becomes severely congested, edematous, and painful. Anuria may result if both kidneys are involved.

DIAGNOSIS

The history and physical examination for acute noncolicky pain should include complete cardiac evaluation and a search for evidence of peripheral embolization. A palpable tender mass in the flank suggests renal vein thrombosis. Edema of both lower extremities or of the penis and scrotum may represent extensive phlebothrombosis with renal vein involvement. Low-grade fever may accompany any of these disorders, but frank sepsis suggests that a renal or perinephric abscess is producing renal vein thrombosis.

Laboratory Examination

Microhematuria of some degree is always observed. Mild proteinuria may be seen with renal artery embolus, whereas heavy proteinuria is the hallmark of renal vein thrombosis.

X-Ray Examination

A plain film of the abdomen and a cross-table lateral view can reveal the calcified wall in an aneurysm of the aorta or renal artery. An emergency pyelogram must be performed to rule out the possibility of an obstructing calculus. The nephrogram phase of the IVP will usually aid in establishing the diagnosis. The nephrogram will be delayed and intensified with a partially obstructing stone; will be normal size with variable splotchy areas of function in the case of embolization; will be diffusely enlarged in renal vein thrombosis; and will be completely absent, as a rule, in renal artery dissection. However, differentiation of a renal artery embolus with extensive vasospasm from a radiolucent calculus causing total obstruction may require emergency arteriography. Early urologic consultation is advised. Since delay in treatment of embolus carries far more serious implications than calculus disease, if there is reasonable suspicion of embolus, emergency arteriography rather than retrograde pyelography or renal scanning will follow the IVP. Emboli are revealed as discrete avascular lesions on the arteriogram.

Arteriography is also necessary to diagnose dissecting aneurysms and renal vein thrombosis. In dissection of an abdominal aortic aneurysm, disruption of the intima and nonfunction of the involved kidney are demonstrated. In renal vein thrombosis, arterial inflow is normal, but renal venography will demonstrate the extent of the lesion.

MANAGEMENT

Renal artery embolus requires emergency surgery in patients who are at low risk for surgical mortality; otherwise, immediate anticoagulation may prevent the thrombus from extending into cortical vessels. Thrombosis of the renal vein should be managed with anticoagulants or surgery, depending upon the primary underlying disease process and the patient's clinical state and prognosis.

Dissection of the renal artery is treated as part of the therapy for aortic dissection (see Chapter 4).

Nonacute Noncolicky Pain

Pain that is neither acute nor colicky is usually a result of swelling within the kidney or of surrounding infection that distorts or irritates the renal capsule. The entity that most frequently produces this type of pain is acute *pyelonephritis,* which is seen more often in women than in men. It usually is the result of infection ascending from the bladder. Reflux through the ureterovesical junction, which permits infection to progress in this pattern, is sometimes caused by a congenital anomaly, but it is frequently secondary to severe cystitis in which the resultant edema compromises the ability of the ureterovesical junction to prevent reflux. Patients with ileal conduit urinary diversions are particularly susceptible to ascending infection owing to reflux and the tendency to stomal obstruction. Patients with neurogenic bladder or indwelling catheters are prone to urinary infections. If pyelonephritis is diagnosed, a predisposing factor such as diabetes, obstruction (e.g., from pregnancy, cancer, or stone), or blood-borne seeding from another site should always be considered.

Renal abscess (carbuncle) is a secondary infection as a result of staphylococci carried by the blood stream from a distant suppurative site. Once established, a carbuncle may drain into the perinephric space where it produces an abscess; but such perinephric abscesses are more often a result of extravasation of infected material (usually gram-negative rods) as a complication of infected caliceal stones or pyonephrosis.

Noncolicky flank pain may also be caused by a hemorrhage into a renal tumor. The onset and severity of pain depends on the rate of bleeding.

DIAGNOSIS

Symptoms of lower urinary tract infection often precede pyelonephritis, and a history of recurrent urinary infections is common. Pyelonephritis may cause flank pain on one or both sides and may be accompanied by fever and chills. Tenderness to percussion in the costovertebral angle and a tender kidney on bimanual examination are frequently found. In particularly severe cases, the patient may complain of abdominal pain and nausea and vomiting.

A renal abscess or a perinephric abscess presents with symptoms such as those of pyelonephritis. Some patients report prior skin infections, which may have seeded through the blood stream to the kidney. Renal tumors may cause flank pain yet be otherwise asymptomatic. Sometimes, however, a patient complains of gross hematuria.

Fever is common with pyelonephritis, abscess, or tumor, and a flank mass may be palpable in any of these conditions. A perinephric abscess may result in retroperitoneal inflammation with such signs as a high ipsilateral diaphragm, pleural effusion, spinal curvature, and flexion of the ipsilateral leg. If an advanced renal tumor has occluded the spermatic vein, a varicocele may develop acutely.

Laboratory Examination

Urinalysis in patients with pyelonephritis reveals many white blood cells, white blood cell casts, mild proteinuria, and often bacteria. For a patient with a renal abscess, the urinalysis may be unremarkable unless the abscess has drained into the collecting system. Perinephric abscesses also may yield unremarkable urine analysis, or they may show contamination with staphylococci. When there is infected calculi or pyonephrosis, the urine contains white blood cells and bacteria, whereas renal tumors produce hematuria without pyuria as a rule. Renal function tests are usually unremarkable, although leukocytosis is common.

X-Ray Examination

In pyelonephritis, the IVP demonstrates somewhat delayed function, and edema is reflected by slightly irregular caliceal outlines. If the renal outline is enlarged and irregular with evidence of a mass lesion, either a renal abscess or a renal tumor is possible. These conditions can be differentiated by nephrotomography, ultrasound, arteriography, or computerized body scan. Tomography and ultrasound demonstrate a thick-walled cystic lesion if an abscess is present or a solid mass if a tumor is present. Although the abscess will be avascular on arteriography, the tumor will demonstrate increased vascular supply with neovascularity.

When there is a perinephric abscess, the IVP will reveal obliteration of the psoas shadow and an elevated hemidiaphragm with a reactive pleural effusion. A caliceal stone may also be demonstrated; inflammatory adhesions fix the kidney so that normal respiratory displacement is absent. Examination with ultrasound may delineate a collection of fluid around the kidney.

MANAGEMENT

Acute pyelonephritis in patients with low-grade fever may be treated with an oral antibiotic, such as ampicillin 500 mg every 6 hours, or trimethoprim/sulfamethoxazole every 12 hours, or nitrofurantoin macrocrystals 100 mg every 6 hours, pending the results of urine culture. Follow-up urologic evaluation is necessary. Patients who are elderly, have significant fever or chills, or have complicating underlying disorders should be hospitalized. These patients should have blood cultures obtained and emergency urography performed. In addition, parenteral antibiotics and prompt urologic consultation are advised. Gram-negative sepsis is dealt with elsewhere (Chapter 28).

Perinephric and renal abscesses must be treated with high doses of systemic antibiotics and early surgical drainage, or even nephrectomy. A patient with a symptomatic renal tumor should be hospitalized for thorough evaluation of the extent of the disease and possible surgery.

HEMATURIA

The causes of hematuria are legion. Even the mildest trauma may produce bleeding from anywhere within the urinary tract, often unmasking an asymptomatic abnormality. However, we shall concentrate on nontraumatic hematuria, the more common causes of which are listed in Tables 37.2 and 37.3. Infection is the leading cause of nontraumatic hematuria, then tumor, obstruction, and calculus. In infancy and childhood, hematuria usually results from infection behind a congenital obstruction. In young adults, infection (cystitis, prostatitis, or pyelonephritis) is a far more common cause of hematuria than calculus, and tumor is rare. In adults older than 50 years old, infection still leads the field, but tumors, benign prostatic hypertrophy, and stones become increasingly common. Of the tumors causing hematuria, those of the bladder are most frequent, followed by the prostate, and then the kidney. Thus

TABLE 37.2 Common Causes of Nontraumatic Hematuria

Source	Setting
Kidney	Glomerulonephritis
	Pyelonephritis
	Papillary necrosis
Renal pelvis or ureter	Calculus
	Carcinoma
	Hydronephrosis
Bladder	Cystitis
	Carcinoma
	Calculus
	Biopsy site
Prostate	Benign prostatic hypertrophy
	Prostatitis
	Carcinoma
	Postprostatectomy
Urethra	Urethritis
	Foreign body
	Calculus
	Condyloma
	Carcinoma

even mild or microscopic hematuria requires a complete urologic investigation.

DIAGNOSIS

History

Gross hematuria should be described as follows: It may be initial, terminal, or total; painful or painless; with or without clots. Initial hematuria, that is, hematuria that occurs as micturition begins, implicates the urethra as the source of bleeding.

TABLE 37.3 Common Etiologies of Nontraumatic Hematuria According to Age

Infancy and childhood
    Infection (usually secondary to obstruction)
Young adults
    Infection (cystitis, prostatitis, pyelonephritis)
    Calculus
Adults older than 50 years
    Infection
    Carcinoma[a]
    Benign prostatic hypertrophy
    Calculus

[a]Carcinoma of the bladder is most common, followed by the prostate, and then the kidney.

Terminal hematuria, on the other hand, usually originates in the prostate, bladder neck, or trigone as the bladder neck contracts to complete voiding. *Total hematuria,* or hematuria throughout micturition, may be a result of active bleeding at any site, but it usually suggests a source of somewhere above the prostate.

Hematuria with pain commonly accompanies inflammatory disorders or calculi, whereas painless bleeding results most often from tumors, benign prostatic hypertrophy, or blood dyscrasias. Large, fresh clots frequently originate in the bladder; in contrast, long stringy clots are casts of the ureter and reflect bleeding in the upper urinary tract. Bleeding is not uncommon 10–20 days after transurethral surgery or fulguration when the original clot dislodges.

Hematuria may occur with certain medical conditions or it may be drug induced. Blood dyscrasias and renal failure, for example, may cause hematuria. Cyclophosphamide may produce a hemorrhagic cystitis, and anticoagulants may provoke bleeding from a previously unsuspected tumor.

Physical Examination

Hematuria in a patient with atrial fibrillation and acute flank pain suggests embolization to the kidney. A palpable mass in the flank may be seen with a renal tumor. Tenderness in the flank and costovertebral angle may be caused by obstruction in the ureter, glomerulonephritis, pyelonephritis, or papillary necrosis. Suprapubic tenderness is common in cystitis. A foreign body, a calculus, or a tumor in the urethra may be palpable. An anterior pelvic mass may represent an invasive bladder cancer. In men, a warm, boggy, tender prostate suggests acute prostatitis, but a rock-hard, nodular gland is usually because of carcinoma. In women, a careful pelvic examination will help eliminate a vaginal source of bleeding. An inflamed urethral caruncle or prolapsed urethral mucosa may be observed. Although any of these findings may be present, the physical examination may be negative.

Laboratory Evaluation

A microscopic analysis of the spun urine is necessary to confirm the diagnosis of hematuria. More than five red blood cells per high-power field is abnormal. Dark urine without red blood cells can result from hemolytic syndromes or occur after ingestion of beets or phenolphthalein laxatives. Red blood cell casts are characteristic of glomerulonephritis; crystals may be associated with calculi; and bacteria and pyuria are usually found with pyelonephritis or cystitis.

Routine blood studies should include a hematocrit to estab-lish a baseline; prothrombin time (PT), partial thromboplastin time (PTT), a platelet count to detect an underlying coagulopathy; and blood urea nitrogen (BUN) and creatinine levels to determine whether the patient has uremia, which can be caused by obstruction or by intrinsic disease. If bleeding is severe, blood should be typed and cross matched in case a transfusion is required. Prostatic carcinoma may be manifested by an elevated titer of fibrin split products, a low fibrinogen level, and an elevated acid phosphatase level. Hypercalcemia may be detected with a renal cell carcinoma.

A urine sample from any patient over 40 years of age who has microscopic hematuria should be sent for a cytology. When hematuria is gross, however, malignant cells are difficult to detect; cytologic examination may therefore be deferred.

All patients with gross hematuria must undergo an IVP as soon as possible unless there is an obvious cause, such as hemorrhagic cystitis, urethritis, or recent transurethral surgery. When there is microhematuria, however, the IVP may be delayed until a later date when the patient has had an appropriate bowel cleansing. The IVP is useful for diagnosing renal masses (Fig. 37.4), papillary necrosis, partial or complete nonfunction resulting from embolism, calculi, hydronephrosis, and bladder tumors or clots. If a patient is allergic to the IVP contrast material, a renal scan may be used to demonstrate obstruction or nonfunction.

MANAGEMENT

The major emphasis in the initial management of hematuria for patients in the emergency room is directed toward preventing or treating clot retention. The urologist should then be consulted to evaluate the necessity for cystoscopy and to control further bleeding.

When hematuria is mild and the etiology is known, as with cystitis or after recent transurethral surgery, management consists of forcing fluids, encouraging frequent voiding, and administering antibiotics, if indicated. However, if clots are being voided with difficulty, or the color of the urine is darker than rosé wine, irrigation is necessary. A No. 22 French three-way Foley urethral catheter with 5 ml balloon is inserted (Procedure 26). Using a wide-mouthed syringe, the bladder is irrigated free of clots with saline. The patient with clot retention is often extremely agitated and in severe discomfort so generous analgesia is necessary while irrigating. As in upper gastrointestinal bleeding, this process may be quite tedious, but it is essential that all clots be evacuated before instituting a continuous saline or Ringer's lactate drip. Once the bladder is clot-free, the bleeding often ceases as relief of bladder distention permits vessel contraction and local hemostasis.

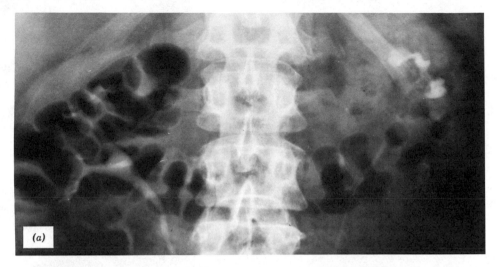

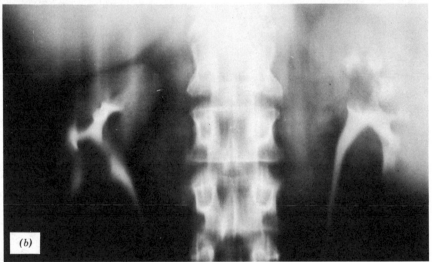

Figure 37.4 Renal pelvis tumor. (a) An IVP in a 58-year-old man with gross hematuria showing a large filling defect in the left renal pelvis. (b) Nephrotomograms 2 weeks later showing persistence of the lesion.

If unable to hand irrigate clots through the No. 22 French catheter, gently insert a No. 24 or No. 26 French "whistle-tip" nephrostomy tube after instilling the urethra with lidocaine (Xylocaine) jelly. Such a tube has a wide lumen, lacks a balloon, and permits more extensive irrigation. When irrigations are clear, the smaller three-way Foley catheter may be reinserted and the continuous drip instituted. If the whistle-tip catheter is unsuccessful, then clot evacuation under anesthesia in the cystoscopy suite is necessary. Broad-spectrum intramuscular antibiotic coverage, for example, kanamycin 500 mg or gentamicin 80 mg, is recommended with the use of such urethral instrumentation.

In handling postprostatectomy bleeding, we must be careful to avoid forceful catheterization that may undermine the bladder neck (Fig. 37.5). If resistance is encountered, a large coudé-tip catheter may aid entry into the bladder. If prostatic bleeding

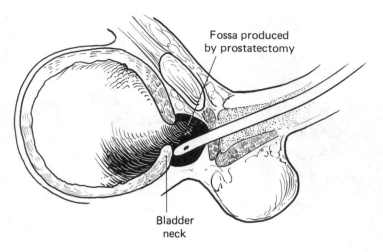

Figure 37.5 Undermining of the bladder neck in the postprostatectomy patient. Gentle manipulation or use of a coudé-tip catheter will prevent this problem.

continues despite continuous irrigation, then a catheter with a 30 ml balloon may be inserted; gentle traction will cause the balloon to occlude the bladder neck and effect tamponade of the prostatic fossa.

Abnormal coagulation parameters must be corrected. In patients with prostatic carcinoma, fibrinolysins may be released locally or systemically, resulting in increased plasmin production, which then promotes the breakdown of fibrin. Elevated titers of fibrin split products and depressed fibrinogen levels reflect this process. ε-Aminocaproic acid inhibits plasminogen activation and therefore controls the fibrinolysis. Dosage recommendations are 5 g in 250 ml 5% dextrose and water administered intravenously over 1 hour, followed by an infusion of 1 g/hr for about 8 hours or until bleeding is controlled. Similar doses are effective orally.

Cystoscopy has both a diagnostic and a therapeutic role in the management of hematuria. All patients with active bleeding of unknown origin should have a urologist perform this procedure in an attempt to localize the source. Bleeding sites and tumors of the bladder may be easily fulgurated. Unilateral upper urinary tract bleeding would require retrograde study and possible arteriography. If bleeding is revealed from both upper urinary tracts, glomerulonephritis is quite likely. Persistent uncontrolled bleeding from any source is an indication for arteriography. In some cases, embolization may control hemorrhage; otherwise, surgery is required.

ACUTE URINARY RETENTION

Acute urinary retention is the sudden inability to void as a result of dysfunction in the lower urinary tract; it must be distinguished from anuria, which is caused by pathology of the upper urinary tract. Retention, characterized by suprapubic discomfort, dribbling, and marked frequency of urination, is the third most common acute urologic disorder, after infection and flank pain. It is primarily a male affliction, with the most common etiologies being prostatism, followed by stricture, prostatitis, and neurogenic bladder (Fig. 37.6). The rare instances of urinary retention in women can usually be attributed to a neurogenic bladder or to psychogenic factors.

Retention can result from penile lesions. *Phimosis* refers to the condition in the uncircumcised male when the foreskin cannot be retracted to expose the glans and meatus (see Fig. 37.11). With extensive preputial adhesions, this may obstruct the meatus. *Paraphimosis* is a situation in which the retracted foreskin has become congested and edematous, producing a circumferential ring (see Fig. 37.12), which may obstruct the distal urethra similar to a constricting foreign body. *Meatal stenosis* may follow circumcision in children, whereas it can be caused by an indwelling catheter or transurethral surgery in adults. Some cases, however, appear to be idiopathic.

Stricture of the more proximal urethra may be the consequence of urethritis, especially gonococcal urethritis; trauma to the penis or perineum; transurethral surgical procedures; or an indwelling catheter. Strictures most commonly form in the submeatal region and in the proximal bulbar urethra just distal to the urinary sphincter.

Occluding objects also can produce urethral obstruction. Most common are urethral stones, which usually lodge at the penoscrotal junction where the urethra narrows. A fascinating array of foreign bodies may be responsible and, rarely, a urethral tumor may be encountered.

The posterior or prostatic urethra is a common site of obstruction. In young men, posterior urethritis and prostatitis may, if edema is severe, produce urinary retention. In elderly men, on the other hand, benign prostatic hypertrophy is the most common cause of retention, which is often precipitated by alcohol ingestion, prostatic infarction, or adrenergic and antihistaminic medications taken for common colds. Transurethral resection of the prostate may result in scarring and consequently contracture of the bladder neck. Prostatic carcinoma may be responsible for recurrent obstruction, even within months after transurethral resection.

A hypotonic, neurogenic bladder may reflect any of a variety of neurologic impairments. The various spinal cord syndromes will present with multiple neurologic deficits, of which failure

to void is only one. In contrast, tabes dorsalis, diabetes mellitus, multiple sclerosis, and syringomyelia may initially be manifested only by urinary symptoms. Many commonly used drugs can precipitate acute retention in patients with borderline bladder function. Anticholinergic (atropinic) drugs, antihistamines, and tricyclic antidepressants decrease contractility of the detrusor muscle. α-Adrenergic agents, such as ephedrine, amphetamines, and proprietary cold medications stimulate closure of the bladder neck, producing increased resistance to voiding.

Psychogenic retention occurs most frequently in young women, especially hospital personnel. But it is occasionally seen in a young man with a history of prostatitis, overwhelming concern about his voiding patterns, and fear of sterility.

DIAGNOSIS

History

Because gradual decompensation of the bladder usually precedes acute retention, the history should focus on symptoms of progressive obstruction such as hesitancy, decrease in the force and caliber of the stream, prolonged micturition, in-

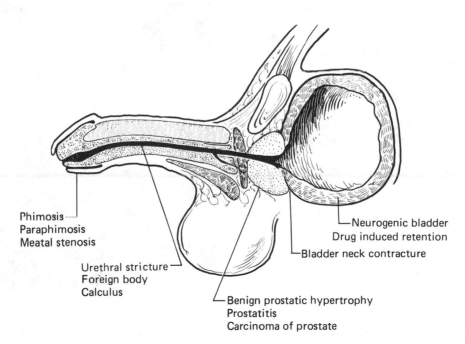

Figure 37.6 Common etiologies of urinary retention.

creased urinary frequency, or nocturia. Often a precipitating event, such as prostatic infarction, excessive alcohol intake, prolonged bedrest, or certain medications, produces acute retention. Concomitant infection may be indicated by symptoms of irritation such as urgency and dysuria. Remember that infection and obstruction are frequent partners in most urologic problems.

In younger men, painful urethral discharge, perineal pain, and fever will precede acute retention from prostatitis or posterior urethritis. A past history of urethritis, penile or perineal trauma, or indwelling Foley catheter suggests urethral stricture. Sudden, painful midstream interruption of voiding, with or without urethral bleeding, may represent a urethral calculus. In older men, prior transurethral surgery may indicate meatal stenosis, urethral stricture, or bladder neck contracture. A past history of prostatic carcinoma may suggest recurrent disease. Peripheral neurologic symptoms may signify progressive or previously undetected neurologic disease and resultant hypotonic neurogenic bladder.

Physical Examination

On physical examination, the patient is usually quite uncomfortable, and a distended bladder is detected by palpation or by percussion in the suprapubic region. Phimosis, paraphimosis, or meatal stenosis can be readily observed, as can a constricting foreign body. A palpable mass along the penile shaft may be a calculus, a foreign body, or a tumor. On rectal examination, if the prostate is warm, exquisitely tender, and possibly fluctuant, the diagnosis of acute prostatitis is fairly certain. Vigorous manipulation *must* be avoided to prevent bacteremia in this situation. If the gland is rubbery, firm, and symmetrically enlarged, benign prostatic hypertrophy is likely, whereas rock-hardness and irregular nodularity imply carcinoma. It is important to emphasize that the palpable size of the prostate bears no correlation to the degree of obstruction.

A neurogenic bladder is very often accompanied by related neurologic signs such as diminished tone in the anal sphincter, reduced sensation in the perineum and around the anus, or other peripheral signs of lower motor neuron injury. An unsuccessful attempt to pass a Foley or coudé catheter may confirm a suspected diagnosis of urethral stricture or bladder neck contracture.

Laboratory Evaluation

The urinalysis is generally unremarkable unless infection is also present. The BUN and creatinine levels may be elevated with

long-standing partial obstruction. If the level of acid phosphatase is high, either prostatic infarction or metastatic carcinoma of the prostate must be considered.

Intravenous urography may be performed after drainage of the distended bladder (Fig. 37.7) on an elective basis, but it is particularly important in patients with hematuria, pyuria, or symptoms related to the upper urinary tract.

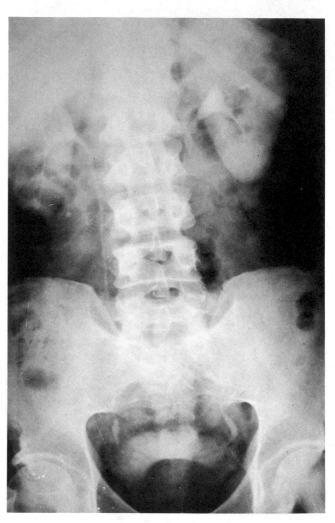

Figure 37.7 Benign prostatic hypertrophy. An IVP in a 60-year-old man with severe voiding symptoms shows the enlarged prostate as a filling defect in the bladder and early J-hooking of the distal ureters from elevation of the trigone by the prostate.

MANAGEMENT

Acute urinary retention produced by phimosis may often be relieved by gentle dilation of the narrow foreskin opening with a hemostat clamp. A dorsal slit procedure (see section on male genital disorders) or circumcision may then be performed on an elective basis. Paraphimosis and constricting foreign bodies must be treated immediately, for delayed treatment results in ischemic necrosis (see section on male genital disorders). Meatal stenosis is best handled by meatotomy under local infiltrative anesthesia (Fig. 37.8).

Urethral stricture can be a frustrating condition to treat, and improper treatment may result in disastrous complications. We recommend that only a urologist attempt to use filiform probes and followers, urethral sounds, or stylets. These instruments can rapidly convert the simple, short stricture into a jungle of false passages; sepsis, abscess formation, additional strictures, or even urethrocutaneous fistulas may result.

We prefer that a Foley catheter (No. 12 French) or a straight infant feeding tube (No. 10 French) be tried first (Procedure 26) while broad-spectrum antibiotics are being given intramuscularly. If successful, this maneuver "softens" the stricture; thereafter, gradually larger catheters may be passed every other day until a No. 22 French catheter is attained.

If even the small catheter is unsuccessful, suprapubic aspiration of the bladder with a No. 20 or No. 22 spinal needle or insertion of a suprapubic catheter should be performed (Procedure 27). Suprapubic aspiration provides several hours of relief during which time urologic consultation can be obtained or the patient can be transferred to another facility.

Urethral calculi, foreign bodies, and tumors must be removed surgically or with a cystoscope. Occasionally, a calculus can be coaxed through the urethra after anesthetic jelly has been instilled, but the rough edges of a stone usually tear the urethral mucosa.

Posterior urethritis or prostatitis should be managed with antibiotics and drainage through a suprapubic catheter. A urethral catheter exacerbates the problem and risks inducing epididymitis or sepsis.

In benign prostatic hypertrophy, the urethra is compressed by the lateral lobes or obstructed by the median lobe. A relatively small Foley catheter (such as a No. 16 French with a 5 ml balloon) can usually pass by the lateral lobes, but it may be unable to ride over a swollen median lobe. In this event, a coudé catheter with an angulated tip may be tried. Should it fail too, either a contracture of the bladder neck or an enlarged median lobe is probable, and a suprapubic catheter must be employed. The risk of perforating the median lobe

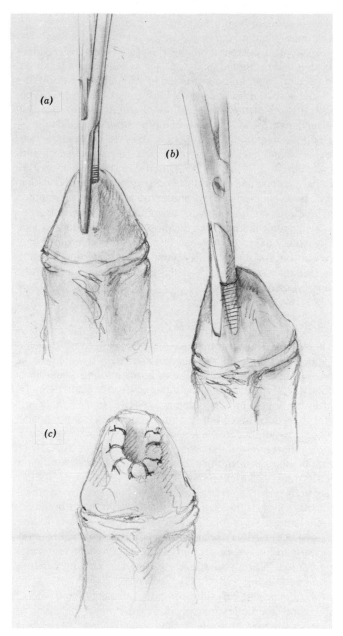

Figure 37.8 Meatotomy for release of meatal stenosis. (a) After infiltration with a local anesthetic either at the meatus or penile base, the ventral meatus is crushed with a straight hemostat to minimize bleeding. (b) The crushed tissue is incised in the midline. (c) The urethral mucosa and glans penis are approximated with several interrupted 4-0 chromic sutures.

with consequent hemorrhage is too great to warrant vigorous blind manipulation.

A patient suspected of having a hypotonic neurogenic bladder should be admitted for neurologic and urologic evaluation. The patient can then be instructed in self-catheterization every 6 hours or so to minimize risk of infection in the residual urine.

Most cases of drug-induced retention can be managed on an outpatient basis. Discontinuing the suspect medication is, of course, mandatory. The patient must be catheterized and begun on an agent such as methenamine mandelate or sulfisoxazole 500 mg every 6 hours orally to suppress urinary infection. The patient should then proceed to have a complete urologic evaluation since a borderline anatomical obstruction that requires correction is not uncommon in this setting.

Psychogenic retention is a diagnosis of exclusion that is made only when neither anatomical obstruction nor neurologic deficit can be uncovered. Reassurance and, if necessary, catheterizations to remove large volumes of residual urine are the appropriate management.

Catheterization and Catheter Care

Whenever a distended bladder must be relieved by catheterization, decompression should proceed slowly to minimize the risk of mucosal hemorrhage with formation and retention of clots. A 400-ml volume should be removed initially then 200 ml every hour until the bladder is empty. Urine output and vital signs must be carefully monitored for several hours after decompression because a postobstructive diuresis may occur. Such a diuresis can be a result of the following factors: (1) an osmotic diuresis from the excess urea accumulated during the partial outlet obstruction preceding acute retention; (2) sodium loss from proximal and distal tubules damaged by hydronephrosis; (3) transitory refractoriness to antidiuretic hormone; and (4) an excess of total body water. Massive output of urine is possible, and if adequate intravascular volume is not maintained with intravenous replacement, hypotension and shock may ensue. Urine and serum electrolytes must be carefully monitored during this phase.

All patients with indwelling urethral catheters should receive either oral antibiotics for specific symptomatic infections or bacterial suppressants (e.g., methanamine mandelate 500 mg four times a day) if the urine is sterile. Try to avoid routine use of bactericidal antibiotics for prophylaxis since there is greater likelihood of the patient developing resistant strains of bacteria while the catheter remains in place. To minimize the risk of infection, the catheter should be carefully maintained. It should be taped securely and washed periodically with an alcohol solution; antibiotic ointment (e.g., polymyxin–bacitracin–neo-mycin) should be applied daily at the meatus; and closed urinary drainage should be meticulously preserved. Generous fluid intake should be encouraged.

FREQUENCY, URGENCY, AND DYSURIA

Irritation of the lower urinary tract (bladder, prostate, seminal vesicles, or urethra) is characterized by urinary frequency, urgency, and dysuria. The most common cause is cystitis, followed by acute urethritis and prostatitis. Seminal vesiculitis, foreign bodies, vesical calculi, and periurethral abscesses are less frequently encountered.

In normal voiding, the stretch reflex, which is stimulated at an intravesical volume of 350–400 ml and mediated by the second through fourth sacral nerve roots (S_2–S_4), may be readily inhibited and regulated by cortical centers. However, inflammation producing mucosal edema decreases vesical elasticity. This causes pain with minimal stretching, resulting in urinary frequency. When the inflammation involves the trigone, urgency may be so severe as to produce involuntary voiding. Dysuria, or painful urination, often occurs with frequency and is usually felt in the distal urethra and less commonly in the suprapubic area. Urethral discharge occurs with infection of the glandular elements (periurethral glands or prostate).

Frequency, urgency, and dysuria may also be produced by upper urinary tract infection with secondary irritation of the lower urinary tract, by a calculus in the intravesical ureter, by radiation therapy to the bladder, or by bladder carcinoma. Frequency without dysuria may represent extrinsic compression of the bladder by a pelvic mass (pregnancy, ovarian cysts, uterine fibroids, tumor) resulting in decreased capacity; partial bladder outlet obstruction with incomplete voiding and more rapid stimulation of the voiding reflex; or may be secondary to renal concentrating defects such as chronic pyelonephritis, hypokalemic nephropathy, uric acid nephropathy, sickle cell disease, glycosuria, or diabetes insipidus.

Upper urinary tract pathology responsible for urinary frequency and dysuria can usually be discounted if the history excludes renal concentrating defects, the urine specific gravity is greater than 1.010, there is no glycosuria, and there is no history of flank pain.

DIAGNOSIS

History

When a patient presents with frequency, urgency, or dysuria, one should inquire about sexual contact, urethral discharge, bloody ejaculate, pain on ejaculation, hematuria, symptoms of outlet obstruction, previous urinary tract infections, and any prior urologic evaluation or instrumentation such as trauma, false passages, indwelling catheters.

Physical Examination

There may be suprapubic tenderness, especially on bimanual examination. A palpable or percussable bladder may be detected if there was prior partial obstruction or if edema of the bladder outlet is severe. Costovertebral angle or flank tenderness suggests upper urinary tract infection or calculus. Examination of the external genitalia should include the meatus with regard to presence of urethral discharge. In women, a careful pelvic examination, with particular attention to masses on bimanual palpation, is important. In men, a gentle rectal examination will supply information regarding the consistency of the prostate and the presence of tenderness, warmth, or fluctuance.

Laboratory Evaluation

The urinalysis should be checked for pyuria, hematuria, and bacteria. Organisms identified on Gram stain of an unspun urine specimen will imply more than 100,000 organisms per milliliter and therefore significant infection (Fig. 37.9). Routine cultures are mandatory. Any urethral discharge should be Gram stained.

In general, intravenous urography may be deferred in acute infection, unless there is suspicion of upper urinary tract disease. Since voiding cystourethrography may demonstrate reflux in a normal bladder with acute inflammation and edema, this study should be postponed until the infection is quiescent.

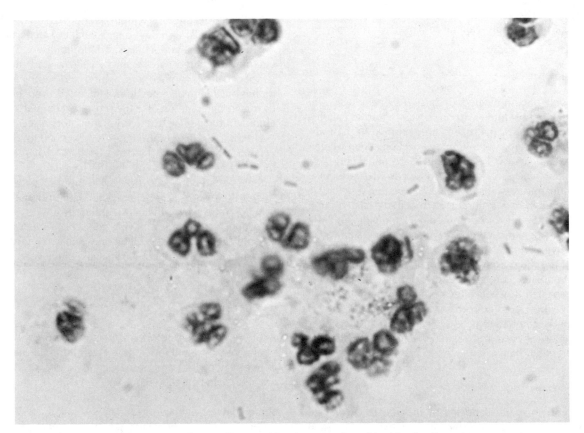

Figure 37.9 Urinary tract infection diagnosed by demonstrating white blood cells and gram-negative bacilli in the urinary sediment.

In patients older than 50 years who have irritative symptoms and hematuria but no bacteriuria, one should consider invasive bladder carcinoma and should obtain urine cytology.

Cystitis

Cystitis is predominantly a female problem because of the short, easily contaminated urethra, but it may occur in males secondary to outlet obstruction or upper urinary tract disease. The typical complaints will be frequency, urgency, dysuria, small voided volumes, suprapubic pain, and sometimes gross hematuria. Lower urinary tract infection may ascend to produce pyelonephritis, at which time fever and flank pain are noted. Cystitis in women is frequently recurrent and often related to sexual intercourse. Coliform bacteria are the common pathogens that colonize the vaginal introitus.

On physical examination, suprapubic tenderness is common. The urethra may be painful, and massage of the peri-urethral glands may express purulence. In older women, urethral stenosis from atrophic vaginal mucosal scarring may be detected.

MANAGEMENT

In women with uncomplicated cystitis, treatment with oral antibiotics may be instituted without obtaining urine cultures since the usual coliform pathogens are sensitive to most antibiotics. However, in men with urinary infection and in women with recurrent infections, urine cultures are mandatory. For therapy of initial infections, we recommend a 7–10 day course of either sulfonamides (sulfisoxazole, 2 g loading dose and 1 g four times a day), or nitrofurantoin (macrocrystals, 100 mg loading dose and 50 mg four times a day). Ampicillin (500 mg four times a day) or tetracycline (500 mg four times a day) may also be effective. Urinary analgesics (phenazopyridine hydrochloride 100 mg three times a day for 2–3 days) will greatly relieve the frequency, urgency, and dysuria. Urine cultures should be repeated 1 week after completing antibiotics. In terms of preventive measures for female patients, proper perineal hygiene is emphasized, as well as voiding after intercourse, treatment of persistent vaginal discharge, and advising showers rather than baths.

RELATED CONDITIONS

Urethral stenosis may be suspected by inability to catheterize the female urethra. Often the stenosis is actually spasm and edema, which resolve with antibiotic therapy. Thus we do not recommend urethral dilatation until after a course of antibiotics.

Certain other types of cystitis require brief mention. *Emphysematous cystitis* is caused by enteric gas-forming bacteria within the bladder wall, often producing a fulminant infection with sepsis. A KUB will demonstrate gas bubbles within the wall of the bladder. This is a serious situation requiring hospitalization, parenteral antibiotics, bladder drainage, and treatment of the underlying obstruction.

Abacterial cystitis may be seen in patients who have tuberculosis, schistosomiasis, or interstitial cystitis (Hunner's ulcer), all of which are rarely seen in an acute situation.

Any man with his first episode of cystitis or women with recurrent episodes of cystitis should be referred for complete urologic evaluation for outlet obstruction.

Acute Urethritis

Acute urethritis presents with frequency, dysuria, and urethral discharge usually 3–6 days after sexual contact. The common organisms are the gonococcus, *Trichomonas,* and *Chlamydia.* Urethral discharge will be thick, yellow, and purulent from gonococcal infection or thin, white, and serous from *Trichomonas* or *Chlamydia* infections. Untreated gonococcal urethritis may progress to involve the prostate, seminal vesicles, and epididymis in men or to pelvic inflammatory disease in women.

Urethral discharge should be Gram stained to identify intracellular gram-negative diplococci (Fig. 37.10) and studied by the hanging drop technique for the flagellated trichomonads. Cultures for gonococcus should be sent in all patients, regardless of the results of the Gram stain. Culturing for *Chlamydia* requires rather sophisticated techniques and is unnecessary. In patients suspected of having gonococcal urethritis, a serologic test for syphilis should be drawn to screen for previously untreated lues, and concurrent anal and oral involvement should be investigated.

MANAGEMENT

Acute gonococcal urethritis is treated with aqueous procaine penicillin G (4.8 million units injected intramuscularly divided between two sites) and probenecid (1 g orally). Patients who are allergic to penicillin receive tetracycline hydrochloride 500 mg four times a day orally for 5 days. An alternative, but somewhat less-effective, regimen is ampicillin 3.5 g, or amoxicillin 3 g, with probenecid 1 g orally. Patients who are unable to tolerate tetracycline may be treated with spectinomycin hy-

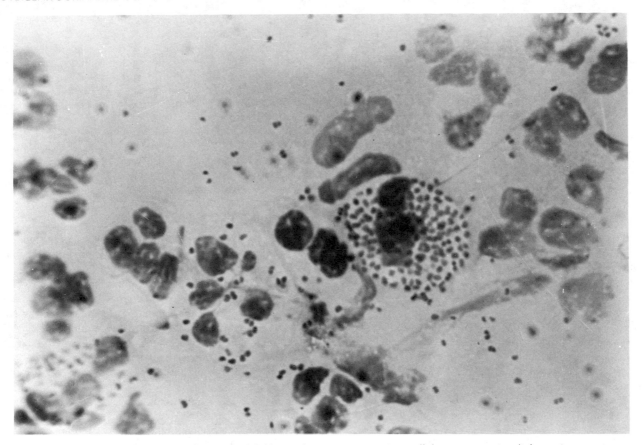

Figure 37.10 Gram stain of urethral discharge showing numerous intracellular gram-negative diplococci characteristic of gonorrhea. Culture for gonorrhea should be obtained regardless of the Gram stain appearance.

drochloride 2 g intramuscularly. These regimens, except for spectinomycin, will cure incubating seronegative syphilis but will probably be inadequate for more advanced diseases; therefore a screening serologic test at the time of treatment, as well as careful follow-up and serology, are important.

Nonspecific urethritis or nongonococcal, nonbacterial urethritis is usually caused by *Chlamydia*. It is effectively controlled with tetraycycline 500 mg four times a day for 10 days, but recurrences are common.

Trichomonas urethritis requires simultaneous treatment of both sexual partners with metronidazole for 10 days (250 mg orally twice a day for the male partner and 250 mg three times a day for the female partner).

Prostatitis

Prostatitis usually occurs in men between the ages of 20 and 40 and presents with irritative symptoms and usually suprapubic pain, malaise, fever, initial or terminal hematuria, hematospermia, and painful ejaculation. There may also be complaints of perineal or referred testicular pain and serous urethral discharge. Prostatitis may produce urinary retention in younger men if edema is severe. Prior episodes of prostatitis or urethritis are common.

On physical examination, we should look for evidence of epididymitis, which may present with prostatitis. The rectal examination will reveal a boggy, tender, warm prostate. A fluctuant area represents prostatic abscess formation. The gentlest examination is mandatory since vigorous massage may produce urinary retention, sepsis, or epididymitis.

Gram stain of the urethral discharge will help in eliminating gonococcus. Cultures are usually sterile, although sometimes *Escherichia coli,* enterococci, or *Klebsiella* is identified.

MANAGEMENT

Treatment with carbenicillin (382 mg every 6 hours) or sulpha/trimethoprim combinations (two tablets twice a day) for 2–3 weeks is effective for uncomplicated cases, but parenteral medications are necessary to control sepsis. Bed rest and sitz baths are helpful. Prostatic massage and sexual intercourse are contraindicated in the acute stage. Urinary retention should be relieved by suprapubic drainage (Procedure 27) since urethral catheters impede drainage of the infected prostatic ducts. Prostatic abscesses should be drained by the urologist, either transurethrally or by needle aspiration.

Seminal Vesiculitis

Seminal vesiculitis will present with identical complaints as prostatitis and therefore may be difficult to differentiate from it. Occasionally, the symptoms are more localized to hematospermia and painful ejaculation and there are few voiding symptoms. An area of tenderness may be localized to the supraprostatic area. Treatment is similar to that for prostatitis.

Foreign Bodies

An incredible variety of foreign bodies have been found in the urinary tract. Such objects within the urethra may cause irritative symptoms, urethral discharge, and urinary retention. They are easily palpable along the penile shaft or sometimes may be demonstrated on plain film of the pelvis. These objects can often be removed by endoscopy, but sometimes open surgery is necessary.

Vesical Calculi

Vesical calculi are the result of chronic infection or bladder outlet obstruction and often present with a long history of obstructive voiding symptoms and the recent onset of abrupt, painful, midstream interruption of voiding. The urine pH is helpful in evaluating such stones. An alkaline urine pH (pH greater than 8) is associated with urea-splitting organisms, such as *Proteus,* and magnesium ammonium phosphate calculi, the so-called "infection stones." An acid urine pH (pH 5–5.5) with-out infection suggests uric acid calculus. Crystals are often seen in the urinary sediment.

The plain abdominal film may reveal a partially calcified infected urinary calculus, but urography is necessary to identify the radiolucent defects of uric acid calculi. Such radiolucent defects may be differentiated from an enlarged median lobe, bladder tumors, blood clots, Foley catheter balloon, or ureterocele.

Vesical calculi may be crushed or extracted by endoscopy if they are smaller than 2 cm. Otherwise, open surgery is advisable. Treatment of the outlet obstruction and infection, if present, will prevent recurrence of bladder stones.

Periurethral Abscess

Periurethral abscess, formerly a complication of postgonococcal stricture and fistula formation, is now more often seen after trauma, careless instrumentation with resultant false passages, or pressure necrosis from indwelling urethral catheters. A history of purulent urethral discharge may be obtained. Postvoid dribbling with irritative symptoms can occur since the cavity fills with urine during voiding and drains afterward.

On physical examination, patients with periurethral abscesses will have a fluctuant mass in the perineum or penoscrotal junction, which may produce purulent urethral discharge upon compression.

Patients who have periurethral abscesses require urgent hospital admission and urologic consultation for temporary suprapubic urinary drainage and systemic antibiotics. Eventual drainage and staged repair of the urethra will be necessary.

MALE GENITAL DISORDERS: PENILE SWELLING

Local trauma or inflammation may cause penile swelling. Penile swelling may also result if venous or lymphatic drainage is obstructed (Table 37.4).

Balanitis

The most common cause of penile swelling is *balanitis,* a nonspecific inflammatory condition of the glans penis in which the foreskin may also be involved (posthitis). Poor hygiene is usually responsible and the condition may be aggravated with phimosis when the glans cannot be cleansed. At first the foreskin is edematous, inflamed, and tender. If untreated, the inflammation may progress to the shaft, producing bullous edema and weeping ulcerations.

TABLE 37.4 Causes of Penile Swelling

Local trauma or inflammation
  Balanitis with or without posthitis
  Phimosis
  Local infection
Obstruction of venous or lymphatic drainage
  Paraphimosis
  Constriction by foreign body
  Penile lymphedema
  Priapism

MANAGEMENT

A mild, localized case of balanoposthitis generally requires only elevation or bed rest, gentle cleansing of the involved area, and topical antibiotic ointment. Oral antibiotics are advisable in diabetics and patients with rather severe inflammation.

Phimosis

Phimosis refers to the situation in which the foreskin meatus is so narrow that the underlying glans cannot be exposed. Dribbling urination, balanitis, and penile carcinoma may be associated with this problem.

MANAGEMENT

When phimosis prevents exposure of the glans, a dorsal slit must be made in the foreskin (Fig. 37.11). The dorsum of the foreskin is infiltrated with 1% lidocaine; then, to limit bleeding, the foreskin should be crushed along the midline with a hemostat. An incision is made to the level of the corona. To prevent injury to the glans, a hemostat should be inserted into the meatus of the foreskin and spread to hold it taut and retract it from the surface of the glans. The free edges should then be approximated with a continuous 4-0 chromic catgut suture.

Local Infections

Superficial abrasions, infections secondary to exfoliative skin disorders, and infection of the suture line after circumcision are other possible causes of penile swelling. Local hygiene and topical antibiotic ointment will promote rapid healing.

Paraphimosis

Paraphimosis is constriction of the lymphatic and venous drainage of the glans penis by the foreskin; it results in edema, venous congestion, and even infarction of the distal penis. This condition may occur whenever an uncircumcised male fails to reduce the retracted foreskin, for example, after intercourse, masturbation, or urethral catheterization. The foreskin then becomes trapped behind the corona of the rapidly engorging glans. Paraphimosis should be differentiated from angioneurotic edema of the foreskin, which is a localized allergic response. Angioneurotic edema is much less common than paraphimosis and is not characterized by constriction bands.

MANAGEMENT

Treatment of paraphimosis requires reduction of the foreskin. While the glans penis is gently compressed, traction should be applied to the foreskin (Fig. 37.12). Failing this, infiltration of a local anesthetic without epinephrine at the base of the penis permits more forceful compression of the edematous tissue. Complete reduction of both compression bands is mandatory since recurrence is more likely if reduction is only partial. If both of these maneuvers are unsuccessful, an emergency dorsal slit must be made.

Constriction by Foreign Bodies

Foreign bodies (soft-drink bottles, tourniquets, rings) used for masturbation or in an attempt to prolong erections can produce significant edema in a fashion similar to paraphimosis. Removing these constricting foreign bodies will test the ingenuity of the physician and the hospital engineers. Generous anesthesia is often required.

Penile Lymphedema

Penile lymphedema virtually always occurs with scrotal edema since the lymphatics of the hemiscrotum and penis anastomose to form a common drainage system through the superficial and deep inguinal nodes to the iliacs. Obstruction anywhere along this chain produces edema of the genitalia. Possible settings include lymphogranuloma venereum, metastatic carcinoma, or filariasis that has involved the inguinal nodes; or pelvic tumors, surgery, or irradiation that has interrupted the iliac drainage. Also thrombosis of deep pelvic veins, anasarca, or extravasation of urine after trauma may produce genital swelling. Treatment of genital lymphedema must be directed at the underlying cause, but scrotal elevation and bed rest are always helpful. Compression dressings should be avoided because they can produce pressure necrosis.

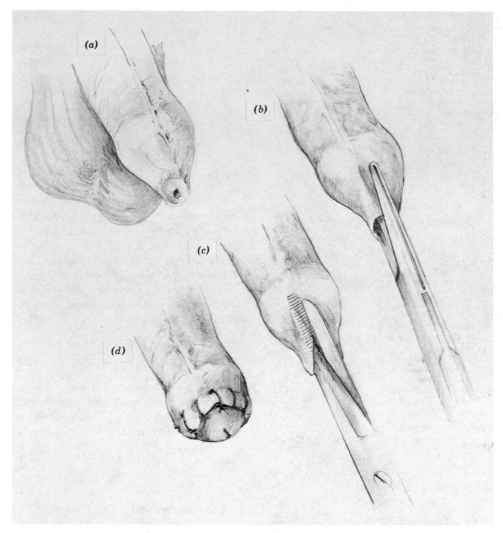

Figure 37.11 Phimosis—dorsal slit procedure. (a) Phimosis is the condition in which the stenotic foreskin meatus prevents retraction over the glans penis. (b) After infiltration with local anesthesia, the dorsal foreskin is crushed in the midline with the hemostat, avoiding the glans. (c) The crushed tissue is incised to procude a V-shaped defect and to expose the glans. (d) The cut edges are oversewn with running 4-0 chromic sutures.

Priapism

Priapism is painful, prolonged erection of the penis. Detumescence is prevented by inadequate drainage of the corpora cavernosa. About 50% of cases are idiopathic; the remainder reflect an underlying disorder such as sickle cell disease or trait, leukemia, metastatic carcinoma, trauma, or instrumen-

tation or may be drug induced (e.g., phenothiazines). The erection may regress spontaneously, but delaying surgery reduces the chance of a successful operation because sludging of blood in the corpora cavernosa leads eventually to thrombosis and fibrosis and impotence as the ultimate consequence.

Priapism is a surgical emergency, but examination and screening (complete blood cell count with differential, sickle

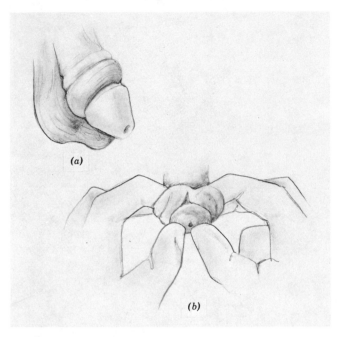

Figure 37.12 Paraphimosis. (a) The retracted foreskin acts as a constricting ring to impede venous and lymphatic drainage of the glans penis. (b) Manual reduction by gentle compression of the glans while sliding the foreskin over the glans using the maneuver depicted is urgent. Failing this, emergency dorsal slit procedure is required.

cell preparation, hemoglobin electrophoresis) for the underlying disorder should not be neglected since early treatment of the primary disorder may prevent recurrence should surgery be successful.

MANAGEMENT

Priapism managed conservatively with sedation, regional anesthesia, ice packs, stilbestrol, anticoagulants, fibrinolytic therapy, corporeal aspiration, and irrigation through large-bore needles has yielded uniformly poor results. Thus if detumescence is not achieved within a few hours, surgical shunting by a urologist is mandatory. The procedure of choice involves shunting venous flow from the poorly drained corpora cavernosa to the corpus spongiosum, which is unaffected. More than 50% of patients are reported to retain potency following such shunts.

MALE GENITAL DISORDERS: SCROTAL MASSES

Scrotal masses are commonly a diagnostic puzzle (Table 37.5). The history should focus on rapidity with which the mass appeared, its duration, the presence of pain, the occurrence of trauma, instrumentation, or antecedent infections—either urinary tract or systemic (mumps, syphilis). The physical exam-

TABLE 37.5 Evaluation of Scrotal Masses

		Pain			
	Age	Degree	Onset	Response to Elevation above Symphysis Pubis	Comments
Hydrocele	Elderly	Absent	—	—	Transilluminates; acute painful hydroceles in younger patients may occur with trauma, inflammation, or tumor
Testis tumor	20–35 yr	Absent	—	—	Does not transilluminate; gynecomastia in 10% of patients; may have acute pain if infarction occurs
Testicular torsion	<25 yr	Severe	Sudden	Increased	Epididymis anterior; surgical emergency
Epididymitis	>20 yr	Severe	Gradual	Decreased	Epididymis posterior; pyuria usual; history of prostatitis, instrumentation, stricture, urinary infection, or recent prostatectomy
Orchitis	>20 yr	Mild or severe	Variable	No change or decreased	Parotitis usually precedes
Varicocele	>20 yr	Absent or mild	Gradual	—	Enlarges when standing; if acute, may represent deep venous obstruction
Incarcerated scrotal hernia	Elderly	Moderate	Sudden	No change	Bowel sounds sometimes audible over mass; bowel gas in scrotum on film; surgical emergency

ination must include careful palpation of the testicles, epididymis, and spermatic cord from the external ring down to the epididymis. Precise localization and orientation of the mass in relation to scrotal contents necessitates examination in both the supine and standing positions. Transillumination using any bright light source will differentiate solid masses from those that are fluid filled. Urine should be checked for pyuria.

Hydrocele

A hydrocele is a collection of serous fluid within the tunica vaginalis. The mass can be transilluminated and may be large enough to prevent the scrotal contents from being palpated (Fig. 37.13). The majority of hydroceles occur in elderly patients, are idiopathic, are relatively asymptomatic, and frequently do not require surgery. However, acutely symptomatic hydroceles, which occur most often in younger patients, may signal an underlying disorder (epididymitis, neoplasm) or may result from trauma. Ultrasonography, Doppler scanning, or radioisotopic scanning may be useful in establishing a diagnosis, but surgical exploration may be required.

Testis Tumor

Any painless mass in the testis of a young adult (20–35 years old) must be regarded as a testis tumor until it is proven otherwise. Tumors usually can be distinguished from the epididymis and cannot be transilluminated. Painful secondary, or "reactive," hydrocele may result from focal infarction and hemorrhage. About 10% of testicular tumors are accompanied by gynecomastia; these are, as a rule, choriocarcinomas producing gonadotropins. The slightest suspicion of a testicular tumor requires that the patient be admitted to the hospital for surgical exploration through an inguinal incision; aspiration or biopsy through the scrotum is contraindicated.

Torsion of the Testicle

In testicular torsion the spermatic cord becomes strangulated; edema and necrosis follow, and testicular atrophy is the eventual outcome in untreated cases. Torsion occurs before puberty in boys with an excessively long spermatic cord enclosed within the tunica vaginalis (the "bell clapper" anomaly) permitting unimpeded rotation. When viewed from the patient's feet, torsion of the left testicle is counterclockwise and torsion of the right testicle is clockwise.

Severe pain and sometimes nausea and vomiting begin acutely in torsion. Several hours later, fever and leukocytosis may develop. Torsion is very difficult to distinguish from acute ep-

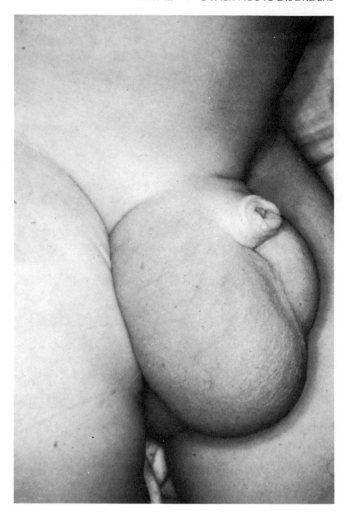

Figure 37.13 Hydrocele in a child with a large, firm, right scrotal mass that transilluminated and did not extend above the cord structures at the level of the external inguinal ring.

ididymitis, but the following generalizations are often helpful: (1) abrupt onset of symptoms is more typical of torsion; (2) a "torted" testis rides high in the scrotum because of the strangulation and cremaster spasm (Fig. 37.14) and the epididymis is located anteriorly, although after a few hours the epididymis may no longer be palpable; (3) lifting the testis above the symphysis aggravates pain caused by torsion, whereas it often provides relief in epididymitis; (4) pyuria is not seen with torsion; (5) radioisotopic scanning of the testis rapidly and reliably differentiates torsion (a "cold" spot) from epididymitis (a "hot"

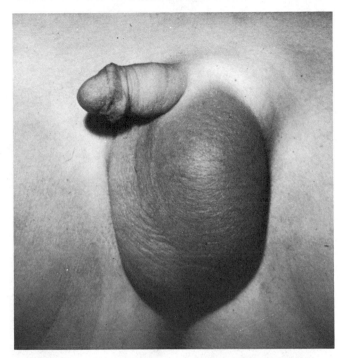

Figure 37. 14 Torsion. The left hemiscrotum is indurated and flushed and the testis is retracted up to the external ring. The edematous, strangulated cord structures produce a visible bulge over the external ring.

spot). Surgical exploration may, nevertheless, be necessary to confirm the diagnosis.

MANAGEMENT

Torsion is a surgical emergency because infarction ensues 4–6 hours after strangulation. Although manual detorsion is possible with local anesthesia, surgical detorsion and bilateral fixation is necessary since there is high risk for bilateral recurrence. The testis should be preserved if at all possible; even if the seminiferous tubules are infarcted, the interstitial cells, which produce testosterone, often survive.

Epididymitis

Eipdidymitis, a chemical or bacterial inflammation of the epididymis, occurs when urine is forced retrograde into the vas deferens. The most dependent portion of the epididymis is involved first, and pain develops gradually. Within several

hours, the pain is severe, the entire epididymis is severely indurated, a hydrocele may form, and the overlying scrotal skin is inflamed (Fig. 37.15). The condition must be distinguished from torsion.

Epididymitis tends to occur in somewhat older patients than does torsion and is often associated with prostatitis, preexisting infection of the urinary tract; urethral instrumentation, urethral stricture, or recent prostatectomy. At times strenuous exertion immediately precedes the onset of symptoms, and what initially seems to be a strangulated hernia proves to be epididymitis.

Physical examination reveals that the epididymis is lying posteriorly, is quite tender, and is indurated. Later the testis and the cord become congested and swollen. Pyuria is quite common, and a urine culture should be obtained before antibiotics are administered. The leukocytosis may be severe. A

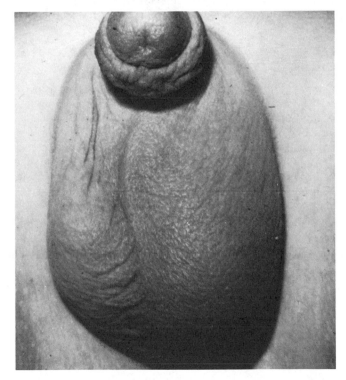

Figure 37.15 Epididymitis. As opposed to torsion, the left testis is well down in the hemiscrotum, and a tender epididymis is palpable posteriorly. The scrotal skin changes, such as induration and loss of scrotal rugae, are similar to torsion. Severe epididymitis often cannot be differentiated from late torsion on physical examination.

tender, boggy prostate, if found, should not be massaged; doing so exacerbates the epididymitis.

MANAGEMENT

Bed rest, scrotal elevation or support, ice packs, antiinflammatory agents, generous analgesics, and a broad-spectrum oral antibiotic, pending the results of urine culture, are the appropriate management. An oral antibiotic, such as ampicillin (500 mg every 6 hours) or tetracycline (500 mg every 6 hours) suffices for an afebrile patient. However, when there is evidence of systemic infection, such as chills and temperature above 38°C (101°F), or of abscess formation with a tender, fluctuant mass, the patient should be hospitalized and treated with systemic antibiotics (aminoglycosides or ampicillin). If the patient shows no improvement, surgical intervention to drain an abscess, open the vas deferens, or even remove the epididymis is necessary. After a severe case of epididymitis, pain may persist for weeks and the induration may not resolve for months. Any patient with voiding symptoms should have urological consultation.

Orchitis

Orchitis, inflammation of the testis, is uncommon; when it occurs, the source may be from a generalized viral infection or from an adjacent acute epididymitis. Mumps orchitis, the most common form, usually occurs after puberty, is most often unilateral, and may present 5–10 days after the onset of parotitis. Discomfort may be mild, with only a slight fever, or the pain may be severe and acute in onset, accompanied by chills, high fever, and nausea and vomiting. In the latter case, the condition may mimic torsion. In such severe cases, the testis is greatly enlarged, hard, and tender; the overlying scrotal skin may be inflamed, and a secondary hydrocele may form. Pyuria does not occur, but microhematuria and proteinuria are common. Leukocytosis, not lymphocytosis, is frequent.

Concomitant parotitis or recent systemic viral disease simplifies diagnosis. In the absence of urinary symptoms or pyuria, epididymitis is unlikely. A testicular scan may be needed to rule out torsion.

MANAGEMENT

Treatment is bed rest, local support or elevation, and analgesia. Neither corticosteroids nor antibiotics have been proven useful. Infiltration of a local anesthetic in the spermatic cord above the testis may relieve swelling and pain. As with torsion, the seminiferous elements may be destroyed, whereas the testos-

terone-producing interstitial cells survive. Sterility may result from bilateral involvement.

Varicocele

A varicocele is a dilated plexus of veins surrounding either testis. The veins of this plexus drain into the internal spermatic veins, which then drain into the inferior vena cava on the right and into the renal vein on the left. Obstruction or incompetent

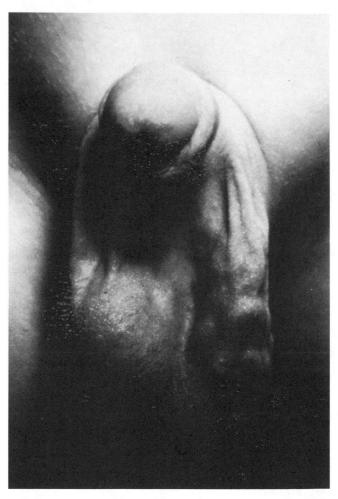

Figure 37.16 Varicocele. The irregular beady outline in the left hemiscrotum is produced by a dilated plexus of veins, which is more pronounced with standing and the Valsalva maneuver. The veins have a rubbery consistency on examination, lying above and posterolateral to the testis.

valves within the veins can lead to a palpable mass of tortuous, dilated veins above and posterior to the ipsilateral testis (Fig. 37.16).

Most commonly, varicoceles are an affliction of younger men, in whom they are chronic, are usually left sided, produce only mild discomfort or sensation of fullness, and may be associated with decreased sperm production. Discomfort can be relieved with scrotal support; surgery is indicated only if there is significant pain or if infertility must be treated.

An acute varicocele in an older man is worrisome since it heralds underlying pathology. If it is right sided, it suggests thrombus in the vena cava or a retroperitoneal tumor. If it is on the left side, the most common cause is renal cell carcinoma that has invaded the renal vein or propagated a thrombus to occlude the spermatic vein. Renal vein thrombosis and lymphoma are other possible causes.

Evaluation of an acute varicocele should begin with an IVP and often proceeds to angiography of the aorta and the vena cava. Treatment should be directed at the underlying disorder.

Scrotal Hernia

An inguinal hernia may extend into the scrotum, producing a scrotal hernia. Reducible hernias pose little problem, but an incarcerated hernia can be mistaken for an abnormality of the testis or epididymis. If a nontender testis can be palpated distinct from the mass, if there are no urinary symptoms or pyuria, and if bowel gas appears in the scrotum on a plain abdominal film, the diagnosis of incarcerated hernia is favored and surgical exploration is necessary.

Other Scrotal Masses

Other scrotal masses include mesenchymal tumors of the spermatic cord, spermatoceles, hydroceles of the cord, and epididymal tumors. They are all painless and asymptomatic and are usually encountered during routine physical examination; only occasionally do they present as acute problems.

SELECTED READINGS

Berger RE, Alexander ER, Harnisch JP et al: Etiology, manifestations, and therapy of acute epididymitis: prospective study of 50 cases. *J Urol* 1979; 121:750.

Corriere JN Jr, Wise MF: Acute cystitis in young women: Diagnosis and treatment. *Urology* 1973; 1:453.

Desautels RE: Managing the urinary catheter. *Geriatrics* 1964; 29:67.

DeWolf WC, Fraley EE: Renal pain. *Urology* 1975; 6:403.

Kunin CM: Detection, prevention and management of urinary tract infections, ed 3. Philadelphia, Lea & Feibiger, 1978.

McHenry MC, Hawk WA: Bacteremia caused by gram negative bacilli. *Med Clin North Am* 1974; 58:623.

Meares EM Jr: Prostatitis syndromes: New perspectives about old woes. *J Urol* 1980; 123:141.

Noble RC: Sexually transmitted disease—A guide to diagnosis and therapy. Garden City, NY, Medical Examination Publishing Co Inc, 1979.

Smith DR: Instrumental examination of the urinary tract, in Smith, DR (ed): *General Urology,* ed 10. Los Altos, Lange Medical Publications, 1981.

Smith DR: Symptoms of disorders of the genitourinary tract, in Smith, DR (ed): *General Urology,* ed 10. Los Altos, Lange Medical Publications, 1981.

Smith DR: Tumors of the genitourinary tract, in Smith, DR (ed): *General Urology,* ed 10. Los Altos, Lange Medical Publications, 1981.

Smith SP, King LR: Torsion of the testis: Techniques of assessment. *Urol Clin North Am* 1979; 6:429.

Tanagho EA: Urinary obstruction and stasis, in Smith, DR (ed): *General Urology,* ed 10. Los Altos, Lange Medical Publications, 1981.

Williamson RCN: Torsion of the testis and allied conditions. *Br J Surg* 1976; 63:465.

38
ACUTE OBSTETRIC AND GYNECOLOGIC DISORDERS

Kirtly Parker Jones
Phillip G. Stubblefield

Ten to twenty percent of all patients who visit a busy city hospital emergency room have gynecologic problems. These problems may be pregnancy related or may involve common gynecologic complaints of vaginal bleeding or pelvic pain. The diagnosis may be as simple as vaginitis or as life threatening as a ruptured ectopic pregnancy. Since primary health care for some areas is provided by the local emergency room, more and more physicians in the emergency room will be faced with obstetric and gynecologic emergencies. Today, more women are willing to seek help for minor gynecologic problems. This, together with an increase in the incidence of sexually transmitted diseases (STD) including gonorrhea, syphilis, vaginitis, and pelvic infections, will bring people with a wide variety of gynecologic problems to the emergency room physician.

In this chapter we will discuss the gynecologic examination, the examination of the pregnant patient, and obstetric and gynecologic problems and will include a section on obstetric emergencies and on the management of a normal vaginal delivery.

GYNECOLOGIC EXAMINATION

The gynecologic physical examination can be somewhat uncomfortable for the patient and her physician and must always be carried out gently. An adequate pelvic examination requires a cooperative and relaxed patient, and a relatively quiet and private examination room can do much to facilitate this. The room must be equipped with a mobile examination lamp or flashlight and a table with stirrups for the proper positioning of the patient. Instruments for examination of the vagina and cervix (gloves, an appropriately sized speculum, swabs, a tenaculum for manipulation of the cervix, a long Kelly clamp or ring forceps for the removal of tissue or foreign objects, slides

and saline for the examination of vaginal secretions) should be on hand before beginning the examination.

The patient is placed in the supine position with her feet in the stirrups, her buttocks at the end of the examination table, and her knees as far apart as is comfortable. A drape covering the patient's knees and abdomen is common, though it is important to maintain voice and eye contact with the patient. The examination begins with a gentle examination of the vulva for lesions or signs of infection. The labia may be gently separated with a gloved hand to view the Bartholin's and periurethral gland openings that are often sites of infection and subsequent abscesses.

The patient is made more comfortable during the speculum examination by choosing a speculum of the appropriate size. A pediatric or Pedersen speculum is advisable for the virginal or preadolescent patient in that the specula are shorter and narrower. The Graves bivalve speculum of average dimensions is adequate for the normal parous patient. A large speculum is necessary for adequate visualization of the vagina and cervix of the obese or multiparous patient. Postmenopausal patients may have a thin, contracted vaginal wall requiring very gentle manipulation with a small speculum. Many emergency rooms are equipped with plastic disposable specula that are convenient but may not be strong enough for adequate visualization in a difficult examination.

The speculum should be moistened with warm water (not a lubricant since this may impair adequate histologic or bacteriologic studies) and placed slowly in the vagina, directed toward the sacrum, and slowly opened and adjusted when the cervix is in view. Papanicolaou smears are taken from a swab in the cervical os and a scrape of the cervix. Cultures for gonorrhea or other pathogens are taken from a swab that has been placed in the cervical os for 15 seconds. A spatula or swab can be used to obtain vaginal secretions for examination under a microscope to evaluate a vaginal discharge. The vagina is examined while slowly removing the speculum.

The bimanual examination of the pelvic organs is performed with one hand on the lower abdomen just above the symphysis pubis and the other hand, which has surgical lubricant on the first two fingers, gently placed in the vagina. The size and consistency of the cervix is felt, and the uterus is felt by placing the lubricated finger in the posterior vagina and gently lifting up in the midline to meet the abdominal hand. Adnexal masses or tenderness are felt by moving both hands to the right and left above the symphysis pubis. Interference from tense rectus muscles can sometimes be overcome by having the patient exhale slowly.

The final part of the pelvic examination is performed with one lubricated finger in the rectum and one in the vagina to assess a uterus that may be flexed posteriorly or a mass in the cul-de-sac.

PHYSICAL AND LABORATORY DIAGNOSES OF PREGNANCY

Frequently, the emergency room physician faces the questions as to whether the female patient is pregnant and, if so, what may be her estimated stage of gestation. The following discussion includes the physical assessment of the pregnant patient, available pregnancy tests, and radiologic and ultrasound diagnoses of pregnancy.

History and Physical Examination

By convention, a pregnancy is dated from the first day of the last menstrual period, and a term gestation is 40 weeks. This convention assumes that the patient has a regular monthly cycle. When questioning a patient who may be pregnant, it is important to know the usual interval between the patient's periods and their normal length, amount of flow, and usual concurrent symptoms (e.g., breast tenderness, cramping). Many women will continue to have bleeding during the first trimester, which can confuse the menstrual history. This bleeding is often not like a normal menstrual period (e.g., lighter, heavier, no cramping). Many young women have irregular menses, and the physician must rely on other physical symptoms of pregnancy (e.g., nausea, vomiting, fatigue, breast tenderness, frequency of urination), the physical examination, or the urine or serum pregnancy test.

The physical examination of the pregnant patient reveals changes in the cervix and in the size of the uterus that may be very subtle in early pregnancy. When the cervix is visualized by speculum examination, it appears softer and has a slight blue cast caused by increased venous flow. The examining hand may feel that the cervix is soft and may feel the pulsations of the cervical branches of the uterine artery at the lateral edges of the cervix. The uterus is relatively softer and more globular in pregnant women. The size of the uterus in the first trimester (first 12–13 weeks) closely correlates with the length of gestation (a uterus the size of a small orange corresponds to 8 weeks, a uterus the size of a grapefruit corresponds to 12 weeks). The uterus can be felt abdominally after 12–13 weeks of gestation; a uterus just above the symphysis pubis corresponds to 12–13 gestational weeks; midway to the umbilicus, 16 weeks; at the umbilicus, 20 weeks; and at the xyphoid, 40 weeks.

The fetal heart can be heard with a portable ultrasonic Doppler device at 13 gestational weeks and can be heard with a stethoscope at 20 weeks (at a normal rate of 120–160 beats/min). Fetal movement can be felt by the mother by 16–18 weeks and by the examining hand by 24 weeks.

Pregnancy Tests

The *urine pregnancy test* has been the standard laboratory method for confirming pregnancy, and it is the most rapid and convenient test. Most emergency rooms will have one of the standard urine test kits. The most widely available pregnancy tests are urine slide tests that require only 2–3 minutes to perform. Methods of performing the test differ from one kit to another, and directions in the package must be followed carefully. The common test kits (Gravindex, Pregnosticon, and Pregnosis) test positive if the concentration of human chorionic gonadotropin (HCG) exceeds 1,500–2,000 mIU/ml urine. This level of HCG is achieved in 95% of normal pregnancies by 6 weeks from last menses, or 4 weeks from conception. Thus a negative test before 6 weeks does not exclude pregnancy. Urine pregnancy tests can be falsely negative or falsely positive because of protein or drugs in the urine.

Diagnosis of early pregnancy and of ectopic pregnancy requires more sensitive pregnancy tests which are increasingly available. The Sensi-Tex test is specific for the beta subunit of the HCG molecule and can detect a level of HCG in the urine of only 250 mIU/ml in 2 hours. More sensitive tests are performed on serum samples. They include the radioreceptor assay (Biocept-G), which is positive at 200 mIU/ml of serum, and the most sensitive and specific of all, the radioimmunoassay for β-HCG, which detects as little as 10 mIU/ml.

Ultrasound and X-ray Studies

The increasing availability of ultrasound diagnostic equipment has made this technique invaluable for the diagnosis of the presence and viability of an intrauterine pregnancy. Ultrasound is available in most hospitals, takes several minutes, can diagnose a pregnancy as early as 5 weeks, and can confirm a missed abortion. Fetal demise, presentation of the fetus, and position and integrity of the placenta are also readily ascertained by pelvic ultrasound. To date, there is no evidence that ultrasound is damaging to maternal or fetal tissues.

A flat film of the abdomen may reveal fetal calcification after 20 weeks. X-ray films of the gravida are discouraged, but in the patient who presents with an acute abdomen, renal stones, or pelvic trauma, the very small risk to the fetus must be weighed against the benefits of the information gained by the procedure.

VAGINAL BLEEDING

When a woman presenting with vaginal bleeding is able to give a history, it is important to obtain information regarding the duration, quantity, and quality of the bleeding. The patient should be questioned regarding the date of her last normal menstrual bleeding and whether the bleeding was of sudden onset or had been gradually increasing; if the blood is coming in clots (significant in that it suggests fairly profuse bleeding); if the bleeding is associated with pain and whether it is constant or cramping in quality; if the patient is pregnant or if there has been a recent instrumentation of the uterus (i.e., biopsy of the cervix, hysterectomy, recent delivery of an infant, or abortion).

In considering the differential diagnosis of vaginal bleeding, the important distinction between bleeding associated with pregnancy and bleeding associated with gynecologic disorders must be made.

Bleeding Associated with Pregnancy of Less Than 20 Weeks Gestation

A history of a delayed menstrual period in a woman who presents with vaginal bleeding and cramping suggests threatened abortion or ectopic pregnancy. A patient may know if she is 3–4 months pregnant; however, the gravida who is less than 8 weeks away from the first day of her last menstrual period may not realize that she is pregnant. An irregular menstrual history; a lack of contraception; and symptoms of cramping, passage of clots, and possibly tissue are all consistent with a threatened or incomplete spontaneous abortion.

THREATENED ABORTION

The physical examination of a woman with a *threatened abortion* reveals blood in the vagina but a cervical os that is closed to the gentle probing of a small ring forceps. The pelvic examination may indicate a tender, soft, globular uterus of dimensions appropriate for gestational age. A complete blood cell count (CBC) must be obtained to assess the patient's hematologic status and possibility of infection. The urine pregnancy test may be positive and should be done to confirm a pregnancy. If a woman is more than 13 weeks pregnant according to history and physical examination, the fetal heart can be heard with a portable ultrasound to verify viability of the pregnancy. The patient should be admitted to the hospital if the bleeding is significant. If the patient's vital signs are stable and bleeding is minimal at the time of the evaluation in the emergency room, she may be sent home with precautions to return if bleeding increases or if tissue is passed. It is important to reassure her that many women have spotting or light bleeding at 6–8 weeks in a pregnancy, and this does not necessarily indicate a poor prognosis for her pregnancy.

INEVITABLE OR INCOMPLETE ABORTION

An *inevitable or incomplete abortion* is marked by profuse bleeding and cramping and the important physical finding of a cervical os that is open. The patient should be started on 10 units of oxytocin in 1,000 ml of lactated Ringer's solution intravenously (oxytocin increases uterine contraction and decreases bleeding). The hematocrit and the patient's blood type must be checked for possible transfusions or blood products, and the patient should be admitted for a dilation and curettage (D&C). The urine pregnancy test may still be positive since the half-life of HCG is approximately 1–2 days.

A *completed spontaneous abortion* may present with a history of bleeding, cramping, and passage of tissue at home or tissue noted in the vagina during the physical examination. The patient's cramping and bleeding will have markedly decreased after complete expulsion of the products of conception. The hematocrit, blood type, and Rh should be obtained. If the uterus is small and firm, the os is closed, and the patient is stable, then the patient may be sent home with precautions regarding a fever or increased bleeding. The patient should, within 2 weeks, have an examination by her gynecologist. The patient may be given methylergonovine (Methergine), 0.2 mg orally three times a day for two days, to assure firm uterine tone and decreased bleeding (methylergonovine is a vasoconstrictor and should not be given to women with hypertension). If the patient is still bleeding or if no tissue is passed, she must be admitted for a D&C.

If the patient is Rh negative, she should be given 1 dose of Rh immune globulin (RhoGAM) intramuscularly. Rh immunization of an Rh-negative mother by an Rh-positive fetus may develop when there is extravasation of fetal blood into the maternal circulation (at term delivery or abortion), and the Rh-negative mother "sees" the Rh antigen and subsequently forms anti-Rh antibodies. These antibodies persist and readily cross the placenta in future pregnancies and can cause hemolysis of the blood cells of an Rh-positive fetus in future pregnancies. Rh immune globulin is an anti-Rh antibody that will bind the Rh antigen from an Rh-positive fetus after an abortion or delivery and can prevent the production of maternal anti-Rh antibodies. Rh immune globulin is routinely given to all Rh-negative women who have had a spontaneous abortion unless they are shown to be already sensitized to the Rh factor.

The prognosis for a woman with a spontaneous abortion in the first 12 weeks of pregnancy is very good with regard to her reproductive potential. As many as 15% of all known pregnancies will spontaneously abort in the first trimester. The vast majority of these women will have normal term pregnancies in the future.

INDUCED ABORTION

The patient may present with bleeding and cramping and a history of a recent *therapeutic abortion*. These may be normal postabortal symptoms, but if the uterus is enlarged and tender and the symptoms are severe, the problem may be retained products of conception and the patient must be admitted for reevacuation. She may be febrile and have an elevated white blood cell count if the products of conception have become infected. Of note is that the sedimentation rate, which is elevated with infections, is also elevated in all pregnancies because of the increase in fibrinogen in the serum during pregnancy.

A patient who presents with acute, severe, constant abdominal pain and an enlarged tender pelvic mass immediately after a therapeutic abortion may have a hematometra (a uterine cavity acutely distended with blood unable to pass through the cervix) or an occult perforation of the uterus. Both of these are emergencies that require hospital admission.

Self-induced or criminal abortion may be complicated by retained products of conception, and the patient may present with cramping and bleeding and may be in hemorrhagic or septic shock. The patient must be stabilized hemodynamically and admitted for broad-spectrum parenteral antibiotics and immediate uterine evacuation. Antibiotic therapy includes a penicillin (ampicillin 2 g every 4 hours, or penicillin 4 million units every 4 hours), an aminoglycoside (gentamicin 1 mg/kg every 8 hours), and anaerobic coverage (clindamycin 600 mg every 6 hours). Cervical culture and Gram stain are important to look for the presence of clostridia, for which the administration of clostridia antitoxin would be required.

MOLAR PREGNANCIES

Rarely (1/1,000 pregnancies), a patient may have vaginal bleeding from a molar pregnancy. Such pregnancies are characterized by a uterus larger than predicted based on the last menstrual period, persistent vaginal spotting of a prune-colored fluid, or passage of tissue that may have a grapelike appearance. These patients may also present with the classic symptoms of toxemia (hypertension, hyperreflexia, and proteinuria) and must be admitted for evacuation of the uterus and supportive therapy.

ECTOPIC PREGNANCY

Any woman of childbearing age who gives a history of persistent vaginal spotting and intermittent or persistent unilateral pelvic pain must be suspected of having an *ectopic pregnancy*.

Many women who present in shock with a ruptured ectopic pregnancy have been seen previously by a physician and have given the above history and symptoms but were misdiagnosed. Ruptured ectopic pregnancies are still a major cause of maternal mortality. A history of a previous ectopic pregnancy, previous pelvic inflammatory disease (PID), previous pelvic or tubal surgery, and contraception using an intrauterine device (IUD) are all risk factors for an ectopic pregnancy. The majority of ectopic pregnancies are found in the fallopian tube; however, ectopic pregnancies can also be found in the cervix, cornua of the uterus, or the abdomen, often growing in the omentum or mesentery of the bowel.

The patient with the *unruptured ectopic pregnancy* may be asymptomatic or may have symptoms of pregnancy (e.g., breast tenderness, nausea). Often, as noted above, there is persistent vaginal spotting and a vague unilateral pelvic pain. The pelvic examination may reveal a normal or slightly enlarged uterus and a tender, thickened adnexa or a discreet adnexal mass. A urine pregnancy test is positive less than 50% of the time, but the β-HCG radioimmunoassay on serum will almost always indicate a pregnancy. The history, physical examination, and laboratory findings can be consistent with an early intrauterine pregnancy with a corpus luteum cyst producing the unilateral mass and pain; however, the diagnosis of ectopic pregnancy must be ruled out through inhospital observation and laparoscopy because the potential sequelae of a ruptured ectopic pregnancy can be so catastrophic.

Patients with the *ruptured ectopic pregnancy* bleed profusely and persistently from the site of implantation. These women are often young and otherwise healthy and may have physiologic compensation for the intraabdominal blood loss that makes the diagnosis more difficult. The patient may complain of unilateral pain, some weakness or dizzyness, or occasional shoulder pain (referred from diaphragmatic irritation by blood in the abdomen). On physical examination, the patient may have postural hypotension and a mildly tender abdomen that may be distended with some subtle signs of peritoneal irritation such as rebound tenderness. The patient is often tender on pelvic examination and may have bulging vaginal fornices from blood in the cul-de-sac. The hematocrit is often acutely depressed; occasionally the white blood cell count is slightly elevated.

It is not difficult to diagnose ruptured ectopic pregnancy when the patient is in shock with a distended abdomen and bulging fornices. It is more important to make the diagnosis in a woman whose ectopic pregnancy is unruptured or in whom there is intraabdominal bleeding but the vital signs are stable and the physical findings are subtle. All patients with ectopic pregnancies, ruptured or unruptured, must be admitted for emergency laparotomy.

The nationwide mortality rates from ectopic pregnancy have been lowered because of the increased use of laparoscopy, more sensitive tests for pregnancy to aid in diagnosis, and aggressive surgical intervention and adequate blood replacement. The incidence of ectopic pregnancy, however, is on the rise. Since the tubal lesions that predispose to ectopic pregnancy are often bilateral, the rate of a subsequent repeat ectopic pregnancy is 15–30%, and about one-half of women fail to conceive after one ectopic gestation.

Bleeding Associated with Pregnancy of More Than 20 Weeks Gestation

The differential diagnosis of vaginal bleeding in a woman with a pregnancy of more than 20 gestational weeks includes labor with bleeding from cervical dilatation, placental abruption, placenta previa, and bleeding cervical lesions.

Confirmation of a pregnancy of more than 20 weeks can be made by history of the last menstrual period, palpation of the uterus above the umbilicus, and (if the fetus is living) a fetal heart rate at 120–160 beats/min heard with a stethoscope. These signs may not be obvious in a very obese patient in whom the diagnosis of pregnancy can be difficult. Again, a history including the quantity and quality of bleeding and the presence or absence of persistent or episodic pain is important.

PLACENTA PREVIA

Painless vaginal bleeding in a pregnant woman of more than 20 weeks (especially after 28 weeks) should be considered a placenta previa (placenta overlying the opening of the cervix) until proven otherwise. No pelvic examination should be undertaken until that diagnosis is ruled out by ultrasound or by pelvic examination in an operating room. Blood flow through the placenta at term is 600 ml/min, and a woman can rapidly exsanguinate from a bleeding placenta previa; a pelvic examination may exacerbate that bleeding. This evaluation is best carried out by an obstetrician in a delivery center. If the bleeding is profuse, the patient must have at least one large-gauge intravenous catheter running and her blood typed and cross matched immediately.

PLACENTAL ABRUPTION

Vaginal bleeding with abdominal or back pain of sudden onset and a firm, tender uterus is consistent with placental separation from the uterine wall (placental abruption). This is an obstetric emergency because a placenta separated from the uterus compromises the fetus, and subsequent bleeding between the uterus and the placenta may result in a woman being in shock out of proportion to her vaginal bleeding. The laboratory findings of decreased platelets, a fibrinogen level less than 300 mg%, and increased fibrin-split products are indicative of placental abruption. As noted previously, fibrinogen is elevated in pregnancy to a level twice normal at term (approximately 400 mg%), and a fibrinogen of 200 mg% (normal in the nonpregnant patient) indicates consumption of clotting factors. Total separation of the placenta leads to fetal demise and a possible disseminated intravascular coagulopathy (DIC) in the mother. Careful observation of the fetal heart rate and maternal clotting factors should be carried out during preparation for admission or transfer to a high-risk obstetric unit.

Disseminated intravascular coagulation is seen more commonly in obstetrics than in any other specialty. It may be a complication of abruption, of amniotic fluid embolism, of toxemia, of long-standing fetal demise, or in the immediate postpartum period. Once the diagnosis of DIC is suspected, blood should be drawn and sent to the laboratory for complete blood cell count, platelet count, prothrombin time (PT), partial thromboplastin time (PTT), and fibrin-split products. The simple observation that an untreated tube of blood from the patient has not formed a firm clot in 10 minutes can all lead the physician to a presumptive diagnosis of DIC. Blood must be sent to the blood bank to type and cross match whole blood, fresh frozen plasma, and cryoprecipitate to replace clotting factors. Obstetric DIC is usually managed adequately with supportive therapy. Termination of the pregnancy is indicated. (Refer to Chapter 40 for discussion of management of DIC.)

CERVICAL LESIONS

Scant spotting to moderate vaginal bleeding may be associated with a bleeding cervical lesion or a *Trichomonas* infection. The history of recent sexual intercourse may be significant since trauma may have exacerbated the bleeding. Again, unless the position of the placenta is known to be *not* low lying, a pelvic examination should be carried out only in controlled conditions.

LABOR

Passage of a small amount of blood mixed with mucus or just mucus with intermittent palpable uterine contractions is consistent with labor. If the patient is pregnant for less than 34 gestational weeks, consultation with a center which has an intensive care nursery regarding transferring of mother and fetus is appropriate. Fetal viability should be assessed by obtaining a fetal heart rate by auscultation. The vaginal bleeding (bloody show) arises from stretching and opening a very vascular cervix.

A woman in labor near term may be transferred to a nearby labor unit. The management of a vaginal delivery is discussed below in the section concerning obstetric emergencies.

POSTPARTUM HEMORRHAGE

Excessive vaginal bleeding in a patient who has delivered a baby within the last 6 weeks should be considered as postpartum hemorrhage. Most frequently, the problem is caused by retained products of conception or uterine atony. The physical examination reveals a boggy tender uterus at the level of or just below the umbilicus. If the patient delivered at home, the physician should ascertain whether the placenta had been delivered. If the placenta had been delivered, oxytocin, 10–20 units in 1,000 ml lactated Ringer's solution in 5% dextrose, should be given intravenously at a rate adequate to maintain firm uterine tone, and/or methylergonovine 0.2 mg intramuscularly may be given. The patient should be admitted for a D&C to rule out retained products of conception. If the placenta is still in the uterus, ergot preparations are contraindicated as they may cause constriction of the cervical canal.

Vaginal Bleeding in the Nonpregnant Patient

In a patient who presents with vaginal bleeding for whom pregnancy has been ruled out, it is helpful to consider age-related causes in the differential diagnosis.

YOUNG CHILDREN

Young children may place foreign objects in the vagina, which leads to injury of the thin vaginal walls and subsequent bleeding. Gentle examination with the finger may reveal a foreign object that may be visualized by a pediatric speculum. Children who sustain a "straddle injury" to the perineum may have a vulvar or vaginal hematoma that may require drainage.

PUBERTAL FEMALE

In the pubertal female, vaginal bleeding accompanied by cramping may be a normal menses. Some women may have scant bleeding at the time of ovulation. Dysfunctional uterine bleeding is common in women soon after the menarche who

have not established regular ovulation. When pregnancy, pathology (cervical lesions), and blood dyscrasias have been eliminated from the diagnosis, dysfunctional uterine bleeding that is profuse may be treated with hormonal therapy or by minisuction curettage. Hormonal therapy diminishes bleeding by stabilizing the endometrium. A combination pill with 0.05 mg ethinyl estradiol and 0.5 mg norgestrel (Ovral), one tablet twice a day for 10 days, will control the bleeding within a few hours and produce a scanty flow when treatment is finished 10 days later.

An alternative therapy is a minisuction vacuum curettage with a small (4–5 mm diameter) flexible cannula using only a special 50-ml syringe as a vacuum source.* This provides immediate control of the bleeding, as well as a tissue diagnosis. If there is a physician available who is experienced in this procedure, it can be performed in a few minutes without anesthesia and using simple instruments.

WOMEN OF REPRODUCTIVE AGE

Women on combination oral contraceptives commonly have "breakthrough bleeding" between menses though it is usually not profuse. Bleeding that occurs early or in the middle of the cycle of oral contraceptives is usually a result of inadequate estrogen to support the endometrium and can be treated with ethinyl estradiol 0.02 mg orally each day for 5 days starting at the onset of the breakthrough bleeding.

Occasional scant bleeding with an IUD in place is not uncommon, and the menstrual period is normally somewhat heavier; however, persistent bleeding between menstrual periods may indicate chronic endometritis. A pelvic infection must be ruled out if the IUD is to be left in place. If there is a history of pelvic pain, if pelvic tenderness is elicited on examination, or if the sedimentation rate is elevated, the IUD should be removed by placing a speculum in the vagina and grasping the IUD string evident at the cervical os with a Kelly forceps and gently pulling it. The complete blood cell count must be obtained and a serum pregnancy test drawn to evaluate a possibly early intrauterine pregnancy or ectopic pregnancy.

PERIMENOPAUSAL WOMEN

Bleeding in the perimenopausal woman may be anovulatory or may be produced by benign or malignant organic lesions. An irregular, firm, enlarged uterus on physical examination is

---

*Gynecologic Aspiration Kit, available from IPAS, 123 West Franklin Street, Chapel Hill, North Carolina.

consistent with uterine myomata (fibroids) that may lead to menometrorrhagia resulting in anemia. If the bleeding is scant, the patient must be referred to a gynecologist for a D&C or endometrial biopsy to rule out malignancy before hormonal therapy is implemented. If the bleeding is profuse, the patient must be admitted for a D&C and may even require an emergency hysterectomy.

POSTMENOPAUSAL WOMEN

In the postmenopausal woman, vaginal bleeding means cancer until proven otherwise. An excoriated thin perineum and vagina in the postmenopausal woman may bleed if irritated. Physical examination may reveal this or a cervical lesion consistent with cervical cancer or a cervical or endometrial polyp. An enlarged uterus suggests uterine cancer. The patient must be seen by a gynecologist for a D&C before any other therapy. The D&C may have to be done immediately if the cancer is advanced and the bleeding profuse. Patients with a known advanced cancer may have bleeding that may be stabilized with a sterile vaginal pack of gauze for compression hemostasis.

PELVIC PAIN

Patients who present with the chief complaint of pelvic pain may have a diagnosis as minor as dysmenorrhea (painful periods) or as serious as an acute abdomen. A history of the nature and duration of the pain, as well as the presence of concurrent physical symptoms such as chills, fever, nausea, weakness, shoulder pain, or vaginal discharge or bleeding, is important. The patient should be questioned regarding recent gynecologic procedures (e.g., abortions, operations).

Pelvic Inflammatory Disease

One of the most frequent causes of pelvic pain seen in an emergency room is pelvic inflammatory disease (PID). This is seen more and more frequently as it is mostly venereal and often gonococcal in origin. Recent studies have shown that 50% of acute PID is gonococcal, and the remainder is a result of a broad spectrum of aerobic and anaerobic bacteria. Gonococcal PID may be the extension of gonococcal cervicitis to the uterus and adnexal structures and into the abdomen. Often, women using IUDs present with PID. The patient may have a history of several days of mild lower abdominal pain that is increasing in intensity. A history of previous PID or recent exposure to gonorrhea may be helpful in making the diagnosis.

The patient complains of anorexia, a vaginal discharge, possibly a fever, and pelvic pain. Physical examination may reveal peritoneal signs of guarding and rebound tenderness. A cervix exquisitely tender to palpation during pelvic examination is the hallmark of PID. Cultures of the cervix plated on a Thayer-Martin medium are important diagnostically and epidemiologically in the diagnosis of gonococcal PID. The white blood cell count and differential may be normal or may reveal only a mild leukocytosis. An elevated erythrocyte sedimentation rate (ESR) may distinguish PID (an inflammatory lesion) from other causes of acute pelvic pain. If the ESR is normal, other pelvic pathology must be seriously considered.

A patient who has difficulty walking, generalized peritoneal signs, a pelvic mass, a temperature over 38°C (100.4°F), or an ESR greater than 40 should be admitted for intravenous antibiotics because inadequate treatment of PID may lead to a pelvic abscess or secondary sterility because of scarring on the fallopian tubes. Broad-spectrum antibiotics should be used (a penicillin, an aminoglycocide, and anerobic coverage or one of the new cephalosporins that covers anerobic organisms). If the signs and symptoms are mild, oral analgesics and antibiotics (tetracycline 500 mg four times a day or ampicillin 500 mg four times a day) may be given and the patient can be followed-up by a gynecologist outside the hospital. Bed rest, analgesics, and a heating pad to the lower abdomen are indicated, and the patient should refrain from intercourse. Pelvic inflammatory disease should be aggressively treated with antibiotics and hospitalization if necessary because the sequelae of possible infertility and increased risk of ectopic pregnancy or recurrent pelvic inflammation and chronic pelvic pain can be devastating to a woman in her reproductive years.

A similar clinical picture with the history of a recent abortion or delivery may signify postabortal or postpartum endometritis, salpingitis, or PID depending on the length of time the infection has been allowed to persist and spread throughout the uterus, parametrium, and pelvis. Similar criteria of physical and laboratory findings indicate hospitalization and intravenous antibiotics (remember the ESR may be moderately elevated in pregnancy and immediately postpartum). Again, less severe cases may be treated with oral antibiotics and methylergonovine 0.2 mg orally three times a day for 2 days.

Occasionally, PID may develop into a pelvic abscess (tuboovarian abscess) and/or septic pelvic thrombophlebitis. An adnexal mass found during physical examination of a woman with PID is an ominous sign since rupture of a tubo-ovarian abscess may lead to septic shock and death. These patients may present in shock and need cardiovascular support with intravenous colloids, antibiotics, and immediate laparotomy.

Ovarian Cysts

A ruptured or leaking ovarian cyst may cause severe pain and an acute abdomen. A ruptured endometrioma (chocolate cyst) or teratoma (dermoid) may spill inflammatory material into the peritoneal cavity causing inflammation of the peritoneum, and therefore a modest elevation of the white blood cell count and ESR. Functional cysts (follicular cyst that ruptures at ovulation or corpus luteum cysts) may rupture with pain and intraabdominal bleeding. In this case, the white blood cell count and ESR are usually normal which differentiates this from PID.

If the symptoms are severe or if the patient has signs of intraperitoneal bleeding, the patient must be admitted for observation and laparoscopy, and often laparotomy, for removal of the cyst. If the symptoms are mild and an ectopic pregnancy is ruled out, the patient may be sent home to be seen by her gynecologist.

Acute onset of unilateral pelvic pain with a mass and exquisite tenderness on palpation may be torsion of an ovarian cyst around the uteroovarian ligament or around the fallopian tube. There may be a low grade fever and slight leukocytosis, but a normal ESR will differentiate this from a tuboovarian abscess. Torsion of an ovary requires immediate surgical intervention.

It is very important to recognize that the symptoms of a bleeding ovarian cyst or torsion of an ovary are also consistent with an ectopic pregnancy. The patient must be thoroughly evaluated and the diagnosis of ectopic pregnancy must be excluded before she is discharged from the emergency room.

Kidney Stones

A patient with a kidney stone may have pelvic pain with radiation to the flank. The abdomen is usually nontender, pelvic organs are nontender, and the urine analysis will usually show red and white blood cells. The treatment includes sedatives, analgesics, hydration, and an intravenous pyelogram (IVP) to confirm the diagnosis. (Refer to Chapter 37 for further urologic causes.)

Dysmenorrhea

Some women may come to the emergency room with the onset of menses and severe dysmenorrhea. This may be accompanied by nausea and vomiting, especially in the teenager or the woman with endometriosis. After the confirmation of a regular menstrual history, a negative pregnancy test, and no evidence of a pelvic infection, analgesics may be prescribed with caution. The potent prostaglandin inhibitors (Motrin, Na-prosyn) have been found to be very helpful for women with dysmenorrhea. They are usually very effective if the first dose is taken a few hours before onset of the cramping, but are still effective even if they are not begun until after the pain is established.

Women with an IUD in place may experience more severe dysmenorrhea and increased menstrual flow than other women. If the IUD is displaced (IUD evident in cervix) or the pain is severe, the IUD should be removed and counseling of the alternative methods of birth control given. Care should be taken to assure that the patient does not have a concurrent infection or an intrauterine or ectopic pregnancy.

Ovulation

Some women regularly experience midcycle pain of ovulation (Mittelschmerz) that may be unilateral or periumbilical. The pain also may be accompanied by anorexia and nausea. The onset of pain at midcycle is diagnostic. Laboratory findings are unremarkable. Midcycle vaginal spotting may accompany ovulation. The pain is self-limited and the patient should be reassured.

Chronic Pelvic Pain

There is a population of women who present to the emergency room with pelvic pain and a history of recurrent pelvic pain of unknown etiology. The chronicity of the pain and the lack of a definitive diagnosis can be frustrating for the patient and her physician. The white blood cell count and differential and ESR are normal, and the pelvic examination may be normal except for generalized tenderness or perhaps lack of mobility of the uterus and adnexal structures. These women may have chronic PID, endometriosis, or adhesions from previous pelvic surgery or inflammation. If the patient has a normal white blood cell count and ESR and a negative pregnancy test (remember to rule out ectopic pregnancy), nonnarcotic analgesics may be prescribed and the patient referred to a gynecologist.

VAGINAL AND PERINEAL INFECTIONS

The reason a significant number of women make gynecologic-related visits to the emergency room concerns vaginal discharge. Although it is technically not an emergency, the patient can be very uncomfortable with severe vulvovaginal inflammation, itching, burning, and a discharge. There are some vaginal infections that have profound medical sequelae. These include gonococcal cervicitis, which, if left untreated, may lead to pelvic inflammatory disease, and vaginal colonization with *Staphylococcus aureus,* which has been implicated in toxic shock syndrome.

Toxic Shock Syndrome

Toxic shock syndrome, described in young menstruating women, is a rare though potentially fatal disease. It has been recognized in men and nonmenstruating women, although the vast majority of patients have been women using vaginal tampons during their menses. The pathogenesis is believed to be a toxin produced by *S. aureus* that is found growing in the vagina. The use of large occlusive tampons is presumed to cause vaginal abrasions that provide an entry site for the toxin.

Toxic shock syndrome has a rapid onset with nausea and vomiting followed by a profuse watery discharge, abdominal pain, and high temperature. Volume depletion leads to progressive symptoms and signs of hypovolemic shock. Accompanying symptoms may include diffuse myalgias, headache, and nonproductive cough. The physical findings include fever, hypotension, a tender abdomen, and, most prominently, an intense diffuse cutaneous erythema. The laboratory reveals a marked leukocytosis with a shift toward immature forms, an elevated hematocrit secondary to dehydration, abnormal liver functions, and an elevated blood urea nitrogen (BUN) and creatinine.

The therapy is immediate volume support with normal saline and colloids (albumen) and parenteral antistaphylococcal antibiotics (oxacillin 2 g every 4 hours). The clinical course may be complicated by myocarditis with congestive heart failure, pulmonary infiltrates, and renal failure. Despite aggressive supportive therapy, the mortality is 18%.

Late developing findings include desquamation of hands, feet, and trunk from 7–10 days after the onset of the disease. The recurrance rate is 20%, and women who have experienced toxic shock syndrome are advised not to use tampons.

Although the incidence of toxic shock syndrome is very low (3–4 cases per 10,000 menstruating women per year), the consequences are profound if the diagnosis is not made and supportive therapy instituted promptly.

Gonococcal Cervicitis

Gonococcal cervicitis may cause a vaginal discharge or may be entirely asymptomatic in women who complain only of a history of exposure to gonorrhea. The cervix may show a purulent odorless discharge, which on Gram stain reveals many intracellular and extracellular gram-positive diplococci. This finding alone is inadequate for a definitive diagnosis. A swab placed in the cervical os for 15 seconds and plated on a Thayer-Martin medium appropriately placed in a candle jar allows the best chance for a positive culture in women with gonococcal cervicitis. A suspicious Gram stain or a history of contact with gonorrhea should lead to treatment with 4.8 million units of procaine penicillin administered intramuscularly. In nonpregnant women with penicillin allergy, tetracycline 1.5 g orally and 0.5 g four times a day for 4 days is recommended. Since tetracycline is contraindicated in pregnancy, erythromycin 1.5 g orally followed by 0.5 g four times a day for 4 days is a safe alternative for pregnant women with a penicillin allergy. For patients in whom compliance with oral medication is questioned, 2 g of spectinomycin can be given intramuscularly.

Monilial Vaginitis

Monilial vaginitis, common in pregnant women, diabetics, and women on oral contraceptives, is caused by an overgrowth of *Candida* that is part of the normal balanced vaginal flora. It can cause an intensely inflamed vulva and vagina and a thick, white, cheesy, nonmalodorous discharge. The hyphae and budding yeast cells can be seen on a wet mount of the vaginal discharge, especially if they are placed in a drop of 10% potassium hydroxide that destroys other vaginal cellular elements. Monilial vaginitis can be treated with miconazole vaginal cream inserted vaginally once a day and applied to the vulva as needed. In severe cases, immediate relief may be given by a providone-iodine (Betadyne) douche or painting the vulva and vagina with a 1% solution of gentian violet.

Trichomonas Vaginitis

A *Trichomonas* infection causes a malodorous frothy green discharge, mild lower abdominal discomfort, severe perineal itching and occasionally dysuria, and a cervicitis manifested by multiple punctate red spots seen on speculum examination. Mobile oval flagellates approximately the size of a white blood cell are seen under the microscope in a preparation of a small amount of the discharge in 2 drops of saline placed on a slide with a cover slip. Metronidazole (Flagyl) 250 mg taken orally three times a day for 7 days is the appropriate treatment. The sexual partner must be treated with a similar regimen. An alternative therapy of 2 g of metronidazole orally at one dose yields approximately the same cure rate (95%). The patient must be warned not to drink alcohol during the course of therapy or she (or he) will experience severe nausea and vomiting. Metronidazole is contraindicated in pregnancy; acid gel applied vaginally or AVC cream may afford some relief.

Bacterial Vaginitis

Nonspecific vaginitis is caused by *Gardnerella vaginalis*. On a wet mount of the malodorous discharge, many bacteria and epithelial cells with bacteria along the edges (clue cells) are commonly seen. Ampicillin 500 mg orally, four times a day for 1 week is the initial therapy. If this fails, metronidazole is prescribed (250 mg three times a day) for the patient and her sexual partner(s).

Foreign Bodies

A patient may present with a foul odor from her vagina, with or without discharge, in which case a retained tampon, condom, or sponge from a gynecologic or obstetric procedures may be discovered. Removal of the foreign body and cleansing of the vagina with providone-iodine lotion is adequate therapy. Children with a malodorous discharge may be brought to the emergency room by their mothers, and examination with a pediatric speculum may reveal a foreign object or piece of toilet paper. The child must be examined carefully for any evidence of sexual trauma and should be questioned gently about the objects found.

VULVAR LESIONS

Herpes Labialis

Herpes infections of the vulva, vagina, or cervix are very common, and a history of the recent onset of a very painful lesion on the vulva accompanied by the symptoms of a viral syndrome (low fever, malaise) may be evidence of a primary herpetic lesion. The lesion consists of multiple vesicles or shallow ulcers, is exquisitely tender, and may be accompanied by inguinal adenopathy. No specific therapy is as yet available. Considerable symptomatic improvement is afforded by warm baths followed by careful drying and application of topical lidocaine (Xylocaine) ointment 2.5% to the lesions. Occasionally, a periurethral herpetic lesion may cause enough swelling to necessitate hospitalization, a Foley catheter to treat urinary retention, and parenteral narcotic analgesics. These lesions are recurrent after the initial infection. The diagnosis is made from the history and by scraping the lesion for cytology (nuclear inclusion bodies can be seen on a Papanicolaou smear) or by viral culture in the appropriate media if a virology laboratory is available. Recent advances in antiviral therapy have included acyclovir (Zovirax). This medication is of use primarily in immunocompromised patients. If it is used at the onset of a primary genital herpes infection, it probably de-

creases the duration of pain, swelling, and viral bleeding. It does not prevent recurrent lesions, and its benefits for the patient with a recurrent herpes lesion are limited.

Syphilis

A syphilitic chancre differs from a herpetic ulcer in that it is larger and is painless. There is a central necrotic area with surrounding edema that may be scraped and examined under a dark-field microscope for *Treponema pallidum*. A VDRL should be drawn and the patient referred to the local epidemiology clinic for identification of sexual contacts. Benzathine penicillin 2.4 million units intramuscularly or tetracycline 500 mg orally four times a day for 15 days is adequate therapy for primary syphilis.

Bartholin's Gland Abscess

Acute or chronic infection of Bartholin's glands may lead to a Bartholin's gland abscess that becomes a tender fluctuant mass in the lower aspect of the labia majora. If the area is merely indurated and not fluctuant, sitz baths four times a day may localize the infection to allow incision and drainage of the abscess under local anesthesia. Culture of the purulent material for gonococci and aerobic and anaerobic bacteria and packing of the cavity with gauze is the appropriate management in the outpatient setting. The patient should continue warm soaks until the wound is healed completely. Antibiotics are not necessary if the abscess is drained adequately, but analgesics are required.

OBSTETRIC PROBLEMS

In addition to vaginal bleeding, there are other problems particular to pregnancy that may be seen in patients in the emergency room (e.g., premature labor, toxemia), and there are symptoms commonly seen that can be a sign of pregnancy (e.g., nausea, fatigue, palpitations). Some of these will be discussed below.

The nausea and vomiting accompanying pregnancy (morning sickness) can be seen as early as 4 weeks from the last menstrual period and can last into the second trimester. The etiology is unknown but it is thought to be perhaps HCG or increased circulating levels of estrogen.

Nausea and vomiting may be severe and lead to dehydration and acetonuria. If a woman of childbearing age, especially an adolescent, complains of protracted nausea and vomiting, a menstrual and contraceptive history should be taken. A pregnancy test and pelvic examination should be done before undertaking an upper gastrointestinal (UGI) series or an oral cholecystogram in the workup of nausea and vomiting. If a patient has nausea during early pregnancy, Chlorpromazine (Compazine) is safe to prescribe. Occasionally, a patient will need to be admitted for intravenous hydration if the specific gravity of the urine is high and the urine is positive for acetone. tor acetone.

Patients with persistent nausea and vomiting after the 20th week of gestation must be investigated for underlying hepatitis, cholestatic jaundice of pregnancy, pyelonephritis, or gallbladder disease. The diagnosis of hyperemesis gravidarum (a psychophysiologic disease) cannot be made until organic causes for nausea have been eliminated.

Toxemia

The triad of hypertension (diastolic pressure greater than 90 mm Hg), hyperreflexia, and proteinuria in pregnant women in the second and third trimesters is the hallmark of toxemia. *Preeclampsia* is the term commonly used for this disease when it is not complicated by seizures; *eclampsia* is the term used if seizures have occurred. Although the pathogenesis of this disease of pregnancy is not clear, the natural history is well known. The patient may present in the emergency room in the end stages of this disease with symptoms that include severe hypertension, headaches, blurring vision, right upper-quadrant pain from a hematoma of the liver capsule, seizures, anuria, stroke, and coma. Occasionally, DIC may accompany severe toxemia. Toxemia is largely a disease of the last 4 weeks of pregnancy, but it may occur earlier in patients who have a molar pregnancy or who have underlying renal or vascular disease (essential hypertension, systemic lupus erythematosis, or diabetic nephropathy).

THERAPY

Toxemia is an obstetric emergency. Therapy is aimed at decreasing the blood pressure, controlling seizures, and transferring the patient to an obstetric facility for immediate delivery. Acute control of blood pressure may be achieved with intravenous hydralazine in 5-mg increments to bring the diastolic pressure to 90 or 100 mm Hg. A Foley catheter should be placed to assess proteinuria and urinary output. The toxemic patient is in a volume-contracted state, and the treatment of oliguria with diuretics will only make the situation more severe. Treatment with volume expansion is controversial.

In the United States, magnesium sulfate is used for seizure control because it has little effect on the soon-to-be delivered infant. Four grams given intravenously over a 10-minute period followed by an infusion of magnesium sulfate at a rate of 1–2 g/hr (10 g magnesium sulfate in 500 ml lactated Ringer's solution at 50–100 ml/hr) is appropriate therapy. Magnesium sulfate may be given intramuscularly, but this is very painful and uptake by the body is less predictable. Magnesium toxicity may be monitored by the briskness of the patellar reflexes, which should be tested every hour. Absent reflexes indicate magnesium toxicity, in which case the infusion should be discontinued until reflexes return to normal. Severe magnesium toxicity may lead to apnea. The actions of magnesium may be reversed by calcium, which acts as a competitive cation.

Toxemia cannot be managed on an outpatient basis since it only becomes more severe with time and the only cure is delivery. Patients may have seizures up to 5 days postpartum and may be treated with diphenylhydantoin (Dilantin) or diazepam (Valium) since fetal toxicity is no longer in question. The disease resolves in the postpartum period.

Premature Labor

As previously described, intermittent lower abdominal or back pain accompanied by tensing of the uterus may be a sign of labor. Patients who are young, are obese, or who have emotional disturbances may not admit or realize that they are pregnant, and the diagnosis may be made by physical examination rather than history. Dilation of the cervix may be assessed digitally if the membranes are intact and there is no vaginal bleeding. Labor before 36 weeks of gestation is termed premature, and arrangements should be made to transfer the patient to a maternity unit with an intensive care nursery.

Recently, the potent beta-sympathomimetics (e.g., terbutaline, ritodrine) have been found to be very effective in stopping or slowing premature labor. Terbutaline is a drug commonly used in asthma, and a dose of 0.25 mg given subcutaneously usually slows uterine contractions within 15 minutes. Since it also causes tachycardia, it should not be given to patients with underlying heart disease or a pulse over 120 beats/minute, and should only be given in consultation with a high-risk obstetric unit to which the patient will be transferred.

TRAUMA

Trauma and the Obstetric Patient

The principles of trauma management are outlined elsewhere in Chapter 12. However, an understanding of some aspects of physiology of the pregnant woman and the fetus are important in the management of trauma in the pregnant patient. These aspects are listed below:

1. In pregnancy, 25% of the cardiac output is delivered to the placenta, which is a low-pressure system, and the gravida may have a normal blood pressure of 90/50.
2. There is dilutional anemia of pregnancy and the average hematocrit near term is 30–36.
3. The average fetal heart rate is 120–160 beats/min. Maternal hypotension leads to inadequate perfusion of the placenta and may result in fetal bradycardia. The weight of the gravid uterus on the inferior vena cava obstructs return flow to the heart and will impair cardiac output. For improved venous return, the ideal position for the pregnant patient (if not contraindicated by her injuries) is the left lateral decubitus position or with a pillow positioned under her right flank.
4. Amniotic fluid protects the fetus from most blunt trauma; however, a severe blow to the abdomen may result in separating the placenta from the uterus and premature labor.
5. In the case of drug toxicity or overdose, it is best to assume that the placenta is protection for the fetus and the maternal liver is better at detoxification than is the fetal liver. Immediate delivery is not warranted, and supportive therapy for the mother is indicated.

Genital Trauma

The perineum is very vascular and lacerations may bleed profusely; hematomas form easily in the loose connective tissue. Genital lesions are seen frequently as a result of straddle injuries in children. Vaginal or vulvar lesions may be repaired with absorbable suture and careful hemostasis. A vaginal pack for pressure may be indicated if the vagina is badly abraded and bleeding. Care must be taken to identify and ensure the integrity of the urethra. A catheterized specimen of urine should be examined for occult blood. Hematomas should be opened and drained if they are expanding and the bleeding vessel is ligated. Nonexpanding small hematomas may be observed and treated with local ice packs.

Postcoital bleeding may be secondary to a tear in the hymeneal ring. If the bleeding continues, careful examination of the bleeding site and a suture with absorbable catgut under local anesthesia is adequate. Occasionally, a cervical lesion may bleed after intercourse and may be identified during speculum examination. The cervix of a pregnant woman is very vascular and may bleed easily after coitus.

Rape

Most reported cases of rape present initially in the emergency room, and many large hospitals have a special team of nurses who make the initial contact with the victim, follow her through the examination by the physician, and have services available for counseling. The physician's role is legal as well as medical, requiring careful documentation of the history and physical and laboratory examinations as follows:

1. Obtain a consent, written and witnessed, for the examination from the patient and, if appropriate, such as for a minor, from the patient's guardian.
2. Obtain the history of the event in the patient's own words. This is the part of the medical record that is most often deficient for medicolegal purposes.
3. Record the physical examination in detail. Describe evidences of trauma on any part of the body and document with photographs if appropriate. Examine clothing for tears or stains.
4. Examine the perineum in detail. Pubic hairs may be combed for foreign objects or semen, which may be placed on a slide or in an envelope. A Wood's light on the perineum and mons may be helpful in identifying semen.
5. A swab from the vaginal pool or areas of the vulva may be used for the analysis of alkaline phosphatase (reliable up to 12 hours after intercourse). Portable kits for the analysis of alkaline phosphatase are available. A wet preparation of the vaginal pool or any area suspicious of semen should be examined for motile or nonmotile sperm.
6. A Papanicolaou smear of the same fluid may preserve evidence of sperm. All evidence should be initialed and placed in a sealed container to be given to the appropriate law enforcement officer.
7. Culture the cervix, anus, and urethra for gonococcus and obtain a serologic test for syphilis. Many experts recommend routine prophylaxis for venereal disease with 4.8 million units of procaine penicillin intramuscularly and 1 g of probenecid orally. This will protect the patient against gonorrhea and early syphilis.
8. Prevent pregnancy. Obtain a pregnancy test to rule out concomittant pregnancy.

A commonly recommended method to prevent pregnancy is the "morning after pill." This consists of a combination pill with ethinyl estradiol 0.050 mg and norgestrel 0.5 mg (Ovral); two pills are given at once and two are given after 12 hours. Patients receiving this regimen may have nausea and should be treated prophylactically with an antiemetic. See Chapter 45 for additional discussion.

SUGGESTED READINGS

Berek SJ, Stubblefield PG: Anatomical and clinical correlations of uterine perforations. *Am J Obstet Gynecol* 1979; 135:181–184.

Gregory GA: Resusitation of the newborn. *Anesthesiology* 1975; 43:225–237.

Hicks JD: Rape: Sexual assault. *Obstet Gynecol Ann* 1978;7:447–465.

International Symposium on Pelvic Inflammatory Disease: *Am J Obstet Gynecol* 1980; 138(7).

Pigani BJ: Ectopic pregnancy. *The Female Patient* 1981; 7:28–33.

Sands RX, Burnhill MS, Hakin-Elahi E: Postabortal atony. *Obstet Gynecol* 1974; 43:595–598.

Smith RP, Ross A: Postcoital contraception using DL-Norgestrol/ethinyl estradiol combination. *Contraception* 1978; 17:247–252.

Strickler RC: Dysfunctional uterine bleeding: diagnosis and treatment. *Postgrad Med* 1979; 66(5):135–146.

Yuzpe AA, Lancer WJ: Ethinyl estradiol and DL-Norgestrol as a postcoital contraceptive. *Fertil Steril* 1977; 28:932–936.

39

VASCULAR EMERGENCIES

Anthony E. Young

Nathan P. Couch

Vascular emergencies result from two mechanisms: acute obstruction and spontaneous or traumatic rupture with hemorrhage. The most common vascular emergencies encountered in the Western world are peripheral arterial occlusions, deep venous thrombosis, pulmonary embolism, ruptured aortic aneurysms, and trauma. Peripheral arteriosclerosis, heart disease, and advancing age are the principal causes of the nontraumatic vascular emergencies. The universal, crucial judgment that the emergency room physicians must form relates to the degree of threat to the patient. High risk vascular emergencies do not permit slow, detailed, time-consuming diagnostic and secondary therapeutic maneuvers.

ACUTE SPONTANEOUS ISCHEMIA OF A LIMB

Whether acute occlusion of an artery is a result of a thrombus or an embolus, failure to diagnose and treat it promptly may result in tissue or limb loss. Prompt action is especially important in patients with an embolism because the source must also be identified and treated to minimize the risk of recurrence.

The paramount diagnostic differences between peripheral arterial embolism and thrombosis relate, first, to the severity and rapidity of symptoms and, second, to the presence of heart disease. Both conditions favor people over 40 years old. It is fortuitous that only about 30% of arterial emboli lodge in the arteries supplying the brain, lungs, kidneys, spleen, or gut (visceral) (Fig. 39.1). Of the "somatic" emboli, comprising the other 70% of arterial emboli, about 75% lodge in the distal abdominal aorta or iliac, and to femoropopliteal arteries; about one-half of somatic emboli lodge in the femoral artery, one-fifth in the popliteal, and one-tenth in the aortoiliac system. The rest lodge in the upper extremities.

The heart is the most common source (85%) for emboli since they usually derive from a mural thrombus on a myocardial infarct, a diseased or artificial valve, a fibrillating atrium, or, occasionally, an atrial myxoma. A clot originating in the arterial tree itself is the next most frequent source. A clot may dislodge from an aortic, femoral, or popliteal aneurysm or from an area of atheroma. The embolus in these situations will occasionally be purely atheromatous. Another common source of embolism is the site of an arterial needle puncture performed for arteriography. Rarely, clots may occur in areas of vasculitis or from subclavian compression by a cervical rib or other thoracic outlet stenosis. Tumor emboli in the vascular tree are rare.

A *paradoxical embolus* is an embolus originating in the venous circulation that reaches the systemic arterial circulation by way of a patent foramen ovale. It is rare, but should be thought of when there is no other identifiable source of the embolus. Pulmonary embolism may precede paradoxical embolism because the subsequent increase in right atrial pressure will induce the right-to-left shunt.

Arterial thrombosis never occurs in healthy people with normal arteries. A great majority of thromboses are superimposed on preexisting atherosclerotic arterial disease, the site usually being the lower limbs (Fig. 39.2). Thrombosis may occur without any obvious precipitating cause or may reflect an episode of dehydration, hypotension, or low cardiac output from whatever cause. Malignancy, oral contraceptives, myeloproliferative disorders, thrombocythemia, homocystinuria, macroglobulinemia, or snake bite (Russell's viper and American copperhead) are sometimes associated with spontaneous arterial thrombosis. Investigations that involve puncturing the brachial artery at the elbow are associated with local arterial thrombosis in approximately 3% of cases. When the site of arterial puncture is the radial artery at the wrist, the incidence of thrombosis is very much higher, though it is only rarely associated with important symptoms.

Thrombosis of the popliteal artery sometimes occurs as a result of popliteal artery entrapment in young people, but this is extremely rare. Arterial spasm with superimposed thrombosis may also occur in inadvertent or intentional drug users from intraarterial or periarterial injection of drugs.

Evaluation

HISTORY AND PHYSICAL EXAMINATION

The most common initial symptom of acute arterial occlusion, whether embolic or thrombotic, is pain, widely ranging in degree. It may be gripping, cramping, or constant and involve variable amounts of the distal leg, that is, the foot alone, the lower leg and foot, or progressively longer segments ranging as high as the groin and buttock. In a matter of hours, paresis and paresthesias appear, signaling ischemic nerve injury. Limb

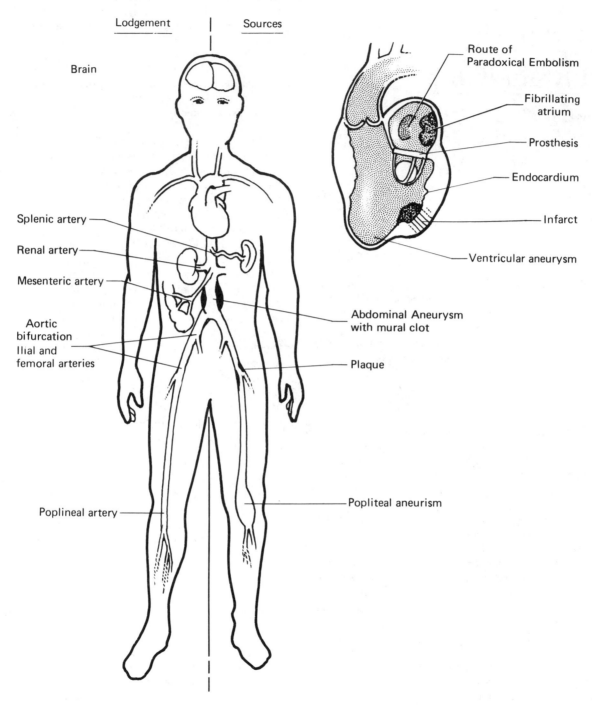

Figure 39.1 Sites of sources and the somatic lodgment of arterial emboli.

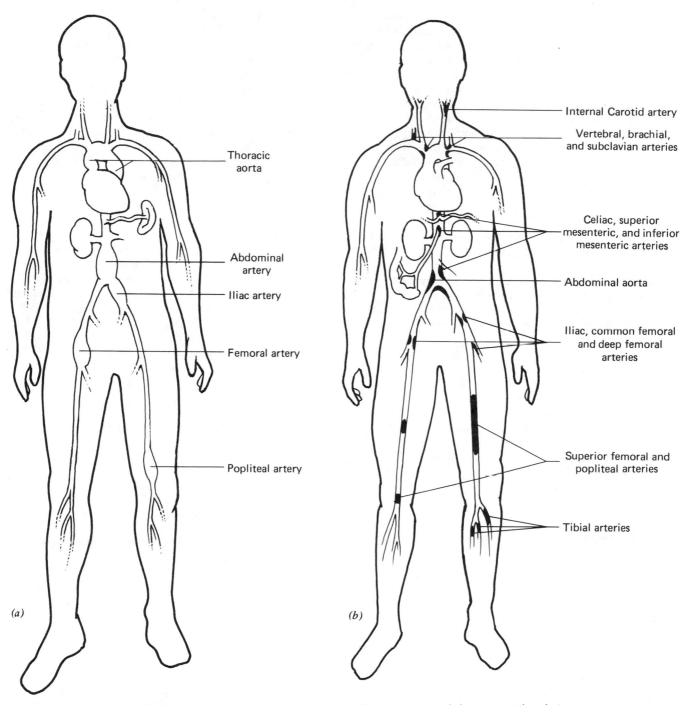

Figure 39.2 (a) Common sites of arterial aneurysm. (b) Common sites of chronic arterial occlusions.

function may be completely lost, and as the process evolves further, the involved limb becomes pallid, then marbled and cold. The extent of cyanosis directly depends on the amount of blood continuing to reach the extremity, however sluggish the flow.

Overall, the severity and extent of the symptoms depend on the level of embolic lodgment or thrombosis, the proportion of arterial cross section that is occluded, and the total length of the occlusion. For example, a large aortic bifurcation embolus may produce extreme ischemia with eventual circulatory collapse because of massive release of potassium or lactic acid from the leg muscles, especially if abrupt reflow is produced by surgical means, whereas a lesser occlusion such as a tibial arterial thrombosis may produce trivial symptoms or only a cool, minimally painful foot. Thrombosis of a previously stenotic superficial femoral artery may result only in shortening of claudication distance. Thus the symptoms and findings of ischemia may be less severe in patients with arterial thrombosis, although the history and physical examination may not enable the emergency room physician to make the distinction.

In severe cases the diagnosis is obvious: the limb is white, pulseless, cold, and motionless. In less severe cases, close examination of the whole vascular tree is essential not only to confirm the diagnosis but also to interpret the present signs in relation to preexisting arterial occlusions. In particular, all pulses must be felt, and discolored or ischemic patches on digits and crack and ulcers on the heel must be noted. Any temperature differences between the limbs must be observed together with deep tenderness or loss of sensation. These signs must be interpreted in relation to any history of claudication, rest pain, palpitations, or previous episodes of acute ischemia. The patient must be closely examined to seek evidence of other small emboli. This will include fundoscopy, careful palpation of the spleen and kidneys, and examination of the urine for red blood cells. A search must also be made for the origin of the embolus; this will particularly involve special examinations of the heart, including continuous electrocardiogram (ECG) monitoring, sequential 12-lead ECG's, and echocardiography.

Certain features enable the clinician to distinguish embolism from thrombosis (Table 39.1). In embolism, the absence of chronic ischemic symptoms and the presence of heart disease are more frequent findings than in thrombosis. The physical examination is less useful in the distinction: in both conditions local findings are similar, although arrhythmias are much more likely to be present in embolism.

OTHER EXAMINATIONS

Diagnosis of acute occlusion is primarily a clinical one, and time should not be spent by the emergency room physician performing angiography merely to confirm the diagnosis before consulting the vascular surgeon. Angiography may be indicated before thrombectomy or embolectomy is undertaken, but it is not always urgent. Doppler ultrasound examination may be useful to follow the pulse distally from its lowest palpable level to the actual point of thrombosis or lodgment of an embolus. Laboratory data may, however, help greatly; the ECG and myocardial enzymes are usually normal in thrombosis but can be abnormal in embolism, and the arteriogram can often make the distinction since collateral arteries, diffuse atheromata, and absence of a meniscoid center contour of the proximal end of the occlusion characterize thrombosis but not embolism.

MANAGEMENT

The treatments of emboli and thrombosis differ. An embolus may cause persistent major ischemia for 12–24 hours before onset of necrosis, but irreversible muscle and nerve damage may occur after only 6 hours. Ischemia as a result of noncritical thrombosis only requires urgent treatment when it is secondary to arterial injury. When it is a complication of long-standing atherosclerosis, investigation and definitive surgery need not be undertaken in the first few hours or even the first day when there is sufficient collateral circulation to preserve the limb. But in all cases in which the emergency room physician notes severe ischemia, early consultation with the vascular surgeon is mandatory.

The objective of treatment is the restoration of blood flow. In the case of small emboli lodged proximally this will sometimes occur spontaneously if the clot breaks up, passes distally, and is lysed. If this does not happen within 3 hours and there

TABLE 39.1 Comparative Clinical Findings: Arterial Occlusions of the Extremities

	Embolism	Thrombosis
Age	40 or older	40 or older
Heart disease (Myocardial infarction, Arrhythmia, Valvular)	+ + + +	+ +
Prior limb symptoms, esp claudication	0	+ +
Severe ischemia	+ + +	+ +
Absent pulses	+ + + +	+ + + +
Arteriographic findings	Useful	Useful

is no return of major pulses, color, and temperature to the limb, then embolectomy will be required if the leg is to be saved or spared from long-term ischemic symptoms. Success of embolectomy is directly proportional to the promptness with which it is undertaken. Even the very sick patient with cardiac disease can withstand an embolectomy performed under local anesthesia using a Fogarty catheter.

In general management, the following principles should be adhered to:

1. *Avoid heat.* The metabolic demands of cool tissue are lower than those of warm tissue. Reheating does not restore circulation. Therefore an ischemic limb should be kept cool. It should be left outside of the bed clothes. Hot water bottles or heating blankets should not, under any circumstances, be applied to the limb.

2. *Avoid elevation of the limb.* Gravity will improve what circulation remains. The head of the bed should be raised 6–10 inches.

3. *Avoid pressure damage to ischemic areas.* The heel should be padded with cotton or wool, or the limb should be placed on a sheepskin.

4. *Any underlying or precipitating disease such as dehydration or congestive cardiac failure should be promptly treated.*

5. *Heparinization is required in patients with emboli to reduce the development of other potential emboli at the source.* There is no clear evidence that anticoagulants significantly reduce the incidence of thrombosis distal to an embolus or arterial thrombosis, and physicians vary as to their use of heparin in this context. In situations in which embolism is a result of bacterial endocarditis, heparinization is contraindicated because of the risk of bleeding from septic microemboli in the cerebral circulation. Vasodilator drugs and sympathectomy are of no value in the early management of acute ischemia.

Additional Clinical Settings of Acute Ischemia

LATE PRESENTATION OF ACUTE ISCHEMIA

Occasionally a patient with an acute embolus or thrombosis will not reach a hospital until irreversible changes have occurred. The limb will then show either developing or established gangrene. How this is to be managed depends on the form the gangrene takes, but ice packing should *not* be performed in the emergency room. Wet gangrene with infection and spreading cellulitis requires prompt amputation. Dry gangrene is followed conservatively until a clear line of demarcation is established. Only then is amputation indicated.

RENAL ARTERY EMBOLISM

Renal artery embolism is uncommon and may be difficult to diagnose clinically. It is sometimes characterized by constant, aching loin pain associated with a tender enlarged kidney, but may also be asymptomatic. There is associated hematuria. It is only rarely possible to salvage the kidney.

MESENTERIC ARTERY THROMBOSIS AND EMBOLISM

Symptomatic mesenteric ischemia occurs after the sudden blockage of the celiac, inferior mesenteric, or, more frequently, the superior mesenteric artery by an embolus. Where the overall mesenteric circulation has been impaired by arteriosclerosis, a low flow state such as cardiac failure or infarction can help to propagate thrombosis and precipitate serious ischemia. Very rarely is the patient persuasively symptomatic before development of catastrophic bowel infarction and necrosis is recognized and surgically treated.

The immediate symptom is acute colicky abdominal pain of sudden onset, which is sometimes associated with vomiting or bloody diarrhea. After several hours this gives way to the symptoms of bowel infarction: continuous pain, peritonitis, and circulatory collapse. Survival of the patient at this stage is almost impossible. Once the condition is recognized, brisk resuscitation with intravenous fluids, antibiotics, and early laparotomy are required. Occasionally it is possible to perform embolectomy or a revascularization procedure, but if the changes are irreversible, salvage is only possible in situations in which resection of the bowel can spare enough absorptive surface to permit survival.

ACUTE PRESENTATION OF SMALL VESSEL DISEASE

Peripheral arterial diseases that predominantly involve the small vessels of the extremities include Raynaud's disease, causalgia, Buerger's disease, ergotism, erythermalgia, scleroderma, systemic lupus erythematosus, and the cryoglobulinopathies. All may present acutely, usually as pain. In general they are differentiated from other vascular disease by presence of peripheral pulses. A discussion of their differential diagnosis is outside the scope of this book; for further information see the Suggested Readings at the end of this chapter. Treatment of all of these conditions when seen in the emergency room can merely be symptomatic since the tissue necrosis that may occur is chronic, of limited and small extent, and cannot be prevented by acute, direct therapy.

ANEURYSMS

Thoracic and dissecting aneurysms are discussed in Chapter 4.

Abdominal Aortic Aneurysms

Most abdominal aortic aneurysms occur in patients over the age of 60, and about 95% are atherosclerotic. Although smoking increases the risk of incurring an abdominal aortic aneurysm, the lesion fairly often affects nonsmokers. Hypertension is also a risk factor in patients with such aneurysms and present in about 50% of patients. The incidence of abdominal aortic aneurysms ranges from 0.6% to 1% of hospital admissions. The male-to-female ratio of incidence is about six. The overall mortality rate from atherosclerotic abdominal aneurysms is about four per 100,000 population.

DIAGNOSIS

The nonruptured abdominal aortic aneurysm may be asymptomatic (but often diagnosable by physical examination) or chronically symptomatic with abdominal or back pain or a sensation of throbbing. The ruptured aneurysm is always symptomatic and there is acute abdominal, back, or groin pain. Whether or not the aneurysm is ruptured, the pain probably arises from stretching of the aortic wall, or the overlying peritoneum, or even the duodenum. The aneurysm need not rupture into the free peritoneal cavity; if it does, survival is unlikely. More often, the hematoma is contained by tamponade in the retroperitoneal space. For this reason, if the containment occurs before 10–15% of the patient's blood volume is lost, the patient may survive many hours or days or long enough to be saved by emergency operation. If the patient has fainted, the blood loss has probably been 20% or more.

Because the patient's only chance for surviving a ruptured abdominal aneurysm is early diagnosis and treatment, the lesion should be thought of in any hypotensive patient who is over age 50 and complaining of acute abdominal or back pain, especially if the patient is a man, is a smoker, or has a history of hypertension. A tender, widely pulsatile abdominal mass should confirm the suspicion, especially if it is in the epigastrium (Fig. 39.3).

If the patient does not receive emergency surgical treatment, death from further hemorrhage is inevitable. If surgery occurs, but only after shock and acute renal failure have begun, the chance for survival is very small.

If the patient has already passed through a syncopal attack or an episode of hypotension, delay for x-rays or any time-

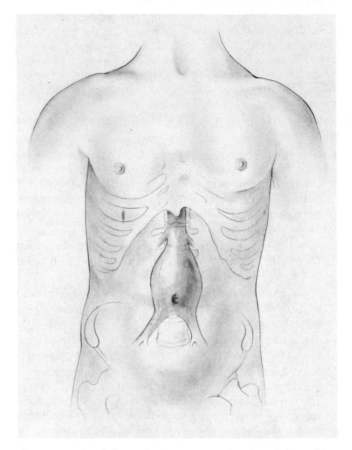

Figure 39.3 The abdominal aortic aneurysm is epigastric in position.

consuming diagnostic work is contraindicated. If the patient has had no evidence of hypovolemia but nevertheless has a tender, wide abdominal pulsatile mass, an emergency abdominal film (anteroposterior and lateral lumbosacral spine film) or ultrasounds can be done, provided that such a study can be performed in less than 2 hours.

But it cannot be stressed too heavily that resuscitation must precede all diagnostic investigations (see below) and patients should never be moved to the x-ray department merely to confirm an obvious diagnosis.

Aneurysms of any size can rupture, although the risk is 35–40% for those of greater than 6 cm in diameter and about 20% for those that are smaller. If rupture or acute expansion of a smaller aneurysm is suspected but the pulsatile mass is impalpable, ultrasound scanning may also be necessary if the vital signs are stable. If the latter test is unavailable, anteroposterior and lateral lumbosacral x-ray films may be made. Only rarely is it advisable to perform aortography since this type of study will be needed only where a question of major aortic branch artery occlusion (e.g., by dissection) is raised.

Because of the extremely high risk of allowing abdominal aortic aneurysms to proceed to rupture, the primary care physician plays a pivotal role by diagnosing such aneurysms earlier in their course. They may then be treated electively by an operation that now carries, in experienced hands, a mortality of 5% or less.

MANAGEMENT

Elective resection of abdominal aortic aneurysms is indicated in any good-risk patient with an aneurysm diameter greater than 5 cm whether or not symptoms are present. On the other hand, it is generally felt that in poor-risk patients, that is, those with important vital organ disease, asymptomatic aneurysms smaller than 7 cm should not be operated upon until they enlarge or become symptomatic. The diameter is usually measured periodically, at 6–12-month intervals, by ultrasound scanning.

For the patient with a suspected ruptured abdominal aortic aneurysm, the first duty of the physician is to treat, or prevent, severe hypotension. At least two large-caliber (14 gauge) intravenous lines are inserted to permit rapid infusion. When hypotension is already present, whole blood is infused as soon as it is available. In this regard, it should be recalled that hypotension is relative; that is, important decreases from the hypertensive levels to which many such patients become accustomed, even if normal in the normal population, may represent serious underperfusion. The use of the gravity, or "G," suit is really of unproven value in resuscitating patients with ruptured aneurysms; if it results in delayed operative control of bleeding, it may be dangerous. As indicated above, delay for diagnostic studies may also be dangerous.

The treatment for expanding aneurysms (i.e., acutely enlarging but unruptured aneurysms) is emergency resection and graft replacement. Nothing will be gained, and perhaps a life will be lost, if surgery is delayed in the hope that further transfusion will reverse the hypotension because the blood pressure can only be supported by decisive control of the aortic bleeding. Obviously, success of aneurysmectomy is inversely proportional to the severity and duration of hypotension pre- and intraoperatively. Patients who are *not* in shock preoperatively have approximately one-half of the 80–100% mortality rate of those who are in shock. Moreover, the prognosis is especially bad if before the surgery the patient is oliguric, has coronary artery or severe pulmonary disease, is physiologically aged, or

has important other vital organ insufficiency. Despite these risk factors, an attempt at emergency surgery is almost always warranted because the result of omitting surgery is uniformly fatal.

Resection and graft replacement for the elective, nonruptured abdominal aortic aneurysm is performed after careful assessment of heart, lung, and kidney function, aortography (to identify aortic branch arterial anomalies), and mechanical bowel preparation. Although diligent support of pulmonary, renal, and cardiac function is necessary for the first 2–3 days, almost all (about 95%) patients make a rapid, smooth recovery and are discharged 8–10 days after their operations.

The long-term prognosis after successful repair of a ruptured aneurysm is similar to that of successful elective aneurysmectomy, namely, about 60% of patients are still alive after 5 years. This is to be compared with an approximately 80% 5-year survival of the "normal" population matched for age and sex.

Iliac, Popliteal, and Femoral Aneurysms

ILIAC ANEURYSMS

Iliac aneurysms are commonly found in association with abdominal aortic aneurysms and are generally impossible to diagnose by physical examination. Precisely for this reason, they are treacherous. That is to say, the patient with a solitary iliac aneurysm that is unassociated with a palpable abdominal aortic aneurysm is at a much less avoidable risk for rupture than is the patient who has the latter. Fortunately rupture of iliac aneurysms occurs in only 1% or 2% of aneurysms that rupture in the aortoiliac system. If diagnosed, their treatment is quite similar to that for abdominal aneurysms.

POPLITEAL ANEURYSMS

Popliteal aneurysms, though much less frequent than abdominal aneurysms, are of serious consequence not because they rupture (which they do not), but because they result in limb loss either through *in situ* thrombosis or repeated popliteotibial embolism of mounting severity to the point of surgically uncorrectable ischemia. Typically such patients give a history of repeated episodes of calf or foot pain, with intervals of spontaneous partial relief, and report for treatment only when the pain or short-range claudication becomes unbearable. Very often the aneurysm is palpable at or above the knee, with or without a pulse, depending upon how thoroughly thrombosis has occurred. In 20–30% of such patients another popliteal aneurysm will be found in the opposite leg. On the symptomatic side, other indications for ischemia, in varying degrees, will be found; these include pallor and coolness of the ankle and foot, muscular weakness, absent ankle pulses, and even hypesthesia or skin ulcers in the more severe cases. Arteriography will indicate the degree of arterial occlusion and, if thrombosis of the aneurysm itself has not occurred, arteriography will usually outline the extent of the aneurysm, especially if there is very little mural thrombus. The treatment is surgical and the urgency depends upon the severity of the ischemia. The preferred technique entails exclusion of the aneurysm with proximal and distal ligatures along with vein bypass grafting. If the aneurysm is so large that size alone results in compression symptoms, all of the clot is evacuated and the medial sac wall is removed.

FEMORAL ANEURYSMS

Femoral aneurysms are fairly rare, are important because they also thrombose or embolize like popliteal aneurysms, and can be treated surgically by resection and interposition grafting or by exclusion, evacuation, and bypass grafting.

With reference to surgical indications in asymptomatic patients, the mere presence of an iliac, popliteal, or femoral arterial aneurysm is usually an indication for repair.

VASCULAR INJURIES

Almost any form of trauma can injure arteries and veins. Knife wounds, gunshot wounds, open or closed fractures, contusions by blunt objects, and dislocations of joints may produce all grades of vascular injury from intimal damage through thrombosis and spasm to arterial disruptions. Venous injury is associated with arterial injury in 40% of traumatic injuries. The arterial injury is the most important.

Arterial injury will be obvious on examination if arterial blood is pulsating from a wound. Arterial bleeding, however, may be occurring when there is only a slight trickle of blood from an open wound, and the diagnosis in the case will be clear from the presence of an expanding, palpable, deep hematoma. Vascular injury may cause loss of peripheral pulses if there is interruption of a main vessel or if there is thrombosis or spasm secondary to injury. Side injury to a vessel or damage to a major tributary will, however, not affect the peripheral pulses, but treatment is nevertheless urgently required. Perivascular hematoma and spasm occasionally play a part in the loss of distal pulses after proximal vascular injury, but this is not a diagnosis to be made in the emergency room. Loss of peripheral pulses in arterial injury is a result of thrombosis or disruption of a vessel until proven otherwise. Posttraumatic arterial spasm is a diagnosis made at operation. In cases of gun shot wounds, remoteness of entry and exit wounds from arteries does not exclude vascular injury. Low-velocity missiles may ricochet or track along tissue planes, and high-velocity bullets cause tissue disruption at a considerable distance from the track of the missile.

DIAGNOSIS

Traumatic arterial injury is a clinical diagnosis and preoperative angiography is not necessarily indicated. A normal angiogram does not exclude significant arterial injury. Spurting hemorrhage from a wound, loss of distal pulse, and the presence of a bruit or a pulsatile or expanding hematoma show that arterial injury has occurred, and exploration is required. If a distal pulse is lost in association with a fracture or dislocation but returns when the fracture or dislocation is reduced, then an emergency operation is not required. The patient's pulse should be carefully watched over the ensuing hours lest posttraumatic arterial thrombosis supervene. The mechanism in this instance is usually an intimal tear occurring at the time of injury or the compressive affect of a perivascular hematoma.

MANAGEMENT

Good access for transfusion must be established in a limb other than the one traumatized. Vascular injuries frequently occur in young people in whom compensation for blood loss is good unless the blood loss is very major when sudden decompensation occurs. It is therefore important to estimate blood loss from the size of the hematoma and descriptions of blood seen at the time of injury. Transfusion should be in proportion to this assessed loss rather than the pulse rate, blood pressure, urine flow, and hemoglobin. The hemoglobin concentration is particularly misleading since it may remain in the normal range for many hours after untreated acute hemorrhage.

The success of the treatment of vascular injuries is measured by the amputation rate. In World War II amputation rate after vascular injury was approximately 50%; in Vietnam it was about 12%. These better results were due to the promptness of definitive surgery. Popliteal arterial injuries carry a higher risk of amputation than iliofemoral injuries because the collateral circulation is less adequate. Successful surgery relies on the anastomosis of divided vessels or the replacement of traumatized vessels by interposed vein grafts or patches. It is important therefore that damage to vessels is not worsened by attempts at direct hemostasis with instruments. Hemostasis in emergency situations should therefore be achieved by pressure over the wound, by proximal pressure over the bleeding artery, or, if the configuration of the wound allows it, by tourniquet.

Delving into wounds with hemostats other than in the operating theater is to be condemned even if the spurting artery can be seen. If an arterial injury has rendered the periphery ischemic, the same care of the periphery (e.g., padding and avoidance of injury) should be taken as after arterial thrombosis or embolism.

Tourniquets

Tourniquets (or blood pressure cuffs) should be avoided if possible. Although they are an effective form of hemostasis, they also act to occlude collateral blood flow into the injured limb. If the use of a tourniquet is inescapable, it must be put on tightly enough to occlude the arterial inflow and as distally as possible. This may be difficult to judge if, at the outset, the hemorrhage is not great. If the tourniquet is not put on tightly enough it will merely occlude the venous outflow while allowing continuing arterial inflow. This worsens the bleeding. If a tourniquet is applied and surgical hemostasis is not quickly available, the tourniquet must be released for a few seconds every half-hour. To ensure that this is done, the time at which the tourniquet was applied should be clearly written on the patient's skin or on a label attached to the tourniquet. If the tourniquet remains in place for several hours, extensive distal thrombosis may occur and, in addition, reflow on release of the tourniquet may flush toxic metabolites into the systemic circulation causing circulatory collapse and even renal failure (akin to the so-called crush syndrome).

Anterior Tibial Compartment Syndrome

If severe ischemia in the territory of the anterior tibial artery exists for more than a few hours, swelling of the anterior tibial muscles often occurs. This also happens after surgical relief of the ischemia. Since the anterior tibial compartment is a closed anatomical structure, this swelling interferes with the function of the anterior tibial muscle and the long extensors of the toes, causing foot drop and inability to dorsiflex the toes. If decompressed early by fasciotomy, function will return. If the compartment is known to have suffered prolonged ischemia, the fasciotomy is best performed prophylactically at the time of arterial repair.

Venous Injury

Venous injury is commonly associated with arterial injury. Hemorrhage may occur early or thrombosis may occur later. An arteriovenous fistula may also develop, but this is less common. Venous thrombosis secondary to trauma is important because it partly jeopardizes the chance of recovery from an arterial injury. It also carries the risk of pulmonary embolism. Traumatic arteriovenous fistulae may develop as a result of a concomitant injury in an adjacent artery and vein. The clinical signs of arteriovenous fistulae—a machinerylike murmur, distended peripheral veins, and a tachycardia—may be absent or attributable to another cause in the first few hours after an injury. A tachycardia as a result of the presence of a distal arteriovenous fistula will disappear if the artery proximal to the fistula is compressed (Branham sign).

Traumatic Aortic Rupture

Rapid horizontal deceleration (such as when the driver of an automobile strikes his or her chest on the steering wheel in a head-on impact) may rupture the aorta. The rupture is the result of differentiated deceleration of the mobile heart and aortic arch from the fixed, descending aorta. The effect of this is to shear the aorta just below the origin of the left subclavian artery. In most instances this results in immediate death, but in about one case in five, clot and the limiting effects of the ribs and pleura prevent catastrophic hemorrhage. These patients are in shock, and a chest radiograph shows a hematoma or a false aneurysm. Without treatment, this progresses to fatal rupture. Surgical repair of the lesion, if undertaken promptly, is usually successful (see Chapter 20).

Iatrogenic Vascular Injuries

The most important and most common physician-induced vascular injury is thrombotic arterial occlusion as a result of retrograde catheter angiography. Where the brachial artery has suffered thrombosis, for example, after the Sones mode of left side of the heart catheterization, the findings include the following: (1) numbness, coolness, or pain in the forearm and hand; (2) prompt fatiguing of the forearm muscles with exercise; and (3) pallor and coolness of the hand with absent wrist pulses. The brachial pulse is usually palpable in the proximal one-third of the upper arm. These findings are virtually always a result of thrombosis, not arterial spasm, and treatment is early thrombectomy.

If the femoral artery has been used for left heart catheterization (Judkins technique), thrombosis will induce much more dramatic findings in the foot and lower part of the leg since there will be marked coldness, numbness, pain, and weakness. Prompt operative correction is always mandatory in the presence of such findings.

Another important iatrogenic cause of acute arterial occlusion is the excessively tight plaster cast. This is a prime reason for the time-honored "cast check" within 24 hours of application and for the deliberate exposure of the fingers or toes for assessment of circulation.

Iatrogenic venous injuries are of lesser importance, and include septic superficial thrombophlebitis as a result of overlong use of a venous access site, escape of an indwelling plastic catheter into the proximal venous system, and popliteal vein compression as a result of prolonged use of a knee rest for procedures performed in lithotomy position. Prevention is the key to the management of all of these conditions.

Treatment of the septic phlebitis is removal of the offending needle or cannula, application of local heat, and antibiotics as determined by cultures. The lost plastic catheter should be extracted by appropriate surgical means or by angiographic devices. The popliteal vein occlusion is treated by elastic support to the calf, elevation, and, if bleeding is not a hazard, anticoagulation.

A special variety of iatrogenic emergencies has appeared in recent years with the everwidening use of percutaneously inserted subclavian or internal jugular intravenous lines. These complications include hemo- or hydrothorax, pericardial tamponade, and pneumothorax. Withdrawal of the offending line is usually sufficient, but when the complication is major, the air or fluid may require evacuation. A later complication, decreasing in frequency, is simple sepsis, which is primarily treated by withdrawal of the plastic catheter.

Strictly speaking, the late complications of arterial reconstructive operations are also iatrogenic. Except for thromboses that result in severe ischemia or false aneurysms that enlarge suddenly or rupture (e.g., the aortoduodenal fistula), these complications do not usually constitute emergencies. In all such cases, however, a vascular surgeon should still be consulted.

VENOUS THROMBOSIS

Venous thrombosis may be presented in one of the following three ways: (1) as pain in the leg, (2) as the effects of venous obstruction, or (3) as pulmonary embolism.

Venous Thrombosis Presenting as Pain in the Leg

There are two categories of venous thrombosis that cause pain in the leg. One is *deep venous thrombosis* in which thrombosis is confined to the deep veins of the calf, thigh, or pelvis; the pain experienced is a dull, deep-seated ache worsened by standing, or dependency, or exercise; the clinical signs may be very few. The other is *superficial thrombophlebitis* in which thrombosis occurs in superficial veins, inflammation of the wall is the primary phenomenon, and therefore tenderness over the vein is easy to elicit.

DIAGNOSIS

Diagnostic tests for venous thrombosis that are noninvasive and can be done in the emergency room may claim to identify significant thromboses. These include Doppler ultrasound studies, impedance plethysmography, and thermography. They are, however, unreliable; all of the techniques have a significant number of false–positive and false–negative results. The most reliable diagnostic measure for venous thrombosis is contrast radiographic phlebography. Phlebography is performed for two reasons. The first is to confirm the presence of venous thrombosis. The second is to determine the extent of the thrombosis and specifically to identify any clot that is loose and capable of embolizing. Ideally, phlebography should be performed bilaterally since venous thrombosis is frequently bilateral—even if there are only unilateral symptoms. But many clinicians compromise and perform unilateral phlebography if the finding is positive.

Deep Venous Thrombosis

The classic signs of *deep venous thrombosis* are unreliable. More than one-half of the cases of significant deep venous thrombosis are completely devoid of positive physical signs. By contrast about one-half of the patients who are investigated by phlebography because venous thrombosis is suspected from signs such as calf tenderness are found to have entirely normal veins. Unilateral ankle edema or distention of superficial veins is, however, suspicious and if associated with tenderness in response to calf palpation should be investigated.

Fully developed iliofemoral thrombosis produces a more dramatic and obvious picture. There is rapid development of thigh and groin pain and gross brawny edema of the limb. The veins are distended and the limb may appear congested to the point of cyanosis. There is often tenderness over the femoral vein in the groin. If severe, and there is thrombosis of collaterals as well as of the iliofemoral system, then the tissue tension in the limb may lead to arterial inflow occlusion with peripheral ischemia that may lead to gangrene. This has been called by the archaic term *phlegmasia cerulea dolens,* whereas the less-severe, nongangrenous form has been called *phlegmasia alba dolens.* Both are merely advanced forms of iliofemoral deep venous thrombosis. Similar severe symptoms may also be produced by spontaneous thrombosis of the inferior vena cava.

These more proximal thromboses may be associated with malaise and fever. If there is ischemia, a primary venous cause is suggested by the gross edema that is always present.

When thrombosis occurs in superficial veins, inflammation of the wall of the vein is usually the primary cause. In deep vein thrombosis, however, inflammation of the wall is a secondary phenomenon and occurs late in the course of the disease. Hence, pain and tenderness on palpation of the calf or over the course of the femoral vein is a late sign.

Patients particularly at risk from venous thrombosis are those who have recently been resting in bed with some other illness, have been subjected to surgery within the previous few weeks, are pregnant, or have neoplasia or other debilitating diseases such as congestive cardiac failure. Women who take oral contraceptives have a higher than normal incidence of spontaneous venous thrombosis, particularly if they also smoke. Venous thrombosis in the axillary vein is uncommon and is most frequently attributable to the hyperabducting effort associated, for example, with chopping wood or hanging pictures. Any of the predisposing causes already mentioned may also be involved.

Superficial Thrombophlebitis

Superficial thrombophlebitis can occur at any site but the most common is in a varicose vein. The diagnosis is usually obvious, the involved vein being palpably thrombosed, hot and tender to touch. The overlying skin sometimes is discolored. There may be malaise with fever. Superficial thrombophlebitis is not normally associated with a risk of pulmonary embolism but embolism from thrombosis in the long saphenous vein has been reported. It may occur when thrombosis occurs high in the long saphenous vein and when a tongue of clot extends into the femoral vein. Superficial thrombophlebitis is only rarely associated with deep vein thrombosis.

When superficial thrombophlebitis occurs at separate sites on separate occasions (thrombophlebitis migrans), underlying neoplasia should be suspected but it is not often found. When it is found it is most likely to be in the bronchus or pancreas.

Pulmonary Embolism

Pulmonary embolism is discussed in Chapters 2 and 3. In at least 50% of cases of pulmonary embolism, no signs of peripheral thrombosis are evident even though the iliofemoral system has been the source of clot. Concern for treating the pulmonary embolism should not detract from a search for the origin of the clot and its treatment since early recurrence of pulmonary embolism is frequent and may prove fatal.

Management of Venous Thrombosis

There are two facets to the management of venous thrombosis. One is the relief of symptoms; the other is the prophylaxis of thromboembolism (Fig. 39.4).

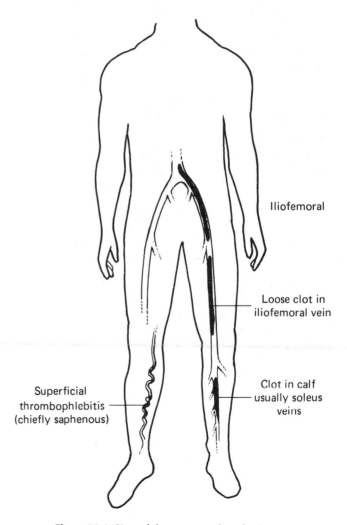

Figure 39.4 Sites of deep venous thrombosis.

SYMPTOMATIC TREATMENT

Superficial thrombophlebitis rarely requires more than symptomatic treatment. Firm elastic bandaging and mild analgesia will often suffice, and the patient should continue to be mobile with elastic (Ace) bandages. This encourages a good venous return and discourages extension of the clot. If deep venous thrombosis is the cause of symptoms in the leg, the patient should also continue to be mobile if the symptoms are mild. If there is swelling and substantial pain, the patient should be instructed to rest in bed with the foot of the bed elevated. Hot packs or towels may relieve the pain. The pain will usually require mild analgesia for its relief. Phenylbutazone (Butazolidine) is not especially effective and because of side effects is contraindicated. Compounds containing aspirin should be avoided if the patient is to be anticoagulated since aspirin may provoke gastrointestinal bleeding and also make smooth anticoagulation difficult.

PROPHYLAXIS OF PULMONARY EMBOLISM AND POSTPHLEBITIC SYNDROME

The risk of pulmonary embolism is greatest when the signs of deep venous thrombosis are the least. Furthermore, postphlebitic syndrome (edema, induration, pigmentation, and ulceration of the lower part of the leg) can occur after apparently minor venous thrombosis. These facts mean that deep venous thrombosis should usually be treated with anticoagulants. An accurate and objective confirmation of the diagnosis is therefore essential because the clinical signs are unreliable, and reliance on them would allow many cases of deep venous thrombosis to go untreated and many instances of trivial superficial thrombophlebitis or even muscle pain to be treated with anticoagulants.

Once the diagnosis of deep vein thrombosis is established, the most common treatment is anticoagulation unless there are specific contraindications. Anticoagulation should initially be with heparin (dose 5,000–7,500 units as a bolus, then 500–1,000 units/hr in continuous IV) and should be commenced with the patient in the hospital. A 3–7-day course of heparin therapy is followed by oral anticoagulants (warfarin), and these should be continued for 2 or 3 months. Anticoagulants will reduce or prevent propagation of the thrombosis and its development at other sites. It may also aid recanalization of clot and reduce damage to venous valves. Both of these latter effects probably reduce the likelihood of the late development of postphlebitic syndrome. Thrombolytic agents such as urokinase and streptokinase may also be used, but they require experienced practitioners and should not be applied in the emergency room.

If phlebography shows a major unattached clot that is judged to be capable of embolizing, some form of surgical venous interruption may be needed. This may take the form of a superficial femoral vein ligation or a nonoccluding clip on the inferior vena cava or iliac veins. The site for interruption is judged from the phlebogram. Heparin can discourage propagation of thrombus, but it will not dissolve clots, hence the need for venous interruption procedures.

Because rethrombosis is so common, venous thrombectomy is not normally used except to save a limb threatened by ischemia in association with severe iliofemoral phlebothrombosis.

SUGGESTED READINGS

Gaspar MR, Barker WF: Peripheral arterial disease, in Ebert P (ed): *Major Problems in Clinical Surgery,* ed 3. Philadelphia, WB Saunders Co, 1981, vol 4, p 504.

Hardy JD: *Critical Surgical Illness,* ed 2. Philadelphia, WB Saunders Co, 1980, p 702.

Hill GJ: *Outpatient Surgery,* ed 2. Philadelphia, WB Saunders Co, 1980, p 1457.

Juergens JL, Spittell JA Jr, Fairbairn JF II: *Allen-Barker-Hines Peripheral Vascular Diseases,* ed 5. Philadelphia, WB Saunders Co, 1980, p 981.

40
HEMATOLOGIC EMERGENCIES

David S. Rosenthal
W.B. Jerry Younger

ANEMIA

Anemia is not a disease but a manifestation of an underlying disorder that causes blood loss, increased red blood cell destruction, or decreased red blood cell production. It is defined in the clinical laboratory as a decrease in the hematocrit or hemoglobin level. The *hematocrit* is a volume measurement that estimates the red blood cell volume as a fraction of the total blood volume. A hematocrit of less than 40% in men or 36% in women indicates anemia. The *hemoglobin* is a concentration measurement and is usually expressed in g/dl of blood. The range of values for normal hemoglobin in men is usually considered to be 14–18 g/dl and in women 12–16 g/dl. Red blood cell (RBC) counts are not as accurate a guide in the diagnosis of anemia as are the hemoglobin and hematocrit because of variations in the hemoglobin content of the individual red blood cells. For example, a patient with classical iron deficiency anemia may have a normal number of red blood cells, but these cells will be smaller than normal (causing a decreased hematocrit) and contain little hemoglobin (decreased hemoglobin concentration).

There are three major mechanisms or categories of anemia:

1. Blood loss: acute or chronic
2. Anemia of decreased production
   a. Iron deficiency
   b. Vitamin B_{12} or folate deficiency
   c. Bone marrow infiltration or aplasia
3. Anemia of increased destruction
   a. Hemolytic anemias

Red cells are (1) lost by excessive bleeding (gastrointestinal, hematuria, etc.), (2) not produced in sufficient amounts by the bone marrow, or (3) lost within the body because of an inherent defect of the red blood cell or an environmental attack on the cell removing it from the circulation well before the end of its normal life span (hemolysis).

Evaluation of the Patient

HISTORY AND PHYSICAL EXAMINATION

Anemia may be recognized by the emergency room physician because of the patient's complaints or physical presentation. Fatigue, weakness, and increasing respiratory or cardiac symptoms are nonspecific complaints and will vary depending on the severity and rapidity of onset of the anemia. Pallor, tachycardia, scleral icterus, and splenomegaly are findings that may alert the physician to anemia. When the hematocrit is reduced below 30% the general symptoms are fatigue, exertional dyspnea, weakness, and dizziness. If the hematocrit is below 18% or the hemoglobin less than 7 g/dl the patient will usually have dyspnea, tachycardia at rest, and a roaring sensation in the ears. If anemia has developed gradually, the patient may be able to compensate sufficiently so that only minimal symptoms will present in spite of hemoglobins less than 10 g/dl. Below 7 g/dl, all patients will have some complaints despite the duration of the anemia.

If anemia develops abruptly as in acute blood loss or acute hemolysis, symptoms are related to the loss in blood volume as well as to reduction in oxygen-carrying capacity. Significantly smaller decreases in red blood cell mass may produce symptoms that would not occur if the anemia developed gradually.

In the patient with acute blood loss, the hemoglobin and hematocrit measurements should not be used as the major or only guide in initial management since these tests are not accurate indicators of total blood volume and do not change until compensatory mechanisms to restore intravascular volume have occurred. Fluid shifts between the intravascular and extravascular compartments occur during the first 4–8 hours after blood loss but may happen more rapidly with the use of intravenous fluid replacement.

In patients with acute blood loss, postural changes in blood pressure and pulse or other evidences of shock are much more accurate indicators of the degree of blood loss. In the normal physiologic situation, there is a slight increase in the blood pressure when the patient is standing. If blood volume has been lost abruptly, the blood pressure will decrease and the pulse rate will increase when the patient assumes a sitting or standing position. A decrease of more than 10 mm Hg in the systolic pressure or a rise in the pulse rate of 10 beats/min or more indicates a significant loss of blood volume. Pallor, sweating, or postural dizziness indicates a loss of at least 15% of the blood volume. A loss of 25% of the blood volume is suggested if postural hypotension is found in the range of 20–30 mm Hg. The loss is probably 50% or more if there are evidences of profound shock when the patient is in the recumbent position.

Specific symptoms in history taking and findings on physical examination may help specify the cause of the anemia. Increased bruising or bleeding associated with significant postural hypotension would suggest acute blood loss. Decreased production anemia states, such as iron deficiency or specific vitamin deficiency, have characteristic findings. For example, a sore, beefy-red tongue, cracking at the angles of the mouth (angular stomatitis), spooning of the nails, a craving for ice, and dysphagia would strongly suggest severe iron deficiency. Lack of vitamin B_{12} may be suggested clinically by a staggering gait, smooth tongue, or early greying of the hair. Many of the hemolytic anemias will present with scleral icterus and/or splenomegaly.

LABORATORY EVALUATION

If acute blood loss has been excluded and the patient is not in need of urgent replacement of blood volume, the clinician should turn to the characterization of the anemia. Anemias can be classified both physiologically (decreased production versus increased destruction) and morphologically. They are characterized by the hemoglobin, hematocrit, red blood cell count, red blood cell indices, reticulocyte count, and red blood cell morphology. The white blood cell (WBC) count, white blood cell differential, and platelet count may add valuable clues in diagnosis.

The reticulocyte count, normally 1–1.5%, is an indirect measure of bone marrow function. It is decreased in anemias caused by lack of production of red cells and is increased after blood loss (hemorrhage or hemolysis). When the bone marrow

is stimulated by a fall in hematocrit, at least a 48-hour lag period is required before the reticulocyte count begins to rise.

Figure 40.1 shows how the reticulocyte count aids the physician in determining whether the anemia is a result of decreased production (absolute decrease in the number of reticulocytes) or increased destruction or hemolysis (moderate to marked increase in reticulocytes).

By evaluating the red blood cell indices and examining the peripheral blood smear, the decreased production anemias can be further subclassified morphologically as hypochromic and microcytic, normochromic and normocytic, or macrocytic (Fig. 40.1). When the complete blood cell count (CBC) is obtained from an automated counter the indices are automatically calculated. The mean cell volume (MCV) indicates the size of the red blood cells and is the most accurate of the indices. If the CBCs are done manually, the indices can be calculated (Table 40.1); the mean corpuscular hemoglobin concentration (MCHC) is the most accurate of the red blood cell indices obtained in this manner. A hypochromic, microcytic anemia would be characterized by a reduced MCV and MCHC; the peripheral blood smear should demonstrate small red blood cells with decreased hemoglobin (Fig. 40.2b). (On peripheral blood smear, the normal red blood cell size is equivalent to the nucleus of an adult lymphocyte) (Fig. 40.2a). An elevated MCV and the finding of large red blood cells in the peripheral blood smear would indicate a macrocytic anemia (Fig. 40.2c).

Hypochromic microcytic anemias are most frequently caused by iron deficiency, which in the adult patient is almost always a result of chronic blood loss (Fig. 40.1). Less commonly,

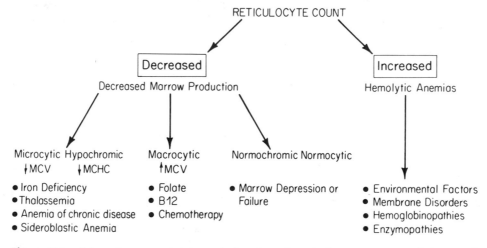

Figure 40.1 Schematic approach to anemia based on the reticulocyte count, morphology, and indices.

TABLE 40.1 Red Blood Cell Indices

Index	Equation	Normal Range
Mean corpuscular volume (MCV)	$\dfrac{\text{Hematocrit} \times 10}{\text{RBC (in millions/mm}^3)}$	80–90 μm^3
Mean corpuscular hemoglobin (MCH)	$\dfrac{\text{Hemoglobin (g/dl)} \times 10}{\text{RBC (in millions/mm}^3)}$	27–31 pg of Hgb per cell
Mean corpuscular hemoglobin concentration (MCHC)	$\dfrac{\text{Hemoglobin (g/dl)} \times 100}{\text{Hematocrit}}$	32–36% (or grams of Hgb per 100 ml of RBC)

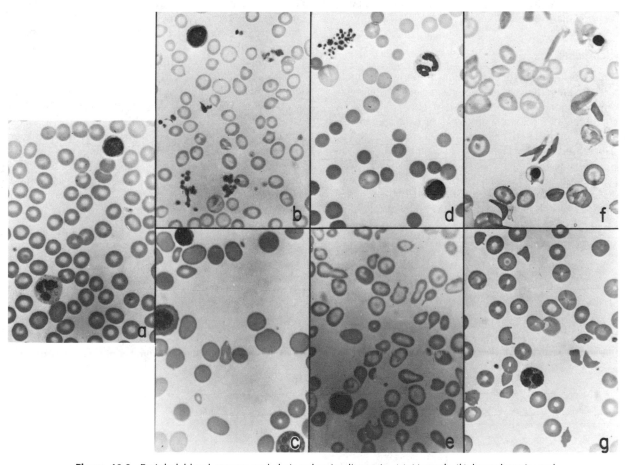

Figure 40.2 Periphal blood smears and their value in diagnosis. (a) Normal; (b) hypochromia and microcytosis of iron deficiency; (c) macrocytosis of megaloblastic anemias; (d) spherocytosis; (e) target cells with hypochromia and microcytosis of thalassemia; (f) sickle cells and targets in sickle cell syndromes; and (g) fragmented cells, schistocytes, helmet cells in microangiopathic hemolysis. (Used with permission from Rosenthal, DS: Problems involving an abnormal blood count. Office Practice of Medicine: Ed Branch, WT, Philadelphia, PA, W.B. Saunders Co., 1982, p. 1030.)

765

microcytic, hypochromic anemias are caused by thalassemia, chronic disease, or sideroblastic anemia.

Macrocytic red blood cells in the presence of decreased reticulocytes suggest folate or vitamin B_{12} deficiency, although it is not unusual for liver disease to cause this. Patients receiving chemotherapy may develop macrocytosis. In the presence of an elevated reticulocyte count, the MCV may be elevated and the cells appear large since young red blood cells (reticulocytes) are larger than older cells. Some anemias associated with a decreased reticulocyte count are normocytic and nomochromic. The red blood cells that are formed are normal, but are reduced in numbers because of marrow depression or failure. The search for a diagnosis usually requires further studies such as a bone marrow examination.

Hemolytic Anemia

The hallmark of a hemolytic anemia is a falling hematocrit associated with an increased reticulocyte count in the absence of bleeding. Jaundice is commonly seen and is caused by increased indirect bilirubinemia produced by hemoglobin degradation. Other associated changes produced by hemolysis include increased serum lactic dehydrogenase (LDH), increased urinary urobilinogen, leukocytosis, thrombocytosis, and nucleated red blood cells in the peripheral blood smear. When red blood cells are destroyed within the circulation, free hemoglobin is released into the plasma. When the level is high there is a pink color to the serum, whereas small amounts can be measured in the laboratory by a spectrophotometer. Brown urine (hemoglobinuria) may occur as a result of the products of hemoglobin metabolism being excreted.

If tests suggest a diagnosis of hemolytic anemia, a search should be made for the etiology (Fig. 40.3). A normal red blood cell has sufficient enzymes and hemoglobin to maintain its shape and allow it to carry out its major function of oxygen transport. If the red blood cell is damaged by environmental factors or has been genetically endowed with insufficient enzymes or an abnormal hemoglobin, it may be destroyed prematurely in the circulation or by the spleen. Table 40.2 lists the major causes of hemolytic anemia: environmental abnormalities, red blood cell membrane disorders, defects in globin structure, and deficiencies of a vital enzyme. All but the environmental conditions are hereditary.

Examination of the peripheral blood smear is often helpful in delineating the cause of hemolytic anemia. In evaluating the peripheral blood smear the clinician should look for the presence of spherocytes (Fig. 40.2d), target (Fig. 40.2c) or sickle cells (Fig. 40.2f), and schistocytes (Fig. 40.2g). Spherocytosis usually implies an autoimmune hemolytic anemia or hereditary spherocytosis; however, spherocytes can occasionally be seen in enzyme defects such as glucose-6-phosphate dehydrogenase (G6PD) deficiency or pyruvate kinase deficiency. Target cells are associated with abnormal hemoglobins, and sickle cells are indications of sickle cell anemia.

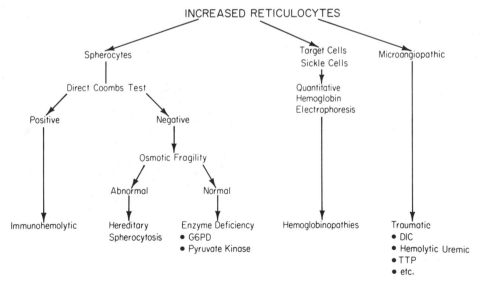

Figure 40.3 Schematic approach to the workup and laboratory evaluation of hemolytic anemias.

TABLE 40.2 Hemolytic Anemias

I. Environmental Factors
    A. Immunohemolytic anemias
        1. Idiopathic or primary
        2. Symptomatic or secondary
            a. Malignant lymphoproliferative disorders
            b. Chronic lymphocytic leukemia (CLL)
            c. Other neoplasms
            d. Medications
            e. Systemic lupus erythematosus (S.L.E.)
            f. Other autoimmune disorders
            g. Infections (infectious mononucleosis, mycoplasmal pneumonia)
        3. Transfusion reactions—incompatibility
    B. Traumatic hemolysis (microangiopathic)
        1. Burns
        2. Disseminated intravascular coagulation
        3. Thrombotic thrombocytopenic purpura
        4. Malignant hypertension
        5. Metastatic carcinoma
        6. Abnormal prosthetic heart valve
        7. Hemolytic uremia syndrome
        8. March hemoglobinuria
    C. Infections
        1. Malaria
        2. Clostridia
II. Abnormalities of the Red Blood Cell Membrane
    A. Hereditary spherocytosis
    B. Paroxysmal nocturnal hemoglobinuria
III. Hemoglobinopathies
    A. Sickle cell anemia
    B. Thalassemias
IV. Red Blood Cell Enzyme Deficiencies
    A. Glucose-6-phosphate dehydrogenase deficiency (G6PD)
    B. Pyruvate kinase

Microangiopathic red cells are caused by a number of disorders, listed in Table 40.2.

Most commonly, spherocytes suggest an immunohemolytic anemia. As can be seen from the schematic approach of Fig. 40.3, the diagnostic test for immunohemolytic anemia is the direct Coombs' test, which detects the presence of either antibody or complement on the red blood cell surface. Performance of an osmotic fragility test should detect patients with hereditary spherocytosis. If the blood smear primarily reveals normal red blood cells with rare spherocytes, an enzyme deficiency may be the etiology of the hemolysis. The two most

common enzyme deficiencies, G6PD deficiency and pyruvate kinase deficiency, can be diagnosed by enzyme assays. Target cells and sickle cells suggest an abnormal hemoglobin; hemoglobin electrophoresis and/or sickle cell preparations should detect most hemoglobinopathies. Determination of the underlying illness should be sought in microangiopathic hemolytic anemias. The Coombs' test and sickle cell screening tests should be readily available to the emergency room physician. Osmotic fragility testing, enzyme assays, and hemoglobin electrophoresis may be scheduled through the hematologist or special hematology laboratories.

SICKLE CELL ANEMIA

Sickle cell anemia is an inherited disorder of the hemoglobin molecule. It results from a single amino acid substitution of valine for glutamic acid in the beta chain. This molecular change causes the hemoglobin to become susceptible to polymerization in the deoxygenated state. This change in the hemoglobin inside red blood cells produces cells that are elongated and crescent in shape (sickle cells). As red blood cells sickle in vivo they become rigid and do not easily pass through the microcirculation, thus producing the symptoms of sickle cell disease.

Patients who are homozygous for hemoglobin S (Hb S) develop sickle cell anemia with all of its clinical manifestations. Patients who are heterozygous for Hb S can be detected in vitro when their red blood cells are exposed to low oxygen tension; however, sickle trait does not usually produce any clinical disease. When Hb S trait is associated with some other hemoglobin abnormality such as hemoglobin C (Hb C) or thalassemia, a clinical picture indistinguishable from homozygous Hemoglobin S may be produced.

Diagnosis

The signs and symptoms of sickle cell anemia may begin in an infant about 6 months of age when the normal switch from fetal hemoglobin to adult hemoglobin occurs. The disease produces both chronic and acute problems. Because the patient has a chronic hemolytic anemia, we may see the manifestations of chronic anemia: cardiomegaly, chronic heart failure, pulmonary disease, and hepatomegaly. Except in infants, splenomegaly is not seen because of repeated splenic infarctions resulting in a small fibrotic organ.

Many organ systems may be affected by sickle cell anemia. In infants and young children, the painful "hand–foot syndrome" (dactylitis) results from the vasoocclusion of nutrient arteries of the metatarsal and metacarpal bones. The child usually presents with painful swelling of hands and feet and may develop bone infarction. In the kidney, necrosis of the renal medulla may occur from hypoxia and hyperosmolarity. Decreased urine specific gravity (less than 1.010) is almost universal. Papillary necrosis may result in occasional episodes of gross hematuria and in rare cases on renal colic. In the eye, retinal infarcts and retinitis proliferans may occur. Aseptic necrosis and bone infarcts may result from vasoocclusive events in bone. Osteomyelitis, especially as a result of salmonellae, is not uncommon. Hepatocellular disease with persistent elevations of the serum glutamic-oxaloacetic transaminase (SGOT) and LDH occur with frequency.

Since hemolysis causes increased indirect bilirubinemia, patients with sickle cell anemia frequently develop calcium bilirubinate gallstones and obstructive jaundice. Central nervous system involvement may result in cranial nerve palsies, hemiplegia, blindness, aphasia, and occasionally coma or convulsions. Other troublesome complications include priapism and recurrent leg ulceration. Pulmonary infarction is commonly encountered and is probably a result of thrombosis in situ rather than embolization. Pneumonia, especially secondary to pneumococcus, is a serious and not infrequent complication of sickle cell disease.

If the diagnosis of sickle cell disease has not been previously made, an evaluation of the blood smear may be satisfactory to make a diagnosis of one of the sickle cell syndromes so that therapy can be initiated. The presence of sickled cells in the peripheral blood smear is almost diagnostic. Recognition of sickle cell disease in the emergency room can be accomplished by the fairly reliable sodium metabisulfate method or by commercially available kits such as the Sickle-dex test. When a drop of red blood cells containing Hb S is mixed with a drop of reducing agent such as sodium metabisulfate on a glass slide the cells will sickle and can be directly observed under the microscope after 15–30 minutes. The Sickle-dex test is based on the decreased solubility of the Hb S in high phosphate buffer solutions. In order to make a definitive diagnosis of homozygous sickle cell disease and to distinguish it from the trait or the other sickle cells syndrome such as sickle cell thalassemia, a hemoglobin electrophoresis is necessary.

Although the patient is susceptible to many acute problems, perhaps the most common and debilitating complication is the "painful crisis" a result of the vasoocclusion of the microcirculation by sickled cells. Patients complain of a sudden pain in muscles, bones, chest, and abdomen. Many patients have typical crises in which their pain is located in the same place each time; however, pain may be located anywhere or in any combination of areas. As may be expected, painful crises can be precipitated by situations in which hypoxia occurs. Crises may also be precipitated by fever, infection, dehydration, or acidosis. Although a precipitating event cannot always be determined, a thorough evaluation for a cause must be made since the precipitating event must be rectified before the patient will recover from the crisis.

A patient who experiences painful crisis frequently presents with fever, leukocytosis, and tachycardia. Since these are the symptoms and signs associated with infection, it may be difficult to exclude infection as a precipitating event. A careful examination and appropriate cultures are mandatory. A leukocyte alkaline phosphatase (LAP), when available, can be a very useful laboratory test. In general patients with sickle cell anemia have a low LAP score and will have an elevation of the score when infection is present. If a baseline LAP is available on the patient for comparison, this test can be particularly helpful.

Therapy

The treatment of painful crisis in sickle cell anemia should be directed at correction of any precipitating event and relief of pain with analgesics; severe pain usually requires narcotics. A combination of meperidine (Demerol) and promethazine hydrochloride (Phenergan) is usually satisfactory. Good hydration is essential. Intravenous fluids should be administered to accomplish this; the amount depends on the degree of dehydration and the age and condition of the patient. Emergency therapies of questionable benefit include oxygen and alkalinization. There is no definite proof that oxygen benefits painful crisis; however, it generally does no harm and in the presence of cardiopulmonary disease or pneumonia may be given liberally. Acidosis can result in precipitation of a painful crisis and when present should be corrected. When acidosis is not present the use of alkalinization has not been shown to be of benefit. Transfusions are recommended if the crisis does not terminate within a reasonable period of time. When necessary, the patient should be transfused with packed red blood cells, which in theory attempts to reduce the patient's sickle cell concentration to less than 40% of the total cells. Investigational approaches designed in the laboratory have offered hope of new treatments. Unfortunately, urea and cyanate as antisickling therapy have not been of clinical help.

Occasionally bone marrow suppression occurs, especially when infection is present. Because patients with sickle cell disease have chronic hemolysis, lack of production of red blood cells can lead to a rapid fall in hematocrit necessitating transfusion. The use of exchange transfusions has been advised in certain clinical settings such as pregnancy and central nervous system complications.

Prognosis

Often the treatment of patients with sickle cell disease has only been by intermittent emergency room care, necessitated by crises, symptoms of anemia, or infections. It is important to recognize that the patient with sickle cell anemia needs coordinated and continued total care by physicians, nurses, and social workers with the goal of preventing complications of the disease. With good supportive care, early therapy for crises, and hypertransfusion when needed, patients with sickle cell disease can live longer.

GLUCOSE-6-PHOSPHATE DEHYDROGENASE DEFICIENCY

Because of the frequency of glucose-6-phosphate dehydrogenase (G6PD) deficiency, it may not be uncommon to see patients with this deficiency in the emergency room. It is especially important to be aware of since many commonly used medications may precipitate hemolysis in a patient with this deficiency.

The enzyme G6PD functions in maintaining the integrity of the red blood cells during stress, primarily from oxidative drugs and infection. In the patient with a G6PD deficiency the hemoglobin in the red blood cell may be oxidized when exposed to oxidant stress, resulting in the cell becoming susceptible to premature destruction (hemolysis). Deficiencies in G6PD activity are not uncommon in African blacks and in people of Mediterranean and Oriental descent. It is a sex-linked inherited disorder carried on the X chromosome. The incidence in black men in the United States approaches 15%. The disorder is less frequent in black women since both chromosomes would have to be affected; however, heterozygous patients may develop hemolysis under sufficient stress.

The G6PD is an age-related red blood cell enzyme, being more abundant in the young red blood cells and having gradually decreasing levels as red blood cells age. When a G6PD deficient patient is exposed to an oxidant stress such as drugs or infection, the older red blood cells will hemolyze, resulting in a marrow stimulus to produce young red blood cells rich in the enzyme and less susceptible to destruction. Hemolysis occurs as a result of the following reactions: (1) an oxidant stress causes hemoglobin to be oxidized to methemoglobin; (2) oxidized hemoglobin forms inclusions within the red blood cell called Heinz bodies; and (3) Heinz bodies adversely affect the red blood cell membrane, increasing its fragility and causing the cell to be removed by the spleen. The end result is similar to other types of hemolysis; there is a drop in the hematocrit, indirect hyperbilirubinemia, dark urine, and the development of reticulocytosis.

Special tests to confirm the diagnosis of G6PD deficiency include a Heinz body preparation and a G6PD assay. The G6PD assay can be performed by a number of laboratory methods; however, it should be remembered that if acute hemolysis has already occurred, the results may be falsely normalized because of the high reticulocyte count.

It is of interest that G6PD deficiency was discovered as a cause of hemolysis during World War II when black soldiers developed anemia and dark urine after receiving primaquine for prophylaxis against malaria. Other oxidizing agents that are commonly associated with hemolysis in this disorder are listed in Table 40.3. Fortunately, in the majority of patients the degree of hemolysis is mild and not life threatening. If hemolysis does occur, any suspicious drugs should be removed from the patient's environment. Transfusions are not usually necessary unless the hemolysis is severe. Adequate hydration is recommended to prevent any renal complications from the hemoglobin release into the plasma. After the diagnosis is confirmed the patient should be warned to avoid the known drug offenders.

Macrocytic Anemias—Vitamin B_{12} and Folate Deficiency

Macrocytic anemias are severe chronic anemias caused primarily by deficiencies of vitamin B_{12} or folate. Folic acid and

TABLE 40.3 Agents and Disorders Associated with Hemolysis in G6PD Deficiency

Antimalarials	Antibacterials
Primaquine	Chloramphenicol
Quinacrine	Nalidixic acid
Chloroquine	Nitrofurantoin
Sulfonamides	Miscellaneous drugs
Diaphenylsulfine	Acetylsalicylic acid
Sulfanilamide	Acetophenetin
Sulfapyridine	Methylene blue
Sulfisoxizole	Ascorbic acid
Chemicals	Infections
Benzene	Hepatitis
Naphthalene	
Diabetic Acidosis	

vitamin B_{12} are both essential cofactors for the synthesis of deoxyribonucleic acid (DNA) so that a deficiency in one of these vitamins affects cells in the body that have a rapid turnover rate, such as bone marrow and intestinal mucosa cells. Under these circumstances, both the myeloid and erythroid cells in the bone marrow have fewer divisions during development and resultant cells are large, appearing as macrocytic red blood cells or hypersegmented polymorphonuclear leukocytes. In many cases, the anemia is part of a pancytopenia since all marrow cells are involved. Even cells from gastric cytology and Papanicolaou smears may be significantly abnormal so as to suggest a class III or IV smear.

The most common cause of vitamin B_{12} deficiency is *pernicious anemia,* an acquired deficiency of gastric intrinsic factor. Vitamin B_{12} deficiency is associated not only with megaloblastic anemia but also with combined systems disease, a neurologic syndrome consisting of central nervous system irritability and depression, together with loss of position and vibratory sense in the hands and feet. Other etiologies of vitamin B_{12} deficiency include absence of the stomach or ileum through surgery and infiltrative or inflammatory disorders of the gastrointestinal tract. (Table 40.4).

The most common cause of folate deficiency is dietary lack of the vitamin. Folate is present in leafy vegetables, meats, yeast, and dairy products and is heat labile so that overcooking may destroy the vitamin. A poor diet can lead to a macrocytic anemia after 6–8 weeks. The causes of folic acid deficiency are outlined in Table 40.4.

TABLE 40.4 Common Causes of Megaloblastic Anemia

Vitamin B_{12} deficiency
   Pernicious anemia—lack of intrinsic factor
   Gastrectomy
   Resected or diseased ileum
   Transcobalmin deficiency (rare)
   Dietary fadist—vegans
Folate deficiency
   Nutritional
   Drugs
      Interfere with absorption (phenobarbital, diphenylhydantoin and contraceptives)
      Competitive inhibition (methotrexate)
   Malabsorption and other diseases of the jejunum
   Increased demand
      Hemolytic anemias
      Pregnancy, infancy
      Malignancies

CLINICAL AND LABORATORY PRESENTATION

High output failure with gradually progressive shortness of breath may be the presenting manifestation in patients with either folate or vitamin B_{12} deficiency. The skin may be lemon colored because of a combination of pallor and indirect bilirubinemia. A depapillated smooth tongue, slight splenomegaly, absence of olfactory sense, and absence of vibratory and position sense in the lower extremities are other characteristics of vitamin B_{12} deficiency. Physical signs in folic acid deficiency are those of a nutritional deficiency such as weight loss or cachexia. In a few patients with vitamin B_{12} deficiency, the neurologic symptoms may be more significant than the degree of macrocytic anemia. Rarely, a patient may have loss of vibratory and position sense because of vitamin B_{12} deficiency in the absence of anemia.

The anemia, often severe with decreased reticulocytes, is characterized by a macrocytosis and often accompanied by neutropenia and/or thrombocytopenia. A bone marrow aspirate is necessary to confirm the diagnosis, and the patient should be referred immediately for this procedure. Morphologic changes in the marrow are diagnostic in megaloblastic anemia, but vitamin B_{12} and folate levels are required to differentiate the vitamin deficiency state; blood samples to determine the levels should be obtained before any treatment is instituted. In vitamin B_{12} deficiency, a Schilling test may also be necessary to differentiate the cause of the deficiency. In this test orally ingested radioactive vitamin B_{12} will appear in the urine if intrinsic factor is present and the ileum is intact. If an abnormally low amount of radioactivity is present in the urine, the defect will be corrected in classic pernicious anemia by the simultaneous ingestion of oral intrinsic factor. Nonspecific abnormalities include increased serum LDH and indirect bilirubinemia.

THERAPY

Unfortunately, therapy is too often "shotgun" in technique; patients are put on vitamin B_{12} and folate with little regard for establishing the mechanism of the deficiency. Historically, this reflects the former "preaching" that newly diagnosed megaloblastic anemia should not be treated with folic acid alone because of the possibility that the combined system disease of vitamin B_{12} deficiency could be made worse by a further depletion of vitamin B_{12} stores caused by folate therapy. With the current, quick reporting of blood vitamin levels, this complication is less likely. Unfortunately, too many patients remain indefinitely on combined therapy for what may be either pure vitamin B_{12} or folate deficiency alone.

Recommended folate replacement is usually 1 mg/day orally, whereas vitamin B_{12} is given subcutaneously in a dose of 100 μg. Initially and especially with combined systems disease, daily vitamin B_{12} injections are recommended for 2 weeks and maintenance therapy is adequately accomplished by 100–1,000 μg subcutaneously monthly or bimonthly.

PROGNOSIS

Therapeutic response in megaloblastic anemias is fairly rapid. Reticulocytes rise within 3–5 days, followed by a gradual increase in the hemoglobin and hematocrit as well as the WBC and platelets. Complications can occur with treatment of older patients. Congestive heart failure may develop as a result of the abrupt increase in hemoglobin and hematocrit since prior to therapy, volume expansion will have compensated for the gradually dropping red blood cell mass. Transfusions are usually withheld for the same reason unless oxygen-carrying capacity has been significantly impaired and producing problems, such as angina. With treatment, the serum potassium may drop because of a sudden transfer of electrolytes into the intracellular space as therapy begins to stimulate DNA synthesis.

Abnormal gastric cytology or cervical Papanicolaou smears should be repeated after completion of therapy. An upper gastrointestinal (GI) series should be performed in any patient with persistently abnormal cytology because of the association of gastric neoplasm with pernicious anemia. In addition, because of the association of myxedema and hypothyroidism with megaloblastic anemias, routine thyroid studies should be obtained.

Much of the workup of patients with macrocytic anemias can be initiated in the emergency room with eventual referral to the specialist for marrow examination or therapy.

Chronic Anemias

One of the most difficult and challenging clinical problems is the persistent anemia that requires long-term follow-up and repeated transfusions. Most of these anemias are normochromic normocytic, but some are mixed morphologically that contain both microcytic and macrocytic cells. The etiologies of such anemias include chronic uremia and liver disease, hypoplastic and aplastic anemia, refractory sideroblastic anemias, preleukemic diseases, and effect of radiation therapy or chemotherapy.

CLINICAL PRESENTATION

The symptoms of patients in the emergency room with chronic anemias may be quite mild considering the degree of anemia.

Compensatory mechanisms have developed over time to increase cardiac output and oxygen delivery to tissues. Almost all patients will, however, become symptomatic when the hemoglobin level falls below 7 g/dl.

THERAPY

Chronic anemias rarely require emergency treatment, and in fact overzealous transfusions may result in volume overload. In most instances chronic anemia should be treated specifically when the underlying etiology can be determined. When transfusion is necessary, tests to determine the etiology should be obtained and sent to the laboratory before transfusion. The emergency use of blood transfusions in these disorders is indicated only for serious symptoms attributable to the low hemoglobin. Possible indications for transfusions include acute myocardial infarctions, severe angina, severe congestive heart failure, acute cerebrovascular insufficiency, and severe dyspnea. Since the blood volume is usually normal in chronic anemias because of the compensatory mechanisms, transfusion when necessary should be done with packed red blood cells in order to increase the oxygen-carrying capacity with less volume. In general, we should aim for a hematocrit of 30%.

Each unit of packed cells contains approximately 250 ml and can be expected to increase the hematocrit in an average adult by approximately 3–4%. Since there is variability in the response, the hematocrit must be followed.

TRANSFUSION REACTION

Transfusion reaction is a general term referring to all of the unfavorable effects of transfusion. These adverse effects may range from the immediate life-threatening hemolytic crisis to the delayed infection of serum hepatitis. Table 40.5 outlines the acute and delayed reactions that may occur.

Hemolytic Crisis

The most devastating transfusion reaction is the acute hemolytic crisis that occurs when mismatched blood is given to a patient. This most often occurs as a result of incompatibilities in the ABO system (e.g., a patient of type B receives type A blood). Most often symptoms will begin after only a small amount of blood has been administered. The patient may have a sense of heat along the vein into which the blood is being transfused followed by flushing of the face, lumbar pain, and constricting discomfort in the chest. Headache, vomiting, and

TABLE 40.5 Acute and Delayed Transfusion Reactions

Acute Reactions
  Hemolytic
    ABO incompatibility
    Other blood group incompatibilities
    Overheating or inadvertent freezing of transfused blood
  Febrile
    Acquired antibodies
      Leukocytes, platelets
    Bacterial contamination
    Pyrogens
  Urticaria and anti-IgA antibodies
    Passive transfer of allergy
    Platelet and leukocyte antibodies
  Asthma
  Pulmonary edema
  Air embolism
  Hyperkalemia
  Hemorrhagic tendency
  Hypocalcemia
  Acidosis
  Hypothermia
Delayed Reactions
  Hemolytic
    Rh incompatibility
    Minor blood group incompatibility
    Old blood
  Infection
    Hepatitis
    Cytomegalovirus
    Malaria and other parasites
    Syphilis
  Allergic: urticaria and asthma
    Passive transfer of antibodies in serum
  Thrombophlebitis
  Hemosiderosis

diarrhea may occur. Pulmonary symptoms—with cough, dyspnea, and wheezing—may be prominent. The patient will frequently develop rigors and high temperatures. Tachycardia and hypotension may occur. If hemolysis is severe hemoglobinemia, hemoglobinuria, oliguria, and renal shutdown may follow.

If any of these signs or symptoms occurs the transfusions should be immediately discontinued. A blood sample should be drawn promptly and the plasma examined for the presence of pink color indicating hemoglobinemia. The urine should be examined for hemoglobin, which can be detected by a benzidine reaction yielding a brownish color. The transfused blood and a freshly drawn blood sample from the patient must be sent to the blood bank immediately, informing the laboratory personnel of the suspicion of a major reaction so that a repeat cross match and Coombs' test can be performed.

After discontinuation of the transfusion, treatment should be begun. Fluids should be administered intravenously to maintain adequate urinary output. Mannitol diuresis (20 g mannitol IV as a 20% solution over 5 min) is generally recommended. This cannot be done if the patient has already developed renal shutdown since fluid overload would probably ensue. If shock is present, it must be appropriately treated.

Febrile Reaction

The most common immediate febrile reaction to transfusion is a result of the leukocytes, platelets, or foreign proteins contained in the blood product. In addition to fever and chills that may occur with this type of reaction, pruritis, urticaria, angioneurotic edema, bronchospasm, and occasionally severe anaphylaxis may occur. If symptoms of this nature occur during the transfusion, the transfusion should be stopped and the patient evaluated as if a hemolytic reaction were occurring. Treatment should be symptomatic; there should be careful monitoring of vital signs and use of antipyretics, antihistamines, and corticosteroids if necessary. If bronchospasm occurs epinephrine may be needed. If the reaction is mild 25–50 mg diphenhydramine (Benadryl) orally or intravenously may be all that is required. If future transfusions are required, washed or frozen red blood cells or prophylactic antihistamines should be used.

Other Reactions

CONGESTIVE HEART FAILURE

Pulmonary edema may occur as a result of volume overload especially in older patients or patients with chronic anemia who had compensatory changes in their blood volume. If pulmonary edema occurs, it should be treated in the usual manner.

URTICARIA

If a patient develops only urticaria during transfusion it is now felt that discontinuation of the transfusion is not necessary. These patients can be managed with antihistamines.

HYPERKALEMIA

Stored blood may contain relatively large amounts of potassium that have been released from red blood cells. Hyperkalemia may result if whole blood has been transfused rapidly, especially in patients with chronic renal failure. Packed red blood cells or fresh blood should reduce the danger of elevation of the serum potassium in these patients.

HYPOCALCEMIA

Because of the acid citrate anticoagulant used in blood transfusion, hypocalcemia and acidosis may occur with multiple transfusions. This can be corrected with calcium gluconate and sodium bicarbonate.

DELAYED REACTIONS

The delayed transfusion reactions are listed in Table 40.5. Urgent treatment is not required although patients may be seen in the emergency room with these complications as a result of a prior transfusion.

HYPERVISCOSITY DISORDERS

When the blood becomes thick or viscous, secondary to elevations of the red blood cell mass (erythrocytosis) or to abnormal or increased level of certain proteins (myeloma, Waldenström's macroglobulinemia or cryoglobulinemia), symptoms such as lethargy, malaise, blurred vision, bleeding, thrombosis, delirium, and occasionally coma may develop. The onset can be acute or insidious but is often life threatening. These disorders can be recognized and evaluated in the emergency room, and therapy can be initiated there.

Polycythemia

Polycythemia is an increase in the red blood cell mass. It can be recognized by the measurement of the hematocrit or hemoglobin. *Polycythemia,* and its synonym, *erythrocytosis,* do not specify a specific disease entity but may be caused by a variety of conditions. As indicated in Table 40.6, a distinction can be made between "relative" and "absolute" polycythemia, as well as between primary and secondary polycythemia. Absolute polycythemia represents those diseases in which there is an absolute increase in the red blood cell mass. Relative polycythemia refers to conditions in which the red blood cell mass

is normal but plasma volume is decreased, producing pseudopolycythemia. Primary polycythemia—polycythemia rubra vera—is one of the myeloproliferative disorders in which an elevated hematocrit occurs as a result of abnormal proliferation of the myeloid compartment of the bone marrow. It is not secondary to increased erythropoietin levels. Secondary polycythemia occur as a physiologic response to increased amounts of erythropoietin. The secondary polycythemias may be further subclassified into those disorders that result from an appropriate increase in erythropoietin secretion (e.g., disorders associated with hypoxia) and those conditions in which erythropoietin is produced inappropriately (e.g., tumors and renal problems).

RELATIVE POLYCYTHEMIA

Relative polycythemia is a distinct and commonly encountered entity that is also referred to as *stress erythrocytosis*. It is not a primary disease process and may be nothing more than a normal physiologic state in which the plasma volume is slightly decreased and the red cell mass is slightly increased.

Clinical Presentation and Diagnosis

Patients are often overweight, nervous, hypertensive, and prone to thromboembolic complications. The hematocrits rarely exceed 60% and usually range between 50–60% although other blood parameters are normal. Clinical manifestations of headache and itching are less severe than may be noted in patients with polycythemia rubra vera, and diagnosis may be distinguished only by red blood cell mass measurement.

The complications are not hematologically related, and reduction of red blood cell volume by means of phlebotomy or chemotherapy is not appropriate. The hypertension, however, may require aggressive management.

SECONDARY POLYCYTHEMIAS

The most common cause of secondary polycythemia is chronic hypoxemia secondary to chronic obstructive pulmonary disease. In some instances, the hemoglobin has been reported to be as high as 24 g/dl and hematocrit as high as 75%. However, most patients with polycythemia as a result of chronic obstructive lung disease do not exceed hematocrits of 57% and hemoglobins of 17 g/dl.

Another cause of secondary polycythemia is cyanotic congenital heart disease. Hematocrits as high as 65% and hemoglobins greater than 20 g/dl may be seen. The most common

TABLE 40.6 Classification of Polycythemia

I. Relative Polycythemia
   Stress
   Dehydration
   Diuretic therapy
   Burns
II. Absolute Polycythemia
   A. Primary
      Polycythemia vera
   B. Secondary
      1. Decreased oxygen transport—appropriate erythropoietin stimulation
         a. High altitude
         b. Impaired ventilation
            Chronic obstructive pulmonary disease
            Pickwickian's syndrome
            Postural hypoxemia
         c. Cardiovascular disorders
            Cyanotic congenital heart disease
            Septal defects
            Fallot's tetralogy
            Atrioventricular (AV) intrapulmonary aneurysms
            Hemangiomata
         d. Impaired hemoglobin function
            Congenital methemoglobinemia
            Congenital hemoglobinopathy with high oxygen affinity
            Intense cigarette smoking
      2. Inappropriate erythropoietin production
         Malignancy: kidney, hepatoma, adrenal, lung
         Benign tumors: uterine fibroids, cerebellar, hemangioma, pheochromocytoma, Cushing's syndrome
         Renal: cysts, hydroneophrosis, Bartter's syndrome, transplantation

cardiac defects producing these elevations are pulmonary stenosis, accompanied by interatrial or ventricular septal defect, complete transposition of the great vessels, Fallot's tetralogy, or persistent truncus arteriosis.

Some hemoglobin variants can cause a shift in the hemoglobin–oxygen dissociation curve such that the hemoglobin molecule does not easily release oxygen to tissues, resulting in relative tissue hypoxia. The shift to the left of the hemoglobin–oxygen dissociation curve results in a marked decrease in oxygen extraction by the tissues. Compensation by increases in the hemoglobin concentration or blood flow are the available mechanisms of the body to maintain oxygen delivery. It appears that the primary response is erythrocytosis mediated by increases in erythropoietin.

Polycythemia may also occur secondary to inappropriate erythopoietin production, for example, due to tumors, renal cysts, hydronephrosis. In some instances, after renal transplantation the hematocrit levels may be quite excessive and threaten kidney rejection.

Clinical Presentation and Diagnosis

Hyperviscosity may occur as the hematocrit increases to above 60%. Although the erythrocytosis may be a homeostatic mechanism compensating for the chronic arterial hypoxemia, unduly increased blood volumes are undesirable. The optimal hemoglobin level in patients with cyanotic congenital heart disease and other chronically hypoxemic states is poorly defined. Cardiac function may be compromised because of both volume load and viscosity of the blood. Ruddy cyanosis, headache, dizziness, roaring in the ears, thrombotic episodes, and bleeding are the major clinical findings.

Most patients with polycythemia can be evaluated as outpatients and the workup can be started in the emergency room. The evaluation should be initiated with a complete history and physical examination and a complete blood count including a platelet count. These studies are most helpful in beginning to separate the secondary polycythemias from polycythemia rubra vera. After these initial studies, a hematologist should be consulted to determine the need for further study such as red blood cell mass or arterial blood gas determinations.

Therapy

When a patient presents with symptoms of hyperviscosity, thrombotic complications, or bleeding complications, urgent therapy may be required. Phlebotomy is the most rapid way to reduce the blood volume and symptoms. Afterward appropriate investigations should be carried out to find the cause of the erythrocytosis. Prognosis depends upon the underlying disorder.

POLYCYTHEMIA RUBRA VERA

Polycythemia rubra vera is a myeloproliferative disorder and results in many laboratory abnormalities in addition to erythrocytosis. Thrombocytosis, leukocytosis, elevated neutrophil alkaline phosphatase activity, elevated levels of serum B_{12} and unsaturated B_{12} binding proteins along with splenomegaly and pruritis may be noted.

Diagnosis

If erythrocytosis is accompanied by increased red blood cell mass, a normal arterial oxygen saturation, and splenomegaly, the diagnosis of polycythemia rubra vera can be confirmed. The following laboratory abnormalities suggest the diagnosis: thrombocytosis, leukocytosis (in the absence of infection), elevated neutrophil alkaline phosphatase activity, or elevated vitamin B_{12} serum and unsaturated vitamin B_{12} binding capacity.

Clinical symptoms of polycythemia rubra vera may be divided into those that are secondary to the increased red blood cell mass and increased blood volume (such as headaches, plethora, pruritis, dyspnea, and bleeding), those due to increased blood viscosity (such as parasthesias and thrombophlebitis), and those due to permetabolism (such as weight loss and night sweats). Angina and claudication are commonly elicited in the history, and arterial hypertension can occur frequently. Although paradoxical, hemorrhage and thrombocytosis are both complications of the disease. Bleeding may be caused by distension of veins and capillaries, by increased blood volume, or by abnormality of platelet function. Thrombosis may be related to increased blood viscosity, thrombocytosis, and perhaps abnormally increased platelet aggregation. Although thrombosis may occur in peripheral blood vessels, cerebral and coronary vessels may be the site of thrombosis. Mesenteric and portal vein thromboses also occur but are less frequent.

Therapy

Phlebotomy is usually performed gradually until the hematocrit falls into the 40–45% range. Thrombocytosis or other abnormalities such as painful splenomegaly may require treatment with an alkylating agent or radioactive phosphorus. Hematologic consultation should be obtained to define these issues.

Prognosis

Polycythemia rubra vera is a chronic myeloproliferative disorder with a fairly favorable long-term prognosis considering the elderly patients involved. Fatal complications include thrombotic episodes and a potential conversion to acute leukemia.

Multiple Myeloma and Waldenström's Macroglobulinemia

Malignancies of the plasma cell and lymphocyte may also be associated with acute hyperviscosity symptoms. Waldenström's macroglobulinemia, multiple myeloma, and occasionally malignant lymphomas may be associated with high levels of serum immunoglobulins causing an increase in plasma viscosity and thus impaired blood flow. Rouleaux formation on the peripheral blood smear and moderate to marked increase in serum total protein (> 8 g/dl) may be the initial laboratory clues in suspecting these disorders. Although there are supportive as well as specific therapies for these disease entities, the acute viscosity symptoms are life threatening and deserve immediate attention and consultation.

Diagnosis

Multiple myeloma is characteristically a disease of older individuals. Back or bone pain is usually accompanied by mild to moderate anemia, elevated sedimentation rate, osteolytic lesions, and osteoporosis. Diagnostic studies include serum protein analysis, bone marrow aspiration, calcium level, and renal function studies. Besides the viscosity problems, hypercalcemia and hyperuricemia may require urgent medical intervention.

Waldenström's macroglobulinemia occurs more frequently in older individuals and is less common than multiple myeloma. It is characterized by anemia, adenopathy, splenomegaly, an abnormal serum protein analysis, and a bone marrow infiltrated by a cell that morphologically is a cross between a plasmacyte and a lymphocyte (a "plymphocyte"). Unlike myeloma, osteolytic disease and bone pain are quite rare. The major symptoms are related to hematologic disease changes because of marrow replacement and viscosity secondary to the abnormal protein.

The hyperviscosity syndrome includes (1) bleeding characterized by bruising, purpura, retinal hemorrhages, epistaxis, and bleeding from mucosal surfaces, (2) retinopathy with retinal hemorrhages, dilatation and segmentation of the retinal vein, and papiledema, (3) neurologic symptoms that may consist of weakness, fatigue, headache, anorexia, vertigo, transient paresis, nystagmus, and coma, and (4) hypervolemia that may result in distention of peripheral blood vessels with increased vascular resistance and cardiac failure. Although the diagnosis can be suspected by elevations in the serum protein, a diagnosis can be made by measurement of the serum viscosity. Symptoms do not usually develop unless the serum viscosity rises above fourfold (relative to water).

Therapy

The development of the hyperviscosity syndrome requires urgent therapy with intensive plasmaphoresis to remove the abnormal protein. After hematologic consultation, chemotherapy to destroy the cells producing the proteins should be initiated. Although slow, plasmaphoresis can be performed by repeated phlebotomies with reinfusion of the packed red blood cells. Only one unit can be safely removed at a time, brought to the blood bank for centrifugation and removal of the plasma, so that the remaining packed red blood cells can be retransfused. Each exchange may take up to 1 hour. Recently machines have become available to allow multiple units of plasma exchange within 1–2 hours. If these machines are available, this is the preferable management of the condition.

Prognosis

Although remissions are made possible by chemotherapy, multiple myeloma and Waldenström macroglobulinemia are potentially fatal, with median survival of 2–5 years.

WHITE BLOOD CELL DISORDERS

The white blood cell count, like the sedimentation rate, is an indicator of underlying disease. As such it may increase or decrease with many stimuli.

Leukopenia and *leukocytosis* are general terms referring to a reduction or an increase, respectively, in the total white blood cell count. Not only is the total white blood cell count of importance, but we must consider the differential diagnosis of neutropenia, eosinophilia, lymphocytosis, monocytosis, and basophilia. Table 40.7 outlines the differential diagnosis of an abnormal white blood count. The two abnormalities of white blood count that are most commonly seen in the emergency room are leukocytosis and neutropenia.

Leukocytosis

The most common cause of leukocytosis is infection. The evaluation and management of the patient with infection are discussed in Chapters 13 and 28.

Of the patients presenting with leukocytosis, those with acute leukemia may also require urgent therapy because of bleeding or infection. Diagnosis requires evaluation of the blood smear and bone marrow by a hematologist. Treatment includes supportive measures and chemotherapy.

Chronic myelogenous leukemia may be confused with a leukemoid reaction. This can usually be separated by performance of a LAP. The LAP is low in chronic myelogenous leukemia and elevated in leukemoid reaction.

Neutropenia

Patients with neutropenia are frequently seen in the emergency room, especially those who have received chemotherapy.

Diagnosis

Pathophysiologically, neutropenia can be secondary to decreased bone marrow production of the myeloid series, peripheral destruction of the cells, or increased use or loss of the cells to the tissues. Most commonly, neutropenia is seen secondary to chemotherapy for malignant diseases. Neutropenia may be seen in patients with various types of infection but is most common in patients with infections of viral etiology. Neutropenia has also been seen in patients with bacteria infections such as typhoid, rickettsial infections such as typhus or Rocky Mountain spotted fever, protozoan infections such as malaria, and overwhelming infections such as tuberculosis or septi-

TABLE 40.7 Evaluation of an Abnormal WBC

I. Leukocytosis
  A. Neutrophilia
    1. Bacterial infection
    2. Inflammation, necrosis, or stress
  B. Lymphocytosis
    1. Viral infections
    2. Mononucleosis
    3. Pertussis
  C. Eosinophilia
    1. Allergic disorders
    2. Parasitic diseases
    3. Tumors, Hodgkin's disease
  D. Basophilia
    1. Myeloproliferative disorders
      a. Polycythemia rubra vera
      b. Myeloid metaplasia
      c. Chronic myelogenous leukemia
  E. Monocytosis
    1. Chronic infections
      a. Tuberculosis
      b. Subacute bacterial endocarditis (SBE)
      c. Rickettsial
    2. Ulcerative colitis
II. Abnormal Response
  A. Acute leukemias, lymphocytic, myelogenous
  B. Chronic leukemias, lymphocytic, myelogenous
  C. Polycythemia rubra vera
  D. Myeloid metaplasia with myelofibrosis
  F. Myelophthisic disorders
III. Neutropenia
  A. Infections
  B. Blood disorders
    1. Megaloblastic anemias, leukemias, aplastic anemias, hypersplenism
  C. Debilitated state or cachexia
  D. Chemicals
    1. Benzene
    2. Dichlorodiphenyltrichloroethane (DDT)
  E. Drugs
  F. Chemotherapy
  G. Irradiation
  H. Rare causes
    1. Cyclic neutropenia
    2. Familial neutropenia
    3. Chronic benign neutropenia
    4. Immune neutropenia

cemia, especially in a debilitated patient. Chemicals and drugs may induce neutropenia. Ionizing radiation, benzene, chemotherapy, antithyroid medications, anticonvulsants, and gold salts are the most commonly implicated. Neutropenia may accompany anemia and thrombocytopenia in the aplastic anemias, megaloblastic anemias, refractory anemias, hypersplenic anemias and myelophthisic marrow disorders such as leukemias and lymphomas, or other tumors. In the absence of infection, drugs, or other associated hematologic problems, neutropenia can occur as an isolated problem. Most commonly this is seen in black patients who normally may have stable neutrophil counts of 1,500 or less per cubic millimeter. There are rare instances of congenital, familial, or acquired disorders such as cyclic neutropenia, chronic benign neutropenia, or immune neutropenia. Most commonly bone marrow examination is necessary to elucidate the cause of neutropenia.

Therapy

Patients with an absolute granulocyte count below 1,000 have a significantly increased susceptibility to infection, especially bacterial. Fever is a rather nonspecific finding but when associated with stomatitis, pharyngitis, or bleeding, the possibility of severe granulocytopenia should be considered.

The patient who presents with significant granulocytopenia *with* fever must be considered to have a life-threatening infection and should be treated as a medical emergency. The patient should be promptly evaluated for areas of specific infection, and all necessary cultures should be taken. The patient should then be immediately started on broad-spectrum antibiotics preferably of bactericidal type; the etiology of the granulocytopenia should be evaluated later.

BLEEDING AND THROMBOSIS

Normal Hemostasis

To understand the mechanisms of disorders that lead to the development of thrombosis or bleeding, it is necessary to understand normal hemostatic mechanisms. The normal sequence of events in clotting can be divided into (1) formation of platelet plug, platelet release reactions, and generation of thrombin; (2) formation of fibrin clot; and (3) dissolution of the fibrin clot by way of the fibrinolytic system.

After a vascular injury, platelets are attracted to the site and will adhere to the exposed tissue. Figure 40.4 illustrates the normal coagulation schema. Activated platelets, as well as the damaged vessel wall, release substances that cause other plate-

COAGULATION AND FIBRINOLYTIC SYSTEM, FOLLOWING TISSUE INJURY.
Ca++, CALCIUM; PL, PHOSPHOLIPID; a, ACTIVATED FACTOR.

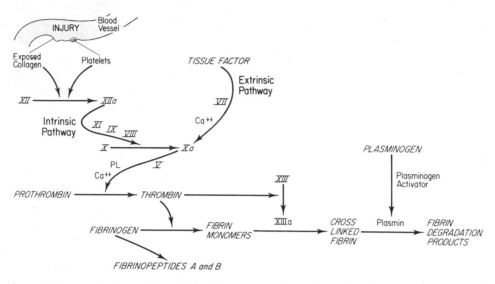

Figure 40.4 Coagulation and fibrinolytic pathways after tissue injury. PL, phospholipid; a, activated factor. (Used with permission from Rosenthal, DS: *Hematologic oncologic disorders and heart disease.* Heart Disease, Ed Braunwald, EB, Philadelphia, PA, W. B. Saunders Co., 1980, p. 1793.)

lets in the circulation to be attracted to the traumatic site, thus beginning the formation of a platelet plug.

As the platelet plug is being formed, exposed collagen from the damaged vessel activates Hageman factor (factor XII). Activated factor XII and its generated by-products stimulate the activation of the intrinsic clotting pathway, which eventually leads to the formation of thrombin. Small amounts of thrombin cause irreversible platelet aggregation and increase the platelet release reactions promoting the formation of more thrombin. Thrombin can also be formed by the extrinsic clotting pathway through a tissue factor released from the damaged vascular endothelium.

Once thrombin has been formed, it attacks the fibrinogen molecule, converting it to fibrin, and there is release of two fragments, fibrinopeptides A and B. As fibrin is laid down, the hemostatic plug is strengthened and stabilized. Release of fibrinopeptide A initiates fibrin polymerization. With activation of factor XIII by thrombin, covalent cross-links are introduced between polymerized fibrin molecules, and the resultant clot becomes mechanically strong and able to withstand the trauma of other events within the vascular system.

Dissolution of the fibrin clot occurs by way of the fibrinolytic system. Plasminogen is incorporated within the clot, ready to

be activated. The exposed endothelial cell serves as the activator during the laying down of fibrin. Fortunately, activation normally does not occur outside the clot, thus restricting the normal extent of fibrinolysis.

Clinical Evaluation of Bleeding Patients

In evaluating a bleeding patient, it should be remembered that localized processes such as a laceration, duodenal ulcers, and poorly sutured wounds, and not disorders of the hemostatic mechanism, account for most bleeding. Certain bleeding manifestations, however, may suggest the presence of a hemostatic disorder. Particularly helpful in this evaluation is the patient's prior experience with surgery, trauma, and dental extractions. A history of prior surgery or trauma without bleeding is evidence against a hereditary hemostatic disorder but does not exclude the possibility of an acquired disorder. The history of easy bruising is difficult to evaluate but may be of significance when the degree of bruising seems out of proportion to the trauma sustained. The development of large superficial ecchymoses or hematomas after minor trauma or a history of hemarthroses may be clues to an underlying coagulation disorder. Recurrent epistaxis and gingival bleeding are most commonly seen in patients with platelet abnormalities. Whenever historical clues to a hemostatic disorder are present, a history of drug intake, especially drugs known to affect hemostasis such as warfarin or aspirin, should be obtained. A positive family history of bleeding may help to define the abnormality.

In examining the patient it is important to search for a local cause to explain the bleeding or for evidence of associated diseases such as jaundice and liver disease that may explain the cause of the hemostatic disorder. The presence and/or absence of hepatomegaly, splenomegaly, lymph node enlargement, and bone tenderness may be helpful in understanding the reason for a hemostatic disorder.

When bleeding is ongoing the patient will require initial management before turning to the laboratory to find a definitive diagnosis. The patient should be kept quiet and should not be exposed to any unnecessary trauma. Careful attention should be paid to problems that may lead to further bleeding such as hypertension. When the bleeding site is accessible, local pressure may be applied to control the bleeding and local vasoconstriction, especially with the use of cold packs, may be of some value. When a hemostatic disorder is suspected, parenteral medication should not be given intramuscularly, unless essential, because of the possibility of causing intramuscular hematoma formation. Drugs such as aspirin that affect the function of platelets should not be administered so as to avoid an added reason for bleeding. Table 40.8 outlines the clinical difference between the types of bleeding seen in patients with coagulation defects versus those with platelet defects.

Laboratory Evaluation of Bleeding

The integrity of the clotting mechanism can be evaluated using various laboratory studies. Platelets are evaluated both numerically and functionally. Platelet function can first be screened by a simple bleeding time and if abnormal by other more sophisticated platelet aggregation studies. Abnormalities of the intrinsic pathway can be detected by the activated partial thromboplastin time (PTT), whereas the extrinsic clotting pathway is screened by the prothrombin time (PT).

PLATELET COUNT

Calculation of platelet number is usually performed by direct counting, similar to the white blood cell count, or by an automated cell counter. A quick but rough estimate of platelet number can be made on a peripheral blood smear by adding the number of platelets seen in each of five oil immersion microscopic fields and multiplying the sum by 2,000. Platelet counts normally range between 150,000 and 450,000/mm^3.

BLEEDING TIME

The bleeding time test has been hampered by the need for standardization and reproducibility. Recently available are templates that allow generally reproducible results. The Ivy bleeding time (template method) is performed on the volar surface of the forearm while a blood pressure cuff inflated to 40 mm Hg is placed on the arm above the test site. A standardized puncture wound 1 mm deep and 9 mm long is made by the template blade, and the time is measured until the bleeding stops. With the new commercially available templates, the normal bleeding time range is 3–9 minutes. Prolonged bleeding indicates a defect in the first phase of clotting, the formation of the platelet plug, and may be because of decreased numbers of platelets or abnormally functioning platelets. Since the bleeding time is affected by thrombocytopenia, doing a bleeding time does not add any additional information when the platelet count is less than 10,000.

PROTHROMBIN TIME

The PT measures the extrinsic pathway. An abnormally prolonged test suggests a deficiency in factors V, VII, X, prothrombin, and/or fibrinogen.

TABLE 40.8 Bleeding Characteristics from Platelet and Coagulation Abnormalities

Coagulation Defect	Platelet Defect
Intramuscular and deep hematomas	Petechiae, pupura
Hemarthrosis	Mucosal bleeding, e.g., epistaxis
Delayed onset of bleeding after trauma	Prolonged bleeding from minor cuts
Rebleeding late after initial episode	Widespread but especially located where capillaries under hydrostatic pressure, e.g., legs
Hemorrhage from venipuncture site if firm pressure not maintained long enough	Superficial ecchymosis around venipuncture sites

PARTIAL THROMBOPLASTIN TIME

The PTT tests the intrinsic pathway factors, such as factors V, VIII, IX, X, XI, XII, prothrombin, and fibrinogen.

SUMMARY

The four tests just described are readily available in all laboratories, and when they are performed as a screening workup for a bleeding disorder they will be sufficient in detecting over 95% of diagnosable bleeding dyscrasias. If an abnormality is found on the screening test, further evaluation is warranted and more specific tests can be done to isolate the problem. Table 40.9 outlines the diagnostic possibilities if one or more of the tests is abnormal and the next step that should be considered.

Platelet Abnormalities

Hemostatic disorders related to platelet abnormalities can be divided into quantitative and qualitative abnormalities. In quantitative disorders, bleeding occurs as a result of a decrease in platelet number. Qualitative disorders occur when the platelet number is adequate but function is abnormal. Both disorders should be associated with a prolonged bleeding time.

Patients who are thrombocytopenic or have abnormally functioning platelets are likely to complain of prolonged bleeding from superficial or minor cuts, easy bruisability, epistaxis, gingival bleeding, and menorrhagia. On physical examination, petechiae, purpura, gingival, and mucosal membrane bleeding are found.

THROMBOCYTOPENIA

In general, major problems with hemostasis do not occur with platelet counts greater than 20,000, and patients with platelet counts over 50,000 should be able to undergo surgical procedures without excessive bleeding. If thrombocytopenia is established, we should carefully question the patient about the use of drugs associated with thrombocytopenia (Table 40.10). The next step in treating any thrombocytopenic patient is to request a hematologic evaluation and determine the need for an urgent bone marrow aspiration and therapeutic intervention.

TABLE 40.9 Laboratory Evaluation—Bleeding Disorders[a]

Platelets	Bleeding Time	PT	PTT	Differential Diagnosis	Diagnostic Tests
↓	ND	nl	nl	ITP, drug sensitivity; bone marrow depression	Platelet antibody, marrow aspirate
↓	ND	abn	abn	DIC	Fibrinogen assays, fibrinogen split products, thrombin time
nl	abn	nl	nl	Platelet function defect, salicylates, uremia	Platelet aggregation, blood urea nitrogen (BUN), creatinine
nl	abn	nl	abn	Von Willebrand's disease	Factor VIII assay, Factor VIII antigen, platelet adhesiveness, ristocetin aggregation
nl	nl	abn	nl	Factor VII deficiency or inhibitor	Factor VII assay (nl plasma should correct PT if no inhibitor)
nl	nl	abn	abn	Factor V, X, II, I deficiencies as in liver disease or with anticoagulants	Liver function tests, F assays (could be a combined deficiency)
nl	nl	nl	abn	Factor VIII (hemophilia), IX, XI, or XII deficiencies or inhibitor	Individual factor assay (nl plasma should correct PTT if no inhibitor)
nl	nl	nl	nl	Factor XIII deficiency	Urea stabilizing test, Factor XIII assay

[a]Abbreviations: nl, normal; ↓, decreased; abn, prolonged; ND, not done (when platelets ↓); F, factor; ITP, idiopathic thrombocytopenic purpura; DIC, disseminated intravascular coagulopathy.

TABLE 40.10 Drug-Induced Thrombocytopenia

Thiazides, diuretics
Ethyl alcohol
Estrogen
Sulfa antibiotics
Diphenylhydantoin
Para-aminosalicylic acid (PAS)
Quinine
Quinidine
Digitoxin
Gold salts
Methyldopa

The thrombocytopenias can be differentiated on the basis of the number of megakaryocytes in the marrow (see Fig. 40.5).

Treatment

When the problem is lack of production of the platelets, platelet transfusion is usually the treatment of choice. For general purposes, the dose of platelet transfusion can be derived by anticipating an increase in platelet count of approximately 10,000/mm^3 for each unit of platelet concentrate infused in the average-sized adult. In treating hemorrhage in thrombocytopenic patients, we should aim to increase the platelet count to approximately 50,000–100,000/mm^3.

Treatment of thrombocytopenia secondary to peripheral destruction is dependent upon the cause of the loss. Although platelet transfusion is not usually harmful, it may be totally useless. Careful questioning of the patient about drugs that may be associated is of prime importance. If any drugs are implicated they should be discontinued. Steroids are usually the therapy of choice in immune thrombocytopenic purpura (ITP), but splenectomy may be required. Proper management requires hematologic consultation.

DISORDERS OF PLATELET FUNCTION

Disorders of platelet function are becoming more common, the increased incidence correlating with the availability of more reliable laboratory tests. These disorders are characterized by an abnormally prolonged bleeding time and can be classified a physiologic platelet defect (Table 40.11). When patients with aggregation defects require treatment for bleeding, they are

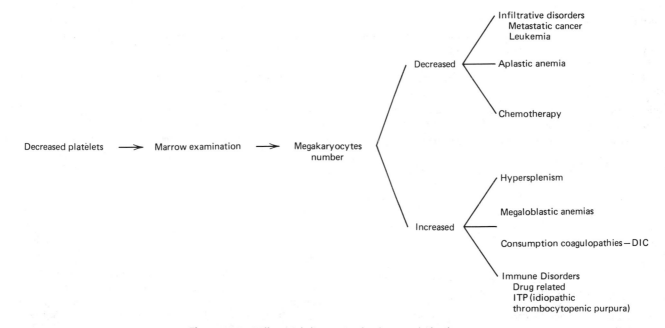

Figure 40.5 Differential diagnosis of a decreased platelet count.

TABLE 40.11 Platelet Function Defects

I. Decreased adhesiveness
    A. Von Willebrand's disease
    B. Bernard-Soulier syndrome
II. Aggregation defects
    A. Thrombasthenia
    B. Storage pool syndrome
    C. Defective release reactions
        1. Uremia
        2. Dysproteinemias—myeloma, Waldenström's
        3. Drugs
            a. Aspirin and aspirin-containing drugs
            b. Chlorpromazine
            c. Diphenhydramine (Benadryl)

given platelet transfusion with platelet concentrates using the same guidelines as in thrombocytopenia.

VON WILLEBRAND'S DISEASE

Von Willebrand's disease is an autosomal dominant disorder in which there is a plasma deficiency of factor VIII, which results in reduction of platelet adhesion to the vessel wall and is associated with a prolonged bleeding time. Diagnostic laboratory tests, ordered by the specialty consultant, include an abnormal ristocetin aggregation, decreased factor VIII, and a decreased factor VIII antigen. There are wide variations in the severity of the bleeding from patient to patient and even from time to time in the same patient. Generally, no therapy is needed, but people are advised to avoid medications such as aspirin. If surgery or dental extractions are required or patients experience trauma, 2 units of fresh or frozen plasma each day are usually sufficient to prevent bleeding complications.

Factor Deficiencies

Over 90% of patients with inherited coagulation disorders have classic hemophilia A (factor VIII deficiency). Christmas disease (hemophilia B or factor IX deficiency) accounts for another 9%, and hereditary factor XI, X, and VII deficiencies the remaining conditions.

FACTOR VIII AND FACTOR IX DEFICIENCIES (HEMOPHILIA AND CHRISTMAS DISEASE)

Factor VIII and IX deficiencies are X-linked recessive disorders, and about 25% of patients have no family history of a bleeding

dyscrasia. The types of bleeding problems encountered are characteristically deep bleeding such as hematomas and bleeding into large joints (hemarthroses). As noted in Table 40.9, the PTT is prolonged, whereas the PT, platelet count, and bleeding time are normal. Specific factor assays are necessary in order to make a diagnosis.

Treatment

Factor levels relate to the severity of the bleeding (greater than 5% is mild, 1–5% moderate, and less than 1% severe). Therapy is required for spontaneous bleeding, trauma, surgery, and dental extractions. There are many available commercial factor VIII and IX preparations, as well as blood bank-prepared cryoprecipitate. The latter is more difficult to prepare and requires a larger volume for replacement, but it carries a lower risk of hepatitis.

All of the coagulation factors are measured in units. Each unit of a specific factor is defined as the amount of that factor in 1 ml of normal plasma. In calculating the dose of factor to be administered, we can expect approximately a 1% rise in factor level for each factor unit infused per kilogram of body weight. The concentrates have been assayed for the amount of factor present. With cryoprecipitate the amount of factor VIII present is usually 70–100 units per unit of cryoprecipitate. For a mild bleed, such as a simple joint bruise, a one-time infusion sufficient to raise the factor level to 5–10% may suffice. For a serious bleed, such as a lacerated tongue, knife wound, or retroperitoneal hematoma, enough units should be given daily to get the level to 25–30% and to maintain it at that level for 2–3 days. If we anticipate a major surgical procedure, levels as high as 50% are needed for 2–3 weeks. Since factor VIII has a half-life of 12 hours it is necessary to infuse it every 12 hours. Factor IX has a half-life of 24 hours and can therefore be administered once daily.

Prognosis

Hematologic consultation should be requested early in the care of the hemophiliac patient, and long-term close follow-ups are strongly recommended. Early treatment may prevent permanent joint damage. New programs of home care and self-care are available for these patients so as to limit their potential frequent emergency room visits.

Although factor VIII and IX deficiencies are the most commonly seen inherited disorders, patients with other factor deficiencies are occasionally seen in the emergency situation. Table 40.12 gives guidelines for therapy for inherited coagulation defects.

TABLE 40.12 Summary of Replacement Therapy for Inherited Coagulation Defects

Deficiency	Factor Replacement	Dosage/kg Body Weight	
		Initial	Maintenance per Day
Fibrinogen	Plasma	25 ml	5–10 ml
(Factor I)	Cryoprecipitate	2–4 bags/10 kg	1 bag/kg every other day
Factor V	Fresh frozen plasma	15–25 ml	10 ml every 12 hr
Factor VII	Plasma	5–10 ml	5 ml four times a day
	Prothrombin complex	5–10 units	5 units four times a day
Von Willebrand's	Fresh frozen plasma	Not necessary	10 ml
	Cryoprecipitate	Not necessary	1 bag/10 kg 1–2 days
Factor IX			
Hemophilia B	Fresh frozen plasma	30 ml	7 ml every 12 hr for 1–4 days
	Purified prothrombin complex	30 units	10 units every 12 hr for 2–4 days
Christmas disease	Fresh frozen plasma	60 ml	7 ml every 12 hr
	Purified prothrombin complex	60 units	10 units every 12 hr
Factor X	Plasma	10–15 ml	10 ml
(Stuart factor)			
Factor XI	Plasma	10–20 ml	5 ml
Factor XIII	Plasma	3–5 ml every 1–2 wk	Unnecessary
Factor VIII Hemophilia A			
	Cryoprecipitate	Not necessary	1.25–1.75 bags/10 kg every 12 hr for 2–4 days
Minor bleed	Purified Factor VIII	Not necessary	10–15 units every 12 hr for 2–4 days
	Fresh frozen plasma	Not necessary	10–15 ml every 12 hr for 2–4 days
	Cryoprecipitate	3.5 bags/10 kg	1.75 bags/10 kg every 8–12 hr
Major bleed	Purified Factor VIII	30 unit	10–15 units every 8–12 hr
	Fresh frozen plasma	30 ml	15 ml every 8–12 hr

Acquired Bleeding Disorders

LIVER DISEASE

Synthesis and degradation of many of the coagulation proteins takes place in the liver. Most of these factors are the vitamin K dependent factors. Impaired vitamin K function and liver failure will result in deficiencies of factors II, VII, IX, X, as well as factor V, and in severe cases fibrinogen decreases. Prothrombin time and PTT will both be abnormal because factors in both intrinsic and extrinsic pathways are affected. In addition, hypersplenism, a common complication of liver disease and portal hypertension, can cause thrombocytopenia.

Treatment

In the patients with liver disease vitamin K should be administered in an attempt to improve the PT and PTT, but if the liver disease is severe, improvement may be only partial. It is not necessary to treat these patients with coagulation factors on a prophylactic basis, but when bleeding occurs it may be necessary to treat the patients with fresh or frozen plasma using 10–15 ml of fresh or frozen plasma per kilogram of body weight.

VITAMIN K DEFICIENCY

Vitamin K deficiency and thus the synthesis of the vitamin K dependent coagulation factors (factors II, VII, IX, and X) usually occur in the setting of liver dysfunction, of abnormalities of vitamin K absorption from the intestinal tract, and with the use of coumarin anticoagulant drugs. Deficiency of vitamin K is manifest by elevation of the PT and PTT; however, in practice the PT is much more prolonged than the PTT.

Treatment

When vitamin K deficiency is suspected the most useful diagnostic test is a therapeutic trial of vitamin K. When 10 mg of vitamin K are administered orally or parenterally (intramuscularly), the abnormal clotting study should return to normal within 12 hours.

MASSIVE TRANSFUSION

Blood stored at 4°C for 48 hours or more becomes deficient in factors V, VII and also in platelets. After transfusions of many units of stored blood, patients can become deficient in these factors on a dilutional basis. It usually requires 10–12 units of blood in a 24-hour period to dilute the patient's normal factors sufficiently to cause significant clinical problems. In most cases major trauma or surgery precipitate this degree of transfusion requirement; however, gastrointestinal hemorrhage or gynecologic or obstetric difficulties may also require massive transfusion.

Diagnosis and Treatment

In patients with this clinical situation, coagulation studies would reveal abnormalities of the PT and PTT and a low platelet count. When bleeding becomes a problem in this situation, the factor deficiencies may be replenished with fresh or frozen plasma and the thrombocytopenia may be corrected with platelet concentrates.

TABLE 40.13 Disorders Associated with DIC

I.   Pregnancy and delivery complications
A.   Abruptio placenta
B.   Amniotic fluid embolism
C.   Septic abortion
D.   Retained dead fetus
II.   Infections
A.   Septicemia, especially with gram-negative organisms
B.   Meningococcemia
C.   Viral infections
III. Hemolytic transfusion reactions
IV.   Metastatic carcinoma, especially prostate, pancreas, lung, stomach, and colon
V.   Extensive tissue damage
A.   Massive trauma
B.   Heat stroke
C.   Burns
D.   Anoxia
VI.   Anaphylactic drug reactions
VII. Acute leukemia, particularly promyelocytic leukemia
VIII. Surgical procedures
A.   Prostatic surgery
B.   Lung surgery
C.   Extracorporeal circulation

DISSEMINATED INTRAVASCULAR COAGULATION

The sudden onset of diffuse hemorrhage in an acutely ill patient who arrives in the emergency room may be the result of disseminated intravascular coagulation (DIC). This disorder results from aberrant release of substances that will activate the coagulation system leading to abnormal thrombin formation and eventual depletion of clotting factors and resultant bleeding. These patients may present with peripheral cyanosis, gangrene of the digits or tip of the nose, and/or diffuse hemorrhage in the skin, in the mucous membranes, and at venipuncture sites. Oliguria or anuria as well as neurologic difficulties are not uncommon. Many disorders have been associated with DIC; the most commonly encountered ones are listed in Table 40.13.

Diagnosis

The clinical suspicion of DIC can be confirmed by laboratory studies. The peripheral blood smear may reveal microangiopathic red cells. The platelet count is decreased and the PT and PTT are both prolonged. In addition, fibrinogen is reduced, causing a prolonged PT, and fibrinogen breakdown products, termed fibrinogen split products (FSP), are found, causing a prolonged thrombin time.

Treatment

Treatment of DIC is directed against both the underlying disease and the resultant bleeding diathesis. These patients are usually acutely ill and require urgent therapy, that is, treatment of septicemia, shock, acute obstetric catastrophe, and so on. If the primary disorder cannot be adequately treated, there may be little success in managing the DIC. If the bleeding is minimal and the underlying disorder is being adequately treated, no therapy may be needed for the DIC. If, however, despite adequate treatment of the primary disorder, bleeding becomes a significant problem, hematologic consultation should be urgently sought regarding the use of fresh or frozen plasma, platelet transfusions, as well as heparin. Heparin's role in this situation is directed against the activation of the coagulation system by the underlying disorder. However, heparin can increase bleeding and in general should not be used without replacements of platelets and coagulation proteins. When heparin is used the usual starting dosage is 500–1,500 units/hr given as a continuous intravenous infusion. Heparin should be discontinued if bleeding increases. The course of the DIC should be closely followed, and there should be frequent observations of the coagulation parameters, including the platelet count, fibrinogen, PT, PTT, thrombin time, and fibrin split products. Improvement in the fibrinogen and reduction of the fibrin split products should occur within 24 hours of control of the DIC. The thrombocytopenia may persist for several days. Improvement of fibrinogen level or reduction of fibrin split products in the patient treated with heparin would be an indication for continuation of the drug.

Prognosis

Since DIC is a result of an acute medical illness, prognosis depends almost entirely upon the speed of the physician in handling the bleeding emergency, as well as the ability to treat the underlying disorder.

FIBRINOLYSIS

Fibrinolysis usually accompanies DIC and rarely occurs as a primary disorder. Use of agents such as ε-aminocaproic acid (EACA), which block fibrinolysis, can be dangerous in patients with DIC since it may lead to widespread and fatal thrombosis. Primary fibrinolysis (i.e., without DIC) has been associated with prostatic manipulation or cancer. In the latter instance, EACA may be indicated.

HYPERCOAGULABLE STATES

In addition to local injury or damage to vessel walls, there are a number of theoretical and clinical mechanisms that have been associated with abnormally increased clotting or what has been termed *the hypercoagulable state*. In many cases, some of the theoretical mechanisms proposed have been difficult to evaluate in vivo as true cause and effect. We should be aware of four mechanisms that may lead to thrombosis: (1) abnormal blood flow and stasis, (2) decreased concentration of clotting inhibitors, (3) abnormal acceleration of platelet release and aggregation, and (4) impaired clearance of activated clotting factors.

Abnormal blood flow or stasis is certainly a contributing factor in thrombosis. Sickle cell disease, polycythemia, and hyperviscosity syndromes are good clinical examples. In addition, oral contraceptives have been repeatedly implicated in thromboembolic disease, in some cases associated with a shortened PTT and increased platelets.

Decreased inhibitors of coagulation proteins prevent the normal inactivation of these proteins and may cause thrombosis. For example, a deficiency of antithrombin III activity has been reported in families with increased thrombosis. Antithrombin III is the principal factor responsible for inactivation of thrombin as well as factors X, XI, and XII. Screening PT and PTT may be shortened or completely normal. Serum levels of antithrombin III are now available.

Although most platelet aggregation defects are associated with bleeding, spontaneous aggregation has been reported to occur in disorders associated with thrombocytosis, such as polycythemia and essential thrombocytosis. Clearance of activated coagulation factors usually takes place in the liver and reticuloendothelial system, and occasionally cirrhosis and viral hepatitis may impair the clearance mechanism and lead to widespread thrombosis.

Anticoagulation Treatment

Anticoagulation is clearly beneficial in the treatment and prevention of thrombosis in the venous side of the circulation. Heparin and oral anticoagulants both have definitive roles in treatment, and platelet suppressive agents are currently being evaluated.

As discussed in Chapters 2, 3, and 39, heparin is the most useful drug available for prophylaxis and treatment of venous thromboembolism. The current recommended dosage for treatment of patients with acute thromboembolism is 30,000 units per day by continuous intravenous infusion or enough to keep the PTT at 1.5–2.5 times the control level. Studies have confirmed that a lower dose of heparin is effective prophylaxis against deep venous thrombosis in postoperative patients. If hemorrhage occurs with heparin therapy, protamine sulfate given about milligram for milligram of heparin should correct the bleeding. The duration of action of heparin is 4 hours. If bleeding occurs more than 4 hours after discontinuation of heparin, protamine is not required.

Oral anticoagulants such as warfarin and its derivatives compete for vitamin K in the liver and interfere with the formation of factors II, VII, IX, and X. The primary indications for long term therapy with these agents are venous thrombosis of the leg and pulmonary embolism after the patient has initially received heparin. In addition, warfarin is useful in prophylaxis in patients with significant mitral stenosis, especially patients with atrial fibrillation, with artificial heart valves, after an acute arterial embolic episode, or after hip surgery. The starting dosage of warfarin is 10 mg/day for 3–4 days and the usual maintenance dosage is 3–8 mg/day. Prothrombin times are usually kept at 2–2.5 times control.

Complications of anticoagulant therapy include significant bleeding or rethrombosis. Both may occur because of the addition or deletion of other medications to warfarin which po-

TABLE 40.14 Drug Effect with Coumarin Derivatives

Potentiate	Antagonize
Phenylbutazone	Barbiturates
Salicylates	Other
Thyroid	Chronic alcohol
Other	Allopurinol
Acute alcohol	Cholestyramine
Anabolic steroids	Diuretics
Antibiotics	Glutethimide
Antiplatelet drugs	Nortriptyline
Clofibrate	Rifampicin
Diphenylhydantoin	
Oral hypoglycemic agents	
Quinidine sulfate	
Sulfonamides	

tentiate or antagonize its action. Physicians should be aware of this combined drug effect. If the patient has to take any of the medications listed in Table 40.14, the physician should be alerted to any change in dosage schedule that may be necessary.

Warfarin overdose is best managed with fresh or frozen plasma transfusions. In general 2 units of fresh or frozen plasma will correct PT sufficiently to stop bleeding. Vitamin K in dosages of 10–25 mg is also effective parenterally, but it takes 12–24 hours to reverse the toxicity and causes temporary resistance to further warfarin treatment.

Platelet suppressive agents such as aspirin, sulfinpyrazone, and dipyridamole are being tested in patients with valvular heart disease, prosthetic valves, cerebral vascular disease, threatened strokes, and coronary artery disease. Preliminary results are encouraging but not definitive.

SELECTED READINGS

Berlin NI: Diagnosis and classification of the polycythemias. *Sem Hematol* 1975; 12:339–351.

Castle WB, Minor GR: *Pathological Physiology and Clinical Descriptions of the Anemias.* New York, Oxford University Press, 1936, p 2.

Handin RI: Bleeding disorders, in Branch W (ed): *Office Practice of Medicine* pp 1049–1062, 1982.

Jones P: Developments and problems in the management of hemophilia. *Sem Hematol* 1977; 14:375–390.

Kaplan AP: Initiation of intrinsic coagulation and fibrinolytic pathways of man. *Prog Hemost Thromb* 1979; 4:127.

Nathan DG, Oski FA: Hematology of infancy and childhood, in Platt O, Nathan DG (eds): *Sickle Cell Disease*, ed 2. Philadelphia, WB Saunders Co, 1981, pp 687–725.

Pirofsky B: Clinical aspects of autoimmune hemolytic anemia. *Sem Hematol* 1976; 13:251–265.

Rosenthal DS: Problems involving an abnormal blood count, in Branch W(ed): *Office Practice of Medicine.* Philadelphia, WB Saunders Co, 1982, pp 1027–1048.

Varat MA, Adolphs RJ, Fowler NO: Cardiovascular effects of anemia. *Am Heart J* 1972; 83:415.

Williams WJ: Principles of coagulation tests, in Williams, WJ (ed): *Hematology,* New York, McGraw-Hill Book Co, 1972, pp 1098–1104.

Williams WJ, Beutler E, Ersley AJ and Rundles RW: *Hematology,* ed 2. New York, McGraw-Hill Book Co, 1977.

Wintrobe MM: *Clinical Hematology*, ed 8. Philadelphia, Lea & Febiger, 1982.

41
PSYCHIATRIC EMERGENCIES

Malcolm P. Rogers
Peter Reich

A psychiatric emergency occurs when there is imminent or actual disruption of the mental system and when there is danger of suicidal or aggressive behavior or of excessive psychological pain or trauma. In this chapter, the psychiatric emergencies most commonly encountered in medical practice will be discussed. These include suicidal states, psychoses, acute overwhelming anxiety and grief, psychological shock, and conditions associated with loss of control of aggressive impulses. The approach to the patient will be presented from the point of view of a physician in a general hospital emergency ward, where expert consultation in psychiatry may not be immediately available. Disturbed patients often seek help in an emergency ward or are brought there by concerned relatives or friends or by the police. A general hospital is one of the few places in most communities where professional help is always available and where a patient in distress can count on receiving comfort and care. In a sense, any medical emergency represents an urgent psychological situation, and it is not surprising to find that many patients on an emergency ward are frightened, depressed, even desperate, or are suffering other acute emotional reactions. It may require some clinical experience before a physician can distinguish these ubiquitous manifestations of stress from psychiatric emergencies in which coping mechanisms start to fail and the psychological apparatus itself begins to break down.

Because the mind is only manifested by the thoughts and behavior of the patient, the recognition of a psychiatric emergency may be one of the most difficult aspects of emergency care. When a patient presents with a major behavioral disturbance, such as a suicide attempt or some form of bizarre or assaultive behavior, or when the patient is having a florid psychotic break, the physician may have no difficulty in defining the situation as a psychiatric emergency. Sometimes psychological crises may present as physical distress or may be masked by concomitant medical or surgical emergencies. At other times, a highly significant mental change may only be seen in the mental content or thought processes of the patient. Some patients may try to conceal their mental disturbances, and it may only be a relative or some other concerned person who provides the crucial data.

Once recognized, a psychiatric emergency, even on a busy Saturday night, can usually be managed by traditional medical measures that are used in any emergency room. The complete etiology of the emergency state does not need to be known in most cases in order for the physician to address the urgent needs of the patient. In some cases in which a psychiatric emergency occurs as the direct result of a medical problem, such as hypoglycemia, head injury, or a toxic state, the underlying medical situation must be managed before the psychiatric emergency will be amenable to treatment. Thus a thorough medical evaluation is always part of the approach to a psychiatric emergency. Beyond this, it is possible to outline a logical approach to the management of emotionally disturbed patients that is well within the expertise of the average physician and can reduce the immediate crisis, minimize psychological morbidity, and open the way to definitive treatment.

APPROACH TO THE PATIENT

General Principles

Although the specific details encountered vary enormously, certain general principles are useful in approaching all psychiatric emergencies.

ESTABLISH RAPID CONTACT

Patients with psychiatric emergencies should not be left standing around, especially patients who are tense, agitated, or ambivalent about asking for help. Rapid contact, for example, an introduction or an expression of genuine concern for the patient's problem, should be made. Then the patient may be led into a room, introduced to the nurse, have vital signs taken, and so on. All of these steps start the process of engagement in the medical system and will allay tension and allow for further waiting if necessary. This process takes only a few minutes and may well be life saving. It may prevent a suicidal patient from fleeing the emergency room to a tragic end.

EXPEDITE TALKING TO REDUCE TENSION

Putting thoughts and emotions into words invariably reduces initial tensions in both the patient and the physician. Problems and issues should be addressed directly. For example, if a patient has just made a suicide attempt, the physician should inquire directly about the suicidal behavior and ask about current suicidal feelings, for example: "Are you still feeling that you want to die"?

MAKE A QUICK FIRST ASSESSMENT

The initial assessment of the patient can proceed rapidly. It is surprising how much clinical information is obtained simply by looking at or briefly listening to the patient, even from across the room. It provides a composite and instantaneous impression of the patient's general appearance, level of consciousness, level of tension, and leading affect or mood. Any obvious neurologic or physical disturbance may also be noted. The value of this rapid initial appraisal grows with experience and guides the clinician's next step.

CHOOSE BEST SETTING FOR THE INTERVIEW

In general a private and relaxed setting for the interview is best. Some patients, especially those who are paranoid and frightened of being trapped or attacked, may do better in a more open space with other people, such as family members or friends or nursing staff, present and not in a small enclosed room. We should attempt to make the patient as comfortable as possible and also as much of a participant in the interview as possible. It often helps, for example, to have a patient who is lying flat sit up together with the physician. Seemingly minor nonverbal communication of this sort goes a long way toward promoting the patient's cooperation and most mature level of functioning. The more we treat the patient as a mature and worthy person, the more we tend to elicit these characteristics.

ALLOW FOR SLOW FINAL EVALUATION

After the initial need for speed in engaging the patient within the medical system or in managing acute behavioral disturbances, the physician should take time to complete the evaluation. Many initially overwhelmed people may reconstitute within a matter of hours when allowed to talk, rest, or even sleep. Often there is no harm in allowing an upset patient to sit a few hours with other people as company. The patient's mental state may change dramatically, so it is important not to be premature in making a disposition based entirely on the initial presentation.

TAKE THE CHIEF COMPLAINT SERIOUSLY

It is important to listen carefully to the patient's chief complaint. Even in psychiatric emergencies, the chief complaint is often a somatic one. The present illness should be elicited with the chief complaint as the starting point, using the language of the patient.

ATTEND TO THE PATIENT'S BODY

A brief physical examination should be performed routinely in almost all psychiatric emergencies, especially when there is a physical complaint. It is much easier to examine a patient who is emotionally upset than most people think. A calm medical approach is reassuring to most patients and tends to bring many situations under control. Physical caring is often the first step in expression of emotional caring and is so interpreted by patients.

APPRECIATE THERAPEUTIC NATURE OF INTERVIEW

Listening is an active and demanding process. Most of the time it means sitting down and giving all of our attention to the patient, even if it is for just 5 or 10 minutes. What patients find most comforting is the feeling of being understood. Unlike most medical interviews, the interview of the patient with a psychiatric emergency not only elicits further information, but is, in itself, therapeutic.

BE NONJUDGMENTAL AND TACTFUL

The physician should be careful to avoid a judgmental or punitive approach, especially toward patients with self-inflicted injuries. The patient may already feel very guilty, and his or her response may be to conceal further a suicidal wish. It is very important to avoid being overheard making snide remarks or joking about other matters. If it is necessary to discuss a patient with another person, whether a member of the family or a professional colleague, the physician should find a separate place out of the range of the patient's hearing, unless the physician specifically wishes to include the patient in the discussion. In that case, the discussion should take place in the immediate presence of the patient and the patient should be offered an opportunity to participate in it. The usual considerations about confidentiality should be observed. The physician should ask permission of the patient to talk with relatives, friends, or outside professionals.

LEARN FROM YOUR OWN EMOTIONS

The physician's own emotional reaction to the patient is of diagnostic value. Feelings are contagious. Depressed patients tend to elicit depression, anxious patients tend to elicit anxiety, and psychotic patients tend to elicit a feeling of strangeness. In this aspect of the examination, the physician is his or her own instrument.

CONTACT FAMILY

It is important to make contact with relatives and outside therapists. The physician should attempt to engage them in caring for the patient in the emergency room and in providing further history. If they are already there, try to have them remain (something they will be more apt to do if they feel their presence is valued). If they are not there, contact them by telephone. If time is a problem, have the nurse or other emergency room personnel make the telephone calls.

ASSESS FAMILY AND SOCIAL SUPPORT

It is important to recognize that relatives and friends may need assistance to help them cope. They frequently feel overwhelmed when dealing with someone in an emotionally distraught or psychotic state. The time spent is well worth it; the physician needs the help of the family. The physician also needs to assess the degree of social support available in the patient's own environment. Any practical and clinically sensible disposition depends on this.

Evaluation of the Patient

HISTORY

Many of the general principles just described are directed toward the special need for rapport in assessing the psychiatric patient. In the realm of personal psychological data, the physician assumes that the patient knows more than he or she does, at least about the conscious mental processes. The knowledge that we gain of the patient's inner world depends in large measure upon the degree of rapport that is established. A genuine wish to understand, together with an open mind, certainly tends to facilitate this exchange of information. Many nonverbal cues can be extremely important. Taking the time to sit down and the care to assure at least some degree of privacy to the patient often speaks louder than words. The more the patient can participate actively and cooperatively in the process, the more information is obtained. Moreover, the very process of eliciting this role in the patient tends to have a potent therapeutic effect.

Sometimes, in spite of the best efforts of the physician, the patient may remain uncooperative. The uncooperativeness may take the form of mute withdrawal or a more subtle kind of secretiveness or sometimes blatant hostility. When resistance is such a predominant force in the interview, it often helps to confront it directly. Find out what is making the patient hesitant to talk or so angry. That becomes a primary focus for the moment rather than any historical content. In so doing, the resistance may be weakened.

Focus on Immediate Crisis

The focus should be on the history of the immediate crisis. Look for a recent event, usually within the previous 24–48 hours, that has precipitated the psychiatric crisis seen in the emergency room. However bizarre the language or emotional state of the patient or confusing the situation may be, we usually find in examining the recent events and changes of the patient's life a far more comprehensible and human explanation for the state of mind. The event may be the loss of a relationship, loss of a job, health related, or any experience that has stressed the psychic equilibrium of the patient. The patient's reaction can be viewed both in terms of the traumatic event and the underlying vulnerability to it. We can usually obtain this history simply by asking the patient to describe what has been happening over the last few days. Sometimes pursuing the principal affect, whether it be sadness or anger, brings the physician to the heart of the matter.

Look for Organic Factors

Always be alert to the possible influence of drugs or alcohol as acute precipitants, as well as of any change in psychoactive medications. Also listen for any somatic symptoms described by the patient that may indicate an underlying organic disturbance. Patients with a mild degree of dementia, for example, may become much more disorganized with an organic stress such as a urinary tract infection or an increase in congestive heart failure.

Establish Baseline

It is necessary to focus on the change in the patient's psychological state and its precipitants, but in doing so we need to have a baseline upon which to measure the change. That requires obtaining a brief picture of the patient's life and interests in its usual state, such as during the weeks or months before the crisis. We can ask patients when they last felt well, or we may look for a period of relative stability in work and interpersonal relationships. In this way we make a brief assessment of the degree of the patient's emotional health under ordinary circumstances, as well as the patient's personality style. This kind of information often comes from family or friends who will describe what the patient used to be like.

Elicit Prior Psychiatric History

The physician also tries to determine whether or not there is any prior psychiatric history. We may ask the patient or friends whether or not the patient has ever seen a psychiatrist before or is currently doing so. Finding out what, if any, psychoactive drugs the patient has taken before and for how long provides a lot of information about the patient's psychiatric history. Knowledge of prior hospitalizations and their length, as well as any specific information about prior suicide attempts or violence, is useful. We can often get the patient to compare the current crisis with previous experience in order to see how he or she has coped in the past and whether or not there is anything really unique about the current problem. If the patient has had contact with other professionals, it is very useful to contact them directly. They can provide a useful perspective on the current crisis in relation to previous levels of functioning. They may also have ongoing clinical responsibility for the patient and may need to be informed of any such crisis. Many difficult disposition problems have been resolved simply by returning patients to their outside ongoing treatment relationships, provided that the emergency room physician and the outside professional are in basic agreement about the best course of action.

Interview Family and/or Friends

In dealing with friends and relatives, the physician is evaluating their capacity to understand and deal realistically with the patient's problems, as well as their role in the psychiatric emergency. Indeed, sometimes we may find that the greater psychopathology lies in a relative and that the shift in the patient's mental status is due to some change in the family's dynamic equilibrium.

MENTAL STATUS EXAMINATION

The mental status is the key to the psychiatric examination of the patient. Briefly, it consists of the patient's appearance and behavior, pattern of speech, mood and affect, predominant concerns, the nature of thought processes, intellectual functioning, and judgment and insight. Most of the information needed in the mental status examination is obtained naturally during the course of taking a history.

Appearance, Behavior, and Manner of Speech

The physician looks in particular for evidence of acute decompensation. For example, a successful executive who appears in the emergency room looking disheveled should alert the physician to the seriousness of the situation. Any evidence of inappropriate or bizarre behavior is noted, as well as any increase or decrease in motor activity. The patient's speech is observed for its rate and for evidence of aphasia.

Mood and Affect

The physician evaluates the mood of the patient, especially with reference to a sense of hopelessness, helplessness, or worthlessness associated with serious depressions. Questions about suicidal thoughts or feelings should be asked, especially when the mood is one of despair. When a patient expresses feelings of rage, the physician should inquire into its source or target. The potential for violent behavior should then be assessed by asking about specific thoughts, plans, weapons, and the prior history of the violence.

Predominant Concerns and Thought Processes

The physician should not overstructure the interview in the beginning by asking too many questions but rather should give the patient an opportunity to organize his or her own thoughts and present his or her own views. The physician listens carefully for the degree of organization and coherence and rationality of the patient's thoughts. Any peculiar ideas or distortions in the patient's sense of reality are noted. If something the patient says seems odd, then it is a good idea to investigate it further. This approach either reveals a well-formed delusion or reassures us that the patient is thinking rationally.

Cognitive Functioning

The cognitive functioning of the patient, especially orientation and recent memory, is observed. This is another reason for trying to elicit the history of the last several days in great detail. If some deficit is suggested, the physician should do more formal testing, such as remembering three objects after 5 minutes, calculating, digit span, serial 7s, and the specific degree of orientation. This assessment of cognitive functioning is critical in the evaluation. When cognitive functioning is impaired, it suggests an organic brain syndrome, provided the patient is cooperating. When not impaired, it suggests a functional disorder.

Insight and Judgment

The best way of determining the level of insight and judgment of the patient is often to ask the patient directly how he or she assesses the situation, what he or she thinks is wrong, and what should be done about it. Asking about future plans can be very useful. Sometimes patients describe the future in very practical and specific terms that clearly imply the intent to go on living and the capacity to cope with returning to their own environment. On the other hand, sometimes patients are either unable to conceive of any reasonable future or else express a wave of hopelessness and despair, as though they could not tolerate further living. As noted above, rapid changes in the mental status of the patient during the course of an emergency room visit are very common. Very often these changes depend on the reactions of those around the patient—friends, family, or the medical staff. If a rapid change has occurred, it is useful to think about the reasons for it. Does the patient's perspective now seem very different from what it was several hours before? And if that is the case, how did the change come about? This is asking, in a sense, whether or not the crisis that has just occurred will be apt to happen again soon after the patient leaves the emergency room or whether at least a partial resolution of the problem has occurred.

PHYSICAL EXAMINATION

The physical examination of the psychiatric patient should be a matter of routine and at times is the best way of establishing psychological rapport. It may provide important clues about drug toxicity or an underlying organic disturbance. Of particular importance in routine screening are blood pressure, pulse, temperature, presence of abnormal movements, signs of autonomic dysfunction, and a brief neurologic examination. If there is any suspicion of drug use, a toxic screen should be obtained.

When to Call the Psychiatrist

As a practical matter, the emergency room physician will have to provide the initial recognition and management of the psychiatric emergency. The psychiatrist is generally called upon to make a more definitive evaluation and disposition, especially in the more serious emergencies such as psychosis or when the patient shows signs of suicidal or violent behavior. Before calling the psychiatrist, the emergency room physician should have made an initial assessment consisting of the pertinent history, both of the presenting problem and of past psychiatric treatment, the mental status, and the social support

available to the patient. Contacting family, friends, or current therapist, if one exists, is especially important and should be initiated before the psychiatrist comes in because recommendations about disposition will depend heavily on the patient's support system. In the case of overdose patients, the psychiatrist should generally be asked to come in *after* the patient has become lucid enough to carry on a reasonable conversation. Consultation should be requested for suicidal or psychotic patients, but as with all consultations, ideally, it should be asked for after the emergency room physician has carried the evaluation as far as possible, depending, in part, on how busy the emergency room is. Sometimes the emergency room physician may call the psychiatrist simply to confirm a decision. In the long run, the emergency room physician will learn far more by using consultations in this manner than as a triage decision.

CLINICAL SETTINGS

Suicidal Patients

The most common type of psychiatric emergency seen in medical practice is the management of the suicidal patient. Most of these cases are patients who have already made suicide attempts. In other cases there may be concern over suicide risk, although overt suicidal behavior has not occurred.

A physician working in a busy emergency room will probably see at least one patient a day who has made a suicide attempt. The incidence of suicide attempts has been rising steadily in the United States and now exceeds 250,000 annually, a rate that approaches epidemic proportions. By far the most frequent form of suicidal behavior seen among patients in an emergency room is ingestion of an overdose of medication. Wrist slashing also occurs, although it is much more unusual than it was 20 years ago. More bizarre suicide attempts are also seen, and some incidents of apparently accidental trauma may also turn out to be self-induced.

Suicide attempts vary in severity from apparently trivial incidents to deadly serious efforts at self-destruction. However, there is no such thing as an inconsequential suicide attempt. Even the ingestion of a few pills in a fit of anger may signal a state of desperation or psychosis.

The most urgent psychiatric question is whether the patient is actively suicidal. After a suicide attempt, most patients are in a state of low suicide potential. They are usually drained of energy, are often regretful of the attempt and are glad to be alive, and they frequently have called attention to their emotional distress and thus have experienced psychological relief. A few patients will go on to make repeated suicide attempts, even while undergoing medical care. Danger signs include psychosis, tension, negativism, such as refusal to talk or resistance to medical treatment, evasiveness, and withdrawal. When a patient appears to be concealing things, it may mean that he or she is continuing to harbor suicidal intent. While examining the patient and attending to medical matters, it is possible simultaneously to assess the mental status of the patient for suicide risk. Spontaneous and uninterrupted comments by the patient are more likely to reveal psychosis than responses to specific questions. Often the physician can encourage the patient to talk by making a sympathetic observation, such as, "You must have been feeling desperate to try to hurt yourself that way." Bizarre methods, such as the ingestion of rat poison or the injection of contaminated water, often reflect underlying psychosis and indicate continuing suicide risk. Suicide attempts made by males, by older people, by patients with a history of schizophrenia or manic–depressive psychosis, or by patients during delirium are more likely to be followed by persistent suicide tension.

EVALUATION AND MANAGEMENT

All patients who have made suicide attempts should be placed on suicide precautions from the moment they arrive in the emergency room. This means that someone other than the physician should be assigned to the patient, who should be kept under close observation. Sharp objects and medication that the patient may still have should be removed. Patients who are unconscious on admission may awaken in a suicidal state. Suicide precautions are indicated until a more definitive evaluation can be made.

Emergency treatment of a patient who has attempted suicide can be divided into three phases. In the first phase, the acute medical and psychological problems are stabilized and the patient is protected from further suicidal behavior. In the second phase, a more searching study of the nature of the suicide attempt is made in order to assess severity, etiology, and prognosis. In the third phase, a treatment plan is worked out to carry the patient beyond the crisis created by the attempt. The overall process need not be time consuming and can readily be carried out in the midst of an active emergency room.

The First Phase—Control

DEAL WITH THE MEDICAL EMERGENCY.   The medical and psychiatric evaluation begin the moment a patient arrives in the emergency room. The medical and surgical aspects of the emer-

gency are managed according to the guidelines described elsewhere in this book. If a patient has taken an overdose of drugs, it is especially important to establish baseline levels of consciousness, vital signs, and neurologic signs because there can be delayed absorption of toxic materials. The stomach contents should be evacuated promptly in every case, even when the patient claims to have ingested only a few pills or when the ingestion occurred several hours ago (see Chapter 42). Information about the nature of an overdose is notoriously unreliable, and lives can be saved by the prompt removal of stomach contents. Ipecac can be given to induce vomiting, providing there is no danger of aspiration. If the patient is obtunded, a stomach tube can be passed and the gastric contents aspirated directly, usually after intubation. The only contraindication to the removal of the stomach contents by mouth is when ingestion of corrosive or highly volatile liquids is suspected. In these situations, an emergency gastrotomy may be indicated. As a matter of routine, an intravenous line should be started in all patients who have made a suicide attempt by ingestion.

SECURE SAFETY.   At this stage, the patient should not be left alone. Sharp objects and pills must be removed from immediate reach, including from the patient's clothing or handbag. Agitated, threatening patients generally require that a security guard be called.

ESTABLISH RAPPORT.   The formal interview should be carried out when the patient's mental status and physical condition have stabilized. However, from the onset of contact, the physician and staff should communicate a sense of sympathy to the patient. There is often a tendency to be aggressive toward patients who have injured themselves intentionally, and patients often feel guilty about their own behaviors. The physician generally sets the tone of the interaction. Direct questions such as, "Did you try to commit suicide?" take on an accusatory note. It may be better to assume with the patient that a suicide attempt has occurred and to make a comment acknowledging the fact rather than raising it as a question that demands an affirmative response.

IDENTIFY THE SUBSTANCE.   The specific substance ingested should be identified as quickly as possible. The police, relatives, or friends may have seen empty bottles in the patient's room. Medicine bottles with the name of the pharmacy and a prescription number can be used to identify the drug if the name of the substance is not on the label. The gastric contents should be examined and materials sent off for analysis, including blood and urine, and if possible, for a toxic screen. If a substance is known and an antidote is available, it should be given as quickly as possible. The patient may not be a reliable source of information regarding the nature and the quantity of the overdose.

SECURE SOURCES OF INFORMATION. The sources of information should be secured. The names and identification numbers of policemen and the names and phone numbers of friends and relatives should be obtained. Otherwise an unconscious patient may be left in an emergency room with little identifying information, and the companions who brought in the patient may disappear while emergency measures are being instituted. Generally friends or family should be urged to stay in the emergency room or to come in if they have not yet arrived.

All of these measures can be accomplished in a few minutes. The patient's situation is stabilized when the gastric contents have been emptied, specific therapy has been initiated if indicated, the patient is under observation, the baseline physical and mental observations have been recorded, and the sources of information have been secured. At this point, the physician can attend to other patients and can return for a more definitive evaluation at a later time. The situation with other forms of suicide attempts, such as slashing or inhalation, is analogous. The injuries are attended to appropriately and the situation is stabilized in the same way.

The Intermediate Phase—Full Assessment

An available psychiatrist is usually called in at this stage, but the nonpsychiatric physician may also develop the skills to complete the entire process. When the acute problems are under control, it is possible to assess the suicide attempt more thoroughly. This is best done after the toxic effects of an overdose are over, although some valuable information on the underlying psychological problems can be obtained by talking to the patient during the twilight phase of consciousness. At such times, a patient may acknowledge a deep-seated suicidal wish whereas later, when the patient is more defended, he or she may deny it. However, a toxic state may be confused with a psychosis. The patient also needs to have a clear mind in order to be able to participate actively in a discussion of follow-up care.

LOOK FOR ORGANIC DISEASE. A physical examination, with special emphasis on the neurologic system, and a toxic screen should always be done on suicidal patients. Although it is unusual, some suicide attempts do occur in response to the early effects of a systemic or neurologic illness. For example,

one woman took an overdose just before the overt onset of systemic lupus erythematosis. Later a mild organic brain syndrome consistent with lupus encephalopathy became apparent. Another patient made a suicide attempt before the diagnosis of an ACTH-secreting tumor of the lungs. Hyperadrenal syndromes, occult malignancies, and disorders of the central nervous system are among the medical conditions most often associated with suicidal behavior, although any condition that disturbs physiological homeostasis can upset psychological controls.

FOCUS ON CONTINUING RISK. Many physicians doubt their ability to conduct an adequate psychiatric evaluation of a patient who has made a suicidal attempt. Actually the evaluation can be limited to the information needed to plan for disposition. The focus is on the question of continuing suicide risk. This determination rests on the seriousness of the attempt, the mental state of the patient both before and after the act, the likelihood of discovery, the availability of emotional supports, the personality and psychological history, and a variety of risk factors, such as age, sex, and marital and occupational status, that have prognostic value. Unemployment, lack of a stable marriage or relationship, advancing age, and being male all increase the risk of suicide. In general, older patients and men have the more serious prognosis. Although women make more suicide attempts than men, there are fewer fatalities among women. Men die by suicide two or three times more frequently than women. Therefore, an older man would constitute a high-risk patient, even though he is rational and appears to have a supportive environment.

A useful concept in assessing the seriousness of a suicide attempt is the risk–rescue ratio. A high-risk attempt is one in which the suicidal behavior itself has grave implications. Jumping from a window, shooting oneself, or ingesting a high dose of a known poison are obvious examples of high-risk attempts. Taking a toxic substance in a lonely setting is an example of a low potential for rescue. This assessment gives some indication of whether the patient intended and expected to die and the patient's attitudes and feelings about the crucial factors. Suicide should be brought up directly through questions such as, "What led you to attempt suicide?" In most cases the direct approach will clear the air and will give the patient relief. If the patient is evasive, it is likely that he or she is concealing a continuing suicide plan. By listening to the patient and observing his or her manner, it is usually easy to determine whether the patient is psychotic or not, once the effects of the suicide attempt itself have cleared. The presence of psychosis after an attempt is always an ominous sign.

SEARCH FOR PRECIPITANTS.   A detailed inquiry into the events immediately preceding the suicide attempt is often a fruitful approach. An impulsive attempt that occurred during a family fight is less ominous than a carefully planned attempt that took place without an obvious precipitant. By recreating the scene it is often possible to determine whether the patient was psychotic before the attempt. Reconstructing the human relationships around the time of increased suicide tension can be helpful in determining whether supportive relationships will be available after discharge and whether the suicide attempt has resulted in a change in the emotional climate that would favor the reduction of suicidal tension.

A brief look at the past history should help to determine whether suicidal behavior is occurring as part of a major decompensation from a previously adequate level of function or whether it is a chronic recurrent form of behavior. In general, a decompensation has more ominous implications and usually means that a major mental disturbance is underway.

ASSESS CONTINUING SUICIDE RISK.   Judging suicide risk is always an uncertain process. The following assessments are helpful:

1. Is the patient psychotic?
2. Was the patient psychotic at the time of the attempt?
3. Was the attempt serious (i.e., did the patient intend to die) and was the attempt of such a nature that death was a serious possibility?
4. Does the patient's life situation suggest continuing tensions of the sort that precipitated the suicide attempt?
5. Does the patient seem to want to live, or is he or she continuing to express hopelessness or an indirect expression of the wish to die?
6. Is the patient significantly depressed?
7. Is the patient undergoing a psychological or medical decompensation?
8. Does the patient acknowledge the suicide attempt, or is the patient hiding something and conveying a feeling of evasiveness?
9. What supports are available in the patient's life, in particular, are there other people who want the patient to live?

It is well not to rush the process of evaluation. The actual contact with the patient need not be excessively long; several brief observations over time are more significant than an extended observation at one point. Decisions are often made prematurely on the basis of the patient's state of mind right after the patient awakens from an overdose. If the patient had been allowed a few hours to recover, the situation may have seemed less grave and an unnecessary hospitalization in a psychiatric facility may have been avoided.

The process of evaluating a patient has important implications for therapy. Often the patient experiences relief by talking freely to a sympathetic physician. Leaving the patient with a positive experience enables him or her to come back for help before suicidal tensions reach a dangerous level again.

The Final Phase—Disposition

DECIDE WHETHER TO HOSPITALIZE.   Whether or not the "suicidal" patient needs in-patient hospitalization for treatment of the psychiatric disorder is the central decision to be made. There are several factors that would lead us to recommend it: continued high risk for suicide; acute psychosis; and depression severe enough to render simple functioning impossible. In making the decision, we should also consider the patient's home environment. What degree of social support is available to the patient? Would family or friends be able to handle any of the above problems—if only for a brief period of time—until effective out-patient therapy can be instituted? The problem is somewhat more complicated when a treatment relationship already exists. In this circumstance, one tends to weigh heavily what the present therapist recommends, but does not necessarily agree if it is in marked conflict with one's own clinical judgment. It is often useful to have the outside therapist come to the emergency room. Often an emergency appointment with the therapist can be arranged, and the patient can be discharged in the company of family or friends to go to such an appointment.

ARRANGE FOR HOSPITALIZATION.   When the physician decides that hospitalization is necessary for the safety of the patient but the patient refuses, then involuntary hospitalization is arranged. This generally requires filling out a specific form and sending the patient to the appropriate facility. At times, private hosptials may be reluctant to accept "involuntary" patients, but state mental hospitals have a responsibility to do so if they agree with the clinical need for hospitalization.

It is important to involve family members in these decisions. Their support greatly facilitates the execution of whatever decision is made. The choice of hospital should be discussed and, if possible, mutually agreed upon. The physician should explain to the patient and family members the reasons for decisions and should avoid premature promises. It is frequently difficult to arrange immediate transfer. Hospitals are often full. Financial issues, such as insurance coverage, often need to be dealt with. Overly specific statements about how long the patient will be in the hospital or what kind of medication will be given should be avoided. General guidelines can be given, pointing out that the physicians in the other hospital will have to make their own decisions. It is important to communicate pertinent clinical details to the other hospital, especially the reasons for deciding upon hospitalization. A patient should never simply be sent to another facility without any prior communication.

ARRANGE FOR TRANSFER. The means of transfer to another hospital should also be carefully considered. When in doubt about the safety of the patient on the way to the other hospital, overtreat rather than undertreat. An ambulance with an attendant accompanying the patient is the most protective. Sometimes an attendant accompanying the patient in a taxicab will suffice. Or sometimes a family member can take the patient to the other hospital. Someone should almost always accompany the patient, and the degree of protection needed depends on the degree of tension, impulsivity, and cooperation of the patient.

ARRANGE FOR OUT-PATIENT FOLLOW-UP. If it is decided that in-patient hospitalization is not necessary, out-patient follow-up should always be offered, although many patients who make suicide attempts may not choose to return for further psychiatric treatment. In general, they will be more apt to return to someplace or someone familiar—the same hospital or the same person who saw them in the emergency room—so if that can be arranged the follow-up will have a higher chance of being successful. Some patients may respond best to the appointment's being made for them at the time of the emergency visit; others should be encouraged to take responsibility themselves for making an appointment after the options and ways of doing so are explained to them. Here again, family or friends may function as important allies in carrying through on recommendations.

BE CAUTIOUS ABOUT MEDICATION. Most suicide patients are already suffering from an overdose of medication, and, in general, any additional drugs are to be avoided. Available antidotes, such as levallorphan for heroin overdoses or physostigmine for atropine psychoses should be given, of course. Occasionally, minor tranquilizers are used when the level of agitation is such that destructive behavior threatens or the patient cannot carry on a conversation.

A suicidal patient should almost never be given a prescription for any drug at the time of the emergency room visit, especially not for antidepressants that require careful out-patient management, take about 2 weeks to work, and are potentially lethal if taken as an overdose. In rare instances, a prescription for a few (about five) minor tranquilizers can be given in the context of helping the patient function until an out-patient appointment can be arranged in the near future. No medication should be given to patients who are frequent drug abusers. Such patients are prone to manipulate, perhaps by threatening further suicide, if they do not get what they want.

Suicidal Patients Who Have Not Yet Made an Attempt

Some patients who come to an emergency room are suicidal, although they have not made suicide attempts and do not express suicidal thoughts overtly. Suicidal behavior is usually preceded by a period of rising tension, during which a patient may be torn between the wish to live and the wish to die and may also be experiencing mounting psychic and physical distress. For such a patient, the arrival in an emergency room is usually an effort to regain control and to find safety from self-destructive impulses. If the patient fails to find the help needed, he or she is likely to leave the emergency room with deepening despair and with an increased suicide potential. Unfortunately, such patients often express their problems indirectly and the clinician needs to be sensitive to the muted messages of depression, despair, or panic.

Some of the patients who constitute this group of psychiatric emergencies are undergoing a psychotic breakdown and are experiencing suicidal impulses along with the panic and chaos associated with a psychotic state. Such patients may complain of bizarre physical symptoms. For example, they may feel that a body part is changing in size or shape. Others may feel that they are dying of an acute episode or that they are suffering from hidden sepsis or cancer. The bizarre quality of these complaints and the psychological tension behind them are sometimes the only clues to the incipient psychosis and its attendant suicide risk. Other patients may be expressing a profound depression in their medical symptoms. Here again the affective quality that is conveyed to the examining physician is often the most valid clinical sign. The findings associated with psychosis are described in more detail in the next section.

Another group of patients that may become suicidal are those with acute organic brain syndromes. In general, any condition that leads to a rapid loss of central nervous system inhibition with consequent emergence of impulses can be associated with self-destructive behavior. Those states of delirium associated with vivid auditory hallucinations are often the most dangerous. For example, during alcoholic hallucinosis, patients often hear accusatory voices that pursue them with devilish persistence until they take desperate action to escape them. The patients may seek sanctuary in an emergency room, only to jump out of a window when they find the voices are following them. Bad trips from lysergic acid diethylamide (LSD) are also notorious in their association with precipitous self-destructive behavior.

Whenever suicide risk is suspected because of psychotic tension, depression, or delirium, the patient should be closely guarded, and potentially lethal objects should be kept out of reach. Even with delirious patients, the clinician should speak directly about suicidal impulses and try to get the patient to verbalize any tension. Often it helps to speak through the symptoms, first talking about how terrible the patient must feel and then moving on to the thought that he or she may feel like killing him or herself to escape or to find relief. At other times, it is wise to suggest that the patient is struggling with suicidal impulses and needs help to support the part that wants to live. Antipsychotic drugs (e.g., haloperidol 2–4 mg) or minor tranquilizers (e.g., diazepam 5–10 mg) can be useful in reducing tension. However, interpersonal contact is the best form of tranquilizer and suicide precaution. Hospitalization in a psychiatric facility is usually indicated for patients who are suicide risks.

PROGNOSIS

In most cases the patient recovers psychologically and medically from an acute episode of becoming suicidal. Impulsive feelings and behaviors pass quickly, and underlying disorders often associated with suicidal issues, such as endogenous depression or acute psychosis, respond within days or a couple of weeks after treatment.

For these reasons, we may point out to suicidal patients who claim that suicide is their decision and that we have no right to stop them, that most patients do change their minds. The role of the emergency room physician is important and often gratifying in aiding this process.

In the long run, however, once the barrier to suicidal behavior is broken, the potential for further attempts and for eventual death by suicide increases markedly. The suicide rate among people who have made one attempt has been found to be 500 times greater than the rate among corresponding people who have made no prior attempts. Although suicide attempts appear as sporadic and acute episodes, in a sense the underlying problem of suicide risk is a chronic disease once it has become manifest, and consideration of long-term treatment is part of the emergency management of every patient who has made a suicide attempt.

Psychotic Patients

Patients are considered psychotic when their psychic apparatus has decompensated to such a degree that they are unable to carry out the ordinary demands of living. Psychosis represents a regression to a more immature level of psychic functioning characterized by primitive defense mechanisms, such as distortion, projection, and a gross denial of reality. The psychotic patient has a significant impairment in his or her sense of reality. There are often delusions, hallucinations, or some type of irrational thought process. Judgment is usually seriously impaired.

Psychosis has many different phases and represents not one disease but rather a final common pathway for many different kinds of functional or organic disturbances. The functional disorders are schizophrenia, manic–depressive psychosis, and transitory stress psychoses. Schizophrenia itself takes many different forms—simple, paranoid, catatonic, or hebephrenic, either in their acute or chronic forms. Manic–depressive psychosis may be either in its manic or depressed phase. There are many different organic disturbances that can produce psychosis. The most commonly encountered are drug states, metabolic encephalopathy, and cerebrovascular disease. Drug states include both excess and withdrawal, such as with alcohol, or the effects of hallucinogenic substances, such as LSD. One of the most important diagnostic tasks of the emergency room physician is to try to differentiate the organic from the functional psychoses. The other crucial diagnostic question is whether the psychosis is acute or chronic. Acute psychoses tend to be unstable and chaotic states in which hospitalization is generally indicated. They are emergencies in several ways. For one thing, they cause enormous pain and suffering. Second, if prolonged, they may produce irreversible damage to the psychic apparatus. Third, they may precipitate unacceptable behavior such as suicide or violence toward others. These issues will be discussed in further detail presently. Regardless of the diagnostic issues, the initial contact and early management of all psychotic patients has much in common.

EVALUATION OF THE PATIENT

Initial Interview and Setting

RELY ON EARLY RECOGNITION.   The first thing a physician in the emergency room is likely to notice is that there is something very strange or inappropriate about psychotic patients. Their dress may be odd. They may have strange stereotyped mannerisms or show extreme body tension. Their irrational thinking may be obvious or it may be hidden. In fact, when dealing with some patients with more hidden psychoses, the physician's first sign of recognition may be that he or she experiences a feeling of strangeness. But early recognition of a psychosis may be life saving. Typically, the psychosis may be overlooked in the process of dealing with the medical complaint and narrowing the focus of concern. Only if the physician pays attention to his or her own intuition and gives the patient an opportunity to talk in more general terms about the patient's life will the psychosis be uncovered. Comments such as, "Is anything else bothering you?" or "You seem kind of tense," may open the door. Also questions about what sort of impact a medical problem has caused on their life will lead rather naturally into a discussion of their psychosocial functioning.

The psychotic patient is usually very frightened, at times to the point of absolute terror. Sometimes the patient's affect is shallow and flat and does not fit with the topic being discussed. Confusion and misperception are common, and there may or may not be impairment in orientation and memory and other cognitive functioning.

MAINTAIN A CALM APPROACH.   It is important to be calm and direct in dealing with psychotic patients. In a sense, we approach them like all other patients but with extra sensitivity to their terror and tendency to misinterpret what is happening. The patient's fear will be augmented by excessive fear in the physician. Conversely, communicating a tolerance for whatever extreme thoughts and emotions the patient may express and not being driven off by them will provide enormous relief to the patient. On the other hand, the physician should not tolerate the threat of violent behavior. If the patient is making a real threat of assault or holding a weapon, we obviously deal with the threat of violent behavior first and swiftly. For more detail, see the section on the violent patient.

ATTEND TO THE CHIEF COMPLAINT.   One of the first things to consider is how the patient got to the emergency room. Is the patient here because of his or her own free will and with some request for help, no matter how bizarre or indirect? For example, one psychotic patient came to the emergency room requesting "an emergency nose job." Another patient came requesting "to examine all patients with psychological troubles." In these instances, the patient wants something from the physician, and this allows for a common ground from which to begin. Or, on the other hand, has the patient been brought in against his or her will? Was the patient, for example, picked up for peculiar behavior and brought handcuffed to the emergency room by the police? If so, being held against his or her will is likely to be the chief complaint of the patient. Even in

this case, we begin with the chief complaint. We may indicate that we would like to be able to let the patient go but that he or she needs to understand a few things first. We may ask, "What is it that made the police think you were dangerous?" Whatever the situation is, we start with the main concern of the patient and begin to talk about it. Talking and listening will immediately begin to relieve the tension and panic. The story will begin to emerge—the specific reasons for coming to the emergency room, the precipants, the background, the identity of key friends and relatives with whom to be in contact, and so forth. We try, for a brief period, to get into the patient's world, to try to understand how the patient really views what is happening to him or her. We may wonder what we would feel if we had the same view of the world. We also wonder what painful truth the psychosis helps the patient to avoid and what sort of life the patient really has. In this way, the "craziness" becomes far more comprehensible and assumes a greater human dimension.

CHOOSE A SECURE SETTING.   Both the patient and the physician need to feel as comfortable as possible during the interview. Paranoid patients, for example, become more tense when crowded into small spaces and blocked off from an exit. Both the physician and the patient may at times feel more at ease if someone else is in the room, either a nurse, an attendant, or perhaps a family member. Physical examinations can usually be performed without difficulty, provided there is some discussion beforehand and provided that it is not forced on the patient without agreement.

Psychotic patients who seem tense and impulsive should always have someone in the room with them. Confused and disoriented patients need to have things explained to them almost continuously. In all cases, a nonthreatening but secure approach and management works best.

DIFFERENTIATE FUNCTIONAL FROM ORGANIC PSYCHOSIS.   One of the central tasks of the emergency room physician is to differentiate the organic from the functional psychosis. The term *functional psychosis* refers in general to schizophrenia, manic–depressive psychosis, and stress psychosis. Strictly speaking, of course, it is believed that both genetic and biochemical factors play an important role in both manic–depressive illness and schizophrenia, but from an operational point of view *organic* means drug-induced, metabolic, circulatory, or other grossly identifiable diseases directly involving brain tissue and manifesting themselves as psychosis. The important point is that all potentially reversible underlying organic disturbances be identified and treated when possible. Meningitis, for example, may present as psychosis and may be rapidly fatal unless treated quickly.

History

There are several factors that help to identify organic psychosis. One is the history. For example, does the patient have a known medical problem, such as chronic renal failure, alcoholism, drug dependency, or metastatic carcinoma, that may predispose toward development of an organic psychosis? Have there been any recent changes in drug use? Some of the antihypertensive medications, for example, reserpine or propranolol, have been associated with psychosis. Is there any evidence of withdrawal from a psychotropic drug? Is there any possibility of hallucinogenic drug use? The physician looks for any prior history of psychosis. As a general rule, patients over the age of 40, with no prior history of psychosis, should be assumed to have an organic psychosis until proven otherwise. In the recent history, the physician looks for the presence of certain organic symptoms, such as fever, seizures, tremulousness, or loss of memory, which may slightly precede or coincide with the onset of psychosis. Much of this history may have to be obtained from other close contacts of the patient, which makes their presence so important during the evaluation of a psychotic patient.

Physical Examination

Of equal importance is the physical examination of the patient. The neurologic examination is of special importance, but the physician also looks thoroughly for evidence of any disease or drug state that may affect brain function—an enlarged liver, dilated or pinpoint pupils, autonomic changes, needle marks, and so forth. The physical examination may also turn up findings that point toward a functional psychosis. For example, one woman who was found to have a red bandage over her back said that it had been there for 3 years and protected her against harmful radio waves. The mental status portion of the examination is especially critical. The level of consciousness, orientation, and other cognitive functions, when impaired, point toward an organic disturbance. Schizophrenic and manic–depressive patients may have strange and delusional thoughts but their intellect is intact. They are generally able to do calculations, to do serial 7's, to remember three objects after 5 minutes, to name the last three presidents, and to tell us what the date is. Visual, as opposed to auditory, hallucinations are also more suggestive of organic psychosis. Whenever a patient is cooperating and appears able to attend to the task at hand but still cannot perform some intellectual function that he or she could have performed before, we should assume the psychosis to be organic. One exception to this general rule is that severe depression, especially in the elderly, may present as a pseudodementia.

Differentiate Acute from Chronic Psychosis

To what extent does the current psychosis reflect a stable and chronic state versus an abrupt change in level of functioning? Often this history is best obtained from friends, relatives, or other professional observers. The physician tries to find out, as with all psychiatric emergencies, what the patient is usually like. Work and social functioning is explored. Inquiries are made about prior psychiatric treatment, hospitalizations, antipsychotic medications, and current treatment relationships. The abrupt development of psychotic symptoms may be occurring for the first time, or it may be an acute decompensation in a previously well-stabilized schizophrenic patient. If it is the latter, the physician always questions whether antipsychotic medication has been discontinued. Some precipitant can almost always be found. Any acute decompensation represents a greater emergency and is associated with greater danger of injury to self or others. The level of tension and panic in the individual patient tends to be higher. Friends and family will also seem more distressed and less able to handle the situation. Acute psychoses require much more vigorous intervention. The physician almost always tends to hospitalize such patients.

Chronicity raises a different set of issues. If the physician learns that the patient's current mental status is not essentially different than it has been over the past several years, then he or she must investigate more closely the exact purpose of the present visit. Perhaps the patient is a chronic schizophrenic who makes regular use of the emergency room for medical complaints. Medical complaints should be taken seriously. Schizophrenics often describe real medical problems in such a bizarre way as not to be seriously considered. For example, one patient complained that glass had been put in her food as her way of accounting for the fact that she had noticed blood in her bowel movements. The way in which such a patient has gotten to the emergency room is important. It may be that someone quite unfamiliar with the patient has overreacted and caused the police to bring the patient to the emergency room. Or perhaps there has been a change in the mental status of someone else living at home, altering the family dynamics such that the patient has been a scapegoat and brought to the hospital. Maybe the family's tolerance has changed. Or perhaps the patient's doctor has gone on vacation or been transferred or has died. Sometimes a chronically psychotic patient will emphasize his or her symptoms as a way of seeking readmission to a hospital. If there is an outside professional involved, the most sensible and time-saving approach is to contact that person.

Management

MEDICATION. We should be quite cautious about giving psychoactive medication to psychotic patients in the emergency room, especially when the etiology is uncertain. When there is an active central nervous system process occurring, in which alertness and consciousness are being monitored as important signs, then we should avoid the use of psychoactive medication. Physical restraints are used if necessary. They are called for when a confused patient is either assaultive, endangering him or herself by trying to get out of the stretcher, or otherwise interfering with needed medical treatment, such as pulling out an intravenous tube or a catheter.

If the diagnosis is less in doubt, however, and the degree of agitation and of disturbance in reality testing is such that interpersonal contact cannot effectively reduce the level of panic, then either chlorpromazine 25 mg intramuscularly (IM), or haloperidol 2–4 mg IM can be given and repeated every half-hour as needed. Haloperidol, which has fewer hypotensive and other cardiovascular side effects, is usually preferable for elderly patients. It is advisable not to give too high a dose initially but rather to repeat smaller dosages frequently as needed.

Sometimes patients request medication. Their own knowledge about what has been most helpful in the past may help the physician to select the best drug and dosage to use. The one specific contraindication for the use of antipsychotic medication is an atropinelike psychosis, which the anticholinergic properties of the antipsychotic drugs will augment. This may occur in either of two situations. The first is the chronic schizophrenic patient who is being treated with a combination of antipsychotic and antiparkinsonian drugs whose combined anticholinergic effect produces a toxic psychosis. The other common situation is a patient who has overdosed either on drugs containing scopolamine, such as one of the proprietary sleeping medications, or drugs possessing anticholinergic properties, such as antihistamines or the tricyclic antidepressants. In both instances there are associated physical findings, such as dilated pupils, tachycardia, flushing, and constipation. The treatment of choice is physostigmine 1 mg IM, followed by close observation.

At times, we may medicate the patient in order to facilitate transfer to another hospital, and some chronic schizophrenics will need a supply of antipsychotic medication to last until their next out-patient appointment.

DISPOSITION. The central issue usually is whether or not to hospitalize the patient. In general, if the psychosis is acute, we would recommend hospitalization. But the decision depends in part on etiologic factors, on the need for further diagnostic evaluation or specific medical treatment, and also on whether the patient's mental and behavioral state exceeds the capacity of his or her family to cope with the patient. If the psychosis is due to a clear underlying medical disturbance that needs further treatment, admission to a medical unit is preferable. Some transient, drug-induced psychoses may be managed best in brief overnight-ward admissions, or even at home, if the patient is medically stable. Bad trips are one example of the latter. This, of course, depends on people being available at home to be with the patient at all times. The patients are managed best by familiar people reassuring the patient that he or she is not "going crazy," but is experiencing the effects of a drug that will not last long. This sort of reassurance should be given to any patient who is experiencing an organic psychosis.

Elderly patients with chronic organic brain syndromes with psychosis who are unable to manage at home may be transferred to psychiatric hospitals or to nursing homes but only if any underlying organic illness in need of acute treatment has been excluded. Acute manic–depressive or schizophrenic patients should be transferred to either mental hospitals or inpatient psychiatric units in general hospitals. Various considerations affect the choice, not the least of which are the patient's and family's own preference and the presence of concomitant medical illness. Disposition planning should be shared with the family, and, at some point, with the patient. The patient's cooperation and motivation are important in every treatment, especially psychiatric treatment.

COMMITMENT. In cases in which the physician decides that hospitalization is essential for the safety of the patient and for society but the patient refuses, then commitment is arranged, usually to a state mental hospital because most private facilities are reluctant to take patients on an involuntary basis. This is arranged by calling the nearest state mental hospital, which will check the patient's address and determine which state hospital has responsibility for patients living in that district. Then the clinical situation is described to the admitting physician at the appropriate hospital. A committal form, a supply of which should be kept in the emergency room, is filled out. In most states any physician may do this, although it is generally advisable to have a psychiatrist involved in the process. The committal form, in most states, represents a request for hospitalization. The state hospital psychiatrist will make his or her own assessment. The specific laws and procedures vary from state to state. The emergency room physician should be familiar with these procedures. Commitment is recommended when the patient is at immediate risk for suicide or serious self-harm or is likely to be harmful to others by virtue of the psychosis and impairment in judgment.

Most chronic schizophrenics can be discharged back into the community, provided adequate follow-up treatment is available.

The Overwhelmed Patient Who Is Not Psychotic

The overwhelmed or psychologically traumatized patient may present as a psychiatric emergency. Acute emotional reactions may be extremely painful and may have long-term psychological morbidity. There may be suicide risk associated with these nonpsychotic states and at times they may be confused with incipient psychosis.

ACUTE ANXIETY STATES

Evaluation

Experienced clinicians are familiar with the patient who arrives at an emergency room in a frightened, agitated state and urgently asks for treatment. The symptoms in such a patient are often the physiologic manifestations of anxiety and may include hyperventilation, paresthesias, chest pain, dizziness, nausea, and faintness. The patient may express the fear of death. These patients are often young, have a history of anxiety episodes, and may have experienced a recent incident of a frightening or disturbing nature. They can be differentiated from the psychotic patients described above in that the panic is not as intense and reality testing is not impaired. They usually have some perception that anxiety may be causing their symptoms. They usually experience relief during the medical workup, and the passage of time usually makes the diagnosis clear.

Management

A serious medical workup directed toward the chief complaint is the best management for patients in an acute anxiety state. If the patient complains of chest pain, an electrocardiogram (ECG) is initially better psychotherapy than is reassurance or an attempt to determine the underlying source of tension. A thorough personal history of the last day or two will usually reveal an acute precipitant. When this event or conflict comes out, there will usually be a reduction of tension.

Definitive Treatment

Untreated, an acute anxiety episode can leave a patient quite shaken and can make him or her more vulnerable to future episodes. Loss of confidence and self-esteem and even clinical depression may follow. It is important not to dismiss these episodes lightly once the physical complaints have been evaluated. The patient needs to master the problem rather than feel like a victim. Psychotherapy, or at least further evaluation in a noncrisis state, is the treatment of choice, and the patient should be encouraged to find follow-up care. Minor tranquilizers should be used sparingly even during an acute episode. The attack will subside if the patient is given sufficient emotional support and the opportunity to interact with a sympathetic listener. Tranquilizers may alleviate anxiety but tend to leave the patient with a feeling that he or she has not mastered the situation and will need tranquilizers for support in the future. The ultimate goal is psychological mastery. The proper role of minor tranquilizers is to facilitate this process when it is blocked by overwhelming anxiety, rather than in sedating patients to the point of their being unaware of the problem or unable to learn new approaches to handling it.

Some anxiety attacks are associated with drugs or alcohol. Diminished control can lead to the breakthrough of unacceptable thoughts or impulses. Substances that interfere with conscious control can also impair a patient's usual defense mechanisms.

ACUTE GRIEF

Evaluation

Grief, the normal response to loss, characteristically includes a sequence of emotional states beginning with disbelief or shock and moving through various painful and, at times, irrational reactions such as anger, guilt, despair, and hopelessness. In most instances, grief ultimately resolves itself within 6 months to 1 year, although depression may persist and some losses are so severe that they can never be fully accepted.

Acute and overwhelming grief can present as a psychiatric emergency. The shock of a devastating loss, such as the death of a child or a spouse, a house fire, or other sudden disruptive event can leave a patient the victim of almost intolerable emotions. Reality testing may be lost in the acute state, and the patient may appear to be psychotic. Agitation, acute suicidal behavior, or simply profound shock can occur in patients suffering acute grief. Medical emergencies can be precipitated at such times. Grieving patients seldom bring themselves to the attention of a physician. More often they are brought to an emergency room by friends or relatives, or they may be the relative who accompanies the victim of a disaster. For example, a patient who is being treated for the effects of an automobile accident may also be suffering from the overwhelming grief of losing a loved one in the same disaster.

Management

Common sense usually shows the way to helping patients with acute grief. Interpersonal support is the mainstay. Someone should sit with the patient and encourage him or her to talk about the loss. Continuing support should be provided with the opportunity to keep contact open after the patient leaves the emergency room. Often the acute reactions will recur at night or when the patient is alone. Relatives and friends should be enlisted as surrogate therapists. Medications, including mild tranquilizers and a few sleeping pills, are useful because they give the patient a sense of continuing support and relief. The patient should be encouraged to stay in the emergency room as long as he or she wishes and should have continuing opportunities to talk to the staff members.

SHOCK STATES FOLLOWING TRAUMA

Evaluation

A person who has been traumatized by an accident, mugging, or a rape, for example, may appear to be detached from the incident or mildly distressed and may not give the appearance of someone who is undergoing a psychiatric emergency. Vigorous intervention in such cases may be needed to prevent posttraumatic psychological disturbances such as depression, nightmares, phobias, and even posttraumatic psychosis. These disturbances may develop weeks later.

Management

Patients should be encouraged to talk about the traumatic event. Often there is amnesia on a psychological basis alone. When the patient has sustained a head injury, the organic effects may add to this amnesia. By talking over the details of the event, the patient may begin to remember some of the frightening aspects and may be able to achieve some degree of mastery and integration, even when in the emergency room. Many such patients would benefit from the opportunity to talk about the incident later, after the initial shock has worn off. Arrangements for follow-up care of patients with physical injuries can include the provision for continuing discussion of the incident.

Violent or Angry, Threatening Patients

Violent behavior rarely occurs in the emergency room. However, the fear of it tends to arouse considerable anxiety in emergency room personnel. Actually, it is surprising that more does not occur because so many intoxicated patients with relatively poor control of impulses are seen in the emergency room. The reason is probably that the hospital is perceived as a neutral, helpful, nonthreatening place, and violence tends to occur in response to a perceived threat of assault. The emergency room is more apt to deal with the many victims of violence in our society rather than with the perpetrators.

EVALUATION—THE UNDERLYING DISORDER

Personality Disorder

Personality disorder is the most common category of threatening patients. These patients have underlying characterologic difficulties with impulse control. Not infrequently they are intoxicated with some drug, usually alcohol, or sometimes barbiturates, which may further suspend their self-restraint and inhibition. They are not psychotic as such. They are provocative, often manipulative about physical complaints, and seem to be looking for a struggle. Here the physician has to guard against his or her own anger and the natural temptation to respond in an angry manner and get into a struggle, which tends only to escalate the problem. The physician should maintain a professional stance, dealing with the medical problem or whatever is needed but refusing to engage in verbal struggles. Fair limits are set, and these patients are treated as having responsibility for their own behaviors. If the patient refuses to leave after being appropriately treated medically or surgically, then security guards and/or the police are summoned to remove the patient.

Delirium

Delirious patients have either acute or exacerbated chronic organic brain syndromes, with clouded sensorium, and are often confused as to where they are and what is happening. They are, therefore, easily prone to misinterpreting events in the emergency room. They may think that people are trying to kill them or that the x-ray machine is a gun, and so forth. They struggle and may take a swing at someone, and they can easily injure themselves or others in their attempts to escape from imagined dangers. They are frequently older people and are easily subdued. It is important to have someone stay with such patients at all times to reorient them to reality and to interpret what is happening. Family, friends, or other familiar people are invaluable in calming these patients and reassuring them of their safety. Careful explanation of any procedure before it is done is important. Restraints are a last resort because they can so easily be perceived as assaultive, thus adding to the patient's feeling of helplessness and panic. The physician should try to make a rapid determination as to the etiology of the organic brain syndrome, whether it is chronic or acute, to what extent it requires immediate treatment, as in a subdural hematoma or meningitis, and so forth. When these issues are clarified, if necessary, haloperidol 2–3 mg, IM, to be repeated every 30 minutes, can be used; it is preferable to chlorpromazine in elderly patients because of its lowered risk to the cardiovascular system.

Acute Functional Psychosis

Physicians generally encounter the threat of violence in a patient who has the delusion that he or she is going to be annihilated. In addition to such paranoia, delusions, catatonic excitement, or manic behavior can also lead to violence. These patients are responding to their frightening distortions and delusions. Generally their orientation, level of consciousness, and intellectual functions are intact, but they are delusional or panicked at their own loss of control.

Calm, nonthreatening interpersonal interventions are frequently able to bring these patients under control. The physician attempts to form an alliance around the purpose of their visit to the emergency room, or, if involuntarily brought in, around the solution of the predicament they find themselves in, namely how did they manage to frighten people so much that they were dragged into an emergency room. There is a certain preselection here. If patients are extremely opposed to coming to the emergency room, they more than likely would already have been physically restrained by the police or friends and family who would then function as important allies in the emergency room. The physician attempts to estimate the amount of control that the patient can exercise. A few minutes of dialogue or interpersonal interaction generally help to decide this question. If it looks as though there is considerable potential for more self-control, then much time and care is taken in a nonthreatening manner to talk the patient back from violence.

Situational Rage Reactions

Most people are capable of acute rage reactions if provoked enough. In the emergency room some patients or family members characteristically express their anxiety or frustration, sometimes with justification, through anger and hostility. Sometimes the anger is projected onto the physician as a convenient and available scapegoat. These people usually are not apt to become violent. By not overreacting but inquiring into the true cause for the anger they can be easily calmed. Just listening to and acknowledging their feelings of anger and frustration helps.

Violence Outside the Emergency Room

Occasionally patients may use the emergency room in an effort to control their own violent impulses in the same way that a suicide patient may come to the emergency room to prevent a suicide attempt. The patient may already have committed some violence or else may be feeling on the verge of further violent behavior. Having enough judgment, he or she may seek out a neutral territory such as a hospital where the behavior and feelings can be better understood and controlled.

Especially when violence is perceived as something alien, uncharacteristic, and out of proportion to the provocation involved, organic etiology should be considered such as temporal lobe epilepsy, brain tumors, or drug states. In any case, it is important to take these cases very seriously. Talking and listening can diffuse a lot of angry feelings that might otherwise be transformed into violence. And patients can be helped to understand that, although angry feelings can be tolerated, violent behavior cannot be.

MANAGEMENT

In addition to the particular management described for the specific types of violence, there are several general guidelines that are important to follow.

Avoid Provocation

Provocation by arguments, sarcasm, ridicule, and so on, or by an indiscreet derogatory remark to a colleague that may be overheard should be avoided. Aggressive threatening patients are protecting their injured self-esteem, and further injury in the emergency room will only inflame their passions. The physician should attempt to cool threatening behavior by dealing with the patient in the usual concerned and respectful professional manner that has been described above. Simply conveying the expectation that a patient will behave appropriately and in a mature way does a great deal to elicit such behavior.

Have Security Personnel Available

When the interpersonal measures described do not significantly reduce the likelihood of imminent violence, the physician should make sure that enough security personnel or attendants are notified to stand by. In most circumstances they should not rush in or provoke the patient at this point but merely be available if needed quickly. Their presence calms other personnel in the emergency room and quite frequently calms the patient. If the patient is threatening to use a weapon, the police should be called immediately. In most cases, hospital personnel should not attempt to approach a patient with a weapon.

Exercise Restraint in Use of Physical Force

In situations in which there is need to subdue the patient physically, enough personnel should be available. One-on-one struggles are dangerous. An effective method is for four or five people to approach the patient behind a mattress and for each person to restrain one of the four limbs and the head, preferably with the patient prone. In this position, medication such as 50 mg chlorpromazine IM or 20 mg diazepam IM can easily be given. The doses can be repeated every 15–30 minutes as needed, provided that the patient's vital signs are closely monitored for evidence of hypotension. An alternative is to use physical restraints around the wrists and ankles while the patient is lying prone on a hospital stretcher. But this method has the drawback of further threatening and enraging patients and should only be used when medication is contraindicated, such as in head injuries, or temporarily until the medication takes effect.

MEDICATIONS

For most cases effective interpersonal management of psychiatric emergencies is preferable to drug management. However, there are two principle categories of psychoactive drugs that may be useful in dealing with some psychiatric emergencies.

Minor Tranquilizers

Minor tranquilizers, also known as anxiolytics, reduce anxiety. The benzodiazepines are the most commonly used anxiolytics, and among them diazepam (Valium) is perhaps the best known. Oral doses of 5–10 mg of diazepam or equivalent doses of one of the other benzodiazepines are recommended in dealing with nonpsychotic patients who are overwhelmed with anxiety, especially when talking alone does not relieve the patient's panic. Oversedation, especially before the problem has been understood, is to be avoided.

Some patients with recurring anxiety attacks may benefit from a prescription of a small number of pills (about 10 or 15) to sustain them until their next psychiatric out-patient appointment.

Antipsychotics

The other principal category of drugs is the antipsychotic medications, also called neuroleptics. These commonly include the phenothiazines, such as chlorpromazine (Thorazine), and the butyrophenones, such as haloperidol (Haldol). These drugs treat the underlying psychosis and are generally used in an emergency room when the patient's level of tension is beyond control. Either chlorpromazine 25 mg, IM, or haloperidol 5 mg, IM, can be used; the former is usually used if more sedation is desired. It is preferable to give the patient his or her usual medication if it is other than these two. The main indications for giving patients doses of these medications in the emergency room are for their uncontrollable agitation and/or significant subjective distress from psychotic symptoms. As with the minor tranquilizers, some patients may need small amounts prescribed to tide them over.

HOSPITALIZATION

Most patients seen in the emergency room as psychiatric emergencies can be sent home with out-patient follow-up provided. Those patients with a major affective disorder or unstable psychosis who are having great difficulty functioning at home are transferred to an inpatient psychiatric unit, which may be in the same hospital, or to an acute medical or surgical unit if there are coexisting medical problems. Patients who are unwilling to accept hospitalization and who are assessed as posing an immediate risk to self or others may need to be hospitalized involuntarily in the designated state hospital or private facility accustomed to receiving involuntary patients. In the transfer itself it is important to provide adequate safety, if need be with members of the nursing staff or family accompanying the patient. It is also important to ensure that the receiving unit be given adequate information.

SELECTED READINGS

Diagnostic and Statistical Manual of Mental Disorders, DSM III (ed. 3) Washington, DC, American Psychiatric Association, 1980.

Glick RA, Meyerson AT, Robbin SE, Talbott JA (eds): *Psychiatric Emergencies*. New York, Grune & Stratton, 1976.

Golden JS, Marchionne AM: Psychiatric emergencies, in Eckert C (ed): *Emergency-Room Care*, ed 2. Boston, Little, Brown & Co, 1971, chap 23.

Kelley RL, Solomon P, Emmanuel HN: Psychiatric emergencies, in Solomon P, Patch VD (eds): *Handbook of Psychiatry*. Los Altos, California, Lange Medical Publications, 1974.

Linn L: *Other psychiatric emergencies* in Kaplan HI, Freedman AM, Sadock BJ (eds): *Comprehensive Textbook of Psychiatry*, Vol 2 (3rd ed). Baltimore, Williams and Wilkins, 1980, pp. 2098–2112.

Resnick HLP: *Suicide* in Kaplan HI, Freedman AM, Sadock BJ (eds): *Comprehensive Textbook of Psychiatry*, Vol. 2 (3rd ed). Baltimore, Williams and Wilkins, 1980, pp. 2085–2098.

Rosenbaum CP, Beebe JE III: *Psychiatric Treatment. Crisis Clinic Consultation*. New York, McGraw-Hill Book Co, 1975.

Shaden RJ (ed): *Manual of Psychiatric Therapeutics*. Boston, Little Brown and Co., 1975.

Shneidman ES, Faberow NL: *Clues to Suicide*. New York, McGraw-Hill Book Co, 1957.

Stengel E: *Suicide and Attempted Suicide*. New York, Jason Aronson Inc, 1974.

Weisman AD, Worden JW: Risk-rescue rating in suicide assessment. *Arch Gen Psychiatry* 1972; 26:553–560.

42
POISONING

Michael A. McGuigan
Frederick H. Lovejoy, Jr.

Acute poisoning in children or adults is a common emergency and a major cause of morbidity and mortality. It is estimated that over 1 million poisonings occur yearly in the United States. Although poison calls encompass a very large number of substances, the most common calls involve patients who have injested salicylates, benzodiazepine sedatives, caustic substances, alcohols, and petroleum distillate hydrocarbons. Fifty percent of all poisonings occur in children 5 years old or younger. Of these patients, 10% develop symptoms, but only 5% of the symptomatic patients require hospitalization. The teenage group accounts for only 5% of all poison calls. Within this group, however, 40% have symptoms, and 15% of these symptomatic patients require hospitalization. Calls concerning adults constitute 20% of all poison calls. Thirty percent of poisoned adults have symptoms, and 10% of these symptomatic patients are hospitalized. Hospitalization for this group is commonly a result of the ingestion of alcohols, tricyclic antidepressants, acetaminophen, salicylates, or benzodiazepine sedatives. Poisoning in the older age groups results in higher morbidity and mortality rates, presumably because adolescent and adult poisonings are often intentional.

The reduction in overall morbidity and mortality from poisonings during the last 20 years is primarily a result of improved diagnosis, therapy, and prevention. Optimal management of the poisoned patient requires that emergency room personnel be familiar with the means for identifying an ingested substance and understand the approaches to management. This chapter supplements information in basic references and offers a general approach to management as well as a review of selected, common overdoses.

A practical approach to the management of the acute overdose may be outlined in five general steps: evaluate, prevent absorption, enhance excretion, inactivate ingested substances, and prevent recurrence.

EVALUATION OF THE PATIENT

The first step in the approach to any poisoned patient should be a brief evaluation of the patient's cardiovascular and respiratory status. These systems should receive needed support before a more complete evaluation is undertaken.

History

Once the patient's physical condition is stable, questions about the poison should be answered: What is the poison? How much was taken? When? What are the contributing factors?

WHAT

Identification of the involved substance is often difficult, particularly in an adult overdose because the history is either unavailable or inaccurate. A class of substances may be ascertained from an awareness of products and medications kept in the home. Definitive identification may be obtained from the container, from the manufacturer, and through drug identification charts such as those found in the *Physicians' Desk Reference*. Another source for identification of unknown products is the regional poison center.

HOW MUCH

The quantity ingested is frequently difficult to determine, especially when liquids are involved. As a useful estimate, a "swallow" in a young child is approximately 4–5 ml. If poisoning occurs from tablets or capsules, it is helpful to know how many were present before the incident. This can be determined from the container label or from the dispensing pharmacy. Treatment should be based on an estimate of the largest possible amount ingested. If more than one child is suspected of having ingested a product, it is wise to assume that each child took the total amount rather than dividing the product among them.

WHEN

The time of exposure should be determined as accurately as possible. A case of poisoning is a dynamic process, and time is required for absorption of the toxin and development of symptoms. If the physician is going to interfere therapeutically or predict the future course, knowing the time of exposure is essential. In general, rapid onset of symptoms is associated with rapidly absorbed drugs whose effects occur quickly, and the severity of the symptoms is often proportional to the amount of poison absorbed. In addition, if drug levels are to be measured, the results can be interpreted accurately only in relation to the time of exposure.

CONTRIBUTING FACTORS

Knowledge of the patient's age and medical history is essential in evaluating a poisoning. Because overdoses in adolescents and adults are more likely to be intentional, the amounts taken are likely to be larger and the substances different from those involved in childhood poisoning. "Toxic doses" may vary with age, as may the toxic effects and the elimination rate of the poison. Past medical history is helpful in establishing normal function of various organ systems and, thus, their ability to withstand toxic effects. The major routes of elimination of toxins from the body involve the liver and kidneys; it is necessary to know that these organ systems are functioning normally.

Physical Examination

Although the findings on examination are generally nonspecific, the presence or absence of physical signs in a poisoned patient may provide a clue to the identity of the toxin. Occasionally, a tentative diagnosis of a toxic agent has to be based on a constellation of nonspecific findings. On the other hand, some poisons produce very characteristic physical signs, and a definitive diagnosis may be made solely on the basis of an examination of the patient (Table 42.1). This outline of physical signs and poisons points out important findings from examinations and some poisons that may cause these findings. The outline is intended as a guide and is not all inclusive. Disease processes that may result in specific physical signs have not been included. They should, however, be considered in every instance of suspected poisoning. Most often, as in any pathologic state, the physical examination yields a limited differential diagnosis, and confirmation comes from laboratory testing.

TABLE 42.1 Signs and Symptoms Associated with Poisoning

I.	Vital Signs		
	A.	Temperature	
		1. Hyperthermia	Belladonna alkaloids, antihistamines, boric acid, dinitrophenol, phenolphthalein, quinine, zinc fumes, monoamine oxidase (MAO) inhibitors, amphetamines, tricyclic antidepressants
		2. Hypothermia	Alcohol, opiate derivatives, chloral hydrate, barbiturates, phenothiazines, tetracycline, glutethimide
	B.	Heart rate	
		1. Arrhythmia	Digitalis, quinidine, tricyclic antidepressants
		2. Bradycardia	Barbiturates, chloral hydrate, opiate derivatives
		3. Tachycardia	Amphetamines, belladonna alkaloids, cocaine, ephedrine, drug withdrawal, xanthines, glutethimide, MAO inhibitors
	C.	Respiratory rate	
		1. Bradypnea	Alcohol, barbiturates, opiate derivatives
		2. Tachypnea	Acetanilid, aromatic oils, carbon monoxide, cyanide, dinitrophenol, nicotine, salicylates, drug withdrawal
	D.	Blood pressure	
		1. Hypertension	Amphetamines, cocaine, ephedrine, phencyclidine, methylphenidate, MAO inhibitors, tricyclic antidepressants
		2. Hypotension	Alcohol, barbiturates, opiate derivatives, phenothiazines, nonbarbiturate hypnotic sedatives (especially meprobamate), antihistamines.
II.	Ocular		
	A.	Pupils	
		1. Dilation	Amphetamines, belladonna alkaloids, chloroform, cocaine, ephedrine, epinephrine, ether, hallucinogens (LSD), isoproterenol, nicotine, pyribenzamine, opiate withdrawal
		2. Constriction	Barbiturates, ethanol, muscarinic compounds, opiate derivatives, organophosphate insecticides, phencyclidine, phenothiazines, physostigmine, pilocarpine
	B.	Optic disc	
		1. Papillitis	Ethylene glycol, methanol
		2. Papilledema	Bromides, heavy metals, vitamin A
	C.	Retinal vessels	
		1. Color changes	Cyanide (arteries and veins same color), methemoglobinemia, carbon monoxide

TABLE 42.1 (Continued)

D. Extraocular movements	
1. Strabismus	Botulism
2. Nystagmus	Phenytoin, phencyclidine, barbiturates, benzodiazepines
III. Oral	
A. Salivation	Caustics, insecticides (organophosphates, carbamates), metals, mushrooms, opiate withdrawal
B. Dry mouth	Antihistamines, belladonna alkaloids, phenothiazines, plants
C. Gums discoloration	Metals (chronic)
D. Odor of breath	Alcohol (phenols, chloral hydrate, ethanol); acetone (salicylates, lacquer, ethanol, isopropanol); wintergreen (methyl salicylate); garlic (phosphorus, arsenic, organophosphate insecticide); bitter almond (cyanide); petroleum distillate hydrocarbons.
IV. Pulmonary	
A. Dyspnea, Rales, Wheezing	Salicylates, opiate derivatives, hydrocarbons, insecticides (organophosphates, carbamates), propranolol
V. Cardiovascular (See vital signs)	
VI. Gastrointestinal	
A. Decreased peristalsis	Opiate derivatives, barbiturates, phenophiazines, antihistamines, alcohol, tricyclic antidepressants
B. Vomiting, pain, diarrhea, bleeding	Metals, alcohol, caustics, phosphorus, muscarine, digitalis, salicylates, xanthines, fluoride, bromide, insecticides (carbamates, organophosphates), plants, food poisoning (mushrooms, staphylococci), drug withdrawal
C. Jaundice	Metals, aniline, nitrobenzene, primaquine, benzene, arsine, mushrooms, quinidine, phosphorus, carbon tetrachloride, phenothiazines, thiazide diuretics, acetaminophen
VII. Renal	
A. Oliguria	Ethylene glycol, metals
B. Urinary retention	Antihistamines, belladonna alkaloids, phenothiazines, tricyclic antidepressants
VIII. Skin	
A. Cyanosis	
1. Methemoglobinemia	Nitrobenzene, aniline dyes, benzocaine, acetanilid, chloralhydrate, amyl or butyl nitrate, nitrites
B. Coloring	Iodine (black); bromide (dark brown); nitric or picric acid (yellow); silver nitrate (blue-black); carbon monoxide (pink); anticholinergic drugs (red)
C. Alopecia	Thallium, radiation, arsenic
D. Sweating	Alcohols, arsenic, aspirin, fluoride, insulin, nitrate, muscarine, mercuric chloride, carbamate or organophosphate insecticides, MAO inhibitors
IX. Neuromuscular	
A. Paresthesias, muscle weakness	Alcohol, organophosphorus compounds (triorthocresylphosphate, insecticides), chlorinated hydrocarbons (methylbromide, polychlorinated biphenyls 2,4-D, pentachlorophenolate), methyl N-butyl ketone, chloramphenicol, disulfiram, gold salts, isoniazid, nitrofurantoin, vinca alkaloids, glutethimide, metals (arsenic, lead, thallium)
B. Fasciculations	Organophosphate insecticides
C. Increased muscle tension; Increased deep tendon reflexes	Phencyclidine, amphetamines, cocaine, ephedrine, MAO inhibitors
X. Central Nervous System	
A. Depression and coma	Ethanol, isopropyl alcohol, barbiturates, tricyclic antidepressants, antihistamines, chloralhydrate, paraldehyde, carbon monoxide, cyanide, hydrogen sulfide, petroleum distillate hydrocarbons, xylene opiates, metals, insecticides (carbamate organophosphate), salicylates, ethchlorvynol, meprobamate, glutethimide, methy prylon, methaqualone, benzodiazapine, bromides
B. Convulsions	Insecticides (carbamate and organophosphate), metals, cyanide, tricyclic antidepressants, strychnine, amphetamines, camphor, plants, mushrooms, propoxyphene, phenytoin, xanthines, methaqualone, MAO inhibitors
C. Hallucination, delerium	Hallucinogens (PCP, LSD, mescaline, peyote, psilocybin), amphetamines, cocaine, belladonna alkaloids, tricyclic antidepressants, alcohol, plants, mushrooms

Laboratory Evaluation

Laboratory investigations are of two general types: clinical laboratory studies consisting of routine biochemical and hematologic determinations, and sophisticated complex drug assays. Clinical laboratory studies are useful in establishing the status of various organ systems and to document that the metabolic and excretory pathways of poison are intact. These studies are accurate, available, rapidly done, and relatively inexpensive. They are essential for the general management of the patient; however, they provide only indirect information about the specific poisoning. Definitive identification of the drug or chemical used in the poisoning requires specific assays. Qualitative screening tests, which often rely on the development of a color in serum, gastric fluid, or urine, have been described for many compounds. Care must be used in reading the test because there are a number of disease states, food substances, and therapeutic medications that may alter the color test results. Thus the results of these qualitative tests are easily misinterpreted and may be misleading.

Laboratories in many hospitals have the ability to do a limited number of relatively easy drug assays. In general, these tests can be done quickly. Among the drug level determinations that are commonly done within a hospital are the alcohols, barbiturates, iron, phenytoin, salicylates, and theophylline. Specific drug level assays and more general toxic screens may not always be accurate, are not often readily available, are time consuming, and are generally expensive. They do, however, provide specific information that needs careful interpretation. A quantitative drug assay alone tells only to what the patient was exposed; but even these are not always accurate for either identifying the drug or determining the level. As with any diagnostic test, the more information with which the laboratory is provided, the more accurate will be the test results. When plasma levels are integrated with the clinical picture, information may be deduced on how much drug was absorbed, when the drug was taken, whether elimination is proceeding as expected, how severe a clinical course to expect, and what the prognosis is. In all instances of poisoning, samples of gastric fluid, serum, and urine should be sent to a laboratory that is capable of doing the desired drug analyses. Although these values will not be helpful in the initial care of the patient, they will play an important role in subsequent management. Saving duplicate samples of body fluids from the acute state is a practice that will allow for confirmation of questionable laboratory results. Regardless of the type of laboratory tests being planned, supportive care and specific therapy should be started on the basis of the clinical diagnosis and should not wait for laboratory results.

MANAGEMENT—GENERAL CONSIDERATIONS

Prevention of Absorption

Systemic absorption of toxins occurs through the gastrointestinal tract, the lungs, and the skin. Because 70% of poisonings occur through ingestion, decontamination of the gastrointestinal tract will be dealt with in detail. Prevention of respiratory and skin absorption will be discussed at the end of the section. Absorption through the gastrointestinal tract can be diminished by several therapeutic maneuvers (see below). The effectiveness of these measures depends on the promptness with which they are instituted as well as on the pharmacologic properties of the ingested agent. Since most drugs are well absorbed from the gastrointestinal tract with peak levels occurring within $1\frac{1}{2}$–2 hours of ingestion, removal from the stomach by emesis or lavage is generally useful only within the first 2 hours after ingestion. Removal after 2 hours is considered for certain drugs that are slowly absorbed (e.g., methyl salicylate, glutethimide, phenytoin) or for drugs that slow gastrointestinal motility and result in delayed absorption (e.g., narcotic or anticholinergic poisonings).

The form in which the drug is dispensed influences the rate of absorption. Liquids are absorbed more rapidly than solids, and enteric-coated, or time-release, products are absorbed more slowly than standard capsules or tablets. The presence of food in the stomach also slows drug absorption. The degree to which a drug is ionized influences its passage through membranes. For example, weak acids, such as salicylate (pK = 3.2), exist in the acid medium of the stomach primarily in the nonionized form and therefore are well absorbed. Thus, the pK of a drug will be an additional factor in determining whether a weak acid is absorbed rapidly in the acid medium of the stomach or slowly in the more alkaline environment of the small bowel. The pK values for individual drugs may be found in standard pharmacology or toxicology texts.

Decisions concerning removal of ingested products from the stomach are among the most common and most critical aspects of initial management. In addition to appreciating the time since ingestion relative to the rate of absorption, the physician needs to consider the patient's clinical status and the risks of leaving the ingested product in the stomach versus the risks of attempting removal.

EMESIS

Emesis is an effective technique for removing ingested poisons of either tablet or liquid form. Syrup of ipecac is used most commonly to induce emesis because it is safe and effective.

After a single dose, vomiting is induced in 85% of patients; and after a second dose, approximately 95% of patients vomit. Forceful emesis generally occurs within 15–20 minutes after oral administration of ipecac syrup. The dose for patients from 1–12 years old is 1 tablespoon (15 ml) of ipecac syrup given orally, followed by 100–500 ml of clear fluids (dependent on age). If emesis has not occurred after 20 minutes, the dose may be repeated. If emesis does not occur in an additional 15–20 minutes and removal of the ingested product is still indicated, lavage should be performed. Traditionally, gentle motion has been recommended as being beneficial in aiding the effects of ipecac syrup, but recent studies have put the usefulness of motion in doubt. There are, however, no adverse effects associated with the use of motion. For the adolescent and adult, 30 ml of ipecac syrup can be given orally twice, in each instance followed by clear fluids. If emesis does not occur within 20 minutes of the second dose and removal is still desired, gastric lavage is indicated. For children 9–12 months of age, a single oral dose (10 ml) of ipecac syrup followed by fluid is recommended. If emesis does not occur after a single dose or if the child is younger than 9 months of age, careful lavage is the preferred method of removal. Emesis should not be induced in a patient with an altered state of consciousness. Because of the risk of aspiration, emesis should not be induced if the patient is obtunded or if the onset of action of the ingested product is sufficiently rapid that obtundation may ensue by the time emesis occurs. The presence of convulsions is a contraindication to emesis. The ingestion of drugs with antiemetic properties is not a contraindication to the use of ipecac.

Ipecac syrup is a remarkably safe product if used properly. Central nervous system and cardiac toxicity have been seen only when the 30-ml limit has been substantially exceeded in a child under 12 years old or when the fluid extract has been used. The fluid extract is 14 times as potent as the syrup and is not available in the United States.

Ipecac syrup is an inexpensive drug, available without prescription, and has a shelf life of 2–3 years, allowing it to be kept in the home for use at the time of a poisoning. It can be administered outside the hospital setting on the advice of a physician or poison center, thereby expediting initial therapy.

A variety of other methods exist for the induction of emesis. Stimulation of the posterior pharynx with a blunt object is generally unsuccessful. Oral copper sulfate may cause hepatotoxicity and is not recommended. Subcutaneous apomorphine is a very rapidly acting, highly effective emetic. Because it frequently causes significant central nervous system depression, its clinical usefulness in the treatment of the acute overdose is limited.

GASTRIC LAVAGE

Gastric lavage is the preferred method of removal of an ingested toxin at any age when appropriate attempts to induce emesis with ipecac syrup have failed. It is also indicated if the patient is younger than 9 months. In the obtunded patient with an intact gag reflex or in the patient who is initially alert but who may become obtunded before emesis is completed, a carefully performed gastric lavage can be done rapidly and safely. When the gag reflex is depressed, lavage should be undertaken only after the patient has been intubated with a cuffed endotracheal tube. After removing any foreign matter from the mouth, the patient should be positioned on the left side with the head slightly lower than the rest of the body. The lavage should be done with small amounts (50 ml in children; 200–300 ml in adults) of half-normal saline and should continue until the return is clear.

Gastric lavage is less effective than forceful emesis. The procedure requires that the patient be brought to a hospital, which delays removal and extends the time for absorption of the ingested product. In addition, the removal of whole or partially dissolved tablets or capsules is possible only with the use of a large-bore orogastric tube (28–36 French). The commonly used 16–18 French tube removes only liquids successfully. The lavage procedure is uncomfortable and is associated with a risk of vomiting and aspiration. Contraindications to lavage include the presence of convulsions and the ingestion of caustic substances or petroleum distillate hydrocarbon products.

ACTIVATED CHARCOAL

Activated charcoal was rediscovered in the last decade as an adjunct to the initial management of the acute overdose patient. It is an odorless, tasteless, fine black powder that, because of its small particle size and large surface area, binds organic compounds and creates a stable complex that does not dissociate. Table 42.2 lists some of the compounds for which activated charcoal has been shown to be effective.

In order to achieve optimal binding of a poison, activated charcoal is best used within 1 hour of ingestion. Charcoal is administered orally at a dose of 5–10 times the weight of the ingested product or at a dose of 1 g/kg. It should be mixed in 30–60 ml of water and may be flavored with 5 ml of cherry syrup or 1 drop of anise to increase its palatability. Because the pediatric patient may not drink this mixture, administration by nasogastric tube may be necessary. Vomiting may occur after the administration of activated charcoal, so appropriate precautions should be taken. Charcoal also serves as a marker

TABLE 42.2 Drugs Absorbed in Vivo by Activated Charcoal

Analgesics and Antipyretics
  Acetaminophen
  Acetylsalicylic acid
  Mefenamic acid
  Methyl salicylate
  Opiates
  Paracetamol
  Propoxyphene
  Salicylamide
  Sodium salicylate
Barbiturates and Sedatives—Hypnotics
  Alcohols
  Barbital
  Ethchlorvynol
  Glutethimide
  Meprobamate
  Phenobarbital
  Secobarbital
Tranquilizers and Antidepressants
  Chlorpromazine
  Imipramine
  Nortriptyline
  Phenothiazines
  Tricyclic antidepressants
Miscellaneous
  Acetylcysteine
  Amphetamine
  Chloroquine
  Chlorpheniramine
  Digoxin
  Ipecac
  Isoniazid
  Phenylpropanolamine
  Phenytoin
  Propantheline

of gastrointestinal motility and provides a general indication of the time at which the ingested product passes from the body.

Activated charcoal is not effective for rapidly absorbed compounds such as cyanide, heavy metals (e.g., iron, lead), agents ingested in gram quantities (e.g., ethanol, glycol), and complex compounds (e.g., petroleum distillates). Charcoal should not be used before or concomitant with ipecac syrup since the charcoal will bind the emetic and prevent vomiting.

SALINE CATHARTICS

Saline cathartics such as magnesium sulfate, sodium sulfate, or magnesium citrate are effective in speeding the rate of transit of a toxic product through the intestinal tract and therefore presumably limiting overall absorption from the small and large bowels. The dosage for each of the sulfate cathartics is 250 mg/kg given orally and repeated every 3 hours until productive of a stool. The oral dose of magnesium citrate is 5 ml/kg for children and 200 ml for adults. This dosage should be repeated every 3 hours until productive of a stool. Saline cathartics are not bound by activated charcoal and may be given after administration of charcoal. Catharsis is recommended for any patient who has taken a potentially toxic dose of a poison. Cathartics are particularly useful in treating ingestions of drugs that slow peristalsis. Because many drugs may be absorbed slowly throughout the bowel, it is recommended that cathartics be used as long as 6–12 hours after ingestion.

Dermal and Pulmonary Absorption

Many toxins such as insecticides or hydrocarbons are absorbed through the skin. Contaminated clothing may provide a reservoir of toxin and should be removed carefully. Thorough washing with soap and water will effectively remove these components from the skin and stop absorption by this route. Care must be taken not to abrade the skin because absorption is rapid through damaged epithelium.

Absorption by inhalation can be halted by removal of the patient from the area of exposure. The use of respiratory therapy is dictated by symptoms.

Enhancement of Excretion

Drugs and other toxins are usually removed from the body by two major pathways. The active compound can be converted to inactive metabolites by the liver and then excreted through the urine or feces, or the active product can be excreted unchanged by the kidneys. For most agents, one pathway predominates, for example, the hepatic route for phenytoin and the renal route for lithium. For a few drugs, such as phenobarbital and salicylates, both pathways are important. Overdoses with drugs that primarily undergo hepatic inactivation are treated by supportive therapy alone, allowing time for the liver to detoxify the ingested product. For some products taken in overdose, hepatic metabolism may produce metabolites that are in themselves toxic (e.g., methanol, glutethimide, acetaminophen). In these cases, the risk of toxicity will persist until the body has eliminated not only the parent compound but the metabolites as well.

DIURESIS

If the predominant excretory route of the active product (parent drug or metabolite) is the kidneys, diuresis may enhance its removal. Fluid diuresis is accomplished by the parenteral administration of large fluid volumes (2,500–3,000 ml/m²/24 hr), as well as by the use of osmotic agents (mannitol or urea) and diuretics (furosemide or ethacrynic acid). This produces an increase in glomerular filtration rate and renal tubular flow, which results in an increased filtration of the drug and a decreased reabsorption in the distal tubules thereby enhancing renal excretion of the toxic compound.

Ionized diuresis is based on the principle that a drug in its ionized form crosses lipid membranes poorly. Alkalinization of the urine (to pH 7.5–8) with parenteral sodium bicarbonate will increase the ionized fraction of weak acids (aspirin or phenobarbital) and decrease their renal tubular absorption. In a similar fashion, urinary excretion of weak bases (amphetamines or phencyclidine) may be enhanced by acidification of the urine (to pH 4–4.5) with parenteral or oral ammonium chloride.

All methods of enhanced excretion carry some risk, and monitoring serum and urinary electrolytes, central venous pressure, electrocardiogram (ECG), and body weight is necessary. The risks involved with enhanced excretion must be weighed carefully against the risks associated with conservative, supportive therapy alone.

DIALYSIS

The severity of the ingestion may place the patient at sufficient risk to necessitate removal of the drug more rapidly than can be accomplished by methods of enhanced excretion other than dialysis. Dialysis is an effective technique for removing certain products or their toxic metabolites from the body. It may also be considered when normal excretory pathways are compromised (e.g., renal or hepatic failure) or when underlying pathology mitigates against forced diuresis (e.g., renal disease, congestive heart failure). Peritoneal dialysis removes many compounds but is less effective than hemodialysis. Hemoperfusion (charcoal or resin) is the newest and most effective method of removing toxins. This method generally accomplishes greater clearance of toxins than does hemodialysis. Adverse effects are minimal, although clinical experience with the procedure is still in a preliminary stage. Refer to a number of compre-

hensive articles listed in the suggested readings at the end of this chapter for more extensive information on the use of these procedures in cases of serious poisonings.

Inactivating Ingested Substances: Local and Systemic Antidotes

The majority of toxic ingestions may be managed by using the general principles discussed in the preceding section. There are, however, a number of toxins for which specific and effective antidotes are available.

Antidotes that exert a local or topical effect include calcium (in the form of calcium lactate, calcium gluconate, or milk) to minimize the caustic effects of fluoride on the gastrointestinal mucosa and 1% sodium bicarbonate to precipitate iron in the gastrointestinal tract and to neutralize its caustic effects.

The following is a review of antidotes that are administered for their systemic effects. The first six are generally needed promptly and are commonly used in the emergency room. The remainder are not usually considered emergency room drugs and can be used after the patient's condition is stable. A drug formulary (Table 42.3) is included to supplement the text and to serve as a rapid reference. Table 42.4 lists some common ingestions for which well-accepted antidotes are available.

NALOXONE HYDROCHLORIDE

Naloxone hydrochloride (Narcan) is a specific narcotic antagonist that is effective in the treatment of acute toxicity from opiate derivatives (codeine, heroin, hydrocodone, hydromorphone, morphine, oxycodone) and synthetic narcotic preparations (diphenoxylate, meperidine, methadone, pentazocine, propoxyphene).

The specificity of action of naloxone allows it to be used in a diagnostic trial as well as in treatment of the acute overdosed patient. In fact, doses of 50 times that recommended have been administered without apparent ill effect.

The recommended intravenous dose for narcotic-induced respiratory and central nervous system depression or hypotension is 0.03 mg/kg in children and 1.2 mg in adults. Desired effects should be seen within 2–3 minutes and consist of pupillary dilation, improved blood pressure, and increased level of consciousness. Because the antagonist achieves its effect by competing with a tissue-bound narcotic, the patient who has taken a large overdose of a narcotic may require multiple intravenous doses of naloxone to produce the desired response. Once a favorable response to the antagonist is obtained the drug should be given as often as necessary to maintain normal

TABLE 42.3 Drugs for the Treatment of Acute Poisoning

Drug	Use	Dosage Pediatric / Adult	Administration	Warnings
Ammonium chloride	Acidification of urine	2.75 mEq/kg/dose / 2.75 mEq/kg/dose	PO or IV q6h prn to urine pH ≤ 5	Use in conjunction with ascorbic acid
Apomorphine	Induction of emesis	0.07 mg/kg / 0.07 mg/kg	Single dose subcutaneously	Use freshly prepared solution; may cause CNS depression
Ascorbic acid	Acidification of urine	1–2 g / 2 g	IV infusion over 6 hr prn urine pH ≤ 5	Use in conjunction with ammonium chloride
Atropine	Carbamate or organophosphate insecticide poisoning	0.05 mg/kg / 2–3 mg	IV or subcutaneously q 2–3 min prn	Repeat until patient shows dilated pupils, tachycardia, or xerostomia
Charcoal, activated	Adsorption of ingested drugs	1 g/kg / 30–50 g	Orally, mixed with 60–90 ml water	May be repeated
Chlorpromazine	Sympathomimetic drug-induced hyperactivity and psychosis	1 mg/kg (max 25 mg) / 25 mg	PO, IM, IV q6h prn	May produce hypotension
Cyanide antidote kit Amyl nitrite Pearls	Cyanide poisoning	1 Pearl / 1 Pearl	Inhale for 30 sec out of each 60 sec; New pearl q 3 min	Use immediately after exposure
Sodium nitrite (3%)		0.3 ml/kg / 10 ml	IV at rate of 2.5–5 ml/min	Administer as soon as possible
Sodium thiosulfate (25%)		1.65 ml/kg / 50 ml	IV at rate of 2.5–5 ml/min	Administer 15–30 min after sodium nitrite
Deferoxamine	Iron poisoning	50 mg/kg (max 2 g) / 1–2 g	IM q6h	
		15 mg/kg/hr / 15 mg/kg/hr	IV infusion	May be given IV if hypotension present; too rapid infusion may cause hypotension
Diphenhydramine	Phenothiazine-induced acute dystonic reactions	1–2 mg/kg / 25–50 mg	IV over 5–10 min	

Drug	Indication	Dose	Administration	Comments
Ethanol (10%)	Ethylene glycol or methanol poisoning	0.7 g/kg	IV × 1 dose	Loading dose only
		0.7 g/kg		
		109 mg/kg	IV hourly to maintain ethanol blood level between 100–150 mg%	Maintenance dose
		109 mg/kg		
Ipecac syrup	Induction of emesis	9–12 months = 10 ml	PO, followed by 90–180 ml H_2O, repeat in 20 min if no emesis	*Contraindications*: Age <9 months coma, convulsions, caustic ingestion
		>12 months = 15 ml		
		30 ml		
Magnesium citrate (NF)	Cathars s	2–5 yr = 20–50 ml	PO q4–6h until stool produced	Contraindicated in renal failure
		6–12 yr = 100–500 ml		
		200–300 ml		
Magnesium sulfate (10%)	Cathars s	2–5 yr = 2–5 g	PO q4–6h until stool produced	Contraindicated in renal failure
		6–12 yr = 5–10 g		
		10–30 g		
Methylene blue (1%)	Methemoglobinemia	1.0 mg/kg	IV over 5–10 min	May produce hemolysis
		10 mg		
N-Acetylcysteine (5%)	Acetaminophen poisoning (not approved for use)	140 mg/kg	PO × 1 dose	Loading dose only
		140 mg/kg		
		70 mg/kg	PO q4h × 17 doses	Maintenance dosages
		70 mg/kg		
Naloxone	Narcotic overdose	0.03 mg/kg	IV push q2–3 min prn	May produce withdrawal in addicted person
		1.2 mg		
Physostigmine	Anticholinergic poisoning (hypertension, coma, irritability, arrhythmias)	0.5 mg	IV over 2–3 min; repeat × 1 in 5 min if no effect	Rapid infusion may cause convulsions
		2.0 mg		
Pralidoxime (2-PAM)	Organophosphate insecticide poisoning	250 mg	IV slowly q8–12h prn	Use after administering atropine
		500–1,000 mg		
Phenytoin	Digitalis-induced arrhythmias	1–5 mg/kg (max 500 mg)	IV slowly q5 min prn not to exceed 50 mg/min	
		250 mg (max 1,000 mg)		

TABLE 42.4 Specific Common Toxins and Their Antidotes

Toxin	Antidote
Morphine, paregoric, meperidine, pentazocine, codeine, methadone, diphenoxylate, propoxyphene	Naloxone hydrochloride (Narcan)
Cyanide salts and gases, insecticides, rodenticides, chemical synthesis	Amyl nitrite, sodium nitrite, sodium thiosulfate
Acetanilid, acetophenetidin (phenacetin), aniline derivatives, antipyrine, benzene derivatives, chlorates, dinitrophenol, dinitrotoulene, hydroquinone, methylene blue, nitrates (if reduced), nitrogen oxide, nitroglycerol, nitrite derivatives, pamaquine, phenetidin, phenylazopyridine, phenylenediamine, phenylhydroxylamine, piperazine, primaquine, pyridium, quinones, resorcinol, sulfa derivatives, trional, toluidine, trinitrotoluene	Methylene blue
Sevin	Atropine sulfate
Bidrin, chlorthion, malathion, parathion	Atropine sulfate and pralidoxime
Carbon monoxide gas	Oxygen
Lead, mercury, arsenic	Calcium disodium, ethylene diamine, tetracetate (EDTA)
Lead, mercury, arsenic	Dimercaprol (BAL)
Lead, copper, mercury, arsenic	Penicillamine
Iron	Deferoxamine
Tricyclic antidepressants (amitriptyline, imipramine, desipramine, doxepin, protriptyline), atropine-like (anisotropine, atropine, belladona, dicyclomine, homatropine, isopropamide, mepenzolate, methantheline, propantheline, pipenzolate, scopolamine), cold medications and sedatives (benactyzine, chlorpheniramine, diphenhydramine, methapyrilene, pyrilamine) plants (amanita muscaria, bittersweet, black henbane, black night shade, deadly night shade, jerusalem cherry, jimson weed, lantana, potato leaves, sprouts, tubers, wild tomato)	Physostigmine (Antilirium)
Ethylene glycol, methanol	Ethanol
Idiosyncratic reaction to phenothiazines (especially piperazine and aliphatic group of phenothiazines)	Diphenhydramine
Amphetamine central nervous system stimulants	Chlorpromazine
Warfarin and dicumarol	Vitamin K_1

blood pressure and respiratory rate, normal or dilated pupils, and an alert sensorium. Careful monitoring of the patient, often for as long as 36 hours, is necessary until the effects of the narcotic have passed.

The older antagonist, levallorphan (Lorfan), has intrinsic agonist properties and may produce respiratory or central nervous system depression in the patient who has not ingested a narcotic. Nalorphine (Nalline), another antagonist with intrinsic agonist properties, is no longer available. The use of these drugs is not recommended.

CYANIDE ANTIDOTES

See the discussion of cyanide under specific poisoning.

METHYLENE BLUE

Methylene blue is used in the therapy of methemoglobinemia. Many compounds, including aniline, benzocaine, chlorates, nitrites, nitrobenzenes, phenacetin, quinones, and sulfonamides, produce methemoglobin by the oxidation of hemoglobin iron from its ferrous to its ferric state. This results in reduced oxygen-transport capacity and decreased release of oxygen to the tissues. Treatment includes the administration of oxygen, which helps to relieve hypoxia, and methylene blue, which reduces ferric iron to its ferrous state. Methylene blue is given intravenously as a 1% solution in a dosage of 1–2 mg/kg over 2–10 minutes. This dose may be repeated in 3–4 hours. Methylene blue itself is capable of causing vomiting, diarrhea, coma, chest pain, and cyanosis. Its use should be reserved for patients with methemoglobin levels above 25%. The effectiveness of therapy should be monitored by serial methemoglobin determinations throughout the course of treatment.

ATROPINE SULFATE AND PRALIDOXIME

Anticholinesterase insecticides consist of two groups: carbamates (Aldicarb, Sevin, Isocarb) and organophosphates (Malathion, Parathion, Chlorthion, Diazinon, Bidrin). Both groups act by inhibiting cholinesterase. The attendant rise in acetylcholine levels produces the characteristic cholinergic (muscarinic) signs of intoxication: miotic pupils, lacrimation, salivation, bradycardia, vomiting, and diarrhea. Other signs of intoxication are nicotinic: muscle fasciculation, respiratory paralysis, and central nervous system depression. Atropine is a competitive blocker of acetylcholine at the receptor sites and reverses the muscarinic signs. Atropine sulfate is given intravenously in an initial dose of 0.05 mg/kg in a child and 2–3 mg in an adult; additional doses are given at 2–5-minute intervals until the toxic (muscarinic) effects have been reversed and cholinergic blockage is achieved (dilated pupils, dry mouth, tachycardia, decreased bowel sounds). Also atropine may partially reverse central nervous system depression. 2-Pyridine aldoxime methiodide (2-PAM), or pralidoxime, regenerates plasma and red blood cell cholinesterase. Note that 2-PAM is used only in the therapy of organophosphate poisoning where it reverses nicotinic effects (muscle fasciculations and respiratory paralysis). This part of therapy should be started as soon as possible but not until an atropinization has been started and the patient's condition is stable. The dosage of 2-PAM is 250 mg–1 g given intravenously, over 2–3 minutes, every 8–12 hours as needed. Atropine should be given whenever a patient has symptoms from either group of insecticides; the 2-PAM should be used whenever a patient is symptomatic from an organophosphate poisoning.

OXYGEN

In patients with acute carbon monoxide poisoning, oxygen is displaced from hemoglobin and carboxyhemoglobin is formed.

Carboxyhemoglobin has a decreased oxygen-carrying capacity and a diminished ability to release oxygen to the tissues, resulting in tissue hypoxia. High concentrations of oxygen are effective in reversing the toxic effects of carbon monoxide. Carboxyhemoglobin levels can be decreased by 50% in 1–2 hours by administering 100% oxygen by a tightly fitting mask.

N-ACETYLCYSTEINE

An acute overdose of acetaminophen results in depletion of hepatic glutathione with a consequent accumulation of acetaminophen metabolic intermediates that are toxic to the hepatocyte. N-Acetylcysteine (Mucomyst) penetrates the hepatocyte and appears to protect against the elevation of liver enzyme levels and hepatocellular damage secondary to acetaminophen overdose.

The use of N-acetylcysteine is indicated if acetaminophen blood levels are in the hepatotoxic range (Fig. 42.1). If an acetaminophen blood level is unavailable, then the need for N-acetylcysteine is dictated by a history of a potentially toxic ingestion (more than 140 mg/kg in a child or more than 7.5 g in an adolescent or adult).

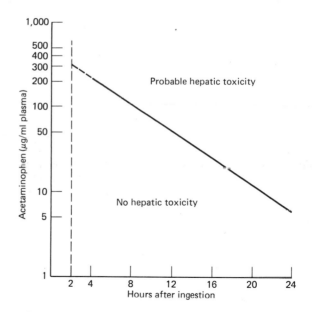

Figure 42.1 Semilogarithmic plot of plasma acetaminophen levels versus time. (*Source:* Rumack BH, Matthew H: Acetaminophen poisoning and toxicity. *Pediatrics* 1975; 55:871–876.)

The initial dose of 140 mg/kg of N-acetylcysteine should be given orally or by lavage tube within 12 hours of a potentially toxic ingestion to assure maximum protection. If treatment is started more than 12 hours after ingestion, less protection is achieved but it is still significantly better than no treatment. Subsequent oral dosages of 70 mg/kg every 4 hours should be given for a total of 18 doses. Recently, the intravenous route has been recommended for the administration of N-acetylcysteine. Until a suitable intravenous preparation is available and until the efficacy has been established, the administration of N-acetylcysteine by the intravenous route cannot be recommended in the United States.

Adverse effects of N-acetylcysteine appear to be minimal and consist primarily of nausea and vomiting. Activated charcoal will bind and prevent absorption of N-acetylcysteine. Therefore the use of activated charcoal in conjunction with N-acetylcysteine is contraindicated.

CHELATING AGENTS

In patients with acute and chronic heavy metal poisoning, the metals bind to organic molecules (especially sulfhydryl groups) that are essential for various enzymatic functions. Chelating agents, by competing with these molecules for the heavy metals, remove the heavy metal from its binding site in the body and the complex is excreted. An excess of the chelating agent must be given to assure that the heavy metal is bound rather than simply redistributed in the body. Characteristics of specific chelating agents and their effectiveness will be reviewed.

Heavy metals that preferentially bind to oxygen and nitrogen (e.g., lead) are effectively chelated by *Calcium disodium ethylenediaminetetraacetate (EDTA) (Versene)*. Because the sodium salt of EDTA will chelate calcium, resulting in hypocalcemia, the calcium disodium salt is used. The dose of CaEDTA is 50–75 mg/kg/day given in 2 or 3 divided doses. Although the intramuscular route is preferred, the drug may be given by slow intravenous infusion. Use of the oral route is not advised. The kidneys offer the only route of excretion for the heavy metal complex so adequate renal function must be established before initiating therapy.

Adverse effects include rash, injection site reaction, fever, hypercalcemia, ECG abnormalities, Fanconi syndrome, and acute tubular necrosis. The ECG, urinalysis, blood urea nitrogen (BUN), and serum calcium and phosphorus should be monitored throughout therapy. These reactions are dose related and reduction or discontinuation of EDTA is required if these complications develop.

Dimercaprol (BAL) is effective in the treatment of heavy metals that bind to sulfur and phosphorus (e.g., lead, mercury,

and arsenic). Dosages, duration of treatment, and the necessity of repetitive courses of therapy depend on the severity of the poisoning. As a general rule, arsenic and mercury require 10–14 days and lead requires 5–7 days of therapy. The drug is given only by the intramuscular route in doses of 3–4 mg/kg. During the first 2–5 days when the body burden of heavy metal is at its highest, BAL is given every 4–6 hours. This frequency is reduced to every 12 hours during the later days of therapy. Iron should not be administered in conjunction with BAL since a toxic complex would be formed. Because the liver is the primary excretory pathway for BAL, compromised hepatic function contraindicates its use. It may, however, be used in the presence of renal failure.

Adverse reactions are dose related and include lacrimation, blepharospasm, paresthesias, nausea, vomiting, tachycardia, and hypertension. Careful monitoring of pulse, blood pressure, and neurologic status should be done throughout the treatment period.

d-Penicillamine (Cuprimine) may be used for both acute and chronic poisoning with lead, arsenic, copper, or mercury. N-acetylpenicillamine has significant advantages over d-penicillamine for mercury poisoning. d-Penicillamine is given only by the oral route and must be taken on an empty stomach at least $1\frac{1}{2}$ hours before meals. For short-term therapy, 100 mg/kg/day in 4 divided doses (with a maximum daily dose of 1 g) may be given for 5 days. For chronic therapy, 30–50 mg/kg/day in 2–4 divided doses is given. Adverse reactions are dose related. At dosages above 50 mg/kg/day rash, fever, nephrotic syndrome, leukopenia, neutropenia, eosinophilia, and coagulation defects may occur. Since the drug is excreted primarily by the kidneys, renal failure is a contraindication to its use. The drug is contraindicated also in patients with penicillin allergy.

Deferoxamine (Desferal) has proved to be a highly effective chelating agent in the treatment of patients with acute iron intoxication. Indications for the use of deferoxamine in patients with acute iron intoxication include the following: (1) a serum iron level exceeding the iron-binding capacity; (2) shock or coma; (3) a positive provocative chelation test with the ingestion of an unknown amount of iron; (4) an absorbed dose in the potentially lethal range.

The chelating dosage of deferoxamine is 50 mg/kg (up to 1–2 g) given intramuscularly every 6–8 hours. The drug may also be given intravenously, but this may produce hypotension if the infusion rate exceeds 15 mg/kg/hr. Deferoxamine binds free unbound iron and the iron–deferoxamine complex is excreted by the kidneys producing a pink or red urine. The iron–deferoxamine complex also may be removed by dialysis or exchange transfusion. Chelation therapy may be discontinued when iron levels fall below the iron-binding capacity or when urine color returns to normal.

Deferoxamine, 50 mg/kg, may also be given intramuscularly as a diagnostic trial. The appearance of pink or red urine (caused by the iron–deferoxamine complex) indicates that the iron-binding capacity has been exceeded by the iron concentration (a positive provocation chelation test) and that a potential for developing systemic toxicity exists. Oral administration of deferoxamine will bind iron remaining in the gastrointestinal tract, however, the cost of the drug and the risk of bolus absorption of chelated iron through damaged intestinal mucosa resulting in hypotension presently limit the use of the oral route.

Adverse effects from deferoxamine include rash, pain at the injection site, hypocalcemia, and hypotension.

PHYSOSTIGMINE

Physostigmine (Antilirium) has been used with increasing frequency in the treatment of anticholinergic poisonings as a result of belladonna alkaloids, antihistamines, tricyclic antidepressants, or various plants. Although it has similar peripheral cholinergic activity as neostigmine, physostigmine has the added ability to pass the blood–brain barrier and exert central nervous system effects. Physostigmine is particularly effective in treating central nervous system excitation or depression, hypertension, signs of atropinization (dilated pupils, dry mouth, tachycardia, hyperpyrexia, bladder and bowel atony), and cardiac arrhythmias (supraventricular tachycardias). Its ability to arrest convulsions and correct hypotension caused by anticholinergic agents is questionable.

Physostigmine may be used as a diagnostic trial in a patient with suspected anticholinergic overdose. If signs of atropinization are reversed, the diagnosis is confirmed. It may also be used in an attempt to alleviate symptoms and signs presenting significant hazard to the patient (cardiac arrhythmias, deep levels of coma, and hypertension). The recommended dose in children is 0.5 mg and in adults and adolescents is 2 mg. Dosages are administered intravenously over 2–3 minutes. If no effect is observed, the dosage may be repeated at 2 minute intervals up to a total dose of 2 mg in children and 4–6 mg in adolescents and adults. Because the effects of physostigmine are usually of shorter duration than the effects of the ingested drug, the antidote may be required as often as every 20–60 minutes until the patient is free of serious anticholinergic effects.

The use of physostigmine carries two risks. First, if the drug is given too rapidly the patient may develop seizures. Second, excessive physostigmine can result in a cholinergic crisis, characterized by miotic pupils, salivation, diarrhea, and vomiting.

This latter effect lasts less than 60 minutes, is rarely serious, and may be reversed by the administration of atropine at a dose one-half that of the physostigmine.

ETHANOL

Methanol is found in antifreeze, paint remover, shellac, and solvents and as a cheap source of alcohol. Methanol overdose causes mild central nervous system depression, metabolic acidosis, and blindness. These findings are the result of the metabolic products of methanol—formaldehyde and formic acid. Both ethanol and methanol are metabolized in the liver by the enzyme alcohol dehydrogenase.

The object of ethanol therapy is to saturate the enzyme thus preventing the metabolism of methanol to its toxic metabolites. Methanol is then excreted slowly by the kidneys over 2–5 days.

In mild overdoses, ethanol may be given orally as 3–4 oz of 90–100 proof whiskey every 3–4 hours. In severe poisoning, a 10% ethanol solution is given intravenously in a loading dose of 0.7 gm/kg followed by maintenance dosages of 109 mg/kg/hr. It is important to maintain ethanol levels greater than 100 mg% until methanol levels have fallen to the nontoxic range (less than 10 mg%).

Methanol and its metabolites are highly dialyzable. Dialysis is indicated when methanol levels exceed 50 mg%, when there is severe uncorrectable acidosis, or when retinal edema and hyperemia are present.

Ethylene glycol (antifreeze) is also metabolized by alcohol dehydrogenase. Poisoning with this compound is treated with ethanol in the same manner as outlined for treating methanol poisoning.

DIPHENHYDRAMINE

Idiosyncratic reactions to phenothiazines produce extrapyramidal effects including opisthotonus, torticollis, oculogyric crisis, rigidity, dystonia, trismus, and tremors. These adverse effects are reversed within 2–3 minutes by the slow intravenous administration of diphenhydramine (Benadryl) at a dose of 1–2 mg/kg. To prevent recurrence of symptoms, diphenhydramine should be maintained for a 24-hour period at a dosage of 1–2 mg/kg given orally every 6 hours. Sedation may be a side effect of therapy, and excessively rapid infusion may produce hypotension. Patients with dose-related signs of phenothiazines toxicity, such as ataxia and lethargy, respond inconsistently to diphenhydramine.

CHLORPROMAZINE

Central nervous system stimulation secondary to amphetamine overdose may be decreased by chlorpromazine given at a dose of 1 mg/kg by the oral or intramuscular route. This dose should be reduced to 0.5 mg/kg when a barbiturate has been taken along with the amphetamine. If the patient has taken dimethoxy methylamphetamine (STP) or dimethyltryptamine (DMT), chlorpromazine may cause hypotension. In these instances, diazepam (Valium) rather than chlorpromazine would be the preferred drug for sedation.

VITAMIN K₁

Vitamin K_1 is used in the treatment of warfarin and dicumarol toxicity. These anticoagulants are common components of rat poisons and exert their effects by inhibiting prothrombin synthesis and producing a hemorrhagic diathesis. Vitamin K_1, given in a dose of 5–10 mg orally or parenterally, will reverse this inhibitory effect on prothrombin synthesis.

Transfer to Hospital

Admission into the hospital should be considered for any poisoned patient who has the potential for developing serious morbidity. The physical condition of the patient as well as the specific poison must be considered. Admission is advised for patients with abnormal or fluctuating vital signs, particularly embarrassment of the cardiorespiratory system. Patients with central nervous system dysfunction should not be released from medical care until their recovery is complete. The presence of significant risk of developing complications related to the poisoning (e.g., pneumonitis, dehydration, hemorrhage) may indicate the need for extended care. If a toxic amount of a poison has been absorbed, the patient should be closely observed until he or she recovers. Admission to the hospital is also recommended when either the identity of the toxin or the clinical course is uncertain. Finally, if the poisoning was the result of a serious psychiatric disorder, hospitalization may be necessary.

Prevention

No therapy for a poisoning is complete until the reasons for its occurrence have been explored and advice for future prevention have been fully explained. In the case of childhood poisoning, the aim should be to make the environment as safe as possible by removing all poisons from the child's access. The use of safety containers, education of the child, and visiting nurses to review potential risks existing in the home with parents are all methods of accomplishing this goal. In the case of the older child, adolescent, or adult, a poisoning should be viewed in the context of a suicide gesture or attempt, and immediate intervention is imperative to prevent a future suicide attempt.

CLINICAL SETTINGS

Acetaminophen

Acute ingestion of acetaminophen-containing products is becoming more common as the therapeutic use of these drugs increase. Although acetaminophen is ingested by all age groups, it appears to have more serious consequences in adolescents and adults. The emergency physician should be aware of the mild early course following ingestion and be able to evaluate and minimize the potential for developing delayed hepatotoxicity.

DIAGNOSIS

The history and physical examination findings of patients who have taken overdoses of acetaminophen correlate poorly with the severity of the poisoning. Acutely toxic doses of acetaminophen are doses greater than 7.5 g in an adult and greater than 150 mg/kg in children. Anorexia, nausea, vomiting, lethargy (no coma), diaphoresis, and epigastric tenderness may occur within the first 12 hours. The more serious problem of liver damage may not manifest itself for 48 hours or more. Liver function test values begin to rise 2–3 days after the poisoning, reach a peak by 5–7 days, and, except in very severe or fatal cases, return to normal over a 2–3 weeks. Fatalities occur as a result of liver failure.

TREATMENT

Initial treatment should be the clearing of residual acetaminophen from the gastrointestinal tract by the use of emesis or lavage and saline cathartics. The most reliable predictor of hepatotoxicity is the acetaminophen blood level. The levels may be interpreted most accurately 4 hours or more after ingestion. Two values obtained at least 4 hours apart allow the physician to evaluate toxicity based on the plasma drug level itself as well as on an acetaminophen half-life (longer than 4 hours in serious poisoning).

If there is a high probability of developing liver damage, the currently recommended treatment is oral N-acetylcysteine (Mucomyst) started as soon as possible after the gastrointestinal tract has been cleared but within 12 hours of ingestion. The initial oral dose of N-acetylcysteine is 140 mg/kg; subsequent dosages are 70 mg/kg by mouth or by nasogastric tube every 4 hours for a total of 18 doses.

PROGNOSIS

The prognosis for an acute acetaminophen overdose is good. Fatalities are rare, and recovery from hepatic damage appears to be complete within 3 months.

Salicylate

Salicylates are found in a large number of medications. These medications are most often meant for oral use, but various dermatologic preparations contain high concentrations of salicylates. Because of the wide availability of salicylates, it is not surprising that salicylate overdose is still one of the most common causes of hospitalization.

DIAGNOSIS

Symptoms of acute salicylate intoxication may occur from single doses greater than 150 mg/kg. Absorption from the gastrointestinal tract is rapid for aqueous solutions, slower for tablet forms (aspirin), and delayed for methyl salicylate (oil of wintergreen), enteric tablets, and aspirin suppositories. In general, absorption of regular aspirin tablets is nearly complete within 2 hours. If patients ingest methyl salicylate and enteric forms of aspirin, absorption may not be complete for 4–6 hours. Absorption will be delayed in the presence of food.

The diagnosis of acute salicylate poisoning is made on the basis of an appropriate history and physical examination, as well as detection of toxic levels of salicylate in the blood. The development and the extent of individual symptoms and signs are variable, but they generally correlate directly with the severity of the poisoning. Tinnitus, vomiting, hyperthermia, and hyperpnea are hallmarks of acute salicylism. A variable degree of central nervous system depression (lethargy, coma) or excitement (irritability, convulsions) is usually present. Laboratory findings include acid–base disturbances (respiratory alkalosis in adults, metabolic acidosis in children), fluid and electrolyte imbalances (loss of water, sodium, potassium), and hypoglycemia.

TREATMENT

Treatment should begin with the removal of salicylate from the gastrointestinal tract. Emesis should be induced with ipecac syrup if it can be done within 2 hours of ingestion. If central nervous system depression is present, gastric lavage should be done. This time limit may be extended to 4 hours if the ingestion was of methyl salicylate, enteric aspirin, or concomitant inhibitors of peristalsis. Activated charcoal will bind salicylates and prevent further absorption. Administration of saline cathartic after the activated charcoal will purge the intestinal tract of remaining salicylates.

Subsequent management consists of correction of metabolic imbalances. Dehydration and electrolyte disturbances should be corrected with adequate volumes of parenteral electrolyte solutions. The fluid also results in a diuresis, enhancing renal excretion of salicylates. Parenteral sodium bicarbonate will correct metabolic acidosis and shift salicylates out of tissues and into the plasma. If the urine is sufficiently alkalinized (pH = 8), salicylate excretion is markedly increased.

Indications for dialysis include a potentially lethal blood level of salicylate (>100 mg%), a deteriorating condition in spite of conservative therapy, or an inability to effect alkaline diuresis.

Caustics

There are many substances that may cause corrosive damage to the gastrointestinal tract. Nonspecific chemicals cause a superficial inflammation of the mouth and esophagus but generally do not result in perforation or stricture. Acidic substances cause a coagulation type of necrosis and thus do not penetrate as deeply as alkalis. Strongly alkaline products produce a liquifactive necrosis, penetrate deeply and rapidly, and result in stricture of the esophagus. The severity of an alkali burn depends on the pH of the substance and the duration of contact with the mucosa. Particles and large amounts of liquids remain in contact with the mucosal surface for longer periods of time and are more likely to cause severe burns.

DIAGNOSIS

Symptoms resulting from a caustic ingestion may not occur immediately. Local pain or burning is almost always present, but severe burns may damage nerve endings, resulting in anesthesia. Dysphagia is common.

A physical examination should be performed on every patient with a history of caustic ingestion. Signs may include fever, agitation, or distress. Mucosal burns appear as whitish-grey or red patches; dermal burns of the face, hands, or trunk appear erythematous. Drooling occurs as a result of dysphagia combined with an outpouring of saliva. Respiratory distress may be present if the larynx is involved or if esophageal perforation has occurred. Leukocytosis may occur.

To evaluate the extent of esophageal damage, further diagnostic procedures are indicated. The absence of mouth burns should not be taken to indicate the absence of esophageal burns. A barium swallow is not useful in evaluating the extent of the esophageal burn in the acute stages since inflammation will obscure the picture. Endoscopy can be used only to document the presence or absence of an esophageal burn.

TREATMENT

If a burn is seen on endoscopy or if symptoms of an esophageal burn are present and endoscopy is not available, the traditional therapy is careful supportive care and corticosteroid therapy. For adults, the corticosteroid dose is equivalent to prednisone 10–20 mg every 6 hours for 2–3 weeks. For children, the dose of corticosteroids is equivalent to prednisone 2–3 mg/kg/day in 4 divided dosages. Dosages should be tapered at the end of therapy.

Broad-spectrum antibiotics given parenterally for prophylaxis are not recommended. Antibiotics should be given if infection can be documented.

PROGNOSIS

The outcome for patients suffering from caustic ingestion depends on the depth and extent of the esophageal burn and the development of esophageal strictures. Follow-up is done by repeated barium swallow or endoscopy.

Cyanide

There are many sources of cyanide. Hydrocyanic (prussic) acid used as a pesticide is a highly toxic form. Cyanide salts found in chemical laboratories and in industry are also very toxic. Cyanide from organic nitrites, cyanamide, medical sources, and plants is of lesser toxicity.

Cyanide acts as a poison by binding to ferric iron in mitochondrial cytochrome oxidase systems. This binding inhibits cellular respiration and results in cellular anoxia.

DIAGNOSIS

Symptoms of cyanide poisoning occur within 15–20 minutes after exposure. Headache, faintness, vertigo, salivation, tachypnea, and bradycardia occur early. Later symptoms include central nervous system depression, respiratory failure, cardiac arrhythmias, and hypotension.

Cyanide can cause death within 15 minutes of ingestion. Since speed in initiating treatment is critical, there is no time for laboratory corroboration of the diagnosis. A history of exposure to cyanide with a rapid onset of bradycardia, coma, and hypotension is adequate for a clinical diagnosis of cyanide poisoning and the initiation of therapy.

TREATMENT

Therapeutic efforts are directed at oxidizing ferrous hemoglobin to a ferric state thereby producing a large circulating pool of methemoglobin, which has a greater affinity for cyanide than does the ferric iron of the mitochondrial system of enzymes.

Methemoglobinemia is created first by the inhalation of amyl nitrite given as a broken pearl held in a cloth over the patient's nose for 30 seconds out of each minute. A new ampule is used every 3 minutes until sodium nitrite becomes available. A 5% concentration of methemoglobin is created by this maneuver. Sodium nitrite, 0.33 ml/kg for children; 10–20 ml for adults, is given intravenously as a 3% solution at a rate of 2.5–5 ml/min. Methemoglobin concentrations should be determined frequently and should not exceed 35–40%.

Cyanide is removed from methemoglobin by administration of a 25% solution of sodium thiosulfate. This leads to formation of a sodium thiocyanate complex that is excreted into the urine. The pediatric dose of sodium thiosulfate is 1.65 ml/kg of the 25% solution; the adult dose is 50 ml of the 25% solution. In both children and adults, thiosulfate is administered 20–30 minutes after sodium nitrite by intravenous infusion at a rate of 2.5–5 ml/min.

If symptoms persist or recur, both sodium nitrite and sodium thiosulfate may be repeated once, 2–3 hours after the first dose. The second dose of sodium nitrite should be one-half the initial dose. Oxygen should be administered throughout the course of therapy.

With sodium nitrite therapy there is a risk of hypotension that is usually transient and is responsive to volume expanders or pressor agents. Sodium thiosulfate is of low toxicity.

Iron

Acute iron poisoning occurs primarily in young children who ingest medicinal iron. Toxicity is based on the amount of elemental iron ingested, not on the amount of iron salt ingested. Ferrous furamate has 33% elemental iron, ferrous sulfate has 20%, and ferrous gluconate has 11.5%. Ingestion of more than 30 mg/kg of elemental iron may result in symptoms.

DIAGNOSIS

Gastrointestinal symptoms resulting from direct irritation of the gastrointestinal mucosa occur within 1–6 hours after the ingestion. Severity ranges from mild epigastric distress and vomiting to marked abdominal pain and hemorrhagic gastroenteritis. In patients who have taken a severe overdose, the serum iron level exceeds the iron-binding capacity and results in free-circulating iron. Free iron causes the systemic symptoms that develop over 24–48 hours. Metabolic acidosis and shock are common and early features of severe overdose. Shock is the most common cause of death in iron poisoning. Coagulation defects and hepatic damage are variable and inconsistent. Miscellaneous effects include fever, leukocytosis, and pulmonary edema. Intestinal scarring and stenosis may occur 3–4 weeks after ingestion.

Confirmation of iron ingestion may be done in several ways. The gastric fluid may be analyzed qualitatively by the Deferoxamine color test. Within 4 hours of ingestion, the development of an orange-red color of 2 ml of gastric fluid containing 2 drops of hydrogen peroxide and 0.5 ml of deferoxamine solution helps to confirm the presence of iron in the gastric fluid. Plain x-ray films of the abdomen may demonstrate radiopaque particles; however, iron tablets may dissolve after 4 hours and solutions of iron are not radiopaque. The provacative chelation test with 50 mg/kg (up to 1–2 g) of intramuscular deferoxamine requires significant absorption of iron to have occurred before a pink-red urine may be produced. Serum iron levels and iron-binding capacity should be determined in any patients who have ingested an unknown or potentially toxic amount of iron. Ancillary laboratory tests include complete blood count, blood glucose, electrolytes, liver function tests, BUN, creatinine, and arterial blood gas determinations.

TREATMENT

If a potentially toxic ingestion of elemental iron is suspected, emptying the stomach should be accomplished as soon as possible. The method of choice is emesis induced with ipecac syrup. If the patient has an altered sensorium or if hematemesis has occurred, gastric lavage is indicated. After gastric emptying, the instillation of 100 ml 1% sodium bicarbonate (orally or by lavage tube) will result in the formation of iron carbonate, which is poorly absorbed and is less irritating than the iron salts.

The goals of treatment are support of the patient's vital functions while enhancing removal of excess iron by administering deferoxamine. Supportive care consists of the maintenance of body temperature, administration of parenteral fluids to main-tain hydration, correction of hypotension with vascular expanders (blood, plasma, albumin), and, if needed, vasopressor drugs. Hypoxia may be corrected with supplemental oxygen; metabolic acidosis may be treated with sodium bicarbonate. Because the iron–deferoxamine complex is excreted through the kidneys, renal function needs to be monitored carefully.

The dosage of deferoxamine is 50 mg/kg (up to 1–2 g) given intramuscularly every 6–8 hours. Deferoxamine may be given intravenously, but it may produce hypotension if the infusion rate exceeds 15 mg/kg/hr. Chelation therapy should be continued until the iron levels fall below the iron-binding capacity or until the urine color returns to normal.

Admission to the hospital for chelation therapy with deferoxamine is recommended for any patient with systemic symptoms or severe gastrointestinal symptoms, for any patient with an ingestion of an unknown amount of iron with a positive provocative chelation test or a serum iron exceeding the iron-binding capacity, or for any patient with a serum iron greater than 400 µg/dl.

Petroleum Distillate Hydrocarbons

Petroleum distillate hydrocarbons include gasoline, lacquer, thinner, furniture polish, kerosene, and lighter fluid. The morbidity associated with these products is usually secondary to pulmonary aspiration, not from absorption from the gastrointestinal tract.

DIAGNOSIS

Gastrointestinal symptoms of ingestion of petroleum distillate hydrocarbons include burning of the mouth and throat, nausea, vomiting, and diarrhea. Pulmonary symptoms arise only from aspiration of petroleum distillate hydrocarbons, not from gastrointestinal absorption. The severity of symptoms ranges from coughing and dyspnea to tachypnea, intercostal retractions, and cyanosis depending on the volume aspirated and physical characteristics of the product. The onset of coughing after aspiration is immediate. Central nervous system symptoms are usually limited to mild depression and may occur with ingestion of large (greater than 10 ml/kg) amounts. Coma and convulsions may occur as a result of hypoxia secondary to massive pulmonary aspiration.

TREATMENT

In the emergency room, the product in question must be identified correctly, and the amount ingested must be estimated.

When a petroleum distillate hydrocarbon is involved, emptying of the stomach is indicated only when large amounts (>10 ml/kg) have been ingested or when smaller amounts have been taken along with more serious toxins (e.g., drugs, insecticides, methanol, heavy metals). If the patient is seen within 2 hours of ingestion and no central nervous system depression is present, vomiting induced by ipecac syrup is recommended. If central nervous system depression is present, the stomach should be lavaged after protecting the trachea with a cuffed endotracheal tube. Activated charcoal, cathartics, and vegetable or mineral oil are not beneficial and are not recommended for use. The course and severity of hydrocarbon pneumonitis are not altered by the use of parenteral corticosteroids. Broad-spectrum antibiotics should be used only if bacterial infection can be documented.

SELECTED READINGS

AMA Drug Evaluations, ed 4. Acton, Massachusetts, AMA Department of Drugs, Publishing Group, Inc, 1980.

Arena JM: Poisoning: Toxicology, Symptoms, Treatment, ed 4. Springfield, Illinois, Charles C Thomas Publisher, 1979.

Bourne PG: Acute Drug Abuse Emergencies. New York, Academic Press, Inc, 1976.

Doull J, Klaassan CD, Amdur MO (eds): Casarett and Doull's Toxicology: The Basic Science of Poisons, ed 2. New York, Macmillan Inc, 1980.

Dreisback RH: Handbook of Poisoning, ed 10. Los Altos, California, Lange Medical Publications, 1980.

Gilman AG, Goodman L, Gilman A: Goodman and Gilman's The Pharmacological Basis of Therapeutics, ed 6. New York, Macmillan Inc, 1980.

Goldfrank LR, Kirstein R: Toxicologic Emergencies: A Handbook in Problem Solving. New York, Appleton-Century-Crofts, 1978.

Gosselin RE, Hodge HC, Smith RP, Gleason MN: Clinical Toxicology of Commercial Products, ed 4. Baltimore, The Williams & Wilkins Co, 1976.

Grant WM: Toxicology of the Eye. Springfield, Illinois, Charles C Thomas Publisher, 1974.

Hardin JW, Arena JM: Human Poisonings from Native and Cultivated Plants. Durham, NC, Duke University Press, 1974.

McGuigan MA, Wason S, Lovejoy FH Jr: Clinical Toxicology Review. Boston, Massachusetts Poison Control System, 1981.

Poisindex. Denver, Colorado, Micromedex, Inc, 1981.

Recognition and Management of Pesticide Poisonings, ed 2. Washington, DC, US Environmental Protection Agency, 1977.

43
DRUG OVERDOSE AND WITHDRAWAL

David C. Lewis
Irving H. Gomolin

This chapter provides basic information on the pharmacology of psychoactive drugs for the diagnosis and management of the problems seen most frequently in the emergency setting. The excessive use, misuse, and abuse of alcohol and psychoactive drugs are responsible for about 20% of the serious problems seen in emergency rooms. The nature and severity of the problems encountered with such a heterogeneous group of psychoactive substances, along with new drugs being introduced, demands a thorough understanding of their pharmacology. Furthermore, emerging patterns of polydrug intoxication and dependence add a further complication to effective emergency care.

The widespread use of psychoactive drugs leads to two major categories of emergency problems. First is the occurrence of the overdose, which is usually intentional. Even with optimal treatment and a knowledge of the specific pharmacology involved, some overdoses are difficult to manage and fatalities occur. Second are the complications of drug abuse and drug addiction. For example, ethanol is not only a cause of fatal overdose but it is also responsible for delirium tremens, the most serious form of addictive drug withdrawal, as well as acute injury from accidents and violence.

Trends both in the patterns of community use and in medical prescribing affect the incidence of drug-related emergencies. For example, as intravenous amphetamine use has declined, so have the complications from this form of stimulant abuse. On the other hand, cocaine abuse is increasing, and since 1980, toxicity from the smoking of cocaine "free base" preparations has been encountered. Although phencyclidine (PCP) intoxication was virtually unheard of 10 years ago, there was a major epidemic of serious complications from PCP abuse from 1977 to 1979 as the drug gained popularity. Its abuse has recently decreased but is still a problem. Another change in usage patterns is the emergence of the abuse of so called "legal stimulants," over-the-counter drugs sold as appetite suppressants. The rise in the availability of these stimulants has paralleled the exclusion of obesity as an approved indication for long-term amphetamine prescribing.

Certain drug abuse patterns may remain stable with a concurrent decrease in emergency room problems as users become more sophisticated about potential problems. Thus there has been a reduction in hospital admissions for "bad trips," although the use of lysergic acid diethylamide (LSD) and other hallucinogens has remained fairly steady since 1970.

Trends in medical prescription of drugs also have a major impact on the incidence of emergencies. Although fatal overdoses from barbiturates and other hypnotics still constitute a major problem in emergency care, the increase in the prescribing of the less toxic benzodiazepine hypnotics has decreased the overall incidence of fatal hypnotic overdoses.

GENERAL CONSIDERATIONS

Factors Affecting the Degree of Observed Drug Effects

Dose is only one factor in determining the degree and prognosis of drug intoxication. The general health of the person and the presence of chronic cardiac, respiratory, hepatic, or renal disease can have diverse effects on the pharmacokinetics and target organ reactions of psychoactive drugs. For ingested drugs, the presence of food in the stomach, the rate of gastric emptying, and the transit time through the gastrointestinal tract can be important determinants of the amount of drug absorbed into the blood stream. Furthermore, the metabolism of acute doses of psychoactive drugs can be affected by the chronic use of the same or a different drug.

Pharmacologic tolerance also plays an important role in determining observed effects since preexisting tolerance protects against some of the toxic effects of drug overdose. Opiates provide the best example of this phenomenon. A record of 5 g of parenteral morphine has been taken by a tolerant person without significant respiratory depression. Although not as pronounced as with the opiates, tolerance to other psychoactive drugs, including barbiturates, nonbarbiturate hypnotics and sedatives, ethanol, amphetamines, and phencyclidine also develops.

In interpreting blood levels of drugs, it is noteworthy that much of the information available concerning toxic serum levels of psychoactive drugs is obtained in nontolerant people and much higher levels may be required to produce toxic effects in patients who have target organ tolerance. It must be emphasized that in the vast majority of overdoses, patient management depends on the clinical status, and blood levels serve merely as confirmatory evidence for the nature and magnitude of the overdose encountered.

Drug Interactions

The mechanisms of drug interactions are multiple and complex. These interactions may occur at any level of drug pharmacokinetics, that is, absorption, distribution, protein binding, metabolism, or excretion. Interactions at receptor sites often result in additive or antagonistic effects. Knowledge of potential drug interactions is important in emergency patient management as well as for following a patient's clinical course. For example, drugs that delay gastric emptying or cause paralytic ileus may delay their own absorption and that of other drugs that may be present. Such drugs include opiates and those drugs possessing anticholinergic properties such as belladonna alkaloids, antihistamines, tricyclic antidepressants, and antipsychotics (phenothiazines, butyrophenones). A waxing and waning state of consciousness as a result of overdose from sedative hypnotic agents such as glutethimide may be explained by such a mechanism.

Another clinically relevant example is the ability of one drug to enhance the hepatic metabolism of another drug. For example, in the chronic alcoholic, the metabolism of barbiturates or meprobamate is increased because of induction of hepatic microsomal enzymes. On the other hand, acute intoxicating doses of ethanol may impair the metabolism of barbiturates or meprobamate because of competition for hepatic enzyme systems.

Drug interactions may be manifest by an antagonism of pharmacodynamic effects. For example, the effects of sedative hypnotics may be partly antagonized by sympathomimetics such as amphetamine and methylphenidate. When such a combined overdose is encountered, knowledge of the amount of each agent ingested and of the pharmacokinetics of both drugs may aid the clinician in predicting the clinical course. The clinician will then be aware of the possibility of excitation followed by depression, or vice versa.

Enhancement of pharmacodynamic effects is a commonly observed feature of multiple drug ingestion. Although the mechanism is unclear, the synergistic effects of multiple central nervous system (CNS) depressants can produce a greater degree of depression than predicted from the individual doses of the drugs taken. Also the delirious patient who has ingested a belladonna alkaloid, antihistamine, or tricyclic antidepressant should not be treated with a phenothiazine or butyrophenone since the anticholinergic effects of these drugs may be additive.

Pharmacodynamics of Psychoactive Drugs

Although each drug has its own unique effects, the following three basic patterns of response to the effects of drug intoxication are seen.

1. *CNS excitatory–sympathomimetic effects:* Agitation, diaphoresis, mydriasis (responsive to light), tremulousness, tachycardia, hypertension, hyperreflexia, and seizures
2. *CNS depressant effects:* Coma of varying degrees, cerebellar dysfunction, respiratory depression, hypotension and hypothermia
3. *Anticholinergic effects:* Agitation, delirium, tachycardia, mydriasis and cycloplegia, diminished sweating, flushed skin, dry mucous membranes, paralytic ileus, and urinary retention

Familiarity with these categories of pharmacodynamic responses will facilitate the clinical diagnostic task.

Table 43.1 lists the salient characteristics of the effects of drug intoxication for specific psychoactive drugs. The signs are listed in a rough approximation to their sequential appearance with increasing toxicity from these drugs.

EVALUATION OF THE DRUG-INTOXICATED PATIENT

History

Although histories from intoxicated patients may be distorted and difficult to obtain, the physician should not assume that such patients are unreliable informants. Drugs purchased illegally are sometimes misrepresented, one drug sold under the name of another, so that the patient may be unaware of what has been taken. The best histories from intoxicated patients are obtained when patients are physically unrestrained, have others present whom they recognize and trust, and perceive the emergency treatment staff as supportive rather than punitive.

The opportunity to obtain history from family, friends, and those who bring the patient for emergency care should not be overlooked. Very often the most useful information on the alcohol and drug use habits, as well as specific information on the amounts and nature of recent drug ingestion, is obtained from these people.

The history should solicit information in the following areas: prescription and nonprescription use of all drugs—type, frequency, duration, and amounts taken; prior episodes of overdose or treatment for drug-related problems; previous suicide attempts; general medical history including diabetes, hypertension, renal or hepatic insufficiency, seizure disorder, chronic pulmonary disease, and trauma.

Physical Examination

The presence of any of the following signs should alert the physician to the possibility of drug intoxication: somnolence,

TABLE 43.1 Characteristics of Drug Intoxication

Barbiturates and alcohol	Opiates
Hyperactivity and irritability	Miosis (reactive to light)
Slurred speech	Somnolence
Nystagmus and ataxia	Decreased bowel motility
Somnolence	Respiratory depression
Respiratory depression	Seizures (rare)
Pulmonary edema (barbiturates)	Hypotension
Loss of consciousness	Pulmonary edema
Hypotension	Hypothermia
Hypothermia	Loss of consciousness
Absent response to noxious stimuli	Absent response to noxious stimuli
Absent deep tendon reflexes	Absent deep tendon reflexes
Amphetamines and cocaine	Belladonna alkaloids and antihistamines[a]
Agitation	Dry mucous membranes
Mydriasis (reactive to light)	Mydriasis and cycloplegia
Sweating	Dry flushed skin
Tachycardia	Tachycardia
Arrhythmias	Urinary retention
Nausea	Paralytic ileus
Vomiting	Agitation
Hypertension	Hallucinations (usually visual)
Hyperthermia	Delirium
Seizures	Hyperthermia
Hypotension	Loss of consciousness

[a]Tricyclic antidepressants show similar signs, as well as cardiac arrhythmias, conduction defects (QRS widening), seizures, respiratory depression, and hypotension.

agitation, delirium, inappropriate behavioral responses, ataxia, nystagmus, abnormal pupil size (miosis and mydriasis), hypotension, and depressed respiration.

In addition to baseline neurologic, cardiopulmonary, and abdominal examinations, the initial physical examination should record pupil size, look for CNS trauma, including ophthalmoscopic examination for increased intracranial pressure, and search for recent needle marks, old scars (tracks), and lymphadenopathy resulting from intravenous or subcutaneous drug use.

The presence of the sequelae of the unsterile parenteral self-administration of drugs can be an important clue that directs the physician's attention to the possibility of a drug abuse problem, and hence, a possible drug etiology as the explanation for the acute presenting problem. These sequelae are many and varied. Whether drugs are injected intravenously (mainlining) or subcutaneously (skin popping), cellulitis and local abscess formation around the injection sites and concomitant regional lymphadenopathy are common. The inflammation may be sterile (chemically induced) or bacterial in origin. Superficial thrombophlebitis may occur secondary to intravenous injections. Inadvertent intraarterial injection may result in ischemic damage. This has been most frequently seen in barbiturate abusers.

Occasionally intoxicated patients do not receive adequate physical examination, either because of their disruptive behavior or because of negative attitudes of the staff toward them. Such patients may be shunted to out-of-the-way niches in the emergency room or released prematurely without being optimally examined or observed. Although a patient's problems may in part be self-induced, this is no justification for errors in diagnosis and management.

The physician should be alert to the possibility that drug intoxication may mask other related or unrelated medical and surgical disorders. Patients should be completely examined for signs of trauma and hidden pathology. The possibility that the overdose is more severe than originally judged should be kept in mind.

Associated Medical Problems

In evaluating patients with drug or alcohol intoxication, the physician should be aware of several complicating medical disorders that occur with greater frequency in such patients.

Early diagnosis of these disorders can affect the treatment and eventual survival of acutely intoxicated patients. Some prominent medical disorders are as follows:

- *Tuberculosis* is seen with increased frequency in alcoholics and heroin addicts.
- *Chronic obstructive pulmonary disease* (COPD) is common in alcoholics who tend to be heavy cigarette smokers.
- *Mixed bacterial infection* and *lung abscesses,* often a result of anaerobic organisms, may complicate aspiration pneumonia, which is frequently seen in obtunded or comatose patients.
- *Streptococcus pneumoniae* (pneumococcal) pneumonia is the most common cause of pneumonia in alcoholics and drug addicts. However, infection with *Klebsiella,* other gram-negative organisms, and *Staphylococcus* may be seen as well.

Medical disorders are frequently encountered secondary to intravenous drug abuse, particularly in heroin addicts. The transmission of malaria and hepatitis virus occurs as a result of needle sharing, and tetanus has been reported in drug abusers who inject subcutaneously. Remote infections that may occur following intravenous drug use include lung abscess, subacute endocarditis, septic arthritis, and osteomyelitis. Pulmonary emboli may be seen as a complication of intravenous drug-induced superficial phlebitis and subsequent deep vein phlebitis. These emboli may be septic if the phlebitis has a pyogenic component. Interstitial or granulomatous lung disease may result from drug contaminants.

Subacute bacterial endocarditis (SBE) (approximately 55% right sided, 5% right and left sided, 40% left sided) can complicate parenteral drug abuse. *Staphylococcus aureus* is the most common offending organism, although *Streptococcus viridans* (α-hemolytic streptococci) and enterococci as well as unusual organisms such as *Escherichia coli, Pseudomonas, Serratia, Klebsiella,* and *Candida albicans* may also be seen. The epidemiology of the drug-abuse associated SBE varies in different areas of the United States.

Underlying chronic brain damage in alcoholics is not uncommon and is usually manifested by impairments in memory, judgment, and cerebellar function. Alcoholics may also have signs of thiamine-deficiency-related Wernicke's encephalopathy and Korsakoff's syndrome.

Acute fatty liver or hepatitis may complicate the management of the alcoholic. Acute and chronic liver damage may give rise to encephalopathy and bleeding diatheses.

Acute and chronic pancreatitis, as well as upper gastrointestinal bleeding because of gastritis, esophageal varices, and peptic ulcer disease, are more common in alcoholics.

Anemia secondary to folate deficiency is common in alcoholics. Direct toxic bone marrow suppression caused by alcohol can also be a cause of anemia, neutropenia, and thrombocytopenia.

In addition to the medical problems secondary to the use and abuse of psychoactive drugs, there are some conditions that can mimic drug intoxication. These include any nondrug cause of coma, delirium, or abnormal behavior. Some of the important differential diagnoses of drug intoxication are in Table 43.2.

Laboratory Drug Identification

Rapid analysis of various body fluids for the identification of many of the drugs taken by patients is becoming increasingly available. The blood sample may provide both qualitative and quantitative information, whereas urine and gastric analyses usually provide only qualitative information.

Drug screening of urine mostly serves as confirmatory evidence for the presence of a drug already identified in the blood. For urinary screening to be of value the drug or at least a measurable metabolite must be excreted by the kidneys. Occasionally urinary screening will identify a drug whose concentration in blood is too low to be detected. For example, drug screening of urine is the standard method to demonstrate the presence of opiates and amphetamines. Gastric contents should also be sent for toxicologic drug screening.

TABLE 43.2 Differential Diagnosis of Drug Intoxication

Category	Condition
Infectious	Meningitis/encephalitis
Immunologic	SLE, vasculitis
Neoplastic	Meningiomas, CNS malignancy
Traumatic	Concussion, subdural and epidural hematomas
Metabolic	Uremic and hepatic encephalopathy
	Hyperthyroidism and myxedema
	Carbon dioxide narcosis
	Hypoglycemia
	Electrolyte disorders
	Diabetic ketoacidosis
	Nonketotic hyperosmolar states
Psychiatric	Acute schizophrenic break
	Acute functional psychosis
Miscellaneous	Intracranial hemorrhage
	Hypertensive encephalopathy
	Postictal states

SLE, systemic lupus erythematosus

There are limitations in relying heavily on laboratory drug identification. Some laboratories may not detect certain drugs because of technical limitations, whereas others may erroneously report drugs that are not responsible for intoxication. Each physician must be aware of the limitations of local hospital and independent toxicology laboratories.

Table 43.3 is a compilation of values obtained from three large clinical laboratories and two published compendia of the therapeutic and toxic blood levels for several psychoactive drugs. Caution must be exercised in applying these data to clinical decision making in a given patient since some data are derived from experience with very few patients. The physician should also be alerted to the fact that assay methods as well as reliability vary from laboratory to laboratory and that most of the available data are derived from nontolerant individuals.

TABLE 43.3 Psychoactive Drugs: Blood Levels Associated with Therapeutic Use and with Severe Intoxication

Drug	Therapeutic Range of Levels[a]	Severe Intoxication Levels[a]
Amitriptyline (Elavil)	50–200 µg/liter	>300 µg/liter
Amobarbital (Amytal)	2–10 µg/ml	>30 µg/ml
Amphetamine (Benzedrine)	0.02–0.04 µg/ml	—
Chloral hydrate (Noctec) (measured as trichlorethanol)	2–8 µg/ml	>100 µg/ml
Chlordiazepoxide (Librium)	1–3 µg/ml	>5 µg/ml
Chlorpromazine (Thorazine)	10–200 µg/liter	>1,000 µg/liter
Cocaine	0.05–0.15 µg/ml	>0.9 µg/ml
Codeine	20–100 µg/liter	>1,600 µg/liter
Desipramine (Norpramin)	20–60 µg/liter	>500 µg/liter
Diazepam (Valium)	0.02–1.5 µg/ml	>5 µg/ml
Ethanol	—	>1,000 µg/ml
Ethchlorvynol (Placidyl)	0.5–6.5 µg/ml	>20 µg/ml
Flurazepam (Dalmane)	10–70 µg/liter	>500 µg/liter
Glutethimide (Doriden)	0.5–7 µg/ml	>10 µg/ml
Imipramine (Tofranil)	20–160 µg/liter	>700 µg/liter
Meperidine (Demerol)	100–1,000 µg/liter	>10 µg/ml
Meprobamate (Equanil)	5–30 µg/ml	>50 µg/ml
Methaqualone (Quaalude)	0.4–4.0 µg/ml	>6 µg/ml
Methyprylon (Noludar)	1–10 µg/ml	>30 µg/ml
Nortriptyline (Aventyl)	30–120 µg/liter	>500 µg/liter
Oxazepam (Serax)	0.2–1.5 µg/ml	>5 µg/ml
Pentazocine (Talwin)	30–100 µg/liter	>200 µg/liter
Pentobarbital (Nembutal)	0.5–2 µg/ml	>10 µg/ml
Phencyclidine	—	>50 µg/liter
Phenobarbital (Luminal)	5–40 µg/ml	>50 µg/ml
Propoxyphene (Darvon)	50–200 µg/liter	>1,000 µg/liter
Secobarbital (Seconal)	0.5–2 µg/ml	>10 µg/ml
Thioridazine (Mellaril)	100–500 µg/liter	>1,000 µg/liter

[a]The concentration units used by laboratories vary widely. Some routinely report values in micrograms (µg) or milligrams (mg) per liter, whereas others report micrograms or milligrams per milliliter or 100 ml. To assist in these conversions the following equivalents should be useful:

10 µg/ml = 1 mg% = 1 mg/100 ml
1 µg/ml = 1 mg/liter = 1,000 µg/liter
1 µg/liter = 1 ng/ml

TREATMENT OF DRUG-INTOXICATED PATIENTS

Treatment of life-threatening intoxication is directed toward the following tasks: support of vital functions, removal of the drug, and institution of specific measures to counteract the adverse effects of the drug. Figure 43.1 is a flowchart illustrating the sequential decision-making process in the management of the patient in whom drug overdose is suspected. Figure 43.2 is a flowchart designed to guide physicians in determination of diagnosis and treatment of specific drug overdoses.

There are some general points about drug-induced unconsciousness that deserve emphasis. A number of classifications for the grading of the degree of coma have been used to classify and follow the course of patients. In these classifications, major disturbances in circulatory and respiratory function are usually associated with the most profound degrees of coma. However, certain drug overdoses may result in relatively intact neurologic function despite profound cardiopulmonary impairment. While there are variations in neurologic responses to drugs, the response to painful stimuli is usually diminished before the loss of deep tendon reflexes in deepening coma. Deeper grades of coma may lessen considerably without indicating sustained improvement. This is particularly apparent with drugs such as glutethimide and in cases in which short-acting antidotes are used (e.g., naloxone for methadone overdose and physostigmine for tricyclic antidepressant overdose). In these cases, the patient may become temporarily alert and then relapse into deep coma. When evaluating the unconscious patient who has taken multiple drugs, some signs may be masked or enhanced by drugs that are not the primary cause of the coma.

ASSESSMENT AND MANAGEMENT OF SPECIFIC DRUG OVERDOSE

Barbiturate and Other Sedative-Hypnotics

Barbiturates and other sedative-hypnotics are abused very frequently and account for a significant proportion of acute medical emergencies encountered in the emergency room setting. Acute intoxication with barbiturates and nonbarbiturate nonbenzodiazepine sedative-hypnotics share similar characteristics. Coma, respiratory depression, and hemodynamic instability are features common to all of these drugs. However, cardiovascular instability in the absence of respiratory depression is more suggestive of the nonbarbiturate nonbenzodiazepine drugs.

BARBITURATES

The barbiturates are chemical derivatives of barbituric acid. Short-acting barbiturates such as secobarbital (Seconal), amobarbital (Amytal), and pentobarbital (Nembutal) have a higher pKa, are more lipid soluble, and are more protein bound than is the long-acting barbiturate, phenobarbital. Because of these physicochemical features, short-acting barbiturates are more rapidly absorbed and hence produce a "disinhibition euphoria" of greater degree than does phenobarbital. Barbiturate abusers therefore prefer the short-acting compounds. Also, as a result of these properties, short-acting barbiturates produce intoxication at doses and plasma levels that are lower than for phenobarbital.

Renal excretion of the parent drug is important only for phenobarbital. Short-acting compounds are largely metabolized by the liver.

Although tolerance to the sedative effects of barbiturates occurs, a proportionate tolerance to the lethal dose is not seen. This reduces the margin of safety of these drugs and contributes to accidental overdose. Most intoxications, however, are due to deliberate overdose. Serious intoxications in adults are associated with ingestion of more than 1 g of a short-acting barbiturate and more than 3 g of phenobarbital. Unlike many of the nonbarbiturate hypnotics, changes in the blood levels of barbiturates correlate well with changes in the levels of coma.

Diagnosis

Acute intoxication is characterized by somnolence, slurred speech, and ataxia. The disinhibition produced by barbiturates causes lability of mood, irritability, and, occasionally, combativeness. Horizontal, as well as vertical, nystagmus is frequently seen. The pupils may be constricted or dilated in patients whose conditions are complicated by prolonged hypoxia. Severe intoxication causes respiratory failure, coma, loss of pharyngeal and deep tendon reflexes, and hypotension. Hypotension is due to central vasomotor depression, direct toxic effects on the myocardium, peripheral vascular effects, and hypoxia. These effects account in part for the pulmonary edema that may be seen. Pulmonary edema may not be recognized on physical examination if spontaneous ventilation is shallow. Hypothermia and cutaneous bullae may be seen in patients who have been lying comatose for several hours. Acute renal failure related to shock or rhabdomyolysis may occur.

Treatment.

There are no specific antidotes for barbiturate overdose, and treatment is primarily supportive. Emesis induced by ipecac

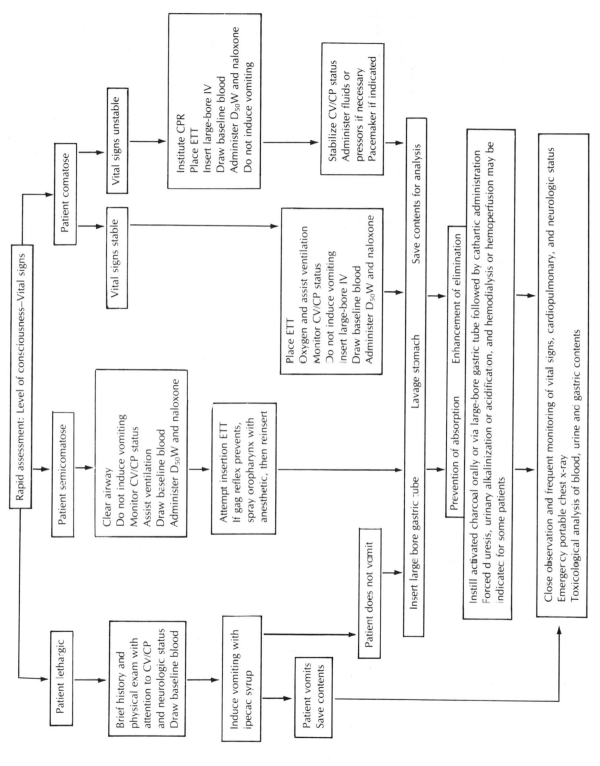

Figure 43.1 General approach to the initial management of suspected depressant drug overdose. (Prepared with the assistance of John Femino, M.D.)

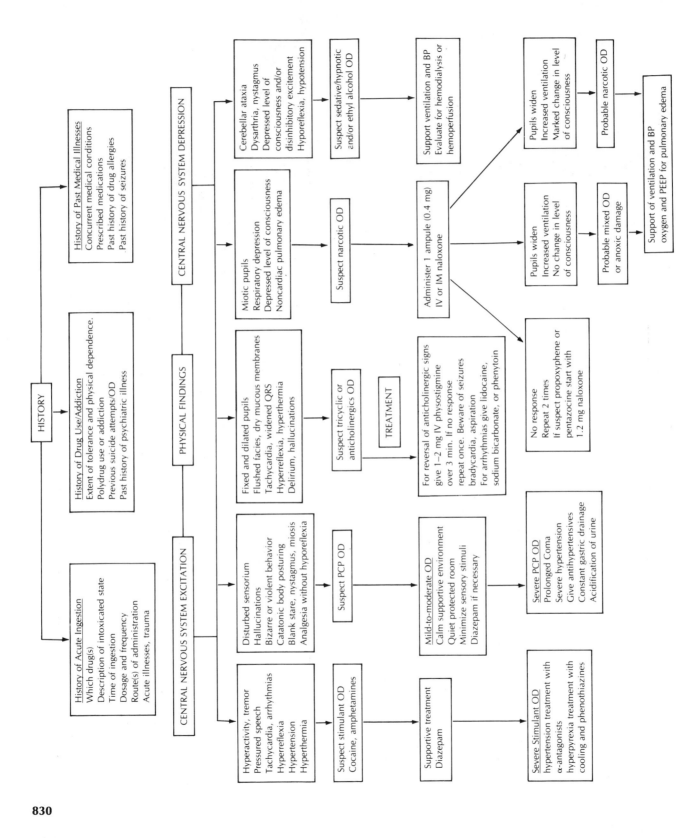

Figure 43.2 Diagram of diagnosis and therapy for specific forms of drug overdose. (Prepared with the assistance of John Femino, M.D.)

syrup should be undertaken in the alert patient. Gastric lavage should be performed up to 4 hours after ingestion in a comatose patient. The airway must be protected with an endotracheal tube during lavage. These procedures should be followed by the instillation of an activated charcoal slurry and saline cathartic by mouth or through the lavage tube.

The major factor in the improved mortality and morbidity from serious barbiturate overdose has been the advent of sophisticated respiratory support measures. Patients in respiratory failure are treated with endotracheal intubation and mechanical ventilation. The use of analeptics is not recommended under any circumstances. Patients with hypotension are treated by elevation of the foot of the bed, volume expansion with intravenous fluids, and vasopressors if required.

Alkalinization of the urine with sodium bicarbonate and forced diuresis accelerate the elimination of phenobarbital, but these procedures should be reserved for patients who are moderately intoxicated since pulmonary edema and electrolyte imbalance may occur secondary to alkalinization. Alkalinization is effective in increasing phenobarbital elimination only if the urine pH is 8 or above and is much less effective for short-acting barbiturates.

Hemodialysis is very effective in clearing barbiturates from the blood, although it is less so for short-acting compounds that are more protein bound and lipid soluble. Resin hemoperfusion is even more effective than hemodialysis. These measures may be considered for patients with potentially fatal blood levels or in whom clinical deterioration or severe complications supervene despite adequate respiratory and cardiovascular support.

An Isoelectric electroencephalogram (EEG) should not be a contraindication to any therapies nor interpreted, at least initially, as evidence for brain death since this finding may occur during overdosage with ensuing complete recovery.

GLUTETHIMIDE (DORIDEN)

In adults serious toxicity is encountered with the ingestion of 5–20 g of glutethimide. Severe glutethimide intoxication has a number of unusual features. Sudden apnea and acute laryngeal spasm can occur without obvious preceeding respiratory depression. Anticholinergic effects including tachycardia, urinary retention, paralytic ileus, and mydriasis are common. Anisocoria may be seen. Hypotension and pulmonary edema are seen more commonly than with barbiturate overdose, and seizures may occur. Cycles of alternating wakefulness and coma occur, and blood levels do not correlate well with levels of coma. In addition to the toxicity of the parent drug, the 4-hydroxy metabolite is active and contributes to central nervous

system depression. Treatment is primarily supportive. Hemodialysis with aqueous solutions is of questionable value. Oil dialysis achieves clearance rates greater than aqueous dialysis. Resin hemoperfusion has also been used.

METHAQUALONE (QUAALUDE)

In adults, severe potentially fatal intoxication occurs with ingestion of 15–25 g of methaqualone. The drug apparently produces less brainstem depression than do barbiturates and other nonbenzodiazepine hypnotics. For this reason the patient may exhibit significant coma with an intact gag reflex. Seizures and delirium can occur with acute intoxication. Extrapyramidal signs such as increased muscle tone, hyperreflexia, and myoclonus may be seen as well. Methaqualone intoxication, like that of glutethimide, may produce anticholinergic effects. Treatment is primarily supportive. Hemodialysis has been used in selected cases, but its value is debatable.

ETHCHLORVYNOL (PLACIDYL)

Acute intoxication by ethchlorvynol may cause prolonged coma and considerable morbidity. In adults, death has been reported with 2.5 g of ethchlorvynol ingested together with alcohol or 5 g ingested alone. Most reported cases of serious intoxication have involved ingestions of 10 g or more, although mild to moderate cases of intoxication may be expected with the ingestion of 4 g.

In addition to producing prolonged coma, severe intoxication by ethchlorvynol also causes hypothermia, hypotension—which may be accompanied by relative bradycardia—respiratory depression, and apnea. Pulmonary edema has been reported infrequently. A pungent aromatic odor of the gastric contents from ingested red capsules is a clue to the diagnosis. Forced diuresis is not recommended. Resin hemoperfusion may be of benefit in severe cases but is limited by the extensive distribution of this drug into fatty tissue.

CHLORAL HYDRATE (NOCTEC)

Chloral hydrate is rapidly metabolized to trichlorethanol and trichloracetic acid. The hypnotic effect is due to trichlorethanol. In adults, death has been reported after the ingestion of 4 g, although survival has been reported after the ingestion of 30 g. The toxic oral dose is approximately 10 g.

Acute intoxication can result in coma, respiratory depression, and hypotension. A wide spectrum of cardiac arrhythmias has been described, including supraventricular and ventricular premature contractions, ventricular tachycardia and fibrillation, and asystole. Ventricular arrhythmias may be resistant to lidocaine. Severe intoxication usually resolves within several days. Prolonged coma may occur in patients with hepatic or renal disease.

MEPROBAMATE (EQUANIL)

In adults, death has been reported after the ingestion of 12 g meprobamate, although survival has occurred after the ingestion of 40 g. The clinical features of intoxication include coma, hypotension, respiratory depression, and pulmonary edema. Hypotension is not well correlated to coma depth and may occur in the absence of respiratory depression.

Treatment of meprobamate intoxication is supportive. In the obtunded patient, gastric lavage is recommended up to 12 hours after ingestion. Although the use of activated charcoal is recommended, a rare complication associated with its use is the formation of meprobamate–charcoal masses in the stomach, which in turn has lead to prolonged and fluctuating grades of coma since meprobamate dissolves slowly in gastric juice. Forced diuresis is not recommended. Resin hemoperfusion appears to be the most effective method for drug removal, although its precise role remains undefined since most cases resolve within 1–5 days.

BENZODIAZEPINES (DALMANE, VALIUM, LIBRIUM)

Benzodiazepine intoxication has become more frequent in the last decade. When ingested alone these drugs are rarely a cause of severe intoxication. Hypotension, respiratory depression, and deep coma are unusual, and fatalities are extremely rare. General supportive measures are indicated, but forced diuresis is not.

ETHANOL

Overdoses with alcohol may cause death. Fatalities occur from the CNS depression caused by alcohol taken either alone or in combination with other sedative-hypnotics, opiates, or tricyclic antidepressants. Severe alcohol intoxication can result in respiratory depression, hypotension, and deep coma. Supraventricular and ventricular arrhythmias are also seen. In people who are not tolerant to alcohol the fatal blood alcohol level is in the range of 400–600 mg%, which correlates with the rapid ingestion of about 0.5 qt of distilled spirits. Chronic drinkers become tolerant to alcohol and can survive higher blood levels (about twice the usual fatal level). Treatment is supportive and primarily directed at respiratory care.

Since alcohol is absorbed and metabolized rapidly, the patient may progress from deep coma to a fully awake state within a period of 6–12 hours. Therefore, treatment with activated charcoal is of limited value. Forced diuresis is not recommended.

Tricyclic Antidepressants

An acute overdose of tricyclic antidepressants is a very serious problem and constitutes one of the most common causes of hospitalization for severe drug intoxication. These drugs are frequently prescribed by psychiatrists and general practitioners. Since the usual indication for their use is depression, it is not surprising that they constitute a significant proportion of overdoses that are intentional.

Available forms of tricyclic antidepressants include amitriptyline (Elavil), nortriptyline (Aventyl), imipramine (Tofranil), desipramine (Norpramin), protriptyline (Vivactil), and doxepin (Sinequan). In therapeutic doses these drugs are rapidly absorbed from the intestine. Because of their local and systemic anticholinergic effects, gastric emptying may be delayed in patients who have taken overdoses. The nonpolar lipophilic highly protein-bound parent drug is metabolized in the liver to polar hydrophilic compounds that are excreted mostly by the kidneys. Some metabolites are pharmacologically active. The half-life in overdose ranges from 25 to 82 hours, and this may play a role in the cardiac deaths reported to occur in some patients as late as 3–6 days after overdose. Serious poisoning has resulted from ingestion of single doses of 7–127 mg/kg (mean 38 mg/kg), and death has resulted from doses of 10–210 mg/kg (mean 65 mg/kg). Symptoms of severe intoxication usually develop within 4 hours of ingestion.

Diagnosis

Tricyclic antidepressants have more powerful anticholinergic effects than do phenothiazines, and these effects account for some of the features of the intoxication from these drugs.

Autonomic nervous system signs result from the anticholinergic effects of tricyclic antidepressants and include mydriasis, dry skin and mucous membranes, flushing of the skin, decreased bowel activity, urinary retention, and fever.

Cardiovascular system signs result from the inhibition of the re-uptake of norepinephrine at sympathetic nerve terminals, cholinergic blockade of vagus nerve, and direct myocardial effects. The result may be rate disturbances, atrial and ventricular arrhythmias, conduction defects, and hypertension or hypotension. Sinus tachycardia is seen in the majority of patients who have taken serious overdoses. Electrocardiographic

(ECG) abnormalities are noteworthy. The PR and QT intervals may be prolonged, and ST segment and T wave changes may occur. In addition the QRS complex may be widened. A QRS complex of greater than 100 ms is correlated with severe toxicity.

CNS signs are probably largely due to competitive antagonism of acetylcholine since both delirium and coma may be reversed with physostigmine, an anticholinesterase, which is capable of penetrating the blood–brain barrier. Inhibition of norpinephrine re-uptake may contribute to the CNS manifestations as well. These effects cause central nervous system excitation manifested by agitation, confusion, delirium, hallucinations, muscular rigidity and twitching, hyperreflexia and seizures, or CNS depression manifest by somnolence and coma. Patients may either show signs of CNS excitation or depression or may vacillate between the two. Respiratory depression may accompany CNS depression.

In some studies tricyclic antidepressant poisoning has been reported to cause death in as many as 7% of patients, although in other studies there have been no observed fatalities. Signs of intoxication usually resolve within 48 hours. Discharge of patients from the hospital when they are free of signs of intoxication is the usual practice.

Treatment

Rapid evaluation of the patient's status should be done in the emergency room. Compromised vital functions should be supported. After stabilization of the patient's condition, the stomach should be emptied of residual drug by gastric lavage or emesis induced with ipecac syrup. The latter is preferred, but the patient must be alert. An activated charcoal slurry followed by a saline cathartic should then be administered in order to prevent absorption of any remaining drug. These interventions are indicated up to 6 hours after ingestion. Forced diuresis is not recommended, and there are no data to suggest that hemodialysis or hemoperfusion alters the course of intoxication.

The presence of an altered mental status, sinus tachycardia, or other arrhythmia in association with autonomic nervous system signs should suggest tricyclic antidepressant poisoning for which hospitalization with cardiac monitoring is recommended.

Patients with respiratory depression should be treated with mechanical ventilation. Patients with hypotension should be treated with elevation of the foot of the bed, volume expanders, and pressors if needed. Pressor therapy should be given with caution since it carries the risk of exacerbating cardiac irritability or, in the case of epinephrine, of exacerbating hypotension. Patients with arrhythmias should first be treated with

sodium bicarbonate in a dose of 0.5–2 mEq/kg followed by phenytoin or lidocaine if arrhythmias persist. Physostigmine may be used for patients with arrhythmias if other measures fail, if there are uncontrollable seizures, or if there is severe hypertension. Patients having seizures should be treated with diazepam or phenytoin.

Physostigmine

Physostigmine is generally recommended for diagnosis and as an antidote for tricyclic antidepressant intoxication since it promptly reverses the anticholinergic toxicity associated with tricyclics, as well as reverses the CNS effects.

The adult dose of physostigmine is 1–2 mg. The drug is given intravenously over 2–3 minutes and may be repeated in 5–10 minutes up to a maximum dose of 4 mg. If there is no response, intoxication with tricyclic antidepressants is in doubt. Signs referrable to the autonomic nervous system, CNS excitation, coma, hypertension, cardiac arrhythmias, and conduction defects may respond well to physostigmine. Temporary reversal of light grades of coma probably adds little to the management of the patient, but reversal of severe coma or delirium may be accomplished with the use of physostigmine. It must be remembered that the duration of action of physostigmine is 1–2 hours and repeat doses may be necessary.

Excessive physostigmine use will result in cholinergic overactivity manifest by miosis, excessive salivation, increased bronchial secretions, diarrhea, bradycardia, and bronchospasm. These latter effects may be reversed by the administration of atropine at a dose one-half that of the physostigmine or of propantheline 15–30 mg intravenously or intramuscularly. Rapid administration of physostigmine can itself cause seizures.

Opiates

Opiates and opiate cogeners such as propoxyphene (Darvon) continue to represent a significant proportion of drug-related emergencies. Apart from intentional overdoses with oral forms of opiates, the emergency room physician is likely to encounter overdoses consequent to intravenous opiate use by addicts.

Diagnosis

The classic triad of coma, constricted pupils, and depressed respirations remains the cardinal feature of opiate toxicity. Opiate overdose should be suspected in any patient presenting with these features. Hypotension consequent to the central effects of these drugs, venous pooling, hypoxia, and acidosis may also be present. Mydriasis does not rule out opiate toxicity since this may result from hypoxia or overdosage with meperidine. Miosis is not diagnostic of opiate effects, and it may also be seen in barbiturate, phenothiazine, and ethanol intoxication.

Pulmonary edema is not infrequently a complicating feature of opiate overdose. It occurs most commonly in the setting of overdose with intravenous heroin, but it may occur after ingestion of propoxyphene, methadone, or sedative-hypnotics. Pulmonary edema is generally of rapid onset and is characterized by frothy sputum that may be bloody. Most patients with opiate-induced pulmonary edema are comatose and have depressed respirations and hypotension. The chest film demonstrates bilateral infiltrates in the absence of cardiomegaly. The pathogenesis of opiate-induced pulmonary edema is not well understood, but increased pulmonary capillary pressure resulting from hypoxia and direct capillary damage appear to be important factors.

Seizures may be seen with meperidine, propoxyphene, codeine, and pentazocine. Overdose with propoxyphene is not infrequently associated with a fatal outcome, particularly when combined with alcohol or other sedative drugs.

Treatment

Support of vital functions and the use of naloxone (Narcan) are the primary approaches to treatment of patients with opiate overdose. When there is evidence of respiratory failure, endotracheal intubation with respiratory support is indicated. Oxygen therapy is indicated for patients with hypoxia and its related acidosis and is the treatment of choice for the complication of pulmonary edema. In addition to oxygen therapy, positive and expiratory pressure (PEEP) may be useful. Pulmonary edema usually resolves within 2–5 days. Since peripheral venous pooling may also contribute to hypotension, raising the legs and the judicious use of intravenous fluids may be necessary. Pressor agents are rarely required once hypoxia and acidosis are corrected and naloxone is administered. Diuretics are relatively contraindicated in the management of pulmonary edema since their efficacy is uncertain and hypotension may be aggravated by their use. If the oral route is responsible for toxicity or if the route of administration is unknown, gastrointestinal (GI) decontamination is undertaken as well. Forced diuresis is not recommended.

Naloxone (Narcan)

As soon as emergency support of vital functions is instituted, the pupil size and respiratory rate should be recorded and therapy with naloxone begun. Unlike earlier antagonists (nalorphine and levallorphan), naloxone is essentially a pure opiate antagonist with no agonist properties. Naloxone counteracts the effects of opiates within seconds to minutes and may precipitate an acute abstinence syndrome if it is given to a currently opiate-addicted patient. It will not affect the respiratory depression caused by alcohol, barbiturates, and other hypnotic sedatives. Its use in the emergency setting is therefore both of diagnostic and therapeutic value. Its use is recommended in all patients with coma and/or respiratory depression in whom the diagnosis is in doubt.

When using naloxone the primary desired effect is reestablishment of effective respiration. Naloxone should be given intravenously but may be used intramuscularly if there is delay in establishing an intravenous site as sometimes is the case if there is extensive venous thrombosis. In patients who have taken pure opiate overdoses the response to parenteral naloxone is immediate, and they show increased respirations and return of pupil size to normal. Coma and hypotension may also respond dramatically but may lag behind the respiratory and pupillary response particularly if hypoxia has been prolonged. Confusion and combativeness may ensue as patients emerge from opiate-induced comas, particularly if an acute withdrawal syndrome is precipitated.

The usual dose is 1 ampule of 0.4 mg or 0.01 mg/kg. This may be repeated every 2–3 minutes if no response occurs. If after 3 dosages have been administered there is no response, the diagnosis of opiate overdose is highly unlikely. However, the possibility of a polydrug intoxication, superimposed head trauma, or other central nervous system event should not be ruled out. Patients with propoxyphene or pentazocine intoxication respond less readily to naloxone. If these drugs are suspected higher (1.2 mg) doses of naloxone should be given. It must be noted that the duration of action of naloxone is 1–2 hours. Therefore, patients must be monitored and naloxone therapy repeated as needed. This is especially true if methadone has been taken since its duration of action is 24–36 hours.

Central Nervous System Stimulants

Central nervous system stimulants include sympathomimetic drugs. The stimulants include amphetamine (Benzedrine), dextroamphetamine (Dexedrine), methamphetamine (Desoxyn), phenmetrazine (Preludin), methylphenidate (Ritalin), and cocaine. Methamphetamine and phenmetrazine are variants of the amphetamine structure. Amphetamines are occasionally encountered in combination with barbiturates (e.g., Dexamyl combines dextroamphetamine and amobarbital). In addition, so-called legal stimulants and appetite suppressants contain various combinations of phenylpropanolamine, ephedrine, caffeine, and phenylephrine, which are also CNS stimulants and can produce intoxication similar to amphetamines.

AMPHETAMINES

The emergency room physician is likely to encounter patients with acute intoxication or amphetamine psychosis.

Severe intoxication has been seen in patients who have ingested 30 mg, yet patients have survived doses of 400–500 mg. Plasma levels of 600 ng/ml have been tolerated by chronic users. The amphetamines are rapidly absorbed from the intestinal tract, and peak levels of 10–50 ng/ml occur 1–2 hours after the ingestion of 10–25 mg. Marked tolerance to repeated amphetamine administration can develop. Amphetamines are metabolized by the liver, and a variable proportion of the parent drug is cleared by the kidney. Renal clearance of the parent drug is pH dependent and is markedly enhanced in the presence of acid urine. The plasma half-life of amphetamine is 16–31 hours when the urinary pH is more than 7.5 and 8–10 hours when the urinary pH is less than 6.

Diagnosis

Symptoms may occur as soon as 30 minutes after an ingestion of amphetamines and include dizziness, headaches, chest pains, palpitations, abdominal cramps, nausea, vomiting, panic states, and auditory and visual hallucinations. Physical findings include confusion, irritability, hostility and assaultiveness, pallor or flushing of the skin, mydriasis, diaphoresis, tachypnea, hypertension, tachycardia, and cardiac arrhythmias. Hyperreflexia and tremor may be noted. In life-threatening intoxications, hyperpyrexia, severe hypertension, and seizures occur and may result in cardiovascular collapse and death. Hyperpyrexia may preceed seizures and indicates severe toxicity. Deaths have been attributed to intracranial hemorrhage or cardiac arryhthmias, but fatalities are infrequent.

Treatment

If the patient has ingested amphetamines, emesis induced with ipecac syrup is preferred over gastric lavage, as long as the patient is alert. This should be followed by an activated charcoal slurry and a saline cathartic.

Mild to moderate intoxications are treated by first placing the patient in a calm environment. Chlorpromazine (Thorazine) in a dose of 1 mg/kg orally or intramuscularly has an excellent calming effect and may reduce associated hypertension. Sedation with a short-acting barbiturate or benzodiaze-

pine is efficacious as well. Acidification of the urine with ammonium chloride in a dose of 12 g daily orally or intravenously is indicated for moderate and severe intoxication.

Severe hypertension should be treated with an α-adrenergic antagonist such as phentolamine or phenoxybenzamine. Diazoxide and nitroprusside have also been successfully used. Hyperpyrexia greater than 39°C (102°F) is an ominous sign and the patient should be treated vigorously. Phenothiazines may be a useful adjunct in treating patients with this complication. Patients with seizures that are not responsive to diazepam should be treated with intravenous barbiturates.

AMPHETAMINE PSYCHOSIS

Although single large doses of amphetamines may produce a toxic paranoid hallucinating state, amphetamine psychosis most often results from chronic abuse. The syndrome resembles paranoid schizophrenia and is characterized by hyperactivity; compulsive behavior; paranoid delusions; visual, auditory, or haptic hallucinations; and a labile affect in which hostility and anxiety may predominate. The syndrome is differentiated from other toxic psychoses in that memory and orientation are preserved. The psychosis generally clears within 1 week. Haloperidol (Haldol) 2–5 mg orally or intramuscularly is preferred in the treatment of patients with psychotic manifestations since there is evidence to suggest that chlorpromazine retards the metabolism of amphetamines.

COCAINE

Cocaine is a naturally occurring stimulant drug that is derived from the leaves of the South American coca plant (*Erythroxylon coca*). The illicit use of cocaine is becoming increasingly prevalent despite the expense of this drug. Cocaine is abused for its ability to induce a euphoric state and a sense of physical vitality. The drug is usually sniffed at 15–30-minute intervals for an average of 3 dosages. Intravenous abusers tend to be those who use other drugs by this route as well. The so-called speedball combines intravenous heroin with cocaine. It had previously been believed that oral cocaine was rendered ineffective because of hydrolysis in the gastrointestinal tract, but recent studies show that the bioavailability of oral cocaine is equivalent to intranasal cocaine and that the euphoric effects are similar.

Cocaine is most commonly obtained as a hydrochloride salt, but it is frequently mixed with lidocaine, procaine, benzocaine, or lactose. A relatively new abuse pattern involves the conversion of cocaine to its "free base" form, which is then combined with tobacco or marijuana and is smoked. The smoking of cocaine free base produces intense effects similar to those from an intravenous injection. Cocaine smoking has a much higher potential for overdose than does intranasal use since intranasal absorption is limited by a fluctuating degree of local vasoconstriction. Cocaine smoking may become compulsive and continuous. Some of the toxicities usually seen with the chronic high dose use of the longer-acting stimulants such as amphetamines are seen with this form of cocaine use.

The acute toxic syndrome resulting from cocaine overdose is virtually indistinguishable from that of amphetamines except that the course is more rapid. The elimination half-life for both intranasal and oral cocaine is approximately 1 hour. Deaths resulting from cocaine are associated with a broad range of doses and have been reported primarily after intravenous use although fatalities from intranasal cocaine administration have been reported. Another cause of fatal cocaine poisoning is seen in smugglers who attempt to conceal plastic or rubber bags containing cocaine in their gastrointestinal tracts. Leakage and subsequent absorption of the cocaine has resulted in some cocaine overdose fatalities. Patients have died within minutes of intravenous injection. Deaths following oral or intranasal overdose have been proceeded by grand mal seizures occurring within 1 hour of ingestion or snorting. Death results from cardiovascular collapse and/or respiratory failure.

Heavy cocaine use may cause a psychosis characterized by paranoid delusions and hallucinations. Hallucinations may be visual, auditory, or haptic (cocaine bugs).

The treatment of patients suffering from cocaine intoxication is similar to that for patients who have taken amphetamines. In animal studies chlorpromazine has been shown to exert a protective effect against cocaine-induced cardiovascular changes. Intravenous barbiturates may be used as well. Urinary acidification is probably of little benefit since the toxicity runs a rapid course and the drug half-life is relatively short.

Phencyclidine

Phencyclidine (PCP) is an easily synthesized dissociative anesthetic agent that has had widespread usage in veterinary medicine. It belongs to the chemical group of cyclohexylamines, is similar to ketamine, and has sympathomimetic and hallucinogenic properties. Phencyclidine has been given various street names including PCP and angel dust. The drug is available in tablets or powder and may be misrepresented to the purchaser as tetrahydrocannabinol (THC), mescaline, or LSD. It may be found as an adulterant of marijuana. Phencyclidine abusers tend to be polydrug abusers.

Phencyclidine is usually smoked with tobacco or marijuana or is ingested. It is occasionally snorted or injected intravenously. Phencyclidine is well absorbed by all means of administration, has high lipid solubility, and has a pKa of 8.5. It is metabolized by the liver, excreted in the urine, and undergoes enteric recirculation. Urinary excretion of phencyclidine is markedly increased in acid urine.

Phencyclidine toxicity is largely dose related. Since toxicologic confirmation of PCP intoxication may not be readily available, the history and recognition of the signs and symptoms are most important for appropriate therapy. Low-dose intoxication tends to occur with doses of 2–10 mg associated with plasma levels of 25–100 ng/ml. High-dose intoxication occurs with doses greater than 25 mg associated with plasma levels greater than 300 ng/ml. In patients with low-dose intoxication, clinical effects begin within minutes of exposure, become maximal in 15–30 minutes, decline after 4–6 hours, and disappear in 24–28 hours. However, severe intoxication may take several days for recovery.

Diagnosis

Mild to moderate intoxication frequently causes agitation and can cause combativeness and violent behavior. Speech is often slow, slurred, and repetitive. The patient's eyes are open with ptosis resulting in blank stare appearance. Pupil size is variable but frequently miotic. Horizontal nystagmus is common; vertical nystagmus may also be seen. Muscle tone is increased, and catatonic rigidity and myoclonus occur. The patient's gait is ataxic. Other prominent features include flushing, hypersalivation, diaphoresis, facial grimacing, grunting and making animallike noises, and vomiting. In patients with mild PCP toxicity, respiratory depression is not seen and pharyngeal reflexes may be accentuated. The patient's pulse and blood pressure are normal or increased. Disorientation and muscular rigidity predispose to accidental death, commonly by drowning.

Severe intoxication results in a coma that may last from hours to days. Comatose patients may display rapid unpredictable fluctuations in their levels of intoxication. In comatose patients the eyes may remain open, periodic respiration or apnea may occur, and hypertension and tachycardia are the rule. Hyperthermia may also occur. Patients with severe intoxication may manifest high output cardiac failure, hypertensive encephalopathy, or cerebrovascular accidents from intracerebral hemorrhage.

Muscular rigidity is usually intense, and opisthotonos, seizures, and status epilepticus may occur. Rhabdomyolysis may occur as a result of muscular spasm and hyperthermia.

Treatment

The patient is placed in a calm, quiet environment since exacerbation of adverse clinical symptoms may occur with minimal verbal or physical stimulation. Induced emesis or gastric lavage are generally not recommended for this reason. Diazepam and haloperidol may help to control agitation. Patients exhibiting violent behavior may require restraints. Treatment of the psychotic behavior associated with PCP overdose may require psychiatric hospitalization. Prolonged psychotic episodes have occurred after PCP use. Haloperidol has been effective in alleviating some of the psychotic symptoms in these patients.

Therapy for severe intoxication is directed toward the management of the potentially lethal effects of cardiovascular stimulation, respiratory depression, and seizures and to the enhancement of drug excretion. In the comatose or convulsing patient endotracheal intubation is indicated with care to avoid aspiration.

Continuous or intermittent nasogastric suctioning or periodic dosages of activated charcoal may remove the enterically recycled drug. Continuous suctioning should be used with caution since it may result in metabolic alkalosis. Urinary acidification with intravenous ascorbic acid 0.5–1.5 g every 4–6 hours or with ammonium chloride in dosages adjusted to maintain a urinary pH of 5.5 or less is also recommended together with a furosemide-induced diuresis. Although gastric suction and urine acidification are in common usage, firm data from controlled clinical trials supporting these interventions are not available. The patient's temperature should be closely monitored and appropriate external cooling measures instituted as indicated. Diazoxide and intravenous propranolol are recommended for the treatment of patients in hypertensive crises. Excessive muscle activity can be treated with intravenous benzodiazepines.

BEHAVIORAL PROBLEMS ASSOCIATED WITH DRUG INTOXICATION

Drunkenness

Patients intoxicated with alcohol may show an extraordinary array of behaviors ranging from a quiet withdrawn depressed affect to gregarious-manic behavior. Some patients will be combative. Generally, intoxicated patients are easily agitated by external stimuli. If the emergency setting is hectic, the likelihood that the intoxicated patient will exhibit disruptive behavior is markedly increased. Staff attitudes are important.

Moralistic or hostile attitudes will exacerbate the patient's own sense of guilt and frustration and make management more difficult. The major management approach combines an accepting attitude with firmness. In general, emergency treatment with psychoactive drugs should be avoided. Possibilities for follow-up treatment should be explored when appropriate. For alcoholics or those addicted to other drugs, placement in a setting in which detoxification can be supervised is indicated. A forceful recommendation for addiction treatment from the emergency room physician can be an important and effective intervention.

Acute Anxiety or Panic Reactions

Acute anxiety reactions may be a manifestation of the drug user not having anticipated the effect of the drug taken. This can occur when the user takes one drug thinking it was another or the user may be inexperienced with the properties of the drug, such as is typically seen in adverse reactions to marijuana. On the other hand, the user may be experienced but the drug may cause unanticipated effects, such as is typically seen in adverse reactions to LSD. In unusual circumstances, the person can be unaware that a drug has even been taken. The most dramatic example of this results from the surreptitious administration of an hallucinogenic drug.

In street jargon the panic reaction has been called a "bad trip." Patients need to be treated in a quiet place by someone who is in constant attendance. The patient should be told that the perceptions that he or she is experiencing are an effect of the drug that has been taken. It is most important to be reassuring since the major fear articulated by those who have had the experience is that they have gone crazy. Medication is rarely indicated; time and reassurance usually suffice. When medication is used, only mild sedation with a benzodiazepine is indicated.

Acute Psychotic Reactions

The organic psychosis complicating drug usage is usually characterized by an abnormal and fluctuating mental status with defects in memory, judgment, and orientation in addition to the thought disorder of an acute psychotic reaction. This form of organic brain syndrome is distinguished from an acute functional psychosis in which the patient is usually oriented and has a constant degree of impairment.

The most important feature of management is to provide a safe, controlled environment for the patient. The psychotic reaction may be mild and short lived. Such patients are often overmedicated, which complicates the evaluation. In the exceptional circumstance when agitation is severe or psychosis is prolonged, mild sedation with benzodiazepines and/or the use of phenothiazines or butyrophenones may be indicated.

Violent Patients

Occasionally violent behavior is a complication of drug intoxication. Patients in whom the potential for violence exists should be positioned so that obstacles or people do not block the room exit since blocking an "escape route" can heighten a patient's anxiety and degree of combativeness. Staff members should position themselves so that they can leave the room quickly for their own protection if necessary. Furthermore, they should not approach these patients alone. There should be adequate personnel present so that if the patient must be restrained, it can be done without injury to the patient or staff. Staff members should avoid threatening talk or action that could incite the potentially violent patient and should be alert to clues that indicate a patient may be losing control and is about to translate impulses into action. Physical restraints and pharmacologic treatment (similar to that used for the agitated psychotic patient) may be indicated for the management of violent patients.

Suicidal Patients

Since drug overdose may represent an intentional suicide attempt, patients should not be left alone in the emergency treatment room in which there is access to sharp instruments or drugs. Whenever the patient confirms that he or she has made a suicide attempt, however ineffectual, a history of previous attempts and underlying depression should be pursued. Psychiatric consultation should be obtained.

DRUG WITHDRAWAL

One of the complications of the compulsive use of some drugs is the occurrence of a drug withdrawal or abstinence syndrome that, in its acute form, may require emergency treatment. Drugs that can produce physical dependence and hence a clearly defined withdrawal syndrome are opiates and opiatelike drugs (e.g., propoxyphene), barbiturates, nonbarbiturate hypnotics, ethanol, and benzodiazepines. A less clearly defined though definite withdrawal pattern is seen in patients who have taken amphetamines and tricyclic antidepressants.

In determining the degree of physical dependence within a particular class of drugs, the amount, duration, frequency of drug use and degree of tolerance are important. The nature and severity of the withdrawal syndrome, however, only partly depends on these factors. Different classes of drugs have their own unique withdrawal patterns. The seriousness of the withdrawal and hence the degree to which its treatment represents a medical emergency depends very much on the class of drug. The most life-threatening forms of withdrawal are seen with alcohol, barbiturates, and the nonbarbiturate nonbenzodiazepine hypnotics. Familiarity with these patterns can help the physician differentiate drug withdrawal from drug intoxication and certain metabolic disorders.

Table 43.4 illustrates patterns of drug withdrawal for two groups of drugs—the opiates and the sedative-hypnotics, including alcohol. The withdrawal characteristics in this table are listed in rough sequential order from the mild to the severe signs of withdrawal.

Alcohol (Ethanol)

Although the withdrawal syndrome is usually triggered by acute abstinence from alcohol, it can also occur with a sharp drop in alcohol consumption or, occasionally, with stable alcohol consumption along with an intercurrent illness, usually infectious. Alcohol withdrawal can produce a variety of clinical syndromes, from a mild hyperadrenergic state called the common abstinence syndrome to delirium tremens (DTs).

COMMON ABSTINENCE SYNDROME

The milder forms of alcohol withdrawal, although not a medical emergency, are still encountered frequently in the emergency treatment setting. Careful evaluation of the patient is necessary in order to rule out complicating medical problems and the possibility that the patient is showing signs of early DTs. Pharmacotherapy may not be indicated. Social setting (nonmedical) detoxification centers in which no psychoactive drugs are used in the detoxification treatment are available for patient referral in many communities.

If pharmacotherapy is used, the benzodiazepines have been found to be safe and effective; chlordiazepoxide and diazepam both have long half-lives and are frequently prescribed. If chlordiazepoxide is used, an initial test dose of 50–100 mg orally is given and the patient observed 2–4 hours later. If the symptoms and signs of withdrawal are not ameliorated or are progressing, the dose is repeated. In most patients, an initial divided dose of 50–200 mg in the first 24-hour period usually provides mild sedation, decreases the tremulousness, and eases the bothersome symptoms of alcohol withdrawal. Occasionally, in severely tremulous and agitated patients dosages as

TABLE 43.4 Characteristics of Drug Withdrawal

Opiates	Barbiturates, Nonbarbiturate Hypnotics, and Alcohol
Agitation	Agitation
Yawning	Tremulousness
Sleeplessness	Sleeplessness
Diaphoresis	Diaphoresis
Tachycardia	Tachycardia
Increased systolic blood pressure	Increased systolic blood pressure
Lacrimation, rhinorrhea	Hyperventilation
Mydriasis	Mild hyperthermia
Piloerection—gooseflesh seen in nipples and skin	Vomiting
Bowel hypermotility	Postural hypotension
Muscle twitches and tremors—seen in peripheral muscles and tongue	Seizures
	Hallucinosis (may occur independently of DTs)
Mild hyperthermia	Delirium tremens
Increased respiration	
Vomiting	
Diarrhea	
Seizures (rare)	

high as 400–600 mg chlordiazepoxide are necessary in the first 24 hours. Once an appropriate initial dosage level is achieved, the drug can be tapered rapidly over 2–4 days.

Benzodiazepines with shorter half-lives, such as lorazepam (Ativan) and oxazepam (Serax), may be preferable for patients with significant liver impairment. Lorazepam can be given in dosages of 1–4 mg orally every 6–8 hours and oxazepam in dosages of 15–60 mg orally every 6–8 hours. Regular 6–8-hour dosage intervals are necessary to maintain constant blood levels, and cessation will result in rapid decreases in levels. During tapering, the 8-hour frequency of administration should be maintained while the dosage is lowered to avoid breakthrough symptoms associated with low trough concentrations.

RUM FITS

Rum fits are grand mal seizures that occur within 7–48 hours of cessation of drinking, with a peak incidence at 24 hours. Fifty percent of the time they occur as a single episode. Only 3% of patients have status epilepticus. The occurrence of rum fits, although usually self-limited and benign, may portend the development of subsequent DTs since in some studies as many as 40% of patients with rum fits have progressed to DTs.

Patients with rum fits often do not require therapy. If the patient has status epilepticus and is unresponsive to diazepam, the use of other anticonvulsants (e.g., barbiturates and phen-

ytoin) is indicated. Alcoholics frequently have concurrent seizure diathesis and are notoriously unreliable in taking medication while they are drinking. If the patient gives a history of prior epilepsy or of discontinuing previously prescribed anticonvulsants, then phenytoin (Dilantin) therapy may be indicated. In the usual case of rum fits, chronic phenytoin therapy is not indicated. Rum fits have been associated with hypomagnesemia and alkalosis, and appropriate replacement therapy may be indicated.

DELIRIUM TREMENS

Diagnosis

The most severe form of alcohol withdrawal is characterized by a symptom complex of profound confusion and disorientation associated with hallucinations and autonomic and motor hyperactivity. The hallucinations of DTs, which are more visual than auditory and are often of a precursory nature, merge with the confusional state. Seizures (rum fits), if they do occur, usually do so before the onset of hallucinations. The confusion is often variable in time and is usually much worse at night. Terrible nightmares aptly described as "horrors" may be the earliest clue to DTs. Delirium tremens are usually accompanied by extreme psychomotor agitation and autonomic hyperactivity. Patients continuously move or make attempts to do so. If they are restrained, excessive isometric contractions can predispose to exhaustion and dehydration. Autonomic hyperactivity is prominent, and the patient has tachycardia, elevated systolic blood pressure, low grade fever, and dilated pupils. Sleep disturbances are common; there is fragmentation of sleep and agitation that may result in patients remaining sleepless for 2–3 days. Patients are usually unable to feed themselves and are often incontinent of urine.

The onset of DTs typically occurs on the second or third day after abstinence, peaks on the fourth day, and gradually subsides during the first week. The duration of DTs is 3–5 days, but prolongation is not uncommon.

Treatment

Aggressive pharmacotherapy early in the course of DTs can markedly contribute to improved patient management and reduce the morbidity and mortality that accompanies the syndrome. Sedating or calming the patient is an essential part of the treatment of DTs. Intravenous diazepam, 10 mg initially followed by 5 mg every 5 minutes until the patient is calm, has proven to be effective. Patients may be switched from parenteral diazepam to oral diazepam, chlordiazepoxide, or the shorter-acting oxazepam or lorazepam as soon as they are able to tolerate oral medication. In addition to the use of benzodiazepines, the use of haloperidol, 2–4 mg intramuscularly every 2–6 hours as necessary, can be used as a supplement to diazepam to control agitation, as well as some of the behaviors secondary to hallucinations. Response to each dosage should be measured before the next one is administered. The addition of haloperidol has been particularly useful for patients who have presented with the common abstinence syndrome and have been treated with adequate doses of chlordiazepoxide but develop DTs. Although some additional sedation with benzodiazepines may be useful for such patients, the addition of another class of drugs has materially aided in their management. Once the patient has stabilized, the dosages of benzodiazepines should be tapered. Haloperidol may be discontinued without tapering.

Physical restraints may be necessary as an emergency measure for the protection of both patient and staff and should be readily available. Early use of restraints should be advocated if any of the staff feels threatened by the patient. Significant injury to staff members has occurred during attempts to apply restraints, and liberal use of security guards and attendants is often warranted.

Attention to vitamin, fluid, and electrolyte replacement and the treatment of complicating illnesses are as important as any drug treatment. Hypokalemia and alkalosis may require im-

mediate attention since they are associated with patients in DTs. Appropriate fluid electrolyte replacement is necessary, especially if insensible losses are prominent. Frequent monitoring of cardiac and renal status is important.

A careful search for infection is essential. Fever is common in patients with DTs, but if it exceeds 39°C (102°F), infection is suggested and must be ruled out. A full fever workup, including a lumbar puncture, chest film, and appropriate cultures, is mandatory. Leukocytosis may be minimal since the bone marrow may still be suppressed by previous alcohol consumption or the presence of hypersplenism. Independent of any measurable parameter, an alcoholic should be considered an immunosuppressed host.

Mortality from classic DTs has leveled off to approximately 10% as compared to 50% in the past, the major improvement being in treating the medical complications and the management of electrolyte imbalance. Older patients with limited end organ reserve or with overwhelming infection have a higher mortality. It should be emphasized that the most important approach to the treatment of DTs rests in the total medical management of the patient, not only in specific pharmacotherapies.

Finally, detoxification from alcohol is not the treatment of alcoholism. It does provide an opportunity, however, to engage the alcoholic in the early stages of treatment. Every effort should be made to couple alcohol detoxification with referral to or the provision of continuing care for the chronic disease of alcoholism.

Barbiturates

Withdrawal from barbiturates is similar to withdrawal from alcohol with the exception that withdrawal seizures are more common and more severe and the occurrence of full blown DTs is relatively rare. Seizures usually have their onset within 72 hours of the last hypnotic dose.

The aim of barbiturate withdrawal treatment is to give enough medication for detoxification to prevent the serious withdrawal signs. The procedure is to give a test dose of a short-acting barbiturate as follows: After withdrawal signs are observed, a 200-mg oral test dose of a short-acting barbiturate (e.g., pentobarbital) is given and the patient is observed for 1 hour. If no signs of drug effect are noted from the test dose in a known barbiturate addict, the first day's total detoxification dose is usually in the 800–1,200-mg range.

After the first 24 hours, the dose is decreased by 100 mg/day until a level of 800 mg is reached; it is then reduced by 50 mg/day. Phenobarbital can be substituted for the short-acting barbiturate after the first 24 hours. Since phenobarbital has a longer half-life, the equivalent dose is one-third to one-half the short-acting barbiturate dose. Phenobarbital can be given orally every 8 hours and the dosage decreased by about 60 mg/day until the 180 mg/day dose is achieved; it is then tapered at the rate of 30 mg/day.

Other Sedative-Hypnotics

The approach to the management of the acute abstinence syndrome is similar to that of barbiturates. A test dose that is approximately twice the usual hypnotic dose is used to gauge the degree of physical dependence. Then a daily dosage schedule based on the test dose findings is instituted, followed by gradual dosage reduction. The drug chosen for detoxification treatment may be the same as the drug that has produced the physical dependence or may be a cross-tolerant barbiturate.

Benzodiazepine Tranquilizers

Discontinuation of therapeutic dosages of diazepam and chlordiazepoxide taken for 4–6 months may result in a minor withdrawal syndrome consisting of agitation, tremor, sweating, and insomnia. Emergency treatment is not required. However, emergency care may be necessary after the abrupt discontinuation of higher dosages taken for longer periods of time. This more serious withdrawal syndrome can result in a toxic psychosis characterized by disorientation, agitation, hallucinations, and delusions. Seizures also occur with the cessation of regular high dose use of benzodiazepines and, presumably because of the long half-life of some of these drugs, may occur weeks after the last dose is taken. Withdrawal is treated by tapering dosages of benzodiazepines.

Opiates

Abrupt discontinuation of opiate intake in a person who is physically dependent on the drug leads to a typical abstinence syndrome that generally does not constitute a life-threatening emergency. In its most severe form, vomiting, diarrhea, muscular twitching, and tremors may occur. In its mild form, there may be few objective signs, but the patient may complain bitterly about symptoms of discomfort and restlessness. Such patients often seek emergency care in spite of their seemingly benign condition.

The onset of withdrawal signs and symptoms depends on the rate of metabolism of the particular opiate used. For heroin, withdrawal signs are observed about 8–12 hours after the last dose and for methadone about 24–48 hours after the last dose.

The opiate withdrawal syndrome may be completely reversed by the administration of any opiate. Detoxification regimens usually use methadone. The procedure to establish the withdrawal medication dose is as follows: After withdrawal signs are observed, give an oral test dose of 10–15 mg methadone and observe the patient 2 hours after administering the test dose. Mild somnolence and the absence of withdrawal signs indicate that this dose is sufficient for the first 24 hours. If no somnolence occurs or if definite abstinence signs persist, an additional 10–20 mg can be given over the next 8–12 hours. Rarely is a methadone detoxification dose of more than 40 mg necessary in the first 24 hours for treating street addiction to opiates. Once the initial level of withdrawal medication is established, methadone can be reduced at a rate of 5 mg/day. Clonidine hydrochloride has also been used to suppress opiate withdrawal signs and symptoms in detoxifying methadone maintenance patients.

SELECTED READINGS

Allen MD, Greenblatt DJ, Noel BJ: Meprobamate overdosage: A continuing problem. *Clin Toxicol* 1977; 11(5):501–515.

American Medical Association Department of Drugs: *AMA Drug Evaluations,* 4th ed. Chicago, American Medical Association, 1980, p 1470.

Barry D, Meyskens FL, Becker CE: Phenothiazine poisoning: A review of 48 cases. *West J Med* 1973; 118(1):1–5.

Becker CE, Morrelli HF: Alcohol and drug abuse in clinical pharmacology, in Melman KL, Morrelli HF (eds): *Basic Principles in Therapeutics.* New York, MacMillan Inc, 1978, p 1008.

Berg MJ, Berlinger WG, Goldberg MJ, et al: Acceleration of the body clearance of phenobarbital by oral activated charcoal. *New Engl J Med* 1982; 307:642.

Biggs JT, Spiker DG, Petit JM et al: Tricyclic antidepressant overdose: Incidence of symptoms. *J Am Med Assoc* 1977; 238(2):135–138.

Bloomer HA: A critical evaluation of diuresis in the treatment of barbiturate intoxication. *J Lab Clin Med* 1966; 67(6):898–905.

Bourne, P. ed: *A Treatment Manual for Acute Drug Abuse Emergencies,* US Dept of Health, Education, and Welfare Publication No. (ADM) 76-230. Rockville, Maryland, National Clearinghouse for Drug Abuse Information, 1976, p 178.

Busto V, Kaplan HL, Sellers EM: Benzodiazepine—Associated emergencies in Toronto. *Am J Psychiatry* 1980; 137:487.

Chazan J, Garella S: Glutethimide intoxication: A prospective study of 70 patients treated conservatively without hemodialysis. *Arch Intern Med* 1971; 128:215.

Cohen S: Amphetamine Abuse. *J Am Med Assoc* 1975; 231(4):414–415.

Cohen S: Cocaine. *J Am Med Assoc* 1975; 231(1):74–75.

Cooper JR (ed): *Sedative-Hypnotic Drugs: Risks and Benefits.* US Dept of Health, Education, and Welfare Publication No. (ADM)79-592.

Rockville, Maryland, National Institute on Drug Abuse, 1977, p 112.

Delgado-Escuetta AV, Wasterlain C, Treiman DM et al: Current concepts in neurology—Management of status epilepticus. *New Engl J Med* 1982; 306:1337.

Done AK: The toxic emergency. *Emergency Med* 1982; p 41–77.

Dreisbach RH: *Handbook of Poisoning.* Los Altos, Lange Medical Publications, 1983, p 632.

Dupont RI, Goldstein A, O'Donnell J (eds): *Handbook on Drug Abuse.* Washington DC, National Institute on Drug Abuse, 1979, p 452.

Espelin DE, Done AK: Amphetamine poisoning: Effectiveness of chlorpromazine. *New Engl J Med* 1968; 278(25):1361–1365.

Finkle BS, McCloskey KL, Goodman LS: Diazepam and drug-associated deaths: A survey in the United States and Canada. *J Am Med Assoc* 1979; 242(5):429–434.

Frand UI, Shim CS, Williams MH Jr: Heroin-induced pulmonary edema: Sequential studies of pulmonary function. *Ann Intern Med* 1972; 77:26–35.

Gold MS, Pottash AC, Sweeney DR et al: Opiate withdrawal using clonidine. *J Am Med Assoc* 1980; 243:343.

Greenblatt DJ, Allen MD, Noel BJ et al: Acute overdosage with benzodiazepine derivatives. *Clin Pharmacol Ther* 1977; 21(4): 497–514.

Greenblatt DJ, Shader RI: Dependence, tolerance and addiction to benzodiazepines: Clinical and pharmacokinetics considerations. *Drug Metab Rev* 1978; 8:13–28.

Gustafson A, Gustafsson G: Acute poisoning with dextropropoxyphene: Clinical symptoms and plasma concentrations. *Acta Med Scand* 1976; 200:241–248.

Gustafson A, Svensson S, Ugander L: Cardiac arrhythmias in chloral hydrate poisoning. *Acta Med Scand* 1977; 201:227–230.

Hollister LE: *Clinical Pharmacology of Psychotherapeutic Drugs. Monographs in Clinical Pharmacology.* New York, Churchill Livingstone, 1978, p. 815.

Ingelfinger JA, Isakson G, Shine D et al: Reliability of the toxic screen in drug overdose. *Clin Pharmacol Ther* 1981; 29:570.

Jaffee JH: Drug addiction and drug abuse, in Gilman AG, Gilman LS (eds): *The Pharmacological Basis of Therapeutics.* New York, MacMillan Inc, 1980, p 535.

Kalant H, Kalant OJ: Death in amphetamine users: Causes and rates. *Can Med Assoc J* 1975; 8:299.

Khantzian EJ, McKenna GJ: Acute toxic and withdrawal reactions associated with drug use and abuse. *Ann Intern Med* 1979; 90:361–372.

Lewis DC, Senay EC: *Treatment of Drug and Alcohol Abuse.* New York, Career Teacher Center, 1981, Vol II, No 2, p 91.

Lorch JA, Garella S: Hemoperfusion to treat intoxications. *Ann Intern Med* 1979; 91:301–304.

Maddock RK, Bloomer HA: Meprobamate overdosage: Evaluation of its severity and methods of treatment. *J Am Med Assoc* 1967; 201(13):999–1003.

Martin WR: Naloxone. *Ann Intern Med* 1976; 85(6):765–768.

Matthew H, Lawson AA: Acute barbiturate poisoning: A review of two years experience. *Q J Med* 1966; 35:(140):539–552.

Matthew H, Roscoe P, Wright N: Acute poisoning: A comparison of hypnotic drugs. *Practitioner* 1972; 208:254.

Misra PS, Lefevre A, Ishii H et al: Increase of ethanol, meprobamate and pentobarbital metabolism after chronic ethanol administration in man and in rats. *Am J Med* 1971; 51:346–351.

National Academy of Sciences: *Report of a Study: Sleeping Pills, Insomnia, and Medical Practice.* Washington DC, National Academy of Sciences, Institute of Medicine, 1979, p 198.

Newton RW: Physostigmine salicylate in the treatment of tricyclic antidepressant overdosage. *J Am Med Assoc* 1975; 231(9):941–943.

NIDA Research Issues: *Use and Abuse of Amphetamine and Its Substitutes.* US Dept of Health, Education, and Welfare Publication No. (ADM) 80-941. Washington DC, US Government Printing Office, 1980, p 558.

NIDA Research Monograph Series: *Cocaine.* US Department of Health, Education, and Welfare Publication No. (ADM) 77-432. Washington DC, US Government Printing Office, 1977, p 220.

Noble J, Matthew H: Acute poisoning by tricyclic antidepressants: Clinical features and management of 100 patients. *Clin Toxicol* 1969; 2(4):403–421.

Petersen RC, Stillman RC (eds): *PCP—Phencyclidine abuse: An appraisal.* NIDA Research Monograph Series, No. 21, US Department of Health, Education, and Welfare Publication No. (ADM) 78-728. Washington DC US Government Printing Office, 1978, p 310.

Quitkin F, Rifkin A, Klein DF: Monoamine oxidase inhibitors. *Arch Gen Psychiatry* 1979; 36:749–760.

Rappolt RT, Gay GR, Farris RD: Emergency management of acute phencyclidine intoxication. *J American College Emergency Physicians* 1979; 8(2):68–76.

Sellers EM, Kalant H: Drug therapy: Alcohol intoxication and withdrawal. *New Engl J Med* 1976; 294:757–762.

Setter HG, Maher JF, Schreiner GE: Barbiturate intoxication: Evaluation of therapy including dialysis in a large series selectively referred because of severity. *Arch Intern Med* 1966; 117:224–235.

Shader RI (ed): *Manual of Psychiatric Therapeutics.* Boston, Little Brown & Co, 1975, p 362.

Sidoff ML: Phencyclidine: Syndromes of abuse and modes of treatment. *Topics in Emergency Medicine* 1979; 1:111–119.

Slovis TL, Ott JE, Teitelbaum DT et al: Physostigmine therapy in acute tricyclic antidepressant poisoning. *Clin Toxicol* 1971; 4(3):451–459.

Smith DE, Wesson DR: Phenobarbital technique for treatment of barbiturate dependence. *Arch Gen Psychiatry* 1971; 24:56–60.

Stewart RD: Tricyclic antidepressant poisoning. *Am Fam Physician* 1979; 19:136.

Sunshine I, Hackett ER: Barbiturate studies: II Correlation between clinical condition and blood barbiturate levels. *Am J Clin Pathol* 1954; 24:1133–1138.

Teehan BP, Maher JF, Carey JJ et al: Acute ethchlorvynol (placidyl) intoxication. *Ann Intern Med* 1970; 72:875–882.

Thompson WL: Management of alcohol withdrawal syndromes. *Arch Intern Med* 1978; 138:238–283.

Uhl JA: Phenytoin: The drug of choice in tricyclic antidepressant overdose? *Ann Emergency Med* 1981; 10:270.

Victor M, Wolfe SM: Causation and treatment of the alcohol withdrawal syndrome, in Bourne PG, Fox R (eds): *Alcoholism: Progress in Research and Treatment.* New York, Academic Press Inc, 1973, p 137.

Wetli CV, Wright RK: Death caused by recreational cocaine use. *J Am Med Assoc* 1979; 241(23):2519–2522.

44
PEDIATRIC EMERGENCIES

Paul H. Wise
Jonathan Bates
John H. Fisher

As children grow and develop, the spectrum of illness and mortality from which they suffer undergoes extensive change in a relatively short time period (Table 44.1). Neonatal conditions, most related to prematurity, account for the majority of deaths to children under 1 year of age. Increasing mobility and independence make the older child more vulnerable to death from injuries sustained from household and, later, motor vehicle accidents. Once children reach the age of 1 year, the chances that they will die from an injury before they are 20 years old is five times more likely than from any other cause. Clearly the treatment and prevention of childhood injuries remains one of the primary challenges of pediatrics in the years to come.

Whereas mortality patterns best reflect the most serious pediatric emergencies, surveys of pediatric morbidity also help us to understand better the types of childhood problems likely to present in an emergency setting. The relative number of children with a specific emergent condition seen at a particular site will vary with community, hospital, and health care delivery system characteristics. In general, however, important childhood morbidity lies in infectious disease, trauma, and allergic disorders, primarily asthma.

EVALUATION OF THE PATIENT

Whereas many critically ill children can be clearly identified as requiring emergency medical attention, the largest group of children presenting to an emergency setting will require careful evaluation before the nature and severity of their illnesses can be properly gauged.

History

A careful history in an emergency setting is a critical, although too often overlooked, aspect of the initial evaluation of the ill child. The length and detail of the interview should reflect the circumstances surrounding the visit. A critically ill child usually requires immediate assessment and intervention, and the initial history must be concise and without great detail. However, a purposeful and directed history may uncover important clues as to the etiology of the presenting problem. Particular attention should be paid to the nature and temporal development of symptoms that have shaped the child's illness. Careful questioning as to the presence of chronic disease or medication is essential. Medic-Alert bracelets or other identification may prove useful, particularly in the unconscious child.

The emergency setting is often characterized by a constellation of human interactions in many ways unique to this area. The clinician often has never met the child or family before; the family is usually presenting in a state of significant crisis; and the physician may not have immediate access to important medical information or records. The history, therefore, is a particularly important aspect of emergency pediatric care since it provides an opportunity to establish a productive rapport with the family and child while gathering critical medical and social information. This relationship has its roots in the ability of the clinician to listen to and address the concerns of the parents or child. Irrespective of their relevance to the ultimate diagnosis, these expressed concerns can often guide the explanation of a particular diagnosis or management plan.

Physical Examination

Most often, the physical examination of a child is a useful and enjoyable experience. Although the child is commonly upset and frightened, a gentle and reassuring approach will usually ensure the cooperation required for a productive examination. Since the young child's response to illness may be nonspecific, the examination should always begin with the careful observation of the child's general state. Posture, movement, and interaction with environmental stimuli should always be noted and can often be best ascertained while the child rests in the parents arms or lap. Vital signs are also critically important and often overlooked. Careful assessment of weight, height, and head circumference for age is also important since it has been shown that poor growth may not be evident on clinical examination alone.

Infants may be difficult to examine because of their increasing fear of nonparental faces and separation from the parent. Performing as much of the examination as possible with the child in the parent's lap is usually helpful. Distraction, such as presenting the child with a colorful object, may also facilitate a more productive examination.

In young children (3–6 years old) it becomes exceedingly important to explain to the child fully and honestly the nature

TABLE 44.1 Major Causes of Death in Children: United States, 1975

Rank	Age (years)				Total
	<1	1–4	5–14	15–24	0–24
1	Neonatal conditions	Accidents	Accidents	Accidents	Accidents
2	Congenital anomalies	Infectious illnesses	Neoplasms	Homicide	Neonatal conditions
3	Infectious illnesses	Congenital anomalies	Infectious illnesses	Suicide	Congenital anomalies
4	Accidents	Neoplasms	Congenital anomalies	Neoplasms	Infectious illnesses

Source: *Vital Statistics: Mortality 1975*. Washington, DC, National Center for Health Statistics.

of all procedures and examinations before performing them. Often it is useful to allow the child to play with a stethoscope or percussion hammer while taking the history. The school age child is usually cooperative and a pleasure to examine. However, this may belie underlying fears or concerns that the child may hold regarding the illness or the clinician's examination. Great care to appreciate fully and to address these anxieties will usually strengthen the clinician's relationship with both the child and parent, ensuring a more productive examination and plan of management.

The adolescent usually appreciates an honest and straightforward discussion of clinical problems and their management. Although it is often useful to speak with and examine the adolescent without the parent present, this method should be discussed with both the parent and child. Adolescents are usually quite concerned with their bodies and often harbor fears regarding their emerging sexuality. It should also be understood that the chief complaint or presenting symptoms may not truly reflect underlying concerns that the adolescent may have difficulty discussing at the outset. For example, it is not uncommon for sexually abused adolescents to present with complaints of headache, abdominal pain, or school problems.

Follow-Up Care

One of the most crucial aspects of pediatric emergency care is a strong commitment to organizing the child's follow-up care. The vast majority of children presenting to an emergency facility do not require hospitalization. Specific and easily understood guidelines for the continuing care of the child must be communicated to the parent or caretaker, preferably in their native language. These guidelines are as follows:

1. Diagnosis
2. General supportive measures (fluids, rest, etc.)
3. Medication (written out in lay terms)
4. Danger signs (fever, decreasing fluid intake, persistent vomiting, etc.)
5. General idea of natural history of illness
6. Specific instructions on how to contact a well-identified clinician for questions or repeat evaluation
7. Specific instructions for follow-up primary care

The last item is of special concern. In general, for all patients presenting to an emergency facility who report no source of primary care, a specific physician or clinic should be identified for follow-up care before the family returns home. Selection of this site is best made by discussing the locally available sources of primary care with the family members and choosing that which seems to best fit their needs. The importance of constructing a sound and specific follow-up plan cannot be overstated. Many of the most tragic cases of unnecessary morbidity and mortality related to medical care received in an emergency facility occur after the child has been evaluated and sent home.

ACUTE PROBLEMS IN THE NEONATE

Some of the more anxiety-provoking and clinically devastating pediatric emergencies occur in the newborn. The normal transition from fetal to neonatal life is usually a smooth, albeit complex, process that rarely fails to be a gratifying experience for the observing clinician. However, despite recent strides in modern obstetrics, medical intervention is sometimes required to assist the newborn in adapting to his or her new environment. The most common problems involve the child's inability to establish adequate lung expansion and gas exchange or to complete successfully the complex shift from a fetal circulatory pattern to that of the air-breathing neonate. Because initiating this process in the first few moments of life is so critical, im-

TABLE 44.2 Conditions Associated with High-Risk Deliveries

Maternal	Fetal	Labor and Delivery
Toxemia	Intrauterine growth retardation	Abnormal length or pattern of labor
Hypertension	Blood group isoimmunization	Breech position
Diabetes mellitus		Transverse or compound position
Pulmonary disease	Meconium staining	Multiple birth
Renal disease	Abnormal fetal heart rate pattern	Cesarean section
Cardiac disease	Prematurity or postmaturity	

Adapted from Cloherty JP, and Stark AR: *Manual of Neonatal Care.* Boston, Little Brown & Co., 1980, p 56.

mediate intervention may be required. The medical response must be thoughtful yet decisive since any significant error or hesitation in providing therapy may have serious consequences in subsequent morbidity or ultimate survival.

Although the importance of prompt intervention cannot be overstated, it must be remembered that this therapy should be provided in a gentle and caring manner. In recent years, a greater appreciation of the social and emotional importance of labor and delivery to both the family and the child has led many to recognize that medical intervention should never preclude gentle handling of the child or supportive communication with observing family members.

One of the most important factors in caring for an ill newborn is adequate preparation for an anticipated problem during delivery. Conditions that place the newborn in a category of high risk are listed in Table 44.2. Required equipment is listed in Table 44.3. Before delivery, all equipment should be tested, oxygen flow and anesthesia bag pop-off valve adjusted, and choice of appropriate endotracheal tube made (Table 44.3).

Evaluation

Upon delivery the child should be placed on a warming table. The mouth, oropharynx, and nostrils should be suctioned with a bulb aspirator. There is some evidence that use of a suction catheter immediately after birth may stimulate cardiac arrhythmias, probably secondary to vagal effects, and therefore should be discouraged until at least 5 minutes have passed and a more stable cardiorespiratory status can be assumed.

TABLE 44.3 Pediatric Equipment for High-Risk Delivery

Respiratory	Drugs	Intravenous Access	Other
Flow through anesthesia bag capable of delivering 100% oxygen	Sodium bicarbonate (0.5 mEq/ml)	Umbilical catheter (No. 3.5 and French)	Radiant warmer
Face mask of appropriate size	Epinephrine (1:10,000)	Umbilical catheterization tray (cutdown tray if not available)	Stethoscope
	Dextrose (50% or 25%)		
Laryngoscope with Miller No. 0 and No. 1 blades		Normal saline flush	Newborn blood pressure cuff
	Calcium gluconate (10%)		
Orotracheal tubes 2.5, 3, and 3.5 mm internal diameter (2 each)		Syringes (1, 3, 5, 10 ml)	Transport incubator with portable oxygen and heat source
	Naloxone		
Oxygen			
	Atropine		

Adapted from Cloherty JP, Stark AR: *Manual of Neonatal Care.* Boston, Little Brown & Co., 1980, p 56–57.

Evaluation of the newborn has been assisted by the use of the Apgar scoring system (Table 44.4). Although it is customary to assign a score at 1 and 5 minutes, it may be more useful to view the Apgar score as a dynamic evaluative tool, guiding the assessment from the time of delivery until stabilization. The child's condition may fluctuate over the course of the first few minutes of life, therefore the relative immediacy and type of intervention required will change as well. A dynamic Apgar scoring system will help shape the level of concern and direction of therapy.

Management

Decisions regarding intervention can be extremely difficult. Concern over the failure to respond adequately must be coupled with an appreciation of the child's inherent ability to improve on his or her own, as well as the significant iatrogenesis associated with many resuscitative techniques.

For children with no significant asphyxia (Apgar 8–10) warming, drying, and gentle suctioning with bulb syringe are sufficient. Evaluation should be continued for at least 5 minutes to assure a stable status. The immediate care of a healthy newborn should also take into consideration the requests of the parents for close initial contact and full participation. It is unusual that the concerns of the parents and those of the pediatrician cannot achieve full harmony in the delivery room.

MILD ASPHYXIA (APGAR 5–7)

Newborns with mild asphyxia usually respond to gentle stimulation and/or oxygen supplementation. Gentle slapping of the feet or stroking of the back are often enough for the child to improve. In addition, 100% oxygen supplied to the face by mask will usually prove helpful. At times gentle provision of intermittent continuous positive airway pressure (CPAP) will evoke an improved respiratory effort.

MODERATE ASPHYXIA (APGAR 3–5)

Newborns with moderate asphyxia will usually be heralded by a heart rate of less than 100 beat/min without response to stimulation. Usually rapid institution of ventilation with appropriate sized bag and mask with 100% oxygen will revive the child. Ventilatory pressure should be adequate to move the chest wall (usually between 20 and 25 cm H_2O), and a rate of between 20 and 40 breaths per minute is recommended. Newborns who fall into this category should be closely observed for at least several hours to rule out underlying pathology, as well as to monitor the child's full recovery from the difficult birth.

SEVERE ASPHYXIA (APGAR 0–2)

Newborns with severe asphyxia demand rapid medical intervention. Full cardiorespiratory resuscitative efforts should be instituted immediately. The approach and mechanics of resuscitation of the newborn are basically similar to those of the child and adult; however, several areas should be emphasized.

Adequate ventilation with 100% oxygen is critically important in trying to resuscitate a newborn. Bag and mask ventilation should be sufficient if the airway is clear and proper technique and mask size are employed. However, if for any reason bag and mask ventilation fails to move the chest adequately or produce good breath sounds bilaterally or if the heart rate remains low, the child should be intubated with an appropriate sized endotracheal tube as follows:

Birth Weight	Oral Cole Tubes	Nasotracheal Portex Tubes
<1,250 g	No. 10, 12	2.5 mm
1,250–2,000 g	No. 15, 16	3 mm
>2,000 g	No. 16, 18	3.5 mm

Cardiac massage should be begun with the heart rate below 60 beats/min. The best technique is to place both hands around

TABLE 44.4 Apgar Scoring System

Sign	Score		
	0	1	2
Heart rate	Absent	Under 100 beats/min	Over 100 beats/min
Respiratory effort	Absent	Slow (irregular)	Good crying
Muscle tone	Limp	Some flexion of extremities	Active motion
Reflex irritability	No response	Grimace	Cough or sneeze
Color	Blue, pale	Pink body, blue extremities	All pink

Source: Apgar V: A proposal for a new method of evaluation of the newborn infant, Current Researches in Anesthesia and Analgesia, 32:260, 1953.

the thorax with compression from the two thumbs placed over each other (see Chapter 1). Care should be taken that the thorax not be squeezed circumferentially. Rather, only the superimposed thumbs placed two-thirds down the sternum should provide the compressive force. Compression should be regular and equal at approximately 100–120 beats/min. Adequacy of the compressions should be judged by the strength of the general femoral pulse.

Intravenous access immediately after delivery is best accomplished by the cannulation of the umbilical vein. This is usually a relatively easy procedure once the umbilical cord has been stabilized by an assistant and the vein is visualized. The saline-filled catheter should be advanced aseptically until the tip lies in the inferior vena cava (approximately 7–10 cm). Care should be taken not to position the tip of the catheter in the liver or portal system. This should be suspected if the tip cannot be passed more than 5–6 cm. In this case the tip should be pulled back until it lies 2–3 cm past the umbilical stump.

MECONIUM ASPIRATION

Meconium-stained amniotic fluid often indicates significant fetal distress and should alert the pediatrician to the possibility of a depressed newborn who may require special attention. Thick meconium if aspirated can cause very serious respiratory compromise by direct plugging action, from chemical pneumonitis, and by providing a conducive environment for bacterial invasion. Pulmonary vascular shunting and persistent fetal circulation may accompany a serious meconium aspiration. Therefore if thick meconium is observed in the amniotic fluid, the obstetrician or midwife should vigorously suction the mouth and nares of the child as soon as the head is free but before the child's first respiration. Upon full delivery an oral endotracheal tube should be inserted and suction applied. This can be repeated several times until no further meconium can be suctioned. Careful observation of heart rate, color, and body tone should be made while suctioning is performed.

UPPER AIRWAY OBSTRUCTION

One area in which children are more highly vulnerable than adults to serious complications is the maintenance of an adequate upper airway. In infants and young children the upper airway is often just a few millimeters wide and can easily be obstructed by swelling of intrinsic tissues or by the entrance of a foreign body. The early diagnosis and emergency management of processes that cause airway compromise must be

of primary concern to any physician dealing with pediatric emergencies.

Congenital Anomalies

Early in life an important cause of upper airway obstruction is the manifestation of congenital anomalies. Choanal atresia, stricture, or total stenosis of the posterior nasal apertures may present with significant respiratory distress. Unilateral atresia is often overlooked since it may only be evidenced by persistent rhinorrhea on the involved side. However, bilateral atresia may produce life-threatening respiratory compromise. Since most newborns are obligate nose breathers, nasal obstruction will produce significant distress with sternal and costal retractions as well as cyanosis. Often attempts at feeding make it more difficult for the infant to breath, and distress becomes more severe. In contrast, crying may cause improved air exchange and thus improve appearance. Diagnosis should be suspected if the above symptoms are present and a small bore catheter fails to pass through the nose to the retropharynx. Initial treatment consists of the placement of a stable oral airway until the infant can mouth breath adequately or until definitive surgical correction can be performed.

Several other congenital conditions that cause considerable upper airway obstruction may present early in life. *Congenital laryngeal stridor,* or *tracheomalacia,* represents a group of congenital disorders caused by absence, malformation, or excessive pliability of the cartilaginous rings that maintain the integrity of the tracheal lumen. Vascular ring anomalies are aberrant vessels from aortic or innominate sources that compress the tracheoesophageal complex. Both tracheomalacia and vascular ring anomalies can present with stridor, wheezing, cyanosis, and significant respiratory distress. It is not unusual that these conditions become clinically more severe when a concomitant upper or lower respiratory tract infection is present. These conditions should always be considered whenever an infant presents with respiratory distress associated with the upper airway.

Definitive diagnosis is aided by neck and chest roentgenograms, a barium swallow, bronchoscopy, and echocardiography; ultimately, angiography may be indicated. However, initially it is imperative to ensure that the child is ventilating and oxygenating well. If significant tachypnea, tachycardia, stridor, retractions, or poor air movement on auscultation are present, arterial blood gas measurements and careful monitoring are imperative. Oxygen by mask may be helpful, but intubation to ensure an intact airway may be indicated when adequate oxygenation or ventilation cannot be maintained.

Laryngotracheobronchitis

Laryngotracheobronchitis (LTB), or croup, is a common affliction in children under 3 years of age. Most urban communities experience fall and late winter epidemics in alternate years. The vast majority are viral (parainfluenza types 1 and 3 and respiratory syncytial virus, RSV) and clinically manifest "typical" viral features such as nontoxic appearance, mild inflammation of mucous membranes, and modest amounts of fever (seldom over 39°C, 102°F rectally for more than a few hours).

DIAGNOSIS

Specific clinical signs of stridor, both inspiratory and expiratory, retractions of the soft tissue of the chest on inspiration, and flaring of the alae nasi develop as viral replication in the subglottic space induces edema sufficient to produce airway obstruction. Typically the clinical course shows waxing and waning symptomatology lasting for several days. The high-pitched stridor or crowing sound in conjunction with a harsh brassy cough is characteristic and is often worse at night.

The principal issues are confirmation of diagnosis and choosing inpatient or outpatient management. Soft tissue anterior–posterior radiographs of the neck readily demonstrate narrowing of the subglottic space to confirm clinical impressions. The inclusion of a lateral view at the same time allows exclusion of the major and most serious alternative diagnosis, supraglottitis (see below), as well as the demonstration of any unsuspected foreign body or other cause of airway compromise (Fig. 44.1).

MANAGEMENT

Relatively few patients with croup need to be admitted to the hospital. The indications primarily center around hypoxia and exhaustion. A good relationship between respiratory rate and arterial oxygen tension has been demonstrated when the patient breaths room air. Patients with croup who breath more than 40 times/min will usually be hypoxic. These patients should be admitted for care unless mitigating circumstances are persuasive. Significant intercostal retractions or cyanosis is a clear indication for admission. Exhaustion of the patient is also an indication for admission, regardless of other factors, since breathing against any upper airway obstruction requires stamina. The child who fails to drink adequate amounts of fluids and who has been sleepless for a night or more is at far greater risk of not meeting his or her respiratory demands than the child who at least drinks well, perhaps eats a little and can sleep somewhat. Whatever assessment is made of either hypoxia or exhaustion, the illness is changeable, and a child with croup who looks good in the emergency room may well have been cyanotic at home. In general it is better to err on the side of admitting the patient.

Basic treatment either at home or in the hospital consists of adequate hydration, either orally or intravenously, and humidification of inspired air. Children with croup require at least 100 ml of water per kilogram of body weight per day, and parents should have a specific goal for oral intake if the patient is discharged home. Humidification in the hospital is easily done. However, particulate water (fog) is *not* indicated because of airway irritation. At home, cool mist vaporizers are safe and effective. Running the shower to increase the humidity in the house is apparently helpful. Since most cases occur in winter when the humidity in most homes is low, use of a variety of measures to promote increased humidity should be emphasized.

Specific therapies are reserved for patients who are admitted. Aerosolized racemic epinephrine (0.5 ml in 2 ml of respiratory normal saline) given as a simple aerosol often can temporarily benefit patients with croup. It is unclear whether racemic epinephrine treatment alters a patient's likelihood of requiring ultimate intubation or tracheostomy. Since some patients have an exacerbation of symptoms within 30–90 minutes of racemic epinephrine treatment, use of the drug mandates admission. Treatments can be repeated hourly as needed provided tachycardia or arrhythmias do not contraindicate. Corticosteroids seem to be of some value. Pending definitive study, common practice is to use brief, high-dose regimens of dexamethasone (Decadron) or methylprednisolone (Solumedrol) for hospitalized patients with moderate-to-severe symptomatology. Antibiotics have traditionally not been advocated; however, recent reports of a clinical syndrome identical to croup in association with *Haemophilus influenzae* type B bacteremia suggest this recommendation may change.

Moderate-to-severely ill patients demonstrating deterioration in the hospital or emergency room merit special attention. Close monitoring of vital signs should be instituted, along with sufficient oxygen to avoid hypoxia. Arterial blood gases may deteriorate in less than an hour. Contingency plans for these patients should be made in advance by contacting the anesthesiologist and surgeon *before* the child experiences a respiratory arrest. If the patient is in *extremis* he or she can be aided by bag and mask ventilation synchronized with his or her own respiratory efforts. High pressures may be required, and a bag and mask arrangement with adjustable pressure release valves should be at the bedside at all times.

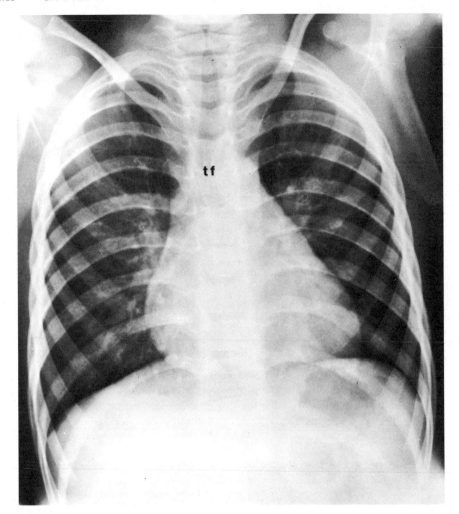

Figure 44.1 Laryngotracheobronchitis: Chest roentgenogram showing narrowing of the subglottic airway.

Supraglottitis (Epiglottitis)

In contrast to the waxing and waning clinical course of croup, supraglottitis is a relentless illness that worsens from onset to airway obstruction in 12–48 hours. Most patients are less than 5 years of age, but illness can strike at any age. Pathologically and anatomically the disease is a local inflammatory process of the entire supraglottic larynx, not just the epiglottis, caused by *H. influenzae*, type B. In most cases the organism can be isolated from blood cultures.

DIAGNOSIS

The illness usually begins abruptly with fever over 39°C (102°F) (rectal) and dysphagia usually manifested by refusal to eat or drink. The child steadily worsens and develops a harsh, guttural inspiratory sound distinct from the "crowing" tone heard in croup. A preference for sitting up with the head and jaw forward becomes increasingly apparent, and a color change is often observed by the family. About 20% of patients have a cough. Late in the course, the patient's dysphagia inhibits swallowing, and saliva is found pooled in the lower jaw and, finally, either drooled by younger children or spat out by older children (Fig. 44.2). From the beginning the patient may indicate substantial pain either in the posterior pharynx or in the midline of the neck above the tracheal cartilage. Thus the triad of fever, dysphagia, and respiratory embarrassment are the features indicative of supraglottitis.

Although supraglottitis is one of the most rapid and feared pediatric emergencies, the patients can initially appear deceptively well. Too often supraglottitis is not recognized for this reason despite the presentation of child with fever, dysphagia, and respiratory symptoms. A less common diagnostic error is to recognize the child as being severely ill but to mistake the head and neck rigidity of supraglottitis for meningismus. The lumbar puncture position in the presence of supraglottitis may fatally compromise the airway.

The diagnosis of supraglottitis is most often made on the basis of the history and the child's clinical appearance alone (Fig. 44.2). As soon as supraglottitis is suspected great care should be taken to disturb the child as little as possible since the child's crying or struggling only increases the likelihood of acute obstruction or exhaustion. Direct visualization of the epiglottitis should not be attempted until control of the airway can be ensured, usually in the operating room. A swollen, raspberry-colored epiglottis is the classic finding; however, inflammation may be confined to the aryepiglottic folds. Therefore a normal appearing tip of the epiglottis should not exclude a diagnosis of supraglottitis. In addition, manipulation of the

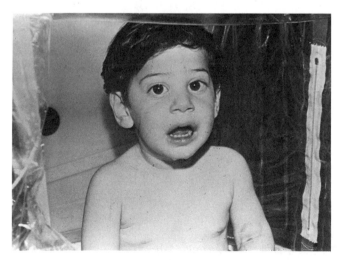

Figure 44.2 Supraglottitis, with characteristic posture, drooling, and protruding jaw.

tongue or posterior pharynx may induce laryngeal spasm, critically obstructing an already compromised airway. All laboratory studies including complete blood cell count (CBC), blood cultures, and blood gases should await the definitive stabilization of the airway.

When the diagnosis is unclear and the child exhibits no evidence of respiratory distress, roentgenographic confirmation of (Fig. 44.3) supraglottitis may be obtained by a lateral neck soft tissue view (Fig. 44.3). If signs of significant or impending respiratory compromise are present, such as stridor, retractions, lethargy, or cyanosis, roentgenographic studies should be omitted. All efforts should once again be directed toward the rapid and controlled placement of a stable artificial airway. When a lateral neck film seems appropriate, it should be carried out rapidly and in the presence of equipment and staff capable of endotracheal intubation or tracheotomy. Characteristic findings of supraglottitis on a lateral neck view are enlarged thumb-shaped epiglottic folds and an enlarged hypopharynx. Straightening of the cervical spine, open mouth, and a protruding mandible are also often seen.

MANAGEMENT

In contrast to croup, supraglottitis requires prompt definitive treatment to avoid a fatal outcome. The foremost concern is the stabilization of the child's airway. All other concerns are of secondary importance. For many years tracheostomy was the primary method of ensuring a patent airway. However, in recent years tracheal intubation has been shown to be both effective and safe in this setting. Nasotracheal intubation is preferred since it tends to be more stable than an oral tube.

The choice between nasotracheal intubation and tracheostomy depends on available resources for initial placement and subsequent nursing care. When both are possible intubation is preferred. Intubation is best done under controlled conditions, usually in the operating room and the patient under general anesthesia. It is useful for an anesthesiologist and otolaryngologist to be called to see the child as soon as the diagnosis of supraglottitis is suspected. They should also accompany the child during transport to the operating room in case the child requires immediate intubation or tracheostomy. Until the child has been transferred to the operating room and intubation carried out, humidified oxygen should be gently administered by mask or funnel. This is often best accomplished by allowing a parent to administer the oxygen when the child is in their arms or close by.

Once the airway is secure, diagnostic studies—CBC, blood cultures, and so on—can be obtained and antibiotics can be started intravenously: chloramphenicol, 25/mg/kg every 6 hours,

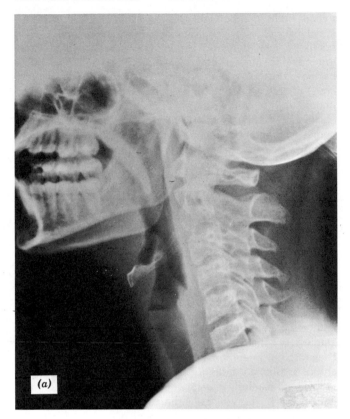 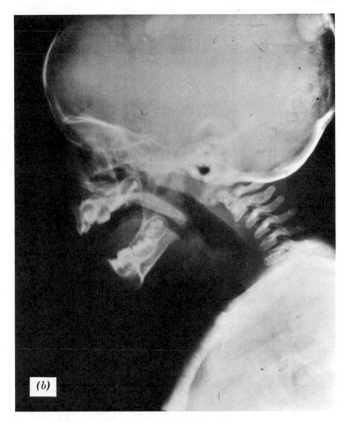

Figure 44.3 Lateral neck soft tissue roentgenograms: (a) normal child; (b) supraglottitis with thumblike enlargement of the epiglottis, enlarged hypopharynx, and obscured vallecula.

if ampicillin-resistant H. influenzae type B are known in the area, or ampicillin, 50 mg/kg every 6 hours, if not. Steroids are not demonstrated to be effective. Extubation can be accomplished in 24–48 hours, and antibiotics can be continued for a total of 7–14 days. Shorter courses of treatment have been demonstrated effective in a small number of cases.

On occasion, a patient with supraglottitis will have a respiratory arrest. It should be remembered that forceful mouth-to-mouth or bag and mask ventilation is almost always effective; it is more likely to be effective, temporarily, than hasty attempts to enter the trachea surgically or with needles, unless the physician is experienced in emergency airway surgery.

Foreign Body Aspiration : *Acute*

A frequent cause of respiratory distress in young children and the leading cause of injury-related deaths in infants is the as-piration of a foreign body. Young children are avid investigators of their environments and tend to place objects in their mouths. Poorly designed or age-inappropriate toys can often be disassembled by the curious toddler, and small parts are frequently placed in the mouth. In addition, foods that the infant or toddler cannot adequately masticate are common aspirated agents. Among the most hazardous are peanuts, hard candy, and gum products.

DIAGNOSIS

The clinical impact of foreign bodies is determined by their nature, size, and the relative degree of airway obstruction they produce. The onset and severity of symptoms depend on the adequacy of subsequent air exchange. Large or oddly shaped foreign bodies may cause severe obstruction, usually occurring at the laryngeal level. The onset of symptoms is sudden and is accompanied by choking, gagging, high-pitched wheezing, or weak cough with dysphonia or aphonia. The child usually appears anxious and in significant distress. In this severe form of aspiration, cyanosis and gradual loss of consciousness usually occur if the foreign body is not expelled or mobilized in a manner that allows more adequate air exchange.

MANAGEMENT

When the acute aspiration is witnessed and subsequent air exchange is inadequate, a series of back blows and chest thrusts usually prove useful. Infants should be supported over the rescuer's forearm with the chin held in the rescuer's hand. The head should be held lower than the body. While the infant is in this position, four sharp back blows should be administered between the infant's scapulae. If this maneuver is not successful, the child should be turned face up and placed on the rescuer's thigh. Four chest thrusts (as in standard cardiopulmonary resuscitation, CPR) should then be delivered. In the older child, the back blows and chest thrusts are performed with the child draped over the rescuer's thighs. Although some physicians still recommend the abdominal thrust (Heimlich maneuver), the latest protocols of the American Heart Association (AHA) discourage this practice in children under 8 years old because of the potential to induce injury to abdominal organs. Blind finger sweeps are usually contraindicated since they often advance the foreign body further down the airway. Instead, if the back blows and chest thrusts prove unsuccessful, the jaw should be lifted and the mouth opened in order to try to visualize the foreign body. If the object is seen, it should be manually removed; if it is not seen, the back blows and chest thrusts should be repeated.

If the child becomes unconscious, artificial ventilation should be begun. Bag and mask ventilation with 100% oxygen should be begun as soon as possible. When there is enough pressure, this method usually provides adequate air exchange since few foreign body obstructions are complete. However, if signs of continued inadequate air exchange persist (poor chest excursion, absent breath sounds, cyanosis), the head should be repositioned and equipment quickly checked. If this provides no improvement, an emergency cricothyrotomy (Procedure 9) should relieve the obstruction on most occasions. A large-bore needle or catheter (14 or 16 gauge) can be inserted into the trachea through the cricothyroid membrane (Procedure 7). If personnel skilled in emergency placement of a tracheostomy tube are available, this procedure should be performed. Again, these invasive procedures are rarely required in managing an aspirated foreign body, and their use is indicated only when the steps outlined above prove unsuccessful.

The above maneuvers should be attempted only when a foreign body prohibits adequate air exchange. If the child is coughing well, can vocalize normally, remains pink, and is not in imminent danger of becoming unconscious, no attempt to remove the foreign body should be made until its location has been documented and definitive removal (e.g., bronchoscopy) under optimal conditions can be attempted. Also, it is important to remember that the presentation of upper airway obstruction may be caused by intrinsic tissues as well as foreign bodies. Supraglottitis, croup, hemangiomas, and aberrant thoracic vessels can also cause airway obstruction. The presence of fever and preceding symptomology usually will differentiate a foreign body aspiration from an intrinsic disease.

Foreign Body Aspiration: *Subacute or Chronic*

Although the acute presentation of severe foreign body obstruction can be catastrophic, the common presentation is more subtle. The chief complaint may reflect symptoms due to complications of the foreign body, and the experience of the actual aspiration may be unwitnessed or forgotten. In this light, the possibility of foreign body aspiration must be considered in both acute and chronic pulmonary conditions in children regardless of whether a history of aspiration can be elicited. Diagnoses of pneumonia (particularly recurrent), bronchitis, croup, or asthma should not be made in children under 5 years old without carefully considering the presence of an aspirated foreign body. The nonacute clinical manifestations of an aspirated foreign body are usually related to the level of the subsequent obstruction. Laryngeal foreign bodies cause hoarseness, recurrent cough (often "croupy" in nature), and at times discomfort. Dyspnea with wheezing or recurrent stridor may occur. Often the severity of these findings is secondary to the increasing inflammatory reaction induced by the foreign body rather than from the foreign body itself.

Tracheal foreign bodies may produce persistent or recurrent cough, bilateral wheeze, dyspnea, and at times hoarseness because of inflammatory changes in the subglottic area. A characteristic audible slap and palpable thump may be found with expiration as the foreign body strikes the subglottic area. Upon inspiration an audible wheeze is usually heard.

Bronchial foreign bodies are the most common form of aspirated foreign bodies. Although it has often been noted that a majority of bronchial foreign bodies reside on the right (since the right mainstem bronchus departs from the trachea at a less acute angle than the left) a left-sided bronchial foreign body is not uncommon. Localized or unilateral wheezing should suggest a foreign body. Localized emphysema or air trapping may occur when the foreign body acts as a ball valve allowing air entry but preventing its exit. This will be reflected on physical examination by a mediastinal shift to the contralateral side with hyperresonance over the obstructed area. Often a foreign body causes distal atelectesis and at times bacterial infection. Here physical findings may mimic those of bacterial pneumonia.

Often a foreign body caught in the retropharynx or esophagus can cause significant respiratory symptoms. A severe inflammatory response can cause swelling and induration which may subsequently compress the airway. Therefore when an aspirated foreign body is suspected, a foreign body lodged in the food passage should also be carefully considered.

DIAGNOSIS

Crucial to the diagnosis of foreign body aspiration is the use of appropriate roentgenographic studies. If the foreign body is radiopaque, its location can be readily identified. However,

many aspirated foreign bodies are not radiopaque, thereby requiring that their existence and location be deduced by indirect means.

If a laryngeal foreign body is suspected both anteroposterior (AP) and lateral neck films are indicated. Views in both planes are helpful in order to distinguish whether the foreign body lies in the airway (anteriorly) or food passage (posteriorly). Tracheal foreign bodies that are not radiopaque can still often be seen from AP chest films since they may be outlined by the lucency of air in the tracheal lumen.

In the case of bronchial foreign bodies, the classical approach has relied upon documenting paradoxical movement of the diaphragms or unilateral obstructive emphysema with a subsequent mediastinal shift to the contralateral side (Holzknecht sign) (Fig. 44.4). Therefore inspiratory and expiratory AP chest films may be diagnostic. However, flouroscopy usu-

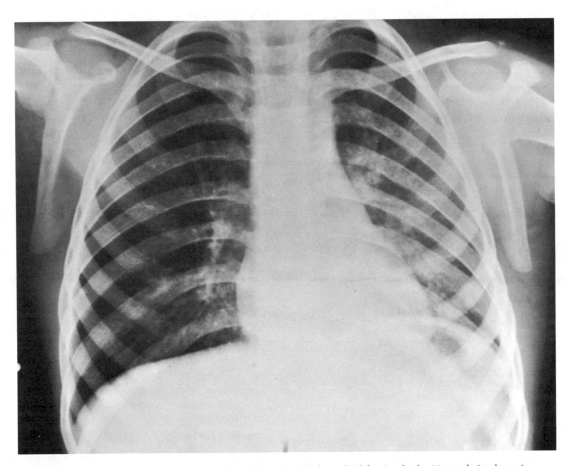

Figure 44.4 Chest roentgenogram of a child with right bronchial foreign body. Note relative hyperinflation of right lung.

ally yields more definitive information particularly in the small child. Lateral decubitus films are often helpful in revealing unilateral air trapping. When the patient is in the lateral decubitis position, the hemidiaphragm of the dependent lung should be higher than the other hemidiaphragms. If the reverse is true, significant air trapping is present.

MANAGEMENT

Aspirated foreign bodies should be regarded as true emergencies only when air exchange is significantly compromised, or when the foreign body may imminently migrate into a more serious position. As stated earlier, emergency mechanical efforts to dislodge a foreign body should be attempted only when air exchange is inadequate to sustain life. In all other cases no attempt to mobilize the foreign body is indicated until definitive bronchoscopy can be performed. It is best that endoscopy be done under the most optimal conditions; therefore proceeding hastily into bronchoscopy as an "emergency" is discouraged unless adequate air exchange is threatened. The development of pediatric fiberoptic bronchoscopes with appropriate tenacula has made the removal of tracheal and bronchial foreign bodies less difficult and should be employed for this purpose. Inhalation and percussive therapy was recommended by some physicians at one time; however, it now is strongly discouraged. Incidents of cardiorespiratory arrest following the migration of the foreign body to the trachea during inhalation and percussive therapy outweigh the minimal documented advantages of this technique. In cases in which a pneumonia process is suspected distal to the foreign body, appropriate cultures during bronchoscopy are advised. Antibiotic therapy is also indicated when such a process is evident.

The prognosis for children in whom aspirated foreign bodies are not removed is not favorable. Persistent infection and deterioration of adequate air exchange will usually occur. Mortality in children in whom aspirated foreign bodies are not removed is quite high. The importance of considering the presence of an aspirated foreign body in all children with respiratory symptoms cannot be overstated.

Children who have had aspirated foreign bodies successfully removed usually have few complications. Infectious conditions may require continued antibiotic therapy after the foreign body has been removed, particularly when the foreign body was long standing. Inflammatory changes may produce fibrotic changes that occasionally will interfere with normal air flow. Persistent atelectasis, pneumonitis, pneumonia, or emphysema should raise the question of a remaining fragment or second foreign body.

FEVER IN INFANTS AND YOUNG CHILDREN

A young child with fever presents a common yet challenging problem for the emergency room physician. Elevated temperature in a child may be a sign of a potentially serious illness; therefore its presence makes a careful and thorough evaluation imperative. At times, recognizable febrile illnesses can be readily diagnosed. Some of the more important of these are discussed below. When localizing symptoms or signs are present, the nature of the evaluation can be concentrated on these findings. However, in recent years the importance of silent, or "occult," bacterial illness in young children has increasingly become more evident. Bacteremia without an apparent source of focus of infection has now become a significant concern when evaluating the young febrile child. In addition, recent data have substantiated the claim that other forms of serious bacterial illness including pneumonia and meningitis often present with a paucity of clinical signs. Therefore in febrile children without evidence of a specific source of infection, the clinician may need to rely on the rational use of laboratory tests to better identify the etiology of the fever. The nature of the evaluation is defined by the dual goals of isolating the source of the fever while not subjecting the child to unnecessary laboratory or radiologic tests.

The complexity of the clinical problem coupled with relative lack of relevant data on the subject has made the evaluation of young children with fever one of the more controversial areas in pediatrics. However, recent work, particularly that by Teele and associates in Boston and McCarthy in New Haven, has provided information critical to the development of a coherent approach. Age of the child is an important factor in assessing the risk of serious bacterial illness. An infant under 3 months of age has an immature immune response, and fever is a dangerous sign of possible bacterial infection. During this period they are at risk for sepsis, pneumonia, and meningitis from gram-negative organisms and group B, β-hemolytic streptococci. Children 3–24 months predominantly suffer from bacteremia and deep tissue invasion from *Streptococcus pneumoniae* (pneumonococcus), and *H. influenza* type B. In children over 24 months of age, bacterial illness usually takes the form of a recognizable local infection and more rarely involves occult disease.

DIAGNOSIS

History

The response of a young child to an illness is usually nonspecific in nature and is manifested by deviations in usual feeding and sleeping patterns and in response to environmental stimuli. Lethargy, poor feeding, and irritability may be important and at times the primary symptoms of serious infectious illness. Careful questioning of the child's usual caretaker can often yield valuable information regarding the relative expression of a febrile illness. The history should ascertain the time, course, and severity of the above symptoms. Objective definition of the scope of the observed alterations, including specific amount of fluid ingested and number of hours asleep, may be helpful. Symptoms related to specific processes should also be reviewed. Nasal congestion, cough, rash, swelling, limp, and other localizing symptoms may provide clues to the underlying etiology of the fever.

The presence of high temperature in a young child increases the chance of a serious bacterial illness. As the temperature elevation increases so does the risk of bacteremia and/or bacterial soft tissue invasion. In one series reported by Teele et al., 3.2% of 600 consecutive febrile children under 24 months old with rectal temperatures of 38.3°C (101°F) were bacteremic. In another study, reported by McCarthy, children under 24 months with temperatures of 40.5–41°C (105–105.8°F), 13% were bacteremic. Twenty-three percent of children presenting with temperatures of greater than 41.1°C (106°F) had positive blood cultures. Therefore the degree of temperature elevation is a primary indicator for serious bacterial invasion.

Physical Examination

On physical examination assessment of the child's general appearance is critical. A lethargic, anxious child with poor posture and a weak cry should alert the clinician to the likelihood that the child is seriously ill. Accurate measurement of vital signs is imperative. A careful blood pressure determination should be taken on any child in whom systemic infection is suspected. Respiratory rate is often somewhat elevated in febrile children. However, a significantly increased respiratory rate may be an important sign of respiratory infection, particularly pneumonia, or respiratory compensation for metabolic acidosis. Tachycardia also may be present secondary to fever, but marked tachycardia or bradycardia suggest a severe stress. Examination of the skin should be extremely thorough. The presence of petichiae, purpura, or diffuse rash may have an important impact on management.

Despite careful examination, serious illness in a significant number of febrile children under 2 years old will not be appreciated by the examiner. A large portion of children with pneumococcal bacteremia and pneumonia and a significant percentage of infants with meningitis may present with silent illness. It is in this light that a number of laboratory and radio-

logic tests have been recommended to assist in the identification of these serious occult illnesses. If the history and/or physical examination reveal meningismus, a swollen joint, rales, or other signs of a specific bacterial illness, appropriate studies can be performed accordingly. However, when the history and examination reveal no specific source of fever, an assessment of the following critical risk factors of occult illness will help decide the nature of further investigation and management.

Laboratory Evaluation

If the child is less than 3 months old and the temperature is 39°C (102°F) or higher or if physical examination or history is suspicious, then a full septic workup including a blood, urine, and cerebrospinal fluid (CSF) examinations and cultures and chest roentgenogram are indicated. Several studies have pointed out the inability of the above tests to identify reliably all infants in this age group who have serious bacterial diseases. Therefore the usual practice is to admit these children after the septic workup for close observation and parenteral antibiotic therapy pending cultures. Some physicians have recently suggested that careful outpatient monitoring is sufficient for some of these infants, however, it is hoped that further studies will substantiate this policy and better identify which children can be managed in this manner.

When an elevated white blood cell (WBC) count and erythrocyte sedimentation rate (ESR) have been performed together, they have been shown to be fairly sensitive indicators of serious bacterial illness. A WBC greater than or equal to 15,000/mm³ and an ESR greater than or equal to 30 suggests such an illness must be ruled out. Therefore in any child less than 2 years of age, whose temperature is greater than or equal to 39.5°C (103°F) rectally, and who has no specific source on examination or history, a WBC and ESR should be done. If both are elevated, a blood culture should be obtained. Several studies have revealed that a large portion of roentgenogram positive pneumonias in this age group are not diagnosed on history or physical examination and are associated with an elevation in WBC and ESR. Therefore in this setting, a chest roentgenogram should also be obtained. If this is negative, a urinalysis and culture should be considered in children in whom symptoms are compatible with a urinary tract infection such as mild gastrointestinal symptoms, abdominal pain, or a lack of respiratory or otic findings. A bagged urine specimen is often adequate; however, when a urinary tract infection is suspected or when a bagged urinalysis is abnormal, a suprapubic bladder aspiration should be performed.

When to perform a lumbar puncture (LP) in these children can often be a difficult decision. Of course, if signs of meningeal irritation or bulging fontanelle are present, the LP should be performed. However, in young children, particularly under 1 year old, meningeal signs including Brudzinzki's and Kernig's signs are often absent; therefore reliance on risk factors becomes important. For children with temperature greater than 39.5°C (103°F) and who have an elevated WBC and ESR, an LP should be seriously considered. Observing the child in a situation more comfortable than on the examining table is often helpful. This period of optimal observation is designed to assess the child's behavioral response to the illness in an effort to rule out meningitis or at least the need for LP. Whether the child is alert and playful on his or her parent's lap or remains inconsolable, irritable or lethargic, should influence the decision. A temperature of 41°C (105.8°F) or greater and/or a WBC of 20,000 or greater in an infant are usually indications for an LP.

MANAGEMENT

If the above examinations reveal no specific source of infection in a child under 2 years old who has high temperature and elevated WBC and ESR, treatment for presumptive bacteremia should be considered. Controversy remains intense on this topic; however, many physicians now advocate antimicrobial therapy. The hope is that this therapy will eliminate any bacteremia that may be present, as well as prevent seeding of deep tissues by the invading organism. Recommendations for treatment are aimed at eradicating the two most prominent offending organisms in this age group—S. pneumoniae and H. influenzae. Therefore amoxicillin at 30 mg/kg/day is usually prescribed. In certain areas, ampicillin-resistant H. influenzae is common, but the standard use of oral chloramphenicol cannot be recommended at this time. Trimethoprim–sulfa methoxazole may be an effective alternative to amoxicillin in penicillin-allergic children. Cefaclor has also been used, although recent case reports of its possible failure to prevent seeding of the meninges may make its use questionable until further studies can definitely determine its use in this regard. It should be remembered, however, that before treatment is considered, blood, urine, and, when appropriate, CSF cultures and a chest roentgenogram should first be obtained. Despite the controversy over treatment, all agree that careful follow-up of children who are not admitted is imperative.

Treatment of the admitted child under 3 months of age should be with penicillin (100,000 units/kg/day) or ampicillin (200 mg/kg/day) intravenously coupled with an aminoglycoside such as kanamycin or gentamicin (5–7.5 mg/kg/day) effective against gram-negative organisms. These should be continued until cultures are confirmed as negative after 72 hours. If the cultures are positive, antibiotic therapy can be altered according to

sensitivity determination of the isolated organism. Children over 4 months old who are admitted for parenteral therapy pending cultures for presumed bacteremia should be treated with penicillin (2–300,000 units/kg/day) or ampicillin (200 mg/kg/day) and chloramphenicol (75–100 mg/kg/day) in situations in which ampicillin-resistant H. influenzae are significant.

SPECIFIC INFECTIOUS CONDITIONS

Otitis Media

Otitis media is the most commonly diagnosed bacterial infection in children. It primarily occurs in children under 2 years old, but may present on into adulthood. Although it is not in itself an emergent condition, it is an important cause of generalized symptoms and fever in young children. In addition, if not recognized, it can progress to cause serious hearing impairment and discomfort, as well as bacteremia and its complications.

Many studies have documented that two organisms—S. pneumoniae (pneumococcus) and H. influenzae—are the predominant causal agents of otitis media. Streptococcus pneumoniae accounts for most cases of otitis media in all age groups. Haemophilus influenzae is responsible for a larger portion of cases of otitis media in younger children than in older children and adults. Other etiologic agents include group A β-hemolytic streptococci, Staphylococcus aureus, Neisseria catarrhalis, Escherichia coli, Pseudomonas aeruginosa, and Klebsiella pneumoniae.

DIAGNOSIS

Symptoms of otitis media may be systemic in nature or specific to the affected ear. In younger children generalized symptoms such as irritability, poor feeding, and vomiting are common. In older children complaints of a painful ear with or without systemic signs are common. Fever often accompanies otitis media; however, it should be remembered that fever may be absent in the presence of active infection. The incidence of high temperature (39.5°C; 103°F) with uncomplicated otitis media remains unclear. It seems apparent that otitis media alone can cause high temperature in young children, but serious bacterial illness may present in conjunction with otitis media. In one study of 49 cases of serious occult bacterial illness unrecognized on physical examination, 16 cases were diagnosed as having otitis media (seven instances of pneumonia with otitis media). Therefore the presence of otitis media should not preclude a careful physical examination or laboratory evaluation if a high temperature or other risk factors are present.

Otoscopic examination should be directed at recognizing signs of active disease. Discharge in the canal can be indicative of an otitis externa without involvement of the middle ear or can indicate a perforation of the tympanic membrane with resultant escape of purulent fluid. The contour and color of the tympanic membrane is often altered by an acute infection. Fullness or bulging of the tympanic membrane is usually a result of increased pressure in the middle ear. If there is an acute infection, the usual pearly gray color of the membrane may appear deep red or whitish. The most sensitive diagnostic sign is a decrease in the mobility of the tympanic membrane to pneumotoscopy. Immobility upon gentle insufflation is indicative of an abnormal tympanic membrane. No one sign is diagnostic of acute otitis media. Rather the grouping of several suspicious findings should guide the clinician in making this diagnosis. Impedence testing, if available, can be useful in confirming the presence of otitis media.

MANAGEMENT

The treatment of otitis media is usually based upon age, which best reflects the relative predominance of S. pneumoniae as a causative agent. Children under 2 months old with otitis media may have significant difficulty in localizing the infectious process. Therefore a child in this age group should be carefully evaluated for evidence of more serious diseases. A child in this age group with otitis media and high temperature should receive a CBC, ESR, blood culture, and LP. Many hospitals admit these children for intravenous therapy at least until blood and CSF cultures are confirmed negative after 72 hours. Antibiotic therapy is similar to that used in cases of suspected septicemia in the neonate. Before therapy is begun, a tympanocentesis by an experienced physician for Gram stain examination and culture is indicated.

Children up to 10 years old who have otitis media should receive ampicillin (100 mg/kg/day), amoxicillin (50 mg/kg/day), or a combination of erythromycin (30 mg/kg/day) and a sulfonamide. Combined trimethoprim–sulfamethoxazole, as well as cefaclor are often used as secondary drugs for patients with otitis media. Further data are presently needed to judge fully the relative effectiveness of these drugs in treating patients with acute otitis media.

Pneumonia

Infection of the lower respiratory tract in a child should be viewed as a serious illness requiring a determined effort to identify the offending organism and close monitoring of the child's clinical course. Pneumonia, particularly in young children, can cause significant respiratory compromise, as well as serve as a site for blood stream and other soft tissue invasion by the infectious agent.

DIAGNOSIS

In an infant or young child pneumonia may present with only nonspecific complaints. Fever, irritability, poor feeding, lethargy, vomiting, and vague abdominal pain may be the only symptoms present. On examination tachypnea should alert the clinician to the possible presence of a pneumonic process. In more severe cases nasal flaring, grunting, subcostal retractions, cyanosis, decreased breath sounds, and rales may be present. However, pneumonia in infants and young children is often clinically silent. Auscultation or percussion of the chest is often unremarkable in young children who have a significant pneumonia present. McCarthy reported that out of 52 cases of pneumonia in children under 2 years old, 27 were not identified by history and physical examination. Therefore it is crucial that a child presenting with fever and nonspecific symptoms and no obvious source of infection be evaluated for pneumonia. An elevated WBC and ESR puts the child at high risk for an occult pneumonia and a chest roentgenogram should be obtained in all such cases.

In older children, pneumonia is more likely to present with more specific pulmonary findings, such as cough, chest pain, abnormal breath sounds, localized dullness, and rales. These symptoms may be accompanied by generalized symptoms including fever, chills, malaise, abdominal pain, or headache.

When pneumonia is suggested a reasonable effort to identify the bacterial etiologic agent should be made. Blood cultures in children under 4 years old or in older children with high temperatures are usually indicated. Sputum Gram stain and cultures can be helpful, though sputum can be difficult to obtain in children. Tracheal aspirate should be obtained if unresponsive or severe infection is evident.

MANAGEMENT

Pneumonia in children under 5 years old is most commonly caused by viral agents. The most common bacterial etiology is S. pneumoniae (pneumococcus). Haemophilus influenzae type B is also a significant cause of pneumonia in children. Penicillin (penicillin G 100,000 units/kg/day or penicillin V 100 mg/kg/day) is the therapy of choice for pneumococcal pneumonia. For a pneumonia of unknown etiology in which H. influenzae must be considered, ampicillin (100 mg/kg/day) should be prescribed. In areas in which H. influenzae shows significant resistance to ampicillin, alternative therapy should be considered for pneumonias unresponsive to ampicillin therapy or for severe pneumonias requiring hospitalization. Trimethoprim–sulfisoxazole and cefaclor have been suggested as efficacious alternatives to ampicillin for oral therapy. For more severe infections intravenous chloramphenicol (100 mg/kg/day) in association with a semisynthetic penicillin effective against *S. aureas* (oxacillin 100 mg/kg/day) should be administered. Again, a strong effort to isolate the offending organism should be made, and antibiotic therapy should be reassessed once the organism and sensitivities are known.

Children over 5 years old who are suspected of having bacterial pneumonia should be treated with penicillin G (100,000 units/kg/day) or penicillin V (100 mg/kg/day). Mycoplasmal pneumonia is a more common causative agent in older children and adolescents. On chest roentgenograms the infiltrates are usually more diffuse, presenting a bronchopneumonic picture. The children are usually less ill appearing, have a low-grade or no fever, and show fewer systemic signs. Cold agglutinins may help to confirm the presence of a mycoplasmal infection. Erythromycin (40 mg/kg/day) is the recommended therapy.

Children under 2 months of age who have pneumonia should be considered at high risk for sepsis and respiratory compromise. Therefore these children should receive a full septic workup and antibiotic therapy (see sepsis).

Hospitalization of children with pneumonia is indicated if there is significant respiratory distress. Tachypnea, retractions, cyanosis, or hypoxia and/or hypercarbia on arterial blood gas should, under most circumstances, warrant admission for close observation, intravenous antibiotics, and, if needed, respiratory support. Additional factors that suggest hospital admission include uncertain observation and medical follow-up, underlying medical conditions making a deep tissue infection especially worrisome (e.g., sickle cell disease, cystic fibrosis, immune deficiency states, cardiac disease), or excessive caretaker anxiety or exhaustion.

Bronchiolitis

Bronchiolitis is a common lower respiratory tract infection that occurs in children under the age of 3. The etiology is viral in nature; it primarily occurs in the winter and spring, often in an epidemic fashion. Respiratory syncytial virus (RSV) is the most common causative agent of bronchiolitis. Inflammation of the small bronchi and bronchioles cause significant swelling and occlusion of the airways. Expiratory obstruction with gas trapping can become severe, and lung volume increases as compliance falls. As the process continues, gas exchange can deteriorate since the child can no longer compensate for the markedly increased respiratory workload. Hypoxia and respiratory failure can occur, particularly in infants.

DIAGNOSIS

The onset of illness usually begins with an upper respiratory tract infection that may last for several days. Breathing subsequently becomes labored with retractions, hyperinflation, and diffuse wheezing. Fever is usually mild, which may help differentiate bronchiolitis from a bacterial process. In mild cases the patient is alert and playful, demonstrating good oxygenation. Oral intake of fluids remains good and the respiratory rate remains below 40 breaths per minute. In more severe cases oral fluid intake falls because of increasing tachypnea (usually above 50 per minute), and hypoxia can be demonstrated on arterial blood gases. Restlessness, agitation, and anxiety are often indications of hypoxia. As the child tires the respiratory rate may fall, which is a sign that respiratory failure is imminent. Roentgenographic studies are useful to help exclude other diagnoses including pneumonia or foreign body aspiration. Chest films in bronchiolitis usually reveal hyperinflation and hyperlucency reflecting air trapping. Blood studies other than arterial blood gases are usually not helpful.

MANAGEMENT

Therapy is primarily determined by the severity of respiratory insufficiency. Mild cases can be managed at home with the parents ensuring good fluid intake and carefully observing for signs of worsening. A cool mist vaporizer may be helpful in this setting. When oral fluid intake is inadequate, retractions are significant, or the respiratory rate is above 50 breaths per minute, hospital admission is probably advised. Arterial blood gases may be helpful in documenting hypoxia.

In the absence of clear bacterial disease, such as pneumonia or otitis media, antibiotics are not indicated. Bronchiodilator therapy remains controversial; however, a trial of bronchodilator therapy similar to that used in patients with asthma is probably useful. Intravenous fluids are required only when the oral route is inadequate. Oxygen therapy should be used in accordance with the relative degree of hypoxia. On occasion, severe respiratory insufficiency requires intubation and mechanical ventilation.

Bronchiolitis may be indistinguishable from early onset asthma. Physical findings and history are quite similar in both illnesses, and their differentiation may have to await the passage of time and the ultimate expression of the disease process. Bronchiolitis may recur; however, multiple bouts of wheezing and respiratory symptoms that respond to bronchodilators suggests a diagnosis of asthma.

Other causes of wheezing should also be considered, particularly if the clinical course is atypical. Localized wheezing suggests foreign body aspiration or an anomalous vessel compressing the bronchus. Persistent wheezing raises the possibility of aspiration syndromes: gastric reflux and aspiration, aspiration while feeding, or tracheoesophageal fistula. Primary congestive heart failure and cystic fibrosis must also be included in the differential diagnosis.

Periorbital Cellulitis

In children, periorbital cellulitis is a serious bacterial infection involving the tissues surrounding the eye. It can present at any age but is more commonly associated with systemic disease in young children.

DIAGNOSIS

Typically the child presents with a warm, red, swelling around one eye. Fever may be present, particularly in young children. A history of recent trauma or break in the continuity of the skin near the eye (laceration, insect bite, varicella lesion) is seen in a number of cases. Conjunctival erythema may also be present. If proptosis, ophthalmoplegia, or impairment of vision is present, orbital involvement is likely and immediate ophthamalogic intervention is required.

In making the diagnosis of periorbital cellulitis, the physician must also consider deeper infections in one of the frontal or ethmoid sinuses that may be related to the surface manifestation. In cases in which there is any doubt about the diagnosis, sinus films or computed tomography (CT) can help elucidate the differential diagnosis.

Cultures of any associated wound or discharge may help identify the offending organism. In febrile or young children, blood cultures are important. In infants, careful consideration of the need for LP is mandatory since meningitis can be associated with a periorbital cellulitis.

MANAGEMENT

Haemophilus influenzae, S. aureas, and group A *Streptococcus* are the most common causative organisms. Therefore antibiotic therapy usually includes ampicillin (100 mg/kg/day) or if ampicillin-resistant *H. influenzae* exist, chloramphenicol (100 mg/kg/day) and a semisynthetic penicillin effective against *S. aureus,* such as oxacillin (100 mg/kg/day). These should be administered intravenously until clinical improvement is evident, at which time oral therapy may be considered. Observation for signs of orbital involvement or associated infectious processes is an important aspect of therapy.

SEIZURES

As many as 4% of all children will have at least one seizure during their first 15 years of life. Whereas the etiology of child-hood seizures is diverse, the most common form is the simple febrile seizure.

Status Epilepticus

DIAGNOSIS

A careful history should be taken to identify underlying disease processes and direct causes for the seizure. Special attention should be paid to the quality and length of seizure activity, the presence of fever or other symptoms (headache, stiff neck, poor feeding, irritability), and the possibility of a history of recent trauma. Past history of seizures or other chronic conditions, prescribed medications and compliance, the possibility of an ingestion, and a family history for seizure disorders should also be covered.

The physical examination is designed to illuminate any direct cause of seizure activity and should be brief but purposeful. Vital signs, air movement, chest wall excursion, and skin color (perfusion, cyanosis, hypopigmented areas) should be carefully reviewed. Evidence of trauma (bruises, lacerations, swelling) or sepsis (petichia, purpura) should be investigated. Pupil size and reaction, disc margins and retinal field findings (papilledema, hemorrhage), muscle tone, reflexes, and cerebellar signs should also be carefully examined.

TREATMENT

The treatment of a child in status epilepticus should begin with the assurance of adequate ventilation and oxygenation. Careful monitoring of vital signs and air movement, as well as subsequent arterial blood gas values, if required, will indicate the adequacy of cardiorespiratory function. If significant compromise is suspected, artificial ventilation with 100% oxygen should be begun by bag and mask or, if required, endotracheal intubation. The primacy of airway management of the seizing child cannot be overstated. Blood for immediate bedside glucose determination (Dextrostix), as well CBC, calcium, urea nitrogen, magnesium, electrolytes, toxic screen, and anticonvulsant levels should be drawn.

The purpose of pharmacologic intervention is the cessation of seizure activity without significant cardiorespiratory suppression. A number of agents are helpful in treating status epilepticus, but some variation exists in their use.

Once adequate oxygenation and ventilation have been ensured, a stable intravenous line can be placed. A glucose-containing solution (5% or 10% dextrose) with 0.25 or 0.5 normal saline may be used, since blood glucose levels 100–150 mg/dl should be maintained.

Diazepam (Valium) is useful for terminating seizures quickly, but it has a short half-life and can be relied upon only for a transient effect. The initial dose is 0.1–0.25 mg/kg given no faster than 1 mg/min. Maximum initial dose is 10 mg. If no response is seen after 15 minutes, a second dose of 0.25–0.4 mg/kg with a maximum dose of 15 mg can be given. Diazepam is capable of causing significant respiratory depression and should never be given until equipment and staff to assist in ventilation are made available.

The mainstay of therapy is the judicious use of diphenylhydantoin (Dilantin). Its effectiveness and relative long duration of action make it a useful adjunct to diazepam administration. In patients with chronic, recurring seizures diphenylhydantoin can be used as the first drug. The onset of action is usually between 20–40 minutes and therefore should not be used if immediate cessation of the seizure is paramount; diazepam is the more appropriate first drug in this setting. If diazepam is given initially, diphenylhydantoin should be begun approximately 15 minutes after the initial diazepam dose. Diphenylhydantoin is given 10–15 mg/kg infused slowly in normal saline over 20 minutes. Since cardiac arrythmias are the most important complication in diphenylhydantoin therapy, careful cardiac monitoring is essential.

If after giving the patient diazepam and diphenylhydantoin seizure activity persists, paraldehyde in a dose of 0.3–0.4 ml/kg diluted with peanut or corn oil (10:1, oil:paraldehyde) can be administered rectally. This can be repeated hourly if necessary. If seizure activity continues, 10 mg/kg phenobarbital may be given intravenously over 10–15 minutes. Care should be taken in using phenobarbital in conjunction with diazepam since respiratory and cardiovascular depression is more common than with each agent alone. If seizure activity continues despite the above outlined therapy, general anesthesia may be indicated. Curarization is sometimes useful to lessen the systemic effects of seizure activity and better allow assistance of ventilation. However, it should be remembered that the use of a paralytic agent does not terminate aberrant cerebral discharge. It is also important that underlying etiologic conditions must be ruled out in patients with prolonged seizures. The possibility of trauma, intracranial infection, increased intracranial pressure, bleeding congenital vascular anomalies, or ingestion of toxic substances or medication should always be considered.

Febrile Seizures

As noted before, simple febrile seizures are the most common form of seizures in young children. They usually occur in children between the ages 3 months and 5 years and are associated with fever but not with a central nervous system infection, metabolic abnormality, or other direct cause. Seizures in febrile children with a past history of nonfebrile seizures cannot be considered simple febrile seizures. In addition, simple febrile seizures are distinct from epilepsy, a condition defined by recurrent nonfebrile seizures.

DIAGNOSIS

A careful history and physical examination will usually identify seizures in children with fevers caused by an underlying metabolic, traumatic, or infectious condition. Electrolyte, calcium, glucose, and other metabolic determinations are probably only useful when the history (e.g., vomiting, diarrhea, dehydration) or physical examination suggests the possibility of metabolic abnormality. Skull films or computed tomography, are not indicated unless a history of physical finding suggests trauma or mass effect.

Since seizure with fever is an important presentation of bacterial meningitis, an LP may be useful. If meningitis is suspected on the basis of history, physical examination, or risk factors (high temperature, elevated WBC and ESR, irritability or lethargy upon optimal observation), then an LP should be performed after a normal retinal examination. Since children under 1 year of age who have meningitis may have few clinical signs, an LP is probably indicated in infants presenting with their first febrile seizure.

Febrile seizures that are longer than 15 minutes, focal in nature, and associated with transient or permanent neurologic abnormalities have a higher probability of being associated with an underlying infection or metabolic or traumatic disorder. Therefore the above laboratory examinations may prove more useful in evaluating these "nonsimple" febrile seizures.

MANAGEMENT

Children who experience a febrile seizure generally enjoy good health and development. A recent National Institutes of Health (NIH) consensus panel found that there are only two important risks associated with febrile seizures: a 30–40% chance of having a second febrile seizure in children not placed on prophylactic anticonvulsant therapy and a slightly increased risk of subsequent epilepsy. More important, they documented no data suggesting subsequent neurologic or developmental impairment as a result of the febrile seizure. Prophylaxis against further febrile seizures, usually with daily phenobarbital, has been a controversial area. It will help prevent subsequent febrile seizures, but there is no evidence that phenobarbital therapy or the prevention of recurred febrile seizures will prevent the development of epilepsy. This, coupled with an appreciation of the side effects of phenobarbital, have led to the panel's recommendation that in patients with simple febrile seizures prophylaxis is not indicated. Intermittent prophylaxis when the child becomes febrile is ineffective in controlling febrile seizures. However, prophylaxis could be considered if any of the following is true:

1. The febrile seizure was longer than 15 minutes, focal, or associated with neurologic deficit
2. There is a family history of nonfebrile seizure disorders
3. Examination showed a preexistent abnormal neurologic condition

Again, there is no evidence that prophylaxis even in the group defined above will prevent subsequent nonfebrile seizure disorders.

The most important therapeutic step is in helping the family members to understand and cope with the emotional concomitants of caring for a child who has experienced a febrile seizure. Commenting on the concensus report, Freeman cogently stated, "Perhaps the most effective prophylaxis is a full discussion with parents and caretakers of the benign nature of febrile seizures, of the management of fever, and of first aid for seizures if necessary. With this management few children will need additional medicine."

ACUTE GASTROINTESTINAL PROBLEMS

Gastroenteritis and Dehydration

Gastroenteric diseases are fairly common among infants and young children and constitute a frequent reason for visiting the clinic or emergency room. The vast majority of these visits will be by patients with viral gastroenteritis, characterized by symptoms of vomiting and diarrhea. However, we must bear in mind the possibility of alternative diagnoses when seeing infants and children with gastrointestinal complaints. Other diseases of the gastrointestinal tract that may be encountered include appendicitis, bacterial enteritis, inflammatory bowel disease anomalies of the intestinal tract, and hepatitis.

DIAGNOSIS

Common gastroenteritis in children typically produces an initial syndrome of vomiting, anorexia, and decreased fluid intake, often followed by diarrhea and crampy abdominal pain. Fever is not usually prominent, and most children recover spontaneously with minimal care. In infants younger than 18 months it is especially important to obtain specific details about the history of vomiting or diarrhea because it is easy to confuse simple spitting up of formula or the normal soft stools of breast-feeding with the symptoms of gastroenteritis. For example, it is not unusual for a breast-fed infant to have a stool, which is often rather soft and unformed in comparison to adult stools, after every feeding.

Most gastroenteritis is presumed to be viral in origin. Epidemics occur within a community at various times of the year, particularly in the fall and winter. Diarrhea and vomiting can be associated with other etiologies (e.g., toxigenic *E. coli*), but the basic therapy remains the same regardless of the cause.

The primary concern in these patients is that they maintain sufficient water and electrolytes despite the losses produced by their illnesses. This can be assessed by historical information about intake and output and from changes in body weight. Clinically, we can determine hydration status from the moisture of the mucous membranes, skin turgor, and urine specific gravity. Note that children have increased elastic tissue in their skin and therefore a search for simple "tenting" may not be sufficient to illustrate decreased turgor. Instead, we have to draw the skin fold upward and twist it in a rotary manner to determine whether or not turgor is abnormal.

MANAGEMENT

For those children with mild dehydration (less than 5% of body weight), simple instructions regarding diet and signs to watch for at home will be sufficient. Chemically simple fluids are better tolerated than more complicated formulas, provoking less nausea and vomiting, and exhibit better retention. Thus soft drinks, liquid gelatin mixtures, and even some of the sugar and electrolyte drinks on the market are easily tolerated as oral fluids by the child. Milk, fruit juices that contain fruit pulp, and most solid foods are not well tolerated and simply provoke more vomiting. If a patient is noticeably febrile, rectal aspirin or acetaminophen may be administered to avoid gastric irritation and further fluid loss.

Dehydration between 5 and 10% of the body weight can usually be managed without intravenous fluid replacement provided that reliable oral replacement can be established. Dehydration beyond 10% of body weight in association with gastroenteritis indicates a substantial risk of shock and altered renal function. Therefore any child at or over 10% dehydration should be hydrated with intravenous fluids.

Pediatricians classify dehydration as one of three kinds: *hypotonic, isotonic,* and *hypertonic.* These terms refer to the relative tonicity of the patient's serum in comparison to the normal osmotic content. A child who loses isotonic fluids through vomiting and diarrhea will therefore have isotonic serum and only require therapy directed at isotonic replacement. Patients who lose hypertonic solutions in their diarrhea may require hypertonic solution replacement because their serum will be hypotonic.

Perhaps the most serious and delicate condition requiring intravenous fluid replacement is that of hypertonic dehydration. For a variety of reasons, patients who develop hypertonic dehydration may have serum osmolality rises from the normal 290 MOSM/liter to values as high as 350 or 370 MOSM/liter. The excessive osmolality of these patients' serum is in most cases due to an increased sodium content. Some will have hyperglycemia in response to their gastroenteritis, which will contribute to the hyperosmolality; in later stages, increased blood urea nitrogen (BUN) will add some additional osmolality to the mixture. Since the serum osmolality rises over some period of time, these patients normally have an increased osmolality intracellularly as well as within the plasma. Thus if free water is administered intravenously and rapidly, the osmotic gradient will draw fluid inside the cells in an effort to return the cellular interior to normal osmolality. The result of such a shift of fluid is a marked cellular edema that can be devastating in certain organs, specifically the brain. Therefore we must provide fluids for patients with hypertonic dehydration very slowly in order to allow for gradual equilibration. Should water be provided too rapidly to these patients they will develop seizures, which can be corrected by administration of a hypertonic fluid to reestablish fluid balance.

Typically, we adjust the rate of intravenous fluid administration in these patients according to their serum sodium levels. Patients with serum sodium values of greater than 150 are defined as having hypertonic dehydration. In this situation, fluids should be administered at a rate calculated to lower the serum sodium no faster than 1 MEq/hr. Thus a child with a serum sodium of 170 (as compared to a normal 135 MEq/liter) would be expected to take at least 35 hours of intravenous therapy before returning to a normal serum sodium value.

Elevated blood sugars are not uncommon and may rise as high as 1,200 mg%. Insulin is not required for these patients because as their fluid balance is corrected with intravenous fluids, the serum glucose will return to normal. The BUN will ultimately return to normal without any intervention but may lag several days behind resolution of the other chemical parameters.

We must always be alert to the possibility that an elevated serum sodium in a patient with gastroenteritis may be because of a feeding error. Historically, boiled skimmed milk was a common home therapy for gastroenteritis; however, in the boiling process the sodium content of the formula was markedly raised and patients who received such a formula were often salt poisoned as a consequence. Similarly, parents who administer formulas that are mixed from concentrated commercial formula preparations may make an error in the dilution and provide their children with excessive salt load.

Because water constitutes a larger part of a child's weight than it does of adult's weight, it is important to remember that correction of fluid and electrolyte imbalances in children must be done smoothly. A child who presents with severe dehydration must initially receive sufficient fluid to restore intravascular volume, blood pressure, and tissue perfusion. A quick but simple way of monitoring tissue perfusion is to monitor the capillary refill time at the heel. By simply pressing the thumb against the child's heel we can produce blanching and measure the time required for that blanching to return to the same hue as the surrounding tissue. Normally it takes 5–10 seconds at the most; however, for severely dehydrated patients it may be minutes before the perfusion is restored. Thus the patient may have a normal blood pressure as measured in the arm although insufficient intravascular volume has been restored and intravenous fluid rates must be adjusted according to the history. A child who has become acutely dehydrated as a result of an injury, for example, a child who has lost large amounts of blood, may receive replacement in a very short period of time to restore normal volume. Patients who have had several days of gastroenteritis before they had become severely dehydrated often cannot tolerate replacement in a matter of hours and may require the first half of the replacement, including calculated deficit, during the first one-third of the replacement period and the second half of the replacement, including deficit, during the second two-thirds. For example, if we estimate that a child needs 1,000 ml of fluid for both deficit replacement and maintenance over a 24-hour period, the rate should be 500 ml in the first 8 hours and 500 ml in the following 16 hours. By adjusting the replacement in this manner, we avoid excessive fluid challenges to the child.

After intravenous fluid therapy and replacement, the child may be started on oral fluid, which are normally clear liquids as discussed above. Once these are tolerated for a period of 24 hours or so, the child may progress to more complex formulas. Typically, the child may go to one-fourth or one-half strength formula, that is to say a normal formula diluted with water. If this is tolerated, the child may then advance to a full-strength formula. Within several days even the most severely dehydrated child should be able to take full-strength formula and within a few days after that return to solid food intake. Note that if the diet is advanced to more complex forms too rapidly, diarrhea may be reprovoked as a result of enzyme changes in the intestinal lining. It is a simple matter to take the diet back one or two stages to the simpler forms. Clear liquids and other simple formulas for more than a few days, however, may paradoxically produce diarrhea known as "starvation stools." Inadequate caloric protein intake may leave the intestinal lining unable to handle any intake without producing diarrhea.

Bacterial diarrheas are less common in children than is viral gastroenteritis. Nevertheless, *Salmonella* and *Shigella* often cause diarrhea in infants and young children, and the possibility of infections with these organisms should be considered. We may recognize such diarrhea states by the presence of many polymorphonuclear leukocytes in the stool, by positive stool cultures, or by extreme values on the white cell blood count particularly with a strong shift to the left. Should bacterial diarrhea be suspected in the younger child, a blood culture is important to exclude the possibility of *Salmonella* bacteremia in association with the bacterial diarrhea. A positive blood culture warrants consultation and probable admission for therapy, whereas the findings of the organism only in the stool without systemic symptoms indicates a more benign prognosis. Antibiotic therapy does not shorten the clinical course of *Salmonella* infections and may prolong the carrier state. *Shigella* infections may be treated in accordance with local antibiotic sensitivities.

Should the gastroenteritis emerge as a chronic problem, either at a low-grade level or intermittently over a period of weeks or months, we must seriously consider the inflammatory bowel diseases (IBD) and cystic fibrosis. Inflammatory bowel diseases have been recognized in children under 2 years of age and therefore must be part of the differential diagnosis in considering chronic diarrhea in a child. Children with IBD or cystic fibrosis will have abnormal stools, will fall off in their growth curves, and will often be small for age. These children will occasionally have severe crampy abdominal pains and may have a fever; those with IBD typically will have an elevated sedimentation rate. However, it is difficult to be certain of the diagnosis using only clinical grounds. Such patients should be assessed with sweat test and barium studies of the intestinal tract and may well warrant referral. Note that many patients with IBD or cystic fibrosis in this age group may not have all of the signs and symptoms that may suggest the diagnosis in an older child.

Congenital Anomalies

There are a variety of intestinal tract anomalies that will produce vomiting or diarrhea and may at times mimic simple infectious gastroenteritis. These conditions may occur anywhere in the gastrointestinal tract, including esophageal web or stenosis, duodenal atresia or stenosis, and duplication of various portions of the bowel, both small and large.

PYLORIC STENOSIS

Congenital hypertrophic pyloric stenosis, an overgrowth of the circular muscle at the outlet of the stomach, presents as progressive vomiting in the first few weeks of life. After several days of increasing frequency, projectile vomiting can occur after each feeding. Characteristically, the vomitus is not bile stained and the infant is hungry. Voiding and passage of stool become infrequent. The stomach is distended with peristaltic waves visible through the upper part of the abdominal wall. The diagnosis is made by palpating an olive-size moveable mass in the upper part of the abdomen or by a gastrointestinal (GI) series. Before a pyloromyotomy, the stomach should be emptied and the water and electrolyte deficit replaced.

MECKEL'S DIVERTICULUM

Meckel's diverticulum is a common gastrointestinal tract anomaly occurring in 1–2% of the population and is usually asymptomatic. It is a 2–8-cm outpocket on the antimesenteric side of the ileum 20–30 cm proximal to the ileocecal valve. It has all of the coats of the ileum and is a persistence beyond fetal life of the intestinal end of the vitelline duct. Gastrointestinal tract bleeding, perforation, or obstruction may occur in the infant or child. The bleeding is usually painless and episodic. The toddler characteristically passes several large grossly bloody stools and appears to be in shock. The bleeding can stop spontaneously and may not recur for several days or weeks. The hematocrit may drop 5% or more and return to normal levels if there is no further bleeding. There is no occult blood in the stool between episodes. The bleeding, which is from a small artery in the crater of a peptic ulcer in the base of the Meckel's diverticulum or adjacent ileum, is a result of a plaque of aberrant gastric mucosa that secretes acid and pepsin. The diagnosis is suspected from the clinical course and may be confirmed with a technetium 99 scan. If the area of gastric mucosa is large enough, it shows as a spot of radioactivity below the stomach. Abdominal exploration for resection of the suspected Meckel's diverticulum is indicated if the scan is positive or a second episode of bleeding occurs.

Intestinal perforation from a Meckel's diverticulum presents either as acute peritonitis with free air and intestinal contents throughout the peritoneal cavity or as a localized walled-off abscess. The ulcer is in the base of the diverticulum near the aberrant gastric mucosa. Proper management requires preoperative preparation with intravenous fluids, antibiotics, and nasogastric suction before emergency resection of the ulcer with the diverticulum. A primary anastomosis is usually possible.

A Meckel's diverticulum may cause intestinal obstruction with the sudden onset of vomiting, cramps, abdominal distention, and dilated loops of bowel seen on plain films of the abdomen. The obstructions are caused by adhesions to the peptic ulcer or aberrant mesenteric blood vessels. In addition, an internal hernia may be formed.

OMPHALOMESENTERIC DUCT

An omphalomesenteric duct presents in infancy as feculent drainage from the umbilicus or acute intestinal obstruction. It is a complete persistence of the vitelline duct with the terminal ileum attached to the umbilicus. If the lumen is open, a few drops of ileal contents may appear intermittently at the umbilicus. Examination with a probe will reveal a mucosal line tract extending into the bowel lumen. The acute obstructive symptoms occur when loops of small bowel twist about the duct as it runs like an adhesive band between the ileum and the back of the umbilicus.

DUPLICATION

Another gastrointestinal tract anomaly is duplication occurring anywhere from the mouth to the anus as a cystic or tubular mass. The mass may be asymptomatic and discovered incidentally or may present with obstruction or bleeding. In the abdomen, a segment of stomach or intestine is isolated from the lumen, lined with mucosa, and has a common muscular coat and blood supply. Partial obstruction of the lumen develops as the isolated segment fills with secretions. If the duplication contains gastric mucosa in its lining, peptic ulceration may lead to bleeding into the duplication or perforation into the lumen of the gastrointestinal tract. The diagnosis may be suspected from the aforementioned symptoms and confirmed during the operation.

INTUSSUSCEPTION

An important cause of abdominal pain and vomiting in young children is intussusception. Here, a segment of intestine invaginates into the lumen of an adjacent portion of intestine causing intermittent and ultimately permanent obstruction and at times intestinal necrosis (Fig. 44.5). Although the true incidence of intussusception has yet to be determined, there is a strong male preponderance and it occurs primarily within the first 2 years of life, most commonly between the fifth and tenth month. The underlying causes of intussusception remain unclear in the majority of cases and are commonly labeled "idiopathic." Of the documented causes the most important is Meckel's diverticulum, which acts as the lead point of the invagination. The idiopathic form accounts for the vast majority of cases in young children, whereas an identifiable lesion is more common in older children. In preadolescents the lead point is often an enlarged mesenteric lymph node as a result of an undiagnosed lymphoma.

Diagnosis

Intussusception usually occurs in healthy well-nourished children. The history usually reveals a dramatic complex of symptoms including intermittent abdominal pain, vomiting, and bloody stools. The pain is characteristically colicky, severe, and intermittent in nature. Often the child is described as experiencing what appears to be violent episodes of abdominal pain causing the child to cry out loudly and draw up his or her legs into a flexed position. Almost all infants and about 80% of older children will vomit during the course of these episodes. The vomiting early in the course of the intussusception seems to be reflexive, whereas the vomiting that is seen later is secondary to the obstructive process. Blood in the stool or rectal discharge is observed in over 95% of infants and 60% of older children. This may occur as the initial presenting symptom or may be observed late in the course of the intussusception. Often the blood is mixed with mucous producing the classic "currant jelly" stools.

A careful physical examination can be critical in making the diagnosis of intussusception. The child may appear normal or quiet, even listless, between colicky episodes. Irritability and restlessness may also be noted. At times a painful episode may be observed in the emergency room, during which the child exhibits all the signs noted above. When the process presents further in its course the child may present with significant prostration, pallor, and a clammy cool perspiration. Occasionally, intussusception in young children may present with an altered mental status characterized by apathy or confusion often mimicking a toxic ingestion or encephalitis. A mass is palpable either abdominally or rectally in the vast majority of reported cases. The mass is classically vague, sausage shaped, and mildly tender and offers virtually a pathognomonic sign in children suspected of having an intussusception. A rectal examination is essential since the mass or bloody stool may only be appreciated in this manner. Fever is common, particularly in infants. The pulse is not usually elevated unless the child is acutely distressed or hypovolemia has developed. Leukocytosis may be present but is of little clinical significance.

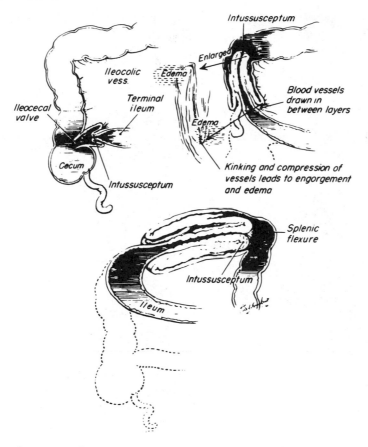

Figure 44.5 Illustration of the development of an ileocecal intussusception. (*Source:* Ravitch MM: Intussusception in infants and children, 1959. Courtesy of Charles C Thomas, Publisher, Springfield, Illinios.

Management

The diagnosis of intussusception is confirmed by barium enema (Fig. 44.6). A characteristic filling defect extends from the cecum into distal parts of the colon. Most intussusceptions can be reduced by the controlled application of hydrostatic pressure of the barium column at the time of the diagnostic barium enema. Recent data have shown that this procedure is both safe and effective and can prevent the need for surgery. It is important, however, that there be close collaboration between surgeons and radiologists in performing this procedure and that careful control be exercised. When hydrostatic reduction is unsuccessful, laparotomy and direct reduction by taxis is required. Resection and anastomosis is necessary if the intussusception cannot be reduced or when necrotic bowel is present.

Throughout the evaluation, required diagnostic procedures and therapy, careful monitoring of blood pressure, pulse, respiration, and urine output are essential. Third spacing of fluid into the bowel may be significant and hypovolemic shock may ensue. Electrolyte disturbances may also develop and should be followed closely. Intravenous infusion of large amounts of volume-expanding fluid including blood may be required and should be carefully monitored.

Prognosis

The prognosis for children undergoing successful reduction or resection is quite good. Early and definitive intervention is the key to good outcome. The problem usually lies in delay subsequent to an erroneous diagnosis of a condition other than intussusception. Physicians inexperienced in evaluating chil-

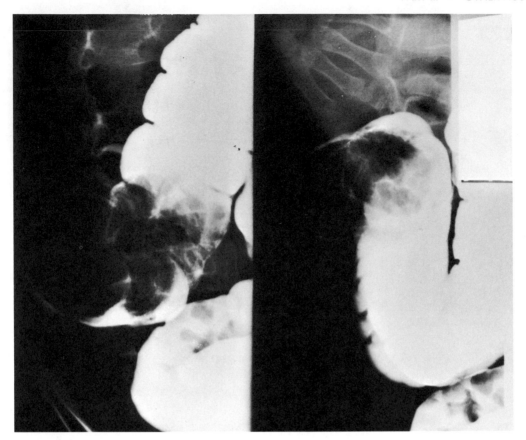

Figure 44.6 Barium enema revealing intussusception. A lobulated obstructive defect is present in the transverse colon.

dren may not suspect intussusception as the underlying cause of vomiting and colicky pain. Often bloody stools are present though missed on physical examination. Before assigning a diagnosis of colic, gastroenteritis, sepsis, or encephalopathy to a young child, intussusception should be considered as a possible alternative cause for the child's clinical presentation.

ASTHMA

General guidelines for the assessment of patients with asthma are discussed in Chapter 2. Of greatest importance for children are a review of medications taken in the preceding 24 hours and a physical examination for signs of cyanosis, air hunger, and/or the use of auxiliary muscles of respiration, pulsus paradoxus, and elevated respiratory rate.

Therapy in children is somewhat varied, reflecting a paucity of good data regarding the relative effectiveness of a number of treatment modalities. Initially, successive injections of subcutaneous epinephrine (1:1,000) at a dosage of 0.01 mg/kg (maximum of 0.4 ml) are given. A dosage should be given every 15–20 minutes until either the patient has cleared or a total of 3 dosages have been administered. Close monitoring for tachycardia and improvement in the respiratory status is essential. Unless home therapy with beta agents has preceded the administration of epinephrine, most patients will show response at some point to these three separate injections. The patient who clears should be given a final injection of long-acting epinephrine (Sus-Phrine) 0.05 ml/kg and be discharged on an appropriate dose of a bronchodilator. Those who fail to clear completely with this regimen can be advanced to a second round of β-adrenergic medication, that is, inhalation of isoetharine (Bronchosol) administered by aerosol without positive pressure. This dose may be repeated up to three times with spacing of 20 minutes between dosages. Again, pulse rates and clinical response to treatment should be closely monitored. The majority of children presenting to emergency rooms will respond at some point to this regimen of β-adrenergic agents.

Patients who have incomplete resolution of their attack at this stage will require intravenous administration of aminophylline. Hydration should be calculated to provide 1.5 times maintenance fluids divided into hourly quantities. Laboratory studies that may be of help in the clinical assessment of the patient include a CBC (with attention directed to the total WBC and the differential for suggestion of bacterial superinfection), blood gases, and theophylline levels of the patient. Admission of the patient should be considered at this time since it will be necessary if aminophylline fails to clear the patient.

Intravenous aminophylline must be based on the previous intake of aminophylline or theophylline derivatives. If no aminophylline or theophylline has been taken in the preceding 12 hours, we may give an infusion calculated at 5–7 mg of theophylline per kilogram of body weight diluted in the intravenous fluids to be administered over at least a 20-minute period. More rapid administration may lead to complications such as seizures or, in very rare instances, cardiac arrhythmias. Monitoring of blood levels of theophylline may help substantially in adjusting the dose for individual patients, if such testing is readily available. If the patient has received aminophylline or theophylline medication within the preceding 6 hours, the initial dose of aminophylline must be adjusted downward. For example, a patient who has received an oral dose of theophylline amounting to 5 mg/kg just before presentation at the emergency room or physician's office would not receive the full dose of aminophylline intravenously; the dose should be adjusted downward substantially to approximately 2–3 mg/kg.

As the intravenous line is placed, hydration is begun, and the aminophylline dose is administered, many practitioners will begin corticosteroid therapy for patients who are having substantial respiratory difficulty. Since it takes 6–8 hours for corticosteroids to have a beneficial effect on the airways, administration at this time offers the earliest possible effect of the drug in the event the patient does not respond to other measures. A suggested dosage would be methylprednisolone 0.25–0.5 mg/kg every 6 hours given intravenously.

For the very severe asthmatic patient who is cyanotic and in substantial distress at presentation, the steps outlined above should be followed simultaneously with frequent monitoring of vital signs and blood gases in order to follow respiratory status changes. Constant aminophylline infusion may be useful in this setting. The dosage for the infusion is 0.9–1.1 mg/kg per hour as a constant intravenous drip. Frequent monitoring of theophylline blood levels is important since certain patients who have slow theophylline metabolism may accumulate toxic levels with this technique.

Another measure, which should be restricted to experienced units and intensive care settings, is the administration of intravenous isoproterenol. Because of the hazards associated with the technique, an arterial line, central venous line, full-support services, and experienced staff are required in the use of this modality. Refractory and severe asthma may require the use of artificial ventilation. Artificial ventilation is normally reserved for patients who demonstrate cyanosis in 40% oxygen and an arterial P_{CO_2} of above 50 that continues to rise. Levels over 65 in an asthmatic child are extremely ominous. Mechanical ventilation using mild myoneural blockade and sedation in a child requires substantial experience to avoid complications and ensure a successful outcome. Pneumothorax and pneumomediastinum are complications of this therapeutic approach.

HEMATOLOGIC EMERGENCIES

Certain hematologic condition of childhood may present as life-threatening emergencies. Others may predispose the child to serious illness. In general these conditions can be grouped into bleeding diathesis, thrombocytopenia, leukemia, and sickle cell anemia. Additional discussion of these conditions can be found in Chapter 40.

Bleeding Diathesis

Bleeding disorders in children may reflect congenital or acquired defects. In either bleeding as a result of these disorders may occur spontaneously or in response to trauma. Congenital disorders include factor VIII deficiency (hemophilia A), factor IX (hemophilia B), or Von Willebrand's disease. These can present with acute bleeding in patients of any age.

The incidence of hemophilia is approximately 1 in 10,000 male births, and often these children require emergency care. Hemophilia A and B are not distinguishable on clinical grounds, but rather their presentation is related to the child's age and severity of factor deficiency. In severe hemophilia (plasma concentration of factor VIII or IX is 1–5% of normal) a history of subcutaneous echymoses, hematomas following intramuscular injection, and prolonged bleeding from minor trauma to the oral cavity can usually be obtained in the first few years of life. Mild disease (plasma concentrations of factor VIII or IX is 5–30%

of normal) can often go undiagnosed until later childhood and even adulthood. Usually significant trauma or a surgical procedure will reveal the presence of abnormally low levels of factors. Prolonged bleeding after minor surgical procedures such as circumcision may indicate a congenital bleeding disorder. However, a history of a normal circumcision does not rule out hemophilia since many patients with mild disease often do not manifest an abnormality in this manner.

DIAGNOSIS

To confirm the diagnosis, tests of platelet count, prothrombin time (PT), and partial thromboplastin time (PTT) should be obtained. In patients with hemophilia only the PTT is elevated. Definitive diagnosis is made by documenting a low plasma factor concentration.

MANAGEMENT

Bleeding episodes in children with hemophilia should be treated immediately. Hemarthrosis or hemorrhage into muscular tissue should be carefully evaluated for severity and loss of function. Soft tissue bleeding, particularly in small children, can pool large quantities of blood extravascularly making careful monitoring of vital signs and blood volume imperative.

The initial symptom is usually pain; later symptoms are swelling and decreased mobility. The most critical aspect of treatment is the immediate infusion of replacement factors. Replacement therapy can usually be based upon the observation that 1 unit of factor VIII per kilogram of body weight raises the plasma levels 1.5%. For mild-to-moderate bleeds correction of plasma levels of factor about 40% is usually adequate to terminate the bleed. Central nervous system hemorrhage is an extreme emergency. Head trauma, headache, alterations of mental status, and abnormalities on neurologic examination are extremely worrisome in children with hemophilia. Neurosurgical evaluation including CT are indicated whenever a central nervous system bleed is suspected. Replacement therapy should aim for an 80–100% increase. For soft tissue and especially central nervous system hemorrhage an effort should be made to begin replacement therapy as soon as possible and not to delay it with diagnostic procedures or tests.

Thrombocytopenia and Leukemia

There are many causes of thrombocytopenia in children, both as a result of decreased production and enhanced destruction. Viral infections can often cause a transient decline in platelet

number. The pathogenesis of this process is not well understood but viral illness can also cause anemia and neutropenia. Bacterial infections, notably meningococcemia, can cause thrombocytopenia both alone and in association with disseminated intravascular coagulation. Thrombocytopenia as a result of bacterial infection is usually, though not always, accompanied by systemic signs of severe illness, whereas viral process is usually more benign.

DIAGNOSIS

Infiltrative diseases of the bone marrow may present with thrombocytopenia. In patients with *leukemia* an accompanying anemia and/or neutropenia or elevation of white blood cells will often be seen. A history of malaise, fevers, and recent weight loss is also common. On examination, lymphadenopathy and splenomegaly are usually evident. Careful review of peripheral blood smear for blasts and, ultimately, bone marrow examination will confirm a diagnosis of leukemia.

Idiopathic thrombocytopenia purpura (ITP) is the most common cause of thrombocytopenia in children. It is an acquired disorder caused by excessive destruction of circulatory platelets, presumably an immunologic basis. Two forms exist—acute and chronic. Over 85% of cases are of the acute form in which a usually healthy child abruptly develops petechiae and ecchymosis. In a majority of cases a history of recent viral illness or immunization can be elicited. The chronic form is usually more insidious in onset. It is more common in older children and, in fact, resembles the ITP course seen in adults.

On physical examination hemorrhagic lesions of the mucous membranes and nonpalpable purpuric and petechial lesions are commonly found. Although some children with ITP present with fever, they usually appear otherwise quite well. The spleen and liver are almost always of normal size and appear unremarkable on abdominal examination. A palpable spleen in this setting would usually imply that an infiltrative process or liver disease exists. The diagnosis of ITP should never be made in a systemically ill or toxic child until infectious, inflammatory, or lymphoproliferative etiology is completely ruled out. In approximately one-third of patients hemorrhagic episodes will occur including epistaxis, hematuria, melena, and menorrhagia.

The diagnosis of ITP is one of exclusion, and other causes of thrombocytopenia must be ruled out. Careful review of the blood smear is mandatory. Abnormal numbers or formed white blood cells, bizarre or fragmented red blood cells, or other finding in addition to low platelet number should raise the suspicion that conditions other than ITP may be present. Prothrombin time and PPT should be normal. As aplastic or infiltrative processes of the bone marrow may present with only thrombocytopenia, a bone marrow examination is usually required before the diagnosis of ITP can be confidently made.

The prognosis for children with ITP is generally quite good. It is difficult to predict whether a particular case of ITP will be of the acute self-limiting type or will develop into one of the 10–15% of cases that are considered chronic in nature. Although the chronic form may present in any age group, it is much more common in children over 10 years old. Almost 80% of all patients with ITP recover completely within 3 months, most within 2. Ninety percent will spontaneously recover within 1 year. However, approximately 1% of children with ITP will sustain a life-threatening gastrointestinal or central nervous system hemorrhage. These severe complications usually occur during the initial few weeks after onset, but it is difficult to predict on presentation which children will in fact develop such problems.

MANAGEMENT

The treatment for children with ITP should be primarily supportive. Activity should be modified to help prevent traumatic injuries, and platelet count and hemoglobin should be followed. Platelet counts can drop to below 10,000/mm³, but prolongation of bleeding time does not usually occur above a count of 20,000/mm³. Packed red blood cells should be transfused when the hemoglobin falls below 7 g/dl or when hemodynamic symptoms are evident. Platelet transfusions are not usually helpful since the evident rise in platelet number is usually quite transient. Platelet transfusions should be administered only in situations of life-threatening bleeding.

Corticosteroids have been used successfully to raise acutely the platelet number of ITP. However, it is still unclear whether the use of corticosteroids will alter the course of the illness or modify its complications. Nevertheless, in the hope of preventing life-threatening hemorrhage, corticosteroids are often employed selectively in children who suffer from continued overt bleeding during the initial 3 weeks of illness. Prednisone is usually prescribed at 4 oral dosages of 3 mg/kg/day with a taper over 2 weeks. The steroid therapy should be tapered and ultimately terminated whether or not the platelet count has risen.

Emergency splenectomy is indicated only for life-threatening central nervous system hemorrhage. In addition, splenectomy should be considered in children in whom thrombocytopenia persists for more than 6 months with evidence of persistent hemorrhage. Splenectomy in children under 4 years old, however, should be avoided if possble in light of the increased risk of serious infection after splenectomy.

Sickle Cell Anemia

The term *sickle cell disease* is generally used to describe a group of *inherited hemoglobinopathies:* homozygous sickle cell anemia (S–S); sickle cell–hemoglobin C disease (S–C); sickle cell β-thalassemia (S–B thal). Each represents a chronic disorder that becomes clinically significant to the emergency room physician because of intermittent cardiovascular crises and predisposition to severe bacterial infection.

DIAGNOSIS

Usually there are no clinical manifestations of sickle cell disease until fetal hemoglobin is substantially replaced by hemoglobin S; this usually occurs by 6 months of age. A common initial presentation is dactylitis or "hand–foot" syndrome, in which painful swelling of the dorsum of the hands and feet reflects ischemia and infarction of the metatarsal and metacarpal bones. Clinical findings that commonly develop are pallor, hepatosplenamegaly, and icterus. Flow murmurs and cardiomegaly secondary to anemia are quite common. Splenomegaly is usually found in early childhood since repeated splenic infarctions and subsequent scarring will gradually shrink the spleen over the first decade of life. By adolescence the child is usually functionally asplenic with Howell-Jolly bodies evident on peripheral blood smear. Hemoglobin levels are usually quite low (5–10 mg/100 ml) with a reticulocytosis commonly between 10 and 25%.

MANAGEMENT

The most common problem in children with sickle cell disease presenting for emergency care is vasoocclusive crisis. These patients present with symptoms related to the site of occlusion. Usually limbs, back, and abdomen are the most severely affected. Common precipitating events may include infection, trauma, dehydration, or exposure to cold.

The primary component of therapy is aggressive hydration. Intravenous infusion of 5% dextrose with 0.25 or 0.5 normal saline 3–5ml/kg/hr (approximately 1.5–2 times maintenance) is usually adequate. Since older patients may have compromised cardiac function, care should be taken to avoid fluid overload in patients with a history of impaired cardiac reserve. Supplemental oxygen may be helpful in some patients and can routinely be administered. Adequate analgesia is a critical goal of emergency management. Acetomeniphen with or without codeine may be helpful in patients with mild cases or those managed in this manner in the past. However, for moderate-to-severe pain from vasoocclusive crisis generous doses of demerol or morphine may be required.

Aplastic crises represent the cessation of red blood cell (RBC) production with subsequent worsening of anemia and drop in reticulocyte and bilirubin levels. Occasionally the resultant drop in hemoglobin may be severe and cause congestive heart failure. Treatment usually includes the careful transfusion of packed RBCs until the hemoglobin level rises to at least 7 gm/100 ml and cardiovascular compromise is alleviated.

The most catastrophic form of sickle cell is the sequestration crisis. Here, blood is pooled in the spleen and liver causing significant hypovolemia and shock. The onset and course of a sequestration crisis can be devastatingly rapid with prostration, shock, and, ultimately, cardiac arrest occurring within minutes. This type of crisis usually occurs in young children since their still functioning spleen is capable of sequestering large volumes of blood. Evidence of hypovolemia (tachycardia, falling blood pressure, poor peripheral perfusion) and prostration in the face of enlarged spleen or liver suggests a sequestration. Hemoglobin levels may fall precipitously. Treatment is directed toward restitution of normovolemia. Infusion of plasma expanders or whole blood should be administered at a rate of at least 20 ml/kg/hr, adjusted to reflect careful central venous pressure measurements.

Patients with sickle cell disease are at increased risk for serious bacterial infection. The underlying defect is not well understood; however, loss of splenic function probably plays a primary role. In fact, children with sickle cell disease should be treated as if they were asplenic. Prophylactic penicillin should be prescribed, and polyvalent pneumococcal vaccine should be administered to all children over 2 years old with sickle cell disease.

Therefore children with sickle cell disease who have a fever without an obvious source must be considered a serious problem. It is usually necessary to draw blood cultures and begin intravenous antibiotic therapy. The most common offending organisms are *S. pneumoniae* (pneumococcus), *Salmonella,* and *H. influenzae.* Therefore ampicillin (50 mg/kg every 6 hours) used alone, or in conjunction with chloramphenicol (25 mg/kg every 6 hours) when ampicillin-resistant *H. influenza* is prevalent, should be administered. Overwhelming sepsis should always be of concern and therefore these children must always be deliberately and cautiously managed.

DIABETIC KETOACIDOSIS IN CHILDREN

Diabetes mellitus is a relatively common metabolic disorder in children; there is a general prevalence of approximately 1.9 cases per 1,000 school-age children. The primary disturbance is a deficiency in circulatory insulin that precipitates a series of complicated metabolic abnormalities. In many ways the resultant state is similar to starvation with significant catabolism, increased lipolysis, ketogenesis, and gluconeogenesis. Hyperglycemia with glycosuria occurs as does ketosis and ketonuria. Accumulation of organic acids, primarily β-hydroxybutyric acid and acetoacetic acid, causes significant metabolic acidosis. The excretion of ketones is associated with cation loss and obligatory osmotic diuresis. The resultant dehydration, acidosis, and electrolyte disturbances can be severe.

DIAGNOSIS

The term *diabetic ketoacidosis* (DKA) is usually used to describe the complex series of disturbances described above. The classical clinical symptoms of diabetes mellitus in childhood are polyuria, polydipsia, and polyphagia. However, there are other important signs and symptoms of juvenile diabetes that must be recognized. Recent weight loss, fatigue, recent onset of enuresis, abdominal pain, vomiting, and prolonged headache can often herald the onset of juvenile diabetes. At times the initial presentation will be one of frank DKA. Here the clinical picture will be one of an obviously ill child, often in extremis, with hyperventilation, tachycardia, stupor or obtundation, dry mucosal surfaces, pallor, and hypotension. The prominent hyperventilation and prostration have been confused for signs of a primary respiratory problem rather than of a compensatory response to an underlying acidosis. Altered mental status or coma secondary to fluid shifts and acidosis involving the central nervous system may also characterize the presentation. A careful history and physical examination with special attention to vital sign measurement will usually reveal many of these clinical findings.

Laboratory findings reflect hyperglycemia, ketoacidosis, dehydration, and electrolyte disturbances. Rapid diagnosis of glycosuria and ketonuria can be made by employing a semiquantitative urine dipstick or clinitest tablet. Dextrostix or chemstrip will quickly assess the blood glucose levels. The importance of this step cannot be overstated. Numerous cases have documented the needlessly tragic outcome of not recognizing severe hyperglycemia by omitting the Dextrostix from the initial evaluation. Ketonuria and ketonemia can be documented by sodium nitroprusside tablets (Acetest). However, caution should be exercised in interpreting the Acetest since it measures only the levels of acetoacetate and acetone and not those of β-hydroxybutyrate. Evidence of acidosis will emerge with a pH and total bicarbonate determination. Hyponatremia is a common finding. However, it usually is not due to true sodium loss but more likely the movement of water extracellularly as a result of hyperglycemia. A simple estimate of true sodium levels can be made by raising the serum sodium by 1.6 mEq for every 100 mg/dl increase in serum glucose. In addition, severe hyperlypidemia (at times with grossly lipemic serum) will artificially reduce measured serum sodium levels. True levels of phosphate and potassium are significantly depleted in DKA. However, because of movement into the extracellular space with severe acidosis, serum phosphate and potassium may be normal or even elevated. In light of significant electrolyte disturbances and acidosis, an electrocardiogram (ECG) should be performed and constant ECG monitoring initiated.

MANAGEMENT

The treatment of DKA consists of several components: (1) fluid and electrolyte replacement; (2) insulin therapy; and (3) metabolic and cardiovascular monitoring. Fluid administration during the emergency phase of treatment is aimed at correcting hypovolemia and its consequent cardiovascular abnormalities. Large-bore intravenous lines should be placed rapidly and securely. Isotonic saline should be infused at 20 ml/kg during the first hour. During the second hour the solution should be changed to half-normal saline with 5% dextrose since the blood glucose level falls subsequent to insulin therapy. Calculation of volume after initial emergency bolus over the first hour depends on maintenance requirements, deficit replacement, and replacement of ongoing losses. Maintenance fluids can be estimated as a daily requirement of 1,700 ml per meter^2(M^2) free water, 50 mEq per M^2 sodium, and 40 mEq per M^2 potassium. Deficits can be calculated as a percentage of body weight. In moderate-to-severe DKA it can be estimated that approximately 10% of body weight has been lost. In this way 100 ml of water, 8 mEq of sodium, 6–10 mEq of potassium, and 6–8 mEq of chloride, each per kilogram of body weight, should be adequate deficit replacement. For example, a 20-kg child with 10% dehydration would require approximately 2 liters of free water, 150 mEq of sodium, 160 mEq of potassium, and 140 mEq of chloride to replace the deficit. Maintenance fluids and electrolytes would be added to this as would replacement of ongoing losses. As a rule, three-fourths of the deficit should be infused over the first 24 hours, making sure that one-half is administered over the first 8 hours. Only one-half of the calculated potassium deficit should be given over the first 24 hours. Initially normal serum potassium levels may drop precipitously since improving pH will allow transfer of potassium to the intracellular space. Therefore as soon as renal function is confirmed, potassium can be added to the infused solution to a maximum of 40 mEq/liter of infused fluid. Careful monitoring of ECG and serum determination will guide potassium therapy. As phosphate deficiency also accompanies DKA, one-half of the potassium should be given as potassium chloride and one-half as potassium phosphate. A low pH often presents the temptation to administer bicarbonate to the child. However, differential permeability of CO_2 and CO_3 across the blood brain barrier may paradoxically lower CSF pH after infusion of bicarbonate. Therefore bicarbonate is probably only indicated when the blood pH is less than 7.10. In this instance moderate dosages of bicarbonate (1–2 mEq of sodium bicarbonate per kilogram of body weight) can be infused slowly over 15–20 minutes. More vigorous bicarbonate therapy will probably be counterproductive. Rather an effort should be made to correct the acidosis by vigorous fluid and insulin administration.

Insulin administration is the keystone of therapy. There are many methods of insulin administration; however, two have been found to be of particular use in this setting. The first depends on an intravenous bolus of regular insulin coupled with the initiation of a constant insulin infusion. The recommended starting dose is 0.1 unit of regular insulin per kilogram of body weight given as an intravenous push. This is best accomplished by first diluting 1 ml of U-100 regular insulin with 9 ml of isotomic saline yielding a final concentration of 10 units/ml. The constant infusion is begun immediately as a dosage of 0.1 unit of regular insulin per kilogram of body weight per hour. This can be calculated by diluting 50 units of regular insulin in 250 ml of normal saline yielding a concentration of 0.2 unit/ml. Plastic tubing will bind insulin, so a few milliliters of the insulin solution should be run through the tubing first to saturate the binding sites before the infusion is begun. An alternative to the constant infusion is the administration of an initial intravenous push of 0.25 unit of regular insulin per kilogram of body weight, followed by a subcutaneous of intramuscular injection of another 0.25 unit of regular insulin per kilogram of body weight. The decision to use the bolus–constant infusion method or the bolus–injection method should be based on the particular capabilities of the staff and facility caring for the patient.

Careful monitoring of cardiovascular stability and metabolic correction is a critical component of therapy. Measurement of vital signs and neurologic examination must be frequent and thorough since hypotension, arrhythmias, mental status alterations, and other abnormalities are frequent complications of DKA and its therapy. Frequent glucose and electrolyte determinations are essential, and insulin and fluid therapy should be modified accordingly. The decrease in serum glucose levels should not exceed approximately 75–100 mg/dl/hr. A rapid decline may provoke significant cerebral edema as a result of the shift of free water from the extracellular space into brain cells. Therefore insulin dosage must be responsive to blood glucose determinations. Total bicarbonate and pH measurements should be followed for improvement. The ECG monitoring should be continuous for at least the first 24 hours of therapy. Central venous pressure monitoring is also usually helpful in ensuring the cautious correction of hypovolemia. In addition careful measurement of input and output can also be helpful in monitoring fluid balance.

Careful attention to these components of care will almost universally result in an active and well-appearing child in just a few days. The task then becomes the education or reeducation of the child and family to the daily care of the diabetic child in the hope of preventing future episodes of ketoacidosis.

SUDDEN INFANT DEATH SYNDROME

Sudden infant death syndrome (SIDS) refers to the unexpected death without an identifiable cause of previously well infants. This syndrome accounts for 2–3 deaths per 1,000 live births and represents the leading cause of death in children between 1 week and 1 year old. Although SIDS has been reported in children under 10 days and over 1 year old, the peak incidence occurs between 2 and 4 months. There tends to be an increased occurrence in the winter months and in males. Several studies have confirmed an increased incidence in low birth weight babies and infants of multiple births.

The causation of SIDS is not well understood. Many theories have been suggested including airway obstruction, infection, and central and metabolic disturbances. Early hypotheses of unobserved asphyxiation, laryngospasm, aspiration, viremia, or allergic reactions have now been fairly well disproved. Recent interest has focused on the identification of an unrecognized chronic condition as the underlying etiology of SIDS. Evidence of chronic underventilation and hypoxemia has been uncovered on postmortem examination of children who have died from apparent SIDS. In addition, researchers have found evidence of significant abnormalities in the control of breathing during sleep in infants who are successfully resuscitated from a SIDS episode. These so-called "near-miss" SIDS infants have revealed alterations in breathing reflexes and, in many, a predisposition for significant episodes of apnea during sleep. Metabolic abnormalities, most recently involving the thyroid, have also been thought to be a possible cause.

The usual case history describes the tragic discovery of a dead infant by a parent who has noticed that the child has slept through a usual awakening or feeding time. In a significant number of cases the deaths have occurred while another person was in the same room. Cases have also been described in which children have died while sleeping in car seats while a parent was driving. Almost always no outcry or agonal motion was noted by the parent. The initial reaction of the parent can vary, but often it is understandably one of great alarm and inaction. Increasing numbers of parents, however, may attempt some form of cardiopulmonary resuscitation and alert emergency personnel. Occasionally, when begun soon after breathing ceases, stimulation or resuscitative efforts may be successful. These near-miss SIDS infants present a complicated management problem.

DIAGNOSIS

The evaluation of an infant presenting with a history of a near-miss SIDS episode should be approached with great care. The clinician should cautiously review the history for evidence of underlying disease and the severity (length of time without respiration, cyanosis, etc.) of the observed episode. Among the issues that should be covered are the possibility of seizure activity, infection, inappropriate feeding mixture, choking or vomiting, recent trauma, and current medications. All of these issues can present in a manner mimicking near-miss SIDS.

The physical examination has the dual goal of ensuring that the child is in no further immediate danger and of ruling out or identifying alternative diagnoses. Careful measurement of vital signs may reveal fever, tachycardia or bradycardia, hypotension, or altered respiratory rate or rhythm. The skin should be examined for signs of trauma (bruises, swelling) or infection (petechiae, rash). The remainder of the examination should include a careful respiratory and neurologic review. Laboratory tests should include a CBC with differential, electrolytes, calcium, BUN, creatinine, blood glucose, and urinalysis. Other tests should reflect particular suspicions based on history and physical examination. This may include an electroencephalogram (EEG) to rule out a seizure disorder or an LP to rule out meningitis.

MANAGEMENT

The management of the near-miss SIDS infant usually includes a period of careful in-hospital observation and monitoring. Not only does this allow a more thorough opportunity to evaluate the infant, but it also provides a time to educate and more fully support the parents. If sepsis is suspected, antibiotic therapy should be administered until cultures are shown to be negative. Once the initial therapeutic decisions have been made, the definitive evaluation of the infant for apnea or other disorders of respiration and arrangements for outpatient management should be coordinated with a medical center with an active program for near-miss SIDS infants. Most areas have access to these centers, and their value as a clinical resource has been well established.

CONGENITAL HEART DISEASE

Congenital heart disease (CHD) refers to developmental abnormalities of the cardiovascular system that are present at birth. It is estimated that CHD affects between 8 and 10 of every 1,000 live births. Of these some 2.2 per 1,000 infants will suffer from critical CHD in which catheterization or corrective surgery will be required in the first year of life. It is this subpopulation of children with critical CHD that is most likely to require emergency care. The most common acute presentation is usually one of congestive heart failure or cyanosis.

Congestive Heart Failure

The nature and timing of presentation of congestive heart failure (CHF) in infants is highly dependent on the underlying etiology. When CHF is present at birth, intrauterine causes are most likely. These would include arrhythmias, anemia caused by erythroblastosis fetalis, hemorrhage, feto-fetal transfusion, or large arteriovenous fistulas, particularly of the brain or liver.

In addition, CHF may present within the first few weeks of life. Hypoplasia of the left ear, coarctation of the aorta, aortic stenosis, total anomalous venous return with pulmonary venous obstruction, transposition of the great vessels with an associated ventricular septal defect, and tricuspid atresia may all cause significant CHF in the first few weeks of life.

A ventricular septal defect (VSD) and other solitary defects that cause left to right shunting may not be apparent until after the first month of life. Pulmonary vascular resistance usually remains elevated in term infants for approximately 4–6 weeks after birth. Therefore significant left-to-right shunts do not usually occur until the end of this time period. An exception, however, is the premature infant in whom pulmonary vascular resistance may be relatively low even during the first few weeks of life.

DIAGNOSIS

Common presenting signs of CHF in infants include tachycardia, tachypnea, and diaphoresis. Often a history of dyspnea and diaphoresis with feeding can be elicited. Cardiomegaly and hyperdynamic precordium can sometimes be appreciated on physical examination. Decreased femoral pulses and low blood pressure relative to upper extremity pressures suggest a coarctation of the aorta. Bounding pulses may indicate the presence of a patent ductus arteriosus (PDA). Heart murmurs should be carefully evaluated (Table 44.5). Hepatomegaly is a common finding, and a careful examination for other congenital anomalies is mandatory whenever CHD is suspected. Unlike in adults, pitting edema and neck vein distention are not usually seen in infants with CHF. Severe CHF may cause hypotension, prostration, and shock.

Chest roentgenogram should help rule out a pulmonary disorder. The heart is usually enlarged because of pulmonary vascular engorgement. Electrocardiogram findings will vary with the nature of the underlying defect (see Table 44.5). Arterial blood gases may be normal or reveal an acidosis with both respiratory and metabolic components.

MANAGEMENT

When CHF is caused by an anemia, the underlying cause must be treated. Packed red blood cells or partial exchange transfusion may prove useful in patients with hemolytic anemias. Hemorrhage should be terminated and volume repleted with whole blood. High output states as a result of vascular anomalies may require surgical ligation or excision when possible.

The medical management of CHF caused by anatomical defects is based upon the use of cardiotonic drugs, diuretics, and fluid and salt restriction. Digoxin is the mainstay of medical therapy. The dosage varies with the age of the child. The route of administration should reflect the severity of the CHF: For mild CHF oral administration is usually adequate, whereas for distressed infants, the intravenous route is preferred. Premature infants should receive a total digitalizing dose (TDD) of 0.03–0.05 mg/kg intravenously or 0.03–0.06 mg/kg orally. The TDD for term infants is 0.03–0.06 mg/kg intravenously or 0.04–0.08 mg/kg orally. Children under 2 years old may receive a TDD of 0.03–0.05 mg/kg intravenously or 0.05–0.07 mg/kg orally. The dose for children over 2 years is 0.02–0.04 mg/kg intravenously or 0.03–0.05 mg/kg orally. Children with signs of significant CHF can be given one-half the TDD initially, followed by one-fourth the TDD 4–8 hours later. Maintenance therapy should be 25–33% of the TDD, usually administered in 2 daily dosages. Electrocardiograms should be taken before each administration of digoxin in order to identify any signs of toxicity. Bradycardia and prolonged P-R interval (greater than 0.16 second) are common indications of digoxin toxicity.

Diuretics should be used when significant fluid retention is

TABLE 44.5 Presenting Signs and Findings in Congenital Heart Disease

Diagnosis	Age	Presenting Signs	Auscultation	Film Findings	ECG Findings
Transposition of the great arteries					
Intact ventricular septum	First hours or days	Cyanosis	Unremarkable	Cardiac enlargement; pulmonary vasculature increased	Right ventricular hypertrophy
Ventricular septal defect	First week	Congestive heart failure	Pansystolic murmur	Cardiac enlargement; pulmonary vasculature greatly increased	Combined ventricular hypertrophy
Ventricular septal defect and pulmonic stenosis	First days or weeks	Cyanosis	Pansystolic and stenotic murmurs	Cardiac enlargement; pulmonary vasculature unremarkable	Combined ventricular hypertrophy
Fallot's tetralogy	First days or weeks	Cyanosis	Early stenotic murmur; single S_2 at upper left sternal border	No cardiac enlargement; pulmonary vasculature decreased	Right ventricular hypertrophy
Pure pulmonary stenosis	First weeks or months or occasionally days	Cyanosis	Late stenotic murmur; widely split S_2, faint P_2	Cardiac enlargement; pulmonary vasculature decreased	Right ventricular hypertrophy
Hypoplastic left heart	First days	Cyanosis and congestive heart failure; all pulses decreased	Late stenotic murmur, single S_2	Cardiac enlargement; pulmonary vasculature greatly increased	Marked right ventricular hypertrophy
Ventricular septal defect	First weeks	Congestive heart failure	Pansystolic murmur narrowly split S_2; loud P_2	Cardiac enlargement; pulmonary vasculature increased	Combined ventrihypertrophy
Coarctation of the aorta	First weeks	Congestive heart failure; decreased femoral pulses	Stenotic murmur across back	Cardiac enlargement; pulmonary vasculature increased (passive)	Right ventricular hypertrophy
Patent ductus arteriosus with pulmonary artery	First weeks	Congestive heart failure; bonding pulses	Crescendic systolic murmur; possibly early diastolic murmur, split S_2; loud P_2	Cardiac enlargement; pulmonary vasculature increased	Combined ventricular hypertrophy

Adapted with permission from Nodas AS: *Heart disease in children*, Hospital Practice, 12:1, 1977, p 107.

observed. Intravenous furosemide (Lasix) is usually effective in producing a rapid duresis. The first dose is 1–2 mg/kg, which may be repeated in an hour if no significant response to the first dose is observed.

When patients with severe CHF are unresponsive to the regimens outlined above, isoproterenol (Isuprel) may be used. It is administered as a constant infusion of 0.1–0.5 µg/kg/min. Monitoring cardiac output, heart rate, and the presence of arrhythmias should guide the rate of infusion.

It should be remembered that fluid and salt loads should be minimized in children with CHF. Therefore all intravenous infusion must be carefully monitored and should reflect only the calculated requirements of each respective patient.

Cyanotic Heart Disease

Patients with central cyanosis because of cardiac defects can be grouped into two general categories. One group is comprised of patients with complex anomalies in whom significant intracardiac mixing of oxygenated and unoxygenated blood occurs. Pulmonary blood flow is usually increased, and congestive heart failure is not uncommon. The leading defects in this group of patients are transposition of the great vessels, hypoplasia of the left side of the heart, single ventricle, and truncus arteriosus. The second group of patients is made up of those with anomalies involving obstruction of pulmonary outflow with secondary right-to-left shunting. The most common lesions in patients in this group are Fallot's tetralogy, pulmonary stenosis with an intact septum, and pulmonary atresia.

DIAGNOSIS

Clinical findings associated with both groups are listed in Table 44.5. Often the leading alternative diagnosis is pulmonary disease. Retraction, grunting, and other signs of lung disease suggest a primary pulmonary process. Right radial arterial blood gases on room air and 100% oxygen will show little difference if a central cardiac defect is present.

Dextrostix and hematocrit determinations should be performed to rule out hypoglycemia and primary polycythemia, respectively. It should also be remembered that cyanosis may represent a manifestation of many underlying disease processes that cause hypoxia or hypoventilation. These include sepsis, shock, central nervous system disease, methemoglobinemia, hypotermia, and toxic ingestion.

MANAGEMENT

In general, when cyanotic cardiac disease is suspected, pediatric cardiologic consultation should be sought immediately. Echocardiography has been an effective tool in evaluating CHD and should be arranged after the chest roentgenogram and ECG have been done. Cardiac catheterization is often required to identify the lesion, however, this is best done in a center experienced in caring for children with CHD. While awaiting evaluation or transfer, careful ECG, vital signs, and blood gas measurements are imperative.

Hypoxic spells with severe cyanosis, tachypnea or apnea, irritability, or loss of consciousness are associated with certain cyanotic congenital heart lesions. Since these spells are most common in Fallot's tetralogy, they are also known as Tet spells. They are usually heralded by significant irritability, cyanosis, and at times a shocklike state that may simulate sepsis or SIDS. Treatment of hypoxic spells consists of administering oxygen, positioning the child in a knee–chest posture, and administering intramuscular morphine (0.1–0.2 mg/kg).

CHILD ABUSE

The abuse and neglect of children can be one of the most difficult and distressing problems facing health workers in an emergency setting. The complex and disturbing emotional responses elicited by a suspected case of child abuse can too often interfere with a careful and reasoned approach to its management. Denial of the possibility that child abuse may be the underlying cause of a presenting injury is, unfortunately, a common response of health care providers in this setting. A poor understanding and subsequent fears of the legal responsibilities related to reporting a suspected case of child abuse can also represent a barrier to high-quality medical practice. In addition, there is often a poor appreciation of the serious sequelae associated with unrecognized or unreported child abuse. It is well documented that abused children presenting with serious injuries have often been medically evaluated previously for abuse-related injuries that were not properly diagnosed or reported as being secondary to abuse.

Child abuse is not a single diagnostic entry. Rather it refers to the following complex of symptoms indicative of maltreatment of children:

1. *Physical abuse:* Physical injury as a result of acts of guardian or caretaker.
2. *Sexual abuse and misuse:* Abuse is the forced sexual contact between a child victim and a perpetrator; misuse is the exposure of a child to sexual stimulation inappropriate for the child's age or role within the family.
3. *Neglect:* This can be further subdivided into four categories:
   a. *Physical neglect* in that the child's requirements for shelter, food, and clothing are not met.
   b. *Emotional neglect* in that the child's need for nuturing and familial environment are not met.
   c. *Medical neglect* in that accessible preventive or therapeutic services are not used on behalf of the child.
   d. *Educational neglect* in that the caretaker does not ensure the level of education mandated by state law.
4. *Inadequate environmental control:* Failure to ensure adequate child care and a safe environment for normal child behaviors.

The clinical manifestations of child abuse can take many forms. Cutaneous manifestations of child abuse may be subtle. Bruising may be generalized or solitary, but the pattern of distribution should always be viewed with the mechanism of injury in mind. For example, bruises or other marks in the shape of a handprint, linear marks consistent with a whipping action, bite marks, or small circular burns from cigarettes are all common cutaneous evidence of child abuse. Distribution of burns often point to possible abuse.

Children under 1 year old with skull and long bone fractures should be carefully evaluated for possible abuse. Occult internal injuries in children should also raise concern. Lacerated liver, spleen, or pancreas; intramural hematoma of the bowel; or bladder contusion or rupture can all be secondary to physical abuse. Occular findings such as retinal or conjunctival hemorrhage, detached retina, or corneal abrasions can also be suggestive of abuse.

Laboratory evaluation can often be helpful. Clearly, film studies will confirm new and old fractures. Technetium bone scan can also reveal areas of bone abnormality and may be useful to replace or supplement a skeletal survey. Urinalysis and CBC may help identify occult injury. Coagulation studies will help rule out a primary bleeding disorder mimicking abuse.

The initial discussion with the family should reflect the special aspects of each individual case. However, Bittner and Newberger have outlined the following general considerations that should guide the interview with family members involved in a suspected case of child abuse:

1. To fully understand the historical and physical antecedents of the child's injury
2. To assess the plausibility of the elicited history
3. To gather past medical history of child and family members
4. To assess the relative ongoing risk to the child in an effort to decide the nature of protective or supportive services
5. To form a relationship with family members that will foster a cooperative and trusting attitude
6. To convey honestly the professional's concerns and requirement to report the case and to explain the general plan for forthcoming management.

Too often the initial interview will be preoccupied with determining the precise individual and motivations responsible for the injury. This approach is usually counterproductive in that it rarely uncovers the desired information and more often alienates the family and undermines subsequent efforts to enlist its participation in an ongoing therapeutic program.

A major task in the management of a suspected case of child abuse is determining the ongoing risk of further abuse if the child returns home. When no serious question of further injury exists, efforts should be primarily aimed at mobilizing the social service and medical resources required by the family and child. A follow-up plan is imperative in order for any abuse case to be followed at home. Reporting the case to appropriate agencies should help ensure adequate follow-up. When the risk of repeated injury to the child seems real, alternative custodial arrangements are required, and admission to the hosptial or other supervised residential placement may be indicated. In-hospital management often offers an opportunity for a more extensive evaluation and initiation of therapy and is recommended for complex cases and for those that are difficult to decipher.

Finally, practitioners should become acquainted with their state laws guiding reporting of suspected cases of child abuse. Although some variation among states does exist, most require reporting to specific state agencies. Failure to report suspected cases of child abuse leaves the practitioner vulnerable to criminal penalties. In all states, statutes regarding privileged communication are abrogated when child abuse is suspected. Reporting not only is mandated by law but can be used to mobilize support services needed by the family in crisis.

Sexual Abuse and Misuse

The term *sexual abuse* is usually used to refer to a child who is the object of aggressive forced sexual contact. The term *sexual misuse* is used in situations in which a child is exposed to stimulation that is inappropriate for the child's age and role in the family. Recent reports have suggested that incidents of sexual abuse and misuse are extremely commonplace in the United States and are vastly underreported. Unlike rape, sexual abuse and particularly misuse are usually perpetrated by a family friend or relative. It is more often chronic and usually does not involve intercourse.

Sexual abuse and misuse may present with a broad range of physical, behavioral, or social symptoms often related to the age of the affected child. Small infants may be the subject of inappropriate manipulation of the genitals. Erythematous or traumatized genitalia may indicate such abuse. Toddlers and school-age children often have difficulty verbalizing disturbing experiences and fears, and nonspecific complaints such as abdominal pain or nausea may represent the response to sexual abuse. Irritation or trauma in the vaginal or penile area requires a careful examination and evaluation of etiology. Sexually transmitted disease (STD) in childhood is being observed in ever-increasing numbers. In all children with vaginal discharge, cultures for gonorrhea should be taken. Although there have been reports suggesting transmission of STD without overt genital contact, evidence to date suggests that this is relatively rare. All children with gonorrhea should be thoroughly evaluated for sexual abuse. Other common presentations of sexual abuse or misuse in children include enuresis, hyperactivity, encopresis, school failure phobias, precocious or aggressive "sexual play." Adolescents are more frequently able to verbalize experiences and concerns than are young children. However, guilt, fear, and anxieties often prevent the adolescent from seeking care. Commonly, sexual abuse in adolescents will be associated with delinquency, leaving home, and school failure. However, there is a growing awareness that sexually abused adolescents are capable of suppressing the impact of such abuse.

Eliciting a history of sexual abuse or misuse from a child

should be approached with great care. The goal is to gather the requisite information to make judgments regarding the need for protective care, support services, and the nature and scope of medical intervention. However, review of the abusive incident or long history of chronic sexual abuse can be a painful and at times traumatic experience for the child and family. Therefore the clinician should tread slowly and with sensitivity during the interview process. Use of sexually explicit dolls may be useful. It may also be helpful for experienced social service or psychiatric personnel to help conduct the interview.

It is important to understand the nature and timing of the abuse. An effort should be made to know whether oral, rectal, penile or vaginal contact took place, as well as an estimate of when the abuse or assault took place. Information regarding the perpetrator may be important in assessing the relative risk inherent in the child's return home. However, as in other forms of child abuse, it may be more productive to delay discussion of the detailed elements of the history for a later time, once the safety of the child in the home has been ensured. The elicited history should be carefully documented in the record.

The physical examination should begin with the usual full pediatric examination. In addition, careful observations and collection procedures should be followed in accordance with medical and evidential concerns in cases of sexual abuse.

A question may arise as to the necessity of performing an internal pelvic examination in a suspected sexually abused child. When a history of vaginal or rectal penetration is elicited or suspected, a careful vaginal examination and appropriate laboratory tests are mandatory. When abnormalities of the external genitalia are present (erythema, echymoses, edema, etc.), an internal vaginal examination is again essential, whether or not the history includes vaginal contact. When the examiner is confident of a history of no contact with the child's genitalia or rectum and no findings on examination suggest such contact, the internal vaginal examination may be deferred. However, when questions arise as to the veracity or completeness of the history, internal examination should be done.

Treatment of the sexually abused child involves the following four major components:

1. Acute medical conditions
2. Sexually transmitted disease prophylaxis
3. Pregnancy prophylaxis, when appropriate
4. Psychiatric and social service management plan

Physical examination should reveal evidence of ongoing medical problems. Bruises, fractures, abdominal trauma, and vaginal lacerations can often be severe. Clearly these condi-

tions must be aggressively dealt with if suspected. Sexually transmitted disease prophylaxis is directed primarily at gonoccocal disease. Some professionals have suggested that such treatment can await positive cultures. However, in light of the disturbed social situation so often evident with these families, we presently feel that follow-up treatment may be difficult and that prophylaxis is indicated upon presentation in any case in which the perpetrator's genitalia have come into contact with the child. Oral ampicillin (50/mg/kg) in one dose (maximum 3.5 gm) or oral amoxicillin (50 mg/kg) in one dose (maximum 3 g) together with oral probenecid (25 mg/kg) (maximum of 1 g) is effective in preventing gonorrhea and does not inflict the pain of intramuscular injection. However, the use of oral antibiotics in this setting does not effectively protect the child from incubating syphilis. Repeat serologic studies for syphilis must be taken 6 weeks and 3 months after the initial sexual contact. Also oral antibiotics do not adequately treat pharyngeal or rectal gonorrhea; therefore if history or physical examination suggests rectal contact, intramuscular therapy is indicated (procaine penicillin 100,000 units/kg with maximum of 4.8 million units, administered half in each buttock intramuscularly together with probenecid 25 mg/kg by mouth). Children who are allergic to penicillin can be given tetracycline (500 mg by mouth every 6 hours for 4 days) if the child is not pregnant and not younger than 9 years old. Spectinomycin intramuscularly can be used in young or pregnant children who are allergic to penicillin.

Pregnancy prophylaxis is an important consideration after intercourse as a result of sexual abuse. Conditions to be met before prophylaxis is attempted include the following:

1. Child should be at risk for pregnancy, including having experienced menarche and not be presently menstruating.
2. Time of unprotected intercourse should be less than 72 hours before treatment.
3. Because of the risk to the fetus of high dose estrogen therapy and the possibility of treating a patient who is already pregnant by previous intercourse, estrogen therapy should be administered only to those patients who would have an abortion if already pregnant from previous intercourse.

Conjugated estrogens (Premarin) should be prescribed at 25 mg, twice a day for 4 days. The use of high dose estrogens is almost universally associated with nausea and vomiting. Therefore prochlorperazine 5–10 mg orally given 2 hours before estrogen is usually prescribed as well.

Decisions as to the relative safety of the child returning home should be carefully weighed. As in other forms of child abuse, if the living situation holds significant risk of continued abuse, admission or alternative placement is indicated. In most states sexual abuse is considered a form of child abuse and those reporting laws will apply. Reporting cases of rape and sexual abuse to the police may be dependent upon the family's wishes, unlike the mandatory reporting of such cases to social service agencies. The variations in local statutes are considerable, and clinicians should become familiar with those of their respective states. Follow-up plans should include medical reevaluation and recultures, when appropriate, after 3–7 days. Ongoing psychiatric therapy is usually indicated since significant psychological problems usually underlie the dynamics between the child and adult in question. In addition, the psychic sequelae of abuse are often severe and long standing.

SELECTED READINGS

Barker G: Current management of croup and epiglottitis. *Pediatr Clin North Am* 1979; 26(3).

Bates J: Epiglottitis: Diagnosis and treatment. *Pediatr Rev* 1979; 1(6).

Bittner S, Newberger E: Pediatric understanding of child abuse and neglect. *Pediatr Rev* 1981; 2(7).

Cloherty JP, Stark AR: *Manual of Neonatal Care.* Boston, Little Brown & Co, 1980.

Concensus Panel: Febrile seizures: Long-term management of children with fever-associated seizures. *Pediatrics* 1980; 66(6).

Gould J: Management of the near-miss infant. *Pediatr Clin North Am* 1979; 26(4).

Graef J, Cone T: *Manual of Pediatric Therapeutics,* 2nd ed. Boston, Little Brown & Co, 1980.

Greensher J, Mofenson H: Emergency treatment of the choking child. *Pediatrics* 1982; 70(1).

Guntheroth W: Initial evaluation of the child for heart disease. *Pediatr Clin North Am* 1978; 25(4).

Haggerty R, Green M (eds): *Ambulatory Pediatrics II.* Philadelphia, WB Saunders Co, 1977.

Heimlich HJ: First aid for choking children. *Pediatrics* 1982; 70(1).

Hochman H et al: Dehydration, diabetic ketoacidosis, and shock in the pediatric patient. *Pediatr Clin North Am* 1979; 26(4)

Illingworth RS: *Common Symptoms of Disease in Children,* 6th ed. Blackwell, 1980.

McCarthy P: What tests are indicated for the child under two with fever? *Pediatr Rev* 1979; 1(2).

Montgomery R, Hathaway W: Acute bleeding emergencies. *Pediatr Clin North Am* 1980; 27(2).

Rothner AD, Erenberg G: Status epilepticus. *Pediatr Clin North Am* 1980; 27(3).

Rovitch M: Intussusception, in Mustard W et al (eds): *Pediatric Surgery.* Year Book, 1980.

Rumsza M, Niggemann E: Medical evaluation of sexually abused children. *Pediatrics* 1982; 69(1).

Teele D: Bacteremia in febrile children under two years: Results of cultures of blood of 600 consecutive febrile children seen in a walk-in clinic. *J Pediatr* 1975.

Winters R (ed): *The Body Fluids in Pediatrics.* Boston, Little Brown & Co, 1973.

MEDICOLEGAL CONSIDERATIONS

PART IV

45

MEDICOLEGAL CONSIDERATIONS OF EMERGENCY MEDICAL CARE

Elliott L. Cohen
Joseph M. Healey, Jr.
Anthony P. Scapicchio

In the emergency situation, knowledgeable and competent physicians should use their skills in a manner consistent with the highest ethical standards of the healing professions. Concern for the injured or dying person should be uppermost in their minds. Hesitation or delay could cause avoidable death or unnecessary suffering. To the full extent of their knowledge and expertise, physicians should act to preserve life and prevent death. Unfortunately, fear of potential legal liability deters some physicians from acting decisively and effectively. This chapter is offered to complement the previous chapters by assisting physicians in understanding their legal rights and duties in the emergency setting. The first part of this chapter, "General Perspectives," is written by a lawyer and sets forth the general principles of medical law regarding emergency care. The second part, "Emergency Department Perspectives," is written by two physicians and discusses potential problem areas for emergency physicians and strategies for avoiding these problems while satisfying legal obligations. Physicians should be reminded that law in the emergency context is deeply rooted in the specific law of each of the 50 states. For this reason, as well as for the equally important reason that the law changes rapidly, physicians are encouraged to use the general guidelines presented in this chapter as a basis for reviewing their practice policies with their attorney–consultants in the specific legal context of their practice.

General Perspectives

Joseph M. Healey, Jr.

The context of emergency care is shaped by two major variables that must be understood and appreciated. First, the term *emergency care* may be used to describe three different settings in which people seek necessary medical care: (1) the *Good Samaritan* situation in which a patient who is injured in an accident needs emergency medical care outside of a health care facility; (2) the *emergency department* situation, in which a patient who is injured outside a health care facility is brought to the facility to obtain emergency care; (3) the *emergency in practice* situation in which a patient who is already receiving medical care becomes in need of emergency medical care. The rights and duties both of physicians and of patients vary according to the setting in which emergency care is sought. The second important variable to be considered is the *legal status of the patient*. Adults of sound mind are regarded by the law as competent to make decisions about their health care. Problems may exist, however, in ascertaining how the health care provider should proceed when the patient is an adult who is not of sound mind, is a minor who has not reached the age of majority, or is a person whose ability to make decisions is compromised by a serious medical condition. Physicians should also take into account the legal status of the patient in evaluating rights and duties in the emergency setting.

SETTINGS IN WHICH EMERGENCY CARE IS PROVIDED

Legal obligations generally commence at the beginning of the physician–patient and hospital–patient relationships. In general, physicians do not have a legal obligation to provide medical care to every person seeking or in need of such care. The law has regarded the relationship between physician and patient as a voluntary relationship in which both parties freely agree to participate. The primary exceptions to this general principle are found in emergency settings. In the Good Samaritan situation, some states have replaced the voluntary dimension of the physician–patient relationship with a statute or regulation requiring that physicians render emergency care. In the emergency department situation, courts have generally held that a health care facility that operates an emergency department has a legal obligation to provide care to those people who come to the facility with an identifiable emergency and are relying upon the implied offer of emergency care. In the emergency in practice situation, by definition a physician–patient relationship existed before the emergency, and therefore legal obligations had already commenced.

Once the relationship is established, physicians have a legal obligation to provide an acceptable quality of medical care. The standard of expected physician performance is derived from the malpractice system. In general, physicians are expected to do what a reasonable physician would do in the same or similar circumstances. It is a standard of ordinary and customary practice that is deeply rooted in the standards of the medical community. Under the theory of malpractice, physicians may be held legally liable for harm directly and proximately caused by a breach of the duty of reasonable care. Physicians who fail to adhere to appropriate standards and who cause injury to their patients are potentially legally liable. The preceding chapters discussed the expected conduct of physicians in all three emergency settings.

Fear of malpractice has become a barrier for some physicians, especially in the Good Samaritan situation. Most states do not require a physician to provide emergency care in this setting. Nonetheless, the highest ethical standards compel a physician to be of assistance to those whose lives are threatened or who suffer pain after an accident. The American Medical Association's *Principles of Medical Ethics* stipulates

> A physician is free to choose whom he [or she] will serve. He [or she] should, however, respond to any requests for his assistance in an emergency.

In general, the members of the medical profession have recognized this obligation to serve their communities by providing emergency care in the Good Samaritan situation. However, some physicians have expressed a reluctance to become involved in such care. This reluctance has been traced in a large measure to fear of malpractice litigation. Such fears are at best excessive and at worst groundless. In 1973, *The Report of the Secretary's Commission on Medical Malpractice* stated the following

> While the fears of physicians about their potential liability for rendering emergency aid are undoubtedly real, they appear to be based on little more than rumor or hearsay, generated and perpetuated in large part by the mass media. . . .
>
> As a Commission, we make no specific findings regarding the real causes behind the reluctance of some physicians to provide emergency aid to accident victims. We do believe, however, that the time has come to set the record straight on at least one issue: the legal risks to render emergency care to accident victims in non-health care settings are minimal if not infinitesimal. Health professionals, as well as the general public, should be so informed.

There is no record of any reported case in U. S. legal history in which a physician acting in the Good Samaritan situation has been found guilty and required to pay damages. It is important that this fear be put to rest as a deterent to providing needed emergency care. The public policy of the vast majority of states has been expressed by the Good Samaritan laws that, though varying significantly from state to state, have the spe-

cific intention of encouraging physicians to provide emergency care by limiting or eliminating the liability of the physician. Physicians should evaluate their potential liability in realistic terms.

INFORMED CONSENT

One particularly important aspect of an existing physician–patient relationship is the requirement that the informed, competent, and voluntary consent of patients be obtained before treatment is provided. Consent represents the mechanism by which patients vindicate their right to self-determination and participate in health care decision making.

Consent is the permission required from the patient before any intrusion into the physical or personal integrity of the patient may be initiated. The standard by which consent is to be evaluated has been undergoing a process of redefinition during the past several years. As a result, there are two standards, each of which is applicable in certain states. The traditional standard is the same as that which is used in malpractice cases in general. A physician is expected to disclose to a patient what a reasonable physician would disclose in the same or similar circumstances. Included in this disclosure should be the nature of the medical condition, the treatment proposed, risks of the procedure, possible side effects, and alternative procedures (if any) and their risks and side effects. After evaluating this information, the patient is free to refuse or accept treatment. An important characteristic of this standard is that it is determined by the medical community. Which side effects and which alternative procedures are to be disclosed depend on the prevailing practice in the medical community. This traditional standard remains the standard in a majority of the states.

In contrast to the traditional standard, a "modern" standard has been recognized in some states. This new standard shifts the focus from the physician to the patient. The modern standard requires that a physician discloses what a reasonable patient would need to know to make an intelligent decision concerning treatment. Included in the disclosure must be the nature of the medical condition, the treatment proposed, significant risks of the procedure, significant possible side effects, and significant alternative procedures and their significant risks and side effects. The standard of *significance* is derived from what a reasonable patient would need to know in the same or similar circumstances. As in the case of the traditional standard, after an appropriate disclosure the patient must make the choice of whether to accept or reject the proposed treatment. Though not yet accepted as the standard in the majority of states, this modern standard has received a good deal of support in recent years.

What makes consent an especially difficult problem in emergency care is not simply the determination of which standard applies, but the very nature of emergency medicine itself, which often does not allow the luxury of detached reflection. Often, steps must be taken quickly to preserve life, to stablize a dangerous condition, or to prevent possible deterioration. We must look at this inherent limitation in terms of special types of patients and special situations.

Good Samaritan Setting

In the Good Samaritan situation, physicians generally have an ethical obligation to provide medical care, but in most states they do not have a legal obligation to do so. If physicians render care in this setting, their potential liability would be affected by the Good Samaritan statute in the specific state. Physicians should review the Good Samaritan statute in their respective states and should act in accordance with its requirements.

If the victim is an adult of sound mind, he or she has the right to consent to treatment and, in most states, to refuse treatment, including life-saving treatment. Although United States courts formerly did not allow patients to refuse life-saving treatment, the prevailing trend of U.S. law during the last quarter of the 20th century has been to recognize the autonomy of a competent adult as more important than the paternalism of the health professional or of the state.

People who have been declared legally incompetent or who are, in fact, incompetent without formal legal recognition of the incompetence, present difficult problems. In such situations, the ability of the individual victim to have or to express a preference for treatment or nontreatment is either suspect or clearly not present. If an adult is rendered incompetent and a life-threatening emergency exists, the law generally permits the physician to imply the consent of the patient, that is, to assume that if the patient were competent she or he would prefer treatment to nontreatment. The physician should concentrate on managing the emergency. In the case of minors, mentally ill people, or mentally retarded people, a parent or legal guardian is generally appointed by the court and has the authority to consent. If such a person is available, his or her consent should be obtained. If a life-threatening emergency exists and the person legally authorized to consent is not available, the physician should imply the necessary consent and proceed with treatment. "Protection" of the autonomy of an incompetent victim in the Good Samaritan setting or fear of liability for performing life-saving interventions should not deter the physician from acting decisively and effectively.

Emergency Department Setting

In the emergency department setting, similar principles to those in the Good Samaritan setting are operative. The consent of adults of sound mind should be sought, and their refusal to accept treatment should generally be respected. Incompetent patients present the same dilemma in this setting as in the Good Samaritan setting. If a life-threatening emergency exists and neither the patient nor the person with legal authority to consent is in a position to give consent, the emergency physician should imply consent and provide treatment. Once again, the unavailability of a consenting person should not be an excuse for allowing a treatable patient to suffer an avoidable death.

Emergency in Medical Practice

The emergency in medical practice situation is among the most complicated and most controversial situations in contemporary medicine. Should a patient be allowed to die either because emergency treatment is not provided or because it is withdrawn from a patient? In recent years, courts have tended to allow adults of sound mind the right to refuse emergency treatment. The most difficult cases involve patients who are not legally competent and are therefore incapable of expressing their wishes. There has been significant discussion about the extent to which a guardian or parent should be allowed to refuse consent in such cases. There has been extended discussion about the extent to which the patient's prior wishes as documented in a living will should determine whether treatment should be provided, not provided, or withdrawn at some point. Determination of the legal rights and duties of physicians in these cases is a matter for the law of the state in which the physician is practicing. Several states have established mechanisms to permit discussions of these issues. Some states have enacted legislation allowing living wills to be legally binding thereby releasing health professionals and institutions who respect the wishes expressed in the living wills from civil or criminal liability. Physicians should explore the laws of their specific states with their attorney–consultants.

Emergency Department Perspectives

Elliot L. Cohen
Anthony P. Scapicchio

Although wide acceptance of the concept of the patient's right to die has led to a great deal of uncertainty, the essential obligation of a physician is to take steps to preserve and protect the life of a patient in a manner consistent with good medical practice, provided the patient consents to accept such treatment. *A physician is responsible for providing medical care in a manner that any reasonable physician would in the same or similar circumstances.*

The standard against which a physician is measured is a medical standard, not an abstract legal standard. The context of the treatment, as discussed in the first part of this chapter, is also important. The phrase "in the same or similar circumstances" allows for the differences that exist in treatment provided in the Good Samaritan setting (e.g., alongside a highway), in an emergency department situation, or in an emergency in practice (e.g., in a hospital). The key word of this standard is *reasonable,* which is evaluated in the context of the decision made. Reasonable treatment is determined by the medical community and the boundaries of medical practice that it recognizes. How the physician in the emergency department, in which most emergency care is rendered, carries out responsibilities is discussed here. The general principles described apply to all physicians and medical personnel who provide emergency medical care.

EMERGENCY DEPARTMENT SETTING

For a variety of reasons, the number of people who visit emergency departments in hospitals has increased steadily since World War II. In 1979 approximately 80 million people visited hospital emergency departments in the United States. In the American College of Emergency Physician Study of more than 10,000 emergency department visits, 44% of the patients stated that they believed their problem required immediate care (within minutes). Of the patients whom the physicians believed required immediate care, 25% had not perceived the same urgency. Emergency department physicians, therefore are faced with patients who have undifferentiated illnesses or injuries. The conditions of many of these patients are not as critical as they believe them to be, yet other patients are more ill than they initially appear.

At one end of the spectrum are patients with acute, life-threatening, and limb-threatening problems that require immediate diagnostic and simultaneous therapeutic intervention. Most of these patients require hospitalization. At the other end of the spectrum are patients with nonacute, noncritical problems for whom timing of diagnostic and therapeutic intervention is not as important. Between the two extremes is the large number of patients with acute and semiacute problems who may require considerable diagnostic study to determine how critical the illness or injury is and whether or not hospitalization will be necessary.

In most emergency departments, the patient is first seen by a triage nurse who takes a brief history and performs a limited examination relevant to the patient's complaint. The triage nurse then assigns a priority status to the patient. Those patients with acute, life-threatening, or limb-threatening symptoms or signs are the first to be examined by the physician. Diagnostic studies are ordered as needed. Resuscitation and stabilization are critical and are begun concurrently. While the patient is being stabilized, the emergency physician mobilizes appropriate specialists and personnel for continued and definitive management.

Patients with acute problems are seen as a second priority, and those with semiacute or nonacute problems are seen as a third priority, usually in the order of their arrival at the emergency department. For these patients, accurate diagnosis is important so initial treatment can be instituted either in the hospital or, more commonly, as an outpatient.

RESPONSIBILITY OF THE EMERGENCY CARE PHYSICIAN

Assessment and Initial Management

The major responsibility of the physician in the emergency department is to establish a minimum data base, which must include history, physical examination, and certain ancillary diagnostic procedures. Sometimes, however, resuscitation and stabilization must begin before completion of the data base. If the patient is unable to give a history, it must be taken by the physician or nurse from a third party. The physician must assess the reliability of the history and interpret it accurately.

Findings of a carefully performed physical examination and results of certain ancillary diagnostic procedures in relation to other elements of the data base are accumulated, assimilated, interpreted, and recorded clearly and legibly on the patient's emergency department record so that this information can be referred to in the future. A working diagnosis is now established, and the diagnosis and potential modes of treatment are discussed with the patient with regard to earlier statements involving consent. Every detail of the therapy, which is compatible with standards of the hospital and the community, should be recorded accurately on the patient's record.

Documentation

THE MEDICAL RECORD

The physician's best source of protection is a legible, well-documented medical record. The law is process oriented and is less frequently concerned with outcome or with the rightness or wrongness of a decision than it is with its justifiability. The standard is what a reasonable physician would do in a similar situation. A judgment error may be defensible, but the thought process that went into the diagnostic or therapeutic decision must be noted on the record.

A medical record should be provided for every patient who is evaluated in the emergency department and should become part of the official hospital record for that patient. It should contain the information that a reasonable physician would need to understand the case and begin treatment effectively. As a minimum, the medical record should contain the following information:

1. Adequate patient identification
2. Time of arrival, means of arrival, and mode of arrival
3. History of injury or illness, including emergency care rendered before arrival, as well as pertinent past medical history, current medications, and allergies
4. Description of physical findings
5. Recording of the laboratory data base
6. Diagnosis
7. Treatment given
8. Condition and time of patient discharge or transfer
9. Final disposition
10. Instructions relative to follow-up care
11. Signature of the attending physician

Discharge of the Physician–Patient Relationship

At the conclusion of treatment in the emergency department, the physician must decide on follow-up care for the patient without abandoning the patient or exposing him or her to additional serious risks. This follow-up care can take three basic forms: (1) admit the patient to the hospital in which emergency care was given, (2) transfer the patient to another facility for follow-up care, or (3) provide for ambulatory follow-up care.

ADMISSION TO THE HOSPITAL

If the patient is admitted to the same hospital in which initial emergency care was provided, it is the legal responsibility of the emergency physician to ensure that the physician or physicians responsible for the patient assume the follow-up care at an appropriate time and place. This means that the emergency department physician must decide whether the attending physician must assume follow-up care in the emergency de-

partment immediately, as in life-threatening situations, or whether the attending physician can assume follow-up care after the patient has been transported to the hospital bed in the event of less urgent situations. Until the attending physician physically assumes responsibility for follow-up care of the patient, the patient remains the legal responsibility of the emergency department physician, the implication being that the emergency physician may be held liable for any undue delay in follow-up care that could result in avoidable complications or aggravation of the original problem.

TRANSFER OF THE PATIENT

If the emergency department physician decides to transfer a patient to another facility, it is his or her responsibility to follow the guidelines set forth by various accrediting agencies. The emergency physician must not arbitrarily transfer a patient from the emergency department to another facility without serious consideration of the medical necessity for the transfer; that is, a transfer should not be done for arbitrary reasons. If sound medical judgment demands the need for transfer to another facility, the emergency physician should proceed as follows: (1) explain to the patient or family or friend the need for the transfer and obtain approval; (2) notify the staff physician (who would have assumed follow-up care of the patient had he or she been admitted to the same hospital) of the proposed transfer, tell him or her the reasons for the transfer, and obtain approval; (3) notify the hospital to which the patient is being transferred, speak to the physician who will assume follow-up care of the patient, state reasons for the transfer, and obtain approval; (4) send a physician or nurse with the patient during the transfer process; (5) send a detailed copy of the medical record including results of radiologic, laboratory, and electrocardiographic tests with the patient to the accepting facility; (6) notify the hospital administrator of the proposed transfer and reasons for it and obtain approval. It is a good idea to verify completion of transfer by telephone or other means of interhospital communication. Remember that even in this situation, the transferring hospital and emergency physician may be held liable for undue delay in essential follow-up care if this is to be provided at another facility.

AMBULATORY FOLLOW-UP CARE

When the emergency department physician decides to provide ambulatory follow-up care, this care can take several forms. However, no matter what form it takes, the patient must understand fully what he or she is to do to continue treatment until the follow-up visit. Instructions should be specific and understandable and should be given in writing with a copy kept as a part of the patient's permanent record. The patient is asked to sign the record, indicating that he or she was given a copy of the instructions. If the physician suspects that the patient will be unable to follow the instructions, appropriate arrangements should be made with a visiting nurse or social worker or the patient should be admitted to the hospital to ensure continuation of proper treatment.

The *"as necessary," or "prn" follow-up care* instructions are for patients with medical problems that are minor, self-limited, those that respond to the treatment outlined in the instructions, and those that usually do not require medical follow-up for reevaluation. These patients must be given written instructions stating that should any questions arise as to the original diagnosis, treatment, or follow-up, they should return to the emergency department or their personal physician as they feel necessary.

The *semiurgent, planned follow-up care* form is designed for a patient whose original problem demands that a follow-up reevaluation be planned at a specific time and place to reassess the patient's progress because there may have been some question as to the exact diagnosis or attendant therapy instituted at the time of the original visit. If necessary, the emergency physician who provided the initial management, or a colleague, should make the reassessment at the appropriate time and in the appropriate place. If the original emergency physician does not provide this follow-up care, he or she must be sure that the original record is available to the emergency department in which follow-up care is administered or to the referral physician.

Nonurgent, planned follow-up means that the patient should have the problem reevaluated or followed-up in a necessary but less urgent fashion. The patient may be instructed to contact his personal physician for a follow-up appointment within a certain period of time or the patient may be instructed to contact one of the staff members of the hospital who, by previous agreement, has consented to accept patients on a follow-up referral basis. Alternatively, the patient may be given an appointment at an appropriate follow-up clinic, which may be provided by the hospital's ambulatory care unit.

Follow-up of Data Base

The emergency department physician is responsible for conducting a follow-up study of the data compiled during the patient's original visit. This applies specifically to laboratory data obtained and interpreted by the emergency physician during the original visit. When the official follow-up interpretations of the various studies are available, these results should be compared with the original interpretations made by the

emergency physician as they appear on the patient's record. Agreement in interpretation of "negative" laboratory studies does not rule out the presence of disease. If the official interpretation indicates an abnormal finding and the original emergency physician's interpretation, as recorded on the patient's record, indicates negative findings, this discrepancy should be clarified by asking the patient to return for reevaluation of the problem. This should be done as soon as possible.

Failure on the part of the emergency physician to provide follow-up care may constitute abandonment. Abandonment is the unilateral severance of the professional relationship between the physician and a patient without reasonable notice at a time when the patient still needs medical attention. It is the responsibility of the emergency physician to provide follow-up care when indicated.

SPECIAL PROBLEMS IN EMERGENCY DEPARTMENTS

Diagnostic or Therapeutic Errors

The emergency department itself often presents problems in logistics. The numbers of patients seen are variable and unpredictable, placing the physician and staff under severe time constraints. Most patients want immediate attention, and often their expectations are not met. The most serious problem is understaffing. Understaffing usually means that the number of physicians and nurses in the emergency department is insufficient for the patient load. However, *understaffing* can also mean that the physicians and nurses who work in the emergency department are either undertrained in most general areas of knowledge or overtrained in specific areas. Both types of understaffing can lead to unintentional diagnostic errors and charges of malpractice. A physician is liable for negligence when his or her conduct fails to meet the legal standard of care and somebody is injured as a result. Negligence, because it is unintentional, cannot willfully be prevented, but a malpractice suit can sometimes be prevented even when a diagnostic error has been committed.

Emergency department physicians must make every attempt to avoid diagnostic errors because their relationships with patients may be a one-time event and they may be unable to correct their errors. Some second meetings do occur, however, and the emergency physician may have the opportunity to explain that a diagnostic error has been made during the first visit. In any case, at the first meeting it is important to establish a meaningful rapport with the patient, which can be developed even during a short emergency department visit. The physician should communicate a true interest in the patient's problem. Often, simple courtesies such as an appropriate introduction, a handshake, an apology, or an explanation for a long wait can go a long way toward developing good rapport.

Realizing that some diagnostic errors are unavoidable, the physician must be prepared to face the patient again at a future date, perhaps under strained circumstances. If the physician has established a good rapport with the patient, he or she can call the patient, correct the diagnostic error, and avoid unnecessary aggravation of a patient's injury. This is an important consideration because although judgmental or diagnostic errors are at times unavoidable, they may be legally defensible. On the other hand, diagnostic errors that are not reconciled may lead to aggravation of injuries. Such situations are legally indefensible.

It is in the area of electrocardiography and radiography that many errors of interpretation are made. These errors can be absolute or relative. An error is *absolute* if a physician interprets results of a diagnostic study as negative when in fact the findings are positive. An error is *relative* if, for example, a physician interprets the results of electrocardiography as showing no abnormality and in fact no abnormality is present but the patient has a cardiac problem. The physician is responsible for recognizing both of these errors.

When physicians go through the careful process of obtaining and documenting the data and arrive at a diagnosis that represents a *judgmental error,* the error may be defensible. An incorrect diagnosis without recorded data is less defensible. If the error is discovered later, it should be pursued either by recalling the patient to the emergency department or by referring the patient to an appropriate specialist. Although judgmental or diagnostic errors based on adequate data may be legally defensible, aggravation of the original injury as a result of undue delay in recognition or rectification of a diagnostic error is less defensible.

Discharge against Medical Advice

A patient may decide to reject the treatment proposed by the emergency department physician. Should this occur, the physician should review with the patient the nature of the illness or injury, the nature of the proposed treatment, and the consequences, if any, of failure to treat the basic illness or injury. If the patient appears to be mentally competent and still refuses the proposed treatment, the emergency physician should ask the patient to formalize the refusal by signing a discharge against medical advice form; the form, then becomes part of the patient's emergency department record.

The patient should be offered an alternative form of therapy,

if one exists. A mode of follow-up care should be arranged by the physician if the patient will accept it. The patient should be told to return to the emergency department should he or she change his or her mind concerning treatment or should the condition deteriorate. Any attempt to hold or treat a mentally competent patient against his or her will could be considered assault and battery and false imprisonment.

If the patient is judged by the physician to be mentally incompetent because of illness, injury, or some other cause (e.g., drug or alcohol intoxication), the physician should err on the side of treatment, particularly in situations in which time is of the essence. The physician should document in the medical record why he or she decided that the patient was incompetent. The patient, after registering in the emergency department for treatment, may decide to leave at any time during diagnosis or treatment. If this is not done formally, as in signing a discharge against medical advice form, the patient's departure is referred to as *elopement.* Obviously, it is best that the patient stay in the emergency department until he or she is seen by a physician.

INTERACTION BETWEEN PHYSICIANS AND LAW ENFORCEMENT OR PUBLIC HEALTH AGENCIES

In the course of emergency treatment of a patient, the physician may find that he or she will have to deal not only with the patient but also with law enforcement or public health officials. Such situations are most likely to occur when there has been an alleged assault or rape, when there has been a gunshot or stab wound, when the patient is in the custody of the police, when the patient is suspected of being under the influence of alcohol or other drugs, when there is suspicion of child abuse or neglect, or when there is a suspected medicolegal death. In addition, many of the communicable diseases, particularly venereal diseases, should be reported to the public health authorities.

Assault or Rape

When a patient seeks medical attention for an alleged assault, the physician should ask the patient if he or she has reported the incident to the police of the town in which the incident is said to have occurred. If the patient has not done so and wants the police to be notified, the physician may call them. The police will usually send an officer to obtain information and investigate the situation. Many victims of alleged sexual assault do not want the incident reported. To the extent permissible by law, the physician should respect the desire of the patient and ensure that all clinical treatment will be kept confidential. In many states sexual assault of a minor must be reported as child abuse.

Unless the patient's injuries require immediate treatment, the patient who wants medical treatment should sign a consent form (after proper explanation) authorizing the physician to perform a complete examination, including a pelvic examination. If the patient also wants to report the incident to the police, the consent form should authorize collection of necessary specimens and release of evidence and other medical information to the police. In any case, a rape victim may benefit from the help of the local rape crisis center, and the center should be called if the patient wishes.

If a patient reports being raped, the physician should take a careful history of the alleged incident noting, in the patient's words, exactly what happened. The history should include date and location; orifices that were penetrated; whether ejaculation had occurred; date of last menstrual period (if more than 6 weeks ago, was a pregnancy test performed and if so, the result); whether the patient has bathed, showered, douched, urinated, defecated, or changed clothes since the alleged incident; date of last coitus; and type of birth control used, if any.

A general physical examination, including evaluation of the patient's emotional state, should be performed after the patient has been undressed and given a hospital gown to wear. A description of all external evidence of trauma (e.g., bites, bruises, abrasions) should be noted on the record. On pelvic examination, any signs of trauma to the vulva should be noted as well as whether the hymenal ring is intact and if there are any lacerations. The vaginal vault and cervix should be examined for lacerations, blood, semen, discharge, or foreign bodies. A careful bimanual and rectal examination should be performed.

Laboratory specimens should include pubic hair that has been combed into a labeled envelope, pubic hair that has been pulled from the roots, samples of any foreign material on the victim's body, scrapings from under the fingernails, a culture for gonorrhea from any orifice allegedly penetrated, blood for typing, and a serum VDRL. Samples of the secretions of any orific allegedly penetrated should be tested for acid phosphatase, and the physician should look at a wet mount of the secretions under a microscope to see if there are any sperm.

The collected evidence and the patient's clothing (if she has not changed clothes since the alleged incident) should be released to the police officer. The officer should sign a release form, and a copy should be placed in the patient's record. The patient can be treated for pregnancy or venereal disease prophylaxis at the discretion of the physician.

Gunshot and Stab Wounds

All gunshot wounds, bullet wounds, powder burns, or other injuries caused by the discharge of a gun must be reported to the police of the town in which the incident occurred, as well as to the police of the town in which the treating physician (and hospital) is located. The same is true of wounds caused by a knife or other sharp object if there is any suspicion that a criminal act was involved. Notification may usually be done by telephone, and an officer will be sent to investigate.

The physician should cooperate with the police who are investigating the case as long as the investigation does not threaten the medical condition of the patient. The medicolegal responsibilities of the physician are to care for the patient, to document the facts, and to preserve the evidence. Physicians should record the facts and refrain from drawing conclusions.

The history of the alleged circumstances of the gunshot or stab wound (i.e., accidental or deliberate) should be recorded, including the time of injury and, if it is a gunshot wound, the range at which the gun was fired. Any known facts about the weapon should be noted (i.e., type, model, caliber, brand name, country of origin), as well as type and caliber of the ammunition.

The appearance of the wound should be described in detail. Avoid using general terms such as "typical gunshot (stab) wound." For stab wounds, the number of wounds, location, length, and depth should be recorded. For gunshot wounds, the entrance wound and exit wound, if any, must be described. In a contact wound (the muzzle of the gun is against the target), the entrance hole will have a surrounding ring of soot, blackened tissue, and possibly some ecchymosis. At close range (less than 1 m), the entrance wound is usually larger than the exit wound. Surrounding the entrance hole may be a halo of the products of discharge and flame burns, depending on exactly how close the muzzle of the gun was to the victim. Gunpowder grains may be imbedded in the skin, causing a tattoolike appearance on the surrounding area. Wounds caused by guns fired from a distance show only the skin wound without tattooing or powder burns. The clothing the victim was wearing can alter the appearance of the wound and harbor important evidence such as powder or flame burns.

Photographs of the wounds are invaluable, and the physician who sees a number of gunshot wounds should document their appearance with photographs. A metric scale should be inserted into the file of each photograph, and the photograph should become a permanent part of the medical record. The evidence to be preserved includes the weapon, its missile, other products of discharge, and the victim's clothing. All such evidence should be given to the police, who should sign a release form. A copy of this form should be maintained in the patient's record. The weapon should be handled carefully to avoid removal of fingerprints and bits of tissue, hair, and clothing. If the weapon is a gun, the physician should not tamper with the firing mechanism.

The bullet or any fragment of the bullet that has been extracted from a patient should be saved since fragments as small as 3 mm can be matched to the involved weapon. With the patient's consent, such a bullet or fragment should be extracted even if it is not a medical necessity if this can be done easily and safely (i.e., the bullet is located just below the skin). Care should be taken not to damage the bullet or fragment with forceps. If the bullet cannot be extracted, radiographs of the involved area and bullet can sometimes give clues as to the caliber or type of weapon.

The clothing of a victim can be valuable evidence and should be preserved. Special care must be taken not to cut through bullet or stab holes. If any clothing was on the victim in an unusual manner (e.g., inside out), it should be noted so that the evidence will not be confusing.

In summary, the medicolegal responsibilities of a physician for a gunshot or stab wound are to care for the patient, report the incident to the police, document appearance of the wound without drawing conclusions, and preserve the evidence and give it to the police.

Patients in Police Custody

When a law enforcement officer brings a patient who is in custody or pending custody to a physician or an emergency department for medical treatment, consent for treatment should proceed in the usual manner. If the patient in custody is a minor, attempts should be made to obtain parental consent. Every attempt should be made to expedite services and discharge the patient as rapidly as possible. The officer should be discouraged from leaving the patient unguarded with the physician or emergency department personnel. If the police do leave the patient unguarded and the patient attempts to leave, the physician should not risk injury by attempting to detain the patient. If the patient leaves, the physician should report this to the police immediately.

Alcohol or Drug Intoxication

Law enforcement officers will be interested in whether a patient is under the influence of alcohol or other mind-altering drugs when a patient has been involved in a motor vehicle accident or has been cited for a motor vehicle violation even if there has not been an accident. In such situations, the police officer

may request that the level of alcohol in the blood be obtained. If the patient consents to having the blood alcohol level tested there is no problem, but the patient may refuse to have a venipuncture performed. To perform a venipuncture against a patient's wishes may leave a physician open to the charge of assault and battery. Therefore, the patient must give consent for this test; some states have implied consent laws that allow the state to revoke the patient's driver's license for a period of time, usually between 3 and 12 months, if he or she refuses to consent to the blood test. Parental consent is not necessary for minors, and the consent of unconscious patients is implied.

A written request for blood alcohol level determination should be signed by the police officer, and consent (oral consent is usually sufficient) of the subject should be obtained. After the site is prepared with nonalcohol-based medium, blood should be drawn by a physician, registered nurse, or registered medical technologist. Results of the test must be made available to the person upon request. A person with an alcohol level above 100–150 mg/dl is considered legally intoxicated in most states.

It is wise to avoid judgmental terms such as "intoxicated" or "inebriated." It is better to describe the patient's physical condition, such as level of consciousness, nystagmus, ataxia, and odor of alcohol on breath and to avoid drawing conclusions.

Law enforcement officials may also be interested in test results of patients suspected of being under the influence of mind-altering drugs such as narcotics, barbiturates, other hypnotic sedatives, amphetamines, or hallucinogens. The procedure used by the police officer to request a blood test to determine presence of such drugs should be similar to that used for a blood alcohol level test. In either case, if the blood levels are needed to help in the medical management of the patient (e.g., unexplained coma, compromise of mental status, seizures), blood, urine, gastric aspirate, or emesis (if available) should be analyzed just as the physician would analyze a specimen for complete blood cell count, blood sugar, or serum electrolytes.

Child Abuse or Neglect

As discussed in Chapter 44, most states now require physicians and other health professionals to report any case of suspected child abuse or neglect. Usually a telephone report followed by a written report to either the local public health or welfare department is required. Failure to report suspected cases is a criminal offense and may be punishable, usually with a fine. On the other hand, most states grant immunity from any civil or criminal action by reason of reporting provided that the report was made in good faith. A child is anyone under the age of majority (usually 18 years old). Whenever possible, the physician should contact the parents (or guardians) of the child and tell them that a report is being submitted.

Child abuse refers to physical injury or sexual abuse, whereas *neglect* means impairment of the child's physical, mental, or emotional condition as a result of the failure of the people (parents or guardians) responsible for care to exercise a minimum degree of care. Examples include severe failure to thrive; malnutrition; lack of medical care; repeated ingestions; repeated accidents as a result of inadequate supervision; inadequate food, clothing, or shelter; poor school attendance; or severe emotional neglect.

The medical record should document evidence of neglect or injury, including the location, size, and age of all bruises and scars or other external findings. Photographs of the lesions are useful. An accurate account of the verbal exchange and an objective assessment of the child's emotional state should be recorded.

Any child who is suspected of being in danger if he or she were to go home with the parent(s) should be admitted to the hospital. These patients usually include children with suspected inflicted injuries, those experiencing severe neglect or failure to thrive, and those who have been sexually abused. If the parents (or legal guardians) refuse to allow the child to be admitted, the presiding judge of the local juvenile or district court can authorize hospitalization of the child until a hearing can be held regarding care and custody of the child.

A physician or other health professional who has reason to believe that a child has died as the result of child abuse or neglect should immediately report the death to the local medical examiner and the local department of public health or welfare.

Medicolegal Deaths

Although laws vary from state to state, most state laws require that a physician notify the local medical examiner when confronted with a suspected medicolegal death. The categories to be reported include death resulting from any act of violence; death resulting from induced abortion; death resulting from chemical, thermal, or electrical burns; people who were found dead; people who died en route to the hospital (dead on arrival); and people who died suddenly in the absence of a recognizable disease or injury. Of course a person with disease may die of that disease or for another reason, so an arbitrary time limit is made at the discretion of the medical examiner. For example, in some states if the person has not been attended by a physician within 14 days, the death must be reported.

Local laws may require that deaths from other causes also be reported. These may include any death within 24 hours after admission to the hospital; any hospital death if the person was unconscious on admission and remained so; any death as a result of a therapeutic misadventure; unexpected death in the course of pregnancy, obstetric deliveries, anesthesia, or surgery; any death pronounced by a physician other than the attending physician; any death occurring under suspicious circumstances; any death of people in police custody; all deaths occurring while at work; and death as a result of cirrhosis. When doubt exists about the medicolegal relationship, the death should be reported to the medical examiner.

When a death is being reported, it is the duty of the reporting physician to notify the medical examiner concerning the time, place, manner, circumstances, and cause of such a death insofar as possible. The fact that a death is to be reported does not mean that the medical examiner will assume jurisdiction. The medical examiner may decline jurisdiction when he or she is satisfied that the death was not related to the categories mentioned.

An autopsy of a person whose death has medicolegal implications is performed by the medical examiner only when it is in the public interest. Autopsies are not ordered for the purpose of medical interest. If the attending physician desires an autopsy and one has been declined by the medical examiner, the attending physician is usually permitted to request permission from the family after getting approval from the medical examiner and from the pathologist who will perform the autopsy. When a death is accepted as medicolegal, the medical examiner will perform the autopsy.

It is not the duty of a medical examiner to pronounce people dead nor to handle the removal of bodies from hospitals, nursing homes, or private residences if the situation does not fall into his or her jurisdiction. A body can be removed only when the medical examiner orders it or when the attending physician has pronounced the patient dead from a recognizable disease and has been attending the patient for a specified period of time, 14 days in some states.

Reportable Diseases

By law, a variety of diseases must be reported to public health authorities. Although states vary as to which diseases are reportable, the list usually includes communicable diseases and almost always includes venereal diseases. The physician should be familiar with the legal reporting requirements of the area in which he or she practices; this list can be obtained from the local public health authorities. Reportable diseases in Massachusetts are listed in Table 45.1.

TABLE 45.1 Reportable Diseases and Conditions in Massachusetts

Reportable to the Local Health Department

Actinomycosis
Animal bite
Anthrax
Chicken pox (varicella)
Cholera
Diarrhea of the newborn
Diphtheria
Dysentery
  Amebic
  Bacillary (shigellosis)
Encephalitis, infectious
  (specify agent)
Food poisoning
  Botulism
  Mushrooms and other poisonous vegetables
  and animal products
  Staphylococcal
German measles (rubella)
Glanders
Hepatitis, viral
Infectious diseases of the eye
  Ophthalmia neonatorum
  Suppurative conjunctivitis
  Trachoma
Impetigo of the newborn
Leprosy
Lymphocytic choriomeningitis
Malaria
Measles
Meningitis
  Meningococcal
  Other
    Pneumococcal
    Streptococcal
    Influenzal (viral)
    H. influenzae

Mumps
Plague
Poliomyelitis
  Paralytic
  Nonparalytic (preparalytic)
Psittacosis
Rabies—human
Rickettsial pox
Rocky Mountain spotted fever
Salmonella infections
  Typhoid
  Paratyphoid
  All other salmonellas
Streptococcal
  Group A infections
    Erysipelas
    Scarlet fever
    Streptococcal sore throat
Smallpox (variola)
Smallpox vaccination reactions
  Generalized vaccinia
  Eczema vaccinatum
Tetanus
Trichinosis
Tuberculosis (all forms)
Tularemia
Typhus fever·(including Brill's disease)
Undulant fever (brucellosis)
Weil's disease (*Leptospira icterohaemorrhagiae*)
Whooping cough (pertussis)
Yellow fever

Reportable to the State Department of Public Health
Chancroid
Gonorrhea
Granuloma inguinale
Lymphogranuloma venereum
Syphilis

CONCLUSIONS

Some of the legal principles involved in the emergency care of patients, as well as common situations in which the physician is likely to be involved, have been described. Every possible medicolegal situation has not been covered, however, in most situations, the practice of good medicine will help prevent charges of malpractice. When in doubt, the physician should apply the general guidelines described. At times the physician may wish to consult an attorney. When it is not feasible to do so, the physician should act in the best interest of the patient.

SUGGESTED READINGS

Annas G: *The Rights of Hospital Patients.* New York, Avon Books, 1975.

Annas G, Glantz L, Katz B: *The Rights of Doctors, Nurses, and Allied Health Professionals.* New York, Avon Discus Books, 1981.

Chayet N: *Legal Implications of Emergency Care.* New York, Appleton-Century-Crofts, 1969.

Curran WJ, Shapiro ED: *Law, Medicine and Forensic Science.* Boston, Little Brown & Company, 1983.

Gifford MS, Franaszek JB: Emergency physicians' and patient's assessments. *Ann Emergency Med* 1980; 9:502–507.

Godley DR, Smith TK: Some medicolegal aspects of gunshot wounds. *J Trauma* 1977; 17:866–871.

Jenkins AL (ed): Legal aspects of the emergency department, in *Emergency Department Organization and Management.* St. Louis, The CV Mosby Co, 1975, pp 159–173.

Vaccarino JM: Malpractice, the problem in perspective. *JAMA* 1977; 283:861–863.

EMERGENCY
PROCEDURES

PART **V**

Airway Management

PROCEDURE 1

CONTROL OF AIRWAY WITH BAG AND MASK

Paul Allen

Control of airway with bag and mask is the most important technique to be mastered in all cases of resuscitation with cardiopulmonary arrest. It tends to be overlooked in situations of in-hospital resuscitations but should not be since it is the basis for proper patient oxygenation. It has a broad application and in some cases may be the only technique required to establish and maintain an airway. It is a simple technique to master and can be lifesaving.

Much time is often wasted in efforts to intubate the trachea of a patient, and the subsequent failure to do so may ultimately end in the patient's demise. As will be seen in the discussion of the technique for proper tracheal intubation, adequate oxygenation is required before attempting this technique, and adequate oxygenation can only be achieved by using the bag and mask. An example of the most common use of bag and mask combination is seen in Figure PR1.1. Its use can be made easier by substituting a compliant anesthesia-type mask for the

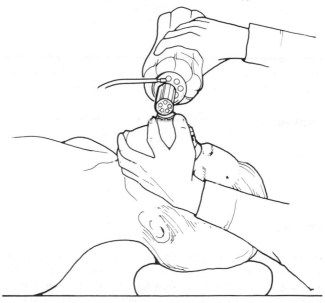

Figure PR1.1 Bag and mask unit. Note position of hands.

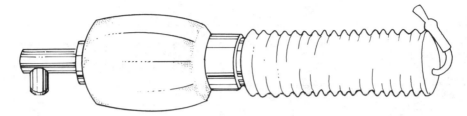

Figure PR1.2 Bag and tail unit to allow 100% oxygen delivery.

more rigid ones frequently supplied as standard equipment from manufacturers. In order to provide a high concentration of oxygen, a 2–3-ft tail made up of large-bore rubber connecting tubing should be applied to the intake end of the bag to prevent entrainment of room air during inspiration (Fig. PR1.2).

INDICATIONS

- Cardiopulmonary failure
- Respiratory failure
- Stridor or other partial obstruction of the upper respiratory tract

CONTRAINDICATIONS

There are no contraindications, but care should be taken with patients who have severe facial trauma or open eye injuries to avoid excessive pressure on the face and/or eyes.

EQUIPMENT

- Bag and mask
- Oxygen with flow meter
- Suction apparatus

POSITION

The key to maintaining an airway with a bag and mask, especially when used without oral or nasal airways, is to position the patient's head so that there is no obstruction in the oral or nasal pharynx to prevent adequate ventilation. This position is

illustrated in Figure PR1.3. Further advancement of the mandible downward and outward, thus translocating the temporal mandibular joint, may be required to move the tongue to a point where it no longer obstructs the natural airway (Fig. PR1.4). Further aid may be obtained by turning the head to either side with the jaw advanced.

PROCEDURE

1. *Clear the airway of dentures and debris.* If the patient is unconscious, clearance can be accomplished by opening

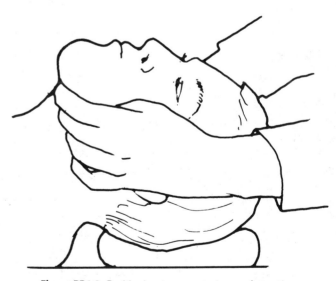

Figure PR1.3 Positioning to correct airway obstruction.

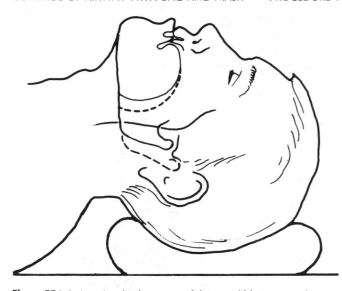

Figure PR1.4 Anterior displacement of the mandible to open airway.

the jaw widely with the thumb and index finger of the nondominant hand (Fig. PR1.5) and removing the debris in the pharynx with the index and third finger of the dominant hand. In the semiconscious patient, one must be careful to avoid any maneuver that may risk one's being bitten by the patient. In all patients the maneuver is most easily accomplished by turning the head to the side.

2. *Select the appropriate-sized mask.* Start out with a No. 3 (small) mask; if it is too small, go up in size until a comfortable fit is achieved. Most frequently the patient will require a smaller mask size than would be predicted since the mask need only cover the nose and mouth and must form a firm seal.

3. *Position the head correctly.* The patient's head should be placed on a thin pillow or folded blanket to provide upward support, which will help to enlarge the airway. This is called the *sniffing position.* Place the mask over the nose and mouth and form a firm seal with the left hand (Fig. PR1.1). A firm seal will be most easily obtained if the physician places the base of the palm of the hand against the patient's cheek bringing it up against the mask and rocking the mask gently to the right side.

4. *Ventilate with the right hand* at a rate of 10–15/min with an inspiratory ratio of 0.5.

5. *Observe* motion of chest and absence of motion of stomach.

6. *Repeat until adequate oxygenation is achieved* and further airway establishment is accomplished or the need for airway assistance has passed.

PITFALLS AND COMPLICATIONS

In *edentulous patients* a proper seal may be difficult to maintain with one hand. This may be solved by holding the mask with two hands and having an assistant squeeze the bag. A second method is to place gauze balls in both cheeks in order to fill out the cheeks to create a good seal. These balls must be removed before further airway management can be accomplished.

Improper positioning of the head or excessive positive bag pressure may cause insufflation of the stomach with inadequate ventilation. This may lead to subsequent regurgitation and aspiration of gastric contents.

The *conscious* or *semiconscious* patient may fight attempts to assist ventilation. This can be overcome with reassurance and very small doses of sedation titrated to prevent obtundation of the patient and further respiratory embarrassment.

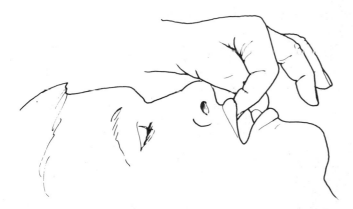

Figure PR1.5 Open the jaw widely by scissoring the thumb and index finger.

PROCEDURE 2

ORAL AIRWAY INSERTION

Paul Allen

An oral airway may be of great assistance in facilitating an unobstructed airway for bag and mask ventilation.

INDICATIONS

- Cardiorespiratory arrest
- Partial or total upper airway obstruction with or without nasal trauma

CONTRAINDICATIONS

- Vincent's angina
- Croup or other pharyngeal infection
- Oral trauma: Oral airway is contraindicated in the totally conscious patient because it may induce vomiting if reflexes are intact.

EQUIPMENT

Use the appropriate-sized oral airway: premature 00–0; neonatal 0–1; 5-year-old child, 2–3; adult female, 5; adult male, 5–6. Do not use too small an airway since it will not keep the tongue forward and may obstruct rather than open the airway.

PROCEDURE

1. Open the patient's mouth by scissoring the jaw open with the thumb and forefinger of the right hand. Do not use the oral airway or other hard instrument to force open the jaw since this may cause unnecessary trauma to the pharynx and mouth and may also break the patient's teeth.
2. Remove dentures and clear airway of debris.

3. Insert airway so that concave portions face away from the tongue (Fig. PR2.1).
4. After insertion to the back of the pharynx, rotate airway 180 deg and slide to its full extent.

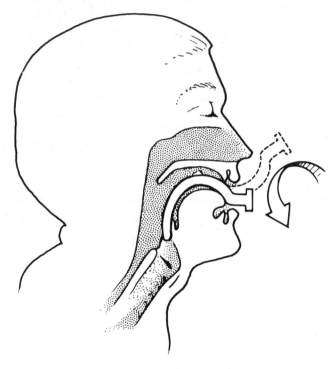

Figure PR2.1 Insert and rotate oral airway.

PITFALLS AND COMPLICATIONS

Failure to clear the airway of foreign material before insertion of the airway may result in aspiration of the material.

In the conscious patient, placement of the airway without topical anesthesia may induce gagging and vomiting; in all patients, placement of the airway may induce *vomiting*.

All patients should be positioned so as to reduce risk of *aspiration* of vomitus (slight head-down position).

Too large an airway may lacerate the palate, especially in children. Conversely, *too small* an airway may increase upper airway obstruction. Most adults require size 5 or larger oral airway.

It is possible to break teeth or lacerate the pharynx by *too forceful placement* of the airway into the mouth of the combative or convulsant patient.

If oral trauma is present, a *nasal airway* is preferred.

PROCEDURE 3

NASAL AIRWAY INSERTION

Paul Allen

A nasal airway may facilitate a clear airway with upper airway obstruction for bag and mask ventilation. It has the advantage over the oral airway in that it is less likely to induce vomiting and can be used in patients with oral trauma.

INDICATIONS

- Cardiorespiratory arrest
- Partial or complete upper respiratory obstruction with or without oral trauma

CONTRAINDICATIONS

- Nasal trauma
- Croup or other infections of the nasopharynx
- Enlarged adenoids

EQUIPMENT

- An appropriate-sized nasal airway
- Water-soluble lubricant

PROCEDURE

1. Examine nose for obstruction, foreign bodies, or septal deviation. Choose the nare that seems to be the larger.
2. Clear mouth and pharynx of dentures and debris.
3. Lubricate the anterior nostril with water-soluble lubricant.
4. Lubricate the nasal airway with water-soluble lubricant.
5. Insert the lubricated airway with the convex surface facing the convexity of the nasopharynx (Fig. PR3.1).

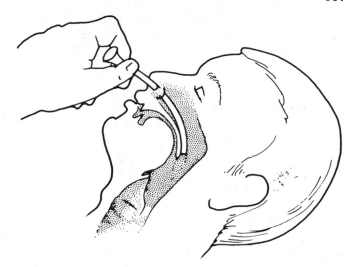

Figure PR3.1 Insert nasal airway.

PITFALLS AND COMPLICATIONS

Vomiting is still a hazard in children; however, the most serious complication following insertion of the nasal airway is the induction of *severe epistaxis*. If severe epistaxis occurs, be careful that aspiration of blood into the trachea does not occur. When appropriate, attempt to stop the epistaxis by using vasoconstrictors and, when necessary, an anterior or posterior nasal pack.

PROCEDURE 4

ENDOTRACHEAL INTUBATION

Paul Allen

Endotracheal intubation establishes definitive airway maintenance in almost all situations in which it is required. It provides good protection of the airway from aspiration and allows spontaneous, assisted, or controlled ventilation. Endotracheal intubation provides us with the additional alternatives of positive and expiratory pressure and/or continuous positive airway pressure.

INDICATIONS

- Airway maintenance
- Cardiorespiratory failure
- Severe airway obstruction of noninfectious nature
- Head and neck injuries with potential for obstruction or respiratory failure
- Superficial airway burns with potential for obstruction or respiratory failure
- Aspiration of gastric contents
- Protection for aspiration in unconscious patients or before lavage of the stomach with Blakemore-Sengstaken tube.

CONTRAINDICATIONS

- Hypoxia: before endotracheal intubation, all patients with *hypoxia* should be adequately oxygenated with face mask or bag and mask assisted ventilation.
- Known cervical spine injury: blind nasotracheal or fiberoptic bronchoscope assisted nasotracheal intubation may be attempted, but if the patient is apneic, cricothyroidotomy and subsequent tracheostomy are indicated.

Orotracheal Intubation

Orotracheal intubation is preferred when a rapid emergency intubation is done. It can be done effectively for urgent and nonemergent cases in which nasotracheal intubation is not possible or desired.

EQUIPMENT

- General
  Intravenous access with running intravenous fluids when time permits
  Working suction with Yaukower suction tip and suction catheters
  Resuscitation drugs
  Oxygen

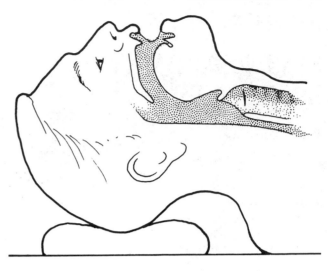

Figure PR4.1 Sniffing position.

- Special
  Laryngoscope with desired blade attached
  Endotracheal tubes of appropriate sizes
  Malleable stylet
  Water-soluble lubricant
  10-ml syringe
  Bite block or oral pharyngeal airway
  Tape for fixation and tincture of benzolin

POSITION

Supine, with patient's head at your midumbilical height. The patient's head should be in sniffing position as for bag and mask ventilation (Fig. PR4.1).

PROCEDURE

1. *Under nonemergent circumstances* the patient's mouth and tongue should first be sprayed with 4% lidocaine (Xylocaine), and the patient should be gently sedated with diazepam and/or narcotics to reduce the emotional trauma.
2. *Select appropriate-sized endotracheal tube* (as described earlier).

3. *Prepare endotracheal tube.* Check cuff for leaks with air. Lubricate the tube and stylet. Insert stylet into the tube and give the tube appropriate curve, not allowing the stylet to protrude from the end of the tube.

4. Choose laryngoscope blade and connect to handle (Fig. PR4.2).

5. Open laryngoscope and check light.

6. *Ensure that the patient is adequately oxygenated.* This can be done by using bag and mask ventilation. Note that endotracheal intubation is always a semielective or elective procedure.

7. Open patient's mouth with right hand, scissoring upper and lower jaw with thumb and index finger, translocating the temporomandibular joint as is done to clean the pharynx (Fig. PR4.3).

8. Hold the laryngoscope in the left hand with the left wrist locked (Fig. PR4.4).

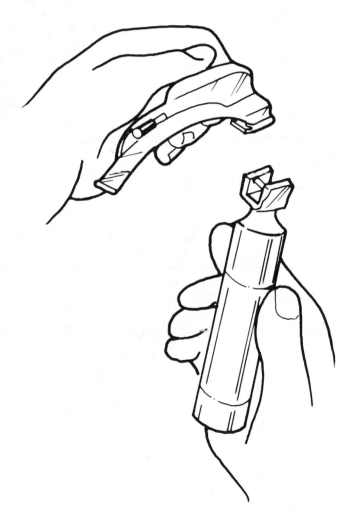

Figure PR4.2 Assemble laryngoscope.

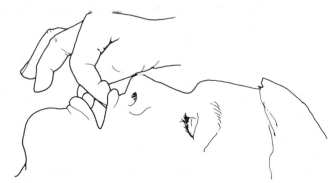

Figure PR4.3 Open mouth.

2. Slide the endotracheal tube between the cords (Fig. PR4.8).
3. Remove the stylet—*it is important to do this before tube is advanced further.*
4. Advance the tube 2 cm.
5. Remove the laryngoscope being careful to avoid the teeth.
6. Inflate the endotracheal tube cuff.

Ascertain Proper Tube Position

1. Hold the tube stable.
2. Attach tube to a positive pressure ventilation bag with 100% oxygen (if possible).
3. Apply intermittent positive pressure ventilation. Note that if the patient is conscious, he or she can take deep breaths attached to a "T" piece with high flow oxygen attached instead.
4. Ascertain bilateral chest expansion.

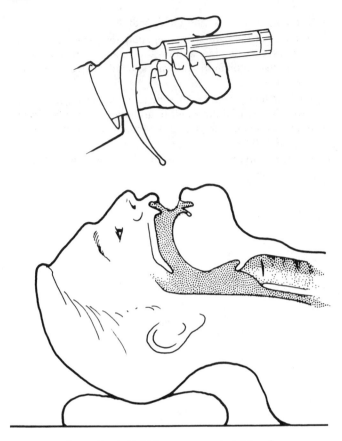

Figure PR4.4 Hold laryngoscope in left hand.

Insert Laryngoscope

1. Insert the blade to the right side of the tongue, pushing the tongue to the left (this is the correct technique for both straight or curved blades).
2. For curved blade technique, advance tip of blade to the groove between the base of the tongue and the epiglottis (Fig. PR4.5). For straight blade technique, advance the blade under the epiglottis (Fig. PR4.6). Visualize the cords (Fig. PR4.7).

Insert Endotracheal Tube

1. Hold the endotracheal tube in the right hand with the bevel facing laterally to provide the minimum profile to pass the cords.

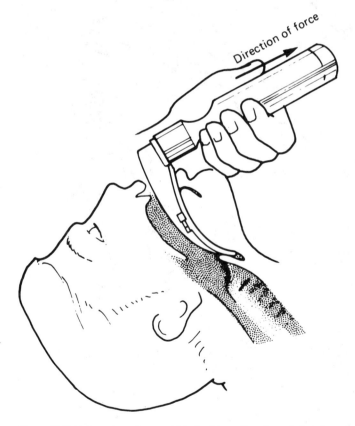

Figure PR4.5 Insertion of curved blade. Note direction of elevation of laryngoscope.

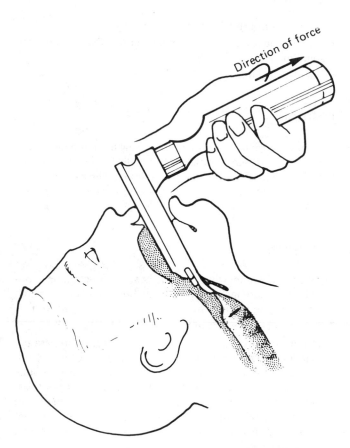

Figure PR4.6 Insertion of straight blade. Note direction of elevation.

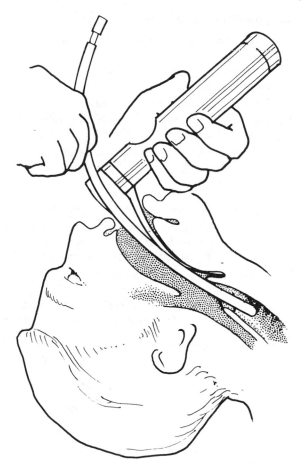

Figure PR4.8 Insert endotracheal tube.

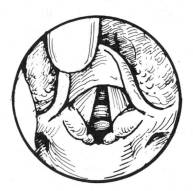

Figure PR4.7 Visualize cords.

5. Ascertain bilateral ventilation by auscultation on both sides near the midaxillary line.

6. Confirm the absence of breath sounds over the gastric area.

7. If unilateral rather than bilateral breath sounds are not heard, deflate the tube cuff, withdraw the tube 1 cm, reinflate the cuff, and repeat steps 1 to 7 of ascertaining proper tube position.

8. If no breath sounds are heard in the chest and sounds are heard over the stomach, stop ventilation, deflate the cuff, suction the mouth, remove the tube, *reoxygenate* the patient with bag and mask, and restart intubation procedure from the beginning.

9. Esophageal intubation increases the risk of regurgitation and aspiration.

Securing the Orotracheal Tube

1. Place a bit block or oropharyngeal airway between the patient's teeth.
2. Cut the tube to an appropriate length so no more than 3 cm protrudes from the mouth.
3. Apply tincture of benzoin to the cheeks.
4. Tape the tube at the level of the exit from the mouth and secure it to the cheeks.
5. Reconnect the tube to an appropriate ventilation device.

Extubation

1. Suction the pharynx with curved mouth suction.
2. Suction the endotracheal tube; limit this suctioning to a maximum of 10 seconds per attempt. Repeated suctioning is unnecessary if there are no secretions present.
3. Ventilate patient; use a breathing bag with 100% oxygen and give several deep breaths.
4. To remove the tube deflate the cuff completely with a syringe and withdraw the tube after a deep inspiration during the subsequent expiration. After it has been removed, apply a face mask to deliver oxygen to the patient.

Nasotracheal Intubation

INDICATIONS

- Nasotracheal intubation is especially indicated in patients with oral trauma.
- Nasotracheal intubation is preferred by many for long-term nursing care. Fixation is more secure than with orotracheal intubation, and good mouth care can be given.
- Blind nasotracheal intubation is less traumatic in the conscious patient in whom urgent rather than emergent airway protection is required.

CONTRAINDICATIONS

Contraindications are the same as for oral intubation and orotracheal intubation. It is contraindicated in cases of nasal or upper facial trauma.

EQUIPMENT

- Same as for orotracheal intubation
- 5% cocaine solution or 1% phenylephrine (Neo-Synephrine) solution
- 2% viscous lidocaine

POSITION

The easiest position for blind nasotracheal intubation is to have the patient in a semisitting position with the head in neutral position and the operator standing in front of the patient. When it is to be done under laryngoscopic visualization, the patient may be in supine position with the operator behind the patient.

PROCEDURE

1. After ascertaining that all equipment is functioning properly, the pharyngeal airway should be cleared of all foreign material and the patient's dentures should be removed.
2. Ensure adequate oxygenation.
3. Administer topical anesthesia. If time allows, prepare the patient's more patent nostril with 5% cocaine. If not, use 1% phenylephrine; use drops and cotton swabs to reduce mucosal swelling and reduce the probability of epistaxis. If cocaine is used, a second benefit is the reduction of pain during the procedure. To be effective, 5–10 minutes are needed for this step with cocaine or 1–2 minutes are needed with phenylephrine.
4. Prepare the tube. Presoften the appropriate-sized endotracheal tube (generally 1 mm smaller in diameter than the corresponding oral tube) by emersing it for 3–5 minutes in warm sterile saline or water. Then lubricate it well with water-soluble lubricant. If no warm saline is available, a water-soluble lubricant is all that should be used.
5. Insert the tube into the more patent nostril and *advance downward rather than backward* into the pharynx (Fig. PR4.9).
6. Advance the tube into the trachea.

Blind Technique

1. Listen for respiratory sounds over the end of the tube and advance the tube slowly until they are heard (Fig. PR4.10). When this occurs, the tip of the tube is at the glottic opening.

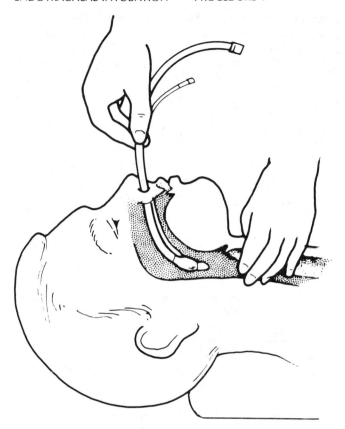

Figure PR4.9 Insert nasotracheal tube.

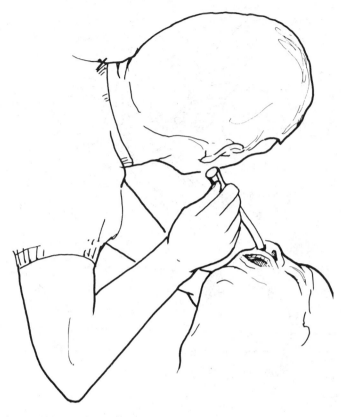

Figure PR4.10 Listen for respiratory sounds.

2. Advance the tube through the glottis into the trachea during inspiration with a single rapid but gentle movement.

3. If the tube will not advance, observe the side of the neck in which the pressure of the tube protrudes outward, and rotate the tube in the opposite direction.

4. If the tube protrudes forward, a 360 deg rotation may facilitate passage through the glottis.

Direct Visualization Technique

After placing the tube into the pharynx, a curved blade laryngoscope is used to visualize the glottis as is done in orotracheal intubation. If necessary, the tip of the endotracheal tube is grasped with Magill forceps and guided into the trachea (Fig. PR4.11). Tube advancement should be done by an assistant. *Caution*—the Magill forceps should not grasp the tube by the balloon cuff since rupture of the cuff may occur if this is done.

After the tube is placed in the trachea, inflate the balloon cuff (Fig. PR4.12) and tape the tube in place after preparing the skin with tincture of benzoin. Alternatively, an umbilical tape may be tied around the tube and then around the head. It should be padded with self-adherent foam padding to prevent pressure on the scalp and face.

Fiberoptic Visualization

An alternative method for direct visualization during nasotracheal intubation is the use of the *fiberoptic bronchoscope*. The bronchoscope is first passed through the tube and then passed through the nares, with tube inside the nose, into the oropharynx under direct visualization. When the tube is placed into the pharynx over the bronchoscope, the bronchoscope is then passed under direct visualization into the larynx. The tube can then be advanced over the bronchoscope into the larynx

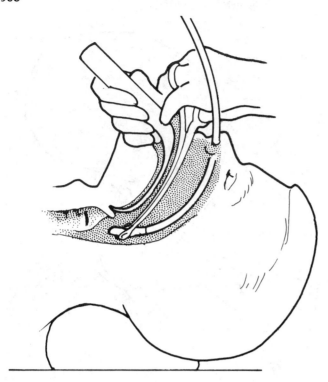

Figure PR4.11 Grasp tube with Magill forceps.

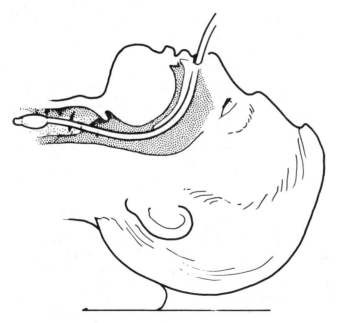

Figure PR4.12 Inflate balloon cuff.

and trachea. This technique is especially useful in patients with cervical trauma. When blind intubation is unsuccessful and causes epistaxis, it is difficult to perform this procedure because active epistaxis obscures the view. This should be considered before attempting a blind technique.

PITFALLS AND COMPLICATIONS

Do not lever the laryngoscope backward using the patient's teeth as a fulcrum. Do not limit access by putting your head into the patient's mouth. *Local trauma* to lips and teeth, gums, pharynx, vocal cords, and trachea can be prevented by adequately protecting these areas by using a gentle technique and not using the laryngoscope as a lever. Removal of the stylet, using an appropriate-sized tube before insertion of the tube past the larynx to the trachea, will also help to prevent these complications.

Failure to visualize the larynx may occur when the airway is not properly cleared with suction and if improper laryngoscopy technique is used.

Vomiting may occur during suctioning of the pharynx because of stimulation of the pharynx. *Aspiration* will occur if proper suction is not immediately available and used properly. The reverse wave can be suppressed by pressure on the cricoid cartilage.

Inadequate visualization of the cords or inability to visualize the tube passing between the cords can cause *esophageal intubation*. This can be prevented by adequate visualization.

Bronchial intubation can occur if the tube is passed too far into the trachea. It usually occurs into the right main stem bronchus. This can be prevented by passing the tube only 1–2 cm past the vocal cords and securing it tightly in place. When bronchial intubation is diagnosed by inadequate breath sounds of one side or the other, it can be corrected by withdrawing the tube after first deflating the cuff.

Injury to the nasal mucosa and subsequent epistaxis is a common complication of nasotracheal intubation. A metal stylet should not be used at any time for nasotracheal intubation.

Nasal intubation can also break the mucosa in the posterior nasopharynx and dissect submucosally into the pharynx with subsequent infection.

If the size of the selected tube is too small, bronchopulmonary toilet may be difficult. The pressure of the balloon cuff on these tubes needs to be high to ensure a proper seal. This may cause pressure necrosis of the trachea in long-term intubation cases. This is a more frequent complication in nasotracheal intubation, in which tube size is by necessity smaller.

PROCEDURE 5

INSERTION OF AN ESOPHAGEAL AIRWAY

Paul Allen

The esophageal airway has been introduced to facilitate airway management without the aid of a laryngoscope and endotracheal tube. The concept is a good one, but in practice, its complications do not make it a substitute for adequate bag and mask ventilation or endotracheal intubation, especially in the in-hospital setting.

INDICATIONS

Use this procedure in situations of respiratory arrest in which long-term bag and mask ventilation is required for an unconscious patient or when endotracheal intubation is not possible because of lack of necessary skills or equipment.

CONTRAINDICATIONS

Do not use this procedure in any situation in which adequate airway management can be maintained by other methods.

EQUIPMENT

- Esophageal airway mask
- Water-soluble lubricant
- Oxygen

POSITION

The patient should be in a supine position with neck flexed. The lower jaw should be extended by the nondominant hand of the examiner, keeping the tongue out of the airway (Fig. PR5.1).

PROCEDURE

Insertion of Airway

1. Clear airway of debris and remove dentures.
2. Advance mandible forward with nondominant hand as shown in Figure PR5.1.
3. With dominant hand, insert lubricated obturate gently into the pharynx and advance slowly into the esophagus (Fig. PR5.2).
4. Advance until the mask fits along the face, then inflate the esophageal balloon cuff (Fig. PR5.3).
5. Ventilate through the mask and check for bilateral breath sounds.

Removal of Esophageal Obturator Airway

1. Obtain a working suction and have it immediately ready.
2. Ventilate the patient with 100% oxygen for six breaths at a rate of 30 breaths/min.
3. Deflate the cuff of the obturator with a syringe.
4. Remove mask and obturator.
5. Suction pharynx.
6. Ventilate with bag and mask.
7. Proceed with endotracheal intubation if required.

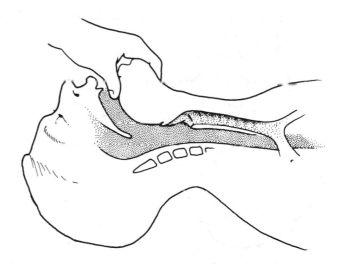

Figure PR5.1 Extend lower jaw.

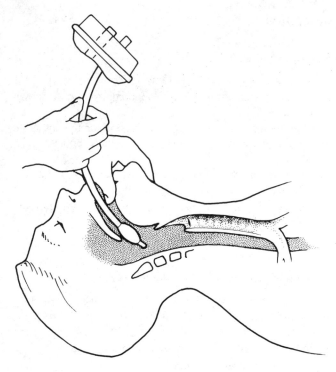

Figure PR5.2 Insert obturator.

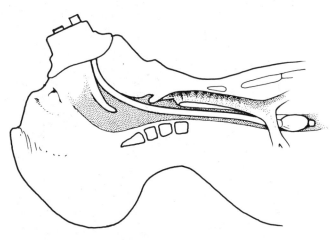

Figure PR5.3 Inflate balloon cuff.

PITFALLS AND COMPLICATIONS

The obturator can be placed inadvertently *into the trachea*. If the point of the obturator is driven too firmly, *perforation of the esophagus* can occur with subsequent mediastinitis. Although the esophageal balloon can protect the airway from regurgitation and the stomach from inflation, this *protection is not complete*. The airway and stomach should be periodically checked for the possibility of this occurrence.

PROCEDURE 6

NASOTRACHEAL SUCTIONING

Paul Allen

Nasotracheal suctioning is a useful method of stimulating coughing and removing tracheobronchial secretions in patients who cannot adequately clear their secretions with normal coughing mechanisms. This sputum is felt to be not as contaminated with oropharyngeal organisms and is useful for cultures of the tracheobronchial tree.

INDICATIONS

- Removal of tracheobronchial secretions
- Stimulating the coughing mechanism
- Obtaining uncontaminated sputum specimens

EQUIPMENT

- Suction catheter with finger occlusion suction vent (No. 14–16 French catheter in adults)
- Suction source
- Sputum trap
- Gloves

- Sterile water or saline
- Specimen container
- Water-soluble lubricant
- Oxygen mask and source

POSITION

Preferred position is patient sitting with the head supported in a neutral position, as for blind nasotracheal intubation. If the above position is not possible, a semisitting or supine position can be used. Selective positioning for intubating both the right and left main stem bronchi independently can be accomplished but is beyond the scope of this discussion.

PROCEDURE

1. Be sure the patient is adequately ventilated.
2. Use gloves and sterile technique.
3. Insert the lubricated tube into the nose by passing the catheter horizontally along the floor of the nose until the tube curves into the hypopharynx.
4. Advance during deep inspiration with finger suction vent open.
5. If intubation is difficult, place the patient's head in the sniffing position. Place a gauze sponge on the tongue and pull the tongue forward gently. This helps to move the epiglottis forward and helps to uncover the glottis. Listen for breath sounds through the catheter and advance the catheter during inspiration at the point of maximum breath sounds.
6. *Confirm endotracheal position.* Passage into trachea will usually cause some coughing. Breath sounds can be heard. The pitch of the voice is changed once the tube passes through the glottis.
7. Apply suction intermittently for a maximum of 10 seconds.
8. Allow reoxygenation before resuctioning. Place oxygen mask over the patient's face for 30–60 seconds. Avoid any suction. Do not remove catheter during reoxygenation.
9. Remove catheter when suctioning is complete.

PITFALLS AND COMPLICATIONS

Cardiac arrhythmias may occur as a result of vagal stimulation and the presence of hypoxia. These may be prevented by en-suring adequate oxygenation before the procedure and by avoiding suctioning for longer than 10 seconds without reoxygenation.

Epistaxis is a common complication. As with all nasal procedures, it can be reduced by proper placement and advancement of the catheter in the nose.

Intratracheal bleeding can occur if suction is too vigorous, resulting in trauma to the trachea.

PROCEDURE 7

NEEDLE INSERTION INTO THE CRICOTHYROID MEMBRANE

Paul Allen

In cases in which there is upper airway obstruction and a contraindication to endotracheal intubation, such as fracture of the cervical spine or an inability to clear the airway of debris, the immediate solution for adequate oxygenation is needle cricothyroidotomy. *This is only a temporary measure* and cannot be used for long-term airway management.

INDICATIONS

Follow this procedure for emergency establishment of an airway in patients with airway obstruction when other remedies are contraindicated or equipment is not available.

CONTRAINDICATIONS

Do not use this procedure *when any other procedure is indicated or accomplishable.*

POSITION

The patient should be supine with head in the neutral position. A small towel roll between the shoulders may be of assistance if the situation permits.

EQUIPMENT

- Prep solution
- Immediately available drugs
- Sterile gloves
- Two large-bore needles (14- or 12-gauge needles with or without a plastic outer cannula)

PROCEDURE

1. Prepare and drape the skin.
2. Locate the cricothyroid membrane by palpatation. This can be found just beneath the inferior prominence of the thyroid cartilage.
3. Insert a large-bore needle, with a plastic catheter over it if possible, through the skin and cricothyroid membrane into the trachea (Fig. PR7.1).
4. Remove the needle, leaving the catheter in place.
5. Tape the catheter (or needle) in place (Fig. PR7.2).
6. Apply oxygen at a rate of 6 liters/min if the patient ventilates spontaneously and ascertain the expiration if possible. An-

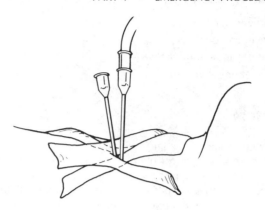

Figure PR7.2 Remove needle and tape catheters in position.

other catheter and needle may be placed along side of the first one to permit both continuous oxygen flow and exhalation.

7. If the patient is unable to ventilate spontaneously, apply flush oxygen to the catheter for 1–2.5 seconds every 5 seconds, then disconnect the catheter from the oxygen source for 2.5–3 seconds. Repeat this cycle until the patient can breathe spontaneously or until this technique can be discontinued.
8. Convert to cricothyroidotomy or tracheostomy as soon as patient's condition permits.

PITFALLS AND COMPLICATIONS

Extreme care must be taken in finding the proper location of the cricothyroid membrane: A needle inserted too low may puncture the thyroid isthmus, which is a highly vascular structure, and there may be subsequent bleeding and further airway compromise. A needle inserted too high may injure the vocal cords. A needle inserted too far may injure the posterior wall of the trachea or perforate the esophagus.

Pneumothorax and pneumomediastinum may be caused by malpositioned needles, especially in children, when the needle penetrates the pleura or mediastinum.

Carbon dioxide retention or *hyperinflation of the lungs* may result from failure to provide an expiratory vent for a patient receiving a continuous flow of oxygen.

This airway should be considered only a *temporary technique.* Failure to provide a more permanent airway is considered an error in patient management.

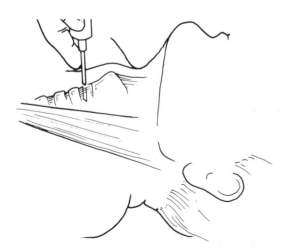

Figure PR7.1 Insert large-bore needle and catheter.

PROCEDURE 8

TRANSTRACHEAL ASPIRATION

Paul Allen

Transtracheal aspiration is a technique that has both diagnostic and therapeutic indications. Since it is not a benign procedure, it should be reserved for situations in which other techniques do not provide adequate results.

INDICATIONS

Therapeutic

Tracheal stimulation will produce coughing in patients with poor cough reflex and inadequate tracheal toilet.

Diagnostic

A sputum specimen uncontaminated by oropharyngeal or nasopharyngeal organisms may be obtained in patients who cannot raise sputum and for whom nasotracheal suctioning is unsuccessful.

CONTRAINDICATIONS

- Bleeding diathesis
- Uncontrollable severe cough
- Unresolved hypoxemia
- Uncooperative patient

EQUIPMENT

- Prepared solution
- Sterile drape
- Sterile gloves
- Local anesthetic with syringe and needle (25 gauge 0.5 in)
- Cannulation equipment, intracath (14 gauge through the needle)

- 5-ml syringe and sterile *nonbacteriostatic* saline
- Culture medium or transport containers
- Sterile dressing

POSITION

The patient should be in a supine position with a pillow or roll under the shoulders to extend the neck.

PROCEDURE

1. Prepare and drape the neck
2. *Infiltrate skin* and subcutaneous tissue down to the cricothyroid membrane with local anesthetic.
3. *Puncture the cricothyroid membrane* using a 14-gauge needle or syringe with the bevel up; aim the needle caudally at a 45 deg angle to the skin. The needle must be held near the point to avoid too deep a puncture.
4. *Aspirate* to confirm position. A free flow of air is characteristic of intratracheal position.
5. Thread the catheter quickly into the trachea (Fig. PR8.1). If the catheter does not thread easily, remove both the needle and the catheter as one unit to avoid cutting the tip of the catheter and repeat the cricothyroid puncture.
6. *Remove the catheter stylet* and slide the needle out over the catheter. Tape catheter in place.
7. *Aspirate* the sputum by attaching a 10-ml syringe to the cannula and aspirating during a voluntary cough. Movement of the intratracheal catheter will usually stimulate the cough reflex if the patient will not or cannot cough spontaneously. If the sputum volume is inadequate or the cough is not well stimulated, inject 2–3 ml sterile nonbacteriostatic saline and aspirate again.
8. *Remove syringe* and inoculate immediately.
9. *Withdraw catheter* and apply dressing; keep pressure on the puncture site for 5 minutes.
10. *Order bed rest for 8 hours.*

PITFALLS AND COMPLICATIONS

All of the complications of cricothyroid needle puncture occur here as well.

A bleeding diathesis can cause *hemoptysis* that could compromise the airway and require endotracheal intubation. This

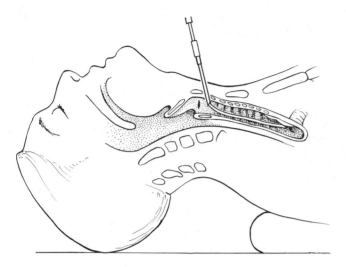

Figure PR8.1 Insert catheter into trachea.

can be prevented by checking bleeding studies before the procedure and assuring that the puncture is between the cricothyroid cartilage. A small amount of blood-tinged sputum is expected for several hours after the procedure.

Subcutaneous and/or mediastinal emphysema is an occasional complication that will occur if air enters the subcutaneous tissue or mediastinum from the trachea or skin surface. This is more likely to occur in patients who are severely coughing on placement of the needle and/or catheter. It can be prevented by careful placement of the needle and by avoiding the procedure in patients with uncontrollable or severe cough.

Postneedle removal subcutaneous emphysema can be prevented by applying pressure to the puncture site until the hole can be sealed. Bed rest after the procedure will also aid in its prevention.

Cardiac arrhythmias or arrest as a result vagal stimulation in a hypoxic patient may occur, as in nasotracheal suctioning. This can be prevented with adequate oxygenation.

Catheter aspiration may occur if the catheter is pulled back through the needle shearing the catheter off with the needle tip. This can be prevented by never withdrawing the catheter through the needle.

PROCEDURE 9

CRICOTHYROTOMY

Nicholas O'Connor

A cricothyrotomy is the simplest and quickest way to gain access to the airway in patients with upper airway obstruction. This procedure can be performed safely by physicians with relatively little surgical experience using simple instruments. There are two favorable anatomical features that contribute to the safety of cricothyrotomy. First, there are no vital structures between the skin and airway in the region of the cricothyroid membrane, only the skin, the platysma muscle, and the membrane itself. Second, the cricoid cartilage, although narrow anteriorly, broadens posteriorly to articule with the thyroid cartilage (Fig. PR9.1). This tough posterior cartilaginous wall prevents inadvertent puncture of the back wall of the larynx. The procedure can be performed without extending the neck, which is contraindicated in patients with suspected cervical spine injuries. Finally, some centers will use the cricothyroid approach for elective insertion of tracheostomy tubes.

INDICATIONS

- Upper airway obstruction from a foreign body lodged in the airway
- Upper airway obstruction from edema, which almost always occurs at or above the level of the vocal chords
- When rapid access to the airway is required and orotracheal of nasotracheal intubation is not feasible
- As a site for elective insertion of a tracheostomy tube when the standard tracheostomy site is not appropriate

CONTRAINDICATIONS

Do not use this procedure when there has been direct trauma to the larynx and the cricoid cartilage has been fractured or crushed.

EQUIPMENT

- Scalpel with a No. 15 blade
- Curved hemostat

- No. 6 or 8 tracheostomy tube with cuff
- If tracheostomy tubes are not available, a 3-inch piece of intravenous tubing
- 4 × 4-inch gauze pad
- Alcohol or povidone-iodine (Betadine) prep (optional)
- 1% lidocaine local anaesthetic (optional)
- 3-ml syringe with a No. 25 needle for anesthesia administration (optional)
- Sterile gloves (optional)
- Suction apparatus with sterile suction catheters (optional)
- Overhead light source (optional)
- Sterile towels (optional)

POSITION

The patient should be lying face up on a stretcher, preferably with arms restrained. The procedure can be performed without extending the patient's neck if cervical spine injuries are suspected. However, the procedure is somewhat easier if the patient's neck is extended.

PROCEDURE

1. If time and conditions permit, prepare and drape the neck.
2. Palpate the cricothyroid space in the midline by running your left index finger along the trachea from the sternal notch toward the chin. Approximately halfway up the neck, the first bump your finger encounters is the cricoid cartilage, and the depression just above this bump is the cricothyroid space (Fig. PR9.2a).
3. If there is time, keeping your left index finger on the cricothyroid space, infiltrate the skin with 1% lidocaine without epinephrine.
4. Keeping your left index finger on the midline of the cricoid cartilage, make a 1.5-cm transverse incision directly through the skin over the cricothyroid membrane. Make the skin incision deep enough so that the wound gapes (a sign that the platysma muscle has been cut, Fig. PR9.2b).
5. Slide the tip of your left index finger into the incision with your fingernail resting on the cricothyroid membrane. Now slide the blade of the scalpel (held so that the blade faces transversely) along your fingernail and poke the blade through the membrane. Give the blade a twist to enlarge the opening (Fig. PR9.2c).

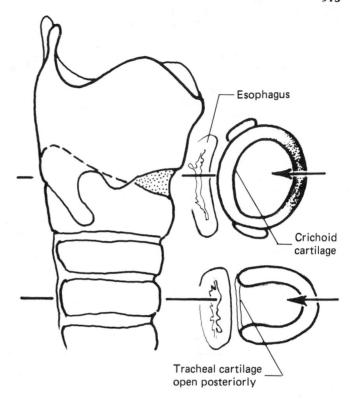

Figure PR9.1 Posterior relationships at level of cricothytoid membrane and level of trachea.

6. Keeping your left finger in position, withdraw the scalpel and insert a curved hemostat in the opening. Spread the blades of the hemostat to enlarge the opening and then insert a tracheostomy tube between the blades of the hemostat (Fig. PR9.2d).
7. Tie the tracheostomy tube in place with tape and place a gauze pad under the tube. The trachea can now be suctioned.

PITFALLS AND COMPLICATIONS

The essential step in this procedure is to identify the cricothyroid space; the identification is easier in men because the cartilage is more prominent than it is in women and children. Making the incision into the thyroid cartilage will not only damage the cartilage but may injure the vocal chords. One of

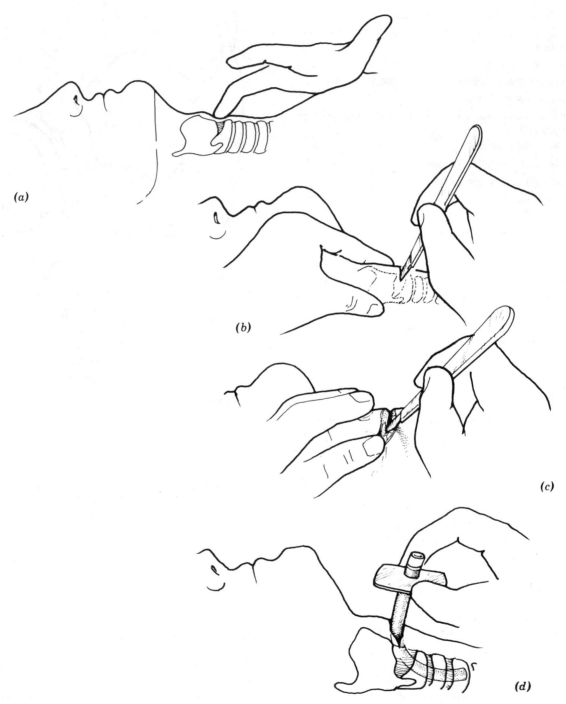

Figure PR9.2 (a) Palpate cricothyroid space; (b) incise skin and platysma; (c) incise cricothyroid membrane; (d) insert tracheostomy tube.

the reasons for keeping the tip of the left index finger in the skin incision is to keep the incision centered over the cricothyroid membrane; this is especially true if the patient is struggling. The membrane is very thin, and the scalpel only needs to be inserted a few millimeters. Insertion of the scalpel too far, especially in a moving patient, could damage the structures of the larynx. One would have to stray quite far from the midline with the incision to injure the superior laryngeal nerves, but this is a possible complication.

PROCEDURE 10

TRACHEOSTOMY

Nicholas O'Connor

A tracheostomy is a surgical procedure, and an emergency tracheostomy should be performed only by physicians who are familiar with and adept at this operation. Good lighting, proper instruments, functioning suction equipment, and a reliable assistant are required. It is preferable that the patient not struggle and be reasonably cooperative. The procedure in an emergency can be frought with complications.

INDICATIONS

- Upper airway obstruction from any cause
- When access to the airway is required and orotracheal or nasotracheal intubation is not feasible
- Crushing injuries to the larynx when a cricothyrotomy is not feasible
- Major injuries to the mandible and maxilla when orotracheal intubation is possible but will obstruct ensuing surgical procedures required to reduce and stabilize the fractures

CONTRAINDICATIONS

- Injuries to the cervical spine because extending the neck will increase the risk of spinal cord injury

- A struggling, uncontrollable patient in whom cricothyrotomy is a safer procedure
- Total upper airway obstruction (e.g., a foreign body lodged in the larynx) and the time required to carry out a tracheostomy favors the use of the swifter cricothyrotomy route.

EQUIPMENT

- Overhead light
- Suction apparatus with sterile tubing
- 1% lidocaine without epinephrine
- 5-ml syringe with a No. 25 needle
- Cuffed tracheostomy tube, No. 6, 7, or 8
- 10-ml syringe
- Tracheostomy tube tapes
- Package of 4 × 4-inch sterile gauze pads
- Prep solution
- Sterile gloves
- Surgical mask
- Scalpel with No. 15 blade
- Four curved hemostats
- Four curved mosquito hemostats
- Two Allis clamps
- Two Kelly clamps
- Two army–navy retractors
- One small self-retaining retractor
- One neurosuction tip
- One vein retractor
- One package of 3-0 plain catgut ties
- One package of 4-0 silk ties
- One package of 4-0 silk sutures
- Straight surgical scissors
- Sterile towels
- Rolled towel
- Two toothed forceps

POSITION

The patient should be lying flat and face up on a narrow table. The patient's arms should be secured to his sides and a restraining strap placed across the upper legs. A rolled towel is placed transversely under the patient's shoulders to extend the neck. An assistant is required on one side of the patient to assist with retraction. Preferably, another assistant will steady the patient's head to keep it in the midline position (Fig. PR10.1).

PROCEDURE

1. Prepare the neck from the mandible to the clavicles and drape the field with sterile towels.
2. Infiltrate the area of the proposed incision with 1% lidocaine.
3. Place the thumb and index finger of the left hand on either side of the trachea to stretch the skin and to steady the trachea.
4. Make a vertical incision over the midline of the trachea 5 cm long from the first to the fourth tracheal ring.
5. Carry the incision down through subcutaneous fat and platysma so that the wound gapes (Fig. PR10.2a). Clamp any bleeding vessels with fine hemostats.
6. Identify any transverse communicating anterior jugular veins; clamp and divide them.
7. Separate the strap muscles in the midline by spreading in a vertical direction with the tips of the scissors; retract the muscles to each side (Fig. PR10.2b).
8. The thyroid isthmus may lie across the trachea and obstruct access to the third tracheal ring. Often the isthmus can be retracted superiorly with a vein retractor. If not, the isthmus should be clamped and divided between two large hemostats. A suture ligature of 4-0 silk should then be placed around each clamp and the clamps removed.
9. Dissect the pretracheal fascia from the trachea using a toothed forceps and scissors.
10. Identify the third tracheal ring and grasp it in the midline with an Allis clamp.
11. Using the scalpel blade at right angles to the trachea, make transverse incisions in the second and third interspaces, then cut across the third tracheal ring on either side of the Allis clamp, and remove the anterior segment of the third tracheal ring (Fig. PR10.2c).
12. Suction the trachea gently and quickly.
13. Remove all clamps on the skin edges. If clamps were placed on communicating veins, ligate the veins with 3-0 catgut and remove the clamps.
14. Insert the tracheostomy tube, usually a No. 8 in adults, and remove the obturator (Fig. PR10.2d).
15. Suction the trachea through the tube.

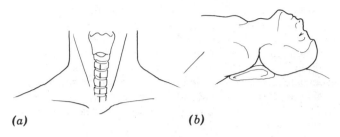

(a)   *(b)*

Figure PR10.1 Position for tracheostomy.

16. If the patient is to be placed on a ventilator, inflate the cuff (Fig. PR10.2e).
17. Suture the skin very loosely.
18. Place a gauze dressing around the tube (Fig. 10.2f).
19. Secure the tube with tracheostomy tapes.

PITFALLS AND COMPLICATIONS

The most common pitfalls can be avoided as follows: Before starting the procedure assemble all the necessary equipment. Check the suction to see that it is working. Preinflate the cuffs on the tracheostomy tubes to be sure they do not leak. Avoid lidocaine with epinephrine, especially in a hypoxic patient, because the epinephrine may potentiate cardiac arrythmias. Have a roll under the shoulders to extend the neck, which positions the trachea more anteriorly. Failure to do this allows the trachea to recede posteriorly and the thyroid to descend over the trachea.

During the procedure it is possible to nick the pleura and cause a pneumothorax. The patient must be checked for this several times after the procedure; this is especially true in children. Failure to clamp communicating veins will lead to bleeding in the field and will seriously impede carrying out the rest of the procedure. Straying from the midline during the dissection can lead to injury to the anterior jugular veins with serious hemorrhage or to the recurrent laryngeal nerves.

When incising the trachea, care must be taken to push the blade in only a few millimeters so that the back wall of the trachea is not injured or the trachea is not transected. If the back wall of the trachea is injured, it is possible to insert the tube into the retrotracheal space with disastrous results. One of the reasons for grasping the third ring with an Allis clamp is to have a firm hold on the excised ring segment so it does not fall into the trachea.

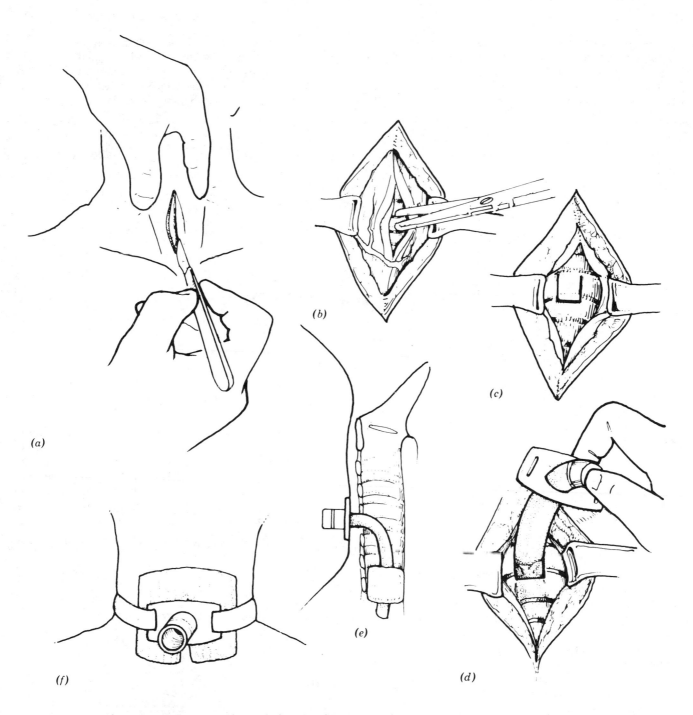

Figure PR10.2 (a) Incise skin and platysma; (b) expose trachea; (c) remove anterior segment of third tracheal ring; (d) insert tracheostomy tube; (e) inflate cuff; (f) place dressing and secure tube with tracheostomy tapes.

A very common problem occurs when the tube is inserted into the lumen of the trachea. This will stimulate the patient to cough; if the operator does not steady the tube, it will be dislodged from the trachea. The cuff on the tube should be inflated gently to prevent pressure necrosis of the tracheal wall.

The skin incision should be sewn up loosely to prevent subcutaneous emphysema from an air leak around the tube. Subcutaneous emphysema can also be a warning sign that the tube is not in the trachea, that the back wall of the trachea has been injured, or occasionally, that the pleura has been injured.

Circulatory Support

PROCEDURE 11

VENOUS ACCESS

David C. Brooks

Gary L. Simpson

Next to the ABC's of resuscitation, venous access is the most important aspect of the initial approach to traumatized or critically ill patients seen in the emergency room. Venous access can be divided into two separate but intimately related procedures: (1) phlebotomy for blood sampling and (2) intravenous catheterization for fluid administration. The overlap will become obvious in the discussion, and although there will be some redundancy, the repetition is worthwhile so that one need not read the entire section to complete one particular task. The importance of being able to obtain either venous access or intravenous catheterization cannot be overstressed, and with one or two exceptions, which will be discussed below, all physicians and nurses working in an emergency room setting should feel comfortable in performing these procedures.

Venipuncture

Venipuncture is such an essential part of the management of all patients in the emergency room that all nurses and physicians working in the emergency room should be able to perform this procedure routinely. The principles and techniques involved are not complicated or difficult to master, and with a rudimentary knowledge of anatomy and minimal confidence, anyone should be able to obtain venous blood from all but the most difficult patients.

INDICATIONS

Venipuncture is indicated for phlebotomy for obtaining venous blood for laboratory determination or culture.

CONTRAINDICATIONS

There are no contraindications.

EQUIPMENT

- 70% isopropyl alcohol swab
- Povidone-iodine swab

- 10-, 20-, or 50-ml syringe
- 20- or 22-gauge 1.5-inch needle
- 20-gauge Vacutainer holder
- Appropriate-sized evacuated tube for desired blood test
- 19- or 21-gauge Butterfly needle
- Tourniquet
- 1-in. tape
- 2 × 2-in. gauze pads
- Adhesive bandage

POSITION

The patient should be supine or sitting comfortably in bed.

PROCEDURE

The procedure should be explained briefly to the patient.

Vein Selection

In order to select a vein, a methodical inspection of the patient's upper extremities is performed with particular attention to the antecubital area (Fig. PR11.1). The median cubital vein, the most prominent vein in this area, is the vein most often selected for phlebotomy for several reasons. It is large, accessible, and unsuitable, in most instances, as an intravenous site because of its location at the bend of the elbow. Since it is the most prominent superficial vein of the extremity, it can be used repeatedly for phlebotomy.

Alternative Veins

If the median cubital vein is not readily visible or palpable, attention is next turned to branches of the median or basilic veins as they course over the volar surface of the forearm. If these veins are indistinct, attempts are made to locate a superficial vein on the dorsum of the hand. In most cases, patients presenting to the emergency room will have at least one of these sites available for access. If all of the aforementioned veins elude detection, alternative sites include the saphenous vein on the medial aspect of the ankle at the medial malleolus, the femoral vein in the groin, or arterial puncture (Fig. PR11.2). These alternatives will be mentioned in the discussion of intravenous sites below.

Tourniquet

Once the proper vein has been selected, a tourniquet is placed proximally on the extremity and tightened sufficiently to impede venous drainage of the extremity but not to halt arterial inflow. The patient should be asked to clench his or her fist. In patients with particularly poor veins several other methods may be used to make the vein more prominent: a warm pack placed over the entire extremity may induce vasodilatation; 70% isopropyl alcohol will provide some cutaneous hyperemia; the vein may be "flicked" with a finger, which is said to paralyze intrinsic vascular tone and make the vein more prominent.

Skin Preparation

The area around the vein and the intended puncture site are well cleansed with either 70% isopropyl alcohol or povidone-iodine. When drawing blood cultures, the skin should always be prepared with povidone-iodine to eliminate any surface contaminents. The top of the blood culture bottles should also be swabbed with povidone-iodine. A 70% isopropyl alcohol skin preparation should be avoided if blood alcohol determinations are to be drawn.

Blood Collection Systems

Several blood collection systems are currently available. Use of either a *Vacutainer* system (consisting of a plastic holder for a double-pointed needle that will allow simultaneous penetration of the vein and an evacuated collecting tube, Fig. PR11.3) or a *sterile syringe* with needle is perfectly acceptable, with each offering certain advantages. Regardless of the system to be used, before beginning the procedure, it is important to ascertain the specific tubes and quantities of blood that will be required. The Vacutainer system is designed to be used when multiple samples are required. Its usefulness is limited, however, by the fact that the unregulated negative pressure within the tubes frequently collapses smaller veins. A sterile syringe with a 20- or 22-gauge needle (smaller needles promote hemolysis) can allow samples to be drawn from small and fragile veins. Equally useful when small or fragile veins are encountered is the winged needle unit (Butterfly) connected to a 5- or 10-ml syringe.

Stabilization

Having selected the vein, placed a tourniquet, and prepared the skin, the operator is now ready to obtain the blood sample. The nondominant hand of the operator is used to place distal traction on the skin to stabilize the vein in the subcutaneous tissue.

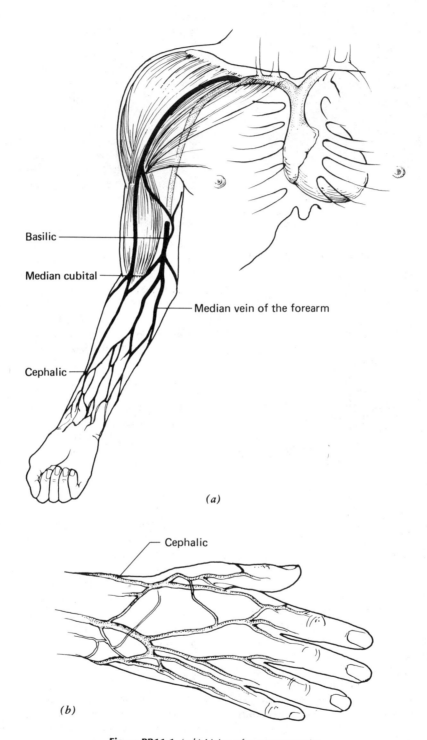

Basilic

Median cubital

Median vein of the forearm

Cephalic

(a)

Cephalic

(b)

Figure PR11.1 (a,b) Veins of upper extremity.

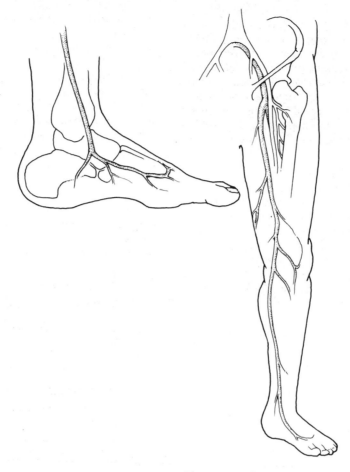

Figure PR11.2 Veins of lower extremity.

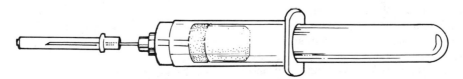

Figure PR11.3 Vacutainer system.

Introducing the Needle

The needle and syringe (or Vacutainer) are held at approximately 10–15 deg to the skin and the needle is briskly introduced beneath the dermis. At this point, the needle is advanced more gingerly into the vein. The flashback of blood into the hub of the syringe indicates successful cannulation of a vein. The needle is then advanced an additional 3–4 mm, and gentle steady aspiration is begun. After the appropriate amount of blood has been withdrawn, the tourniquet is released and the needle removed.

When using the Vacutainer system, care must be taken to prevent backflow into the bloodstream of the nonsterile chemical additives contained in the tubes. The patient's arm should be held downward with the collecting system dependent. The collecting tube should not be seated on the needle until after the external needle has entered the vein. If seated prematurely, the collecting tube may lose its vacuum. When withdrawing multiple blood samples, care should be taken to stabilize the Vacutainer when changing tubes lest the needle lacerate the vein.

Dressing

A small piece of sterile gauze is placed over the puncture site and gentle pressure is applied for 2–3 minutes. The patient's arm should be elevated to decrease venous pressure.

PITFALLS AND COMPLICATIONS

Fortunately, problems associated with venipuncture are relatively few and far between. Care should always be taken to compress the vein adequately after the blood sample is drawn, particularly in patients with anticoagulated blood. When particularly small and fragile veins are encountered, it may be advantageous to use a scalp vein needle, as discussed in the section on intravenous catheters.

Venous Catheterization

Venous catheterization naturally follows venipuncture. When it is known that a patient will require both venipuncture and venous access, the two procedures may be combined, thus obviating the need for two separate needle punctures. Two important considerations should be kept in mind when performing venous catheterization. First, the operator must select a vein based either on visualization or palpation of the vein. Nothing is accomplished by blindly stabbing the patient in an effort to find an elusive vein. Ultimately, time will be saved by making a thorough examination of the patient's extremities before attempting to place an intravenous catheter. Second, the operator should always consider the purpose of the line. In resuscitation from hypovolemic shock, the largest and shortest line will provide the most rapid instillation of fluid. Alternatively, the patient who requires an intravenous solely for parenteral antibiotics should receive a line commensurate with those requirements. And as a final caveat, it should be remembered that a small volume of fluid can be given through a large line, but a large volume cannot be given through a small line.

In this section five types of venous access are presented: peripheral percutaneous lines, peripheral central line placement, venesection or cutdowns, subclavian lines, and internal jugular lines.

Peripheral Percutaneous Venous Catheterization

EQUIPMENT

- Appropriate venous catheter (Angiocath, Argyle, Quik-cath, Medicut, etc.), gauge 12–20
- IV solution
- IV tubing and anesthesia extension set
- Tourniquet
- Iodophor ointment
- 2 × 2-inch sterile gauze
- 70% isopropyl alcohol or povidone-iodine swab
- 1-inch tape
- Arm board
- Lidocaine 0.5% or 1% a in tuberculin (TB) syringe with 25-gauge $^5/_8$-inch needle

POSITION

The patient should be comfortably supine on the bed or on a stretcher.

PROCEDURE

Always explain the procedure to the patient before proceeding.

Vein Selection

The two most important considerations when placing an intravenous cannula are the location of the vein and the size of the catheter. These decisions must be made promptly since access may be necessary instantaneously. The following are commonly used intravenous sites.

1. The median forearm or basilic veins are two moderately large veins located on the medial aspect of the volar surface of the forearm. They represent two excellent sites for venous catheterization in situations in which moderate to large amounts of fluid are to be given (see Fig. PR11.1a).

2. The superficial dorsal hand veins are a network of veins that represents an easy and convenient site for catheterization when minimal to moderate amounts of fluid are to be given (Fig. PR11.1b). Venous catheterization in these veins is well tolerated by the patient because it causes little interference with normal extremity function. When possible, it is best to place these lines in the nondominant hand since this will be the most useful configuration for the patient. They can be easily fitted with a heparin lock to allow intermittent drug administration.

3. The cephalic or "anesthetist's" vein is a prominent vein located on the radial aspect of the wrist. It is a large-caliber vein that drains the hand and into which a fairly good-sized catheter (16 or 18 gauge) can be placed. Catheterization of this vein is usually well tolerated by the patient but generally requires an arm board.

4. The volar wrist veins are smaller veins located distally on the volar surface of the wrist. They offer a less desirable alternative to the above mentioned veins because of their small size and relative fragility. Catheterization of these veins also requires an armboard and may be uncomfortable since the wrist must be held in slight extension. It has also been suggested that these sites are prone to injury of the median nerve if infiltration or extravasation occur. Nonetheless, they may be tried when other veins are not available.

5. The median cubital vein is a very large vein in the antecubital space running from the radial to ulnar aspects. Catheterization should only be performed when large fluid volumes are needed rapidly and no other site is available. Its main usefulness, as noted above, is for repeated phlebotomy. This usefulness is negated if it has been used for catheterization.

6. The external jugular is a moderate-sized vein located on the lateral portion of the anterior neck running medial to lateral across the clavicular belly of the sternocleidomastoid. When the patient is in a slight Trendelenburg, or even supine position, it can generally be found in all except the most obese patient. In some instances when an 18-gauge, or larger, short catheter has been introduced into the external jugular, the needle can be replaced by an appropriate-sized J-wire which, in experienced hands, can be threaded into a central position. Once this is done, the short 18-gauge catheter can be removed and a longer (12-inch) catheter can be threaded over the J-wire. This gives a central line without resorting to either an internal jugular or subclavian line and their attendant risks.

7. The saphenous vein is a large vein located on the medial aspect of the ankle just anterior to the medial malleolus (the artery nearby is the posterior tibial and is located posterior to the medial malleolus) (Fig. PR11.2). When upper extremity veins are not available, this is often a satisfactory alternative. Although it may be cannulated percutaneously, it often requires venous cutdown.

Catheter Selection

At present the following types of catheter systems, all using triple-bevelled needles are available (Fig. PR11.4):

1. Winged needle units (scalp vein, Butterfly, etc.) are available in ¾-inch length, gauged 16–25. These sets are particularly useful for infants and children, elderly patients, simple hydration, and intermittent intravenous injections when the heparin lock modification is used. The cannula is usually inserted with a sterile syringe attached to the female Luer-Lok of the unit to provide negative pressure.

2. Catheter-over-needle units (Angiocath, Medicut, Quikcath, etc.) are available in ¾–2-inch lengths, gauged 12–22. These sets have become increasingly popular because of their stability and relative long life expectancy as venous conduits. The units are useful in the administration of blood products and drugs and when rapid infusion of fluids is necessary.

3. Catheter-inside-needle units (Intracath, Deseret subclavian set, etc.) are available in catheter lengths of 8–28 inches. The introducing needle ranges in size from 14 to 21 gauge. The inner cannula is from 16 to 22 gauge. These catheters can be used wherever the catheter-over-needle units are used. Because of their length, they are particularly useful for central line placement and are generally reserved for this purpose.

Gauge Selection

Once the type of catheter has been selected, the size of the catheter lumen must be chosen. This decision should be individualized to each patient. Bear in mind that flow in a fluid-

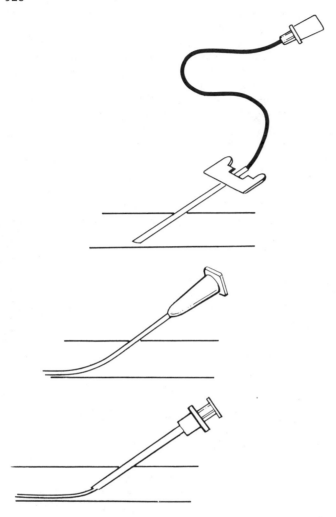

Figure PR11.4 Triple-bevelled needles: (a) winged needle unit; (b) catheter-over-needle unit; (c) catheter-inside-needle unit.

Inspection

The vein should be inspected and palpated. A soft ballotable feel assures the operator that the vein is not phlebitic or sclerosed. The procedure should be explained to the patient.

Preliminaries

Before starting the procedure, the operator should ensure that all of the equipment and solutions to be used are readily at hand. The proper intravenous solution should be connected to the tubing and all air should be flushed from the line. It is also wise to have one or two extra catheters on hand. Place three 3-inch pieces of adhesive tape close at hand to be used when securing the catheter.

Local Anesthesia

If the patient is unduly anxious or concerned, local anesthesia may be provided with an intradermal wheal of plain 0.5 or 1% lidocaine placed with a TB syringe. Local anesthesia is generally not necessary if the catheter is 20 gauge or smaller. Nonetheless, large catheters (18 gauge and larger) are painful and a small amount of lidocaine may ease the patient's discomfort.

Tourniquet

The tourniquet is placed proximally and the area of the intended catheterization is thoroughly prepared with a 70% isopropyl sponge or povidine-iodine solution. Ordinarily, gloves are not required when placing a peripheral short line.

Stabilization

The nondominant hand of the operator is used to place distal traction on the skin, thus firmly anchoring the vein in the subcutaneous tissue.

Needle Introduction

If a large-gauge catheter is to be used, the patient's skin may be prepunctured with an 18-gauge needle. This will facilitate passage of the plastic catheter through the dermis. The catheter is grasped between the thumb and forefinger with its attached syringe resting against the palm of the operator's hand. The vein may be approached from above, at a venous junction, or from the side, but most people find that lateral entry (particularly when using the catheter-over-needle unit) is the most frequently used (Fig. PR11.5). The skin adjacent to the vein is then briskly punctured with the needle held approximately

filled conduit is proportional to the radius of the conduit raised to the fourth power and is inversely proportional to the length of the conduit. Thus, a large-bore catheter of short length will deliver far more fluid per unit time than a similar catheter of greater length. A central line is, therefore, not the optimal line for delivering large amounts of fluid during the initial portion of resuscitation from hypovolemia. The fluid to be infused must also be considered. Blood and blood products will flow with difficulty through catheters smaller than 18 gauge.

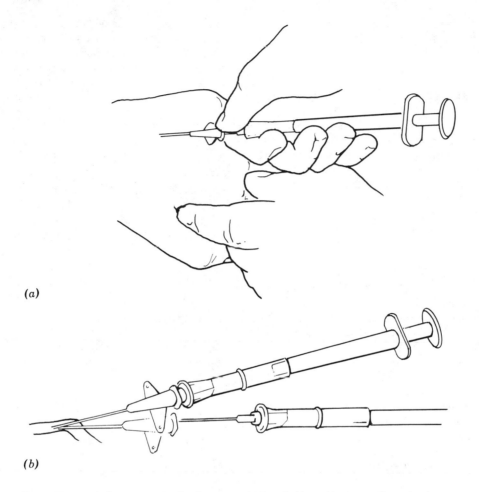

(a)

(b)

Figure PR11.5 Catheter-over-needle placement. (a) Stretch skin and insert needle and catheter; (b) release syringe and needle.

10–15 deg to the axis of the arm. Once beneath the dermis, the angle is narrowed so that the catheter is nearly flush with the axis of the arm and the catheter is gingerly advanced into the vein with the bevel up. Once flashback of blood is seen in the needle hub, the catheter and needle are advanced along the course of the vein an additional 2–3 mm. If a syringe is supplied with the catheter, it is aspirated to ensure free return of blood, and the plastic catheter is advanced completely into the vein while the needle is held stationary. Pressure is placed at the tip of the catheter to prevent backflow of blood, the tourniquet is released, the needle is completely removed from the catheter, and the intravenous solution is attached.

Dressing

Iodophor ointment is applied to the puncture site and a small piece of gauze is placed over the entry point including the catheter hub. The catheter is securely taped into place and an armboard is attached if necessary. Armboards should be used whenever the catheter crosses a joint or when undue movement of the catheter is anticipated.

PITFALLS AND COMPLICATIONS

Immediate pain or swelling at the site of insertion indicates *extravasation,* and the solution should be held until confirmation of the catheter's position can be made. Because some swelling can result from local tissue trauma, extravasation can be confirmed by occluding venous return proximally and noting the infusion rate. If the infusion continues despite proximal venous compression (i.e., it is running out of the vein) infiltration has presumably occurred. The development of a *hematoma* signifies that the vein has been lacerated or the catheter has exited the back wall. In this situation the vein cannot be salvaged for an intravenous line and another site will have to be selected. If the new site is to be in the same general area, the first catheter, with its needle removed, should be left in place until a new intravenous line has been established. This will generally minimize bleeding from the lacerated or punctured vein. Once the second intravenous line is established, remove the failed catheter and apply pressure to the lacerated vein.

Phlebitis occurs when irritating or hypertonic infusions are used. The maximal concentration to be infused should be commensurate with the location of the catheter. Catheters placed in the lower extremities should never be used to administer irritating or hypertonic solutions and should be reserved for infusions of saline or dilute dextrose solutions.

Sepsis is caused by inattention to aseptic technique. The operator should ensure strict asepsis during the catheterization and until the dressing has been applied. The dressing should be inspected and changed daily, and catheters should not be maintained for more than 72 hours without being changed.

Peripheral Central Line

In certain circumstances, a short peripheral line will not be sufficient for the patient's needs. An indication for a central line may be present but the operator wishes to avoid a subclavian or internal jugular line. Central lines are helpful from both a therapeutic and diagnostic standpoint. Not only can cardiotonic drugs be given with assurance that they are reaching the target organ, but measurements of central pressures

may be useful in patient management. Some of the complications of using a subclavian or internal jugular line can be obviated by placement of a percutaneous central line. This section deals with percutaneously placed central lines in the upper extremities.

INDICATIONS

- Central venous pressure monitoring
- Swan-Ganz line placement
- Hyperalimentation access. (Because of the strict asepsis and tight adherence to accepted protocol involved in placing a hyperalimentation line and, moreover, because there is no conceivable reason why a hyperalimentation line should be placed in an emergency setting, this topic will not be addressed.)

CONTRAINDICATIONS

This procedure should not be performed in patients with known superior vena cava syndrome.

EQUIPMENT

- All of the equipment mentioned in percutaneous venous catheterization
- Sterile towels or paper sheets
- Gloves
- Mask
- 4-0 suture on cutting needle
- Needle holder
- Suture scissors
- 14-, 19-, 20-gauge catheters (generally long lines of the catheter-inside-needle type)

POSITION

The patient is placed supine on a stretcher or bed. The patient's arm is positioned fully extended and abducted 90 deg from the shoulder in the same plane as the patient's trunk in order to straighten the course of the axillary vein and facilitate unobstructed passage of the catheter.

PROCEDURE

Vein Selection

When indicated, a central venous pressure (CVP) line can usually be established through catheterization of the median vein or basilic vein distal to the antecubital fossa. The cephalic vein should be avoided. Although it is a large vein, it takes a tortuous route as it travels centrally and makes a 90 deg turn in the shoulder and thus may be difficult to thread. On the other hand, the basilic vein and its tributaries are in continuity with the great veins of the thorax and generally provide no anatomical obstruction to passage of the catheter. If the basilic vein, the median forearm vein, or any of their direct tributaries cannot be visualized or palpated in the antecubital fossa after placing a tourniquet, it is best to proceed directly to venesection.

Tourniquet

A tourniquet is applied to the upper arm as previously described.

Preparation

Because the placement of a central line is more prone to septic complications than a short intravenous line or simple venipuncture, stricter attention to asepsis is mandatory. The skin in a wide perimeter around the vein (8–10 cm) should be thoroughly prepared with povidone-iodine. Sterile towels or paper sheets should be used, and the operator should wear sterile gloves. Needle holder, skin sutures, and scissors should be arranged in a convenient position on the sterile field.

Catheter Selection

A catheter-inside-needle unit of the appropriate size is selected. The normal catheter selected for an adult is a 16-gauge catheter with a 14-gauge introducing needle. For pediatric patients or patients with small superficial veins, a 19-gauge catheter (17-gauge needle) may be selected. An assistant will be necessary to remove the catheter from its nonsterile container and pass it to the operator in an aseptic fashion.

Anesthesia

Using a 25-gauge needle, the operator raises a small wheal of 1% lidocaine without epinephrine at the site of catheterization. Although anesthesia is optional when placing peripheral short lines, the gauge of most central line needles is large enough so that anesthesia should routinely be used.

Needle Introduction

Before beginning, the introducing needle should be loosened and then reattached to the hub of the plastic sleeve that guards the catheter. This eases the removal of the sleeve after the catheter has been introduced into the vein (Fig. PR11.6). The introducing needle is held in a similar fashion as in the catheter-over-needle unit technique, the skin is pierced, and the needle is gently introduced into the vein. When the needle has successfully entered the vein, the operator will see the return of blood along the entire length of the catheter.

Threading

The introducing needle is advanced an additional 1–2 mm to ensure that it is well into the vein. The needle is stabilized by the operator, and with the other hand the operator then advances the plastic catheter through the needle and into the vein from within the plastic sleeve. The plastic sleeve will bunch up as this is being done and the operator may need to pause now and then to straighten it. Once the catheter is well into the vein, the tourniquet is released. When the catheter has been fully advanced, the plastic sleeve is removed from the needle hub and the thin wire stylet is discarded. The needle is removed from the vein and seated firmly into the catheter hub. A needle guard is provided in each set and should be placed over the junction of the needle tip and catheter. This prevents inadvertent laceration of the tubing or the patient. The catheter is then connected to the intravenous solution directly or with an intervening three-way stopcock, depending on whether the line will be used for CVP monitoring or simple fluid administration. The needle guard and hub of the catheter should be sutured to the skin after the instillation of additional lidocaine. This precaution prevents inadvertent dislodgement of the catheter.

Confirm Position

The intravenous bottle should be lowered below the edge of the bed to check for blood return before starting the infusion. A chest film should be obtained to verify location of the catheter.

Dressing

The catheter should be dressed with iodophor ointment and covered with a 2 × 2-inch sterile gauze. The catheter should

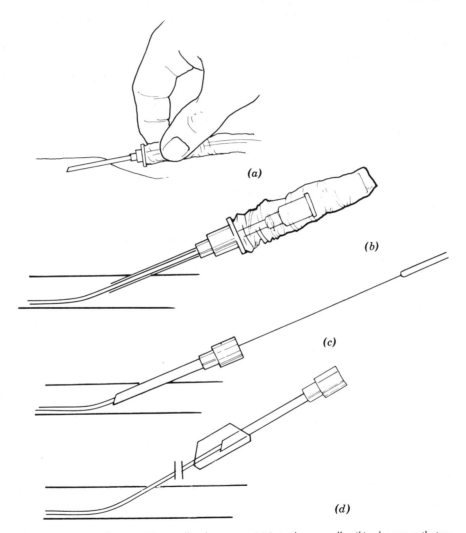

Figure PR11.6 Catheter-inside-needle placement. (a) Introduce needle; (b) advance catheter; (c) remove wire stylette; (d) withdraw needle, attach to catheter hub, attach needle guard.

then be securely taped into place and an armboard attached, as necessary.

PITFALLS AND COMPLICATIONS

Several problems can be encountered when placing a long line. If cannulation fails, the catheter and needle should be removed as a unit so as to prevent *catheter embolus* if the catheter tip is sheared. *Difficulty advancing* the catheter is usually caused by valves or venous tortuosity. The arm may be further abducted to straighten the vein. Alternatively, the head can be rotated to the opposite side, which may further straighten the vessel. One final method is to remove the wire stylet from the catheter and begin infusion. This may serve to dilate the vein and facilitate passage.

Hematomas are caused by lacerations of the vein. They can be prevented by selecting veins of adequate size to accept the catheter and by stabilizing the catheter once the vein has been entered. The rigid needle should not be advanced more than 2–3 mm into the vein once the return of blood is seen. Because of the long length of these lines, they are more prone to develop *phlebitic or septic* complications. Strict attention to aseptic technique, continuous dressing surveillance, and the avoidance of irritating or hypertonic solutions will lessen these problems. Catheters that just match the size of the vein are more irritating than small catheters; therefore smaller catheters should be selected whenever possible. When blood products are infused or blood samples are taken from the line, the line should be *flushed thoroughly* with saline to prevent the buildup of clot at the tip.

Venesection (Cutdown)

When the antecubital veins cannot be visualized, it is often safer to attempt venous cannulation by venesection than to proceed directly to a percutaneously placed subclavian or internal jugular line. Venesection may be used for placement of a central line through the basilic or median forearm vein or it may be used as a short line to give a rapid fluid volume. The technique for exposure of the vein is the same for both.

POSITION

Position of the patient is the same as for percutaneous central catheter.

EQUIPMENT

In addition to the equipment for a peripheral central line, a small dissection set should be available. This should include the following items:

- Three fine curved snaps
- Needle holder
- Fine scissors
- Suture scissors
- Fine smooth forceps
- Adson toothed forceps
- Self-retaining retractor
- Vein retractor
- Scalpel with No. 10, 15 and 11 blades
- 3-0 and 4-0 silk sutures (ties)
- 4-0 nonabsorbable skin sutures with cutting needle
- Vein introducer
- 10-ml normal saline in sterile syringe

PROCEDURE

Tourniquet

Tourniquet application is identical to that described for the percutaneous approach. A tourniquet placed before the procedure is begun may help visualize the vein. It should not be left on during the venesection procedure, however, since it will cause excessive bleeding at the cutdown site.

Vein Selection

In addition to the median basilic and median veins already mentioned in the section on percutaneous central lines, several other veins are available for cutdown. Access to the central venous circulation will not always be obtained with these lines; nevertheless they should be kept in mind as sites for rapid venesection placement of lines.

1. *Cephalic vein.* When forearm veins such as the median cubital or basilic are not available for cutdown, the *cephalic vein* in the upper arm or deltopectoral groove can be approached and catheterized in a fashion similar to permanent pacemaker insertion.
2. The *external jugular* is an equally good alternative if it is not suitable for percutaneous catheterization.
3. The *origin of the saphenous vein* in the ankle may be used

for venous cutdown if it is not suitable for percutaneous catheterization.

4. The landmarks for the *saphenofemoral junction* are the inguinal ligament, the pubic tubercle, and the femoral artery. The vein is easily found two fingerbreadths lateral and two fingerbreadths inferior to the pubic tubercle. It is medial to the femoral artery (remember N.A.V.E.L.—nerve, artery, vein, empty space, lacunar ligament). The catheter length should be selected by measuring from the incision site to the umbilicus. This will ensure that the catheter lies in the inferior vena cava. *Warning:* It is imperative that the catheter be placed and secured in the very proximal saphenous vein, not in the femoral vein. A catheter that is placed directly into the femoral vein and is secured will occlude all venous return from the leg. This procedure should only be attempted by experienced personnel.

Skin Preparation and Draping

Skin preparation and draping are identical to that described for the percutaneous approach. A wide sterile field covering the entire volar surface of the forearm and extending proximally and distally 8–10 cm should be provided in order to allow the operator ample space. The area draped should allow the operator sufficient room to manipulate the vein and incision site. A sterile field adjacent to the incision site on which to set out the sterile instruments should be available.

Anesthesia

Because an actual skin incision will be made, anesthesia will necessarily be more extensive than the simple wheal used in the percutaneous approach. The operator should have 5–10 ml of 1% lidocaine available. An *assistant* who is out of the sterile field is most helpful.

Technique

The procedure is explained to the patient. After the sterile field has been placed, lidocaine is infiltrated into the area of the proposed incision.

Incision

Incisions transverse to the axis of the vein should be used for all vessels with the exception of the saphenofemoral junction. This area is best approached through a longitudinal incision about 10 cm long. In the upper extremity and ankle an incision of 3–4 cm should suffice. The incision is gingerly extended through the skin until the subcutaneous tissue is free.

Dissection

The loose areolar tissue is bluntly dissected aside, and the tissue spread with a curved hemostat along the axis of the vein so as not to disrupt the vein or any of its branches. Two levels of structures exist in the forearm. The superficial level contains subcutaneous fat and superficial veins. Deep to this, beneath the muscular fascia, are the arteries, nerves, and deep veins of the forearm. Initially, venesection should be confined to the superficial compartment above the fascia and well away from the deep neurovascular structures.

Identify the Vein

The vein is identified as a pulseless, thin-walled vessel whose blue color blanches when distal traction is applied. Care should be taken to avoid nerves and arteries. It is always wise to palpate the structure for a pulse before proceeding. If a vein is not easily identified, the assistant may briefly tighten the tourniquet. This will increase the filling in the veins and make them more readily apparent. The position of the basilic vein is indicated in Figure PR11.7.

Isolation of the Vein

The vein is dissected free of the surrounding tissue for a distance of 4 cm along its axis, and fine ties are passed proximally and distally. The distal tie should be secured and left long; the proximal tie should not be secured. Traction is placed on the proximal tie.

Venotomy

Pierce the midsection of the vein with a No. 11 scalpel blade, blade up (Figure PR11.8 illustrates cutdown of saphenous vein at the ankle.) A fine hemostat inserted a short distance into the vein will dilate the venotomy. An alternative method for those with some surgical experience involves a small transverse venotomy made with the tips of fine dissecting scissors. The tips may then be gently insinuated into the vein and the vein dilated. It may be helpful to grasp the vein with fine forceps before incising it.

Insertion

The catheter tip is then inserted into the venotomy and is gently advanced. The wire stylet is removed and the catheter is connected to an intravenous solution. The proper length for a central line placed through cutdown of the basilic vein can be determined by measuring the distance from the incision to the

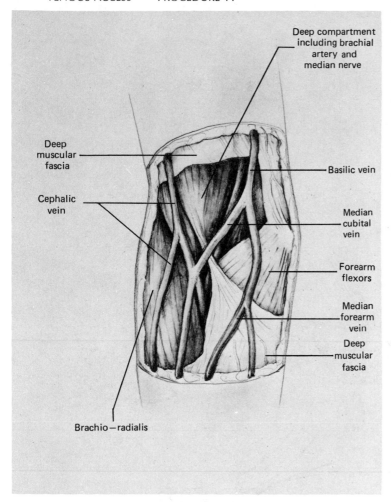

Figure PR11.7 Relations of the basilic vein.

Labels on figure:
Deep compartment including brachial artery and median nerve
Deep muscular fascia
Cephalic vein
Basilic vein
Median cubital vein
Forearm flexors
Median forearm vein
Deep muscular fascia
Brachio—radialis

needle through the skin from inside out. Thread the catheter into the needle from outside in. Remove the needle and proceed as above. The catheter will now exit the skin adjacent to the skin incision. This technique may lessen the incidence of infection at the incision site. This alternative takes somewhat longer to perform and should not be attempted in the emergency situation.

Closure

Once the catheter is in place and the infusion fluid is running easily, the proximal tie is secured around the vein, including the catheter. It should not be so tight as to occlude the catheter. The wound is inspected for bleeding and the skin incision is closed with three or four interrupted simple sutures of 4-0 nonabsorbable material. For additional security, the catheter hub should be sutured to the underlying skin.

Dressing

The wound is dressed, taped, and secured as previously described. An armboard is routinely used to stabilize the catheter. X-ray confirmation of position is required.

PITFALLS AND COMPLICATIONS

Difficulties in passing the catheter may be encountered. The various maneuvers to help pass the catheter that are described in the percutaneous approach are applicable here as well. On occasion, a particularly small or vasospastic vein may be encountered. A small amount of lidocaine (1–2 ml) dripped directly onto the vein will cause slight vasodilatation and thus facilitate entry of the catheter. The vein may also go into spasm while threading the catheter; wiping the catheter in a sponge soaked in lidocaine will overcome this obstacle. If none of these techniques succeeds, the catheter should be pulled back to the point where it flows most easily and secured in place. Never abandon a cutdown in which some flow is available. A small *vein introducer* may also be useful to hold open the venotomy while introducing the catheter to the vein. During dissection great care should be taken to identify the *brachial artery* in the arm and the *femoral artery* in the groin. Frequent palpations of the field before sharp dissection of any tissue will reveal the pulse. Arterial lacerations should be immediately repaired with interrupted 5-0 or 6-0 Prolene vascular sutures.

Additional complications and problems are similar to those encountered with other lines. These include infection, phlebitis, and hematoma. Because an actual skin incision is made,

suprasternal notch when the arm is fully abducted. When the line is in place, the tip will lie in the superior vena cava. Most catheter tips are blunt. Beveling the tip with scissors before insertion is not routinely encouraged. When this is necessary because of the size of the vein, the operator must be sure that the tip is not left too sharp since it may then lacerate or penetrate the vein wall. Flush the catheter with 5–10 ml of saline before attaching the infusion tubing.

An *alternative method* allows the catheter to be brought out through a separate stab wound rather than through the incision. After the vein has been isolated and the distal ligature has been tied but before the venotomy has been made, pass a 14-gauge

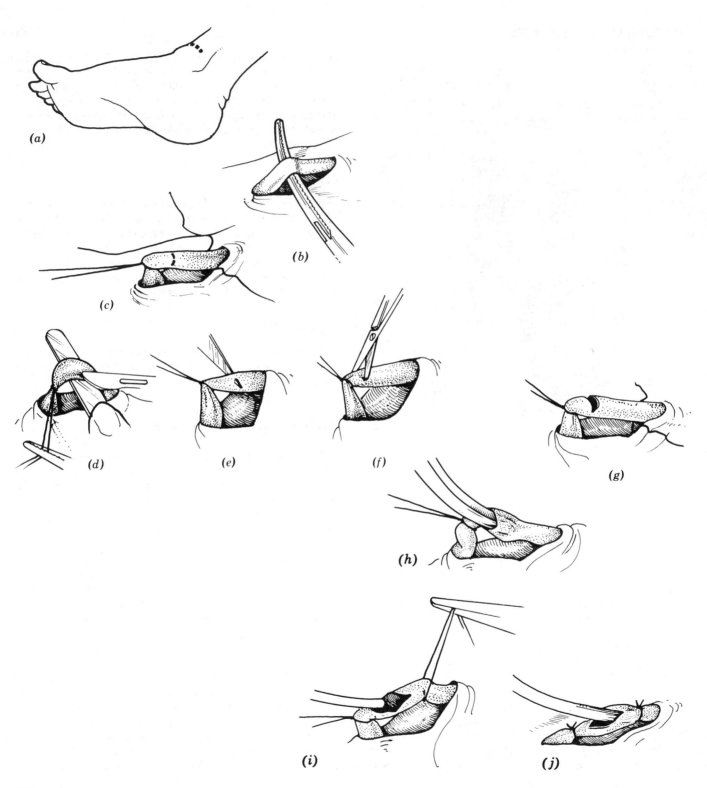

(a)

(b)

(c)

(d)

(e)

(f)

(g)

(h)

(i)

(j)

934

the operator must carefully follow aseptic technique. The catheter dressing should be changed frequently and new intravenous tubing placed daily. Catheters should not be left in place for extended periods of time and should be removed at the first sign of infection.

Lower extremity cutdowns should be reserved for patients who are in extremis and in whom large volumes of fluid are rapidly needed. Because of their hypertonicity or irritating nature, they should not be used routinely for infusion of substances that may precipitate thrombophlebitis.

Subclavian Vein Catheterization

The subclavian vein is one of the mainstays of intravenous access in the critically injured or ill patients seen in the emergency room. All physicians should have some familiarity with the procedure and should feel comfortable in attempting catheterization in the emergency setting. The subclavian vein is the preferred route in the resuscitated patient for several reasons. First, it does not interfere with attempts to obtain an airway; second, the landmarks for this catheterization are easier to see and appreciate in the injured patient; and third, after resuscitation there is far more patient acceptance of the subclavian line sutured to the upper thorax than of the internal jugular line sutured to the neck. The venous anatomy of the upper thorax, neck, and great vessels is shown in Figure PR11.9.

INDICATIONS

This procedure is performed when it is necessary to have central vein access for placement of central venous pressure line, Swan-Ganz line, or percutaneous pacemaker.

CONTRAINDICATIONS

- Superior vena cava syndrome
- Thrombocytopenia
- Abnormal clotting studies

EQUIPMENT

- Sterile towels
- Povidone–iodine (Betadine) solution
- Deseret subclavian set or similar 14-gauge needle-over-catheter set (8 or 12 inch length)
- IV solution and tubing
- Small dissection kit (see above)
- 3-0 silk on a cutting needle
- Scissors
- Povidone-iodine ointment
- 2 × 2-inch sterile gauze
- 1-inch tape

POSITION

The patient is placed in slight Trendelenburg position (10–20 deg) to distend the vein. The patient's shoulders should be hyperextended with a rolled towel between the shoulder blades to elevate the vein more anteriorly. The patient's head is rotated to the contralateral side.

PROCEDURE

Unless a specific unilateral contraindication exists, such as emphysematous blebs, radical neck dissection, or preexisting contralateral pneumothorax, one can safely approach either the right or left subclavian vein. The left subclavian vein has a slightly straighter course into the superior vena cava, but most operators find both sides equally effective. The potential hazards of the technique are such that the operator should be thoroughly familiar with the anatomy of the area before attempting the procedure.

Anatomy

The subclavian vein lies immediately posterior to the medial segment of the clavicle. The vein follows a course running from the axilla, over the first rib, and behind the clavicle at the junction of the medial and middle thirds of the clavicle

Figure PR11.8 Saphenous cutdown. (*a*) Incise skin transversely; (*b*) isolate vein; (*c*) pass proximal and distal ties under vessel; tie distal suture; (*d,e,f,g*) incise vein with scalpel or fine scissors; (*h*) gently dilate vein; (*i*) advance catheter; (*j*) secure proximal tie.

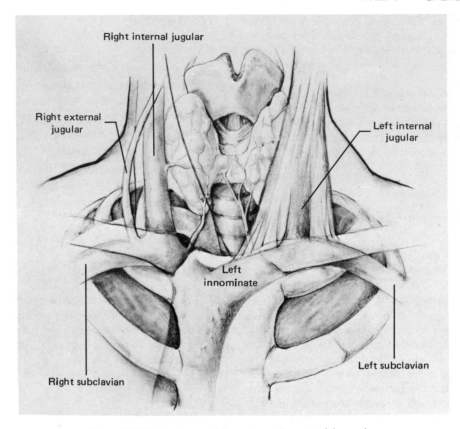

Figure PR11.9 Anatomy of the veins at the root of the neck.

(see Fig. PR11.9). The vein continues in the thorax to join the internal jugular vein and form the innominate vein. The subclavian artery lies deep to it and is separated from it by the scalenus anterior muscle. The pleura lies approximately 5 mm posterior to the vein and represents the greatest potential hazard in percutaneous catheterization.

Skin Preparation

The areas above and below the clavicle are thoroughly prepared and draped. The sterile field should extend from the nipple inferiorly to the midneck superiorly and from just beyond the midline to the acromioclavicular joint laterally. The operator should wear a mask and gloves. In emergency situations when the need for intravenous access is paramount, strict attention to asepsis may be set aside, if necessary.

Landmarks

The first rib dives beneath the clavicle at the junction of the middle and the medial third of the clavicle. This junction can

often be appreciated by firmly palpating for the angle formed by this intersection. The subclavian vein is best located at this point, posterior to the clavicle and anterior to the rib. Moving 1 or 2 cm laterally and inferiorly to this allows the operator to sneak under the clavicle and locate the vein.

Use of Finding Needle

It is prudent to use a small-caliber (18- or 20-gauge, 2-inch long) needle to localize the vein before proceeding with the 14-gauge introducing needle. The needle should be directed in a plane 30–35 deg to the axis of the thorax toward a point 2 cm above the suprasternal notch (Fig. PR11.10). It is often said that the vein will be found by directing the needle to the suprasternal notch itself. The vein's course actually takes it somewhat higher in the neck and will be more reliably found by directing the needle above the notch. The smaller finding needle, attached to a 10-ml syringe, is advanced along this

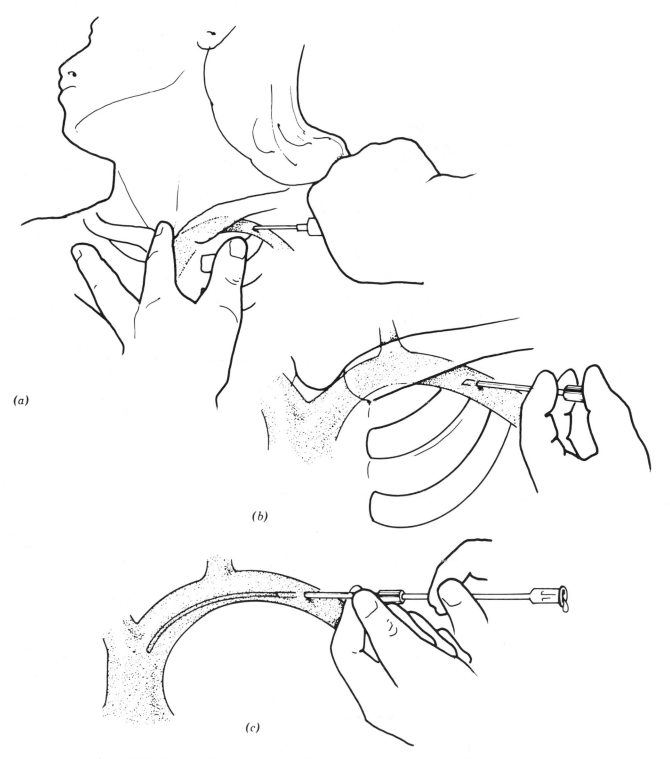

Figure PR11.10 Subclavian catheterization. (a) Insert needle; (b) protect needle hub after removing syringe; (c) insert catheter; (d) withdraw needle; (e) attach needle, suture to skin, and apply dressing.

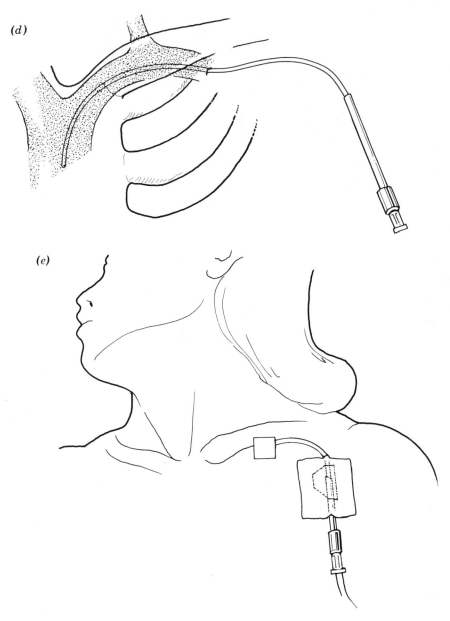

Figure PR11.10 (continued)

course to the inferior margin of the clavicle. When this is located the needle should be walked downward until it will just pass beneath the clavicle. Staying as close as possible to the inferior margin of the clavicle lessens the chance of pneumothorax. When the needle tip is beneath the clavicle, the angle formed by the needle shaft and the chest wall should be lessened so that the syringe and needle lie nearly parallel to the chest wall as possible. The needle is then advanced toward the supraclavicular notch. Gentle negative pressure should be maintained so that the operator knows with the first flashback of blood that he or she has entered the vein.

Inserting Catheter

Once the vein has been located, the finding needle is removed (Fig. PR11.10) and the 14-gauge needle and syringe are advanced along the same three-dimensional course, again maintaining gentle negative pressure on the syringe until the vein is entered. When the vein is entered and blood freely returns into the syringe, the needle and syringe are advanced an additional 2–3 mm and are held firmly in place at the hub to prevent movement and laceration of the vessel. While the needle is still firmly stabilized by the operator's nondominant hand, the syringe is removed, the thumb of the nondominant hand is placed over the open hub of the needle to prevent air aspiration, and the catheter is introduced into the needle and advanced until it is in a central position. The needle is then withdrawn over the catheter. Most currently available sets allow the needle to be completely removed and discarded and an adapter attached to the catheter. On older sets in which the needle cannot be completely removed, the needle guard is snapped into place and the intravenous solution is attached. If the catheter will not advance, both needle and catheter should be removed in tandem since the catheter tip may shear off at the end of the needle and embolize if it is pulled through the needle.

An alternative method has recently been introduced that uses the Arrow or the Cordis set. Complete prepackaged sets are provided that include a small-gauge needle (18 gauge) and a flexible wire. This needle is used to locate the subclavian vein as done in the previously described method. Instead of proceeding to the larger-gauge introducing needle, the flexible guide wire is introduced through the needle into a central position. The needle is then completely removed and the catheter to be used for solution administration is threaded over the wire into a central position. The guide wire is then removed and the catheter is connected to the solution and sutured to the skin. The advantage of this technique is that the large 14-gauge needle is never used and thus cannot injure adjacent structures.

Regardless of which method is used, the catheter must be sutured to the skin of the chest wall midway between the clavicle and nipple and dressed with iodophor ointment and sterile gauze.

Confirming Position

Placement can be ascertained by lowering the solution bottle below the edge of the bed and observing the return of blood. A chest film should always be obtained at the earliest possible moment after subclavian or internal jugular catheterization to ensure both position and the lack of pneumothorax.

PITFALLS AND COMPLICATIONS

The two major complications associated with subclavian catheterization are *laceration of the artery* and *pneumothorax*. The former is less likely to occur when a subclavian approach is used than when the internal jugular is catheterized. By exerting a small amount of negative pressure on the syringe after it has pierced the skin, the operator will know the moment the vein has been entered. Because the artery is located posterior to the vein, the vein should always be entered first.

In contradistinction, *pneumothorax* is more common with a subclavian approach than with a high internal jugular approach. This is because the dome of the pleura lies much closer to the subclavian vein. A certain number of pneumothoraces will occur, but these can be minimized by staying right beneath the inferior border of the clavicle as the needle is advanced. When *air is aspirated* into the syringe, the operator should have a high index of suspicion that he or she has lacerated the pleura. The needle should be removed, the chest auscultated, and a chest film promptly obtained. This will rule out the possibility of pneumothorax.

Hematoma can be caused by laceration of the vein or inadvertent entry into the subclavian artery. When this occurs the needle and catheter should be gently removed as a unit and pressure placed on the area of the hematoma. The operator should always be alert to the sensation of pulsations as he or she advances the needle. If pulsations are felt, the needle should be withdrawn and redirected. The direction of the needle should not be changed unless the tip has been withdrawn and lies just beneath the skin. Moving the needle while it lies beneath the clavicle can easily incur damage not only to the vein but to the artery and pleura as well. The needle and catheter should never be advanced against resistance.

Other complications include *hydrothorax* if the catheter tip exits the vein and fluid is infused into the thoracic cavity, or *hydromediastinum* if the catheter perforates the cava in the chest. Both can be obviated if care is taken to ensure that blood returns into the catheter when it is lowered below the level of the right atrium. *Thrombophlebitis* or its late sequellae, *subclavian vein thrombosis,* can occur if aseptic technique is not followed and the catheter is left in place beyond its period of usefulness. If the catheter is to be used to draw blood samples, it should be *thoroughly flushed* to prevent clot developing at the tip.

Internal Jugular Catheterization

The internal jugular vein is a reasonable alternative approach to the great venous vessels in certain situations. Because the right internal jugular catheter represents a straighter course to the superior vena cava than the left, it is particularly well suited for procedures such as placing pacemakers and inferior vena cava occluding umbrellas. Nonetheless, it, too, is fraught with potential complications and as a general rule is more difficult to catheterize in the emergency situation. This is due to the fact that simultaneous attempts to establish an endotracheal airway during resuscitation will interfere with the venotomist at the head of the bed. In general, in emergency situations the subclavian vein is preferable to the internal jugular.

The indications, contraindications, equipment, and position are the same as for subclavian catheterization.

PROCEDURE

Anatomy

The internal jugular vein exits at the base of the skull through the posterior compartment of the jugular foramen and joins the subclavian vein to form the innominate vein posterior to the medial end of the clavicle (Fig. PR11.9). Its course runs initially lateral to the internal carotid artery and then anterolateral to the common carotid. Nearly its entire length is covered by the sternocleidomastoid muscle. The right internal jugular vein is straighter and usually larger than the left and should be the first vein attempted.

Skin Preparation

The entire side of the patient's neck, extending across the midline, the anterior chest, and the sweep of the shoulder, is prepared with povidone-iodine solution and sterilely draped. The operator should wear a mask and gloves.

Approach

Two approaches to the vein are possible. As with subclavian vein catheterization, a finding needle (18 or 20 gauge, 2 inches) should be used to localize the vein before inserting the 14-gauge needle.

In the *high approach* the operator aligns the needle and syringe parallel to the anterior border of the sternocleidomastoid and adjacent to the triangle formed by the junction of the two bellies of the muscle, elevates his or her hand, and directs the needle point approximately 30 deg posterior to the coronal plane and toward the ipsilateral hip (Fig. PR11.11a,b). This motion directs the needle through the muscle belly, into the vein and lateral to the carotid artery. The pulse of the carotid should be palpated and the needle always directed slightly lateral to this.

In the *low approach* the puncture site is located 1 cm lateral to the lateral border of the sternal head of the sternocleidomastoid and 1 cm above the clavicle between the sternal and clavicular heads (Fig. PR11.11c,d). The axis of the needle and the syringe is maintained at 45 deg angle to the skin. The tip of the needle is directed toward the xyphoid process.

In both methods, slight negative pressure is applied to the syringe once the needle has pierced the skin; the flashback of blood indicates that the vein has been entered. Once the vessel has been entered, the needle is advanced an additional 2 mm before removing the syringe and threading the catheter.

After the catheter has been threaded centrally, its position is checked by lowering the intravenous bottle below the level of the patient and observing for blood return. An x-ray film should be obtained immediately.

Dressing

When the line is in place and good return has been obtained, the hub should be sutured to the skin with two 3-0 nonabsorbable sutures (Fig. PR11.11e). Iodophor ointment and gauze are applied and the catheter is firmly secured with adhesive tape.

PITFALLS AND COMPLICATIONS

The potential complications are discussed in the section on subclavian catheterization but will be reiterated here. *Hematoma* can be caused by laceration of either the internal jugular vein or the carotid artery. Injury to the carotid artery can be best avoided by placing the tips of the nondominant hand along the course of the artery's pulsations and always directing the needle lateral to this. If the vein is not found initially, the needle should be withdrawn before attempting to search in another

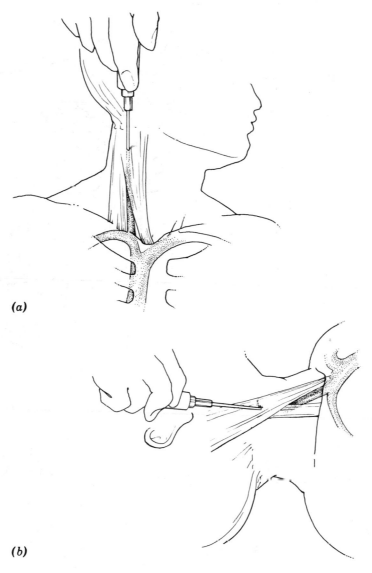

(a)

(b)

Figure PR11.11 Internal jugular catheterization. (a,b) High approach; (c,d) low approach; (e) suture catheter to skin and apply dressing.

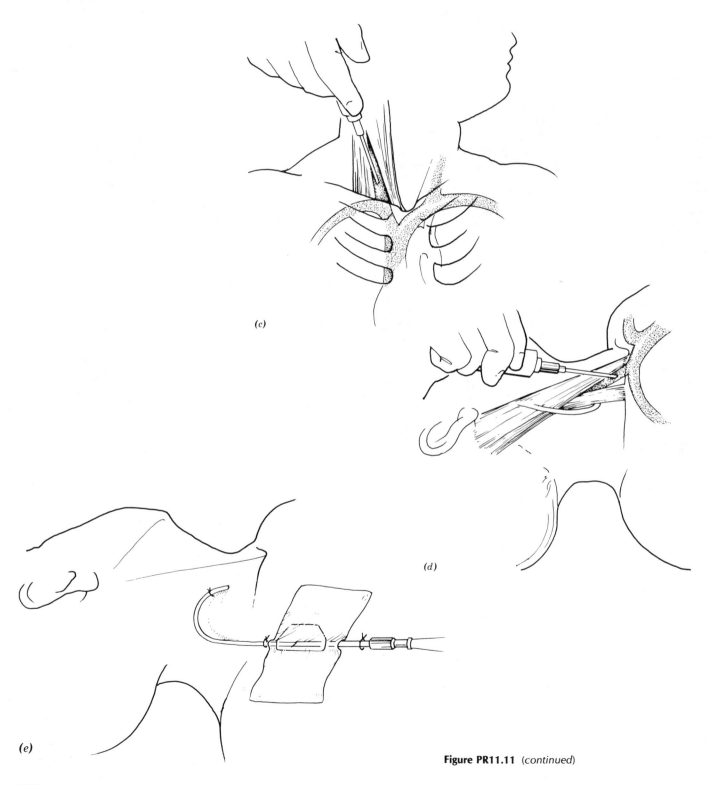

(c)

(d)

(e)

Figure PR11.11 (continued)

area. If a hematoma does develop, firm pressure should be placed over the site of bleeding. *Hydrothorax* and *hydromediastinum* can be prevented by checking for blood return into the catheter before the infusion is begun. Never advance the catheter against resistance. *Phlebitis and sepsis* are best dealt with prophylactically. Pay strict attention to asepsis, change dressing and tubing regularly, and remove the catheter at the first sign of infection. *Air embolism* can be avoided by putting the patient in 10–20 deg Trendelenburg position and by placing a gloved thumb over the needle hub before introducing the catheter.

PROCEDURE 12

CENTRAL VENOUS PRESSURE MONITORING

David C. Brooks

Gary L. Simpson

Assessment of cardiac output is an integral part of the evaluation and management of critically ill patients. Within the limits of this discussion, *cardiac output* can be defined as the interaction between venous return (which describes a function of mean capillary pressure, venous resistance, and right atrial pressure) and cardiac performance (which translates literally as left ventricular function).

The clinician can approximate the patient's cardiac output at the bedside by gauging blood pressure, urine output, and tissue perfusion. This rough estimation, however, cannot be quantified, and though all physicians routinely assess all of these aspects when inspecting a patient, these parameters do not allow precise definition of cardiac output. Currently there are two methods for quantifying central pressure and thus aiding in evaluating cardiac function. They are the central venous pressure (CVP) line and the pulmonary artery catheter (Swan-Ganz line). The Swan-Ganz line unquestionably provides more

information than the CVP line. Nonetheless, it is not without its drawbacks. It has a higher complication rate, is more difficult to place accurately, and requires more sophisticated interpretation. Finally, it is an inappropriate line for placement in the emergency room in the vast majority of cases. Conversion kits are available (Cordis sheath, Arrow, etc.) that contain a guide wire and an appropriate-sized sheath for a Swan-Ganz catheter and allow subclavian of internal jugular lines to be converted to Swan-Ganz lines in a more leisurely setting. For these reasons this section will deal exclusively with the traditional CVP line.

The CVP is measured directly from the tip of any centrally placed catheter. If the catheter has been threaded centrally, the tip lies in the superior vena cava (SVC). Because there is virtually no gradient between the superior vena cava, the right atrium, and the right ventricle, the CVP effectively approximates right ventricular filling pressure. It should be emphasized here and always remembered that the CVP only measures *right-sided* pressures and that no statement about *left-sided function* can reliably be made from CVP measurements.

DECISION TO USE A CENTRAL VENOUS PRESSURE LINE

The decision to use a CVP line must include considerations of both the acute pathologic process and any underlying factors that could affect cardiopulmonary hemodynamics. When cardiac function is normal, the *CVP is reduced* in hypovolemic states such as hemorrhage, vomiting, or diarrhea. *Pressure elevations* are primarily seen in right ventricular failure of any sort (e.g., secondary to pulmonic stenosis; chronic obstructive pulmonary disease (COPD); pulmonary embolism) and in pericardial tamponade and tricuspid regurgitation. The CVP may be normal in patients with acute myocardial infarction and pulmonary edema. In such patients, left ventricular failure may lead to pulmonary edema in the face of normal right ventricular function. An elevation of the CVP in this setting is more indicative of right ventricular failure.

In the emergency room setting, several guidelines for the use of a CVP line should be established. Any young, previously healthy patient brought to the hospital after suffering trauma generally does not require CVP measurement as a part of the initial resuscitation. The important consideration for such a patient is maximal volume infusion until normalization of clinical hemodynamic data is obtained. On the other hand, a patient presenting with cardiovascular collapse in the setting of known cardiovascular disease may benefit from CVP measurements early in the course of resuscitation. Thus, the physician must decide whether there is a reasonable chance of finding an abnormal CVP in any particular patient and, if so, will the patient's management be altered by these findings.

INDICATIONS

- Suspicion of biventricular failure when pulmonary artery monitoring is not available
- Suspicion of cor pulmonale
- Suspicion of cardiac tamponade
- Management of fluid resuscitation in the fragile patient

CONTRAINDICATIONS (relative)

Do not perform this procedure on patients with uncomplicated hypovolemia.

EQUIPMENT

- Central venous line placed either percutaneously or by venesection
- Three-way stopcock
- Water manometer

POSITION

The patient is placed in the bed in a supine position and completely flat. The position of the bed should be recorded.

PROCEDURE

CVP cannot be determined without a catheter in a central position. This can be accomplished as a subclavian or internal jugular line or as a peripheral long line. These lines were described in previous sections.

Preparation

The intravenous solution should be temporarily halted and the three-way stopcock inserted between the intravenous tubing and the catheter. A water manometer tube is then attached to the free arm of the three-way stopcock. After the patient has been comfortably positioned, the exact reference point for the measurement must be located. The following are two methods for doing this:

1. The standard point of reference is designed as a point midway between the anterior and posterior chest walls and this level is marked clearly on the patient's thorax in the axilla with a skin pencil.
2. The standard reference point is determined by "leveling" (with a carpenter's level) the sternal prominence at the second intercostal space (angle of Louis) with the 5-cm mark on the manometer scale (since the right atrium is assumed to be approximately 5 cm posterior to the sternal angle). Alternatively, the manometer can be standardized at zero by placing the level at a point on the lateral thoracic wall 5 cm below the sternal prominence and leveling with zero on the manometer scale.

Although the latter method is used most frequently, the crucial factor is standardization of the technique whenever measurements are performed. The method for determining the point of reference should initially be recorded and this same method should be used throughout the care of a specific patient.

Once the monitoring system has been standardized, the manometer is filled with intravenous fluid by closing the stopcock to the patient and diverting the infusion into the manometer. The stopcock is then turned off to the intravenous bottle (thus establishing continuity between the patient and the manometer tube). The meniscus will slowly fall until it has reached a level reflecting the CVP. The CVP (measured in centimeters of water), the time, the exact position of the bed, and the standard reference point should be recorded.

The criteria for acceptance of the CVP measurement are as follows:

1. Free flow of the intravenous infusion through the CVP line and/or demonstration of the free return of blood through the catheter.
2. Intrathoracic catheter tip position confirmed by film. The catheter should ideally be placed in the SVC.
3. Respiratory variation of meniscus during measurements.

PITFALLS AND COMPLICATIONS

If the stopcock is turned off to the intravenous bottle for long periods of time (more than 15 minutes), the catheter may *clot*. Be sure to return the three-way stopcock to its normal position after measurements are taken. Make sure that the tubing from the manometer to the catheter is as short as possible. The CVP should be measured with *saline or dextrose* to minimize damping due to viscosity. Care should be taken to note any diminution or damping of the meniscus. This represents small clot at the end of the catheter and requires flushing of the catheter to prevent thombosis. *Blood products* should not be routinely run through CVP catheters since they tend to sludge the lumen. Note any *respirator settings* that may tend to obscure the actual reading from the manometer.

ARTERIAL PUNCTURE AND BLOOD GAS DETERMINATION

Reed E. Pyeritz

Blood sampled from an artery provides the most informative and reliable source for measurement of partial pressures of oxygen (PO_2) and carbon dioxide (PCO_2), oxygen saturation, systemic pH, and serum ammonia and lactate concentration. Moreover, in clinical situations, particularly emergencies, in which obtaining blood specimens from a vein is impossible, one of several arteries can usually be punctured and blood withdrawn. Because of the relative importance of the results from determinations made on arterial blood specimens, the influence of patient agitation on some results and on the success of the procedure itself, and the potential complications, the physician or technician must be capable of quickly and atraumatically performing arterial puncture from one of several sites and of handling the sample properly to ensure accurate results.

INDICATIONS

Arterial Puncture

- Determination of arterial blood gases
- Determination of serum ammonia
- Determination of serum lactate

- Obtaining blood specimens for other purposes when a vein cannot be punctured

Blood Gas (PO_2, PCO_2, oxygen saturation, pH) determination

- Newly stuporous or comatose patients
- Ventilatory insufficiency, cyanosis, or focal or diffuse pulmonary disease
- Acid–base disorders
- Cardiac dysrhythmias
- Severe anemia
- Carbon monoxide poisoning or inhalation of other toxins or smoke
- Cardiopulmonary resuscitation

CONTRAINDICATIONS

- Inability to palpate arterial pulsation
- Known or suspected severe arterial occlusive disease of either an atherosclerotic or vasospastic nature
- Positive Allen test (described subsequently)
- Anticoagulation, pathologic or iatrogenic

EQUIPMENT

- 5-ml syringe with a freely movable plunger
- No. 22 2-inch needle
- About 1 ml sterile heparin solution, 100–1,000 units/ml
- Cap for syringe or a rubber stopper
- Skin prep solution
- Dry gauze pad
- Container of crushed ice

SELECTION OF ARTERIAL SITE

The three arteries that we should be comfortable puncturing are the radial just proximal to the wrist, the brachial just proximal to the antecubital fossa, and the femoral just distal to the inguinal ligament. Each site has advantages and risks, and the site chosen should take into account the operator's experience, the clinical situation, and relative contraindications. For example, during cardiopulmonary resuscitation or severe hypotension, the femoral artery affords the largest target and the strongest pulse and should be the preferred site for arterial puncture, even though the risks of arterial bleeding subsequent to the puncture or of atherosclerotic plaque dislodgement are greater than at other sites. If the clinical situation is more stable, however, the radial artery generally is the site affording the best collateral flow, the least pain, and the least risk of occult hemorrhage. If radial artery puncture is contraindicated or is unsuccessful in the nonemergency situation, then brachial artery puncture should be attempted next.

POSITION

For femoral artery puncture, the patient should be supine with the hip in the neutral position. For radial artery puncture, the wrist should be supinated and supported in mild hyperextension, such as over a folded towel. For brachial artery puncture, the elbow should be supinated and supported in full extension.

PROCEDURE

Locate the Arterial Pulse

In elderly patients, the radial artery may be superficial and not well anchored in subcutaneous tissue or may be quite hard, suggesting atherosclerosis.

Perform the Allen Test

If radial artery puncture is planned, the Allen test should be performed (Fig. PR13.1). In this modification of this test, the patency of the anastomotic arches of the hand is assessed. Raise the patient's arm well above heart level, have the raised hand actively or passively clenched, and firmly occlude both the ulnar and radial arteries at the wrist. After about 5 seconds, lower the arm and relax the hand, which should by then appear cadaveric. Release pressure on the ulnar, but not the radial, artery and observe the palm closely for the flush that indicates return of arterial flow. The entire hand should regain color in less than 15 seconds (negative test). A longer delay suggests that perfusion of part of the hand—usually the thumb, index finger, and thenar eminence—depends on radial circulation.

Prepare the Skin

The skin overlying the pulse should be cleansed with an io-dophor solution. Local anesthesia is rarely necessary but may prove useful in particularly anxious patients. They will hyperventilate during instillation of the lidocaine and tend to breathe more near their baseline several minutes later when the arterial puncture is performed, resulting in a more informative P_{CO_2} and pH.

Prepare the Syringe

The heparin solution should be drawn into the syringe, the inside of the entire barrel wetted, and the heparin expelled through the needle to be used for the puncture.

Perform the Arterial Puncture

The syringe should be grasped as if holding a pencil. At the radial and brachial arteries, palpate the pulse just proximal to the intended puncture site with one finger of the other hand. Direct the needle, with the bevel up, under the skin at a 45–60 deg angle, aiming for the palpable pulse (Fig. PR13.2). Slowly advance the needle; the pulsation is often transmitted to the syringe as the needle contacts the artery. On puncturing the artery, the syringe should fill with blood without aspiration. This will not necessarily happen in patients with severe hypotension, although blood should appear spontaneously in the needle hub and appear arterialized unless hypoxemia is also present. Gentle aspiration will then produce the required sample.

Femoral Artery Puncture

The femoral artery should be palpated 2–3 cm distal to the inguinal ligament; the second and third fingers can straddle the artery such that the force of the pulsation is equal in the two fingers. The space between the fingers should thus be centered on the artery and provide a target for the needle puncture. The needle should be advanced slowly, perpendicular to the artery, until the pulsation is transmitted to the syringe. The needle should *not* be advanced completely through the artery, as some physicians recommend, and then pulled back until blood flow begins.

Compress the Site for 5 Minutes

Whenever arterial puncture is attempted, the site should be compressed with dry, sterile gauze, even in those instances when no arterial blood was obtained. Steady pressure should be maintained for 5 minutes or longer if coagulation abnormalities are present.

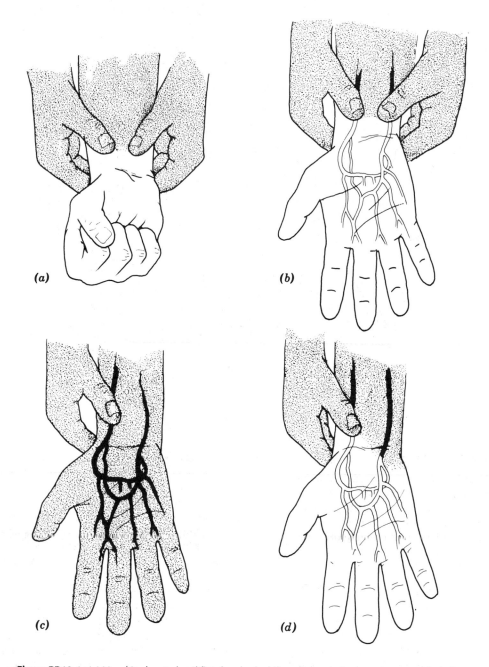

Figure PR13.1 (a) Hand is elevated and fist clenched while radial and ulnar arteries are occluded. (b) Hand is lowered and fist is unclenched. Hand is cadaveric. (c) Ulnar artery compression is released while radial artery compression is continued. The entire hand should regain color in less than 15 seconds. (d) Positive test. In the presence of ulnar artery occlusion, hand remains cadaveric while radial artery compression is maintained.

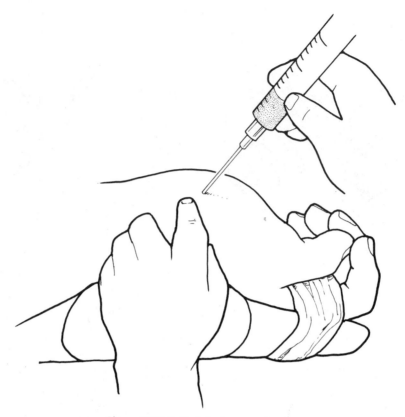

Figure PR13.2 Radial artery puncture.

Handle the Sample Properly

All air bubbles should be immediately expelled and either the syringe should be securely capped or the needle impaled into a rubber stopper. The syringe is first gently rotated to ensure mixing of heparin with the blood and is then placed on ice and transported without delay to the laboratory.

PITFALLS AND COMPLICATIONS

Hemorrhage is usually readily apparent at the radial site; when it is extensive, a pressure palsy of the radial or median nerve can occur. Bleeding from a brachial or particularly a femoral puncture may go unnoticed, even when several hundred milliliters of blood has extravasated into the thigh. This complication can be avoided by using a narrow-gauge needle, conscientiously compressing the artery after puncture, and not repeating punctures at the same site.

Thrombosis must obviously occur in any arterial puncture, but the occurrence of an occlusive thrombus is uncommon in a normal artery. In arteries stenosed by atherosclerosis and possessing noncompliant walls, distal flow may be compromised by even minimal thrombosis. This complication is most common at the radial site. Cyanosis or ischemia developing distal to an arterial puncture must not be taken lightly; vascular surgical consultation should be considered.

Spurious laboratory results most often result from venous admixture in the sample. This is more likely to occur when the sample is aspirated and during femoral puncture—particularly if the needle is first passed completely through the artery—because the femoral vein lies just lateral and often under the artery. Failure to expel bubbles from the specimen will result in measured P_{O_2} and P_{CO_2} that have shifted toward those found in ambient air; at sea level these are a P_{O_2} of 160 mm Hg and a P_{CO_2} of 0 mm Hg. Failure to chill the specimen permits leukocyte oxygen consumption with a reduction in P_{O_2} and erythrocyte glycolysis with production of carbon dioxide.

PROCEDURE 14

PERIPHERAL ARTERIAL CANNULATION

Reed E. Pyeritz

As techniques and equipment have improved, the indications for and the frequency of arterial cannulation in all hospitalized patients have expanded. Many of the current indications, such as angiography, cardiac catheterization, hemodialysis, and drug administration, which require specialized equipment and techniques, are beyond the realm of the emergency room and will not be discussed in this book.

INDICATIONS

- Continual monitoring of arterial pressure in shock (particularly situations requiring intravenous pressor agents), major surgery, and administration of parenteral hypotensive drugs
- Determination of cardiac output by the dye-dilution method
- Need for repeated sampling of arterial blood

Any patient who requires five or more arterial punctures per day is a candidate for an arterial cannula. Factors that influence the decision to place a catheter include the suitability of peripheral arterial sites, the technical competence of the operator, the ability or willingness of the patient to tolerate repeated arterial punctures, and the presence of the contraindications discussed below. By using an arterial cannula, the decrease in Pco_2 that often occurs secondary to hyperventilation at the time of arterial puncture is avoided; moreover, blood gases can be accurately determined during sleep or excerise.

CONTRAINDICATIONS

Absolute

- Cannulation of an artery that is the sole source of perfusion to any distal site
- Positive Allen test

Relative

- Severe atherosclerosis
- Vasospastic arterial disease
- Hypercoagulable states
- Anticoagulation, pathologic or iatrogenic

SITES FOR PERIPHERAL ARTERIAL CANNULATION

- Radial artery at the wrist
- Dorsalis pedis artery
- Brachial artery
- Femoral artery—only for emergency, short-term monitoring of pressure when other sites unacceptable

Short catheters (4–15 cm) placed in a peripheral artery are satisfactory for most blood sampling and pressure-monitoring functions. Occasionally, the blood pressure and pulse tracing obtained from a peripheral arterial cannula will differ significantly from the more meaningful situation in the central arterial system. This most often occurs in patients with hypotension accompanied by severe vasoconstriction, in patients whose arteries are rendered noncompliant by atherosclerosis, and in patients in hyperdynamic circulatory states. In these situations, a catheter that passes into the intrathoracic aorta or subclavian artery is indicated (this subject is not discussed here).

The distal *radial artery* is the most frequently cannulated site because of its superficial location, which enables percutaneous insertion in many instances, and the usually excellent collateral circulation about the wrist.

The *dorsalis pedis artery* shares characteristics with the radial artery that make it an acceptable second choice for percutaneous or cutdown cannulation.

The *brachial artery* just proximal to the cubital fossa should be avoided if at all possible. The artery lies deeper than either the radial or dorsalis pedis, is closely surrounded by major tendons, veins, and nerves, requires a cutdown approach, and has been proven to have a substantially higher rate of complication.

Because the *femoral artery* just distal to the inguinal ligament is the largest peripheral artery in the body, it is relatively easy to cannulate percutaneously, even in clinical situations in which the pulse is barely palpable or absent. The complications associated with the femoral site are considerable, limiting its use to emergencies in which other peripheral sites are unsuitable.

EQUIPMENT

- Sterile gloves
- Sterile drapes
- Short arm board
- Gauze roll, about 3-inch diameter
- Six 4 × 4-inch gauze sponges
- Iodophor skin preparation solution
- 1% lidocaine, about 5 ml
- No. 25 needle
- Two 2-0 silk ties or ¼-inch umbilical tape
- No. 15 scalpel blade and handle
- Toothed and plain forceps, one each
- Two curved mosquito snaps
- Iris scissors
- Catheter-over-needle unit, No. 16, 18, or 20 (e.g., Angio-cath, Argyle Medicut, Quick Cath, or Longdwell), 5–8 cm long
- Pressure transducer tubing, 4–6 inches long
- 5-ml syringe
- Heparinized saline, 100 units/ml, about 10 ml
- Three-way metal stopcock
- Tincture of benzoin
- Antiseptic ointment

Attach the stopcock to one end of the transducer tubing and the syringe containing heparinized saline to the sampling port of the stopcock; completely fill the tubing with the solution.

PROCEDURE

Approach to Radial Artery

POSITION THE WRIST

If the patient's nondominant arm passes scrutiny by the Allen test (described under arterial puncture), it is positioned with a gauze roll under the supinated extended wrist, tape over the proximal interphalangeal joints excluding the thumb, and tape over the forearm in a nonconstricting fashion (Fig. PR14.1). The arm board is secured to the stretcher or bed with tape to prevent motion at an inconvenient time.

PREPARE THE SKIN

The iodophor is applied to the entire flexor forearm and wrist three times and allowed to dry after each application. The site is then draped to expose just the region over the radial pulse.

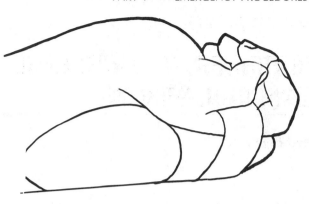

Figure PR14.1 Position for radial artery cannulation.

ANESTHETIZE

Using a No. 25 needle, 1% lidocaine without epinephrine is infiltrated intradermally directly over the pulse about 3–4 cm proximal to the styloid process of the radius. Extend the skin wheal along the axis of the artery for 1–2 cm. Carry the infiltration deeper along the lateral (radial) side of the pulse, through the volar fascia, nearly to the periosteum. Take care not to administer anesthetic into the artery or so much as to obliterate the pulse. The site is thus prepared for either percutaneous cannulation or cutdown; if the percutaneous approach proves unsuccessful, a cutdown can be immediately begun without waste of time or equipment.

Percutaneous Cannulation

INCISE THE SKIN

Make a 1–2-mm incision over the pulse to prevent fraying the catheter tip.

INTRODUCE THE CATHETER

Hold the catheter unit by the needle hub at a 60 deg angle to the skin (Fig. PR14.2). While palpating the pulse, advance the unit completely through the artery. Advance the catheter along the needle 3–5 mm to ensure that the end of the catheter is also through the posterior arterial wall (Fig. PR14.3a). While stabilizing the catheter, remove the needle and set it aside on the sterile field.

CANNULATE THE ARTERY

Depress the hub of the catheter flat against the wrist and slowly withdraw. Appearance of blood *pulsating* from the hub indi-

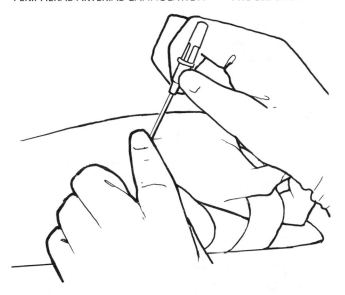

Figure PR14.2 Position for radial arterial cannulation.

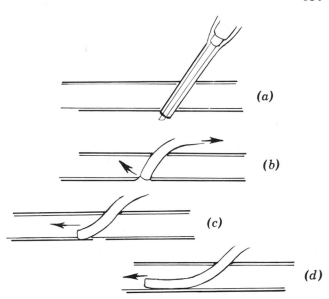

Figure PR14.3 (a) Transfix artery; (b) withdraw gently until there is flashback of blood; (c) depress end of catheter, withdraw slightly, then advance gently; (d) advance.

cates that the tip is within the arterial lumen and is the signal to advance the catheter (Fig. PR14.3b,c,d). If flow stops while advancing, the catheter should again be withdrawn until pulsatile blood flow appears and then 1–2 mm further before readvancing. If no blood appears at all while the catheter is withdrawn to the skin, the artery was not punctured. Remove the catheter entirely, reinsert the needle, and repeat the procedure. To avoid damage to the arterial wall, the number of unsuccessful attempts at percutaneous puncture should be limited to three or four before performing a cutdown.

ATTACH THE TUBING

Attach the transducer tubing through the Luer Lok to the catheter hub (Fig. PR14.4). The stopcock should be attached to the other end of the tubing and a syringe containing the heparinized saline attached to the stopcock. First, aspirate the catheter to ensure ready blood flow and to remove any air bubbles; then, *slowly* flush the tubing and catheter and close the stopcock.

SECURE THE CATHETER

Pass a 4-0 suture through the skin just beside the catheter hub and secure it. Then tie the suture around the hub or through suture holes, if present. Swab the surrounding skin with tincture of benzoin and place a dab of antiseptic ointment over the

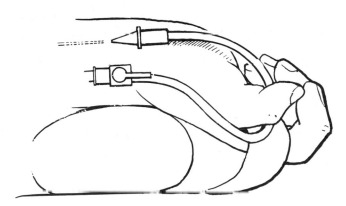

Figure PR14.4 Attach to catheter and fix in position.

catheter insertion. Securely tape the proximal tubing to the wrist and tape the distal tubing and the stopcock to the arm board.

FLUSH THE CATHETER

Studies have shown the ease with which retrograde embolization from radial artery cannulae can occur because of vigorous flushing. All that is required to maintain catheter patency is 2–5 ml of heparinized saline per hour infused continuously by pump.

Cutdown Approach

When attempts at percutaneous cannulation fail or when a patient is so poorly perfused that a pulse cannot be felt, a cutdown to expose the artery is required. Positioning and preparation is the same as described directly above.

MAKE THE INCISION

Make the incision along the course of the artery a distance of 1.5–2 cm. This coincides with the direction of travel of most wrist structures and reduces the chance of injuring them.

BLUNTLY DISSECT TO THE ARTERY

Once the volar fascia is incised, use the curved snap to dissect bluntly down to the artery, which should appear whitish and pulsatile.

ISOLATE THE ARTERY

Pass a curved snap under the artery; gently dissect the radial nerve (usually lies medial), the venae communicans, and all extraneous tissue away from the artery. Pass two pieces of 2-0 silk or umbilical tape under the artery and manipulate one to the proximal extent and the other to the distal extent of the incision (Fig. PR14.5).

CANNULATE THE ARTERY

While exerting gentle traction on the distal tie, puncture the artery with the catheter-over-needle unit and advance fully into the lumen (Fig. PR14.6). Pulsatile blood flow signals success. The needle can be withdrawn and the catheter advanced fully into the lumen.

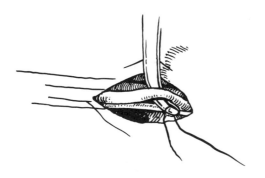

Figure PR14.5 Isolate artery.

CONNECT THE TUBING

Proceed as described above to attach the transducer tubing and flush the cannula.

CLOSE THE SKIN INCISION

Usually two 4-0 silk sutures are all that are necessary to close the incision around the catheter hub. If bleeding from the hole in the artery does not stop after several minutes of compression, the first and most proximal skin suture should be passed *deep* to the artery and tied snugly by completing a vertical mattress stitch. The most distal suture, once tied, can then be tied around the catheter hub. Dress the incision and securely tape the transducer tubing and stopcock to the arm board.

Approach to the Dorsalis Pedis Artery

The techniques for percutaneous and cutdown cannulation of the dorsalis pedis artery are parallel with those described above for the radial artery.

Approach to the Brachial Artery

The brachial artery should only be cannulated after isolation of the artery by means of cutdown. The technique is similar to the cutdown approach to the radial artery with the exception that the skin incision should be made parallel to the flexion creases in the cubital fossa.

Approach to the Femoral Artery

By using the principles described for percutaneous radial artery cannulation and a long (6-inch) catheter-over-needle unit, the femoral artery can be easily cannulated by puncturing the artery directly under the pulse. During the time that the cannula remains in place, which should in any event be short, the patient's hip must be maintained in the neutral position.

A preferable alternative technique involves using a Seldinger needle, guide wire, and introducer, but such equipment is seldom available when emergency cannulation is needed.

PITFALLS AND COMPLICATIONS

Hemorrhage results from accidental disconnection of the cannula or tubing; rarely from the arterial puncture site while the cannula is in place; and frequently, though usually to a minor

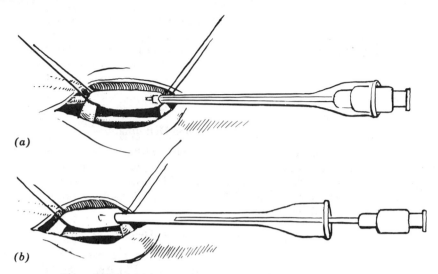

Figure PR14.6 (a) Insert catheter- over -needle; (b) withdraw needle.

degree, when the cannula is removed. Because dislodgment or disconnection of the cannula risks exsanguination, the patient should never be unattended and great care should be used in securing the catheter to the skin.

Any arterial cannulation causes intimal injury and subsequent scarring, both of which serve as a nidus for *thrombosis*. At the radial site, loss of pulse and decrease in blood flow are common occurrences immediately after catheter removal, and they increase in frequency the longer the artery is cannulated. Most occlusions recannalize to some degree, but this process may take months. If at any time after insertion of a radial cannula some part of the hand becomes ischemic, the cannula must be removed. Any serious thrombotic episode should be managed vigorously with anticoagulation and vascular surgical consultation.

Retrograde embolization to the cerebral circulation as a result of a vigorous flush of a radial or brachial cannula is an underappreciated risk about which the nursing staff must be educated. If a pressure tracing becomes damped or if blood cannot be withdrawn, a gentle flush of 1–2 ml should be attempted. If this is unsuccessful, the cannula should be removed. Antegrade embolization to the end arteries of the fingers is an indication for systemic anticoagulation and cannula removal.

Infection should be extremely uncommon but may involve the soft tissues at a cutdown site and would usually be because of gram-positive bacteria.

PROCEDURE 15

DEFIBRILLATION

William Strauss

The last three decades have produced an explosive development and growth of the disciplines of critical care and emergency medicine. The institution of basic cardiac life support—cardiopulmonary resuscitation (CPR)—and electrical defibrillation has been central to the successful therapy for the most critically ill patient, the cardiac arrest victim. While the former made it possible to sustain life, the development of alternating current (AC) defibrillators followed by direct current (DC) devices permitted definitive therapy for the most common fatal cardiac rhythm disorder.

The impetus for the development of electrical defibrillation stems from the fact that cardiovascular disease, which is related primarily to ischemic coronary heart disease, is the leading cause of death in the United States. Approximately 60% of these deaths occur suddenly—most occur before the patient reaches the hospital. Of these, 60–70% are due to ventricular fibrillation; thus, defibrillation provides a potentially life-saving mechanism for many thousands of sudden death victims. Despite the apparent simplicity of this technique, certain factors can improve or reduce the likelihood of success.

INDICATIONS

The exclusive indication for defibrillation is ventricular fibrillation (VF). The techniques and equipment for defibrillation may also be used for the electrical conversion of supraventricular tachyarrhythmias and ventricular tachycardia, the only difference being synchronization to the QRS complex. Elective synchronized cardioversion will not be specifically discussed further.

EQUIPMENT

All current *defibrillators* are DC devices that have replaced the heavier, less portable AC units. An adjustable high-voltage DC power supply charges a capacitor that delivers a brief (4–12 msec) monophasic charge to a pair of paddles. The only other required equipment is a *paste* or other material to reduce the electrical resistance of the skin (see below).

PROCEDURE

The procedure for defibrillation, as discussed below, is relatively standard and simple: Turn defibrillator on, set desired charge, place paddles, and discharge. The basic set up of all defibrillators is the same, but each is organized slightly differently. The physician should become familiar with the commonly available units.

Initiate Basic Life Support

If, in a monitored situation, fibrillation is observed to occur while a defibrillator is at hand, defibrillation should be performed at once before initiation of basic life support (BLS). If this is not the case, BLS must be instituted and continued in optimal fashion until the defibrillator arrives.

Turn on Power and Establish Rhythm

Almost all current devices integrate a monitor with the defibrillator, which allows rapid diagnosis of cardiac rhythm. Monitor and defibrillator on/off switches may be combined or sep-

arate. Most monitor–defibrillator units are able to monitor the electrocardiogram (ECG) by means of either patient leads or paddle electrodes—so called "quick-look paddles." If the latter are used, conductive gel or paste must be applied initially. Use of patient cables provides the advantage of continuous monitoring.

Blind Defibrillation

Time is of the essence! If the defibrillator at hand does not contain a monitor, a cardiac arrest victim should receive an immediate DC shock as soon as a defibrillator is available without ECG confirmation of ventricular fibrillation.

Turn on Defibrillator Power

Once again, this may be a separate control from the monitor on/off switch. Ensure that the unit is not in the synchronous mode used for cardioversion.

Apply Conductive Material

Saline-soaked pads or an appropriate paste should be applied to minimize burns to the patient's skin and to reduce the skin's electrical resistance. Certain materials, for example, Redux paste, have been found to be effective in lowering resistance. Other materials, such as ultrasonic gel, should not be used.

Select Energy Level and Charge the Capacitor

Most defibrillators have a dial to set the desired energy level. Early units measured the level as *stored*; however, it has been determined that the actual output of units indicating 400 J stored ranged from 155 J to 340 J. Most current devices now indicate actual *energy delivered* and have consistent outputs of 320–400 J.

While a controversy exists as to initial energy levels (see below), current American Heart Association recommendations are to attempt defibrillation with an initial setting of 200–300 J delivered energy; a second attempt at the same energy level should be made if the first is unsuccessful.

Apply Paddles to the Chest, Clear the Area, and Deliver Countershock

The overwhelming clinical practice today is to use *anterior or anterior–apical paddle placement*. The anterior paddle is placed just beneath the right clavicle along the right sternal edge (Fig. PR15.1). (This paddle has erroneously been labeled by some manufacturers as the "sternal" paddle. The electrical resistance of bone is high, and effectively delivered energy will be reduced if the paddle is actually placed over the sternum.) The second electrode is placed over the apex of the heart, that is, at the anterior axillary line.

The second pattern of paddle placement is *anterior–posterior* (AP) with one paddle over the precordium and the other in back under the left scapula. The AP approach, which was once used for emergency as well as elective procedures, has largely been abandoned because of the ease of application of the anterior placement. However, some studies have demonstrated improved success at lower energy levels for ventricular defi-

brillation with the AP approach, presumably because of more efficient current flow.

Whichever placement is chosen, the paddles should be placed on the chest with a slight twisting motion to distribute the electrode paste evenly. Rechecking the monitor confirms the continued presence of VF. The operator clears the area and *ensures that no personnel are in contact with the patient.* Firm pressure is applied to the paddles and the unit is discharged. Discharge buttons may be on both paddles requiring simultaneous depression, on a single paddle, or on the defibrillator itself. Evidence of effective discharge of the unit is manifested by skeletal muscle contraction.

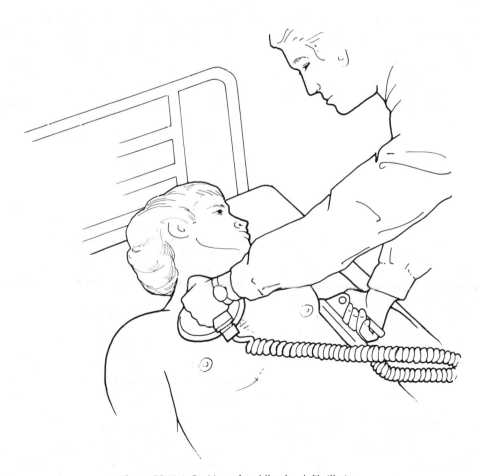

Figure PR15.1 Position of paddles for defibrillation.

Reassess Rhythm and Effective Circulation

Check the monitor for rhythm. If VF persists, repeat the above procedure immediately. If an organized rhythm is present, check for the presence of a pulse. If no pulse is present, resume CPR.

PITFALLS AND COMPLICATIONS

Several factors affect the likelihood for successful defibrillation. Some, such as underlying disease status, are not modifiable. In other cases, the potential for success can be changed. Many of these factors have a reverse side as well: The potential for electrically induced myocardial tissue damage increases as larger and repetitive shocks are applied.

Electrocardiographic Misdiagnosis

At times, low-amplitude or fine VF has been diagnosed as asystole and treated pharmacologically without attempt at defibrillation. Additionally, it has been demonstrated that VF may occasionally appear to be asystole if only a single ECG lead is monitored. To minimize this situation, varying ECG leads should be viewed if a multiple-lead ECG machine is available. In the case of quick look paddle electrodes, it is hoped that shifting the paddle position will afford a look at a different electrical vector.

Interval from Onset of Arrhythmia to Defibrillation

Several investigators have suggested the critical importance of duration of the rhythm disturbance to application of definitive therapy. The longer VF persists, the less likely defibrillation will be successful; however, it should be emphasized that the many cases of success after a more prolonged delay mandate an attempt at electrical defibrillation whenever the defibrillator becomes available. The need for rapid delivery of definitive therapy prompted some physicians in the early 1970s to recommend blind defibrillation of cardiac arrest victims if ECG confirmations of VF were not available.

Underlying Disease and Type of Ventricular Fibrillation

The underlying status of the patient has been found to be critically important to the success of defibrillation. Ischemic heart disease patients, either with acute myocardial infarctions and VF or with out-of-hospital primary VF in the absence of myocardial infarction, have a high likelihood for success. In contrast, patients fibrillating in the setting of profound left ventricular failure or major noncardiac organ system derangements have a much poorer defibrillation rate.

Obviously, we cannot modify the actual disease state of any patient to be treated; however, such considerations should be kept in mind when analyzing studies reporting adequacy or inadequacy of an aspect of the defibrillation technique. Such an example may be the reported reduced ability to defibrillate very obese patients. The suggestion has been made that this is secondary to the difficulty in providing adequate CPR rather than insufficient energy doses.

Current Density and Transthoracic Resistance

The final group of factors that can affect success involves the interrelationship between delivered energy and the tissue's resistance to electrical flow.

The energy delivered by a defibrillator is a factor of power (watts) applied for a duration (seconds) and is expressed as watt-seconds or joules. The electrical discharge is measured in both voltage (potential) and current flow (amperes);

$$\text{potential drop} \times \text{amperes} = \text{watts}.$$

It has become apparent that it is the current density or flow that defibrillates the heart rather than simply the energy delivered. Thus, the standard electrical equation,

$$\text{resistance (ohms)} = \frac{\text{potential}}{\text{current}},$$

assumes great importance.

The current flow for any given energy setting is dependent on the amount of resistance encountered. An arbitrary resistance of 50 Ω is used to test defibrillators, but studies have documented that the transthoracic resistance (TTR) can range up to several times greater than this. Certain factors may modify this with resultant increase or decrease in effective current flow.

PADDLE SIZE AND LOCATION

Although the current standard paddle is 8–9 cm in diameter, there is accumulating evidence that use of one or both paddles that are 13 cm will significantly reduce TTR. Similarly, studies of VF as well as of electrical conversion of atrial fibrillation suggest a lower TTR when the AP placement is used.

SKIN-PADDLE INTERFACE

The skin can provide a very high electrical resistance if the electrodes are bare or if inappropriate conductive material is used. Laboratory evaluation of such materials has been conducted, and recommendations for H-P redux paste, G.E. gel, Cor-gel, and American Writer have resulted. Commercially available defibrillator electrode pads and saline soaked four-by-fours are also appropriate.

PHASE OF VENTILATION

Recent animal studies have documented an increased TTR and significantly lower success rate of defibrillation when the discharges were delivered during inspiration as opposed to expiration.

PADDLE CONTACT PRESSURE

Similarly, animal studies have documented as much as 30% decrease in TTR when firm pressure is applied. This may be related in part to decreasing lung volume with firm pressure.

RECOMMENDED ENERGY LEVELS

For several years, a major controversy has raged as to the appropriate energy requirements for adults—especially those weighing more than 100 kg. An extensive discussion is beyond the limits of this section, but a brief review may be useful.

Retrospective analyses of defibrillation success and animal studies suggested an inverse relationship between body weight and successful defibrillation. The concern was raised that available defibrillators were not powerful enough to defibrillate large adults. Subsequent studies were unable to document a correlation between successful defibrillation and body weight. Some groups were able to demonstrate high percentages of successful defibrillation—up to 95%—using energy doses of less than 200 J, irrespective of body weight. Additionally disturbing was work that suggested a reduced effectiveness when higher energy levels were used (see below, "Complications").

These studies suggest that a reasonable approach would be an initial attempt at 200 J delivered. If this is unsuccessful the same energy level should be repeated because of the reduction of TTR, albeit small, that can occur with repeated shocks. If still unsuccessful, epinephrine and sodium bicarbonate should be administered while effective BLS continues. After an interval appropriate to allow for circulation of the above medications, a shock with 340–360 J (delivered) should be administered.

Complications

The gravest complication associated with defibrillation is inability to defibrillate. As described above, certain procedures should be followed to optimize the chances for success. However, intimately associated with this is the risk of myocardial tissue damage if repeated shocks are necessary or if higher than required energy levels are used.

MYOCARDIAL TISSUE DAMAGE

Electrocardiogram ST changes, elevated cardiac isoenzymes, and abnormal technetium pyrophosphate scans have been reported in animal studies of defibrillation, as well as in clinical series. Additional investigations have revealed pathologic changes and reduction in indices of left ventricular performance. Each of these abnormalities appeared to have an increased incidence as the number of shocks and dose of energy used was increased. However, none of the findings is specific for damage secondary to electrical injury. In a retrospective analysis of patients, it was suggested that there was an increased rate of failure to defibrillate at energy levels greater than 3 J/kg or 240 J total. Potentially, these findings may simply reflect the application of maximum available energy at the unsuccessful conclusion of arrests; nonetheless, the potential for postchock arrhythmias at high energy levels is real. Using chick embryo myocardial cell sheets, it has been reported that immediate postshock arrhythmias occurred increasingly as administered energy was increased, suggesting that the reduced rate of successful defibrillation at higher energies may be related to secondary arrhythmias produced by the shock.

PERMANENT PACEMAKER DAMAGE

With the ever-increasing prevalence of permanent pacemakers (PPM) in our population, reports of pacemakers destroyed by the high-density current flows attendant to defibrillation are not surprising. Although this problem is not entirely surmountable, use of the AP paddle placement or at least positioning the anterior paddle as near to the right sternal border as possible may reduce the current flow across the pacemaker. All patients with PPM who are defibrillated should have evaluation of the pacemaker function after stabilization.

SUGGESTED READINGS

Adgey et al: Ventricular defibrillation: Appropriate energy levels. *Circulation* 1979; 60:219.

Crampton R: Accepted, controversial, and speculative aspects of ventricular defibrillation. *Prog Cardiovasc Dis* 1980; 23:167.

Gascho JA et al: Determinants of ventricular defibrillation in man. *Circulation* 1979; 60:231.

Tacker WA, Ewy GA: Emergency defibrillation dose: Recommendations and rationale. *Circulation* 1979; 60:223.

PROCEDURE 16

INSERTION OF PACEMAKERS

William Strauss

Electrical stimulation of the heart has been used since it was first introduced by Zoll in 1952 to provide artificial stimulation to the atria or ventricles with resultant depolarization. Over the years, this technique has gained wide acceptance as treatment of bradyarrhythmias. It can be used prophylactically for patients who are in certain acute myocardial infarction states and as acute overdrive suppressive therapy for patients with several tachyarrhythmias.

In the emergency room or other similar settings, cardiac pacing is reserved for the treatment of marked bradycardic states that are resistant to pharmocologic therapy and are associated with hemodynamic compromise. The subsequent discussion will focus on such situations and the techniques for emergency pacemaker insertion. Although an occasional emergency room has fluoroscopy immediately available, the techniques described here will deal exclusively with insertion without the assistance of fluoroscopy.

INDICATIONS

Many situations require the semiemergent introduction of a pacemaker system: high-degree atrioventricular block or intraventricular block in the face of an acute myocardial infarction, Stokes-Adams attacks secondary to bradyarrhythmia or heart block, symptomatic sick sinus or tachycardia–bradycardia syndrome, and supraventricular tachycardias. Our discussion will emphasize the treatment of profound bradycardia, heart block, or asystole—conditions most flagrantly displayed by the patient in cardiac arrest.

Although there is often a very fine dividing line between the different situations, generally the semielective case will permit transfer to a radiology suite for fluoroscopically guided insertion. The need for pacemaker therapy as well as the urgency will obviously reflect on the type of rhythm disturbance, hemodynamic status, and, finally, the response to drugs.

The success of this technique will depend greatly on the situation in which it is attempted: The response to institution of artificial pacing of bradycardia or heart block associated with hypoperfusion or hypotension can yield dramatic restoration of cardiac output. On the other hand, when a pacemaker is tried as a last resort in the situation of asystole, the results can be abysmal. Experiences with a series of patients undergoing cardiopulmonary resuscitation (CPR) and refractory to the usual physical and pharmacologic interventions have been reported. Seventy-seven percent of bradycardiac patients were able to be captured and paced. In contrast, only 31% of patients with asystole were able to be paced, but the pacemaker-induced complex was not associated with a palpable pulse in any of the patients and no patient survived.

CONTRAINDICATIONS

There are essentially no contraindications to the institution of pacemaker therapy, although each of the methods of electrode insertion has the potential for complications.

EQUIPMENT

The pacemaker system is comprised of a generator and an electrode system. Additionally an electrocardiogram (ECG) machine is needed to confirm electrode location and ventricular capture.

Generator

External generator boxes are made by several companies; all basically share the following features.

ON/OFF SWITCH

Many units have a mechanism, such as depressing a lock button, to prevent the generator from being inadvertently turned off.

ADJUSTABLE OUTPUT

The adjustable output switch, which is measured in milliamperes, permits the power output to be varied, generally over a range from a fraction of a milliampere to 20–25 mA. Additionally, this setting can be adjusted to assess the power threshold necessary for capture at the time of insertion and subsequently to ensure the adequacy of the system.

VARIABLE RATE

The variable rate control permits adjustment of the pacing stimulus firing rate. Ventricular pacemakers have rate capabilities as low as 35 or as high as 180/min. Atrial generators used to treat atrial tachyarrhythmias have the capacity to pace at 500 and even 800/min. Such units should never be used for ventricular pacing.

VARIABLE SENSITIVITY

Adjusting this control varies the pacemaker from a fully asynchronous mode to full demand function. In the asynchronous or fixed-rate setting, the pacemaker will continue to fire despite any native QRS complexes. This may create competition between the pacemaker and the patient's underlying rhythm. Although this may be tolerated in many patients, it can reduce cardiac output as would any premature beat, such as a premature ventricular contraction (PVC). Even more worrisome is the potential for an electrical impulse landing on the portion of the T wave (repolarization) that represents the supernormal phase of excitability. In patients with myocardial ischemia, this can induce ventricular fibrillation (VF).

When the pacemaker is set on the demand mode, intrinsic complexes are sensed by the pacemaker and an internal circuit inhibits the pacemaker from firing. If, on the other hand, an interval of time passes without a native beat dependent on the rate set, the pacemaker fires stimulating the ventricle. The ability to vary the sensing threshold permits the assessment of electrode function and placement. It also provides a means of compensating for electrical interference or artifact.

PACING/SENSING INDICATORS

Many units have lights or needle indicators that signal each time the pacer senses a QRS as well as each time it fires.

Pacing Electrodes

All pacemaker systems require a closed electrical circuit. This may be accomplished by a bipolar system in which both the positive and negative leads are on the end of the catheter and are separated by a small distance, for example, 1 cm. Most transvenous pacing wires are bipolar. Unipolar catheters use a single electrode at the tip of the catheter in contact with the heart; the other electrode is a subcutaneous ground.

There is little difference between the two systems; however, a unipolar system is more sensitive in its ability to sense intrinsic complexes and is more able to pace when the power threshold is high. A bipolar system that is functioning inadequately can be converted to a unipolar system by disconnecting the proximal electrode from the generator and attaching it with alligator clips to either a metal suture needle through the skin or frequently a disposable ECG electrode.

Several catheters are available for temporary pacing. The choice of an electrode is dependent on the site chosen for vascular access and the method of blind insertion.

BALLOON-TIPPED FLOATING CATHETERS

Ballon-tipped floating catheters are 3F and 5F flexible catheters that have bipolar electrodes separated by a balloon. The 3F catheter is used for internal jugular, subclavian, and brachial veins, whereas the 5F catheter is preferred for femoral vein insertion. After the vein is entered, the distal lead is attached to an ECG, the balloon is inflated, and the catheter is advanced until an intraventricular ECG is obtained. At this point, the balloon is deflated and the catheter is advanced until a "current of injury" pattern is seen. (See below, "Procedure.")

Since its introduction a decade ago, this flow-directed catheter has become a popular choice for semielective procedures because of the rapidity and ease of proper positioning. It also has been found to be effective in emergency situations. The balloon-tipped system was compared against fluoroscopically guided semirigid catheters (see below) in both semielective and emergency situations. The balloon-tipped system took significantly less time and was associated with less ventricular arrhythmias at time of insertion. The superiority of the balloon-tipped system was apparent even for the emergency insertions—cases of high degree or complete heart block as well as frank cardiac arrest. Many feel the balloon-tipped system is the safest and quickest catheter and requires the least experience to master.

SEMIFLEXIBLE CATHETER

Semiflexible catheters are relatively flexible and have a slightly curved hockey-stick shaped distal end. They are most successfully advanced blindly from the left subclavian or right internal jugular vein. The left median basilic may also be used, but there is somewhat less likelihood for success. Which vein is chosen is dependent on the skill and experience of the person performing the procedure.

RIGID PACING CATHETERS

The fairly rigid 6F or 7F catheters are typically introduced under fluoroscopic guidance. They may be introduced from the femoral veins blindly if other catheters are unavailable or unable to be passed secondary to lack of blood flow during cardiac arrest.

TRANSTHORACIC PACING STYLET

The transthoracic pacing stylet unit consists of a stainless steel wire that is introduced through a needle into the left or right ventricle. The distal end is bent back upon itself in the shape of a "V" or "J" so that as the needle is withdrawn, the catheter tip remains in contact with the endocardium. The other lead (anode) may be either located more proximally on the wire, maintaining contact with the chest wall, or a separate lead attached to the subcutaneous tissue as with any unipolar system.

Because its insertion does not require blood flow, this electrode is easily inserted during a cardiac arrest. However, since its introduction nearly 20 years ago, it has frequently been used as a last measure during cardiac arrests with the expected dismal success rate. Its use should be reserved for those most urgent cases where time does not permit transvenous placement.

PROCEDURE

The basic procedure for pacemaker insertion is the same for all catheter systems: enter the vein, advance the catheter into contact with ventricular endocardium, and adjust the rate and threshold settings. Specific modifications for the catheter electrode chosen are discussed below.

Skin Preparation

Cleanse the insertion site with povidone-iodine solution. Even in full arrest situations, at least a modicum of attention to aseptic technique should be followed. Drape a wide area around the insertion site with sterile towels.

Entering the Vein

Multiple sites are available, each with advantages and disadvantages. The right internal jugular can be easily entered and provides a direct and quick route into the right ventricle (RV). After insertion the catheter position remains fixed, providing stable pacing. Either subclavian vein can be used for balloon-tipped catheter placements. The semiflexible catheter can be more easily placed blindly through the left subclavian. Although the femoral vein is most commonly used for fluoroscopically guided rigid pacing catheters, such catheters can be at times blindly advanced from this route. The larger (5F) balloon-tipped catheter can be introduced through the femoral vein, although with difficulty in low-flow states. Finally, the antecubital (median basilic) veins can be used to introduce balloon-directed catheters. The blind insertion of semiflexible catheters is generally only possible from the left arm. This site has the disadvantage that movement of the arm by the patient will likely change the location of the electrode tip.

Advancing the Tip

Advance catheter with electrocardiographic monitoring of tip location.

With the exception of the transthoracic technique, blind pacemaker insertion is guided by means of the ECG. The limb leads of a properly grounded ECG machine are attached, and the "V" lead is connected by an alligator clip to the distal electrode of the pacing catheter. The V lead is monitored as the catheter is advanced; the balloon is inflated if this system is being used.

The pattern seen from the superior vena cava (SVC) resembles that of lead aV_R on a 12-lead cardiogram: negative P waves and QRS complexes. As the right atrium (RA) is entered, the P waves become much larger, gradually becoming upright as the electrode advances from high to low RA. As the tricuspid valve is crossed, large intercavitary QRS complexes are seen. As the catheter is further advanced (with balloon deflated), marked elevation of the ST segment (current of injury pattern) will be seen. This should be the proper position for ventricular pacing. If the QRS size is seen to be diminished, the catheter has probably passed into the pulmonary artery.

The technique for insertions of the transthoracic pacing stylet is somewhat different. The intracardiac needle should be inserted at the apex of the triangle formed by the xiphoid and left costal margin (Fig. PR16.1). The needle is directed cephalad, slightly to the left of midline and at a 20–30 deg angle to the skin. Once the needle is fully inserted, the inner obturator is removed and a syringe is attached. Aspiration of blood indicates intraventricular position. If there is no blood return, gradually withdraw the needle, aspirating continually, until blood is free flowing. At that point, introduce the pacing stylet into the needle. Remove the needle while fixating the stylet position. Attach the electrode adapter to the stylet and connect it to the generator. If capture of the ventricle is not present, gently manipulate the stylet until successful capture is seen.

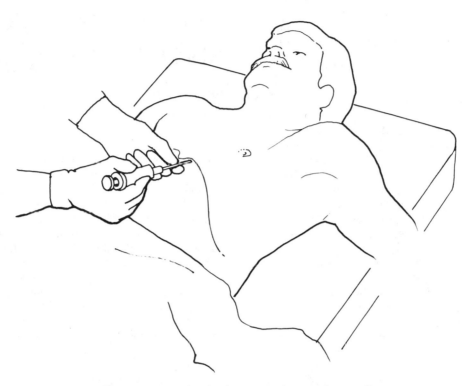

Figure PR16.1 Subxiphoid insertion of intracardiac needle.

Adjustment of Threshold and Rate Setting

Contact with the endocardium will be manifested by ventricular capture by the pacemaker. The rate initially should be set well above the intrinsic rate (e.g., 20 beats/min) to minimize competition. The power output should gradually be diminished until evidence of loss of capture is seen on the surface ECG. This represents the pacing threshold and should be less than 1 mA. If not, the electrode location is not ideal and should be changed. The need for such a change is relative, of course, and repositioning should be performed only when the patient is stabilized. After determining the pacing threshold, the output should be set at two to three times the threshold, generally 3–3.5 mA. The pacer should be set on synchronous or demand mode.

If an intrinsic rhythm is present, the sensing threshold should also be tested. After reducing the pacer rate to slightly less than the intrinsic rate, the demand–asynchronous dial should be gradually turned from demand toward fixed rate. The level of sensing threshold should be recorded and tested daily along with pacing threshold.

Finally, the final rate setting is made. This is dependent on the underlying rhythm and desired output. Optimal cardiac output is generally achieved at a rate of 70–90 beats/min.

Confirming Position

A chest film must be obtained to ensure proper electrode position—just to the left of the spine on the posterior–anterior (PA) film and pointing anteriorly on the lateral. Also, pneumothorax must be ruled out if a subclavian or internal jugular approach was used.

PITFALLS AND COMPLICATIONS

Many of the complications associated with pacemaker insertion are related to the technique of venous access and the presence of any catheter in a blood vessel, for example, sepsis and pneumothorax. Such complications can be minimized by using the optimal technique at the time of insertion and by being vigilant throughout the use of the pacemaker.

Use of the transthoracic system carries with it the potential for laceration of a coronary artery, cardiac tamponade, and pneumothorax.

Additional problems are related to the pacemaker systems themselves. Perforation of the RA or RV may occur with use of the stiffer catheters. It may be detected by loss of ventricular capture, intercostal or diaphragmatic stimulation, and occasionally a pericardial friction rub. Changes in the ECG from the typical LBBB pattern or posterior direction of the catheter on lateral chest film are also suggestive of perforation.

A final complication is ventricular ectopic activity, either at the time of insertion or secondary to competition with the patient's native rhythm. The former is usually self-limited and does not require suppressive therapy. The latter is handled by ensuring that the sensing (demand) mode is fully operational and by setting the pacer rate well above or below the intrinsic rate.

SELECTED READINGS

Furman S, Escher DJW: Temporary cardiac pacing, in *Principles and Techniques of Cardiac Pacing.* New York, Harper & Row Publishers Inc, 1970, p 62–112.

Hazard PB, Benton C, Milnor JP: Transvenous cardiac pacing in cardiopulmonary resuscitation. *Crit Care Med* 1981; 9:666.

Lang R et al: Use of the balloon-tipped floating catheter in temporary transvenous cardiac pacing. PACE 1981; 4:491.

Roe BB: Intractable Stokes-Adams disease: A method of emergency management. *Am Heart J* 1965; 69:470.

Rosenburg AS, Grossman JI, Escher DJW: Bedside transvenous cardiac pacing. *Am Heart J* 1969; 77:697.

Schnitzler RN, Caracta RN, Damato RN: Floating catheter for temporary transvenous ventricular pacing. *Am J Cardiol* 1973; 31:351.

PROCEDURE 17

USE OF MILITARY ANTISHOCK TROUSERS

Russell Nauta

Military antishock trousers (MAST) (G Suit) serve three basic functions for the traumatized patient. The first is to provide hemostasis by increasing the pressure in the tissues surrounding a bleeding vessel, thereby decreasing flow from the inside of the vessel to the outside. This also allows elastic tissue of the arterial walls to contract and make the arteriotomy smaller, thus slowing the bleeding. The second function is related to autotransfusion of the hypotensive patient, whereby application of the suit returns approximately 2 units of blood to the heart by way of the venous channels draining the legs and pelvis. The third advantage is related to splinting of lower extremity and pelvic fractures, particularly in those patients who have comminuted or unstable injuries.

Adequate benefit from the garment can only be achieved by an understanding of its application to the patient and proper inflation of the garment's pressure chambers. Although the emergency room physician often finds the garment in place upon transport of the patient to the hospital, he or she should be familiar with its application as an adjunct to the treatment of fractures below the waist and of bleeding in the traumatized patient.

INDICATIONS

- Abdominal hemorrhage from blunt or penetrating trauma that does not resolve with routine volume resuscitation
- Severe lacerations or external blood loss in the areas covered by the garment, pending surgical attention to those areas
- Leaking or ruptured abdominal aneurysm with hemodynamic compromise
- Unstable femoral, pelvic, and other lower extremity fractures in the multiply-traumatized patient

CONTRAINDICATIONS

- Pulmonary edema is an absolute contraindication.

- The MAST suit should be applied to the pregnant woman with reluctance since the fetus may be endangered.
- Congestive heart failure and cardiogenic shock are relative contraindications.

EQUIPMENT

A pair of antishock trousers is the only equipment needed.

POSITION

The patient should be supine.

PROCEDURE

1. Place the suit under the patient. The suit is ideally positioned with the upper aspect of the abdominal portion at the costal margin. The trousers should be adjusted to come to the level of the patient's ankle.

2. Secure the leg tabs or leg fasteners to encircle the limbs with the garment and secure in place (Fig. PR17.1).

3. Connect the MAST suit to the inflation apparatus (Fig. PR17.2). Inflate the trousers first, monitoring the patient's blood pressure and continuing inflation until the patient's blood pressure begins to respond. The garment can exert a maximum pressure of 100 mm Hg, but most of the salutory effect is felt between 0 and 30 mm Hg.

4. Some garments are equipped with a pressure gauge that monitors the pressure applied by the garment for each section. If the inflation of the leg panels is not sufficient to correct the hemodynamic abnormality, the abdominal portion of the garment should be inflated. For maximal auto-transfusion effect, pressure in the abdominal panels should not exceed the pressure in the leg panels. Insufflation of the garment beyond that which it is designed to tolerate is decompressed through a pressure relief valve; there is negligible hemodynamic advantage beyond 100 mm Hg in most patients.

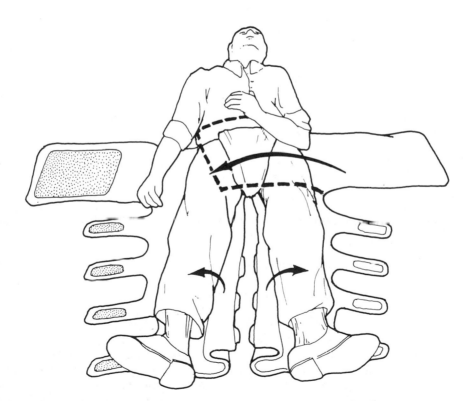

Figure PR17.1 Encircle the patient's legs and secure the trousers in position; then encircle the abdomen.

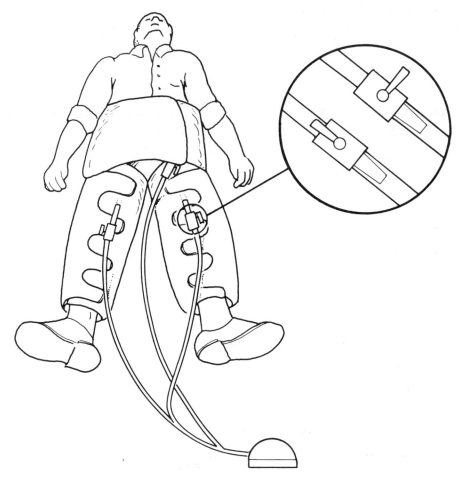

Figure PR17.2 Connect the suit to the inflation apparatus and inflate trousers first.

PITFALLS AND COMPLICATIONS

Inability to ventilate the patient may result if the garment is applied higher than the costal margin. *Inadequate securing* of both the limb and abdominal portion of the garment will not provide the desired splinting effect for below the waist fractures, and maximal pressure cannot be achieved. Hyperinflation of the abdominal component relative to the limb components will inhibit maximum autotransfusion. Overestimation of the volume deficit may lead to *pulmonary edema* or *congestive heart failure* when the garment is overzealously inflated. Underestimation of volume deficit and false complacency with the hemodynamic status of the patient in the inflated suit may lead to *cardiovascular collapse* when the garment is deflated. Moving the patient when applying the MAST suit may *exacerbate other injuries*. It is necessary to pay careful attention to pelvic fractures and to the cervical spine while applying the device. In pregnant patients, *fetal blood flow may be decreased* when inflating the abdominal panel. *Loss of pressure* may result from leaky valves, failure to lock valves, loose tubing, leaky chambers, or a disconnection.

The garment should be viewed as an adjunctive measure and should not take the place of careful assessment of the patient, adequate volume replacement, and attention to skeletal and soft tissue injuries. Once inflated, the garment should only be deflated in situations in which adequate respiratory support and blood transfusion capabilities are present.

ASPIRATION AND DRAINAGE TECHNIQUES AND DIAGNOSTIC PROCEDURES

PROCEDURE 18

THORACENTESIS

John H. Sanders

Thoracentesis is performed to remove fluid or air from the pleural cavity without injury to the heart, lung, liver, or chest wall vessels. Unless a collection is loculated in an inaccessible location, most fluid and air can be removed by a sixth or seventh intercostal space approach (Fig. PR18.1). Fluid is best obtained posteriorly, one or two fingers breadth below the tip of the scapula.

Air is traditionally sought in the second intercostal space anteriorly. This approach is favored by many, but the internal mammary artery and great vessels are not far away. The fifth or sixth intercostal space can easily be entered just lateral to the border of the pectoralis major, even with the nipple, with greater safety and equal yield.

Thoracentesis may be diagnostic or therapeutic, depending upon the condition suspected.

INDICATIONS

- Hydrothorax
- Hemothorax
- Stable pneumothorax
- Empyema

CONTRAINDICATIONS

- Patient is known to be taking anticoagulants
- Chest tube will most likely be required anyway
- Pneumonia—needle injury may cause empyema

EQUIPMENT

- Antiseptic preparation solution
- Sterile gloves
- 4 × 4-inch gauze sponges
- Towels or sterile draping sheet
- 1 or 2% lidocaine without epinephrine
- 3-ml syringe with 25-gauge needle for local anesthesia

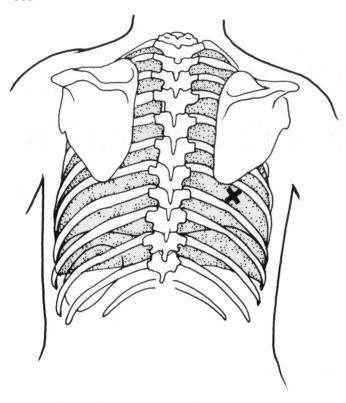

Figure PR18.1 Common site for needle insertion.

- 22-gauge, 1.5-inch needle
- Three-way stopcock
- 50-ml syringe
- 12-inch long, large (16-gauge) catheter-through-needle intravenous placement system
- Appropriate containers for fluid for diagnostic tests
- Hemostat
- Adhesive dressing

POSITION

If fluid is expected, the patient is best seated sideways on a chair with arms draped over a pillow placed on a bedside stand. This allows easy access to the back and a dependent position for the fluid. If air is sought, the patient may recline supine with the back up at a 30 deg angle and place his or her hand behind the head.

PROCEDURE

Before preparation and draping, the region to be tapped should be percussed to locate the air or fluid level. In addition, the patient's name, the date, and the involved side should be double checked on the x-ray film for certainty. A needle scratch or a convenient skin blemish can serve as a marker.

Preparation and draping must be thorough and wide enough to allow access to an interspace above and below the intended mark. Sterile technique, including a surgical mask, should be observed throughout the procedure.

Anesthetize the Site

The small syringe and needle should be filled with lidocaine and a skin weal should be raised. The syringe is then refilled and the 22-gauge needle is attached. The needle is advanced to touch the rib *under* the desired site and 0.5–1 ml of local anesthesia is placed. The needle is then walked off the *top* of the rib border until it is free and advances toward the pleura (Fig. PR18.2) Small amounts of anesthetic are placed, the syringe is aspirated, and if no material returns, the needle is again advanced 0.5–1 cm. This is repeated until entry into the pleural space occurs, heralded by the return of air or fluid upon aspiration. The needle is then backed out until it is just outside of the pleural surface. The remaining anesthetic (1–2 ml) is then injected to provide good pleural anesthesia, and the needle is removed.

Thoracentesis

The needle is next removed from the intravenous catheter system. The small syringe is then attached to this large needle, it is filled with local anesthesia, and it is advanced into the pleural space in the same way as was the anesthetic needle (Fig. PR18.2b). When matter is returned (Fig. PR18.2c) the syringe is removed while the patient holds his or her breath and bears down against a closed glottis. The end of the needle is covered by a gloved finger and the patient is again allowed to breathe (Fig. PR18.2d). The catheter unit, with its stylet removed, is then advanced through the needle, again with the patient holding a Valsalva maneuver (Fig. PR18.2e). The needle is removed over the catheter and the stopcock is attached to the catheter hub. Plastic protection against shearing the catheter with the needle is placed properly, as for an intravenous unit (Fig. PR18.2f). Fluid or air may now be withdrawn slowly for as long a period as necessary using the large syringe. Specimens from the early return should be sent to the laboratory. The catheter may be moved in and out a bit for optimal position.

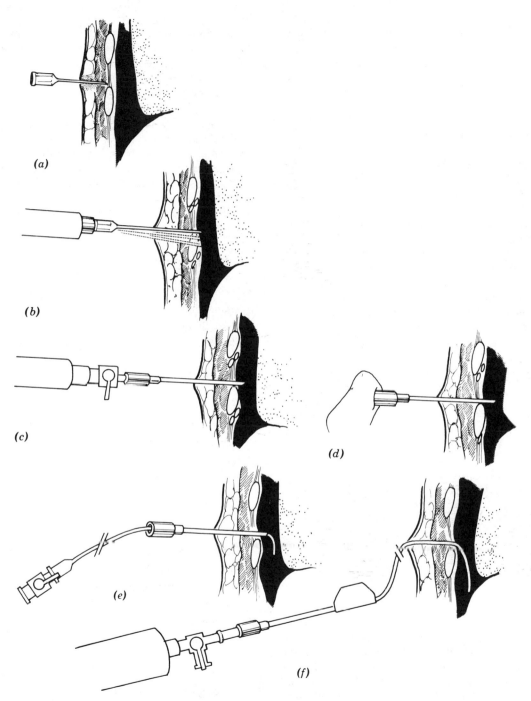

Figure PR18.2 (a) Anesthetize, using top of rib as reference point; (b) insert thoracentesis needle; (c) withdraw fluid; (d) remove syringe and cover end of needle with finger; (e) insert catheter; (f) remove needle, attach stopcock, and attach needle guard.

The stylet, which was removed earlier, may be used to judge how much of the catheter is inside the chest.

When the procedure is complete, the entire unit is removed and discarded. The wound is covered with an adhesive dressing.

PITFALLS AND COMPLICATIONS

If the needle is removed from the chest as soon as the catheter is introduced and the plastic guard is placed over the catheter, a *severed catheter* is very unlikely to occur.

Pneumothorax may occur if the lung is injured or care is not taken to have the patient hold a Valsalva maneuver with needle changes. Lung injury usually requires placement of a chest tube. *Injury to abdominal organs* may occur if the puncture is made too low. *Empyema* may occur if thoracentesis is inappropriately performed on a patient who has a consolidated lung and no free chest fluid. *Hemorrhage* may occur if the patient is on anticoagulants or if the intercostal or internal mammary vessels are injured. A lateral position on the chest wall and on top of the rib should obviate these pitfalls.

PROCEDURE 19

CHEST TUBE INSERTION

John H. Sanders

Chest tube insertion is frequently carried out in the emergency room as a therapeutic procedure for patients with pneumothorax, hemothorax, or hydrothorax. The purpose is to provide an appropriate-sized drainage tube in an appropriate location that will provide continuous evacuation of the chest cavity and allow reexpansion of the lung. There are several ways that this may be accomplished and a larger number of possible drainage systems to provide safe egress of fluid or air from the chest cavity without allowing an open pneumothorax to occur.

Chest tube insertion can be an extremely painful procedure for a patient; therefore it is especially important to pay attention to the proper means of accomplishing local anesthesia.

CHEST TUBE MANAGEMENT

Because there are a number of subtleties regarding the function of chest tubes and their drainage systems, as well as the care of patients who have them, it is advisable to enlist the help of an experienced surgeon in the care of such a patient. In many centers it is the policy to notify the involved surgeon when a chest tube is going to be placed. In this way it will be possible to satisfy partially the idiosyncrasies of a given institution and surgeon.

INDICATIONS

- Spontaneous pneumothorax
- Traumatic pneumothorax
- Hemothorax
- Hydrothorax

CONTRAINDICATIONS

- Systemic anticoagulation
- Small, stable spontaneous pneumothorax
- Empyema caused by acid-fast organisms
- Loculated hydrothorax or pneumothorax

EQUIPMENT

- Sterile gloves
- Surgical mask
- Antiseptic solution
- Two curved hemostats or Kelly clamps
- Gauze
- Sponges
- Sterile towels or draping sheets
- 10-ml syringe
- 25-gauge needle
- 22-gauge, 1.5-in. needle
- No. 15 scalpel blade with handle
- Appropriate-sized intercostal catheter: 20 French for pneumothorax; 28–32 French for fluid collections or blood

- Large silk or other nonabsorbable suture material on a cutting skin needle (0-0, 1-0, or 2-0)
- Appropriate drainage system

POSITION

Chest tube insertion is easily accomplished with the patient supine with the appropriate hand behind the head or with the torso elevated at a 30 deg angle. This prevents the tube from being placed too far posteriorly, which is exceptionally uncomfortable for the patient. If it is desired to place the tube somewhat more posteriorly than usual, a small roll may be placed under the patient's side to allow better exposure.

PROCEDURE

Preparation and Draping

Chest tube insertion must be accomplished with the same rigid adherence to surgical technique as any other surgical procedure. Sterile gloves must be worn throughout, a surgical mask should be worn, and great care must be taken to avoid contamination of the pleural cavity. It is important to select an appropriate site for chest tube insertion. For practical purposes we recommend that all chest tubes be inserted into the lateral chest wall behind the border of the pectoralis major muscle. The fifth or sixth intercostal space is generally lateral to the nipple and is an excellent site for insertion of tubes for either air or fluid drainage (Fig. PR19.1). If large volumes of blood or other fluid are anticipated, the more posterior chest wall should be chosen, but in no case should a tube be inserted so far posteriorly that a patient will be obliged to lie upon it for a prolonged period of time. Many groups recommend the insertion of an anterior chest tube for pneumothorax. This is generally accomplished in the second intercostal space in the midclavicular line. We strongly recommend against this because of the possible hazard to the mediastinum and great vessels. In addition, it is an unsightly location for a scar. Lateral chest tube placement is equally effective, more comfortable, and ultimately more cosmetic.

Local Anesthesia

Proper application of local anesthesia will make this procedure almost painless for the patient. Inappropriate application of local anesthesia makes it an excrutiating ordeal. After the appropriate site has been selected, prepared, and draped, a skin wheal should be raised using a 10-ml syringe and 25-gauge

needle. In a relatively thin person this same needle may be used to anesthetize the periosteum of the rib under the insertion site and occasionally the pleura itself. In most people it will be necessary to use the 22-gauge, 1.5-inch needle to advance local anesthesia to the periosteum and the pleural surface. Once the pleural surface has been pierced and it is possible to aspirate fluid or air from the thorax, the needle is gradually withdrawn until aspiration ceases. At this point, a relatively large volume (5–10 ml) of local anesthesia is injected immediately exterior to the pleural surface. This anesthetizes a relatively broad area of pleura sufficient to allow insertion without undue pain. It also may block the intercostal nerve of the selected interspace to a certain extent. Up to this point, the local anesthetic application is identical to that used for thoracentesis.

Chest Tube Insertion

The appropriate-sized chest tube should be selected. An 18–20 French catheter is large enough for air drainage but is not adequate for fluid or blood drainage. In cases of large fluid collections or hemothorax from trauma, a 28–32 French catheter should be selected. The scalpel is used to make a small transverse incision 1.5 cm in length overlying the rib below the selected interspace. Using blunt dissection with the hemostat or Kelly clamp, the pleural space is entered, taking care to grasp the hemostat in such a fashion that it cannot accidently enter more than 1 inch into the pleural space (Fig. PR19.2). The hemostat is spread to provide a satisfactory tract for the tube, and a finger may then be inserted along the tube tract to ensure that the pleural space has been entered freely and that there is no adherent lung or diaphragm in the region of the selected placement. In such a fashion it is occasionally possible to feel evident pleural pathology such as tumor studding. With the patient holding his or her breath in full inspiration and bearing down slightly to increase intrathoracic pressure, the finger is removed and the catheter is placed (Fig. PR19.2c). It is helpful to have a suture tied around the catheter to mark the desired length of insertion. This ensures that the last side hole of the catheter is, in fact, within the pleural space and acts as a frame of reference until a chest film can be taken. If a pneumothorax is present, the tube may be directed anteriorly; if fluid or blood is present, the tube should be directed posteriorly. The hemostat or Kelly clamp is placed on the tube to prevent excessive air entry into the chest or fluid drainage into the bed. The tube is then sutured in place using heavy, nonabsorbable suture material. This stay suture should perform two functions. It should anchor the tube thoroughly to the skin so that it cannot be pulled free or moved inadvertently. It

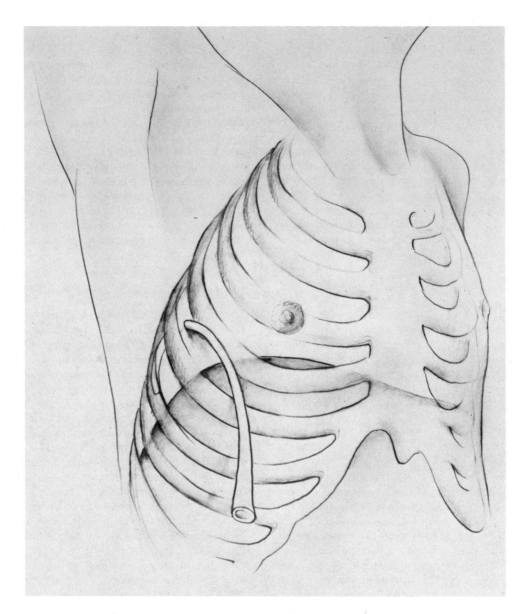

Figure PR19.1 Recommended site for insertion of most chest tubes.

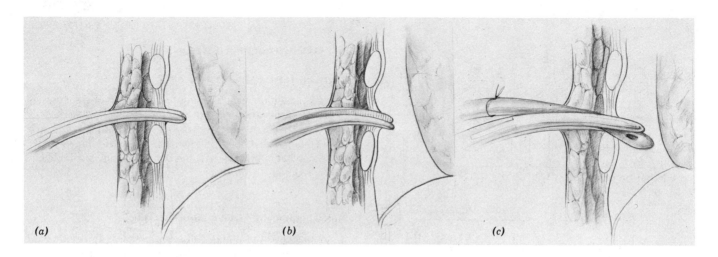

Figure PR19.2 (a) Insert Kelly clamp; (b) open clamp; (c) insert tube.

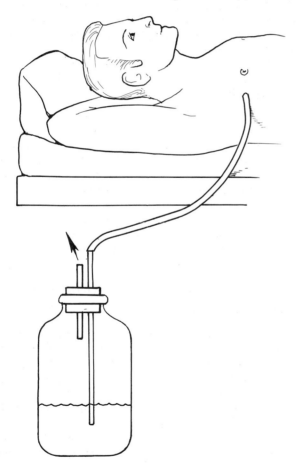

Figure PR19.3 Underwater seal.

should also close any redundancy in the skin incision made for insertion and prevent leakage of air and fluid around the catheter. After the tube placement is completed, the tube is connected to a suitable drainage system. A dressing is placed around the catheter and the tube is taped securely to the patient's chest wall. All connections to drainage systems must also be taped to prevent disconnection and air leakage.

Drainage Systems

Several satisfactory drainage systems have been designed for the purpose of providing safe pleural fluid evacuation. Because intrathoracic pressure varies from positive to negative throughout the inspiratory and expiratory cycle, the only essential requirement to successful pleural evacuation is some sort of one-way valve that allows fluid and air to exit but prevents its return. There are mechanical systems that do this, but the safest and simplest system is the underwater seal (Fig. PR19.3). This consists of a bottle that is open to air and has a tube that rests 1–2 cm below the surface of the saline-filled chamber. Air and fluid easily exit through this, but drawing fluid up to the chest cavity would necessitate an inspiratory force greater than 100 cm H_2O, which cannot be achieved by the diaphragm. Many institutions use other forms of underwater seals in conjunction with some sort of vacuum applied to the system. The oldest of these is the three bottle suction system shown in Figure PR19.4a. The first bottle in line from the patient is a reservoir for collecting fluid or blood as it drains from the pleural cavity. The second bottle, to which this is connected, is the underwater seal; and the final bottle is the suction-regulating bottle. The last bottle acts to prevent too high a negative pressure

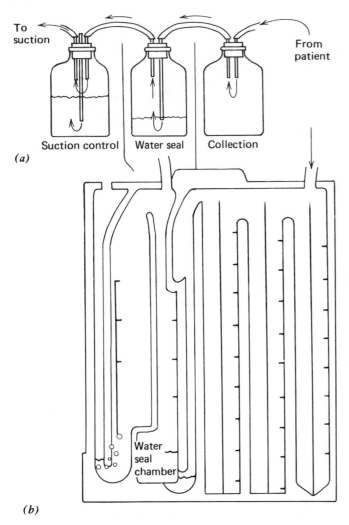

(a)

Suction control | Water seal | Collection

To suction

From patient

Water seal chamber

(b)

Figure PR19.4 (a) Three bottle suction; (b) disposable suction unit.

being applied to the patient. When an unregulated vacuum is applied to the suction-regulating bottle, air enters through the longest tube, thereby keeping the suction at the present level. There are a number of disposable systems that incorporate all three chambers into a plastic, disposable unit that works quite well. One of these is shown in Figure PR19.4b.

Regardless of the system available at a given hospital, it should be thoroughly investigated and understood by any who may use it—before the need arises. Improper use of drainage systems can be dangerous.

PITFALLS AND COMPLICATIONS

Injury to Heart and Great Vessels

The most common reason for injury to the heart or great vessels by chest tube insertion is the use of catheter-over-trocar devices that are 35–40 cm long and can easily penetrate any organ within their reach if not properly used. For this reason we prefer the somewhat more cumbersome but universally available hemostat method.

Subdiaphragmatic Placement of the Tube

If low placement of a chest tube is attempted, it is quite easy to place it through or below the diaphragm and into neighboring soft organs. For this reason, it is better to insert a chest tube at the level of the fifth or sixth intercostal space and direct it inferiorly than to try and place it low in the first place. Once again, the hemostat and finger method of placement is far safer than the trocar system.

Open Pneumothorax

Once the chest tube has been placed, an open pneumothorax has by definition been created. This is easily limited by clamping the tube with the patient bearing down in maximal inspiration. This will expel some air and fluid from the chest and partially reexpand the lung until connection to a drainage device can be made. Open pneumothroax also occurs if disconnection of the underwater seal to the patient occurs. This can sometimes be subtle and take the form of a large hole in the back of a plastic drainage system. Unless one looks for and finds proper function of the drainage system at all times, such accidents can easily be overlooked.

Unexplained Air Leakage

Air leakage is seen by observing bubbles occurring in the underwater seal portion of the drainage system. Although the leakage may be from the surface of the lung, it may also be from any hole, however minute, anywhere along the drainage tract. One of the least obvious forms of air leakage occurs when the needle used to suture the chest tube in place inadvertently perforates the tube just below the surface of the skin. This is not seen on the x-ray film and acts in the same fashion as a continued air leak from the surface of the lung. Prevention is the only means of diagnosing and treating this particular pitfall.

Tension Pneumothorax

Once placed, a chest tube should never be clamped unless it is to make a final check for air leak before removal of the tube. A patient who has even a small air leak can develop a tension pneumothorax when the tube is clamped. For this reason, we would prefer to have a patient develop an open pneumothorax if some accident causes loss of the underwater seal than to have a patient develop a tension pneumothorax that could be fatal.

Dislodgment of the Tube

Unless a tube is properly attached to the patient, it is very easy to dislodge it. This may also take somewhat subtle forms. Although the tube is securely attached to the patient's chest wall, the skin is elastic. A tube that has been placed rather shallowly in the chest can easily be pulled into a subcutaneous position where it fails to perform properly. From all outward appearances and most radiographic appearances, it still appears to be in place. Awareness of this pitfall is once again the only means of prevention.

Subcutaneous Emphysema

With a properly functioning chest tube there should be very little subcutaneous emphysema around the insertion site. If the tube is not functioning properly or has ceased to function at all, air and fluid from the chest cavity will leak around the chest tube into the subcutaneous tissues and present as subcutaneous emphysema.

PROCEDURE 20

PERICARDIOCENTESIS

John H. Sanders

Pericardiocentesis is performed to remove blood, pus, or other fluid from the pericardial space. Occasionally it is performed as a diagnostic procedure, in which case it may be desirable to perform it in a suite that has fluoroscopy and other helpful equipment available. Many times, however, pericardiocentesis will be required as the immediate and life-saving therapy for a condition that has caused cardiac tamponade.

Properly performed, pericardiocentesis carries very little risk and should certainly be among the skills of any practicing physician.

INDICATIONS

Diagnostic

Pericardiocentesis is indicated for patients with pericardial effusion of unknown origin.

Therapeutic

- Cardiac tamponade
- Malignant pericardial effusion
- Uremic pericardial effusion
- Traumatic hemopericardium
- Ruptured thoracic aortic aneurysm

CONTRAINDICATIONS

Do not perform pericardiocentesis if there is systemic anticoagulation

EQUIPMENT

- Direct current defibrillator
- Electrocardiograph unit or cardiac monitor
- Antiseptic preparation solution
- Gauze sponges
- Draping towels or sheet
- Sterile gloves
- 10-ml syringe
- 25-gauge needle
- 22-gauge, 1.5-in. needle
- 1 or 2% lidocaine (Xylocaine) without epinephrine
- Three-way stopcock
- 50-ml syringe
- Catheter-over-needle unit, 16-gauge, at least 3.5-inches long
- Appropriate tubes for hematocrit, culture, or other desired tests

POSITION

Generally speaking, the patient should be positioned with the head and torso elevated at a 30 deg angle (Fig. PR20.1). Occasionally, if the patient is in shock he or she may be aspirated supine, but the awake patient with cardiac tamponade will generally not tolerate being supine. Nasal oxygen or an oxygen mask may provide some comfort. The leads of the electrocardiogram (ECG) should be attached in such a fashion that a satisfactory tracing is obtained, and a properly functioning defibrillator should be present.

PROCEDURE

Prepare the lower chest, upper abdomen, and epigastrium widely with a satisfactory antiseptic solution. After this, the drapes should be applied in such a fashion that all of the tissues within a 4-in. radius of the xyphoid process can easily be palpated. It is helpful to have a more extensive drape to cover the lower abdomen and knees, as well as the upper thorax, in order to allow some motion of both the patient and the operator without contamination.

Anesthetize the Skin and Subcutaneous Tissues

Using the small syringe and needle, a local anesthetic is used to raise a skin wheal 2 cm below to 1 cm to the left of the xyphoid process. The 22-gauge needle is then attached and advanced to contact the costal margin on the left side, and local anesthesia is infiltrated along this track to and including the costal margin.

Pericardiocentesis

The 10-ml syringe is next attached to the plastic catheter-over-needle unit. It is helpful to have 4 or 5 ml of local anesthetic in the syringe during the pericardial puncture. The catheter-over-needle unit with the attached syringe is then advanced to contact the left costal margin. This requires a course that

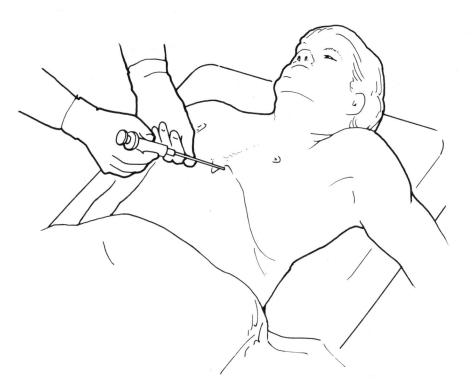

Figure PR20.1 Advance catheter-over-needle unit with attached syringe aiming approximately for the middle of the left scapula.

would aim approximately for the middle of the left scapula. After contacting the costal margin, the needle is walked off the costal margin and advanced 0.5 cm at a time (Fig. PR20.2, PR20.3). After each advancement, a small amount of local anesthesia is infiltrated to clear the needle of tissue or thrombus and aspiration is attempted. In an average-sized adult, the pericardium will be entered approximately 3 inches from the skin puncture site. Once fluid is aspirated from the pericardium, the catheter-over-needle unit should be advanced another 0.5–1 cm and the needle removed. The plastic catheter is then aspirated using the large syringe and three-way stopcock.

Many cardiologists advocate the attachment of an ECG lead directly to the advancing needle. This has the advantage of

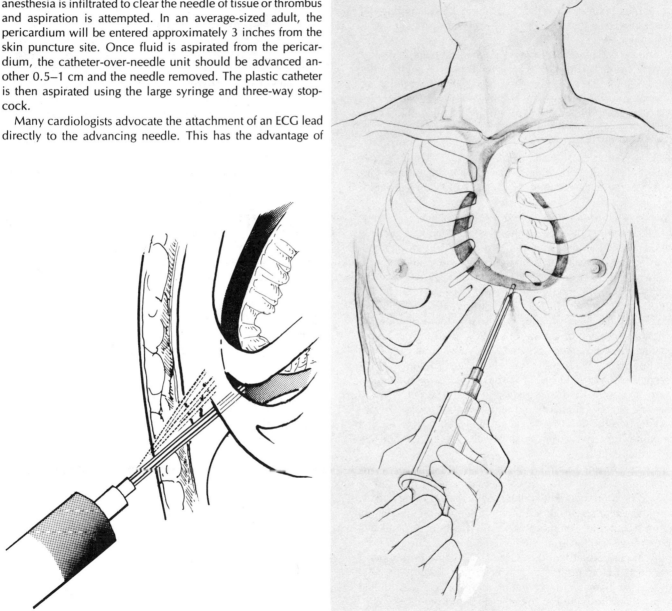

Figures PR20.2 and PR20.3 Walk needle off costal margin and advance .5cm at a time, infiltrating a small amount of local anesthesia and attempting aspiration after each advancement.

displaying an injury potential if the heart is directly contacted and may prevent entry into the right or left ventricle. However, an improperly shielded ECG apparatus can easily cause ventricular fibrillation under these circumstances. It is therefore our recommendation that the ECG simply be watched for the appearance of ventricular arrhythmias that also will herald cardiac puncture.

Some people have recommended a parasternal approach to the pericardium. This carries a far higher risk of injury to the pleura, lung, internal mammary artery, or left anterior descending coronary artery than the subxyphoid approach. Other texts have shown a needle course from the subxyphoid route that is directed toward the right scapula. This course would carry an increased risk of injury to the right atrium or vena cava. The ventricular walls are thicker and therefore more tolerant of needle injury than are the venous chambers of the heart. We therefore recommend a course directed toward the left side.

When pericardiocentesis is performed to relieve tamponade caused by trauma, it is frequently possible to obtain complete hemodynamic recovery after removal of 75–100 ml of blood. It may well be possible to aspirate a larger quantity than this, but in trauma it is frequently difficult to be certain that the needle is not positioned within the right or left ventricle. Because of this, we should not continue to remove blood from the pericardium without limit. We usually stop aspiration following the removal of 200 ml of blood if a satisfactory hemodynamic result has been obtained. The catheter may be left in position for removal of more fluid should it accumulate. In the presence of tamponade from chronic fluid accumulation, a larger volume of fluid is present and it will be necessary to remove a larger volume of fluid to obtain a satisfactory hemodynamic result. Amounts as large as 1,200–1,500 ml can sometimes be removed in patients with malignant or uremic pericardial effusions.

If there is doubt about the origin of blood obtained by pericardiocentesis, there are several bedside checks that can be made to be more certain that the blood is not coming directly from a vascular space. Blood that has been in the pericardial sac for 10 minutes or more is usually defibrinated and will therefore fail to clot in a suitable container. A check for the ability of pericardial blood to clot can be carried out faster if an activated clotting time tube is used. In bloody pericardial effusion, the hematocrit of the fluid in the pericardium should be less than the patient's hematocrit. Blood within the pericardium may sometimes clot completely, without defibrination. This prevents aspiration altogether and may necessitate urgent or bedside thoracotomy for relief of tamponade.

If catheter placement has been successful, it may prove help-ful to leave the plastic catheter in place to allow subsequent aspiration or the placement of a larger unit by the Seldinger technique at a later time.

PITFALLS AND COMPLICATIONS

Ventricular fibrillation may occur as a result of needle contact with the heart or leakage current if an ECG lead is attached to the needle. For this reason, a properly functioning defibrillator should always be present before this procedure is attempted.

Ventricular perforation may occur during any attempt at pericardiocentesis. If the needle is slowly advanced, this is less likely to occur, especially if the local anesthetic solution is used to clear the needle before each attempt at aspiration. This complication is more likely to occur in conditions in which a small amount of fluid exists in the pericardium than when there is a large chronic accumulation. Because the walls of the right and left ventricle are relatively thick, penetration by a 16-gauge needle seldom causes serious bleeding.

Pneumothorax may occur if the pleural cavity is entered and the lung is injured. This can easily occur if the puncture is made too far lateral and the pericardial cavity is missed altogether.

Peritoneal penetration may occur if care is not taken to walk the needle off the rib margin before attempting to advance into the pericardium. This is generally not a serious problem unless a hollow viscus is also penetrated.

PROCEDURE 21

NASOGASTRIC TUBE INSERTION

Edmund B. Cabot

Nasogastric (NG) intubation is one of the simplest and most common forms of bedside intervention for the critically ill patient, both in the emergency room setting and on the hospital ward. The properly placed nasogastric tube can be of critical diagnostic value, as well as an important therapeutic modality in numerous situations referred to in previous chapters.

Since this procedure is most frequently performed on the awake and alert patient, the greatest obstacle is in overcoming the patient's apprehension. Few patients will readily accept the notion of a tube being inserted into the nose and down the back of the throat into the stomach without some concern for their own discomfort. Thus, the inexperienced physician's approach to the patient will, to a large extent, govern initial success, as well as the patient's subsequent reactions to the procedure. Reassurance will go a long way toward eliciting the patient's cooperation and the success of the whole maneuver.

These remarks do not apply to the unconscious patient, for whom the procedure may be even more critical and perhaps life-saving. In such cases a somewhat different approach may be necessary.

INDICATIONS

- Any multiple trauma involving the trunk (chest and/or abdomen)
- Any unconscious patient in the acute setting
- Before any elective or semielective endotracheal intubation on a full stomach or when the state of gastric contents is unknown
- When acute gastric dilation is known or suspected
- When gastrointestinal (GI) hemorrhage of any sort (upper or lower GI bleeding, excluding obvious hemorrhoidal bleeding) is known or suspected
- When intestinal obstruction at any level is known or suspected
- To remove recently ingested toxic substances
- When perforation of any intraabdominal hollow viscus is known or suspected
- Any penetrating injury to the abdomen in which violation of the peritoneal cavity is known or suspected
- Any significant blunt abdominal trauma in which injury to any viscus is known or suspected
- Obvious peritonitis, regardless of etiology
- Significant retroperitoneal injury or inflammation
- Paralytic ileus, regardless of etiology
- Protracted vomiting
- To facilitate radiographic (contrast) evaluation of the upper GI tract in the unconscious or uncooperative patient, when indicated

- Failure of previously placed nasogastric tube because of occlusion or inadequate size
- Recent endotracheal intubation

CONTRAINDICATIONS

- Complete obstruction of the nasopharynx
- Major facial trauma
- Suspected cervical spinal cord injury
- Presence of functioning gastrostomy tube

EQUIPMENT

- Nasogastric tube—preferably *large-bore* (18F for adults) Salem Sump (Fig. PR21.1) (rather than single lumen Levin) and preferably well chilled (e.g., stored in refrigerator or packed in ice water) to stiffen tube

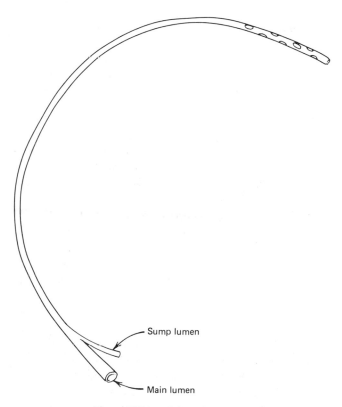

Sump lumen

Main lumen

Figure PR21.1 Salem sump tube.

- Suction apparatus—preferably intermittent Gomco device on high setting or equivalent wall suction (with calibrated water trap) on low setting (80 mm Hg or 100 cm H_2O)
- 50-ml catheter-tip (Toomey) syringe
- Emesis basin
- Water-soluble lubricant (Lubrifax, Surgilube)
- 1-inch adhesive tape—preferably Dermicel cloth tape
- Stethoscope
- Suction tubing with connector
- Facial tissue (optional)
- Cup of tap water with flexible straw
- Cetacaine spray (optional)
- Examining gloves (optional)

POSITION

The patient should be sitting upright or semireclining (if possible) with the neck slightly flexed (if uninjured).

PROCEDURE

1. *Assemble equipment* and explain to the patient *why* the tube is necessary, *how* we plan to proceed, and *what* to expect. Explain that if excessive gagging occurs, we will anesthetize the back of the throat (Cetacaine spray). Do not mention vomiting.
2. *Test the equipment* ahead of time by connecting the NG tube to the suction apparatus and immersing the end of the tube in water. Then disconnect tube from suction.
3. *Measure the distance* from the xyphoid to the top of the patient's head, and note the distance on the tube relative to the black markers that are usually present (Fig. PR21.2).
4. *Examine the nasal passages* and select the most widely patent nostril.
5. *Instruct the patient* to breathe through the mouth.
6. *Lubricate* the distal 3 inches of the NG tube *liberally* with water-soluble jelly.
7. *Introduce the tip* of the NG tube into the nostril, and with one hand gently supporting the back of the patient's head, slowly advance the tube *straight back* (posteriorly, *not* cephalad) into the posterior nasopharynx (Fig. PR21.3).
8. *Rotate* the tube slowly if it will not easily advance further.
9. *Ask the patient to swallow* repeatedly as the tube advances past the soft palate and down the posterior pharynx. This may be facilitated by having the patient sip water from a straw as you advance the tube (Fig. PR21.4). Once the patient has swallowed the tube past the glottis and into the upper esophagus, the tube usually passes more readily. Continue to have the patient swallow as the tube is more rapidly passed into the stomach, supporting the head with one hand and advancing the tube with the other.

10. *Advance the tube* until the previously noted marker is at the level of the nose. A good rule of thumb, in most adults, is to have two black markers still showing (on a standard Salem Sump tube). Advancing the tube too far may cause it to coil up in the stomach, preventing proper function, to pass down into the duodenum, or even to turn back up into the esophagus.

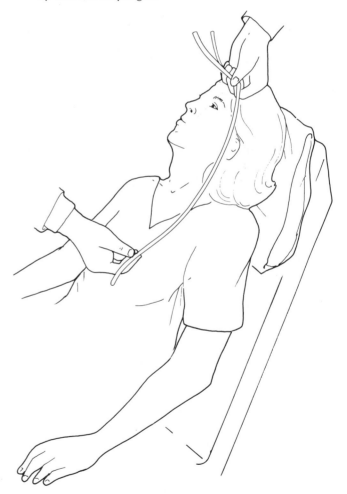

Figure PR21.2 Measure distance to xiphoid.

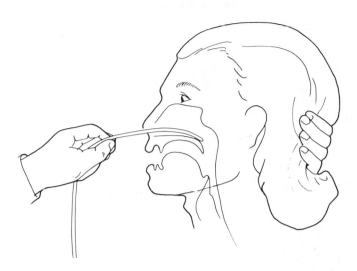

Figure PR21.3 Introduce tube.

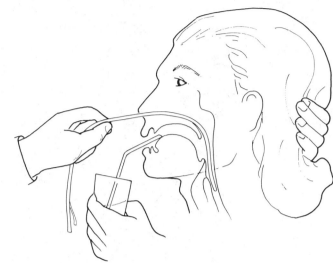

Figure PR21.4 Have patient swallow.

11. *Check the proper position* of the tube by aspirating obvious gastric contents with the catheter tip syringe and/or injecting 20 ml of air into the stomach by means of the same syringe, while listening over the epigastrium with a stethoscope for a bubbling sound (Fig. PR21.5).

12. *Affix the tube* to the nose using a 6–8 inch length of 1 inch adhesive tape running longitudinally from the forehead and down the nose out onto the long axis of the tube. Use a second piece of tape across the nose and out onto the zygomatic regions to further secure the first piece as necessary (Fig. PR21.6). Do *not* secure a loop of tube up to the forehead in such a way as to cause pressure on the nasal ala.

13. *Connect the tube* to the suction apparatus and check again for proper function.

PITFALLS AND COMPLICATIONS

The unconscious patient obviously cannot cooperate by swallowing the tube voluntarily. In this case, introducing the tube past the glottic region blindly may be made somewhat more difficult because of coiling of the tube in the oropharynx. This problem is detected by resistance to passage of the tube and by visualizing the coiled tube through the opened mouth. The solution to the problem may require introducing two fingers of a gloved hand into the mouth to pull the base of the tongue forward and direct the tip of the tube back against the posterior pharynx, while continuing to introduce the tube gently with the other hand at the nose. It may also be helpful to obtain a second tube that has been well chilled and is stiffer.

The intubated patient may present similar difficulties because of partial glottic obstruction arising from the endotracheal tube in the adjacent airway. The solution may again involve manipulating the NG tube through the mouth, and passage may be facilitated by temporarily deflating the balloon cuff of the endotracheal tube.

Excessive gagging is rarely a problem in the routine insertion of an NG tube. Should this be a problem, the pharynx can be anesthetized with either Cetacaine spray or a viscous lidocaine gargle and the patient instructed in panting through the mouth.

Complete nasal obstruction may occasionally make NG intubation impossible, in which case the tube can be introduced orally, following removal of any dentures.

Long tubes, such as the Miller-Abbott and Cantor tubes, are rarely, if ever, indicated in the emergency room setting. They are introduced in an analogous fashion but usually require proper positioning through the pylorus in the fluoroscopy suite. A properly functioning Salem Sump tube that is well positioned in the stomach under almost all circumstances will adequately decompress not only the stomach but eventually the bulk of the small bowel.

Epistaxis as a result of traumatic introduction of the NG tube through the nasal passage is an occasional complication; it is

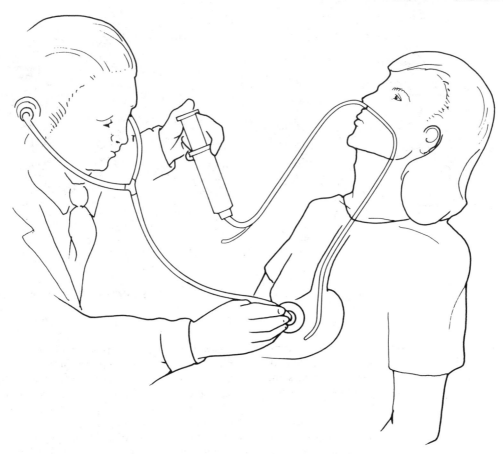

Figure PR21.5 Check position of tube.

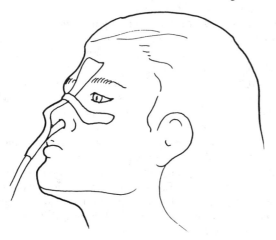

Figure PR21.6 Tape tube securely and comfortably.

best prevented by thorough lubrication of the tube and gentle introduction in a horizontal plane (straight back).

Failure to drain properly may result from improper positioning of the tube in the stomach, occlusion of the lumen of the tube because of kinking or particulate matter, or a malfunctioning suction apparatus. The suction can easily be tested by inserting the connection tubing in water and observing its ability to raise a column of liquid. If the suction is too vigorous, the tube will be occluded by the gastric mucosa being sucked against the openings at the tip of the NG tube. This is remedied by moderating the amount of suction applied and/or gently moving the tube in or out 2–3 in.

The use of a double lumen Salem Sump NG tube of adequate bore (No. 18F) greatly improves both the management of these problems and the ability to evaluate the upper GI tract. The smaller sump lumen should be open to the atmosphere to allow proper sumping action. All too often, when the main (suction) lumen becomes occluded gastric contents back up the sump lumen. Annoyed personnel (or the patient) will then clamp the sump tube, further compounding the problem. The solution to this problem is to instruct those caring for the patient in the proper management of a sump tube, including irrigation of *both* lumens with either air or tap water and aspiration of the main lumen by means of a catheter-tip syringe. When a double lumen sump tube is hooked up to proper suction and functioning properly, we should be able to hear air being sucked into the sump lumen. Temporary occlusion of this lumen should visually retard flow of liquid into the main suction tubing.

Other, more *long-term complications* of NG intubation include *otitis media* from obstruction of a eustachian tube, *esophageal erosion* because of mechanical irritation and malfunction of the lower esophageal sphincter with reflux esophagitis, *gastric erosion* with low-grade GI bleeding because of prolonged intubation and mechanical erosion of the gastric mucosa, and *ulceration* of the nasal alae because of pressure necrosis. These are all preventable by careful attention to detail and removal of the tube as soon as possible.

PROCEDURE 22

GASTRIC LAVAGE

Edmund B. Cabot

The principle purpose of gastric lavage is to remove any contents from the stomach that cannot readily and/or rapidly be removed by regular nasogastric (NG) intubation (see Procedure 21). This may include large volumes of fluid, particulate matter, clotted blood, or toxic substances.

The procedure involves introduction of a large-bore Ewald tube into the stomach, through which large volumes of saline can be rapidly instilled and removed. Most commonly this maneuver is performed in the patient who has massive upper gastrointestinal (GI) hemorrhage when much of the stomach may be filled with partially clotted blood.

Although it is common practice in this setting to lavage the stomach with iced saline on the theory that this will promote vasoconstriction in the gastric submucosa and thus diminish

the bleeding, there is little experimental evidence to suggest that rapid cooling within the gastric lumen actually accomplishes significant changes in gastric blood flow. It may, in fact, predispose the gastric mucosa to further acid-peptic damage. It is clinically apparent, however, that in many instances, removal of large amounts of clotted blood helps to diminish gastric hemorrhage, particularly when it is a result of diffuse erosive gastritis. This may be explained by the damping down of the gastric phase of acid secretion that is secondary to distention of the gastric antrum.

The technique of proper gastric lavage requires at least two people—one to lavage and one to manage the lavage solution. The procedure should generally be regarded as temporary since bleeding will either be controlled to a level manageable by more long-term NG intubation or be obviously uncontrolled and require emergency surgical intervention. Gastric lavage for removal of poisonous substances is similarly a short-term therapy.

INDICATIONS

- Massive GI hemorrhage uncontrollable or unassessable by routine NG intubation
- Removal of known or suspected blood clot from the gastric lumen—especially in the setting of major bleeding from erosive gastritis
- Removal of any particulate matter not adequately aspirated by routine NG intubation

CONTRAINDICATIONS

- Known or suspected esophageal rupture, perforation, stricture, or obstruction
- Excessive facial trauma
- Cervical spinal cord injury

EQUIPMENT

- Ewald tube
- Four or more 60-ml catheter-tip (Toomey) syringes
- Two large basins
- Six or more liters of saline for irrigation
- Ample supply of crushed or cube ice (if indicated)

- Six or more large bottles of liquid antacid (e.g., Mylanta II) (as needed)
- Water-soluble lubricating jelly
- Large emesis basin
- Towels or chucks
- Kelly clamp and heavy scissors
- Cetacaine spray or viscous lidocaine
- Activated charcoal (as indicated)

POSITION

In the conscious, alert, cooperative patient who is not in shock, the Ewald tube should be passed when the patient is in the sitting or semireclining position. The obtunded patient should first undergo endotracheal intubation and may therefore be supine.

PROCEDURE

1. The procedure for *inserting an Ewald tube* is essentially the same as for inserting a regular NG tube (Procedure 21) with

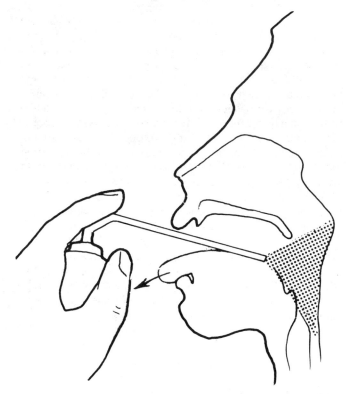

Figure PR22.2 Anesthetize oropharynx.

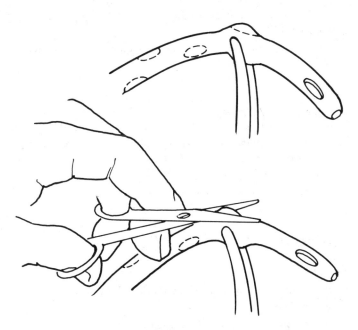

Figure PR22.1 Create extra holes.

the exception that the caliber of the tube may prevent insertion in the nasal passage. As a result, Ewald tubes are commonly passed per os. It is often advisable to *create extra holes* near the tip of the Ewald tube to facilitate removal of particulate matter or clotted blood. It is important to create smooth holes of the proper size. Too large a hole will allow gastric mucosa to be sucked in, obstructing the hole, whereas an irregular hole may injure the mucosa further. A simple technique for creating additional holes involves clamping the tube partway across so the protruding portion can be snipped off (see Fig. PR22.1).

2. *Topically anesthetize* the oropharynx to avoid excessive gagging (Fig. PR22.2). Passing a large tube down the throat of a patient whose stomach may be full of blood or toxic

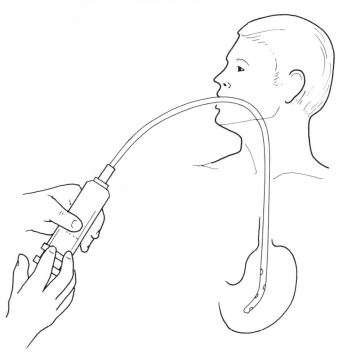

Figure PR22.3 Aspirate.

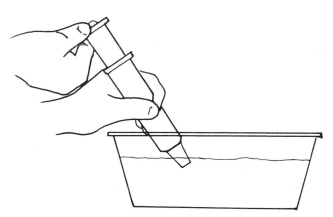

Figure PR22.4 Instill saline, iced saline, or saline–antacid slurry; then aspirate.

materials may produce vomiting. It is wise to have a large emesis basin ready. If the patient is unconscious or obtunded, endotracheal intubation should precede passage of the Ewald tube to prevent aspiration, although deflation of the balloon may be necessary to initiate passage down the esophagus.

3. *Check the position of the tube.* Aspiration of blood or gastric contents usually determines that the tube has entered the stomach (Fig. PR22.3). This can be further confirmed by instillation of air and auscultation over the epigastrium.

4. *Instill* 100–200 ml lavage fluid (saline, iced saline, or saline–antacid slurry, as indicated) into the stomach through a series of catheter-tip syringes prepared by an assistant (Fig. PR22.4).

5. *Aspirate* the stomach by syringe or bulb–pump mechanism (supplied with some tubes); discard the effluent in a second basin.

6. *Repeat* this process of instillation and aspiration until the aspirate is clear or longer if necessary. In cases of ingestion, it may be advisable to instill a slurry of activated charcoal in saline as the final step before removal of the tube.

PITFALLS AND COMPLICATIONS

As mentioned above, passage of such a large tube may well produce vomiting. In neurologically impaired or obtunded patients with depressed gas reflexes, there is a real risk of *aspiration of gastric contents.* The physician must be ready to turn the patient rapidly on his or her side during passage of any tube, and endotracheal intubation should precede passage of an Ewald tube in the high-risk patient.

Bleeding from laceration of the nasopharyngeal or oropharyngeal mucosa is not uncommon. This is best avoided by gentle manipulation of the tube, adequate lubrication, and care in creating any extra holes to avoid rough surfaces.

Gagging in the conscious alert patient is to be expected because of the large size of the tube unless the posterior pharynx is adequately anesthetized.

Failure to drain or aspirate properly implies either that the tube is not properly positioned in the stomach or the lumen of the tube is obstructed by large particulate matter such as clotted blood.

Other more *long-term complications,* such as those described for routine NG tube (Procedure 21), are uncommon with Ewald tubes provided that the tube is removed promptly after lavaging the stomach. If continued gastric decompression is indicated, as it usually is, the Ewald tube should be replaced by a Salem Sump NG tube.

PROCEDURE 23

SENGSTAKEN-BLAKEMORE TUBE INSERTION

Edmund B. Cabot

The Sengstaken-Blakemore (SB) tube has very limited application. Its insertion is basically similar to that of a nasogastric (NG) tube (Procedure 21), but the tube itself is much more complicated. The positioning of an SB tube is critical to its proper function, and once it is in place, it requires constant attention by properly trained medical personnel.

The SB tube has three separate lumens. The *main lumen* is for aspiration of gastric contents. The two *balloon lumens* are for inflating the lower or gastric balloon and for inflating the upper or esophageal balloon. The primary function of a tube such as the SB is to provide balloon tamponade of the distal esophagus and gastric cardia. Thus the tube must be precisely positioned and the balloons must be properly inflated. Failure to do this not only negates the purpose of the SB tube but also endangers the patient. A clear understanding of the function of the SB tube, the indication for its use, and its potential hazards are mandatory before attempting its insertion.

INDICATIONS

- Continued upper gastrointestinal (GI) hemorrhage *known* to be from esophageal or gastric varices
- Massive and uncontrolled upper GI hemorrhage from suspected varices in the known cirrhotic
- Continued bleeding from a documented Mallory-Weiss tear of the distal esophageal and/or proximal gastric mucosa

CONTRAINDICATIONS

- Gastrointestinal bleeding from any site other than the distal esophagus or gastric cardia
- Known or suspected esophageal rupture or perforation (e.g., Boerhaave syndrome)
- Known or suspected esophageal stricture or obstruction
- Obstructed nasopharynx
- Facial trauma
- Cervical spinal cord injury

EQUIPMENT

- Sengstaken-Blakemore tube
- Suction apparatus with water trap—intermittent Gomco on high setting, or low (80 mm Hg) wall suction
- Mercury manometer, such as standard sphygmomanometer, with inflation bulb and suitable tubing
- Y connector
- Three rubber shod clamps (Crile, Kelly, etc.)
- 50-ml catheter-tip (Toomey) syringe

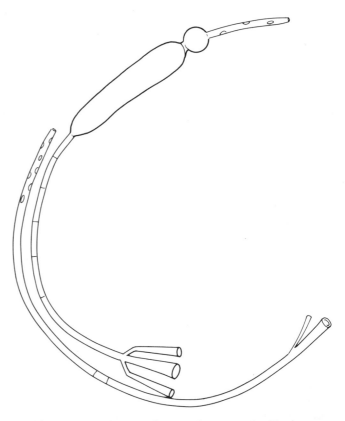

Figure PR23.1 Measure the NG tube against the SB tube.

- Water-soluable lubricating jelly
- Cetacaine spray
- 1 inch adhesive tape
- Cup of water with flexible straw
- Emesis basin
- Examining gloves (optional)
- Parenteral sedative such as injectable meperidine (Demerol)
- Cube of foam rubber (usually supplied with SB tube)
- Heavy scissors—dressing variety
- No. 18F NG tube—Levin tube or Salem sump—with secondary suction apparatus

POSITION

The preferred position is for the patient to be sitting up, perhaps with the help of an assistant. If the patient is in shock, the tube can be passed when he or she is in the supine position with slight elevation at the head.

PROCEDURE

1. *Sedate the patient.* The SB tubes are not always easy to pass and may cause considerable patient discomfort. Therefore adequate sedation with injectable narcotics (e.g., meperidine) is mandatory. The use of such drugs, however, must be tempered in patients with hepatic encephalopathy or in hemorrhagic shock.

2. *Assemble the equipment* and try to explain the procedure to the patient while the sedation is taking effect. Some cooperation on the patient's part can make insertion and maintenance of the SB tube much easier and safer.

3. *Test the SB tube* by inflating each balloon with air under water and checking for any leaks. Then completely deflate both balloons.

4. *Measure the NG tube* against the SB tube so that the tip of the NG tube is at the upper end of the esophageal balloon on the SB tube. Mark the NG tube with adhesive tape at the confluence of the three lumens at the outer end of the SB tube (Fig. PR23.1).

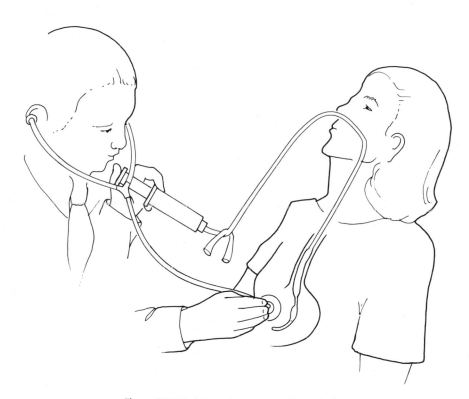

Figure PR23.2 Inject air to test position of tube.

5. *Anesthetize the nasal passages* and the posterior pharynx with Cetacaine spray.
   Thoroughly lubricate the nasal passage by injecting water-soluble jelly into the nostril; lubricate the SB tube and balloons as well.

6. *Insert the tip* of the SB tube in the nose *and gently advance* it straight back (not cephalad) into the pharynx. (See "Insertion of Nasogastric Tube," Procedure 21). If the patient can cooperate, passage of the tube into and down the esophagus is facilitated by having the patient swallow sips of water from a straw. Continue to advance the tube into the stomach until the 50-cm mark (on tube) is *at least* at or in the nose.

7. *Aspirate the gastric lumen.* Aspiration of blood from the gastric lumen of the tube does not necessarily mean the tip is in the stomach in this setting. Injection of air (20 ml)

into the gastric lumen with audible bubbling over the epigastrium provides better reassurance (Fig. PR23.2). If there is any question as to the position of the tube, partially retract it and reinsert it as far as possible. It is mandatory that the *gastric balloon* be *well within the stomach* before its inflation.

8. *Slowly inflate the gastric balloon* with only 50 ml of air (Fig. PR23.3). Be sure the correct lumen is being used (note markings on tube). Clamp the conical portion of the gastric balloon lumen with a rubber-shod clamp, and gently withdraw the tube until resistance is felt, indicating engagement of the gastric balloon at the gastroesophageal junction.

9. *Verify the position* of the tube once again by injecting air in the main lumen and listening for bubbling over the epigastrium.

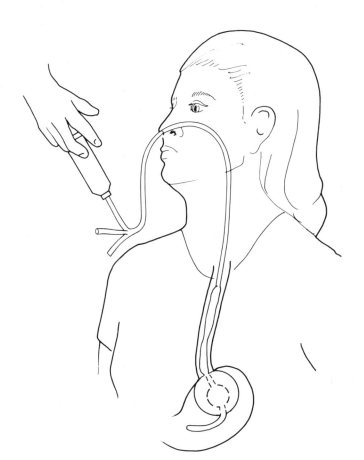

Figure PR23.3 Slowly inflate gastric balloon.

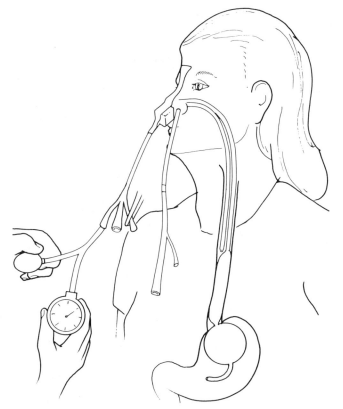

Figure PR23.4 Slowly inflate esophageal balloon, if necessary.

10. *Advance the tube* further down into the stomach before fully inflating the gastric balloon with an additional 200 ml of air and reclamping this lumen.

11. *Withdraw the tube* again until mild resistance is felt as the gastric balloon compresses the cardia.

12. *Place the foam rubber cube* around the tube and against the nose; tape it in place with a circumferential band of adhesive tape.

13. *Lavage the stomach* through the gastric lumen to remove clots, and connect this lumen to gentle suction.

14. *Insert the NG tube* through the opposite nostril and pass it into the esophagus to the predetermined level.

15. *Connect the NG tube* to a second suction apparatus to remove blood and secretions from the now occluded esophagus.

16. *Ascertain the rate of bleeding.* Gentle traction on the gastric balloon at the gastroesophageal junction may well gain control over the bleeding varices. Check the esophageal aspirate (NG tube) for fresh blood, and lavage the stomach through the gastric lumen of the SB tube to see if it clears. If bleeding continues, connect the esophageal balloon lumen to the mercury manometer through the Y connector (Fig. PR23.4) and slowly inflate the *esophageal balloon* with air to 30 mm Hg pressure. Clamp the esophageal balloon lumen to maintain this pressure and recheck at frequent intervals (every 30 minutes). If bleeding persists, the esophageal balloon may be inflated to a *maximum* of 45 mm Hg of baseline pressure.

17. *Additional traction* can be placed on the gastric balloon by attaching it to a traction helmet (e.g., football helmet with face guard) if bleeding is still uncontrolled. This maneuver should be considered *only* in patients with *exsanguinating hemorrhage* as a means of temporary control before surgical intervention. This degree of pressure on the gastric mucosa will cause necrosis within hours.

PITFALLS AND COMPLICATIONS

Most of the problems described for NG intubation in Procedure 21 also apply to SB intubation. The SB tubes pose the additional major threat of *dislodgement* and *major airway obstruction.* For this reason, a pair of sturdy scissors should be at the patient's bedside at all times. If at any time the patient develops obvious upper airway distress, the entire SB tube should be immediately transected to decompress both balloons and should be rapidly withdrawn (Fig. PR23.5).

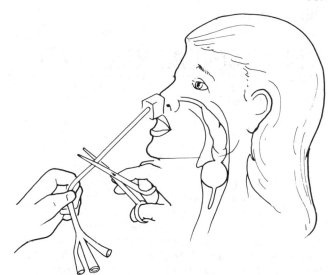

Figure PR23.5 Cut tube if airway distress ocurs.

Since SB tubes are not sump tubes, they are more prone to occlusion of the main gastric aspiration channel. They need to be frequently irrigated to ensure proper function. If the stomach is not thoroughly lavaged before insertion of the SB tube, this lumen is doomed to fail because of plugging with clotted blood.

Pulmonary aspiration is a common complication of SB tubes. It is best prevented by emptying the stomach before insertion of the SB tube and properly placing an NG tube above the esophageal balloon to remove blood and secretions from the esophagus. Prophylactic antibiotics should be considered.

Esophagogastric erosions readily occur with SB tubes because of mucosal sloughing in the regions of the two balloons and pressure necrosis. Thus the esophageal balloon should not be inflated at all if bleeding is controlled by the gastric balloon alone. The tube should not be put on tension unless absolutely necessary to control bleeding from gastric varices. If at all possible, removal of the SB tube should be accomplished within 48 hours; if not, the patient should be considered a candidate for emergency surgery.

Esophageal rupture is a catastrophic complication of SB tubes and is usually a result of inflation of the gastric balloon in the esophagus. For this reason, proper positioning of the tube before inflation of either balloon is absolutely mandatory. If there is any doubt as to the position of the tube, radiographic confirmation should be obtained *before* balloon inflation.

PROCEDURE 24

PERITONEAL LAVAGE

Edmund B. Cabot

Diagnostic lavage of the peritoneal cavity is the single most important tool in the evaluation of potential intraperitoneal injury following blunt abdominal trauma. Its principle use in this setting is the detection of hemorrhage into the free peritoneal cavity, which is most commonly the result of a ruptured spleen or laceration of the liver. The technique may also be used to detect leakage of bile following disruption of any portion of the biliary tree, free rupture of the bladder, and, in some cases, major pancreatic injury.

The diagnosis of significant intraabdominal injury as a result of blunt trauma, particularly in the multiple-trauma victim following, for example, a motor vehicle accident, may be difficult and is all too frequently delayed until the patient is in hypovolemic shock or diffuse peritonitis has become well established. Early recognition of potentially life-threatening injuries for which prompt surgical intervention is indicated is obviously in the patient's best interest, but many factors may obscure the need for immediate laparotomy. When there is an obvious penetrating injury to the abdomen or when plain films easily demonstrate free air in the peritoneal cavity, the decision to explore the abdomen is easy, and peritoneal lavage is a waste of time and may serve to spread contamination. On the other hand, the victim of multiple trauma may be comatose or in shock for any of a variety of reasons. In this setting, significant injury to an intraabdominal viscus may be overlooked, and diagnostic peritoneal lavage should be considered as a part of the initial evaluation.

The technique, although basically simple, requires some understanding of anatomy and considerable attention to detail in order for it to be useful and safe. This procedure should generally not be attempted alone without some prior experience.

INDICATIONS

- Multiple-trauma victims who may have sustained concomitant abdominal trauma
- Patients who have sustained potentially significant blunt abdominal trauma
- Presence of hypovolemic shock in the traumatized patient for whom there is no other obvious cause of significant blood loss

CONTRAINDICATIONS

- Obvious penetrating abdominal trauma
- Obvious free air in the peritoneal cavity on plain films (KUB, upright, or lateral decubitus)
- Patients for whom immediate laparotomy is otherwise indicated
- Patients who had previous abdominal surgery, particularly with lower abdominal incisions or known peritoneal adhesions
- Massively distended bowel on plain films
- Full urinary bladder
- Pregnancy

EQUIPMENT

- Surgical prep solution (e.g., povidone-iodine)
- Sterile gauze
- Sterile towels
- Mask, sterile gown, sterile gloves
- 1% lidocaine, preferably *with* epinephrine
- 5-ml syringe with 25- and 22-gauge needles
- Scalpel, preferably No. 15 blade, with handle
- Two curved hemostat clamps
- Peritoneal dialysis catheter with trochar
- Intravenous administration tubing and pole
- 1,000-ml bag or bottle of sterile Ringer's lactate for infusion
- 2-0 silk suture on cutting needle
- Gauze dressing
- Adhesive tape
- Blood specimen tubes with stoppers
- 20-ml syringe

POSITION

The patient should be in a supine position. Good lighting and a comfortable height provide a definite advantage.

PROCEDURE

1. *Decompress the bladder* by means of a Foley catheter placed to constant drainage using the usual sterile technique.

2. *Put on gown and gloves* in a sterile fashion with mask in place.

3. *Widely prepare* the lower abdomen with povidone-iodine or similar solution. The infraumbilical region is sterilely draped with towels or a fenestrated sheet.

4. *Infiltrate the skin* in the midline of the lower abdomen one-third the distance from the umbilicus to the pubis, using a 25-gauge needle on a 5-ml syringe, and 1% lidocaine with epinephrine.

5. *Infiltrate the subcutaneous tissues* down to the midline facia with additional 1% lidocaine, using a No. 22 needle.

6. *Make a vertical incision* in the skin approximately 2–4 cm in length, depending on the size of the patient and the amount of subcutaneous fat (Fig. PR24.1).

7. *Divide the subcutaneous fat,* usually by blunt dissection using the curved hemostats, until the midline facia (linea alba) is identified. This may be facilitated in the cooperative patient by asking him or her to lift his or her head off the stretcher. Care should be taken to avoid bleeding since this will subsequently produce false positive results.

8. *Incise the facia* vertically under direct vision (Fig. PR24.2).

9. *Expose the peritoneum* beneath the underlying fat and gently grasp it with both curved clamps.

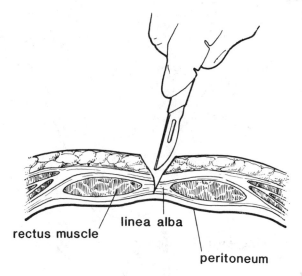

Figure PR24.2 Incise fascia.

10. *Elevate the peritoneum* by gentle upward traction on the clamps using the nondominant hand.

11. *Insert the dialysis catheter* with protruding trocar tip approximately 1 cm into the peritoneal cavity using a firm grasp with the dominant hand (Fig. PR24.3). Alternatively, a small (5-mm) nick can be made in the tented-up peritoneum and the catheter introduced without the trocar.

12. *Withdraw the trocar* once the tip of the catheter has clearly entered the free peritoneal cavity (Fig. PR24.4).

13. *Advance the catheter* alone until all of the holes are well within the abdominal cavity—approximately one-half the total catheter length. During this maneuver, the catheter may be directed toward the side of greatest clinical suspicion. If the patient experiences additional pain, withdraw the catheter slightly and readvance it in a slightly different direction (Fig. PR24.5).

14. *Attach an extension tube* to the catheter with an L connector (supplied with dialysis catheter) after sliding the fixation device down the catheter to the abdominal wall.

15. *Aspirate* with a 20-ml syringe (Fig. PR24.6). If gross blood, bile, or bowel contents are aspirated, the test is definitive and the catheter may be removed.

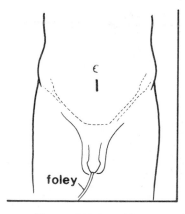

Figure PR24.1 Incision.

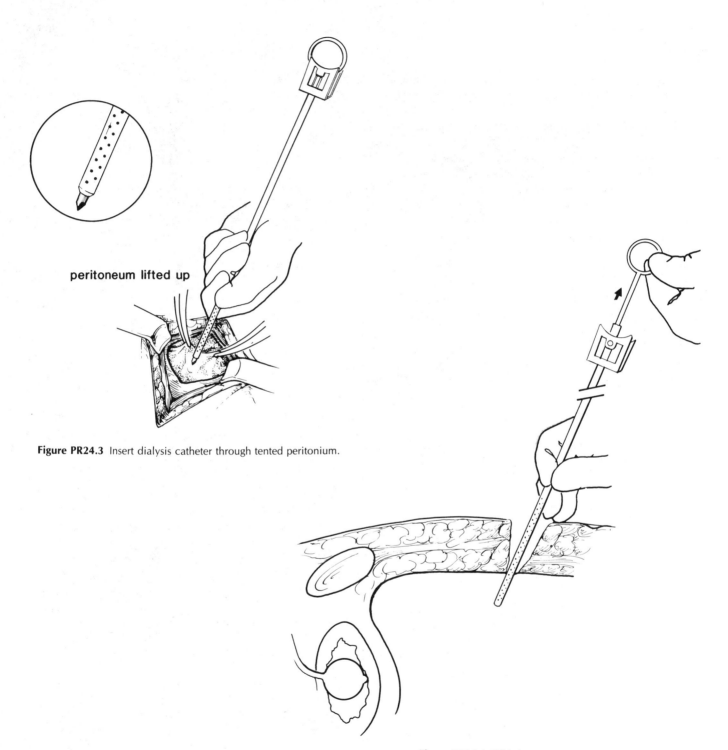

peritoneum lifted up

Figure PR24.3 Insert dialysis catheter through tented peritonium.

Figure PR24.4 Withdraw trocar.

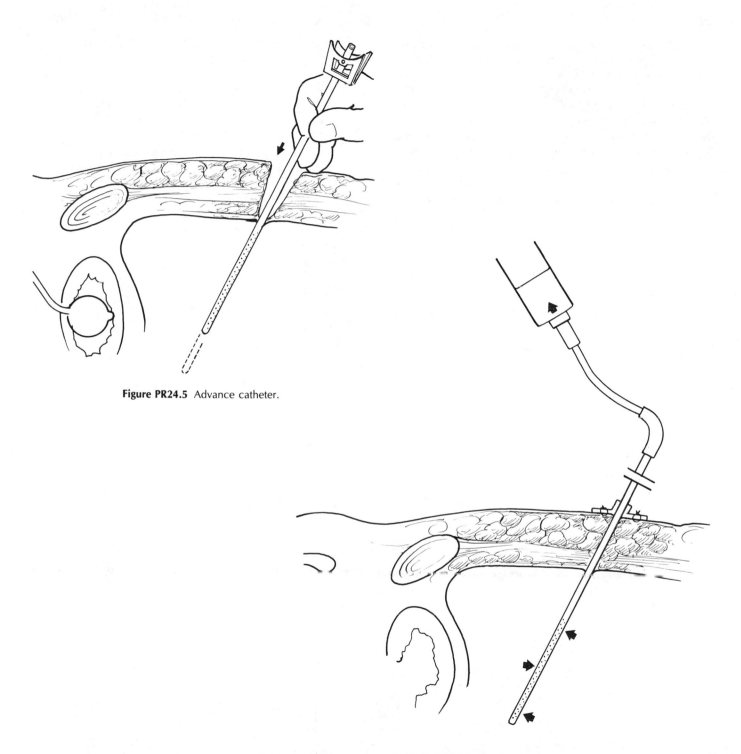

Figure PR24.5 Advance catheter.

Figure PR24.6 Attach tube and aspirate.

16. *Rapidly infuse* 1 liter of lactated Ringer's solution (assuming the initial aspirate is minimal or nondiagnostic) by replacing the syringe with intranveous administration tubing connected to an infusion bottle or bag on an intravenous pole (Fig. PR24.7).

17. *Suture the fixation device* to the skin with 2-0 silk suture.

18. *Roll the patient* from side to side, if possible, to disperse the fluid within the peritoneal cavity following infusion.

19. *Siphon the fluid* back out of the patient, when instillation and dispersal have been completed, by placing the solution bag or bottle below the patient (e.g., on the floor) while it is still connected to the dialysis catheter. Be sure to vent the solution bottle as needed.

20. *Evaluate the effluent.* If the unspun fluid is so red that newsprint cannot be read through it, there is a high probability of significant intraperitoneal bleeding requiring emergency laparotomy. Bloody fluid through which newsprint can be read is equivocal.

21. *Decant effluent* into several specimen tubes and send for red blood cell (RBC) count, hematocrit (HCT), white blood cell (WBC) count, total bilirubin, amylase, urea nitrogen, and culture (Table 24.1). An RBC count greater than

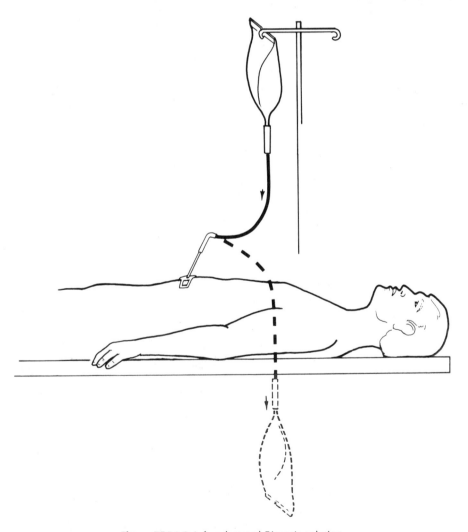

Figure PR24.7 Infuse lactated Ringer's solution.

100,000/mm³ of unspun fluid implies significant intra-peritoneal bleeding.

22. *Repeat the lavage* 1 hour later if the initial evaluation is equivocal.

TABLE 24.1 Positive Peritoneal Lavage

Qualitative
  Initial Aspirate
    Gross blood
    Obvious bile
    Bowel contents
  Lavage effluent
    Cannot read newsprint
    Bacteria on Gram stain
Quantitative
  RBC > 100,000/mm³
  HCT > 2%
  WBC > 500/mm³
  Amylase > 175 units/100 ml
  Increasing bilirubin
  Decreasing urea nitrogen

Alternative Technique

Another technique for performing diagnostic peritoneal lavage has recently been described and may prove to be even safer and simpler than the open technique described above. This method uses a guide wire for the introduction of a polytetrafluoroethylene (PTFE) (Teflon) catheter into the peritoneal cavity and is available commercially as a prepackaged kit (Lazarus-Nelson Peritoneal Lavage Tray, Kormed).

The indications, contraindications, basic equipment, position, insertion site, and preparation of the patient are the same as described above. The technique, illustrated in Figure PR24.8, is as follows;

1. *Decompress the bladder* by catheter drainage.

2. *Prepare and drape* the lower abdomen.

3. *Anesthetize* the skin and subcutaneous tissues at a point one-third the distance from the umbilicus to the pubis with 1% lidocaine with epinephrine.

4. *Incise the skin* 4–5 mm transversely. If a No. 11 blade is used, it may be possible to incise the linea alba blindly with the tip of the blade.

5. *Advance the 18-gauge needle* (supplied with the kit) through the skin incision and linea alba, aiming slightly inferiorly. A slight popping sensation may be noted as the peritoneum is punctured. This may be facilitated by having the patient lift his or her head to produce some tension of the abdominal wall.

6. *Introduce the guide wire* (supplied with the kit) through the needle, floppy end first. If it does not easily fall into the abdominal cavity, it should be pulled back and the needle advanced again into the free abdominal cavity. Once the guide wire is clearly well within the abdomen (roughly half its length), the needle is removed over the outer end of the wire.

7. *Advance the PTFE (Teflon) catheter* (supplied with the kit) over the wire and into the abdomen, while holding the outer end of the guide wire and using a twisting motion on the catheter.

8. *Remove the guide wire* once the catheter has been fully introduced and is being firmly held in position.

9. *Aspirate* the peritoneal cavity with a 10- or 20-ml syringe and proceed as necessary with peritoneal lavage as described above.

PITFALLS AND COMPLICATIONS

Perforation of a hollow viscus, such as a loop of bowel or the bladder, is an obvious catastrophy that will in and of itself require emergency laparotomy. This can usually be avoided by prior catheter drainage of the bladder, extreme caution in the presence of surgical scars, preliminary films to detect distended bowel, and attention to detail in introducing the catheter. Although blind insertion of the trocar–catheter apparatus through a tiny skin incision is used in some hospitals, it is clearly safer to identify the peritoneal surface visibly, as described above. Use of the alternative guide wire technique largely obviates this danger since the only sharp object entering the abdomen is an 18-guage needle, which carries minimal morbidity even if the bowel is punctured.

Intraperitoneal bleeding, iatrogenically caused, may be because of laceration of an omental vessel, a mesenteric vessel, or even the inferior vena cava or aorta. This will, at the very least, confuse the situation by resulting in a false-positive tap and may obviously result in an otherwise unnecessary laparotomy, both to control the bleeding and to rule out other sources. This catastrophy can be avoided by not advancing more than the tip of the trocar–catheter apparatus into the peritoneal cavity before withdrawing the trocar at least part way or by not using the trocar at all.

Bleeding from the incision is not only an annoyance but may result in an equivocal tap. This is best avoided by using the true midline approach and paying attention so as to avoid subcutaneous vessels when exposing the linea alba.

Pneumoperitoneum can be induced at the time of catheter insertion. This presents no great hazard by itself but may confuse subsequent evaluation of the patient. It is easily avoided by running Ringer's lactate into the administration tubing before its attachment to the dialysis catheter.

Peritonitis is an extremely rare complication of peritoneal lavage. Proper attention to aseptic techniques, use of the correct solution (lactated Ringer's for infusion), prompt removal of the dialysis catheter following diagnostic lavage, and compliance with the appropriate indications and contraindications (see above) will largely eliminate this risk.

Wound infection is also rare and can usually be avoided by aseptic techniques and prompt wound closure.

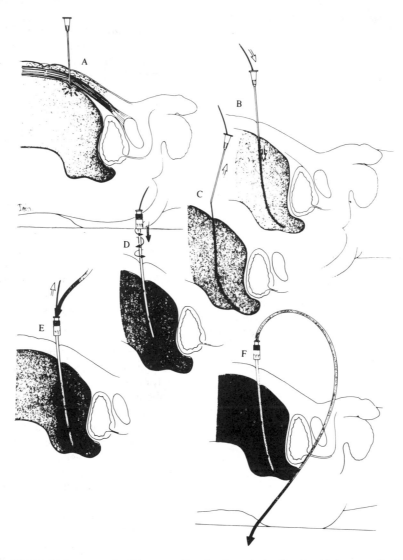

Figure PR24.8 (a) Insert needle; (b) pass guide wire through needle; (c) withdraw needle, leaving guide wire in place; (d) advance PTFI (Teflon) catheter over wire; (e) withdraw guide wire and infuse salt solution; (f) break seal on intravenous solution and allow peritoneal fluid to drain into infusion container. (Danto LA, Paracentesis and diagnostic peritoneal lavage, in Blaisdell FW, Trunkey DD (ed): Trauma Management, Vol I-Abdominal Trauma. Courtesy of Thieme-Stratton Inc., New York.)

PROCEDURE 25

ABDOMINAL TAP

Edmund B. Cabot

In patients with blunt abdominal trauma, diagnostic needle paracentesis, or the four-quadrant tap, has largely been replaced by the far more accurate technique of peritoneal lavage to detect significant intraabdominal injuries (Procedure 24). If, on the other hand, a patient has an obvious large collection of fluid in the free peritoneal cavity (i.e., ascites), the need may arise to obtain an aliquot of this fluid for diagnostic purposes. In such cases, needle aspiration of the fluid is clearly preferable to the more complicated and somewhat more hazardous technique of introducing a peritoneal dialysis catheter, as described for peritoneal lavage.

Occasionally, in the setting of obvious tense ascites with respiratory embarrassment as a result of inadequate diaphragmatic excursions, it may be desirable to decompress the abdomen slowly through a small catheter (as opposed to the relatively large dialysis catheter) introduced percutaneously. This will relieve the problem only temporarily since the offending ascites will usually reaccumulate. Conversely, rapid removal of large amounts of ascitic fluid, which may be possible through a dialysis catheter, may result in a sudden fall in blood pressure, particularly in patients with low serum oncotic pressure due to hypoalbuminemia.

In the nontrauma patient, paracentesis of any sort is rarely an emergency procedure. Few patients requiring this level of invasive diagnostic procedure would not be admitted to the hospital where the procedure could be performed on a more elective basis. Nonetheless, the physician in the emergency room will be able to perform the procedure just as safely and accurately as anyone else, provided certain simple principles of the technique are followed. Success is based on good judgement and some knowledge of anatomy.

INDICATIONS

Diagnostic

- Peritonitis of uncertain etiology with no localizing signs and obvious free peritoneal fluid (i.e., suspected infected or chemical ascites)
- Suspected primary peritonitis
- Suspected tuberculous peritonitis
- Suspected pancreatic ascites
- Suspected chylous ascites
- Suspected malignant ascites

Therapeutic

- Massive ascites causing respiratory embarrassment

CONTRAINDICATIONS

- Distended loops of bowel on x-ray study
- Known peritoneal adhesions
- Multiple previous abdominal incisions
- Obvious surgical pathology requiring laparotomy

EQUIPMENT

- Surgical prep solution (e.g., povidone-iodine)
- Sterile gauze
- Sterile towels
- Sterile gloves
- 1% lidocaine for injection
- 5-ml syringe with 25- and 22-gauge needles
- 18-gauge short-bevel Luer-Lok spinal needle
- 10-ml glass syringe
- 50-ml glass syringe
- Three-way stopcock
- Intravenous administration set (tubing)
- Empty, sterile, 1-liter bottle(s)
- 16-guage catheter-inside-needle unit (Intracath) (14-gauge needle)
- Blood specimen tubes with stoppers

POSITION

Usually the patient is supine or semirecumbent. The procedure may also be performed with the patient sitting up.

CHOICE OF SITE

The choice of site for paracentesis depends somewhat on the situation. Areas of previous abdominal surgery should obviously be avoided. An enlarged liver or distended gallbladder may make the right upper quadrant more hazardous. The left upper quadrant should be avoided if there is palpable splenomegaly. The lateral flank regions are unsafe because of the fixed position of the colon along the right and left gutters. Generally speaking, the safest sites for abdominal tap are either the right of left lower quadrant anteriorly, just lateral to the margin of the rectus muscle, or the infraumbilical midline (Fig. PR25.1).

PROCEDURE

1. *Obtain films* of the abdomen, including KUB and upright or cross-table lateral, to rule out the presence of distended loops of bowel or free air in the peritoneal cavity.
2. *Prepare the skin.* Wearing sterile gloves, the physician should prepare the selected area with povidone-iodine, using a circular motion moving away from the central point, and drape the area with sterile towels.
3. *Anesthetize the skin by infiltrating* it with 1% lidocaine, using 5-ml syringe and 25-gauge needle.
4. *Assemble the equipment.* Attach a 50-ml glass syringe to one arm of a three-way stopcock and intravenous tubing

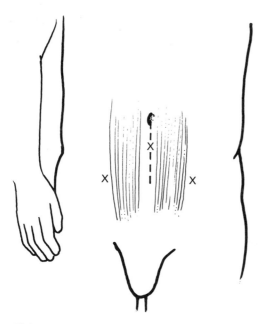

Figure PR25.1 Usual positions for abdominal tap.

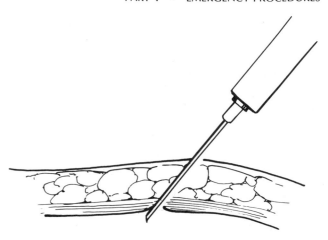

Figure PR25.2 Withdraw fluid.

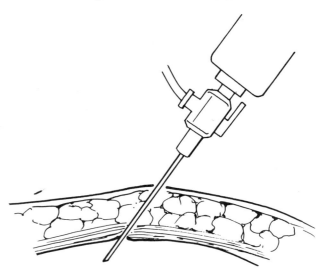

Figure PR25.3 Stopcock assembly for withdrawal of a large amount of fluid.

(with collection bottle) to a second arm. Be sure to understand how the three-way valve works, and have this all assembled and ready to attach when needed.

5. *Perform paracentesis.* A short-bevel 18-gauge Luer-Lok spinal needle is advanced bimanually, with stylet in place, through the anesthetized skin and abdominal wall. Entry into the free peritoneal cavity is usually easy to detect by the sudden decrease in force needed to advance the needle. Remove the stylet and attach a 10-ml glass syringe to the spinal needle. Withdraw fluid to confirm the needle's position within the peritoneal cavity (Fig. PR25.2). If a diagnostic

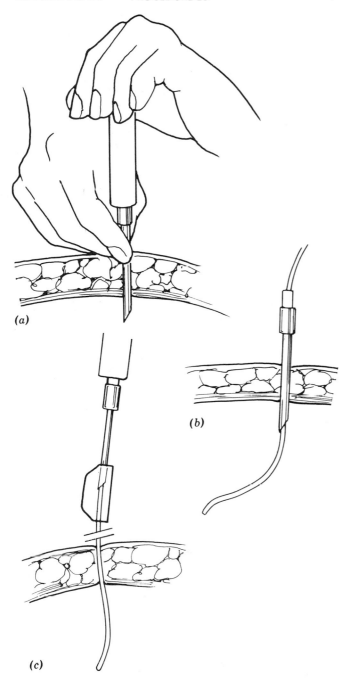

(a)

(b)

(c)

Figure PR25.4 (a) Insert 16-gauge catheter-inside-needle unit; (b) insert catheter; (c) withdraw needle, attach needle guard, and attach to intravenous tubing.

tap is all that is indicated and only a small aliquot (10 ml) of fluid is all that is needed, then *withdraw* the needle and syringe as a unit and place the fluid in the appropriate tube(s).

6. *If a therapeutic tap* is indicated or a large amount of fluid is required (as for cytology), remove the 10-ml syringe and replace it with the preassembled stopcock apparatus. By proper operation of the stopcock valve, fluid can be aspirated from the peritoneal cavity and expelled into the collection bottle (Fig. PR25.3).

7. *An alternative method* for the removal of large amounts of fluid (500 ml or more) is to use a 16-gauge catheter-inside-needle unit in lieu of the spinal needle, provided the patient is not too obese to permit penetration of the full thickness of the abdominal wall with this relatively short needle (Fig. PR25.4a). After positioning the catheter well within the abdominal cavity and withdrawing the needle, the catheter stylet is removed and the catheter is connected to intravenous tubing (Fig. PR25.4b,c). Fluid can then be syphoned off by placing the collection bottle below the patient and readjusting the position of the catheter from time to time to ensure continued flow.

PITFALLS AND COMPLICATIONS

Puncturing the bladder is easy to avoid by requiring the patient to void beforehand, percussing the lower abdomen, or placing a Foley catheter beforehand, if needed.

Puncturing other organs is also usually avoidable by a thorough physical examination, adequate plain films of the abdomen, and avoidance of obvious adhesions, scars, organomegaly, and distended loops of bowel. Thinking about the possible hazards of a procedure goes a long way toward avoiding complications.

Peritonitis as a result of the introduction of pathogens is an uncommon complication of routine paracentesis provided adequate aseptic technique is used.

Failure to obtain fluid suggests either an incorrect diagnosis of ascites or malposition of the paracentesis needle. The latter can either be because of failure to penetrate the entire abdominal wall and enter the peritoneal cavity or because of obstruction by intraabdominal tissues, such as omentum or bowel wall, in which case the needle should be withdrawn and reintroduced.

Laceration of an intraabdominal organ with resultant bleeding or spillage of bowel contents can be avoided by never moving the needle in any direction other than along its main axis.

PROCEDURE 26

URETHRAL CATHETERIZATION

Peter T. Nieh

Urethral catheterization is a frequently used procedure that provides great relief with negligible discomfort when performed properly. On the other hand, it may induce injury and pain when attempted precipitiously or recklessly. The basic urethral catheters are illustrated in Figure PR26.1. The standard *Foley catheter* is a single lumen, blunt-tipped straight catheter with a retaining balloon lumen. The irrigating Foley catheter, so-called *three-way catheter,* has in addition another lumen for irrigating solutions. The *coudé catheter* has a more narrow and angulated tip to permit insertion over an obstruction, such as a median lobe or posterior bladder neck. The protuberance at the drainage end indicates the direction of the angulated tip to aid in guiding the catheter. The *whistle-tip catheter* is a large-bore, single lumen tube with a generous end hole, making it ideal for irrigation removal of larger clots. With any of the catheters, undue force will traumatize the urethra. Proper positioning of the catheter is essential before balloon inflation.

INDICATIONS

- Urinary retention
- Gross hematuria with clots
- Sterile urinary collection for culture specimen
- Intermittent catheterization in neurogenic bladder

CONTRAINDICATIONS

- Acute prostatitis
- Acute epididymitis
- Pelvic fracture with blood at the urethral meatus, as there may be incomplete urethral disruption
- Recent transurethral resection of the prostate—should be approached with great caution since traumatic catheterization may easily undermine the bladder neck

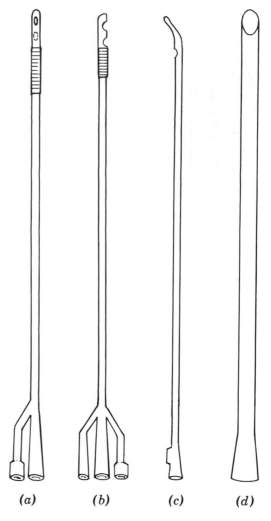

(a)   **(b)**   **(c)**   **(d)**

Figure PR26.1 The commonly used urethral catheters: (a) Foley catheter (b) irrigating (3-way Foley catheter); (c) Coude catheter; (d) Whistle-tip catheter.

EQUIPMENT

- Urethral catheter
- Antiseptic solution for cleansing, for example, povidone-iodine solution
- Sterile gloves
- Sterile drapes
- Water-soluble lubricating jelly
- Culture vial

- Syringe with saline to inflate retaining balloon
- 2% lidocaine jelly—may be used in the anxious patient for urethral instillation, providing excellent topical anesthesia within 5 minutes to facilitate catheterization
- Urinary drainage bag
- Adhesive tape

POSITION

The patient is placed supine with the thighs partially abducted. Access to the female urethral meatus is improved by having the patient draw up the knees into a frog-leg position.

PROCEDURE

Male

1. *Apply sterile drape* around penile shaft.
2. *Prepare glans*—retract foreskin, if necessary, to expose meatus; prepare with the antiseptic solution (Fig. PR26.2).
3. *Lubricate catheter tip* generously.
4. *Introduce catheter* into meatus (Fig. PR26.3).
5. *Advance catheter* up to balloon sidearm. With the penis pulled taut and almost horizontal, the catheter glides easily with only slight resistance and some discomfort just as the catheter traverses the external sphincter. *Never force a catheter in attempting to bypass an obstruction.*

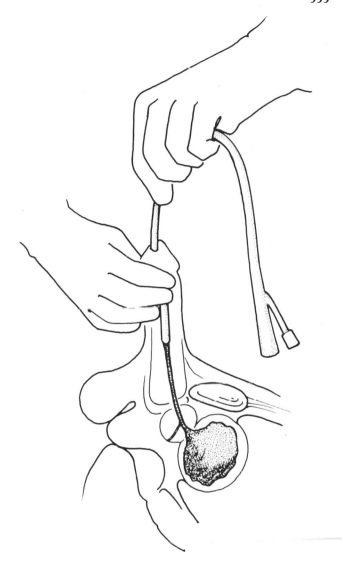

Figure PR26.3 Introduce lubricated catheter.

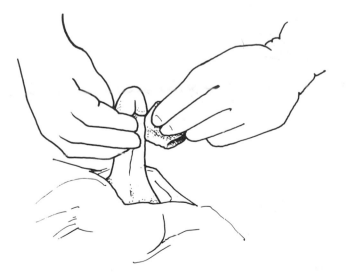

Figure PR26.2 Retract foreskin and prepare area.

6. *Obtain urine specimen.* Gentle irrigation with sterile saline may be required to establish flow and verify catheter position.
7. *Inflate retaining balloon* with sterile saline (usually 5 ml) (Fig. PR26.4). If pain is encountered, the catheter may well be in the prostatic urethra. Deflate the balloon and reposition the catheter. If this is unsuccessful but the catheter still drains, secure the catheter to the penile shaft with tape, leaving the balloon deflated.

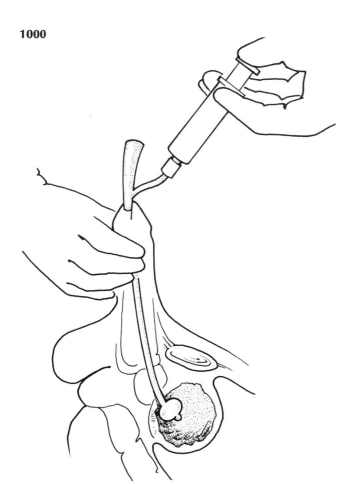

Figure PR26.4 Inflate balloon.

8. *Withdraw catheter* gently to seat balloon against bladder neck.
9. *Connect catheter to drainage bag.*
10. *Secure drainage tubing* with tape to medial thigh to prevent accidental dislodgement. (Fig. PR26.5)

Female

1. *Prepare the perineum and vaginal introitus* with antiseptic solution.
2. *Expose urethral meatus* by spreading the labia. Gauze sponges packed into the posterior vagina can facilitate exposure in difficult cases of obesity, redundant vaginal mucosa, or a recessed meatus (Fig. PR26.6).
3. *Lubricate catheter tip* generously.
4. *Introduce catheter* into meatus.
5. *Advance catheter* about half-way.
6. *Obtain urine specimen.* Gentle irrigation with sterile saline will help ascertain proper positioning within bladder.
7. *Inflate retaining balloon* with 5 ml sterile saline.
8. *Withdraw catheter gently* to position against bladder neck.
9. *Connect to drainage bag.*
10. *Secure drainage tubing* with tape to medial thigh to prevent accidental dislodgment.

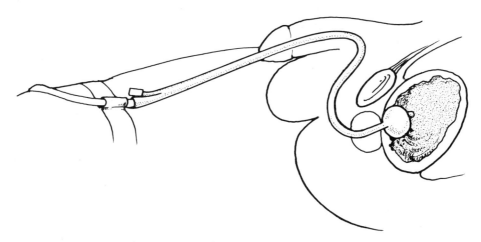

Figure PR26.5 Secure drainage tubing.

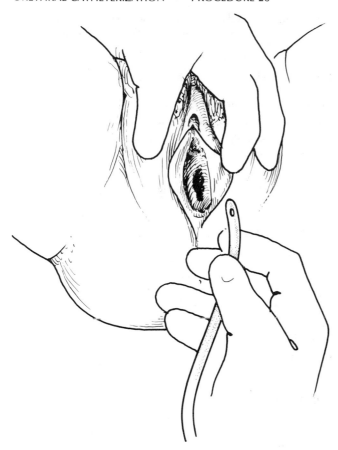

Figure PR26.6 Expose urethral meatus in preparation for catheterization of a female patient.

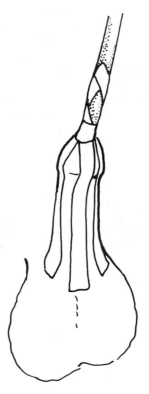

Figure PR26.7 Catheter can be taped to penile shaft in uncooperative patient and the balloon left deflated.

PITFALLS AND COMPLICATIONS

In *anxious patients,* especially younger men, 2% lidocaine jelly instilled in the meatus is an excellent topical anesthesia for any urethral instrumentation.

In *uncooperative patients,* especially those who are confused or combative, one must carefully secure the drainage tubing to the medial thigh to prevent its withdrawal. Restraints may be necessary to prevent the patient from removing the catheter with the balloon inflated. In some instances, we may consider leaving the balloon deflated and merely using tape along the penile shaft to secure the urethral catheter (Fig. PR26.7).

In cases of *meatal stenosis,* the narrowed meatus may be enlarged by a meatotomy with local anesthetic (see Chapter 33).

In cases of *urethral obstruction,* a small pediatric No.5F or 8F feeding catheter may bypass a urethral lesion. Lidocaine jelly is often helpful. Urethral sounds, filiforms, and follower catheters should be left to the urologist, but a suprapubic catheterization (Procedure 27) could be easily performed when unable to catheterize urethrally.

In patients with *recent prostatectomy* use a No.18F or 20F coudé-tipped catheter to get over the posterior bladder neck. Gentle elevation with the finger in the rectum may assist in this maneuver.

Traumatic catheterization may occur with inflation of the balloon in the prostatic urethra or with forceful insertion of a catheter, resulting in a false passage, such as perforation of the urethral mucosa or undermining of the bladder neck. Bleeding and the increased risk of infection are to be expected. A single gentle attempt at repositioning or replacing the catheter may be attempted, but suprapubic catheterization may be necessary. Broad-spectrum antibiotics are recommended for prophylaxis.

Hematuria may occur with traumatic catheterization or decompression of an overdistended bladder. Some advocate that slow drainage of the bladder will diminish the bleeding from ruptured submucosal veins. Usually a generous fluid intake is sufficient to prevent clots from occluding the catheter.

Sepsis is a danger with any difficult catheterization or when urethral or prostatic infection is present. In any case except simple catheterizations, a parenteral antibiotic (e.g., aminoglycoside or cephalosporin) followed by oral suppressive medications (e.g., methenamine, sulfisoxazole) are good precautions.

Urethral stricture is a long-term complication that is caused by urethral mucosal injury or pericatheter urethral infection. It is best avoided by a gentle catheterization technique, minimizing traction on the catheter by securing the drainage tubing, and using a polytetrafluoroethylene (PTFE)-coated (Teflon-coated) or silicone catheter of small caliber (No.16F or 18F).

PROCEDURE 27

SUPRAPUBIC CATHETERIZATION

Peter T. Nieh

Suprapubic catheterization is a technique that has simplified the management of urinary retention in situations in which urethral instrumentation is neither feasible nor advisable. Simple suprapubic aspiration of the distended bladder will provide rapid temporary relief when awaiting arrival of a urologist or during transfer to another facility. The technique described below uses the readily available intravenous catheters that are used for access through the subclavian or internal jugular route.

Dow Corning markets a silastic cystocatheter (No.8F and 12F) apparatus with a stopcock and faceplate to secure tubing.*

INDICATIONS

- Failed urethral catheterization
- Known urethral strictures or false passage
- Urinary retention with prostatitis–epididymitis in which case a urethral catheter will aggravate the infection
- Periurethral abscess
- Urethral rupture following pelvic fracture

CONTRAINDICATIONS

- Previous intraabdominal surgery involving the pelvis since small bowel may be encountered beneath the inferior portion of the incision. Prior extraperitoneal surgery, however, usually will not affect the procedure.
- Gross hematuria with clots since the suprapubic catheter lumen is inadequate to evacuate clots.
- Contracted, or decompressed, bladder.

EQUIPMENT

- Prep razor
- Antiseptic prep solution
- Sterile gloves
- Sterile drape and sponges
- 1% lidocaine 5ml
- 6-ml syringe
- 20-gauge spinal needle
- No.11 scalpel blade and handle
- No.14- or 16-gauge intravenous catheter with needle (catheter-inside-needle units), 8-in. long
- 0-0 or 2-0 silk suture
- Drainage tubing (intravenous tubing)
- Drainage bag (ureteral or biliary drainage device or empty intravenous bottle)
- Povidone-iodine ointment
- Adhesive tape

*Dow Corning Cystocath Suprapubic Drainage System, Dow Corning Corporation Medical Products, Midland, Michigan 48640

POSITION

The patient must be supine.

PROCEDURE

1. *Palpate or percuss the bladder* (Fig. PR27.1).
2. *Shave and prepare* the suprapubic area.
3. *Inject local anesthetic,* using spinal needle after wheal has been raised. Select a site one to two finger breadths above the symphysis pubis in the midline. Infiltrate widely.
4. *Localize bladder* directing the spinal needle roughly 30 deg from the vertical in the midline, aiming for the tip of the coccyx (Fig. PR27.2). Aspirate frequently to ascertain entry into bladder. If we are unable to enter bladder and the bladder can not be percussed, after about 1 hour reassess the need for drainage. Otherwise the risk for inadvertent perforation of the bowel is increased.
5. *Incise skin* making a 2–3-mm stab incision with a No. 11 blade.
6. *Insert catheter-inside-needle unit into bladder.* Attach the syringe onto the needle and carefully guide it toward the bladder as with the spinal needle previously. There will be a slight resistance as the rectus fascia is penetrated, and the urine will be aspirated into the syringe as the

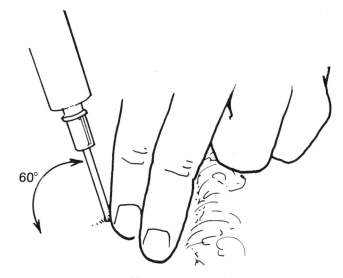

Figure PR27.2 Localize bladder.

bladder is entered. Advance the needle another 2 cm to be sure this is well within the bladder.

7. *Insert the catheter* through the needle after removing the syringe. Twist and lock the catheter and needle hubs (Fig. PR27.3).
8. *Withdraw needle and catheter together* from bladder and apply protective clip to needle tip (Fig. PR27.3).
9. *Ascertain proper position* in bladder by aspirating.
10. *Secure catheter* with silk sutures (Fig. PR27.4).
11. *Attach catheter to urinary drainage tubing and bag.*
12. *Apply sterile dressing;* use povidone-iodine ointment around entry site.
13. *Secure drainage tubing* with tape.

PITFALLS AND COMPLICATIONS

Minor degrees of *hematuria* are common after suprapubic catheterization; it is related to the bladder entry site and bleeding from ruptured submucosal veins following decompression. Generous hydration minimizes the risk of clotting.

If prior surgical adhesions fix the bowel into the pelvis, the *bowel may be penetrated.* Localized pain and low-grade fever may occur. Placement of the catheter may be confirmed by

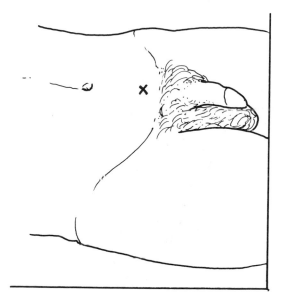

Figure PR27.1 Palpate distended bladder.

injecting contrast medium through the catheter; if the tubing is outside of the bladder, it should be removed. This complication is avoided by staying in the midline close to the pubis aiming carefully for the coccyx, and waiting until the bladder is palpable.

Poor drainage may occur if the catheter tip migrates into the prostatic urethra, thus occluding the lumen. Or else the catheter may become lodged against a mucosal fold, thus impeding drainage. Gentle irrigation with 25–50 ml saline may be necessary to establish flow. Injection of contrast material may be required to check for position. If the catheter is flexible enough, extra side holes near the tip may be added to improve drainage before advancing through the needle.

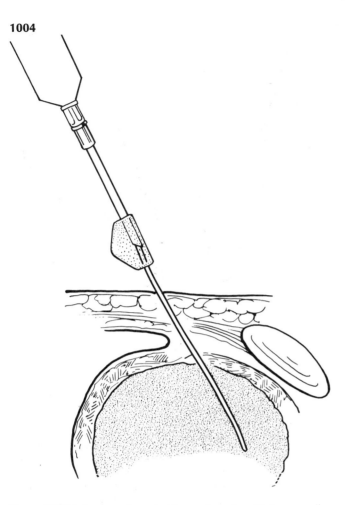

Figure PR27.3 Insert catheter-inside-needle unit, withdraw needle, and attach needle guard.

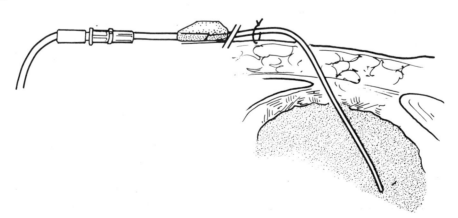

Figure PR27.4 Secure catheter with suture and attach to drainage tubing.

PROCEDURE 28

PROCTO-SIGMOIDOSCOPY

Edmund B. Cabot

Although sigmoidoscopy is often thought of as a procedure performed only by colorectal specialists in elective situations after adequate cleansing of the lower bowel, it can often be of important diagnostic and/or therapeutic value in the emergency room setting (Chapter 35).

The indications for sigmoidoscopy in the emergency room vary considerably with the availability of time and equipment and the experience of the physician. In many cases that are neither chronic nor urgent, the patient may best be served by a course of enemas or cathartics and elective examination under ideal circumstances, such as in the endoscopy suite at a later date. This is often the situation with both outpatients and patients being admitted to the hospital.

When necessary, the procedure, which is not very demanding, can be done when the patient is in bed or on a stretcher, that is, any place that has some privacy, and with only a few essential items of equipment. There are certain relatively urgent situations confronting the emergency room physician when proctoscopy is an important part of the diagnostic evaluation and may be the format for therapeutic intervention as well.

The decision to perform this procedure in the emergency room depends on the circumstances. There are no hard rules concerning the indications. The physician must decide on the basis of the patient's history and physical examination, which must include a careful anorectal examination (Chapter 35).

INDICATIONS

Diagnostic

- Rectal bleeding
- Rectal pain
- Rectal trauma
- Palpable rectal mass
- Tenesmus

- Obstipation
- Large bowel obstruction
- History of inflammatory bowel disease
- History of rectal tumor

Therapeutic

- Sigmoid volvulus
- Fecal impaction
- Rectal foreign body

CONTRAINDICATIONS

- Colonic perforation
- Impending barium enema
- Massive ongoing rectal bleeding

EQUIPMENT

- Proctosigmoidoscope (25 cm) with obturator, light source, occlusive eyepiece, and insufflation bulb
- Rubber examining gloves
- Ample water-soluble lubricating jelly
- Long, rigid suction cannula with tubing
- Long, large cotton swabs
- Long biopsy forceps
- Specimen bottle(s), 10% formalin
- Source of constant suction with trap

POSITION

From the examiner's standpoint, the patient is best placed in the knee–chest position. This position allows the abdominal contents to fall away from the pelvic floor and facilitates passage of the sigmoidoscope beyond the peritoneal reflection (15–17 cm from the anus) and into the sigmoid colon to its maximum length (22–25 cm). The examiner stands directly behind the patient at the foot of the examining table with unobstructed maneuverability.

However, the knee–chest position is often poorly tolerated by elderly, debilitated, obese, or acutely ill patients, and it may be difficult to execute in cramped quarters or in a regular hospital bed. Under these circumstances, the left lateral (Sims) position may be more appropriate (Fig. PR28.1). If the hips are fully flexed with the knees drawn up as far as possible and the patient's buttocks positioned beyond the edge of the stretcher or bed, the lateral decubitus position with the examiner sitting down usually permits satisfactory examination.

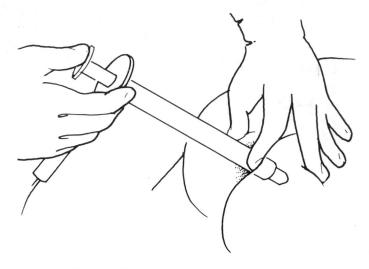

Figure PR28.2 Introduce the sigmoidoscope.

PROCEDURE

1. *Set the stage.* Explain the procedure to the patient, including the possibility of experiencing a cramping or bloating sensation associated with the insufflation of air. Drape the patient and take whatever steps are possible to ensure the patient's sense of modesty. Examining gloves should be worn, and the equipment should be placed within easy reach of the examiner. It is often helpful to have an assistant or nurse available to hand things to the examiner and to reassure the patient.

2. *Perform the physical examination.* Inspect the perineum and perianal region (Chapter 36). Perform thorough digital rectal examination with a well-lubricated, gloved index finger.

3. *Prepare the equipment.* Check the light source and insufflation balloon for proper function before introducing the sigmoidoscope. Place the obturator in the sigmoidoscope and generously lubricate the tip of the obturator and distal end of the sigmoidoscope.

4. *Insert the sigmoidoscope.* Separate the buttocks with the nondominant hand, while holding the sigmoidoscope by its proximal end, using the thumb to support the obturator (Fig. PR28.2). Gently insert the sigmoidoscope in the anal canal until the distal end of the scope is judged to be just within the rectal ampulla (4–6 cm). Remove the obturator (Fig. PR28.3) and attach an eyepiece with a light source and insufflator (Fig. PR28.4). *Do not* under any circum-

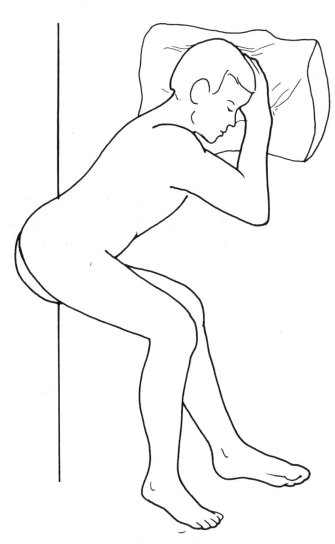

Figure PR28.1 Left lateral (Sim's) position.

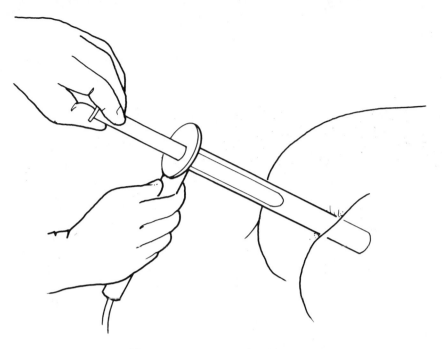

Figure PR28.3 Remove the obturator.

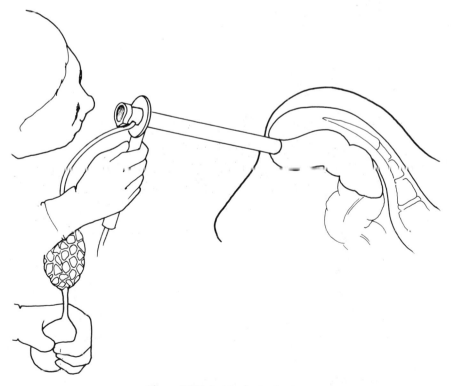

Figure PR28.4 Attach eyepiece.

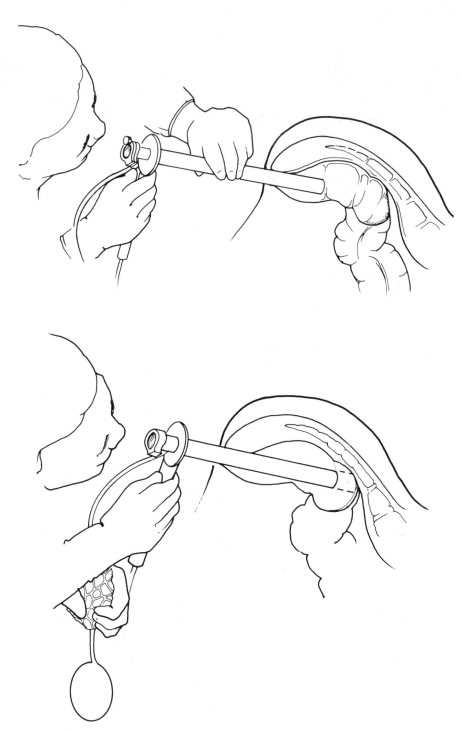

Figure PR28.5 Advance sigmoidoscope, always under direct vision.

stances advance the sigmoidoscope unless the bowel lumen is clearly visible.

5. *Advance the sigmoidoscope under direct vision* with the eyepiece closed and the light source on; initially aim it posteriorly toward the sacrum. Insufflate air only as necessary to distend the bowel slightly and visualize the lumen. This is done by steadying the shaft of the sigmoidoscope with one hand resting on the buttock while the other hand pumps air into the insufflator balloon and then gently compresses the balloon, while observing the lumen of the rectum (Fig. PR28.5). Slowly advance the scope in this manner until resistance is met, or the lumen can no longer be visualized, or the patient complains of increased pain. *Do not force the scope beyond this point.* In the well-prepared bowel, the experienced examiner is usually able to pass the scope above the peritoneal reflection. At this point, the bowel usually takes a fairly sharp turn, but by gentle insufflation and angulation of the scope, it is possible to negotiate the turn with minimal patient discomfort (Fig. PR28.5 bottom). If the view is obscured by blood, mucous, enema fluid, or liquid feces, the eyepiece is opened (releasing the air), and suction or swabs are used. It may be helpful to wipe off the window in the eyepiece in order to remove condensation or other fluid obscuring the view.

6. *Inspect the lumen.* Having reached the limit of insertion, the sigmoidoscope is very slowly withdrawn while the bowel mucosa is examined circumferentially. This is best accomplished while one hand supports the scope at the anus and serves as a fulcrum while the other hand moves the scope in gentle circles and slowly withdraws. Note the appearance of the rectal mucosa generally, and record the level (from the anus) of any specific lesions. Obtain biopsy specimens when appropriate, using the long biopsy forceps. Open the eyepiece to release residual air before completing removal of the sigmoidoscope from the rectal ampulla.

PITFALLS AND COMPLICATIONS

Bowel perforation is an uncommon, but catastrophic, complication of proctosigmoidoscopy that is generally avoidable by meticulous attention to the above techniques. Above all, *do not* advance the scope blindly or use excessive force. Be sure the lumen is in view as the scope is advanced. Avoid the use of excessive insufflation of air. Obtain biopsy specimens of lesions only when they are clearly seen, and avoid a tearing motion with the forceps or excessive depth within the bowel wall. Sigmoidoscopy should not be performed if perforation is already suspected.

Bleeding into the lumen makes an examination impossible. Sigmoidoscopy should not be attempted in the face of overt, ongoing hematochezia. Avoid taking a biopsy specimen of vascular appearing lesions. Avoid excessive angulation of the scope that may tear the mucosa. Avoid the use of force. If electrocautery is available; it may be used very gingerly for brief periods to control bleeding from biopsy sites, but it is usually unnecessary. A previous history of coagulation defects is a contraindication to rectal biopsy.

Patient discomfort is highly variable. Gentleness and reassurance are paramount. Avoid excessive use of insufflation that may produce considerable cramping sensations.

Failure to visualize the lumen of the well-prepared bowel is usually a function of inexperience. It is helpful to think anatomically while advancing the sigmoidoscope, remembering the initial posterior angulation of the rectum along the cup of the sacrum and its sharp angulation at the peritoneal reflection (usually to the left).

PROCEDURE 29

LUMBAR PUNCTURE

Lewis Sudarsky

The examination of cerebrospinal fluid (CSF) and the measurement of intracranial pressure are important in the diagnoses and management of a wide range of neurologic and systemic diseases. Information gained through lumbar puncture (LP) is vital in the diagnoses of infections and inflammatory and neoplastic diseases involving the nervous system. Prompt LP and early initiation of therapy directly affect the outcome of patients with bacterial meningitis. Lumbar puncture is thus imperative in cases of suspected meningitis and in septic patients in general, especially neonates. Although the widespread availability of computed tomography (CT) has replaced LP as a first diagnostic procedure in many neurologic situations, determination of intracranial pressure and the knowledge of bleeding into the subarachnoid space may require a spinal tap. In a community hospital, a psychiatric facility, or even in a teaching hospital, LP is often done incorrectly; and as a general rule, the technique is grossly underutilized.

INDICATIONS

Diagnostic

It is difficult to catalogue the indications for diagnostic and therapeutic LP fully. Common indications for LP as an accident floor procedure are considered below.

CLINICAL SUSPICION OF MENINGITIS

Prompt LP for culture, blood cell count, and chemical examination is imperative.

TO RULE OUT INTRACRANIAL INFECTION

Lumbar puncture is particularly indicated in the septic patient, the febrile patient with abnormal mental status, and the immunoincompetent patient with altered mental status (even in the absence of fever). Patients in the latter category should include alcoholics, neonates, and the elderly. It is difficult to generalize about such cases, and LP should be considered as part of a thoughtful assessment of the individual problem.

CLINICAL SUSPICION OF INTRACRANIAL HEMORRHAGE, ESPECIALLY SUBARACHNOID HEMORRHAGE

CT has largely replaced LP as the first procedure of choice in patients suspected of having an intracranial hemorrhage, especially the somnolent patient with focal signs. However, subsequent LP is often necessary to confirm bleeding in such patients. In small aneurysmal hemorrhages, the CT scan may fail to demonstrate blood. Lumbar puncture should thus be considered before dismissing the patient with the acute onset of "the worst headache of my life" as a benign headache disorder. Lumbar puncture is also done to rule out intracranial bleeding in stroke patients before initiation of anticoagulation. Start of anticoagulent therapy should be deferred 4–6 hours after LP to prevent lumbar extradural or subdural bleeding (see below).

TO DIAGNOSE IMMUNE MEDIATED ACUTE NEUROLOGIC DISEASE

Particular cases of immune mediated acute neurologic disease include acute multiple sclerosis, which may show lymphocytosis and abnormal immunoglobulins in the spinal fluid. Guillain-Barré syndrome may be diagnosed by finding high CSF protein and a minimal cellular response in patients with an early acute neuropathy (gait unsteadiness, distal weakness and vibratory loss, absent ankle reflexes). Such patients require hospitalization in a unit specialized for respiratory care. Acute

psychosis is a common presenting feature of central nervous system (CNS) lupus, the activity of which can be assessed by monitoring pleocytosis, protein, and complement in CSF.

CANCER PATIENTS

Cytologic examination of the spinal fluid is often important in patients with neoplastic disease, that is, patients with leukemia, lymphoma, or systemic cancer who develop neurologic illness. Examination of the CSF is essential to diagnoses of leptomeningeal cancer and may provide a clue to parenchymal involvement of nervous structures. LP is not always the first study in such cases; it should be undertaken in conjunction with neurologic consultants.

FEBRILE PATIENTS WITH SEIZURE

LP is often indicated as a general diagnostic test in patients with a variety of acute conditions. The onset of seizures in a febrile patient, including the first febrile seizure in a child, warrants LP since meningitis or encephalitis commonly present as childhood seizures. Acute change of mental state in an adult is another such situation, though many of the acute confusional states have toxic or metabolic bases.

THERAPEUTIC LUMBAR PUNCTURE

Removal of spinal fluid may be used as a therapeutic procedure in patients with compensated adult hydrocephalus, meningitis, or pseudotumor cerebri who have become acutely symptomatic. Lumbar puncture is also done as part of other acute diagnostic and therapeutic procedures (e.g., myelography, intrathecal chemotherapy).

CONTRAINDICATIONS

Absolute

In the presence of suspected bacterial meningitis, there are no absolute contraindications to LP. There are, however, a number of strong relative risks that should be taken into account in a balanced clinical decision regarding LP.

Relative

BLEEDING RISK

Patients with fewer than 20,000 platelets and patients on full therapeutic anticoagulation are at risk for hemorrhagic complications of the procedure. Lumbar extradural and subdural hematoma may complicate the procedure even if no obvious traumatic tap is encountered. This infrequent complication of LP is serious and may result in persistent saddle anesthesia and sphincteric disturbance. An LP should be undertaken only after thrombocythemia is corrected with platelet transfusion; anticoagulation may be partially reversed with fresh frozen plasma when the prothrombin time exceeds 18/12.

PAPILLEDEMA OR INTRACRANIAL MASS

The most feared complication of LP is the possibility of aggravating or precipitating a herniation syndrome in patients with an intracranial mass. There is controversy about the degree of risk involved. Most studies on the subject suggest that the risk of herniation after LP in such cases is low, probably less than 3%. Before the advent of CT scanning, LP and pneumoencephalography were done routinely in patients with brain tumors. Most neurologists, however, are familiar with a case or two in which deterioration occurred within 12 hours of the procedure.

In theory, the risk derives from the displacement of brain within the intracranial compartment, which can be facilitated by the acute removal of CSF from below, the creation of a dural "leak," and the creation of a pressure gradient across the tentorium or foramen magnum.

The preferred procedure is to obtain a CT scan when a patient with papilledema or suspected intracranial mass requires an LP. (Papilledema may take 12–24 hours to emerge after an acute event; its absence does not imply normal pressure.) If there is no evidence of midline shift or displacement of the ventricular system, LP should be done to record the pressure and facilitate diagnosis. In patients with midline displacement or an intracranial mass deforming the brain and ventricles, we prefer to avoid routine studies of CSF. It is occasionally necessary to perform LP in such patients, for example, the patient with known brain metastases and suspected bacterial meningitis. In such cases, LP should be done with extreme caution, in the hospital, under neurologic or neurosurgical supervision. A No.22 or smaller needle is preferred.

SOFT TISSUE INFECTION IN THE LUMBAR REGION

Pyogenic infection of the skin or soft tissue overlying the lumbar spinal canal is a contraindication to LP. To puncture the subarachnoid space through infected tissue would risk spreading microorganisms and causing meningitis. In such cases the procedure should be done by cisternal puncture or lateral cervical puncture at C1–2. The latter is routinely done under fluoroscopy, although it can be done as a bedside procedure by someone trained in its use.

SPINAL TUMOR, ARTERIOVENOUS MALFORMATION, SPINAL FUSION OR DEFORMITY

In the patient with a dorsal tumor, spinal arteriovenous malformation, or an anatomy that precludes LP, the examination of CSF should be done through cisternal or lateral cervical puncture. Lumbar puncture may cause clinical deterioration in patients with spinal cord compression who have complete block to CSF.

EQUIPMENT

- Four sterile collection tubes for CSF
- 3½-inch needles with stylet, No. 18, 20, or 22 (The No. 22 needle is preferred when high pressure is a concern. The smaller needles may cause less headache, although dynamics are damped through the No. 22 or smaller needles.)
- 2-ml syringe
- No. 22 1-inch needle and intradermal needle
- Sterile lidocaine
- Manometer for measurement of pressure
- Three-way stopcock
- Drape for back (optional)
- Alcohol and povidone-iodine (Betadine) or similar skin preparation solution
- 4 × 4-inch gauze pads for skin preparation
- Sterile gloves

POSITION

The procedure is best carried out when the patient is in the lateral recumbent position, parallel to the bed, cot, or table, with head flexed and knees up. The sitting position will also be described here for future reference.

Lateral Recumbent Position (Preferred)

Correct positioning of the patient is the major determinant of how easy the procedure will be. The proper position is illustrated in Figure PR29.1. Stated in another way, the major reason for lack of success with this procedure is incorrect placement of the patient (Fig. PR29.1a). A firm flat surface is best; a pillow under the head will help keep the patient's spine horizontal. The patient's back and shoulders must be squared and perpendicular to the table, otherwise the needle will be

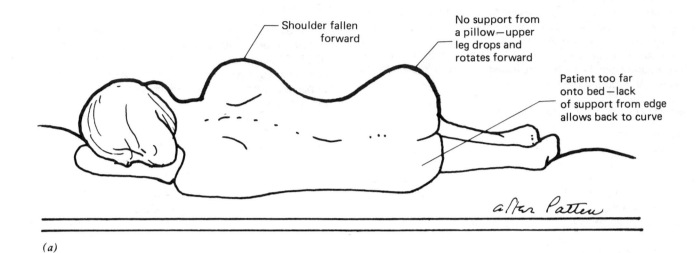

(a)

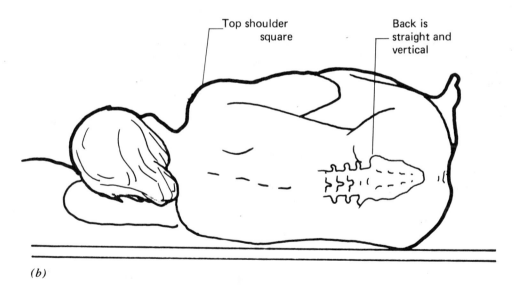

(b)

Figure PR29.1 (a) Incorrect position for LP; (b) correct position for LP. (Adapted with permission from Patten J: *Neurological Differential Diagnosis*. Harold Starke Limited, 1977.)

oblique to the midsagittal plane (Fig. PR29.2). An inspection of the bony relations demonstrates that the width of the interspace increases as the patient flexes his or her back. To maximize the opening, the head and neck should be flexed forward and the knees brought up to the chest. (Recheck to be sure the patient's top shoulder has not slipped forward from the vertical.) The assistance of another person to hold the patient in position is helpful and is vital if the patient is uncooperative. (Agitated patients may have to be sedated with short-acting drugs.)

Sitting Position

Patients may be approached for LP as they sit over the side of the bed. The patient's head and trunk should be flexed forward. The arms and shoulders are best supported over a bedside table, as is commonly done for thoracentesis. Accurate determination of pressure is not possible when the patient is in the sitting position.

PROCEDURE

Prepare the Skin and Anesthetize Soft Tissues

Before preparation of the skin, it is important to palpate the bony landmarks. The L3–4 interspace is roughly parallel with the patient's iliac crest. The spinous process of the lumbar vertebrae and interspaces can be palpated and marked by a scratch, if necessary. In an obese patient, proper positioning and attention to the skeletal landmarks are even more important. LP may be performed at L3–4, L4–5, or the L5–Sl interspaces. Higher punctures should not be attempted. The conus medullaris of the spinal cord terminates at L1–2 in 94% of patients but occasionally terminates at L2–3. A sterile field is created for the instruments, and the back is prepared and draped with a sterile cloth (draping is optional; it permits palpation of the landmarks but obscures their direct vision). Alternating washes of povidone-iodine and alcohol are a suitable preparation. Aseptic technique is essential. At this point gloves are

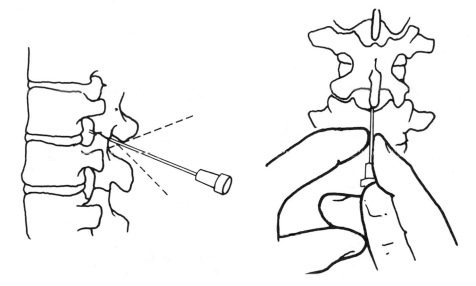

Figure PR29.2 Correct and incorrect angulation of needle for LP. (Adapted with permission from Patten J: *Neurological Differential Diagnosis.* Harold Starke Limited, 1977.)

put on. A subcutaneous wheal is raised with lidocaine, and the deeper tissues are infiltrated with 1–2 ml local anesthetic using a standard 1-inch needle. The area may be massaged to facilitate diffusion of the anesthetic.

Insertion of Needle

A puncture needle with a stylet is inserted into the interspace in the midline, and orientation is maintained in the midsagittal plane. A palpating thumb can be maintained on the interspace or the spinous process below to help guide the needle by feel. Aiming for the umbilicus will often produce the correct spatial attitude in a thin patient. Advance the needle about 1½–2 inches, at which point a slight resistance is evident.

With a slight additional penetration (a few millimeters), a give or pop is felt as the needle enters the subarachnoid space. Remove the stylet and check for the emergence of fluid. If no fluid is seen, reinsert the stylet, advance it several millimeters further, and repeat the procedure. If bone is encountered, retract the needle nearly completely, reorient it, and try again. If a nerve root is encountered, the distribution of the radicular pain will indicate to which side of the midline the needle deviates. If the flow of fluid is intermittent or minimal, replacing the stylet and rotating the needle 90 deg may free the orifice from the dura or nerve roots.

Pressure Recording

When fluid is obtained, the manometer and stopcock are attached, and the manometer is open to the needle. Initial (opening) pressure is recorded. The meniscus should fluctuate with respirations and increase after abdominal pressure. The stopcock is now opened from the needle to the outside to allow the collection of fluid. Two to three milliliters of fluid are obtained for each of the following: initial cell count (tube 1), chemistry (tube 2), bacteriology (tube 3), and miscellaneous studies and final blood cell count (tube 4). Label the tubes immediately. A closing pressure is recorded, the stylet is reinserted (to avoid withdrawing radicular tissue), and the needle is withdrawn. Most physicians recommend that the patient rest in a prone or supine position with the head down for 1–4 hours after the procedure to minimize the risk of LP headache.

Failures

If repeated attempts at LP fail, it may be useful to do the following:

1. Reposition the patient on his or her other side.
2. Have a colleague try the procedure.

3. Try the procedure with the patient in the sitting position. (Measurement of pressure is not obtained in the sitting position.)

Extreme Scoliosis or Back Deformity

Lumbar puncture may be necessary in a patient with deformity of the back or bony landmarks. A review of plain films of the back may help to plan the strategy. Failure to obtain entry into the subarachnoid space may necessitate LP under fluoroscopic control or puncture from above. (See below.)

Lumbar Puncture in Infants

A technique similar to this discussed may be used in children and infants. A shorter needle is used, but a needle with a stylet is desirable. The practice of using a butterfly (scalp vein) needle for LP in an infant has been abandoned because of concern about implanting tissue that may potentially grow as an epidermoid tumor. This late complication of the procedure is rare. Proper head positioning is important; if flow is not encountered with good position of the needle, reposition the patient's head. When the fontanelles are collapsed, the pressure may be low or even negative.

Counting the Fluid

Errors are sometimes encountered when blood cell count is entrusted to the laboratory; it is best to count the fluid yourself. A cubic milliliter of fluid is introduced into a clean counting chamber with a capillary tube or pipette. If the fluid is bloody, prior dilution may facilitate counting, but it is important not to forget to correct for dilution. The total number of cells under the grid is counted. White blood cells are larger and differ in appearance from red blood cells. Recounting fluid to which a drop (less than 2% by volume) of glacial acetic acid has been added is often helpful when red blood cells are numerous. Red blood cells are lysed, and white blood cells pucker so that polymorphonuclear leukocytes are identifiable from lymphocytes. Wright's stain may also be used for this purpose. A good differential of the white blood cells is best obtained from a cytocentrifuge preparation of spun fluid.

Cisternal Puncture and Lateral Cervical Puncture

These procedures are detailed in the older texts. Generally, they should only be performed by neurologists, neurosurgeons, or radiologists who are familiar with their use, since the needle comes within millimeters of vital neural structures in the medulla.

PITFALLS AND COMPLICATIONS

Pressure is Too High

The first thing to appreciate is that we have already created a dural hole and potential CSF leak. *Do not panic and do not remove the needle.* Nothing is gained by removing the needle and important information may be lost. First, check that the pressure is valid by relaxing the patient's legs and freeing constraints on the abdomen or neck. Collect a small amount of fluid (0.5–1 ml should be adequate) for bacteriologic studies and blood cell count; often these studies can be done on the volume of CSF from the manometer without any further removal. From 80 to 150 mm H_2O is the normal range of CSF pressure. Pressure in excess of 190 mm H_2O is clearly elevated, and pressure in excess of 300 mm H_2O is disturbingly high. If there is concern about an intracranial mass lesion with displacement of brain tissue, it may be helpful to reduce the pressure by intravenous infusion of a dehydrating agent, such as urea or mannitol (1–1.5 g/kg) before removing the needle. When the pressure is lowered, the needle may be removed with less potential for CSF leak. Finally, inform the neurologic or neurosurgical consultant about the case so that follow-up care can be arranged. As mentioned earlier, the risk for fatal brain herniation or marked neurologic deterioration after LP is not high, but such complications have been reported.

The Bloody Tap

In situations of the bloody tap, the priority is to decide whether bloody CSF has resulted from a traumatic tap or an intracranial or spinal hemorrhage. A traumatic tap need not be a difficult procedure with repeated thrusts. A clean, first pass, effortless puncture may nick a dural or arachnoid vein. Several simple clinical observations are helpful in distinguishing the traumatic tap from a genuinely hemorrhagic CSF. A traumatic tap often clears measurably between the first and final tube since clear CSF washes out the bleeding. Always count first and last tubes in such cases, although failure to clear is inconclusive. A thin stripe of blood is often seen in traumatic LP; this should be noted. The pressure is elevated in most conditions with gross subarachnoid bleeding; a careful pressure should be recorded. Blood from genuinely hemorrhagic CSF should not clot.

The CSF should be spun down to compare supernatant fluid with water. Xanthochromia resulting from heme pigments indicates bleeding before the procedure. Subarachnoid blood excites an inflammatory cellular response. The ratio of white blood cells to red blood cells in genuine subarachnoid hemorrhage is in excess of that seen in peripheral blood (generally 1:700).

Finally, if the data are important, repeat the tap immediately at the next higher interspace. The bleeding induced by traumatic puncture will often diffuse slowly so that a clean tap may be had at the next higher interspace.

Dry Tap

A dry tap may be evidence of intradural pathology and obliterations or loculation of the subarachnoid space. This occurs, for example, in adhesive arachnoiditis. If fluid does not appear when the needle feels as if it is properly placed, rotate the bevel. If there is still no success, try the adjacent interspace. Repeated failure should elicit neurologic and neurosurgical consultation.

Pus

If gross pus is encountered, presumably the needle has entered a loculated infection, such as an epidural abscess. Do not advance the needle further so as not to penetrate the subarachnoid space. Aspirate pus for culture, begin appropriate antibiotic coverage, and obtain consultation to arrange cervical puncture and myelography.

Lumbar Puncture Headache

Headaches complicate 10–30% of lumbar punctures, depending on the caliber of the needle and the expertise of the person performing the procedure. Classic LP headache occurs when the patient is sitting up or standing and is minimized by having the patient lie down. In theory, LP headaches are due to CSF leak created by the needle, low-pressure dynamics, and traction on intracranial structures. The headache is usually self-limited, lasts 1–7 days, and is adequately treated with bed rest and analgesics to minimize discomfort. Persistence beyond 2 weeks indicates persistent CSF leak and may require intradural injection of autologous blood serum or primary repair. Laceration of the dura during LP can be minimized by avoidance of any lateral movement of the needle during the procedure. (Do not attempt to redirect the needle while it is deep in the patient's back.)

PROCEDURE 30

CULDOCENTESIS

Kirtly Parker Jones

The *cul-de-sac*, the anatomical space between the uterus and the rectum, is the lowest point in the abdomen to which fluid can drain (Fig. PR30.1). Placing a needle transvaginally into this space is termed *culdocentesis*. The technique is simple, of only moderate discomfort, and of minimal risk when appropriate precautions are taken. It can be very helpful in diagnosing free intraperitoneal blood, primarily from a source in the pelvis.

INDICATIONS

- To evaluate the presence of significant intraperitoneal bleeding in patients in whom an ectopic pregnancy is known or expected.
- Female patients with sudden onset of pelvic or lower abdominal pain with hemodynamic instability (orthostatic changes, low hematocrit).
- To diagnose a ruptured ovarian cyst (culdocentesis would yield straw-colored fluid, perhaps slightly blood tinged, and the patient could be treated with observation) versus a bleeding ovarian cyst or ectopic pregnancy (yielding nonclotting blood and requiring laparotomy).

CONTRAINDICATIONS

- An acutely retroverted uterus that is immobile and will not allow entry into the cul-de-sac.
- A pelvis that on preliminary examination reveals a mass in the cul-de-sac.
- Patients not in the reproductive years—premenarchal or postmenopausal women. This procedure may be too traumatic for a child; furthermore the possibility of a pelvic source of bleeding is highly unlikely. The postmenopausal woman with lower abdominal pain has a high probability of a primary bowel problem, which is a contraindication to the procedure.
- Occasionally culdocentesis is used to obtain fluid for culture in a patient with pelvic inflammatory disease or a pelvic

abscess; however, this is not a procedure that is necessarily done by the emergency room physician.

EQUIPMENT

- A comfortable table with examination stirrups
- Bivalve speculum
- Cervical tenaculum
- 10-ml syringe
- 18- or 20-gauge spinal needle
- Sterile sponges
- Antiseptic prep solution
- Long dressing forceps

POSITION

The patient should be comfortable in the lithotomy position with her shoulders higher than her hips for adequate collection of fluid in the cul-de-sac. The physician must be comfortably seated with good spot lighting to observe the posterior fornix of the vagina.

PROCEDURE

The *patient is adequately informed of the procedure*, the information hoped to be gained, and the possible discomforts, which are similar to a sharp menstrual cramp. A bimanual examination is performed to assess the position, size, and mobility of the uterus and the presence of adnexal masses and to rule out a mass in the cul-de-sac or a frozen pelvis in which pelvic organs and bowel are firmly adherent in the cul-de-sac.

A *speculum is placed in the vagina* and is widely opened with the cervix well in view. A *cervical tenaculum is placed on the posterior* portion of the cervix after the cervix and posterior vagina have been swabbed with antiseptic solution (Fig. PR30.2). The cervix is lifted anteriorly with the tenaculum and the *spinal needle is thrust firmly and quickly through the vagina* in the midline posterior to the cervix slightly posterior to the vaginal reflection on the cervix. The needle should be placed no more than 2.5 cm through the vaginal wall.

Fluid is aspirated with a 10-ml syringe. If blood is obtained, it is observed for clotting over 5 minutes. If the blood clots, it is most likely from a vaginal or pelvic vein. Nonclotting blood confirms significant intraabdominal bleeding that has clotted and the clot has lysed. If serous clear fluid is obtained, the culdocentesis was successful and rules out intraperitoneal blood.

If cloudy fluid or pus is obtained, it should be cultured anaerobically and aerobically and for *Neisseria*. If no fluid is obtained, the procedure may be repeated once. The needle is withdrawn and the speculum is removed.

PITFALLS AND COMPLICATIONS

A culdocentesis that yields no fluid does not rule out intraperitoneal bleeding. The procedure may have been technically inadequate or the amount of intraperitoneal fluid may be small.

Acute onset of bleeding will create blood in the cul-de-sac that is clotted and will not aspirate. A ruptured ectopic pregnancy that has been bleeding for several hours during which the patient has orthostatic changes or a low hematocrit will usually yield nonclotting blood.

Aspiration of air or feces indicates placement of the needle posteriorly into the rectum or a sigmoid colon obliterating the cul-de-sac. This can be avoided by a careful pelvic examination before the procedure and by directing the needle in the axis of the uterus. Laceration of pelvic veins can be avoided by placing the needle in the midline.

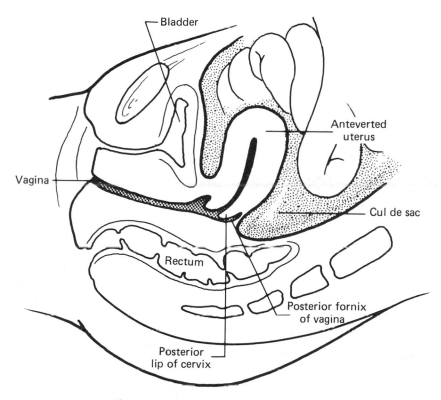

Figure PR30.1 Pelvic structures—sagittal view.

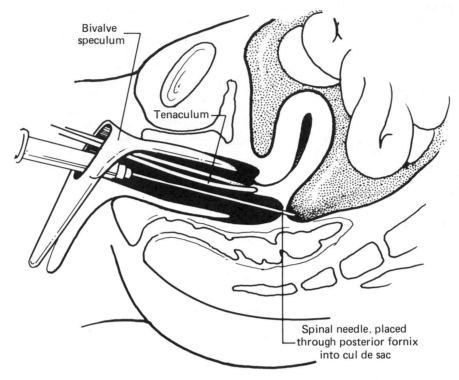

Figure PR30.2 Perform culdocentesis while tenaculum grasps posterior lip of cervix.

Procedure 31

JOINT ASPIRATION

Donald T. Reilly

Synovial fluid is the product of the synovial lining of a joint. *Arthrocentesis,* or joint aspiration, is a diagnostic tool that may reflect local or systemic processes affecting the synovium. An effusion, by definition, is an increase in the joint fluid and must first be diagnosed before aspiration is attempted. The loss of normal bony contours and landmarks can occur both with an effusion and soft tissue swelling. An effusion will usually show a fluid wave and will be confined to the anatomical limits of the joint.

Trauma to a joint may cause an immediate effusion in the form of a hemarthrosis from tearing vascular structures or subchondral bone fracture. An occult fracture may therefore be diagnosed when bloody joint fluid observed in a shallow dish is noted to contain fat globules. This is one of the fairly rare indications for traumatic effusion aspirations. Immobilization is usually sufficient treatment of a traumatic effusion. Decompression aspiration is an even rarer indication. The presence of a traumatic effusion is not an indication for aspiration.

Trauma or degenerative changes may also result in a synovitis and gradually appearing effusion by disrupting the normally smooth mechanical function of a joint.

INDICATIONS

- Effusion with suspicion of an occult fracture
- Acute, painful, nontraumatized joint
- Suspected septic arthritis

CONTRAINDICATIONS (RELATIVE)

Cellulitis over a joint is a contraindication for this procedure.

EQUIPMENT

- Hypodermic needles (25 gauge; 20 or 18 gauge, depending on joint size)
- Syringes (3 ml and 20 ml)
- Povidone-iodine (Betadine) prep solution
- Sterile towels
- Sterile gauge sponges
- Sterile gloves
- 1% lidocaine
- Culture tubes
- A plain glass tube (for crystal and chemical analysis)
- An anticoagulant tube (ethylenediaminetetraacetic acid—EDTA—for blood cell count)

PROCEDURE

Under sterile conditions prepare the skin over the regions for aspiration and landmarks that are to be palpated. The prepared field is then sterily draped and the skin is anesthetized with lidocaine using the 25-gauge needle and 30-ml syringe. The subcutaneous tissue should also be anesthestized down to the capsule of the joint. The 18-gauge needle on the 20-ml syringe is then introduced through the lidocaine wheal. Gentle steady pressure through the subcutaneous tissue will be met with a change in resistance when the needle point reaches the joint capsule. A perceptible give will be encountered once the joint capsule is entered and the needle is in the joint space. Gentle aspiration is important since hypertrophic synovium and debris will obliterate the needle lumen and make full evacuation difficult. The joint aspirate can be sent for Gram stain, protein and glucose level, crystals, blood cell count with differential, and culture. A dry sterile dressing should be placed over the aspiration site.

Specific Joint Aspirations

ELBOW

With the elbow held flexed at a 90 deg angle the radioulnar aspect of the elbow can be entered just below or above the palpable radial head (Fig. PR31.1).

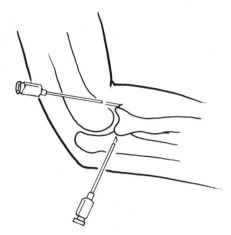

Figure PR31.1 Elbow aspiration above or below the radial head laterally.

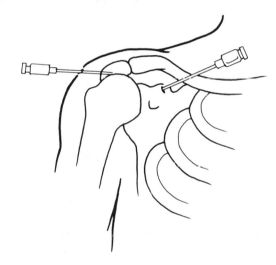

Figure PR31.2 Shoulder aspiration shown anteromedially or posterolaterally.

SHOULDER

With the patient's arm at the side, the shoulder joint may be aspirated anteriorly and lateral to the caracoid process (Fig. PR31.2). Posteriorly, the shoulder may be aspirated inferior to the acromium.

KNEE

With an effusion, the knee is held most comfortably in slight flexion. Full extension makes aspiration easiest. The joint area

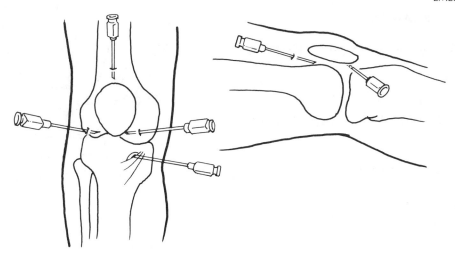

Figure PR31.3 Knee aspiration shown with pes bursa injection inferomedially.

under the inferior pole of the patella can be approached either medially or laterally (Fig. PR31.3). Occasionally, a large effusion can be aspirated from the suprapatellar pouch.

ANKLE

The ankle joint is usually best entered anterolaterally with the bulging joint capsule felt anterior to the fibula (Fig. PR31.4). This point is about 1–2 cm proximal to the tip of the fibula.

WRIST

The dorsum of the wrist just distal to the radioulna joint offers the safest entry for aspiration (Fig. PR31.5).

Specific Disease Processes

TENOSYNOVIAL OR BURSA INFLAMMATIONS

The tenosynovium surrounding tendons or bursa can be involved in the overuse syndromes or processes of inflamming joints mentioned above. The technique described above for joint aspiration can be used for instillation of medication or diagnosis. Lidocaine mixed with a long-acting steroid preparation is injected for both immediate diagnosis and subsequent treatment. The olecranon and prepatellar bursae are usually only aspirated when a septic bursitis is suspected, and usually the patient requires only rest and possibly oral antiinflammatories for treatment.

DE QUERVAIN'S DISEASE

The first dorsal wrist compartment containing the abductor pollicis longus and extensor pollicis brevis is often involved in stenosing tenosynovitis. Injection and splinting are the first choice of treatment, but chronic involvement may require surgical release.

SUBACROMIAL BURSITIS AND BICEPS TENDONITIS

The shoulder is commonly involved because of its unique anatomy of the rotator cuff and biceps tendon gliding between the humeral head and the acromium. The subacromial bursa can be entered laterally just inferior to the acromium. The long head of the biceps can usually be palpated between the greater and lesser tuberositis. Instillation of a lidocaine and steroid mixture can be done directly anterior, but care must be taken to instill into the tendon sheath and not the tendon. This can be accomplished by feeling the resistance to injection if the needle is in the tendon substance and withdrawing slightly until easy free flow is encountered. The subacromial bursa is best entered laterally (Fig. PR31.2).

GREATER TROCHANTERIC BURSITIS

Direct palpation over the greater trochanter that causes pain is diagnostic of this painful entity. Direct injection in a conelike fashion will ensure instillation in a sufficient region for good results. In obese patients, a spinal needle may be required.

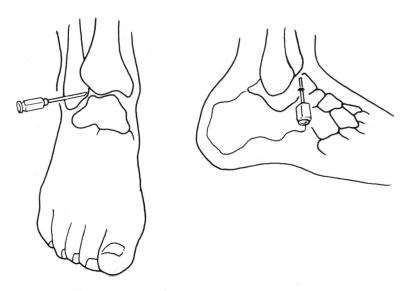

Figure PR31.4 Ankle aspiration at the anterolateral portal.

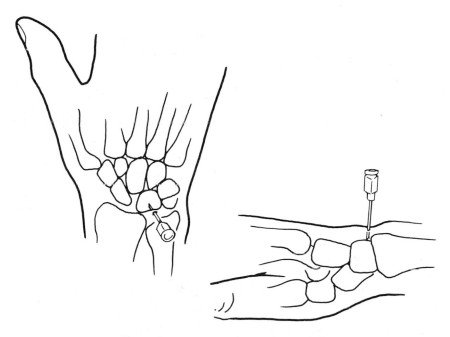

Figure PR31.5 Wrist aspiration dorsoradially.

PES ANSERINUS BURSITIS

Often pes anserinus bursitis is confused with intraarticular knee joint pathology. The bursa can be palpated distal to the medial joint and injected directly anteromedially (Fig. PR31.3).

PITFALLS AND COMPLICATIONS

Introduction of sepsis into a sterile joint because of skin contamination can be obviated by careful attention to strict aseptic technique. Cellulitis can usually be avoided by alternative aspiration sites. Fluid in overlying structures should not be confused with a joint effusion. A prepatellar bursitis will give the impression of fluid in the subcutaneous tissues and is not connected to the knee joint. Similarly, the fluid in an olecranon bursa is not in the elbow joint. With easily palpable joints, the presence of the arthrocentesis needle in the joint is relatively easy to determine. A false-negative aspiration of the hip can only be avoided with the use of fluoroscopy and radioopaque dye and therefore is not amenable to the emergency room situation.

PROCEDURE 32

SCHIÖTZ TONOMETRY

Alfredo A. Sadun

Open-angle glaucoma, a leading cause of blindness in the United States, develops without pain and with an insidious visual loss. It occurs in about 0.5% of the population and it is seen primarily among the elderly.

The pathophysiology of open-angle glaucoma is thought to be an obstruction of aqueous outflow producing an elevated intraocular pressure that leads to loss of axons in the optic disc and subsequent visual field loss. The visual field losses may occur after 20 years of elevated intraocular pressure at which time it is felt the optic disc has become more vulnerable. Treatment usually succeeds in lowering intraocular pressure but not in reversing visual field losses. It is therefore extremely beneficial to diagnose the disease early by screenings. Mea-

surement of intraocular pressure by tonometry also helps differentiate serious angle-closure glaucoma from other more benign causes of red eye.

The Schiötz tonometer is a relatively inexpensive and durable instrument that is easy to use in a 1-minute examination. The instrument is composed of a footplate through which a plunger falls (Fig. PR32.1). Various weights can be rested on this plunger, which moves independently of a sleeve used to hold the instrument. Scale readings are taken and, based on the weight used, converted to millimeters of mercury of pressure using a conversion table. With the footplate resting on the cornea, the plunger indents the cornea to a degree dependent on the intraocular pressure. This technique is quite accurate and reliable probably more so than the expensive air puff machine used by optometrists.

INDICATIONS

- Routine screening of all patients over age 35 or with a positive family history of glaucoma
- Anyone suspected of having high intraocular pressure
- Differential diagnosis of red eye to rule out angle-closure glaucoma
- To monitor patients with angle-closure glaucoma to test the efficacy of medical treatment
- To follow patients on topical or systemic steroids who may develop steroid responsiveness (reversible rise in intraocular pressure with steroid use)

CONTRAINDICATIONS

- Infectious conjunctivitis is a relative contraindication for this technique, since a variety of viral and bacterial agents can be spread by Schiötz tonometry.
- Corneal ulcer, which may thin the cornea to the point at which tonometry is dangerous.
- Immediate postoperative period after intraocular surgery.

EQUIPMENT

- Schiötz tonometry kit (tonometer, additional weights, zeroing platform, conversion table)
- Alcohol or alcohol prep pads
- Cotton or gauze
- Proparacaine (Ophthaine) 0.5%

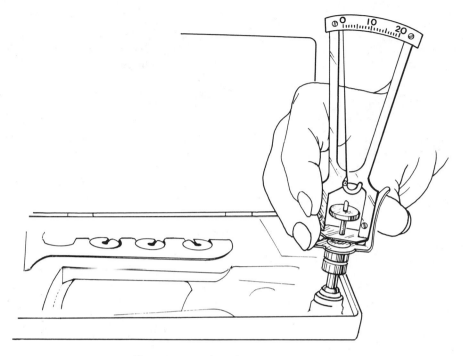

Figure PR32.1 The Schiæotz tonometer.

POSITION

The patient should be comfortable with head tilted back and eyes looking to a spot on the ceiling. This is usually best accomplished with the patient on a flat bed or cot without pillows. Young patients have supple enough necks to tilt their heads back from a sitting position. The examiner can approach the patient from above the head or to one side.

The wheelchair bound patient represents a challenge. If transfer to a cot is difficult, the examiner can sit on a chair behind the wheelchair bound patient. He then tilts the wheelchair backwards onto his own lap with the wheels as fulcrum, resting the back of the wheelchair on his legs and using his feet to stabilize the wheels. The patient's head is then tilted into the correct position.

PROCEDURE

Zero Tonometer

The tonometer should be checked to make sure that the plunger moves freely through the base plate. When the tonometer is fixed on the zeroing platform, the needle should point to the zero on the scale (Fig. PR32.1). The thin metal needle can be bent slightly as an adjustment.

Clean the Base Plate

Alcohol-soaked cotton balls or alcohol preparation pads can be used to clean and disinfect the base plate and plunger. The alcohol should be allowed to dry or be wiped off with sterile gauze to prevent denuding the corneal epithelium.

Apply Anesthesia

One drop of proparacaine, 0.5%, or similar topical anesthesia, should be instilled in each eye (Fig. PR32.2). Allow 30 seconds for anesthesia to develop.

Apply the Tonometer

The patient is asked to stare at a spot on the ceiling or at his or her own finger held outstretched above his or her head. The examiner uses the nondominant hand to open the patient's lids widely apart. The tonometer is gently placed squarely on the central cornea. It rests on the eye such that the finger grip sleeve no longer supports any of the weight of the tonometer. The tonometer scale is read, and the procedure is repeated on the patient's other eye. The tonometer in Figure PR32.3 is about to be placed in position.

Additional Weights

If the scale reading is 4 or less, a more accurate measurement can be taken with heavier weights. The 7.5-g weight should be placed on top of the standard 5.5-g weight in the tonometer astride the central column. The tonometry reading is repeated. If the scale reading is again 4 or less, repeat the measurement with the 10-g weight (after removing the 7.5-g weight).

Reading Results

The scale readings can be recorded directly together with the weight used. For example, OD (right eye): 7/5.5 (7-scale reading, 5.5-weight); OS (left eye): 3/5.5, 6/7.5. It is usually necessary, however, to translate these scale/weight readings to pressure in millimeters of mercury (mm Hg). A table is enclosed in each tonometer kit. Simply find the column for the weight used and record the pressure in millimeters of mercury beside the scale readings just taken. Intraocular pressures between 10 and 20 mm Hg are normal. Pressures of 20–30 mm Hg are characteristic of open-angle glaucoma. Acute, angle-closure attacks of glaucoma often result in pressures of 30–60 mm Hg. Pressure readings below 8 mm Hg may also indicate significant pathology.

PITFALLS AND COMPLICATIONS

The tonometer needle may have become bent by rough handling. This should be noted and corrected when zeroing the instrument. Similarly, a poorly maintained tonometer may have a plunger bar that sticks. When the plunger is not resting on any surface, it should descend and the reading on the scale should be maximum (> 20). If the plunger does not slide easily it can be removed and cleaned with acetone, ether, or alcohol.

During the process of applying the instrument to the eye, care should be taken that the base plate does not rest on or touch the lids.

Tonometry should not be attempted on patients with any form of eye infection since it may easily become the vehicle for the spread of a communicable disease.

Tonometry should not be done on patients within the first 2 weeks after any intraocular surgery. This is to prevent disturbing the wound or creating a source of eye infection.

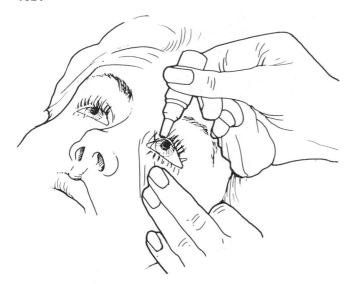

Figure PR32.2 Anesthetize the eye.

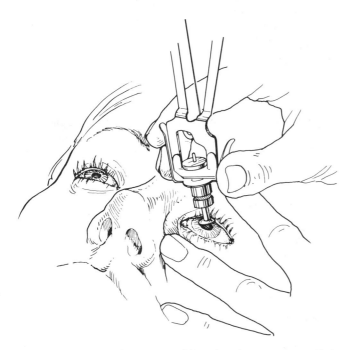

Figure PR32.3 Spread patients eyelids and apply tonometer gently to the surface of the eye. It must not be angulated in relation to the cornea.

PROCEDURE 33

VAGINAL DELIVERY

Kirtly Parker Jones

The occasion to do a vaginal delivery in an emergency room arises most often with the multiparous patient who has a history of rapid labor. Most normal vaginal deliveries occur spontaneously and, given adequate light and exposure to monitor the events of childbirth, the least intervention is the best.

EQUIPMENT

- A comfortable table with examination stirrups
- Bulb syringe
- Two sterile Kelly clamps
- Umbilical clamp or umbilical tape
- Vial of 10 units oxytocin (Pitocin)
- Sterile sponges
- Sterile towels
- Sterile gloves
- Warm sterile or clean blanket

POSITION

If possible, place the mother in the lithotomy position to allow adequate exposure and room to aid in delivery of the infant (Fig. PR33.1).

PROCEDURE

1. Care should be taken to protect the vaginal and perineal tissues from an explosive delivery; gently controlled guidance of the infant without an attempt to obstruct or delay the delivery is optimal. Maternal expulsive forces will deliver the *head,* which *should be gently guided through the introitus* to avoid lacerations of the perineum (Fig. PR33.1*b*). A bulb syringe should be used to suction the infant's mouth and nose after birth of the head and before the first breath. Attention should be directed to the infant's neck; reduce any nuchal cords gently over the head. A very tight nuchal cord may be doubly clamped and cut and the infant delivered immediately.

2. The shoulders are allowed to rotate into an anterior–posterior position: then, using gentle downward pressure on the head and maternal expulsive forces, the *anterior shoulder is delivered* (Fig. PR33.2).

3. The *posterior shoulder is delivered* by lifting the infant upward and subsequently delivering the body (Fig. PR33.2*b,c*).

4. The infant should be held below the level of the mother's uterus while the *oropharynx is suctioned* again with a bulb syringe. The *cord is doubly clamped* with sterile Kelly clamps

and a sterile scissors is used to cut between them (Fig. PR33.3). The infant's umbilical stump may then be tied with umbilical tape, an umbilical clamp if available, or any narrow, sterile, nonadhesive gauze tape. The infant should be dried and kept warm, preferably in its mother's arms. Oxygen should be administered by pediatric mask if the infant is cyanotic and responding poorly.

5. The *delivery of the placenta* is potentially the most dangerous time for the mother; it is when most postpartum hemorrhages due to retained placenta or uterine atony occur. After delivery of the infant, the clamped cord should be allowed to rest on the perineum. The placenta should appear at the introitus within 20 minutes; massage of the uterus may aid in the separation of the placenta. Traction

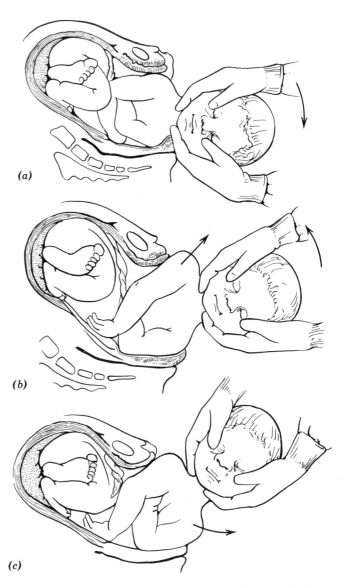

Figure PR33.2 (a) Deliver anterior shoulder, applying gentle downward pressure on the head. (b, c) deliver posterior shoulder by gently lifting the infant upward.

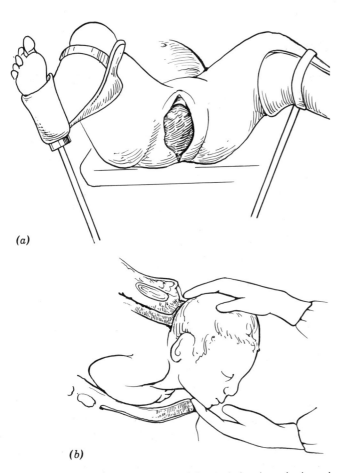

Figure PR33.1 (a)Lithotomy position; (b) Guide head gently through the introitus.

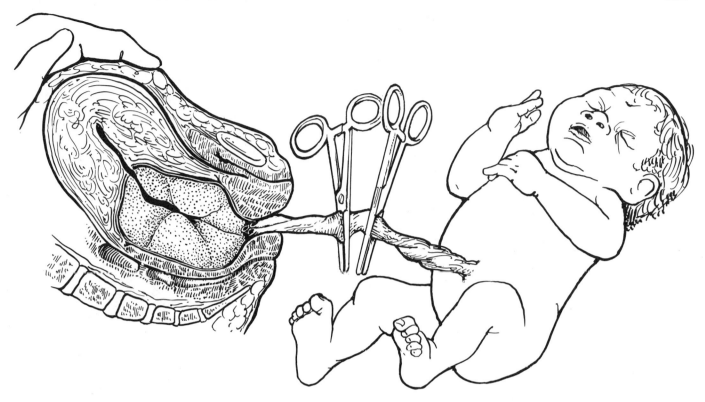

Figure PR33.3 Cut the cord between the Kelly clamps.

on the cord may only lead to rupture of the cord or eversion of the uterus. If the patient is bleeding profusely or if the placenta is not seen after $\frac{1}{2}$ hour, the patient must be transferred to the operating room for manual removal of the placenta by trained personnel under sterile conditions.

6. After delivery of the placenta, oxytocin (10 units in 1,000 ml of 5% dextrose in lactated Ringer's solution) of methylergonovine (Methergine) (0.2 mg intramuscularly) may help maintain uterine tone and decrease blood loss. Any vaginal or perineal laceration may be repaired in layers with absorbable sutures.

PITFALLS AND COMPLICATIONS

On examining a patient in labor or with ruptured membranes, if an umbilical cord is felt in the cervix or vagina, the patient must immediately be placed in Trendelenburg position. The examining hand should lift the presenting part of the fetus off the prolapsed cord. The mother must be taken for immediate cesarean section. A prolapsed limb (foot or arm) should not be delivered vaginally if there is a viable fetus; the mother should be taken for a cesarean section.

Breech presentation (buttocks or feet presenting first) occurs in 3 to 4 percent of deliveries. The maneuvers of a breech delivery are difficult and not appropriate for presentation here. If a breech delivery is imminent and no experienced person is present or available for telephone consultation, the best approach is to allow maternal forces to deliver the body of the infant up to the head. If the head does not deliver spontaneously,, the infant is held horizontally with the back up (an assistant is necessary) and one hand gives firm suprapubic pressure while a finger of the other is placed in the infants mouth to flex and deliver the head. A wide episiotomy may be necessary.

INDEX